YOUR GUIDE TO

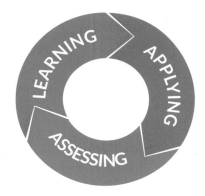

Maternal-Newborn Nursing

The Critical Components of Nursing Care

Everything you need to succeed...
in class, in clinical, on exams, and on the NCLEX®

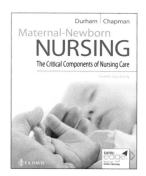

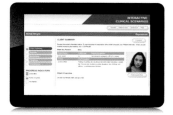

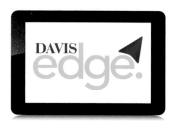

LEARNING

Your text provides the foundational knowledge you need to know.

APPLYING

Interactive Clinical Scenarios show you how theory applies to practice.

ASSESSING

Davis Edge is the online Q&A review platform that evaluates your mastery of the material and builds your test-taking skills.

Your journey to success
BEGINS HERE!

Your text works together with Interactive Clinical Scenarios and Davis Edge to make this often-intimidating, but must-know content easier to master.

Don't miss everything that's waiting online to make learning less stressful... and save you time. Follow the instructions on the inside front cover to use the access code to unlock your resources today.

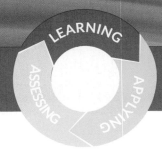

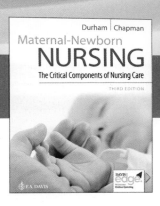

Durham | Chapman

Maternal-Newborn

NURSING

The Critical Components of Nursing Care

THIRD EDITION

F.A. DAVIS

DAVIS edge

LEARNING

STEP #1

Build a solid foundation.

Critical Component Boxes highlight essential information in each chapter.

Evidence-Based Practice Boxes focus on current research-based and practice guidelines related to nursing care.

CRITICAL COMPONENT

The Importance of Patient-Centered Pregnancy Care

Women experiencing pregnancy complications are especially physiologically, psychologically, emotionally, and spiritually vulnerable. Nurses are in a unique position to explore a woman's needs and advocate for the woman's participation in management of pregnancy complications. It is essential to recognize the patient or designee as the source of control and full partner in providing compassionate and coordinated care based on respect for the patient's preferences, values, and needs.

Some suggestions to foster respect for a woman's prefere[nces], values, and needs include:

- Elicit patient values, preferences, and expressed needs [as] part of clinical interview, implementation of care plan, [and] evaluation of care.
- Communicate patient values, preferences, and express[ed] needs to other members of the health care team.
- Value the patient's expertise with her own health and symptoms.
- Respect patient and family preferences for degree of a[ctive] engagement in care process.

Evidence-Based Practice: Venous Thromboembolism Bundle

Obstetric venous thromboembolism is a leading cause of severe maternal morbidity and mortality. Maternal death from thromboembolism is amenable to prevention, and thromboprophylaxis is the most readily implementable means of systematically reducing the maternal death rate. Observational data support the benefit of risk-factor-based prophylaxis in reducing obstetric thromboembolism. This bundle, developed by a multidisciplinary working group and published by the National Partnership for Maternal Safety under the guidance of the Council on Patient Safety in Women's Health Care, supports routine thromboembolism risk assessment for obstetric patients, with appropriate use of pharmacologic and mechanical prophylaxis. Safety bundles outline critical clinical practices that should [be imple]mented in every maternity unit. The bundle is divided into four domains: [The] *Readiness* domain, which supports establishment of risk-assessment [protocol]s throughout pregnancy. Risk assessment should occur at four time points [in preg]nancy: (a) during the first prenatal visit, (b) during all antepartum admis[sions, (c)] immediately postpartum during a hospitalization for childbirth, and (d) [on disch]arge home after a birth. The *Recognition* domain, which reviews clin[ical reco]mmendations from major existing guidelines for patients recognized to be [at increa]sed risk for thromboembolism. The *Response* domain, which outlines [the r]ecommendations for prophylaxis for at-risk patients from the NPMS work[ing grou]p; and (d) the *Reporting and Systems Learning* domain, which [outlines] recommendations for quality assurance and surveillance.

SAFE AND EFFECTIVE NURSING CARE: Understanding Medication

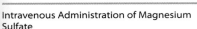

Intravenous Administration of Magnesium Sulfate

Magnesium sulfate is indicated for women with severe features of preeclampsia. Although the exact method of action in seizure prophylaxis is not clearly understood, therapeutic levels of the drug will result in cerebral vasodilation, thereby reducing ischemia caused by vasospasm. Magnesium sulfate also slows neuromuscular conduction, depresses the vasomotor center, and decreases central nervous system irritability (Poole, 2014). Continuous intravenous administration:

- Loading dose: 4–6 g diluted in 100 mL of IV fluid administered over 15–20 minutes
- Continuous infusion: 2 g/hr in 100 mL of IV fluid for maintenance
- Laboratory evaluation: Measure serum magnesium level at 4–6 hours, after onset of treatment. Dosage should be adjusted to maintain a therapeutic level of 4 to 8 mg/dl
- Duration: Intravenous infusion should continue for 24 hours post-delivery.
- The antidote for magnesium toxicity is calcium gluconate or calcium chloride 5–10 mEq given IV slowly over 5–10 minutes.

Safe and Effective Nursing Care Boxes summarize important safety concepts, such as understanding medications and patient education.

Case Study

As a nurse in an antenatal clinic, you are part of an interdisciplinary team that is caring for Margarite Sanchez during her pregnancy. Margarite is a 28-year-old G3 P1 Hispanic woman here for her first prenatal care appointment. By her LMP she is at 8 weeks' gestation. She is 5 feet, 7 inches tall and her weight today is 140 (states pre-pregnancy weight was 137, BMI = 21.5). Margarite reports some spotting 2 weeks ago that prompted her to do a home pregnancy test that was positive. The spotting has stopped. She tells you that she is very tired throughout the day and has some nausea in the morning and breast tenderness. She is happy to be pregnant but a bit surprised.

Outline the aspects of your initial assessment.
Outline for Margarite what laboratory tests are done during this first prenatal visit and rationale for the tests.
Detail the prenatal education and anticipatory guidance appropriate for the first trimester of pregnancy.
What teaching would you do for Margarite's discomforts of pregnancy?
Discuss nursing diagnosis, nursing activities, and expected outcomes related to this woman.

At 18 weeks' gestation, Margarite comes to the clinic for a prenatal visit. She states she thinks she felt her baby move for the first time last week and that the pregnancy now feels real to her. She states, "I feel great! The nausea and fatigue are gone." She is concerned she is not eating enough protein, as she has little interest in red meat but eats beans and rice at dinner. She remembers discussing with you at her first visit some screening tests for problems with the baby but now is unsure how they are done and what they are for.

Outline for Margarite nutritional needs during pregnancy, highlighting protein requirements.
Outline for Margarite the screening tests that are done in the second trimester and what they are for.
Detail the prenatal education and anticipatory guidance appropriate for the second trimester of pregnancy.
Discuss nursing diagnosis, nursing activities, and expected outcomes related to Margarite.

Margarite comes to your clinic for a prenatal visit and is now at 34 weeks' gestation. She states she feels well but has some swelling in her legs at the end of the day, a backache at the end of the day, and difficulty getting comfortable enough to fall asleep. She is also having difficulty sleeping, as she gets up to go to the bathroom two or three times a night.

She remembers from her first pregnancy some things she should be aware of that indicate a problem at the end of pregnancy but is not sure what they are.

Detail the prenatal education and anticipatory guidance appropriate for the third trimester of pregnancy.
What teaching would you do for Margarite's discomforts of pregnancy?
What warning signs would you reinforce with Margarite at this point in her pregnancy?
Discuss nursing diagnosis, nursing activities, and expected outcomes specific to Margarite.

Case Studies at the end of the chapter let you test your understanding and apply your knowledge in a clinical context.

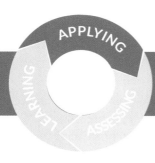

APPLYING

STEP #2

Practice in a safe environment.

- Psychosocial Adaptations During Pregnancy
- Pregestational Diabetes Mellitus
- Breastfeeding
- Postpartum Hemorrhage
- Nutrition
- Normal Postpartum Assessment
- Placenta Previa
- Perinatal Loss
- Pharmacological Pain Relief Measures
- Postpartum Teaching/Knowledge
- Preterm Labor
- Deep Vein Thrombosis

Interactive Clinical Scenarios walk you through the nursing process with client summaries, multiple-choice questions with rationales, drag- and drop activities, and so much more.

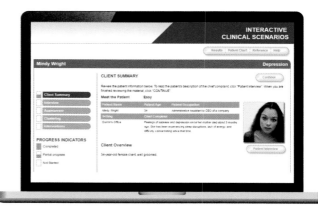

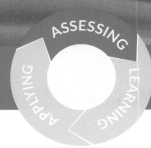

ASSESSING

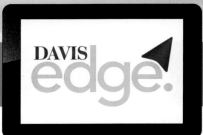

STEP #3

Study smarter, not harder.

Davis Edge is the interactive, online Q&A review platform that provides the practice you need to master course content and to improve your scores on classroom exams. Access it from a laptop, tablet, or mobile device for review and study on the go.

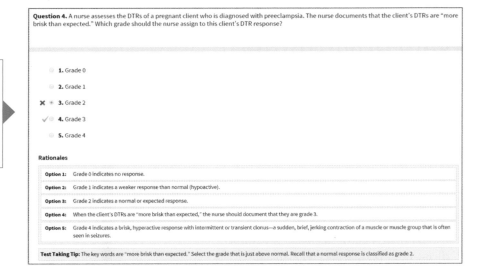

Assignments are made by your instructor. Or, create your own practice quizzes to review before an exam.

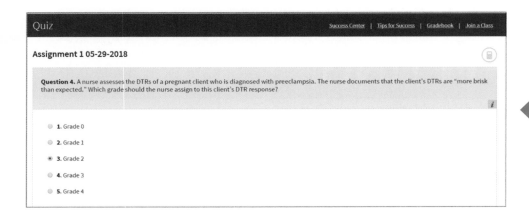

Comprehensive rationales explain why your responses are correct or incorrect. Page-specific references direct you to the relevant content in *Maternal-Newborn Nursing*.

Test-taking tips help you understand how to tackle difficult questions.

The Success Center offers a snapshot of your progress and identifies your strengths and weaknesses.

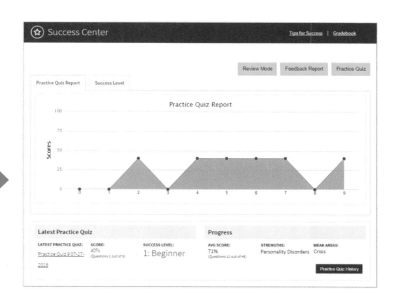

The Feedback Report drills down to show your performance in individual content areas. It's easy to create new practice quizzes that focus on your areas of weakness or to select the topics or concepts you want to study.

★ ★ ★ ★ ★

"Davis Edge is the reason why I passed my course."

– Sakina Anderson, Student at La Grange College

95%

of students surveyed received a B or higher in their class using Davis Edge.

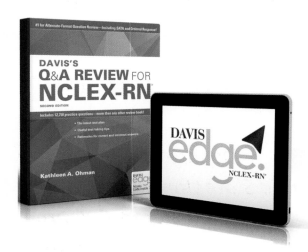
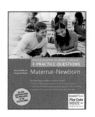
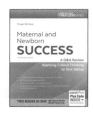
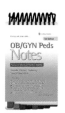

THIRD EDITION

Maternal-Newborn
NURSING

The Critical Components of Nursing Care

Roberta F. Durham, RN, PhD

Professor
Department of Nursing
California State University, East Bay
Hayward, California
Professor Alumnus
Samuel Merritt University
Oakland, California

Linda L. Chapman, RN, PhD

Professor Emeritus
Samuel Merritt University
Oakland, California

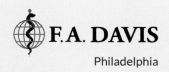

F.A. DAVIS

Philadelphia

F.A. Davis Company
1915 Arch Street
Philadelphia, PA 19103
www.fadavis.com

Printed in the United States of America

Last digit indicates print number: 10 9 8 7 6 5 4 3

Acquisitions Editor: Jacalyn Sharp
Developmental Editor: Andrea Miller
Manager of Project and eProject Development: Catherine Carroll
Content Project Manager: Amanda Minutola
Design and Illustration Manager: Carolyn O'Brien

As new scientific information becomes available through basic and clinical research, recommended treatments and drug therapies undergo changes. The author(s) and publisher have done everything possible to make this book accurate, up to date, and in accord with accepted standards at the time of publication. The author(s), editors, and publisher are not responsible for errors or omissions or for consequences from application of the book, and make no warranty, expressed or implied, in regard to the contents of the book. Any practice described in this book should be applied by the reader in accordance with professional standards of care used in regard to the unique circumstances that may apply in each situation. The reader is advised always to check product information (package inserts) for changes and new information regarding dose and contraindications before administering any drug. Caution is especially urged when using new or infrequently ordered drugs.

Library of Congress Cataloging-in-Publication Data
Names: Durham, Roberta F., author. | Chapman, Linda L., author.
Title: Maternal-newborn nursing: the critical components of nursing care/
  Roberta F. Durham, Linda L. Chapman.
Description: Third edition. | Philadelphia, PA: F. A. Davis Company, [2019]
  |Includes bibliographical references and index.
Identifiers: LCCN 2018025213 (print) | LCCN 2018025999 (ebook) | ISBN
  9780803690103 | ISBN 9780803666542
Subjects: | MESH: Maternal-Child Nursing | Perinatal Care
Classification: LCC RG951 (ebook) | LCC RG951 (print) | NLM WY157.3 | DDC
  618.2/0231--dc23
LC record available at https://lccn.loc.gov/2018025213

To my parents Raymond and Virginia "Ducky" Durham, husband, Douglas Fredebaugh and sisters, Ginny Durham and Dr. Patricia Durham Taylor. Thank you for your love and support. Aloha

To my husband, Chuck; my son, Mike; my daughter-in-law, Rachel; and my granddaughters, Cassidy and Kelsie. Thank you for being a big part of my life and this book. Love Linda, mom, and grandma

Preface

FOCUS

In this third edition of *Maternal-Newborn Nursing: The Critical Components of Nursing Care*, we continue to emphasize the basics of maternity nursing, focusing on evidence-based practice for all levels of nursing programs. Because we realize that today's students lead complex lives and must juggle multiple roles as student, parent, employee, and spouse, we developed this textbook, with its accompanying electronic ancillaries, to present the critical components of maternity nursing in a clear and concise format that lends itself to ease of comprehension while maintaining the integrity of the substantive content. It may be particularly useful for programs designed to present the subject of maternity in an abbreviated or condensed way.

We revised the textbook based on the recommendations of those who have used it—faculty from various states and students in all types of programs—and our own experiences. Revisions include enhanced rationale for nursing actions in all chapters, increased content in pathophysiology in many areas, and expanded high-risk content. We have updated content to keep current in standards in practice, including new guidelines for management of pregnancy complications, management of postpartum hemorrhage, management of intrapartal fetal heart rate abnormalities, assessment and care of the late preterm infant, and assessment and care of the newborn with hyperbilirubinemia. We have expanded sections on patient education, patient teaching resources, and complementary and alternative therapies. Professional standards of care for maternity nurses are based on current practice guidelines and research.

CRITICAL COMPONENTS

This textbook focuses on the critical components of maternity nursing. Critical components are the major areas of knowledge essential for a basic understanding of maternity nursing. The critical components were determined from the authors' combined 50 years of teaching maternity nursing in both traditional and accelerated programs and years of clinical practice in the maternity setting. Current guidelines and standards are integrated and summarized for a pragmatic approach to patient- and family-focused care. This focus is especially evident when discussing complications or deviations from the norm.

The focus of the text is on normal pregnancy and childbirth. Chapters on low-risk antenatal, intrapartal, postpartum, and neonate are followed by chapters on high risk and complications in each area. Complications germane to the nursing domain and childbearing population focus on understanding and synthesizing the critical elements for nursing care.

ORGANIZATION

This evidence-based text utilizes theory and clinical knowledge of maternity nursing. The conceptual framework is based on family developmental theory, and substantive theory that forms the foundation for maternity care is presented. The book is organized according to the natural sequence of the perinatal cycle, pregnancy, labor and birth, postpartum, and neonate. We have taken a biopsychosocial approach dealing with the physiological and psychological adaptation, and the social and cultural influences impacting childbearing families, with emphasis on nursing actions and care of women and families. We believe childbirth is a natural, developmental process.

Nursing is an ever-changing science. New research and clinical knowledge expand knowledge and change clinical practice. *Maternal-Newborn Nursing: The Critical Components of Nursing Care* reflects current knowledge, standards, and trends in maternity services, including the trend toward higher levels of intervention in maternity care. These standards and trends are reflected in our chapter on tests during the antepartal period, as well as a chapter devoted to fetal assessment and electronic fetal monitoring. We have devoted a chapter to the care of cesarean birth families, as nearly one-third of births in the United States are via cesarean.

This textbook clusters physiological changes, nursing assessment, and nursing care content in each chapter. Typically, a chapter is divided into systems in which the physiology; nursing care, including assessment and interventions; expected outcomes; and common deviations of one subsystem are presented. Psychosocial and cultural dimensions of nursing care are highlighted in each chapter.

FEATURES

This textbook presents the critical components of maternal–newborn nursing in a pragmatic, condensed format by using the following features:

- Bulleted format: For easy-to-read content
- Figures, tables, boxes, concept maps, and clinical pathways: Summarizes information in a visual way
- Learning Outcomes: Identifies what the reader will know and be able to do by the end of the chapter

x

- Critical Components: Highlights critical information in maternal–newborn nursing
- Evidenced-Based Practice: Highlights current research and practice guidelines related to nursing care
- Case Studies: Ties it all together by applying critical components in clinical context
- Safe and Effective Nursing Care (SENC): Highlights SENC concepts as they apply to the chapter content:
  - Cultural Competence: Stresses the importance of cultural factors in nursing care
  - Understanding Medications: Highlights commonly administered medications used during pregnancy, labor and birth, postpartum, and neonatal periods
  - Patient Education: Reflects current evidence-based practice guidelines and recommendations

APPENDICES

The appendices include:

- Association of Women's Health, Obstetric and Neonatal Nurses (AWHONN) guide to breastfeeding
- Recommended immunization schedule for infants and children aged 0 to 23 months
- What Does a Safe Sleep Environment Look Like?
- Common and standard laboratory values for pregnant and nonpregnant women and the neonate
- Immunization and pregnancy table
- Cervical dilation chart
- Temperature equivalents
- Newborn weight-conversion chart

RESOURCES AVAILABLE

Student

Use the unique code from the inside front cover to access the following student resources:

- Interactive Clinical Scenarios: Experience real-world challenges while working through each step in the nursing process
- Teaching Cards: Covers different topics focusing on the care and discharge of postpartum families formatted into cards that can be easily printed out and used to study
- Davis Edge + e-book: An online Q&A review platform with integrated interactive e-book that seamlessly blends into the classroom to give students the additional practice questions they need to perform well on course and board exams

Instructor

Instructors will have access to:

- Active Classroom Instructor's Guide: Maps, resources, and activities for an active classroom approach
- PowerPoints: Fully customizable slides summarizing key concepts from each chapter
- Test Bank: NCLEX-style questions with rationales for correct and incorrect answers in ExamView Pro
- Davis Edge + e-book: Create assignments, track your students' progress, and access the complete text online with our online Q&A review platform
- Image Bank: Includes all images from the text

Authors

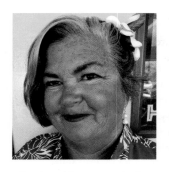

Roberta Durham

Roberta Durham, RN, PhD, is professor at California State University, East Bay, in Hayward, California, and a professor alumnus at Samuel Merritt University in Oakland, California. She received her bachelor's degree in nursing from the University of Rhode Island and her master's degree in nursing as a perinatal clinical specialist from the University of California, San Francisco. Dr. Durham received her PhD in nursing from the University of California, San Francisco, where she studied grounded theory method with Drs. Anselm Strauss and Leonard Schatzman. Her program of research has been on the management of premature labor and the prevention of premature birth. She has conducted international research and published her substantive and methodological work widely. She was previously a visiting professor at the University of Glasgow and is currently involved in international research in Central America to improve perinatal outcomes. She is a founding member of Hands for Global Health and serves as the vice chair on the board of directors and director of research. She has worked for over 25 years in labor and delivery units in the San Francisco Bay Area.

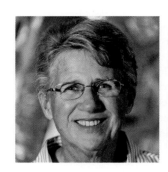

Linda Chapman

Linda Chapman, RN, PhD, has recently retired from University of Arizona College of Nursing and is a professor emeritus at Samuel Merritt University in Oakland, California. She received her diploma in nursing from Samuel Merritt Hospital School of Nursing, her bachelor's degree in nursing from University of Utah, and her master's degree in nursing from the University of California, San Francisco. Dr. Chapman received her PhD from the University of California, San Francisco, where she studied with Drs. Ramona Mercer and Katharyn May. Her program of research has been on the experience of men during the perinatal period. She has conducted research and published her substantive work in practice and research journals. She worked for 25 years in nursery, postpartum, and labor and birthing units at Samuel Merritt Hospital/Summit Medical Center in the San Francisco Bay Area.

Contributors

Sabine O. Balden, BSN, RN
OR Staff Nurse
Sutter Health California Pacific Medical Center
San Francisco, California

Sylvia A. Fischer, RN, MSN, CNM, FNP-C
Clinical instructor
University of Arizona
Tucson, Arizona

Melissa M. Goldsmith, PhD, RNC-MNN
Clinical Associate Professor
University of Arizona College of Nursing
Tucson, Arizona

Scout Emersen Hebnick, RNC-OB, MSN
Lecturer, Nurse Educator
California State University, East Bay
Hayward, California

Nancy Irland, DNP, MSN, CNM
Perinatal Clinical Specialist
Providence Health System, Oregon Region
Portland, Oregon

Kara L. Johnson, DNP, RNC-OB, CNS
Perinatal Clinical Nurse Specialist/Regional Program Manager
    Clinical Standardization-Perinatal
Providence Health & Services
Portland, Oregon

Patrick Kilgallen, BSN, RN
Staff Nurse Intermediate Intensive Care (IICU)
U.S. Department of Veterans Affairs
VA Palo Alto Health Care System
Palo Alto, California

Megan Elise Levy, BSN, RN, PHN
High-Risk Clinical Nurse II; Lecturer
Highland Hospital; California State University, East Bay
Oakland, California

Connie Miller, DNP, RNC-OB, CNE, CCCE
Clinical Associate Professor and Director, General Nursing
    and Health Education Division
University of Arizona College of Nursing
Tucson, Arizona

Rachael Miller, RN, BSN
Labor and Delivery Staff Nurse
University of California San Diego Health
San Diego, California

Janice J. Stinson, RNC, PhD
Labor and Delivery Staff Nurse
Alta Bates Summit Medical Center
Berkeley, California

Darice Taylor, MSN, RNC-NIC
Clinical Instructor
University of Arizona
Tucson, Arizona

Cecilia Urbina, RN, BSN
Graduate
California State University, East Bay
Hayward, CA

Reviewers

Karen M. Bennett, RN, MS, CCE
Associate Professor
Bill and Sandra Pomeroy College of Nursing
    at Crouse Hospital
Syracuse, New York

Tammy Bryant, RN, MSN
Program Chair—Associate of Science of Nursing
Southern Regional Technical College
Thomasville, Georgia

Carol Caico, NP, PhD, CS, OGNP-BC
Associate Professor
New York Institute of Technology
Old Westbury, New York

Julie C. Chew, RN, MS, PhD
Associate Professor
Dixie State University
St. George, Utah

Beth Desaretz Chiatti, PhD, RN, CTN, CSN
Assistant Professor
Drexel University
Philadelphia, Pennsylvania

Angela Clark, RNC-OB, MSN, BSN
Senior Clinical Faculty
Eastern Kentucky University
Richmond, Kentucky

Georgina Colalillo, MS, RN, CNE
Professor
Queensborough Community College/CUNY
Bayside, New York

Theresa Dubiel, MSN, RN
Faculty
Washtenaw Community College
Ann Arbor, Michigan

Susan Ellison, MSN, RNC, CNE
Course Coordinator
Middlesex County College Nursing Program
Edison, New Jersey

Nkonye Ezeobah, RN, MSN, RNC-MNN, FNP, PhD
Professor of Nursing, Assistant Program Director
Los Angeles Southwest College
Los Angeles, California

Jeffrey Fouche-Camargo, DNP, APRN, WHNP-BC, RNC-OB, C-EFM
Assistant Professor of Nursing
Georgia Gwinnett College
Lawrenceville, Georgia

Sharlene Georgesen, PhD, MSN, RN
Associate Professor
Morningside College
Sioux City, Iowa

Susan Golden, MSN, RN
Nursing Faculty
Eastern New Mexico University, Roswell
Roswell, New Mexico

Maria Grandinetti, PhD, RN, BSBA, CNE
Associate Professor
Wilkes University Passan School of Nursing
Wilkes-Barre, Pennsylvania

Elizabeth Hartman, PhD, MSN, RNC-OB, CNE
Associate Professor, Nursing Curriculum Committee Chairman
West Coast University, Los Angeles Campus
North Hollywood, California

Holly Howard, MSN-Ed, RNC
BSN Faculty
Arizona College
Mesa, Arizona

Susan Ihlenfeldt, RN, MSN, CNS
Nursing Faculty
Front Range Community College, Larimer Campus
Fort Collins, Colorado

Barbara Jared, PhD, MSN, RN, WHNP-BC
Assistant Professor of Nursing
Tennessee Technological University
Cookeville, Tennessee

Tina L. Koch, MS, RN, RAC-CT
ADN Assistant Professor
College of Southern Idaho
Twin Falls, Idaho

Maria D. Krol, DNP, RNC-NIC
Assistant Professor
Southern Connecticut State University
New Haven, Connecticut

Kathleen N. Krov, PhD, CNM, RN, CNE
Professor Health Science
Raritan Valley Community College
North Branch, New Jersey

Barbara Lane, MSN, RN-BC
Program Coordinator
Lincoln University, Ft. Wood Campus
Ft. Leonard Wood, Missouri

Cindy Lutkenhaus, MSN, RNC-OB
Professor
North Central Texas College
Gainesville, Texas

Bernita Missal, PhD, RN
Professor
Bethel University
St. Paul, Minnesota

Matthew Moore, JD, MPH
Assistant Professor
California State University, East Bay
Hayward, California

Wendy Moore, PhD-C, RNC-MNN, CNE
Assistant Professor of Nursing
Hartwick College
Oneonta, New York

Paula Moreau, PhD, RN
Professor of Nursing
Quinsigamond Community College
Worcester, Massachusetts

Jill Morsbach, MSN, RNC-MNN
Assistant Professor of Nursing
Missouri Western State University
St. Joseph, Missouri

Daisy G. Mullassery, DrNP, MSN, RN, WHNP- BC
Assistant Professor
University of Texas Health Science Center, School of Nursing
Houston, Texas

Margaret O'Neil, MN, RNC-OB
Nursing Faculty
Yakima Valley College
Yakima, Washington

Cecelia O'Neill, MSN, RNC-OB, C-EFM
Co-Course Director; Nursing of Women and Infants Across the
    Life Span
University of Pennsylvania
Philadelphia, Pennsylvania

Jan Pinheiro, RNC-OB, MSN
Senior Clinical Instructor
Eastern Kentucky University
Richmond, Kentucky

Theresa Puckett, PhD, RN
Professor of Nursing
Cuyahoga Community College, Metro Campus
Cleveland, Ohio

Colleen M. Quinlan, PhD, APRN
Associate Professor
University of Toledo
Toledo, Ohio

Marisue Rayno, RN, EdD
Nursing Professor
Luzerne County Community College
Nanticoke, Pennsylvania

Nancy Reno, MSN, APRN, FNP-BC
Nursing Faculty
Front Range Community College
Fort Collins, Colorado

Linda L. Rider, EdD, RN, CNE
Chairperson and Associate Professor
University of Central Oklahoma
Edmond, Oklahoma

Paula Rolfe BSc (hons), MSc, RN, BN, MN
Nurse Educator
Western Regional School of Nursing
Corner Brook, Newfoundland

Cynthia Rothenberger, DNP, RN, ACNS-BC
Assistant Professor, Nursing; Prelicensure Program
    Coordinator
Alvernia University
Reading, Pennsylvania

Donna Sandretto, MS, RN, CNE
Assistant Professor of Nursing, Course Coordinator
Niagara County Community College
Sanborn, New York

Barbara Stoner, RN, MSN
Faculty
Arapahoe Community College
Littleton, Colorado

Lisa Storck, MSN, RN
Faculty, Instructor
St. Luke's School of Nursing
Bethlehem, Pennsylvania

Jennifer Storer, MSN, RN
Associate Professor of Nursing
Kirkwood Community College
Cedar Rapids, Iowa

Bridget Sunkes, MS, RN
Assistant Professor
Pomeroy College of Nursing at Crouse Hospital
Syracuse, New York

Judy Wattman, MA, RNC, CLE
Instructor
Normandale Community College
Bloomington, Minnesota

Marcie Weissner, MSN, RNC-OB
Assistant Professor, Emeritus
University of Saint Francis, Fort Wayne
Fort Wayne, Indiana

Barbara L. Morrison Wilford, DNP, MBA/HCA, RN, CKC
Associate Professor of Nursing
Lorain County Community College
Elyria, Ohio

Acknowledgments

We are grateful to the following people, who helped us turn an idea into reality:

- Our husbands, Douglas Fredebaugh and Chuck Chapman, for their ongoing support and love
- Our colleagues at Samuel Merritt University, who helped us develop from novice to expert teachers
- Our current and past colleagues at the California State University, East Bay, and University of Arizona College of Nursing for their suggestions and support

- Our teachers and mentors Katharyn A. May, RN, DNSc, FAAN, and Ramona T. Mercer, RN, PhD, FAAN
- Our F.A. Davis team, Jacalyn Sharp, Amanda Minutola, and Andrea Miller, for their guidance
- Our contributors for sharing their expertise

Contents in Brief

Table of Contents

Maternity Nursing Overview

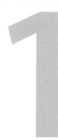

Trends and Issues

Linda L. Chapman, RN, PhD

LEARNING OUTCOMES

Upon completion of this chapter, the student will be able to:

1. Discuss current trends in the management of labor and birth.
2. Discuss current trends in maternal and infant health outcomes.
3. Identify leading causes of infant death.
4. Discuss current maternal and infant health issues.
5. Identify the primary maternal and infant goals of *Healthy People 2020*.

TRENDS

During the past 100 years, care of the childbearing family has undergone numerous changes in response to advances in technology, medicine, and nursing, as well as the individual desires of childbearing couples. As noted in Table 1–1, childbirth moved from the comfortable surroundings of the home to the unfamiliar surroundings of the hospital. In 1900, fewer than 5% of births took place in the hospital. By the late 1930s, this had increased to 75% of births (Wertz & Wertz, 1979). In the 1980s, hospital-based birthing suites were developed to reflect the homelike environment couples desired. Other notable birthing trends include:

- Fetal monitoring during labor began in the 1970s.
- Use of lactation consultants as part of the postpartum hospital team started in the late 1980s and early 1990s.
- The Baby-Friendly Hospital Initiative was developed by the World Health Organization (WHO) and the United Nations Children's Fund (UNICEF) in 1991. This initiative focuses on hospital practices that protect, promote, and support breastfeeding (see Chapter 16).
- The Back to Sleep campaign was initiated by the National Institute of Child Health and Human Development (NICHD) in 1996 to educate parents about the importance of placing infants on their backs to sleep to reduce the risk of sudden infant death syndrome.
- In 2012, the NICHD's Safe to Sleep campaign built on the Back to Sleep campaign (see Chapter 16).

Advances in obstetrical care and medicine have tremendously impacted the number of maternal and infant deaths, with maternal mortality rates declining from 607.9 per 100,000 live births in 1915 to 14 per 100,000 live births in 2015, and infant mortality rates declining from 50.1 per 1,000 live births in 1915 to 5.8 per 1,000 live births in 2017 (Bureau of the Census, 1917; CIA, 2018a; CIA, 2018c; WHO, 2018a). In contrast, cesarean births increased from 20.7% in 1996 to 32.9% in 2009 (Hamilton, Martin, & Ventura, 2011). By 2016, however, the cesarean rate decreased to 31.9% (Martin et al., 2018). Induction of labor rates have increased from a low of 5% in 1970 to 23.3% in 2012 (Osterman & Martin, 2014).

Fertility and Birthrates

Total fertility rate (TFR) is "the average number of children that would be born per woman if all women lived to the end of their childbearing years and bore children according to a given fertility rate at each age" (CIA, 2018a). TFR is an indicator of population change; greater than 2 indicates that the country's population is growing, while less than 2 indicates a population decreasing in

TABLE 1–1   Past and Present Trends

PAST TRENDS	PRESENT TRENDS
Nursing: Focus on physiological changes and needs of the mother and infant	Family-centered maternity nursing: Focus on both the physiological and psychosocial changes and needs of the childbearing family
Primarily home births	Primarily hospital births
Women labored in one room and delivered in another room	Women labor, deliver, and recover in the same room
Delivery rooms cold and sterile	Birthing rooms warm and homelike
Expectant fathers and family excluded from the labor and birth experience	Expectant partner, family, and friends involved in the labor and birth experience
Expectant fathers or family members excluded from cesarean births	Expectant partner or family members in the operating room during cesarean births
Labor pain management: Amnesia or "twilight sleep" to natural childbirth	Labor pain management: analgesics, epidurals, and nitrous oxide
Hospital postpartum stay of 10 days	Hospital postpartum stay of 48 hours or less
Infant mortality rate of 50.1 per 1,000 live births in 1915 (Bureau of the Census, 1917)	Infant mortality rate of 5.8 per 1,000 live births in 2017 (CIA, 2018c)
Diarrhea and enteritis: Number one cause of infant death in 1915 (Bureau of the Census, 1917)	Congenital malformations and abnormalities: Number one cause of infant mortality in 2015 (Martin et al., 2018)
Maternal mortality rate of 607.9 per 100,000 live births in 1915 (Bureau of Census, 1917)	Maternal mortality rate of 14 per 100,000 live births in 2015 (WHO, 2015)
Induction of labor rate of 9.5% in 1990 (Martin et al., 2006)	Induction of labor rate of 23.3% in 2012 (Osterman & Martin, 2014)
Cesarean section rate of 20.7% in 1996 (Martin et al., 2006)	Cesarean section rate of 31.9% in 2016 (Martin et al., 2018)
Low probability of survival for infants born at or before 28 weeks of gestation	Increased survival rates for infants born between 24 weeks and 28 weeks of gestation

size (CIA, 2018a). In 2017, the United States ranked 143 out of 224 countries with an approximate TFR of 1.87 children born/woman. This shows that the population is decreasing in size and that its members are growing older. Table 1–2 provides information from select countries and their 1960 and 2017 TFR, which indicates a decrease in each country's TFR. Singapore has the greatest decrease, from 5.5 to 0.83 children born/woman.

Birthrate is the number of live births per 1,000 people. In 2017, the United States was ranked number 158 out of 226 countries with an estimated birthrate of 12.5 (CIA, 2018b). Table 1–3 provides data on U.S. birthrates from 1960 to 2017. The following is a sample ranking of other countries:

- Angola is ranked 1 with a rate of 44.20.
- Egypt is ranked 40 with a rate of 29.60.
- Mexico is ranked 94 with a rate of 18.30.
- Australia is ranked 165 with a rate of 12.10.
- The United Kingdom is ranked 166 with a rate of 12.10.
- Canada is ranked 190 with a rate of 10.30.
- Japan is ranked 223 with a rate of 7.70.
- Monaco is ranked 226 with a rate of 6.60 (CIA 2018a).

The United States saw decreases in both the fertility rate and the birthrate between 1960 and 2017. During this period, the TFR decreased 49%, from 3.7 to 1.87 children born/woman. The birthrate during this same period decreased 47%, from 23.7 to 12.5 live births per 1,000. This decline may be attributed to:

- Availability of a variety of highly effective contraceptive methods.
- More women delaying reproduction to pursue careers, having fewer children, or choosing to remain child-free.
- Legalization and availability of elective abortions.
- The rising cost of raising children, leading to smaller families.

An interesting trend is noted regarding birthrate and the mother's age for the 26-year period from 1990 to 2016 (Table 1–4). The birthrates decreased for women aged 15 to 29 but increased for women aged 30 to 45 and older. The greatest increase was seen in women aged 40 and older. The greatest decrease was in women aged 15 to 19. This trend is influenced by the increasing number

TABLE 1-2 Total Fertility Rate (TFR) 1960 and 2017

COUNTRY	1960	2017	COUNTRY	1960	2017
Afghanistan	7.5	5.12	Israel	3.9	2.64
Niger	7.4	6.49	Canada	3.8	1.6
Brazil	6.1	1.75	United States	3.7	1.87
Mexico	6.8	2.24	United Kingdom	2.7	1.88
Egypt	6.6	3.47	Denmark	2.6	1.61
Singapore	5.5	0.82	Russia	2.5	1.61
New Zealand	4.1	2.02	Germany	2.4	1.45

CIA, 2018a; World Bank, 2016a.

TABLE 1-3 Birth Rates, United States of America, 1960–2015

	1960	1970	1980	1990	2000	2010	2015	2017
Birthrate	23.7	18.4	15.9	16.7	14.4	13	12.5	12.5

CIA, 2018b; Hamilton et al., 2007b, 2009b, 2011, 2016.

TABLE 1-4 Birth Rates by Age of Mother (per 1,000)

	15–19	20–24	25–29	30–34	35–39	40–44	45 +
1990	59.9	116.5	120.2	80.8	31.7	5.5	0.2
2000	47.7	109.7	113.5	91.2	39.7	8.0	0.5
2005	40.5	102.2	115.5	95.8	46.3	9.1	0.6
2010	34.1	90.0	108.3	96.6	45.9	10.2	0.7
2015	22.3	76.9	104.3	101.4	51.7	11.0	0.8
2016	22.3	73.8	102.1	102.7	52.7	11.4	0.9
Change from 1990 to 2016	↓62.7%	↓36.7%	↓15%	↑27.1%	↑66.2%	↑107%	↑350%

Hamilton et al., 2007b, 2009b, 2011, 2016; Martin et al., 2018.

of women who have delayed childbirth due to career choices or socioeconomic reasons and the increased availability of contraceptives for younger women.

The United States had a total of 3,945,875 births in 2016, a birthrate of 12.2. The percentages of these births by race are:

● American Indian or Alaska Native: 0.8%.
● Asian: 6.4%.
● Native Hawaiian or other Pacific Islanders: 0.2%.
● Hispanic: 23%.
● Non-Hispanic black: 14%.
● Non-Hispanic white: 52% (Martin et al., 2018).

These percentages reflect the multicultural population of the United States and present an exciting challenge to health care workers, who must adapt the care they provide to reflect an understanding of the beliefs and cultural practices of a wide variety of childbearing families.

Preterm Births

Preterm births are divided into three classifications:

- Very premature: Neonates born at less than 32 weeks of gestation
- Moderately premature: Neonates born between 32 and 33 completed weeks of gestation
- Late premature: Neonates born between 34 and 36 completed weeks of gestation

Globally, it is estimated that in 2015 there were 15 million premature births. Complications related to preterm birth are the leading cause of death for children younger than age 5 (WHO, 2018a). In the United States from 2000 to 2015, preterm births decreased by 24% to a total preterm birthrate of 9.62, but in 2016 it increased to 9.95% (Hamilton, Martin, & Osterman, 2016; Hamilton, Martin, & Ventura, 2011; Martin et al., 2018). The 2016 increase in total preterm rate is attributed to an increase in late preterm births (Martin et al., 2018). Despite widespread advances in perinatal care, the preterm birthrate remains high compared to that of other high-income countries, such as Canada, Japan, Australia, Israel, and Norway. Table 1–5 provides information on the percentages of preterm births in the United States in 2005, 2010, 2015, and 2016.

The 2016 percentages of premature births based on the mother's race are:

- Hispanic: 9.45%.
- Non-Hispanic black: 13.77%.
- Non-Hispanic white: 9.04% (Martin et al., 2018).

These percentages substantially contribute to racial and ethnic disparities in infant health outcome, discussed later in this chapter. Premature birth impacts both the emotional well-being of parents and the length and quality of life for the preterm infant. A shorter gestational period increases the risk of complications related to immature body organs and systems that can have lifelong negative effects, including but not limited to:

- Respiratory disorders
- Cerebral palsy
- Vision and hearing disorders
- Developmental delays

TABLE 1–5 Percentages of Preterm Births in United States, 2005, 2010, 2015, 2016

	2005	2010	2015	2016
Very Preterm	2.03	1.97	1.58	1.59
Moderately Preterm	1.6	1.53	1.17	1.17
Late Preterm	9.09	8.49	6.87	7.09
Total Preterm	12.73	11.99	9.62	9.85

Hamilton et al., 2011; Hamilton et al., 2016; Martin et al., 2018.

Of all infant deaths, 36% are related to preterm birth (CDC, 2016a). Parents of preterm infants must also contend with increased health care costs.

Neonatal Birth Weight Rates

Neonatal birth weight rates are reported by the Centers for Disease Control and Prevention (CDC) in three major categories: low, normal, and high. Normal birth weight is between 2,500 and 3,999 grams; high birth weight is 4,000 grams or greater; low birth weight is below 2,500 grams. Low birth weight is divided into two categories:

- Low birth weight (LBW) is defined as birth weight that is less than 2,500 grams but greater than 1,500 grams. The percentage of LBW neonates has increased from 8% in 2014 to 8.17% in 2016 (Hamilton et al., 2016; Martin et al., 2018).
- Very low birth weight (VLBW) is defined as a birth weight of less than 1,500 grams. The percentage of VLBW neonates has remained stable at 1.4% in 2014 and 1.4% in 2016 (Hamilton et al., 2016; Martin et al., 2018).

The weight of neonates at birth is an important predictor of future morbidity and mortality rates (Martin et al., 2011):

- Neonates with birth weights between 4,000 and 4,999 grams have the lowest mortality rate during the first year of life.
- VLBW neonates are 100 times more likely to die during the first year of life than are neonates with birth weights greater than 2,500 grams.
- VLBW neonates account for 1.45% of all births and 54% of all infant deaths (Martin et al., 2011).

Infant Mortality Rates

Infant mortality is defined as a death before the first birthday. Globally, infant mortality has decreased from 64.8 deaths per 1,000 live births in 1990 to 30.5 deaths per 1,000 live births in 2016 (WHO, 2018b). Infant mortality rates in the United States decreased from 26 per 1,000 live births in 1960 to 5.8 in 2017 (CIA, 2018c; Kochanek, Murphy, Xu, & Tejada, 2016). This decrease in the United States is related to:

- Improvement and advances in knowledge and care of high-risk neonates, notably:
  - Advances in medical technology such as extracorporeal membrane oxygenation therapy (ECMO), used for respiratory distress in preterm infants (see Chapter 17).
  - Advances in medical treatment such as exogenous pulmonary surfactant (see Chapter 17).
- Improved prenatal care.
- Increased infant sleep safety education.

Although this is a significant decrease, the infant mortality rate remains too high for a nation with the available wealth and health care resources of the United States. The leading causes of infant deaths are listed in Table 1–6. Infant deaths related to SIDS and respiratory distress syndrome (RDS) of newborns significantly

TABLE 1–6   Leading Causes of Infant Deaths and Mortality Rates (Rates per 100,000 Live Births)

CAUSE OF DEATH	1995 RATE	CAUSE OF DEATH	2010 RATE	CAUSE OF DEATH	2015 RATE
Congenital malformations and chromosomal abnormalities	168.1	Congenital malformations and chromosomal abnormalities	126.9	Congenital malformations and chromosomal abnormalities	121.3
Disorders related to short gestation and low birth weight	100.9	Disorders related to short gestation and low birth weight	103.2	Disorders related to short gestation and low birth weight	102.7
Sudden infant death syndrome	87.1	Sudden infant death syndrome	47.2	Sudden infant death syndrome	39.4
Respiratory distress of newborns	37.3	Newborn affected by maternal complications of pregnancy	38.9	Newborn affected by maternal complications of pregnancy	38.3
Newborns affected by maternal complications of pregnancy	33.6	Accidents	26.1	Accidents	32.4
Newborns affected by complications of placenta, cord, and membranes	24.7	Newborns affected by complications of placenta, cord, and membranes	25.7	Newborns affected by complications of placenta, cord, and membranes	22.9
Infections specific to the perinatal period	20.2	Bacterial sepsis of the newborn	14.2	Bacterial sepsis of the newborn	15.1
Accidents	20.2	Disease of the circulatory system	12.5	Respiratory distress of newborns	11.6
Pneumonia and influenza	12.6	Respiratory distress of newborns	12.4	Disease of the circulatory system	10.8
Intrauterine hypoxia and birth asphyxia	12.2	Necrotizing enterocolitis	11.7	Neonatal hemorrhage	10.2

Anderson, Kochanek, & Murphy, 1997; Kochanek et al., 2016; Martin et al., 2018; Murphy, Xu, & Kochanek, 2012.

decreased between 1995 and 2015. The decrease in SIDS can be attributed to Safe to Sleep, a public education program led by NICHD and other initiatives to teach parents safe newborn sleep habits, such as placing the child in the crib on his or her back. The decrease in deaths related to RDS reflects advances in medical and nursing care of preterm infants.

Maternal Death and Mortality Rates

The Department of Health and Human Services uses several definitions of maternal death:

- Maternal death is defined by WHO as the death of a woman during pregnancy or within 42 days of pregnancy termination caused by conditions aggravated by the pregnancy or associated medical treatments. This category excludes death from accidents or injuries.
- Direct obstetric death results from complications during pregnancy, labor, birth, and/or the postpartum period, including deaths caused by interventions, omission of interventions, or incorrect treatment. An example of this category is death caused by postpartum hemorrhage.
- Indirect obstetric death is caused by a preexisting disease or a disease that develops during pregnancy without direct

obstetrical cause but is aggravated by the pregnancy. One example is death related to complication of systemic lupus erythematosus that was aggravated by pregnancy.
- Late maternal death occurs more than 42 days after termination of pregnancy from a direct or indirect obstetrical cause.
- Pregnancy-related death is the death of a woman during pregnancy or within 1 year of the end of pregnancy from a pregnancy complication, a chain of events initiated by pregnancy, or the aggravation of an unrelated condition by the physiological effects of pregnancy (Hoyert, 2007). An example is a pulmonary embolism related to deep vein thrombosis that leads to death during or after pregnancy.

Maternal mortality ratio (MMR) is defined as the number of maternal deaths per 100,000 live births. In the United States, MMR significantly decreased from 607.9 in 1915 to 12 in 1990 (Hoyert, 2007; WHO, 2015); however, as of 2015, MMR has increased by 14% to 14. Table 1–7 provides international MMR data and lifetime risk of maternal death. Note that the United States is one of a few countries whose MMR has increased. Lifetime risk is the probability that a 15-year-old woman will eventually die from a maternal cause (WHO, 2015). The United States has a high lifetime risk of maternal death, at 1 in 3,800,

TABLE 1-7   Trends in Estimates of Maternal Mortality Ratio (MMR), 1990–2015, and Lifetime Risk of Maternal Death, 2015

COUNTRY	MMR 1990	MMR 2000	MMR 2010	MMR 2015	% CHANGE IN MMR BETWEEN 1990 AND 2015	LIFETIME RISK OF MATERNAL DEATH (2015): 1 IN
Afghanistan	1,340	1,100	584	396	70.4	52
Argentina	72	60	58	52	27.8	790
Australia	8	9	6	6	25.0	8,700
Austria	8	5	4	4	50.0	18,200
Bahamas	46	61	85	80	–73.9	660
Brazil	104	66	65	44	57.7	1,200
Burundi	1,220	954	808	712	41.6	23
Canada	7	9	8	7	0.0	8,800
China	97	58	35	27	72.2	2,400
Congo	603	653	509	442	26.7	45
Cuba	58	43	44	39	32.8	1,800
Czech Republic	14	7	5	4	71.4	14,800
Denmark	11	9	7	6	38.8	9,500
Egypt	106	63	40	33	68.9	810
Finland	6	5	3	3	50.0	21,700
El Salvador	157	84	59	54	65.5	890
Ethiopia	1,250	897	353	353	71.8	64
France	15	12	9	8	46.7	6,100
Georgia	34	37	40	36	–5.9	1,500
Germany	11	8	7	6	45.5	11,700
Greece	5	4	3	3	40	23,700
Guyana	171	210	241	229	–33.9	170
Haiti	625	505	389	359	42.6	90
Hungary	24	15	15	17	29.2	4,400
India	556	374	215	174	6.7	220
Iran	123	51	27	25	79.7	2,000
Iraq	107	63	51	50	53.3	420
Israel	11	8	6	5	54.5	6,200
Italy	8	5	4	4	50	19,700
Jamaica	79	89	93	89	–12.7	520
Japan	14	10	6	5	64.3	13,400

TABLE 1-7 Trends in Estimates of Maternal Mortality Ratio (MMR), 1990–2015, and Lifetime Risk of Maternal Death, 2015—cont'd

COUNTRY	MMR 1990	MMR 2000	MMR 2010	MMR 2015	% CHANGE IN MMR BETWEEN 1990 AND 2015	LIFETIME RISK OF MATERNAL DEATH (2015): 1 IN
Jordan	110	77	59	58	47.3	490
Kenya	687	759	605	510	25.8	42
Kuwait	7	7	5	4	42.9	10,300
Libera	1,500	1,270	811	25	51.7	28
Mexico	90	77	45	38	57.8	1,100
Netherlands	12	14	8	7	41.7	8,700
New Zealand	18	12	13	11	38.9	4,500
Pakistan	431	306	211	178	58.7	140
Philippines	152	124	129	114	25	280
Poland	17	8	4	3	82.4	22,100
Republic of Korea	21	16	15	11	47.6	7,200
Romania	124	51	30	31	75	2,300
Russia Federation	63	57	29	25	60.3	2,300
Saudi Arabia	46	23	14	12	73.9	3,100
Serbia	14	17	16	17	−21.4	3,900
Singapore	12	18	11	10	16.7	8,200
South Africa	108	85	154	138	−27.8	300
Syrian Arab Republic	123	73	49	68	44.7	440
Tonga	75	97	130	124	−65.3	58
Turkey	97	79	23	16	83.5	3,000
United Arab Emirates	17	8	6	6	6	7,900
United Kingdom	10	12	10	9	10	5,800
United States of America	12	12	14	14	−16.7	3,800
Zimbabwe	440	590	446	443	−0.7	52

World Health Organization, 2015.

compared to other developed countries; for example, Greece's risk is 1 out of 23,700 and Poland's is 1 out of 22,100. Worldwide, there were an estimated 303,000 maternal deaths in 2015:

- 99% of these deaths occur in developing countries.
- 66% occur in the sub-Saharan Africa region.
- Maternal deaths worldwide have decreased by 44% from 1990 to 2015.

The decrease of maternal deaths in developing countries is attributed to increased female education, increased use of contraception, improved antenatal care, and increased number of births attended by skilled health personnel (WHO, 2015). Primary causes of maternal deaths worldwide are:

- Severe hemorrhage
- Infections

- Eclampsia
- Obstructed labor
- Complications of abortions
- Other causes, such as anemia, HIV/AIDS, and cardiovascular disease (WHO, 2015)

ISSUES

Primary issues affecting the health of mothers and infants include Teen Pregnancy, tobacco and electronic cigarette use during pregnancy, substance abuse during pregnancy, obesity, and health disparities.

Teen Pregnancy

As shown in Table 1–8, the birthrate for teenagers in the United States has been declining since 1990:

- The birth rate for teenagers aged 15 to 17 has decreased 76.5% from 1990 to 2016, with a decrease of 49.1% from 2010 to 2016.
- The greatest percentage of change occurred in ages 10 to 14, with a decrease of 85.7% from 1990 to 2016.
- Massachusetts has the lowest teen birthrate, at 8.5, and Arkansas has the highest teen birthrate, at 34.6 (Table 1–9).
- The teen birthrate in the United States in 2016 was higher than other developed countries, with 21 births per 1,000 females aged 15 to 19 compared to Switzerland's rate of 3 and Canada's rate of 9. Teen birthrates of selected countries are:
  - Denmark—3
  - Japan—4
  - Saudi Arabia—9
  - Australia—14
  - India—23
  - Russia—27
  - South Africa—44
  - Mexico—62

- Democratic Republic of the Congo—122 (World Bank, 2016b)

Table 1–10 provides information on the change in pregnancy rates of females aged 15 to 19 by race/ethnicity. All race/ethnicity groups have experienced a decline, with Asian/Pacific Islanders having the greatest decrease of 75% since 1991. The birthrate among Hispanic girls aged 15 to 19 is more than twice the rate of non-Hispanic white births for that age group.

Parity and Marital Status

Teen mothers are more likely to have additional children and to be unmarried (Hamilton et al., 2016):

- 83% of all births for teens are first births, 15% are second births, and 2% are third or more births.
- 17% of all teen mothers will have at least one more birth before age 20.
- 89% of teen mothers are unmarried.

Implications of Teen Pregnancy and Birth

Teen births have adverse long-term effects on both the mothers and children, presenting a variety of issues for both teen parents and society. For teen mothers, these include:

- Poverty and income disparities
  - 66% of teen mothers are poor and 25% begin receiving welfare within 3 years of the birth of their first child (National Conference of State Legislators, 2016).
  - 17% of teen mothers will have a second child before age 20, which further decreases their ability to complete school and qualify for well-paying jobs (National Campaign to Prevent Teen Pregnancy, 2016a).
- Risk of sexually transmitted illnesses, including HIV, as well as hypertensive problems during pregnancy
  - Chlamydia causes increased risk of neonatal conjunctivitis and chlamydial pneumonia.
  - Syphilis increases the risk of neonatal blindness and maternal and neonatal death.
  - Gonorrhea increases risk of neonatal conjunctivitis and blindness.

TABLE 1-8 Birthrates for Teen Females: Births per 1,000 Live Births

AGE	1990	2005	2010	2015	2016	PERCENTAGE OF CHANGE 1990–2016	PERCENTAGE OF CHANGE 2010–2016
10–14	1.4	0.7	0.4	0.2	0.2	↓85.7%	↓50%
15–17	37.5	21.4	17.3	9.9	8.8	↓76.5%	↓49.1%
18–19	88.6	69.9	58.3	40.7	37.5	↓57.7%	↓35.7%

Hamilton et al., 2011; Hamilton et al., 2016; Martin et al., 2018.

TABLE 1-9 Teen Birthrate 2016: Births per 1,000 Girls Age 15-19

STATE	BIRTHRATE	STATE	BIRTH RATE	STATE	BIRTH RATE
Alabama	28.3	Louisiana	30.6	Oklahoma	33.4
Alaska	25.8	Maine	14.7	Oregon	16.6
Arizona	23.6	Maryland	15.9	Pennsylvania	15.8
Arkansas	34.6	Massachusetts	8.5	Rhode Island	12.9
California	17.0	Michigan	17.7	South Carolina	23.7
Colorado	17.8	Minnesota	12.6	South Dakota	25.1
Connecticut	9.4	Mississippi	32.6	Tennessee	28.0
Delaware	19.5	Missouri	23.4	Texas	31.0
District of Columbia	24.0	Montana	23.7	Utah	15.6
Florida	19.3	Nebraska	19.1	Vermont	10.3
Georgia	23.6	Nevada	24.2	Virginia	15.5
Hawaii	19.2	New Hampshire	9.3	Washington	16.6
Idaho	20.1	New Jersey	11.0	West Virginia	29.3
Illinois	18.7	New Mexico	29.8	Wisconsin	15.0
Indiana	23.6	New York	13.2	Wyoming	26.1
Iowa	17.2	North Carolina	21.8		
Kansas	21.9	North Dakota	20.3		
Kentucky	30.9	Ohio	21.8		

HHS, 2018.

TABLE 1-10 Teen Pregnancy Rate by Race/Ethnicity, 2015: Pregnancies per 1,000 Girls Age 15-19

RACE/ETHNICITY	RATE 2015	RATE 2016	CHANGE SINCE 2013	CHANGE SINCE 1991
Non-Hispanic Black	31.8	29	↓ 8%	↓ 75%
Hispanic	34.9	32	↓ 9%	↓ 70%
Non-Hispanic White	16	14	↓ 10%	↓ 67%

National Campaign to Prevent Teen Pregnancy, 2016b.

● Educational issues, with only half of teen mothers earning a high school diploma by age 22 and less than 2% finishing college by age 30 (National Conference of State Legislators, 2016).

Children born to teen mothers are at increased risk for:

● Health problems related to prematurity and/or low birth weight, including infant death, respiratory distress syndrome, intraventricular bleeding, vision problems, and intestinal problems.

- A higher mortality rate for infants of women younger than age 15 compared with infants born to women of all ages.
- Behavioral problems.
- Placement in foster homes.
- Lower school achievement and dropping out of school.
- Incarceration during adolescence (Youth.Gov, 2016).

Teen fathers have a 30% lower probability of graduating from high school than boys who are not fathers (Youth.Gov, 2016). In addition, teenage males without an involved father are at higher risk for being incarcerated, dropping out of school, and abusing drugs or alcohol.

CRITICAL COMPONENT

Teen Pregnancies

Teen pregnancies have short-term and long-term adverse effects for teen mothers, teen fathers, their children, their community, and society.

Tobacco and Electronic Cigarette Use During Pregnancy

Tobacco use during pregnancy is associated with an increased risk of LBW, intrauterine growth restriction, miscarriage, abruptio placenta, premature birth, SIDS, and respiratory problems in the newborn.

- Cigarette smoking during pregnancy declined from 19.5% in 1989 to 8.4% in 2014 (Curtain & Mathews, 2016).
- Women who smoke during pregnancy are less likely to breastfeed their infants.
- Of women who smoked prior to pregnancy, 20.6% quit during pregnancy (Curtain & Mathews, 2016).
- Based on age, the highest smoking prevalence rate is among women aged 20 to 24 (Table 1–11).
- Based on race, the highest percentage of female smokers is among American Indians and Alaska Natives (see Table 1–11).
- Based on educational level, the highest percentage of female smokers are women with less than high school education (see Table 1–11).

Electronic cigarettes (e-cigarettes) are increasingly prevalent in the United States, but their effects when used during pregnancy are not fully understood. E-cigarettes are not controlled by the Food and Drug Administration (FDA) and may contain carcinogenic and toxic compounds. Nicotine, which is present in e-cigarettes, is a health danger to both the pregnant woman and her fetus. It can adversely affect the developing fetal brain and lungs.

CRITICAL COMPONENT

Tobacco and E-Cigarettes

- Nicotine is a health danger for pregnant women and their developing fetuses.
- Pregnant women should not use any tobacco product or e-cigarettes, since nicotine is toxic to developing fetuses and impairs fetal brain and lung development (CDC, 2018a).

TABLE 1–11　Prevalence of Maternal Smoking During Pregnancy by Maternal Characteristics	
MATERNAL CHARACTERISTICS	**SMOKING PREVALENCE RATE (PERCENT)**
Age	
Under 20	10.1
20–24	13
25–29	9
30–34	5.7
35 and over	4.5
Marital Status	
Unmarried	14.7
Married	4.1
Race	
White	12.2
Black	6.8
Asian	0.7
American Indian or Alaska Native	18
Hispanic	2
Education	
Less than high school	14.1
High school and some college	11
Bachelor's degree or higher	0.9

Curtin & Mathews, 2016.

Substance Abuse During Pregnancy

In the general U.S. population, the use of illicit drugs and marijuana is greatest in people aged 18 to 25 and the use of alcohol is greatest for people aged 26 to 34 (Table 1–12). Asian Americans have the lowest use of illicit drugs and marijuana and Native Hawaiian and Pacific Islanders have the lowest use of alcohol. American Indians and Alaska Natives have the highest use of illicit drugs and marijuana, and non-Hispanic white women have the highest use of alcohol.

The use of alcohol and illicit drugs during pregnancy can have a profound effect on the developing fetus and the health of the neonate. Ten percent of women report use of alcohol during pregnancy and 3% of women report binge drinking during pregnancy (CDC, 2016b). Exposure to alcohol during pregnancy

TABLE 1-12   Use of Selected Substances Among Persons Aged 12 and Over 35 by Age and Race, 2014 (Percent of Population)

CHARACTERISTICS	ANY ILLICIT DRUG	MARIJUANA	NONMEDICAL USE OF ANY PSYCHOTHERAPEUTIC DRUG	ALCOHOL USE
Age				
12–13	3.4	1.1	1.8	2.1
14–15	7.6	5.5	2.6	8.5
16–17	16.5	15	3.4	23.3
18–25	22	19.6	4.4	59.6
26–34	15.1	12.7	4.1	66
35 and over	6.7	5.2	1.7	54.4
Race				
Non-Hispanic white	10.4	8.7	2.5	57.7
Non-Hispanic black	12.4	10.3	2.7	44.2
American Indian or Alaska Native	14.9	11.8	4.8	42.3
Native Hawaiian or Pacific Islander	15.6	12.1	6.2	37.9
Asia	4.1	2.8	1.1	38.7
Hispanic or Latina	8.9	6.7	2.5	44.4

NCHS, 2016.

places the developing fetus at risk for fetal death; low birth weight; intrauterine growth retardation; mental retardation; and fetal alcohol spectrum disorders (FASDs), which is "a group of conditions that can occur in a person whose mother drank alcohol during pregnancy" (CDC, 2017). For more information on FASDs, which have physical, behavioral, and cognitive effects, see Chapter 17.

Exposure to illicit drugs during pregnancy is associated with preterm birth, abruptio placenta, drug withdrawal for the neonate, and congenital defects.

● Cocaine use during pregnancy can cause strokes and seizure in the developing fetus and can affect cognitive performance, information processing, and attention to tasks in children (WebMD, 2014).
● Marijuana use during pregnancy may have a negative effect on the neurological development of the fetus (NIDA, 2016).

Obesity

Obesity is defined as a body mass index (BMI) greater than or equal to 30. In the United States, the percentage of adult and youth who are obese is increasing. In 2000, 30.5% of adults and 13.9% of youth were obese. In 2014, 36.5% of adults and 17%

of youth aged 2 to 16 were obese, 34.4% of women aged 20 to 39 years were obese, and 21% of females aged 12 to 19 years were obese (Ogden, Carroll, Fryar, & Flegal, 2015).

CRITICAL COMPONENT

Obesity

In the United States, obesity is a major health concern for both adults and youth. Pregnant women who are obese are at higher risk for complications such as diabetes and cesarean birth. Infants born to woman who are obese are at higher risk for complications such as intrauterine fetal death and birth injuries related to macrosomia.

Obesity in childbearing women has adverse effects on both the woman and her child. Pregnant women who are obese are at higher risk for:

● Gestational hypertension
● Preeclampsia
● Gestational diabetes

TABLE 1–13   Racial Health Disparities

	AMERICAN INDIAN OR ALASKA NATIVE	ASIAN OR PACIFIC ISLANDER	BLACK	HISPANIC OR LATINA	WHITE
Preterm Birth by Gestational Age					
34–36 weeks	6.8%	5.2%	7.2%	5.7%	5.3%
32–33 weeks	1%	0.7%	1.3%	0.8%	0.7%
Less than 32 weeks	1.2%	0.9%	2.6%	1.2%	0.9%
Infant Mortality Rate	7.72	3.9	11.11	5.00	5.06
Cesarean Births[a]	21.5%	27.6	29.9%	25.8%	25%
Women Receiving Late or No Prenatal Care	10.8%	5.7%	9.7%	7.5%	4.3%
Obesity[b]					
2–5 years	N/A	N/A	10.4%	15.6%	5.2%
6–11 years	N/A	9.8%	21.4%	25%	13.6%
12–19 years	N/A	9.4%	22.6%	22.8%	19.6%
Hypertension[c]	N/A	25%	44%	28.6%	28%
Cigarette Smoking[c]	N/A	5.1%	13.7%	7.4%	18.3%
Influenza Vaccination					
18–64 years	N/A	41.3%	30.8%	27.9%	38.5%
65 years and over	N/A	72.7%	57.4%	60.8%	72.4%
No Health Insurance Coverage					
Under 18 years	N/A	4.3%	2.9%	8%	3.6%
18–64 years	N/A	7.3%	14.5%	27.2%	8.8%

NCHS, 2016.
[a]*Low-risk births delivered by cesarean section*
[b]*Children and adolescents with obesity*
[c]*Women only*

- Thromboembolism
- Cesarean birth
- Wound infections
- Shoulder dystocia related to macrosomia (birth weight more than 4,000 grams)
- Sleep apnea
- Anesthesia complications

Fetuses and infants of obese pregnant women are at higher risk for:

- Fetal abnormalities, including spina bifida, heart defects, anorectal atresia, and hypospadias.
- Intrauterine fetal death.

- Birth injuries related to macrosomia.
- Childhood obesity and diabetes.

Health Disparities

The topic of health disparities addresses differences in access, use of health care services, and health outcomes among various ages, sexual orientations, races, ethnicities, disabilities, socioeconomic levels, and geographic groups. Table 1–13 provides information on racial health disparities, the greatest of which are experienced by those who are black and Hispanic. Infant mortality rates in the United States are highest for black children.

TABLE 1–14 Sexual Orientation Health Disparities, Women Aged 18 and Over (Reported in Percentages)

	GAY OR LESBIAN	BISEXUAL	STRAIGHT
Sexual Orientation	1.5	0.9	97.7
Health-Related Behaviors			
Current cigarette smokers	25.7	28.5	15
Five or more alcoholic drinks in 1 day at least once a year	25.8	33.8	14.3
Met federal guidelines for aerobic physical activity	47.9	55.5	45.1
Health Status			
Health status described as excellent or very good	53.4	55.5	59.8
Experienced serious psychological distress in past 30 days	5.3	10.9	4.2
Obese	36.7	40.9	28.3
Health Care Services			
Received influenza vaccine during past year	42.9	32.2	44.9
Ever tested for HIV	51.6	52.6	40.2
Health Care Access			
Has a usual place to go for medical care	77.5	72.5	87.8
Failed to obtain needed medical care for past year due to cost	14.3	16.2	8.2
Currently uninsured	16.6	24.1	14.9
Currently with public health plan coverage	21.8	23.5	33.9
Currently with private health insurance coverage	67.8	53.7	61.9

Ward, Dahlhamer, Galinsky, & Joesti, 2014.

CRITICAL COMPONENT

Health Disparities and Infant Mortality
Infant mortality is an indicator of maternal health, community health status, and availability of quality health care services (CDC, 2018b).

Health care disparities based on sexual orientation are experienced by lesbian, gay, bisexual, and transgender (LGBT) individuals. Table 1–14 provides information on health care disparities based on sexual orientation. Less than 3% of the adult female population self-identifies as lesbian/gay or bisexual. According to data collected by National Health Statistic Reports, LGBT women are more likely to smoke cigarettes, drink heavily, and be obese than heterosexual women. They are less likely to have a relationship with a regular health care provider and more frequently fail to obtain medical care due to cost (Ward et al, 2014).

MATERNAL AND CHILD HEALTH GOALS

The health of a nation is reflected in the health of expectant women and their infants. Diseases and illness related to complications during pregnancy and the neonatal period can have a lifelong impact on the health of that individual. LBW and premature neonates are at higher risk for chronic respiratory diseases and abnormalities in neurological development. The CDC and Health Resources and Services have set national health goals published in *Healthy People 2020* (Table 1–15). Improving the health of women before and during pregnancy and the health of infants will have lifelong effects on the health of the nation.

TABLE 1–15   *Healthy People 2020* Maternal and Infant Health Goals

OBJECTIVES	BASELINE	2020 TARGET
Reduce the rate of fetal deaths at 20 or more weeks of gestation	6.2 per 1,000 live births and fetal deaths	5.6 per 1,000 live births and fetal deaths
Reduce the rate of fetal and infant deaths during the perinatal period (28 weeks of gestation to 7 days after birth)	6.6 per 1,000 live births and fetal deaths	5.9 per 1,000 live births and fetal deaths
Reduce rate of all infant deaths	6.7 per 1,000 live births	6 per 1,000 live births
Reduce the rate of neonatal deaths	4.5 per 1,000 live births	4.1 per 1,000 live births
Reduce rate of postnatal deaths (between 28 days and 1 year)	2.2 per 1,000 live births	2 per 1,000 live births
Reduce rate of infant deaths related to birth defects (all birth defects)	1.4 per 1,000 live births	1.3 per 1,000 live births
Reduce rate of infant deaths related to congenital heart defects	0.38 per 1,000 live births	0.34 per 1,000 live births
Reduce the rate of infant deaths from sudden infant death syndrome (SIDS)	0.55 per 1,000 live births	0.50 per 1,000 live births
Reduce the rate of infant deaths from sudden unexpected causes (includes SIDS, unknown cause, accidental suffocation, and strangulation in bed)	0.93 per 1,000 live births	0.84 per 1,000 live births
Reduce the 1-year mortality rate for infants with Down syndrome	48.6 deaths within the first year of life per 1,000 infants diagnosed with Down syndrome	43.7 deaths within the first year of life per 1,000 infants with Down syndrome
Reduce the rate of maternal mortality	12.7 maternal deaths per 100,000 live births	11.4 maternal deaths per 100,000 live births
Reduce maternal illness and complications due to pregnancy (complications during hospitalized labor and delivery)	31.1% of pregnant females	28%
Reduce cesarean births among low-risk women with no prior cesarean births	27.4% of low-risk females	23.9%
Reduce cesarean births among low-risk women giving birth with a prior cesarean birth	90.8% of low-risk females giving birth with a prior cesarean	81.7%
Reduce low birth weight (LBW)	8.2% of live births	7.8%
Reduce very low birth weight (VLBW)	1.5% of live births	1.4%
Reduce total preterm births	12.7% of live births	11.4%
Reduce late preterm or live births at 34 to 36 weeks of gestation	9% of live births	8.1%
Reduce live births at 32 to 33 weeks of gestation	1.6% of live births	1.4%
Reduce very preterm or live births at less than 32 weeks of gestation	2% of live births	1.8%
Increase the proportion of pregnant women who receive prenatal care beginning in first trimester	70.8% of females delivering a live birth	77.9%

TABLE 1-15 *Healthy People 2020* Maternal and Infant Health Goals—cont'd

OBJECTIVES	BASELINE	2020 TARGET
Increase the proportion of pregnant women who receive early and adequate prenatal care	70.5% of pregnant females	77.6%
Increase abstinence from alcohol among pregnant women	89.4% of pregnant females aged 15 to 44 reported abstaining from alcohol in the past 30 days	98.3%
Increase abstinence from binge drinking among pregnant women	95% of pregnant females aged 15 to 44 reported abstaining from binge drinking during the past 30 days	100%
Increase abstinence from cigarette smoking among pregnant women	89.6% of females delivering a live birth reported abstaining from smoking cigarettes during pregnancy	98.6%
Increase abstinence from illicit drugs among pregnant women	94.8% of pregnant females aged 15 to 44 reported abstaining from illicit drugs in the past 30 days	100%
Increase the proportion of women of childbearing potential with intake of at least 400 mcg of folic acid from fortified foods or dietary supplements	23.8% of nonpregnant females aged 15 to 44	26.2%
Reduce the proportion of women of childbearing potential who have lower red blood cell folate concentrations	24.9% of nonpregnant females aged 15 to 44	22.4%
Increase the proportion of women delivering a live birth who took multivitamins/folic acid prior to pregnancy	30.3% of females delivering a live birth	33.3%
Increase the proportion of women delivering a live birth who did not smoke prior to pregnancy	79.8% of females delivering a recent live birth did not smoke in the 3 months prior to pregnancy	87.8%
Increase the proportion of women delivering a live birth who did not drink alcohol prior to pregnancy	50.6% of females delivering a recent live birth did not drink alcohol in the 3 months prior to pregnancy	55.6%
Increase the proportion of women delivering a live birth who had a healthy weight prior to pregnancy	52.5% of females delivering a recent live birth had a normal weight (i.e., a BMI of 18.5 to 24.9) prior to pregnancy	57.8%
Increase the proportion of women delivering a live birth who used contraception postpartum to plan their next pregnancy	88.6% of women delivering a live birth used contraception postpartum to plan their next pregnancy	97.5%
Reduce the proportion of women aged 18 to 44 who have impaired fecundity	12.7% of females aged 18 to 44 had impaired fecundity	11.4%
Reduce postpartum relapse of smoking among women who quit smoking during pregnancy	42.4% of postpartum women who quit smoking during pregnancy relapsed	38.2%
Increase the proportion of infants who are put to sleep on their backs	68.9% of infants were put to sleep on their backs	75.8%
Increase the proportion of infants who are ever breastfed	74% of infants	81.9%

Continued

TABLE 1–15   *Healthy People 2020* Maternal and Infant Health Goals—cont'd

OBJECTIVES	BASELINE	2020 TARGET
Increase the proportion of infants who are breastfed at 6 months	43.5% of infants	60.6%
Increase the proportion of infants who are breastfed at 1 year	22.7% of infants	34.1%
Increase the proportion of infants who are breastfed exclusively through 3 months	33.6% of infants	46.2%
Increase the proportion of infants who are breastfed exclusively through 6 months	14.1% of infants	25.5%
Increase the proportion of employers that have worksite lactation support programs	25% of employers reported providing an on-site lactation/mother's room	38%
Reduce the proportion of breastfed newborns who receive formula supplementation within the first 2 days of life	24.2% of breastfed newborns received formula supplementation within the first 2 days of life	14.2%
Increase the proportion of live births that occur in facilities that provide recommended care for lactating mothers and their babies	2.9% of live births occurred in facilities that provide recommended care for lactating mothers and their babies	8.1%

Healthy People 2020, 2016.

REFERENCES

Anderson, R., Kochanek, K., & Murphy, S. (1997). Report of final mortality statistic, 1995. *Monthly Vital Statistics Reports, 45*, 11, sup 2. Hyattsville, MD: National Center for Health Statistics. Retrieved from https://www.cdc.gov/nchs/data/mvsr/supp/mv45_11s2.pdf.

Bureau of the Census. (1917). Statistical abstract of the United States: 1917. Retrieved from https://www.census.gov/library/publications/1918/compendia/statab/40ed.html

Centers for Disease Control and Prevention (CDC). (2016a). *Preterm birth*. Retrieved from www.cdc.gov/reproductivehealth/maternalinfanthealth/pretermbirth.htm.

Centers for Disease Control and Prevention (CDC). (2016b). *Heath, United States, 2015*. Retrieved from www.cdc.gov/nchs/data/hus/hus15.pdf#050.

Centers for Disease Control and Prevention (CDC). (2017). *Basics of FASDs*. Retrieved from https://www.cdc.gov/ncbddd/fasd/facts.html

Centers for Disease Control and Prevention (CDC). (2018a). *E-cigarette information*. Retrieved from https://www.cdc.gov/tobacco/basic_information/e-cigarettes/

Centers for Disease Control and Prevention (CDC). (2018b). *Infant mortality*. Retrieved from https://www.cdc.gov/reproductivehealth/maternalinfanthealth/infantmortality.htm

Central Intelligence Agency (CIA). (2018a). *Total fertility rates*. Retrieved from https://www.cia.gov/library/publications/resources/the-world-factbook/rankorder/2091rank.html

Central Intelligence Agency (CIA). (2018b). *Birth rates*. Retrieved from https://www.cia.gov/library/publications/resources/the-world-factbook/rankorder/2054rank.html

Central Intelligence Agency (CIA). (2018c). *Infant mortality rates*. Retrieved from https://www.cia.gov/library/publications/resources/the-world-factbook/rankorder/2091rank.html

Curtain, M., & Mathews, M. (2016). Smoking prevalence and cessation before and during pregnancy: Data from birth certificate, 2014. *National Vital Statistics, 65*, 1.

Hamilton, B., Martin, J., & Osterman, J. (2016). Births: Preliminary data for 2015. *National Vital Statistics Reports, 65*(3).

Hamilton, B., Martin, J., & Ventura, S. (2007a). Preliminary data for 2006. *National Vital Statistics Reports, 56*, 1–28. Hyattsville, MD: National Center for Health Statistics. Retrieved from www.cdc.gov/nchs/data/nvsr/nvsr56/nvsr56_07.pdf.

Hamilton, B., Martin, J., & Ventura, S. (2007b). Births: Preliminary data for 2005. *National Vital Statistics Reports, 55*(11). Hyattsville, MD: National Center for Health Statistics.

Hamilton, B., Martin, J., & Ventura, S. (2009a). Preliminary data for 2007. *National Vital Statistics Reports, 57*, 1–23. Hyattsville, MD: National Center for Health Statistics.

Hamilton, B., Martin, J., & Ventura, S. (2009b). Births: Preliminary data for 2006. *National Vital Statistics Reports, 56*(7). Hyattsville, MD: National Center for Health Statistics. 2007.

Hamilton, B., Martin, J., & Ventura, S. (2011). Preliminary data for 2010. *National Vital Statistics Reports, 60*, 1–25. Hyattsville, MD: National Center for Health Statistics. Retrieved from www.cdc.gov/nchs/data/nvsr/nvsr60/nvsr60_02.pdf.

Health and Human Services (HHS). (2016). *Trends in teen pregnancy and childbearing*. Retrieved from: www.hhs.gov/ash/oah/adolescent-development/reproductive-health-and-teen-pregnancy/teen-pregnancy-and-childbearing/trends/index.html

Healthy People 2020. (2016). *Maternal, infant and child health*. Retrieved from www.healthypeople.gov/2020/topics-objectives/topic/maternal-infant-and-child-health.

Hoyert, D. (2007). Maternal mortality and related concepts. *National Center for Human Statistics. Vital Health Stats, 3*.

Kochanek, M., Murphy, S., Xu, J., & Tejada, B. (2016). Deaths: Final data for 2014. *National Vital Statistics Reports, 65*(4).

Martin, J., Hamilton, B, Sutton, P, Ventura, S., Menacker, F., & Kirmeyer, S. (2006). Final data for 2004. *National Vital Statistic Report, 55*. Retrieved from www.cdc.gov/nchs/data/nvsr/nvsr55/nvsr545_11.pdf

Martin, J., Hamilton, B., Ventura, S., Osterman, M., Kirmeyer, S., Mathews, T., & Wilson, E. (2011). Birth: Final data for 2009. *National Vital Statistic Reports, 57*(1). Hyattsville, MD: National Center for Health Statistics.

Martin, J., Osterman, M., Driscoll, A., & Drake, P. (2018). Births: Final Data for 2016. *National Vital Statistics Reports, 67*(1). Hyattsville, MD: National Center for Health Statistics.

Murphy, S., Xu, J., & Kochanek, K. (2012). Deaths: Preliminary data for 2010. *National Vital Statistics Report, 60*(4). Hyattsville, MD: National Center for Health Science.

Murphy, S., Xu, J., Kochanek, K., Curtin, M., & Arias, E. (2017). Deaths: Final data for 2015. *National Vital Statistics Reports, 66*(6). Hyattsville, MD: National Center for Health Statistics.

National Campaign to Prevent Teen Pregnancy. (2016a). *Counting it up: The public costs of teen childbearing.* Retrieved from www.thenationalcampaign.org.

National Campaign to Prevent Teen Pregnancy. (2016b). *State and national data, 2015.* Retrieved from www.thenationalcampaign.org/data/landing.

National Center for Health Statistics (NCHS). (2016). *Health, United States, 2015.* Retrieved from www.cdc.gov/nchs/data/hus/hus15.pdf#050.

National Conference of State Legislatures. (2016). *Teen pregnancy prevention.* Retrieved from www.ncsl.org/research/health/teen-pregnancy-prevention.aspx#proverty.

National Institute on Drug Abuse (NIDA). (2016). *Marijuana.* Retrieved from www.drugabuse.gov/publications/research-reports/marijuana/can-marijuana-use-during-pregnancy-harm-baby.

Ogden, C., Carroll, M., Fryar, C., & Flegal, K. (2015). *Prevalence of obesity in the United States, 2011–2014. NCHS data brief, no. 219.* Retrieved from www.cdc.gov/nchs/data/databriefs/db219.pdf.

Osterman, M., & Martin, J. (2014). *Recent decline in induction of labor by gestational age.* NCHS data brief, no. 155. Retrieved from www.cdc.gov/nchs/data/databriefs/db155.htm.

Ward, B., Dahlhamer, J., Galinsky, A., & Joesti, S. (2014). Sexual orientation and health among U.S. adults: National health interview survey, 2013. *National Health Statistic Reports, 77.*

WebMD. (2014). *Drug use and pregnancy.* Retrieved from www.webMd.com/baby/drug-use-and-pregnancy.

Wertz, R., & Wertz, D. (1979). *Lying-in: A History of Childbirth in America.* New York, NY: Schocken Books.

World Bank. (2016a). *Fertility, rate, total (births per woman).* Retrieved from http://data.worldbank.org/indicator/SP.DYN.TFRT.IN?

World Bank. (2016b). *Adolescent fertility rate (births per 1,000 women ages 15–19).* Retrieved from https://data.worldbank.org/indicator/SP.ADO.TFRT

WHO, UNICEF, UNFPA, World Bank Group and United Nations Population Division. (2015). *Trends in maternal mortality: 1990 to 2015: Estimates by WHO, UNICEF, UNFPA, World Bank Group and the United Population Division.* Geneva: WHO Document Production Services.

World Health Organization. (2018a). *Key facts.* Retrieved from www.who.int/en/news-room/fact-sheets/detail/preterm-birth

World Health Organization. (2018b). *Infant mortality.* Retrieved from http://www.who.int/gho/child_health/mortality/neonatal_infant_text/en/

Youth.Gov. (2016). *Adverse effects of teen pregnancy.* Retrieved from www.youth.gov/youth-topics/teen-pregnancy-prevention/adverse-effects-teen-pregnancy.

Ethics and Standards of Practice Issues

2

Roberta F. Durham RN, PhD
Sabine Balden RN, BSN

LEARNING OUTCOMES

Upon completion of this chapter, the student will be able to:
1. Debate ethical issues in maternity nursing.
2. Explore standards of practice in maternity nursing.
3. Describe legal issues in maternity nursing.
4. Analyze concepts related to evidence-based practice.

INTRODUCTION

Maternity nursing is an area of nursing practice that is both exciting and dynamic. There are unique ethical challenges in maternity nursing, with an obligation to practice safe, evidence-based nursing care that is responsive to the needs of women and their families.

This chapter presents the foundational principles set forth by the American Nurses Association (ANA) Code of Ethics and addresses specialty practice standards from the Association of Women's Health, Obstetric and Neonatal Nurses (AWHONN), which outline duties and obligations of obstetric and neonatal nurses. Ethical principles are reviewed within the context of perinatal dilemmas and ethical decision making, and common issues in maternity nursing litigation are presented. Finally, evidence-based practice and challenges in research utilization in the perinatal setting are explored.

ETHICS IN NURSING PRACTICE

The terms ethics and morality are often used interchangeably, but they have different meanings. Morality is very personal and can be adaptable over time; in a pluralistic society, there are many different standards of morality. Ethics, however, are the results of a disciplined study of morality expressed in systemic norms (Stephenson, 2016). In nursing, current professional ethical standards are codified in the ANA Code of Ethics (2015). These standards are based on universal ethical principles and are binding to nurses, regardless of whether they agree with nurses' personal morality.

ANA Code of Ethics

The ANA Code of Ethics describes the goals, values, and obligations of nursing. This code applies to all nurses and is intended to be adaptable to areas of specialty nursing. The purpose of the Code of Ethics is to be a:

- Nonnegotiable ethical standard for the profession;
- Reflection of the profession's own understanding of its commitment to society;
- Statement on the ethical duties and obligations of every nurse;
- Resource for nurses confronted with ethical dilemmas.

Table 2–1 lists the fundamental values and ethical principles of the nursing profession as described in the ANA's 2015 Code of Ethics. The ANA offers interpretive statements to further clarify the nine basic provisions outlined in the table and how they should be applied (www.nursingworld.com).

TABLE 2-1   Overview of American Nurses Association Code of Ethics

Provision 1	The nurse practices with compassion and respect for the inherent dignity, worth, and uniqueness of every person.
Provision 2	The nurse's primary commitment is to the patient, whether an individual, family, group, or community.
Provision 3	The nurse promotes, advocates for, and strives to protect the health, safety, and rights of all patients.
Provision 4	The nurse has authority, accountability, and responsibility for nursing practice, decisions, and actions consistent with the nurse's obligation to promote health and provide optimum care.
Provision 5	The nurse owes the same duties to self as to others, including the responsibility to promote health and safety, to preserve wholeness of character and integrity, to maintain competence, and to continue personal and professional growth.
Provision 6	The nurse, through individual and collective effort, establishes, maintains, and improves the ethical environment of the work setting and provides quality health care.
Provision 7	The nurse, in all roles and settings, advances the profession through research and scholarly inquiry development of professional standards and policy.
Provision 8	The nurse collaborates with other health professionals and the public to promote human rights and health diplomacy and to decrease health disparities.
Provision 9	The profession of nursing, collectively through its professional organizations, articulates nursing values, maintains the integrity of the profession, and integrates the principle of social justice into nursing and health policy.

Ethical Principles

In addition to medically sound care, nurses are called on to provide compassionate and ethically sound care. This is not always an easy task. Maternity nursing is unique in that the nurse is caring for two patients at the same time, the woman and fetus, and decisions are often complicated by the timeline of fetal development. Medical decisions that were ethical in the 12th week of gestation may no longer be ethical at 35 weeks' gestation and vice versa. Technological advances in the neonatal intensive care unit (NICU) blur the line of viability, defined as the moment when a fetus is developed enough to survive outside of the uterus with a reasonable probability of growing and developing as a human being; this definition adds another dimension of complexity (Stephenson, 2016).

Understanding the ethical principles that form the basis of a code of ethics can help guide nurses confronted with ethically complex situations (ANA, 2015). While the principles are not difficult to define, they can become complicated and mutually contradictory in some circumstances:

Beneficence: The obligation to do good. In maternity nursing, this applies to both the woman and the fetus and is usually uncomplicated. Educating your patient about interventions and behaviors that benefit both her and her fetus are examples of beneficence.

Nonmaleficence: The obligation to do no harm to either the woman or the fetus. For example, helping a mother understand the potential consequences of drug abuse or alcohol ingestion during pregnancy.

Fidelity: Being accountable for your responsibilities and loyal to your commitments, such as ensuring your patient is being appropriately cared for by your relief nurse before going off shift.

Veracity: Being truthful. This can mean being honest with your patient about risks and benefits of a caesarean or admitting that you need assistance to give appropriate care.

Autonomy: The right to self-determination. It is related to free choice and personal decisions and is the basis for informed consent in health care (Stephenson, 2016). This applies only to the pregnant woman, as the fetus is not able to conceive of or express preferences.

Justice: This is related to allocation of resources and ensures that resources are used equitably. What is considered equitable, however, may be subjective and cause conflict. For example, at the societal level it relates to which initiatives or programs are funded, while at the individual level it may be who receives an organ transplant (Stephenson, 2016).

Ethical Approaches

Ethical principles can compete in every area of nursing. In maternity nursing, this is compounded by the nurse's responsibilities to both the woman and the fetus. A woman's autonomy can include her right to make decisions that are not in the best interest of the fetus. Or in contrast she may forgo needed therapies for herself until after her delivery, such as chemotherapy treatment for malignant cancer that would harm the fetus, which may not be in her best interest. A nurse is not in a position to voice approval or disapproval of the decisions the woman makes but should advocate for a woman to make informed decisions.

When considering the best approach to managing limited resources, there are three primary philosophies to consider (ANA, 2015): utilitarianism, libertarianism, and egalitarianism. Each has its own strengths and weaknesses, and they can all be effective decision-making strategies in various situations:

Utilitarianism: This is the principle of distributing resources to produce the greatest good for the most people and opposes using large amounts of resources for the benefit of a few.

Libertarianism: This philosophy promotes the idea that some people are more valuable to society than others and thus need to be given the resources they require to survive. To do otherwise is to waste resources.

Egalitarianism: This moral principle focuses on the belief that all people are equal. This principle emphasizes distributing resources according to need to protect those in society who are marginalized and vulnerable.

Consider the situation of a premature but healthy infant who needs extensive and expensive technological support to survive for the first few weeks. Should the infant's access to lifesaving support be dependent on the family's ability to pay? What if the infant is not healthy and will likely be severely disabled if he or she survives, requiring lifelong care and intensive resources? Does that change the decision to provide resources for the child to survive infancy? Should it change the decision? These situations can be very challenging to nurses as they advocate for both mothers and infants and navigate ethical dilemmas.

Ethical Dilemmas

Ethical dilemmas occur in all areas of life and while they can be addressed in many ways, nurses must consider their clear obligations and duties to their patients. And because maternity nurses must advocate for both maternal and fetal well-being, it may not be possible to "do the right thing" for both.

Some ethical dilemmas are easily avoided. Implementing safe practices according to evidence-based practice (EBP) guidelines, helping to establish a culture of safety and professionalism and safety in your workplace, and reporting both individual and system errors can prevent many ethically challenging situations (Lachman, 2007; Simpson, 2014). But consider the example from earlier in which the mother requires chemotherapy that may harm the fetus or the ethics of deciding to terminate a severely abnormally developed fetus. Is it ethical to delay treatment for a pregnant woman with cancer, potentially shortening her life or in the other situation continue a pregnancy with a nonviable fetus that results in a painful, short life for the newborn? How does one balance advocating for the mother and the fetus if the mother insists on continuing with high-risk behaviors during her pregnancy? There are no simple answers to such situations, yet maternity nurses must help mothers and families navigate these and other ethical dilemmas. Practice dictates that the primary advocacy role of maternity nurses is on behalf of the mother. Obligations to the fetus are tempered by the context of the mother's

decisions, and that can be complicated. As individuals with their own ideas of morality, maternity nurses may not agree with the mother's choices, yet their duty to respect her autonomy will help guide them in managing the consequences. Adding to the challenge is the fact that while caring for women and their families, nurses encounter diverse cultural practices, spiritual beliefs, and attitudes toward health and health care. Patterns of communication and decision making are influenced by culture, so cultural awareness can help nurses navigate decision making with patients and families.

Other issues in which maternity nurses will be required to help educate, guide, and ultimately advocate for patients include:

- Court-ordered treatments that infringe on the pregnant woman's right to autonomy.
- Criminalization of pregnant women with substance use disorders.
- The difficult decision to withdraw life support from the infant or the mother.
- Treatment of genetic disorders or fetal abnormalities.
- Systemic inequities that prevent or delay allocation of resources in pregnancy care during the previable period.
- Equal access to prenatal care.
- Genetic engineering, cloning, and surrogacy.
- Navigating difficult decisions such as sanctity of life versus quality of life for extremely premature or severely disabled infants, including whether to resuscitate borderline-viable infants.
- Fetal reduction and preconception gender selection.

Evidence shows that nurses who understand and internalize professional nursing ethics are less likely to suffer from a loss of confidence and self-esteem as a result of facing these difficult situations (Iacobucci, 2013). Nurses can experience moral distress from situations in which their core beliefs conflict with providing care. Moral distress occurs in the day-to-day setting and involves situations in which one acts against one's better judgment due to internal or external constraints. Putting aside one's values and carrying out an action one believes is wrong threatens the authenticity of the moral self. Unfortunately, situations of moral distress are common in health care, and damage to providers' moral integrity occurs with alarming frequency (Epstein & Delgado, 2010) (see Box 2–1). The goal is to preserve moral sensitivity and integrity by recognizing, valuing, and hearing staff.

Ethics in Neonatal Care

Care of extremely premature infants is especially challenging. Maternity and NICU nurses have an ethical obligation to care for the infant and respect parental decisions regarding the infant, but they also have a duty to do no harm (Fig. 2–1). Categories for neonates in the NICU may include:

- Infants for whom aggressive care would probably be futile, where prognosis for a meaningful life is extremely poor or hopeless.
- Infants for whom aggressive care would probably result in clear benefit to overall well-being, where prevailing

knowledge and evidence indicate excellent chances for beneficial outcomes and meaningful interactions.

● Infants for whom the effect of aggressive care is mostly uncertain.

An especially important related ethical issue concerns futility (Chervenak, McCullough, & Burke Sosa, 2013). Families sometimes request inappropriate or futile care. This does not relieve nurses of their ethical duty to advocate for appropriate care. Identifying the neonate's status will help guide the maternity nurse's parental counseling and decision making. It is critical to remember that veracity is one of the ethical principles binding the nurse; keeping parents fully informed supports their ability to make the best choices for themselves. Withholding information, even to protect or spare the parents from emotional pain and disappointment, may be well intentioned, but it makes assumptions about what is best for the mother and her family without giving

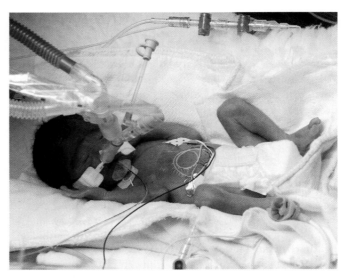

FIGURE 2–1 Extremely premature baby in the NICU.

BOX 2–1 | Clinical Examples of Perinatal Ethical Dilemmas

Ethical dilemmas occur in all areas of nursing. However, because maternity nurses must advocate for both maternal and fetal well-being, there is not always a clear path for doing the right thing for both the mother and the fetus. Examples include:

● Court-ordered treatment

● Withdrawal of life support

● Harvesting of fetal organs or tissue

● In vitro fertilization and decisions for disposal of remaining fertilized ova

● Allocation of resources in pregnancy care during the previable period

● Fetal surgery

● Treatment of genetic disorders or fetal abnormalities found on prenatal screening

● Equal access to prenatal care

● Maternal rights versus fetal rights

● Extraordinary medical treatment for pregnancy complications

● Using organs from an anencephalic infant

● Genetic engineering

● Cloning

● Surrogacy

● Drug testing in pregnancy

● Sanctity of life versus quality of life for extremely premature or severely disabled infants

● Substance abuse in pregnancy

● Borderline viability: to resuscitate or not

● Fetal reduction

● Preconception gender selection

them a chance to participate in that decision. This represents a form of paternalism, in which an authority figure, in this case health care personnel, makes choices for others; this is considered to be very disrespectful and inappropriate (Chervenak et al., 2013; Stephenson, 2016).

Parents often lack the expertise to make fully informed decisions regarding the care of their neonate, so communication and collaboration are critical. The parents are the ones who must manage the long-term consequences of decisions, whether that means grieving over the death of their child or adapting to the difficult realities of having a child who may require lifelong care. Developing a consensus for the plan of care that incorporates parental wishes, ethical standards, and realistic assessments of available resources requires a team approach between the appropriate health care professionals and parents, in which parental concerns are acknowledged and validated. Such a plan will minimize needless harm or suffering for the neonate and ethical dilemmas for the NICU nurse, as well as give parents a sense of participation and control.

Nurses are required to keep parents fully informed of all developments and respect parental decisions, but they also have a duty to the neonate. This may require counseling the parents, offering support, and referring them to additional resources. At times, balancing these obligations can lead to an ethical dilemma. Nurses are the primary link between neonates in the ICU and their parents, and they interact more with families than any other health care professional, putting them in a unique position to help identify and ensure the best possible outcome (Mattson & Smith, 2016). Being sensitive to the ethical contexts and receptive to parental concerns can help the nurse navigate these situations.

Ethical Decision-Making Models

Clinical situations that raise ethical questions are a challenge to navigate, with multiple clinical facts to consider. In addition, patient and family values, concerns, and preferences must be considered. In some cases, a decision is needed quickly. When faced with these difficult clinical situations, a systematic approach can help health care providers reach an ethical decision or recommendation (Schumann & Alfandre, 2008). One common approach for ethical decision making in clinical settings is the Jonsen model, widely referred to as the "four topics method" (Jonsen, Siegler, & Winslade, 2002).

The four topics method was developed to provide clinicians with a framework for sorting through and focusing on specific aspects of clinical ethics cases and connecting the circumstances of a case to their underlying ethical principles. Each topic—medical indications, patient preferences, quality of life, and contextual features—represents a set of specific questions to be considered in working through the ethical conflict or case. The purpose of the four topics method is to sort out data so that one can determine what is central to the discussion (Jonsen et al., 2002). The boxes do not give us an answer, but instead point us to areas of confusion or contention. When you finish sorting the data, ask, "In which quadrant does the problem seem to lie?" This provides guidance for physicians and nurses on where to gather more resources and how to intervene. The next sections review the four topics, relate them to ethical concepts, and present relevant questions.

Medical Indications

Clinical ethics case analysis using the four topics method begins with an articulation of the medical facts of the case, including the diagnosis, prognosis, treatment options, and how the patient can benefit, if at all, from treatment (Schumann & Alfandre, 2008). This topic relates to the ethical principles of and consideration of beneficence and nonmaleficence. Relevant questions include:

- What is the patient's medical problem? History? Diagnosis? Prognosis?
- Is the problem acute? Chronic? Critical? Emergent? Reversible?
- What are the goals of treatment?
- What are the probabilities of success?
- In sum, how can this patient benefit from medical and nursing care, and how can harm be avoided?

Patient Preferences

This topic focuses on the expressed or presumed wishes and values of the patient, including respect for patient autonomy. While the United States prioritizes the autonomy of the individual, most cultures value the family, the community, and the overall population in concert with the individual. Relevant questions include:

- Has the patient been informed of benefits and risks, understood this information, and given consent?
- Has the patient expressed prior preferences, such as advance directives?
- Is the patient unwilling or unable to cooperate with medical treatment? If so, why?
- In sum, is the patient's right to choose being respected to the extent possible in ethics and law?

Quality of Life

In clinical ethics case analysis, it is important to consider what effect the indicated treatment will have on the patient's quality of life (Schumann & Alfandre, 2008). However, how does one define quality of life? Clearly, quality of life is defined by one's perspective, and perceptions of quality may vary significantly from one person to the next. To honor a patient's idea of quality of life, the principles of beneficence, nonmaleficence, and respect for autonomy should be considered. Relevant questions include:

- What are the prospects, with or without treatment, for a return to normal life?
- What physical, mental, and social deficits is the patient likely to experience if treatment succeeds?
- Are there biases that might prejudice the provider's evaluation of the patient's quality of life?
- Is the patient's present or future condition such that his or her continued life might be judged as undesirable?
- Are there plans for comfort and palliative care?

Contextual Features

The final step in the four topics method is to consider the larger context in which the case is occurring and determine whether any contextual features are relevant to the case and its ethical analysis (Schumann & Alfandre, 2008). The context of a case is determined by multiple social factors, including (among others) the dynamics of the family, the living situation of the patient, and the cultural and religious beliefs of the patient and the family. This includes consideration of the concepts of loyalty and fairness. Relevant questions include:

- Are there family issues that might influence treatment decisions?
- Are there financial and economic factors?
- Are there religious or cultural factors?
- Are there problems of allocation of resources?
- How does the law affect treatment decisions?

In summary, the four topics approach helps to highlight areas of controversy and clarify the principles underlying the circumstances of a clinical ethics case, which in turn guides discussion among care team members, patients, and families toward achieving a resolution that respects the patient's values and preferences.

Ethics and Practice: Nurses' Rights and Responsibilities

The Association of Women's Health, Obstetric and Neonatal Nurses (AWHONN) is the professional nursing association representing nurses in neonatal nursing. AWHONN supports the protection of an individual nurse's right to choose to participate in any reproductive health care service or research activity. Nurses have the right under federal law to refuse to assist in the performance of any health care procedure in keeping with personal moral, ethical, or religious beliefs (AWHONN, 2016a).

However, as AWHONN considers access to affordable and acceptable health care services a basic human right (AWHONN, 2016b), it also advocates that nurses adhere to the following principles:

● Nurses should not abandon a patient nor refuse to provide care based on prejudice or bias.
● Nurses have the professional responsibility to provide high-quality, impartial nursing care to all patients in emergency situations, regardless of nurses' personal beliefs.
● Nurses have a professional obligation to inform their employers of any attitudes and beliefs that may interfere with essential job functions.

The core values as defined by AWHONN (2009), aligned with the Code of Ethics, are as follows:

Commitment to professional and social responsibility

Accountability for personal and professional contribution

Respect for diversity of and among colleagues and clients

Integrity in exemplifying the highest standards in personal and professional behavior

Nursing excellence for quality outcomes in practice, education, research, advocacy, and management

Generation of knowledge to enhance the science and practice of nursing to improve the health of women and newborns

These core values, denoted by the acronym CARING, are foundational to excellence in nursing practice and support work environments that promote optimal patient outcomes and staff engagement.

STANDARDS OF PRACTICE

In addition to a Code of Ethics from the ANA (2015), practice standards from AWHONN help to guide professional nursing practice using the ANA (2015) scope and standards of practice as its foundation. The standards summarize what AWHONN believes is the nursing profession's best judgment and optimal protocol based on current research and clinical practice (Box 2–2). AWHONN believes that these standards are helpful for all nurses engaged in the functions described. As with most or all such standards, certain qualifications should be borne in mind:

● These standards articulate general guidelines; additional considerations or procedures may be warranted for particular patients or settings. The best interest of an individual patient is always the touchstone of practice.
● These standards are but one source of guidance. Nurses also must act in accordance with applicable law, institutional rules and procedures, and established interprofessional arrangements concerning the division of duties.
● These standards represent optimal practice. Full compliance may not be possible at all times with all patients in all settings.

● These standards serve as a guide for optimal practice. They are not designed to define standards of practice for employment, licensure, discipline, reimbursement, or legal or other purposes.
● These standards may change in response to changes in research and practice.
● The standards define the nurse's responsibility to the patient and the roles and behaviors to which the nurse is accountable. The definition of terms delimits the scope of the standards (Table 2–2).

The standards of practice set forth are intended to define the roles, functions, and competencies of the nurse who strives to provide high-quality service to patients. The Standards of Professional Performance delineate the various roles and behaviors for which the professional nurse is accountable. The standards are enduring and should remain largely stable over time because they reflect the philosophical values of the profession (ANA, 2015).

LEGAL ISSUES IN DELIVERY OF CARE

Due to an ever-changing practice care environment and the ethical and legal dilemmas inherent in the profession, nurses are at increased risk of being named in a malpractice litigation process (Watson, 2014). Current trends in medical malpractice lawsuits suggest that the gold standard is evidence-based practice.

The charge of "failure to communicate" is a major issue in most malpractice suits against nurses. Nurses have been found negligent for placing patients in harm's way by failing to communicate issues and concerns to colleagues, charge nurses, and physicians (Brown, 2016). One landmark analytical report based on data from obstetrical-related malpractice cases asserted errors in clinical judgment were cited in 77% of obstetrical medical malpractice cases; the next most prevalent areas of causation were miscommunication (36%), technical error (26%), inadequate documentation (26%), administrative failures (23%), and ineffective supervision (15%) (Crico Strategies, 2010). For example, intrapartum care is inherently dynamic and nuanced, and crucial evidence gaps exist. As a result, road signs may be unclear or change quickly, leading providers to have completely different interpretations of the right course of action.

Conflicting approaches are easily exacerbated by the dynamic nature of labor. Differences of opinion and prioritization are bound to occur. Data suggest that despite encouraging progress in developing cultures of safety in individual centers and systems, significant and necessary work will be required to reverse overt disruptive behaviors in labor and delivery and to correct more subtle forms of systemic disrespect. It has been suggested that hospitals need to transparently address deficiencies in interpersonal interaction and clinical performance to achieve optimal care of childbearing women (Lyndon et al., 2014).

BOX 2-2 | Standards for Professional Nursing Practice in the Care of Women and Newborns

Standards of Care

Standard I. Assessment

The nurse gathers health data about women and newborns in the context of woman-centered and family-centered care.

Standard II. Diagnosis

The nurse generates nursing diagnosis by analyzing assessment data to identify and differentiate normal physiological and developmental transitions form pathophysiological variations and other clinical issues in the context of woman-centered and family-centered care.

Standard III. Outcome Identification

The nurse individualizes expected outcomes for the women and newborns in the context of woman-centered and family-centered care.

Standard IV. Planning

The nurse generates a plan of care that includes interventions to attain expected outcomes for women and newborns in the context of woman-centered and family-centered care.

Standard V. Implementation

The nurse implements the interventions identified in the woman's or newborn's plan of care in the context of woman-centered and family-centered care.

Standard V(a). Coordination of Care

The nurse coordinates care to women and newborns in the context of woman-centered and family-centered care and within her or his scope of practice.

Standard V(b). Health Teaching and Health Promotion

The nurse uses teaching strategies that promote, maintain, or restore health in the context of woman-centered and family-centered care.

Standard VI. Evaluation

The nurse evaluates the progress of women and newborns toward attainment of expected outcomes in the context of woman-centered and family-centered care.

Standards of Professional Performance

Standard VII. Quality of Practice

The nurse evaluates and implements measures to improve quality, safety, and effectiveness of nursing for women and newborns.

Standard VIII. Education

The nurse acquires and maintains knowledge and competencies that utilize current evidence-based nursing practice for women and newborns.

Standard IX. Professional Practice Evaluation

The nurse evaluates her or his own nursing practice in relation to current evidence-based patient care information, professional practice standards, and guidelines, statutes, and regulations.

Standard X. Ethics

The nurse's decisions and actions on behalf of women, fetuses, and newborns are determined in an ethical manner and guided by a framework for an ethical decision-making process.

Standard XI. Collegiality

The nurse interacts with and contributes to the professional development of other health care providers.

Standard XII. Collaboration and Communication

The nurse collaborates and communicates with women, families, health care providers, and the community in providing safe and holistic care.

Standard XIII. Research

The nurse generates and/or uses evidence to identify, examine, validate, and evaluate interprofessional knowledge, theories, and varied approaches in providing care to women and newborns.

Standard XIV. Resources and Technology

The nurse considers factors related to safety, effectiveness, technology, and cost in planning and delivering care to women and newborns.

Standard XV. Leadership

Within appropriate roles in the setting in which the nurse functions, she or he should seek to serve as a role model, change agent, consultant, and mentor to women, families, and other health care professionals.

Association of Women's Health, Obstetric and Neonatal Nurses (AWHONN), 2009.

Maternity nursing is the most litigious of all practice areas. Contributing to this is the complexity of caring for two patients at once. Five clinical situations account for most fetal and neonatal injuries and litigation in obstetrics (Simpson, 2014):

- Inability to recognize and/or inability to appropriately respond to intrapartum fetal compromise.
- Inability to perform a timely cesarean birth (30 minutes from decision to incision) when indicated by fetal or maternal condition.
- Inability to appropriately initiate resuscitation of a depressed neonate.
- Inappropriate use of oxytocin or misoprostol, leading to uterine tachysystole, uterine rupture, and fetal intolerance of labor and/or fetal death.
- Inappropriate use of forceps/vacuum and/or preventable shoulder dystocia.

The expectation of obstetrics is a perfect outcome. Obstetrics malpractice can cause morbidity and mortality that may lead to litigation (Adinima, 2016). The number of obstetric malpractice claims represents only about 5% of all malpractice claims, but the dollar amount for the claims represents up to 35% of the total financial liability of a hospital or health care system

TABLE 2-2　Terms Related to Standards

TERM	DEFINITION
Assessment	A systematic, dynamic process by which the nurse, through interaction with women, newborns, families, significant others, and health care providers, collects, monitors, and analyzes data. Data may include the following dimensions: psychological, biotechnological, physical, sociocultural, spiritual, cognitive, developmental, and economic, as well as functional abilities and lifestyle.
Cultural consciousness	The acceptance of and respect for the attributes of diversity and includes the acknowledgment of both similarities and differences. Culturally competent care includes recognition and awareness of the cultural perspective of those who are served. Within the scope of law and institutional policies, providers should consider how best to adapt their treatment approach in light of the values and cultural preferences of the client.
Childbearing and newborn health care	A model of care addressing the health promotion, maintenance, and restoration needs of women from preconception through the postpartum period, and low-risk, high-risk, and critically ill newborns from birth through discharge and follow-up, within the social, political, economic, and environmental context of the mother's, her newborn's, and the family's lives.
Diagnosis	A clinical judgment about the patient's response to actual or potential health conditions or needs. Diagnoses provide the basis for determination of a plan of nursing care to achieve expected outcomes.
Diversity	A quality that encompasses acceptance and respect related to but not limited to age, class, culture, people with special health care needs, education level, ethnicity, family structure, gender, ideologies, political beliefs, race, religion, sexual orientation, style, and values.
Evaluation	The process of determining the patient's progress toward attainment of expected outcomes and the effectiveness of nursing care.
Expected outcomes	Response to nursing interventions that is measurable, desirable, and observable.
Family-centered maternity care	A model of care based on the philosophy that the physical, sociocultural, psychological, spiritual, and economic needs of the woman and her family, however the family may be defined, should be integrated and considered collectively. Provisions of Family Centered Care (FCC) require mutual trust and collaboration between the woman, her family, and health care professionals.
Guideline	A framework developed through experts' consensus and review of the literature, which guides patient-focused activities that affect the provisions of care.
Implementation	The process of taking action by intervening, delegating, and/or coordinating. Women, newborns, families, significant others, or health care providers may direct the implementation of interventions within the plan of care.
Outcome	A measurable individual, family, or community state, behavior, or perception that is responsive to nursing interventions.
Standard	Authoritative statement defined and promoted by the profession and by which the quality of practice, service, or education can be evaluated.
Standards of practice	Authoritative statements that describe competent clinical nursing practice for women and newborns demonstrated through assessment, diagnosis, outcome identification, planning, implementation, and evaluation.
Standards of professional performance	Authoritative statements that describe competent behavior in the professional role, including activities related to quality of practice, education, professional practice evaluation, ethics, collegiality, collaboration, communication, research, resources and technology, and leadership.
Standards of professional performance	Authoritative statements that describe competent behavior in the professional role, including activities related to quality of care, performance appraisal, resource utilization, education, collegiality, ethics, collaboration, research, and research utilization.
Women's health care	A model of care addressing women's health promotion, maintenance, and restoration needs occurring across the life span and relating to one or more life strategies: adolescence, young adulthood, middle years, and older within the social, political, economic, and environmental context of their lives (AWHONN, 1999).

Association of Women's Health, Obstetric and Neonatal Nurses (AWHONN), 2009.

(Simpson, 2014). The literature indicates that patients who are more dissatisfied with the interpersonal interaction with health care providers are more likely to pursue litigation (Lagana, 2000). It has also been suggested that increased use of technology may interfere with a nurse's ability to engage with women and families in a therapeutic and caring interaction.

Fetal Monitoring

Interpretation of fetal heart rate (FHR) monitoring is often a key element of litigation; this clinical issue is related to the nurse's ability to recognize and appropriately respond to intrapartal fetal compromise. For that reason, this example will serve to illustrate how nursing standards, guidelines, and policies should be the foundation of safe practice. Common allegations related to fetal monitoring are:

- Failure to accurately assess maternal and fetal status.
- Failure to appreciate a deteriorating fetal status.
- Failure to treat an abnormal or indeterminate FHR.
- Failure to reduce or discontinue oxytocin with an abnormal or indeterminate FHR.
- Failure to correctly communicate maternal/fetal status to the care provider.
- Failure to institute the chain of command when there is a clinical disagreement.

Nurses are accountable for safe and effective FHR assessment, and failure to do so contributes to claims of nursing negligence (Gilbert, 2007; Mahlmeister, 2000; Pearson, 2011; Simpson, 2014). AWHONN (2015) provides a position statement on fetal assessment that states:

- AWHONN strongly advises that nurses complete a course of study that includes physiological interpretation of electronic fetal monitoring (EFM) and its implications for care in labor.
- Each facility should develop a policy that defines when to use EFM and auscultation of FHR and specifies frequency and documentation based on best available evidence, professional association guidelines, and expert consensus.

Effective, timely communication and collaboration among health care professionals is central to providing quality care and optimizing patient outcomes and to ensuring Category II (indeterminate) or Category III (abnormal) FHR patterns are managed appropriately. Organizational resources and systems should be in place to support timely interventions when FHR is indeterminate or abnormal (Simpson, 2014; Simpson & Knox, 2003). Uniform FHR terminology and interpretation are necessary to facilitate appropriate communication and legally defensible documentation (Lyndon & Ali, 2015).

Interpretation of FHR data can sometimes result in conflict. There may be agreement about ominous patterns and normal patterns, but often care providers encounter patterns that fall between these extremes (Freeman, 2002). Such conflicts in the

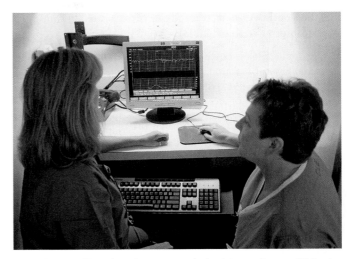

FIGURE 2-2 Together the nurse and physician review an EFM strip.

clinical setting need to be resolved quickly but sometimes cannot be resolved between the caregivers immediately involved. When this occurs:

- The nurse must initiate the course of action when the clinical situation is a matter of maternal or fetal well-being.
- In a case of a primary care provider not responding to an abnormal FHR or a deteriorating clinical situation, the nurse should use the chain of command to resolve the situation, advocate for the patient's safety, and seek necessary interventions to avoid a potentially adverse outcome.
- At the first level, notify the immediate supervisor for assistance. Further steps are defined by the structure of the institution, and a policy outlining communication for the chain of command should exist (Fig. 2–2).

Risk Management

Risk management is a systems approach to litigation prevention that involves the identification of systems problems, analysis, and treatment of risks before a suit is brought. There are two key components of a successful risk-management program:

- Avoiding preventable adverse outcomes to the fetus during labor requires competent care providers who use consistent and current FHR-monitoring language in practice environments with systems in place that permit timely clinical intervention.
- Decreasing risk of liability exposure includes methods to demonstrate evidence that the provision of appropriate, timely care accurately reflects maternal fetal status before, during, and after interventions occurred.

Not all adverse or unexpected outcomes are preventable or result from poor care. Some suggest the risk of liability can be reduced and injuries to mothers and neonates can be reduced when all members of the perinatal team follow two basic tenets (Simpson, 2014; Simpson & Knox, 2003):

1. Use applicable evidence and/or published standards and guidelines as the foundation of care.
2. Make patient safety a priority over convenience, productivity, and costs.

All nurses need to bear in mind that the most—and sometimes the only—defensible nursing actions are those whose sole focus is on the health and well-being of the patient.

EVIDENCE-BASED PRACTICE

Health care professions increasingly strive to make practice decisions with the best available knowledge or evidence. Evidence-based practice (EBP) and terms such as *evidence-based medicine* (EBM) and *evidence-based nursing* (EBN) reflect a very important global paradigm shift in how to view health care outcomes, how the discipline is taught, how practice is conducted, and how health care practices are evaluated for quality. In the early 1990s, agencies were established with interdisciplinary teams to gather and assess available research literature and develop evidence-based clinical guidelines. Now the Agency for Healthcare Research and Quality (AHRQ) is a clearinghouse for clinical guidelines (www.guidelines.gov). This public database is an important resource for clinicians. For a clinical practice guideline to be included by the National Guideline Clearinghouse, it must meet four rigorous criteria:

1. Contains systematically developed recommendations, strategies, or other information to assist health care decision making in specific clinical circumstances.
2. Produced under the auspices of a relevant professional organization.
3. Development process included a verifiable, systematic search and review of the existing literature published in peer-reviewed journals.
4. Is current—that is, developed, reviewed, or revised within the last 5 years.

Most health professionals view the EBP movement as a systematic approach to determine the most current and relevant evidence upon which to base decisions about patient care (Melnyk & Fineout-Overholt, 2005). However, as nurses, it is important to remember that even if rigorously conducted research reports "good evidence" findings, this may not always translate to the "right" decisions for an individual patient. Most authors and clinicians have extended the definition of EBP to include the integration of best *research evidence, clinical expertise,* and *patient values* in making decisions about patient care. Clinical expertise comes from knowledge and experience over time and includes professional practice opinions and position statements. Patient values are the unique circumstances of each patient and should include individual preferences. Best research evidence includes current findings from both quantitative and qualitative research methods.

CRITICAL COMPONENT

Evidence-Based Practice in Nursing

EBP definition: Integrate best current evidence with clinical expertise and patient/family preferences and values for delivery of optimal health care.

Nurses are in a unique position to explore a woman's preferences and advocate for the use of best current evidence and clinical expertise for delivery of optimal health care. Some suggestions to foster EBP in clinical settings include the following:

- Describe and locate reliable sources for evidence reports and clinical practice guidelines.
- Question rationale for routine approaches to care that result in less-than-desired outcomes or adverse events.
- Base individualized care plan on patient values, clinical expertise, and evidence.

Evidence-Based Practice: Cochrane Reviews

An important resource for EBP is systematic reviews. One such source is Cochrane Reviews (www.cochrane.org). The Cochrane Review is an international consortium of experts who perform systematic reviews and meta-analysis on all available data, evaluating the body of evidence on a clinical topic for quality of study design and study results. These reviews look at randomized clinical trials of interventions related to a specific clinical problem and, after assessing the findings from rigorous studies, make recommendations for clinical practice. They consider the randomized controlled trial (RCT) the gold standard of research evidence.

Although not absolute, a hierarchy can be helpful when evaluating research evidence. When considering potential interventions, nurses should look for the highest level of evidence (LOE) relevant to the clinical problem. A hierarchy of strength of evidence for treatment decisions is presented in Figure 2–3, indicating unsystematic clinical observations as the lowest level and systematic reviews of RCTs as the highest level of evidence. There are many LOE hierarchies, and they have continued to evolve and change with time (Hokanson Hawks, 2016).

Evidence-Based Nursing

Evidence-based nursing (EBN) has become an internationally recognized although sometimes contested part of nursing practice. While EBN is central to the knowledge base for nursing (Fain, 2017), its critics dislike the central role of RCTs in providing evidence for nursing, claiming that the context and experience of nursing care are removed from evaluation of evidence. The principles of evidence-based health care have been driven by requirements to deliver quality care within economically constrained conditions.

Some nurses have adopted a predominantly medical model of evidence, with RCTs as the central, methodological approach to defining good evidence. EBN has been criticized for this stance,

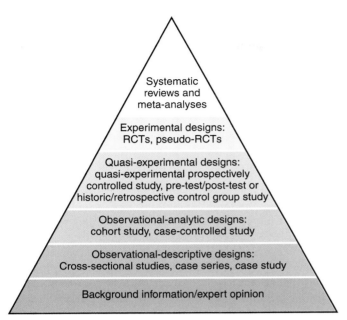

FIGURE 2–3 Levels of evidence.

citing the lack of relevance of RCTs for some important areas of nursing practice. Criticisms stem from the fact that RCTs are given an illusionary stance of credibility when there may not be credible evidence relevant to nursing practice and theory (Fawcett & Garity, 2009). Most experts now believe both quantitative and qualitative research findings are relevant to inform the practice of nursing.

Utilization of Research in Clinical Practice

To enhance EBP and support the choices of childbearing women and families, we must utilize quantitative *and* qualitative research findings in practice (Durham, 2002). Although nursing has developed models for assisting practitioners in applying research findings in practice (Cronenwett, 1995; Stetler, 1994; Titler & Goode, 1995), these models only assist in applying quantitative research findings for utilization in practice.

Qualitative research is increasingly recognized as an integral part of the evidence that informs EBP. Qualitative researchers investigate naturally occurring phenomena and describe, analyze, and sometimes theorize on these occurrences. They also describe the context and relationships of key factors related to the phenomena. This kind of work is conducted in the "real world," not in a controlled situation, and yields important findings for practice. Reports of qualitative research are conveyed in language that may be more understandable to practitioners. Story lines from qualitative research are often a more compelling and culturally resonant way to communicate research findings, particularly to staff, affected groups, and policy makers (Sandelowski, 1996). Guidelines for utilization of qualitative research findings are outlined by Swanson, Durham, and Albright (1997) and include evaluating the findings or proposed theory for its context, generalizability, and fit with one's own practice; evaluating the concepts, conditions, and variation explained in

the findings; and evaluating findings for enhancing and informing one's practice.

In the current era of cost containment, nurses must know what is going on in their patients' lives, because practitioners are limited to interacting with clients within an ever-smaller window of time and space. Qualitative research can assist in bringing practitioners an awareness of that larger world and its implications for their scope of practice (Swanson, Durham, & Albright, 1997). Qualitative research describes and analyzes our patients' realities. The research findings have the capacity to influence conceptual thinking and cause practitioners to question assumptions about a phenomenon in practice (Cronenwett, 1995). Incorporating qualitative research as evidence to support research-based practice can enhance nursing practice and can resolve some of the tensions between art and science with which nurses sometimes find themselves struggling (Durham, 2002). Experts have presented guidelines for utilizing qualitative research in practice that can enhance clinicians' ability to use qualitative findings for EBP (Miller, 2010; Sandelowski, 1996; Sandelowski & Barroso, 2003; Thorne, 2009).

Research Utilization Challenges

Health care often falls short in translating research into practice and improvement of care. While adopting EBP has resulted in improvements in patient outcome, large gaps remain between what we know and what we do (Scott, 2010). Failing to use the latest health care research is costly and harmful, and can lead to ineffective care. Many innovations have become common practice in perinatal nursing, such as electronic fetal monitoring and family centered care. These changes in care were influenced by factors such as medical and technological innovations and social context of the time and families' preferences.

The increasing use of technology during birth, threats of litigation, and providing the best care under time and cost constraints are the realities facing perinatal nurses today. Continuous EFM in labor is one of the most common interventions during labor. However, there is little evidence to support the use of continuous EFM, especially with low-risk patients. A recent Cochrane Review compared the efficacy and safety of routine continuous EFM of labor with intermittent auscultation (Alfirevic et al., 2017). The reviewers concluded that use of routine EFM has no measurable impact on infant morbidity and mortality. In the latest review, the authors concluded continuous EFM during labor is associated with a reduction in neonatal seizures but no significant differences in cerebral palsy, infant mortality, or other standard measures of neonatal well-being. However, continuous EFM was associated with an increase in caesarean births and operative vaginal births. They noted the real challenge is how best to convey this uncertainty to women to enable them to make an informed choice without compromising the normality of labor.

Although EBP is the goal of nursing care and has become the standard of care in the United States, the evidence about EFM has not been used in practice. Research evidence does not support the use of continuous EFM. Its use can instead be attributed to habit, convenience, liability, staffing, and economics. It is no longer acceptable for nurses to continue doing things the way they have always been done without questioning if it is the best approach. One way nurses can ensure EBP in their setting is by participating in multidisciplinary teams that generate research-based practice guidelines.

Barriers to Evidence-Based Practice

Despite concerns that the rise of EBP threatens to transform nursing practice into a performative exercise disciplined by scientific knowledge, others have found that scientific knowledge is by no means the preeminent source of knowledge within the dynamic settings of health care (Angus, Hodnett, & O'Brien-Pallas, 2003).

Nurses may face challenges in translating research into practice due to a number of factors, including a lack of time, training, and mentoring (Johnston et al., 2016; Mazurek et al., 2016; Simpson, 2014). Barriers commonly cited focus on areas of knowledge, skills, and attitudes:

- Inadequate knowledge and skills in EBP by nurses and other health care professionals.
- Lack of cultures and environments that support EBP.
- Misperceptions that EBP takes too much time.
- Outdated organizational politics and policies.
- Limited resources and tools available for point-of-care providers, including budgetary investment in EBP by chief nurse executives.
- Resistance from colleagues, nurse managers, and nurse leaders.
- Inadequate numbers of EBP mentors in health care systems.
- Academic programs that continue to teach baccalaureate, master's, and doctor of nursing practice students the rigorous process of how to conduct research instead of taking an evidence-based approach to care.

Strategies to Enhance Evidence-Based Practice

Authors describe a strategic approach to engaging, empowering, and supporting a nursing workforce to participate in EBP (McKeever et al., 2016). This can be facilitated through the formation of a committee dedicated to developing and implementing evidence-based clinical guidelines that support nursing practice. Other strategies to improve EBP in clinical practice include initiatives driven by an organizational desire to reduce variation in nursing care delivered to patients and families. Recognizing that some nurses do not possess requisite skills to conduct a literature search, critically appraise pertinent literature, and synthesize evidence into a clinical guideline, the Nursing Clinical Effectiveness Committee established processes to support nurses in activities to foster the development, implementation, and evaluation of clinical guidelines. Support provided to the staff should include identifying areas of practice requiring clinical guidance, evidence identification and evaluation, clinical guideline development, and strategic development of an education-based implementation plan to promote guideline adoption into practice (McKeever et al., 2016).

Resistance to change can be difficult to overcome. Therefore, strategies that target knowledge, skills, and attitudes must be utilized for successful implementation of EBP clinical guidelines. These can include:

- Grand rounds
- Simulation training
- Learning/skills fairs
- Posters
- One-on-one meetings
- Case conferences

Tools have been developed to guide nurses and students through the basic steps to locate and critically appraise online scientific literature while linking users to quality electronic resources to support EBP. As the world becomes increasingly digital, advances in technology have changed how students access evidence-based information, yet some research suggests a limited ability to locate quality online research and a lack of skills needed to evaluate the scientific literature (Long et al., 2016). Earlier publications outline a general attitude and offer specific suggestions to promote EBP (Melnyk & Fineout-Overholt, 2011). They include:

- Cultivating a spirit of inquiry within an EBP culture and environment
- Asking the burning clinical question in PICOT (i.e., **P**atient population, **I**ntervention or **I**ssue of interest, **C**omparison intervention or group, **O**utcome, and **T**ime frame) format.
- Searching for and collecting the most relevant best evidence.
- Critically appraising the evidence (i.e., rapid critical appraisal, evaluation, synthesis, and recommendations).
- Integrating the best evidence with one's clinical expertise and patient preferences and values in making a practice decision or change.
- Evaluating outcomes of the practice decision or change based on evidence.
- Disseminating the outcomes of the EBP decision or change.

AWHONN Perinatal Quality Measures

AWHONN advances the nursing profession by providing nurses with evidence-based education and practice resources, legislative programs, research, and interprofessional collaboration to help them deliver the highest quality care for women and newborns. Because the actions of nurses have significant impact on patient outcomes, measuring the quality of care provided by registered nurses is a vital component of health care improvement. Nurses' expert knowledge can and should shape the care environment and influence decisions of patients. Since 2012, AWHONN has developed an introductory set of nursing care quality measures. These measures, also referred to as *nurse-sensitive measures*, align with The Joint Commission's Perinatal Care Core Measures Set. This is one of many steps AWHONN is taking to lead and support efforts to improve the quality of health care provided to women and newborns (2014). Initiatives reflect current priorities and EBP and are listed in Box 2–3.

BOX 2-3 | AWHONN Nursing Care Quality Measures

AWHONN Nursing Care Quality Measures

Triage of a Pregnant Woman and Her Fetus(es)

The purpose of this measure is to increase the percentage of pregnant women who present to the labor and birth unit with a report of a real or perceived problem or an emergency condition who are triaged by a registered nurse or nurse-midwife within 10 minutes of arrival.

Second Stage of Labor: Mother-Initiated, Spontaneous Pushing

The purpose of this measure is to support mother-initiated, spontaneous pushing in the second stage of labor.

Skin-to-Skin Is Initiated Immediately Following Birth

The purpose of this measure is to increase the percentage of healthy, term newborns who are placed in skin-to-skin contact with their mothers within the first 5 minutes following birth.

Duration of Uninterrupted Skin-to-Skin Contact

The purpose of this measure is to increase the percentage of healthy, term newborns of stable mothers who receive uninterrupted skin-to-skin contact for at least 60 minutes.

Eliminating Supplementation of Breast Milk–Fed, Healthy, Term Newborns

The purpose of this measure is to reduce the percentage of healthy, term, newborns fed any breast milk who also receive supplementation with water, glucose water, or formula without medical indication during their hospital stays.

Protect Maternal Milk Volume for Premature Infants Admitted to the NICU

The purpose of this measure is to increase the percentage of mothers of premature newborns admitted to the neonatal intensive care unit (NICU) who receive a breast pump, receive the appropriate instruction and support from a registered nurse, and have the nurse remain with them throughout the first pumping session within 6 hours postbirth.

Initial Contact With Parents Following a Neonatal Transport

The purpose of this measure is to increase the percentage of mothers who receive a phone call from the referral hospital's NICU nurse within 4 hours of infant arrival to the referral hospital.

Perinatal Grief Support

The purpose of this measure is to increase the percentage of women who are offered support for grief responses after perinatal loss.

Women's Health and Wellness Coordination Throughout the Life Span

The purpose of this measure is to increase the percentage of women who are offered annual health and wellness screening in the ambulatory care setting.

Continuous Labor Support

The purpose of this measure is to increase the percentage of women in labor who receive continuous, non-pharmacological labor support customized to meet their physical and emotional needs provided by a registered nurse (RN) or by a certified doula who follows the guidance of the RN.

Partial Labor Support

The purpose of this measure is to increase the percentage of women who receive non-pharmacological labor support from an RN at least once every hour during intrapartum labor care.

Freedom of Movement During Labor

The purpose of this measure is to increase the percentage of women with term pregnancies who experience freedom of movement during labor.

Association of Women's Health, Obstetric, and Neonatal Nurses (AWHONN, 2014).

REFERENCES

Adinima, J. (2016). Litigations and the obstetrician in clinical practice. *Annals of Medical and Health Sciences, 6*(2), 74–79.

Alfirevic, Z., Devane, D., Gyte, G., & Cuthbert, A. (2017). Continuous cardiotocography (CTG) as a form of electronic fetal monitoring (EFM) for fetal assessment during labour. Cochrane Database of Systematic Reviews 2017, Issue 2. Art. No.: CD006066. DOI: 10.1002/14651858.CD006066.pub3.

American Nurses Association (ANA). (2004). *Nursing: Scope and standards of practice.* Washington, DC: Author.

American Nurses Association (ANA). (2015). *Code of ethics for nurses with interpretive statements.* Silver Spring, MD: American Nurses Publishing.

Angus, J., Hodnett, E., & O'Brien-Pallas, L. (2003). Implementing evidence-based nursing practice: A tale of two intrapartum nursing units. *Nursing Inquiry, 10*(4), 218–228.

Association of Women's Health, Obstetric and Neonatal Nurses (AWHONN). (2009). *Standards for professional nursing practice in the care of women and newborns* (7th ed.). Washington, DC: Author.

Association of Women's Health, Obstetric and Neonatal Nurses (AWHONN). (2014). *Women's health and perinatal nursing care quality refined draft measures specifications.* Washington, DC: Author.

Association of Women's Health, Obstetric and Neonatal Nurses (AWHONN). (2015). *AWHONN position statement: Fetal heart monitoring.* Washington, DC: Author.

Association of Women's Health, Obstetric and Neonatal Nurses (AWHONN). (2016a). *Rights and responsibilities of nurses related to reproductive health care.* Washington, DC: Author.

Association of Women's Health, Obstetric and Neonatal Nurses (AWHONN). (2016b). *AWHONN position statement: Ethical decision making in the clinical setting.* Washington, DC: Author.

Brown, G. (2016). Averting malpractice issues in today's nursing practice. *ABNF Journal, 27*(2), 25–27.

Chervenak, F., McCullough, L., & Burke Sosa, M. E. (2013). Ethical challenges. In N. Troirano, C. Harvey, & B. Flood Chez (Eds.), *High-risk & critical care obstetrics* (3d ed.). Philadelphia, PA: Lippincott, Williams & Wilkens.

Crico Strategies. (2010). *2010 Annual Benchmarking Report: Malpractice risks in obstetrics.* Cambridge, MA: Author.

Cronenwett, L. (1995). Effective methods for disseminating research findings to nurses in practice. *Nursing Clinics of North America, 30*(3), 429–438.

Durham, R. (2002). Women, work and midwifery. In R. Mander & V. Flemming (Eds.), *Failure to progress* (pp. 122–132). London, England: Routledge.

Epstein, E. G., & Delgado, S. (2010). Understanding and addressing moral distress. *Online Journal of Issues in Nursing, 15*(3), Manuscript 1.

Fain, J. (2017). *Reading, understanding and applying nursing research* (5th ed.). Philadelphia, PA: F.A. Davis Co.

Fawcett, J., & Garity, J. (2009). *Evaluating research for evidence based nursing practice.* Philadelphia, PA: F.A. Davis.

Freeman, R. (2002). Problems with intrapartal fetal heart rate monitoring interpretation and patient management. *American Journal of Obstetrics and Gynecology, 100*(4), 813–816.

Gilbert, E. (2007). *Manual of high risk pregnancy and delivery.* St. Louis, MO: C. V. Mosby.

Hokanson Hawks, J. (2016). Changing the level of evidence. *Urologic Nursing, 36*(6), 265–281. doi:10.7257/1053-816X.2016.36.6.265.

Iacobucci, T. A., Daly, B. J., Lindell, D., & Griffin, M. Q. (2013). Professional values, self-esteem, and ethical confidence of baccalaureate nursing students. *Nursing Ethics, 20*(4), 479–490. doi:10.1177/0969733012458608.

Johnston, B., Coole, C., Feakes, R., Whitworth, G., Tyrell, T., & Hardy, B. (2016). Exploring the barriers to and facilitators of implementing research into practice. *British Journal of Community Nursing, 21*(8), 392–398.

Jonsen, A. R., Siegler, M., & Winslade, W. J. (2002). *Clinical ethics: A practical approach to ethical decision in clinical medicine* (5th ed.). New York, NY: McGraw-Hill.

Lachman, V. D. (2007). Patient safety: The ethical imperative. *MedSurg Nursing, 16*(6), 401–403.

Lagana, K. (2000). The "right" to a caring relationship: The law and ethic of care. *Journal of Perinatal & Neonatal Nursing, 14*(2), 12–24.

Long, J., Gannaway, P., Ford, C., Doumit, R., Zeeni, N., Sukkarieh-Haraty, O., & Song, H. (2016). Effectiveness of a technology-based intervention to teach evidence-based practice: The EBR tool. *Worldviews on Evidence-Based Nursing, 13*(1), 59–65.

Lyndon, A., & Ali, L. U. (2015). *Fetal heart monitoring: Principles and practices* (5th ed.). Dubuque, IA: Kendall Hunt Publishing.

Lyndon, A., Zlatnik, M. G., Maxfield, D. G., Lewis, A., McMillan, C., & Kennedy, H. P. (2014). Contributions of clinical disconnections and unresolved conflict to failures in intrapartum safety. *Journal of Obstetric, Gynecologic & Neonatal Nursing, 43*(1), 2–12.

Mahlmeister, L. (2000). Legal implications of fetal heart rate assessment. *Journal of Obstetric, Gynecologic, & Neonatal Nursing, 29*, 517–526.

Mattson, l., & Smith, J. (2016) *Core curriculum for maternal-newborn nursing* (5th ed.). St. Louis, MO: Elsevier.

Mazurek Melnyk, B., Gallagher-Ford, L., & Fineout-Overholt, E. (2016). Improving healthcare quality, patient outcomes, and costs with evidence-based practice. *Reflections on Nursing Leadership, 42*(3), 1–8.

McKeever, S., Twomey, B., Hawley, M., Lima, S., Kinney, S., & Newall, F. (2016). Engaging a nursing workforce in evidence-based practice: Introduction of a nursing clinical effectiveness committee. *Worldviews on Evidence-Based Nursing, 13*(1), 85–88. doi:10.1111/wvn.12119.

Melnyk, B. M., & Fineout-Overholt, E. (2005). *Evidence-based practice in nursing and healthcare: A guide to best practice.* Philadelphia, PA: Lippincott Williams & Wilkins.

Melnyk, B. M., & Fineout-Overholt, E. (2011). *Evidence-based practice in nursing & healthcare. A guide to best practice* (pp. 1–24). Philadelphia, PA: Wolters Kluwer/ Lippincott Williams & Wilkins.

Miller, W. R. (2010). Qualitative research findings as evidence: Utility in nursing practice. *Clinical Nurse Specialist CNS, 24*(4), 191–193. http:doi.org/10.1097/ NUR.0b013e3181e36087.

Pearson, N. (2011). Oxytocin safety. *Nursing for Women's Health, 15*(2), 110–117.

Sandelowski, M. (1996). Using qualitative methods in intervention studies. *Research in Nursing and Health, 19*, 359–364.

Sandelowski, M., & Barroso, J. (2003). Classifying the findings in qualitative studies. *Qualitative Health Research, 13*, 905–923.

Schumann, J. H., & Alfandre, D. (2008). Clinical ethical decision making: The four topics approach. *Seminars Medical Practice, 11*, 36–42.

Scott, S. D. (2010). *Achieving consistent quality care. Using research to guide clinical practice* (2d ed.). Washington, DC: Association of Women's Health, Obstetrics and Neonatal Nursing.

Simpson, K. (2014). Perinatal patient safety and professional liability issues. In K. Simpson, P. Creehan, & AWHONN (Eds.), *Perinatal nursing* (4th ed.). Philadelphia, PA: Lippincott Williams & Wilkins.

Simpson, K., & Knox, E. (2003). Common area of litigation related to care during labor and birth: Recommendations to promote patient safety and decrease risk exposure. *Journal of Perinatal and Neonatal Nursing, 17*(2), 110–125.

Stephenson, C. (2016). Ethics. In S. Mattson & J. Smith (Eds.), *Core curriculum for maternal-newborn nursing* (5th ed.). St Louis, MO: Elsevier.

Stetler, C. (1994). Refinement of the Stetler/Marram model for application of research findings to practice. *Nursing Outlook, 42*, 15–25.

Swanson, J., Durham, R., & Albright, J. (1997). Clinical utilization/application of qualitative research. In J. Morse (Ed.), *Completing a qualitative project: Details and dialogue* (pp. 253–282). Thousand Oaks, CA: Sage.

Thorne, S. (2009). The role of qualitative research within an evidence-based context: Can metasynthesis be the answer? *International Journal of Nursing Studies, 46*(4), 569–575.

Titler, M., & Goode, C. (1995). Research utilization. *Nursing Clinics of North America, 30*(3), xv.

Watson, E. (2014). Nursing malpractice: Costs, trends, and issues. *Journal of Legal Nurse Consulting, 25*(1), 26–31.

The Antepartal Period

Genetics, Conception, Fetal Development, and Reproductive Technology

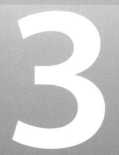

3

Linda L. Chapman, RN, PhD

LEARNING OUTCOMES

Upon completion of this chapter, the student will be able to:

1. Discuss the relevance of genetics within the context of the care of the childbearing family.
2. Identify critical components of conception, embryonic development, and fetal development.
3. Describe the development and function of the placenta and amniotic fluid.
4. List the common causes of infertility.
5. Describe the common diagnostic tests used to identify causes of infertility.
6. Describe the most common methods used in assisted fertility.
7. Discuss the ethical and emotional implications of assisted reproductive therapies.

GENETICS AND THE CHILDBEARING FAMILY

Genes, the basic functional and physical units of heredity, are composed of DNA and protein. The human genome—the complete set of an organism's DNA—contains approximately 30,000 genes. Each human cell contains 46 chromosomes, including 22 homologous pairs of chromosomes and one pair of sex chromosomes designated as either XX (female) or XY (male). Each chromosome contains numerous genes. Genotype is a person's genetic makeup, while phenotype is the ways in which these genes are outwardly expressed, such as eye color, hair color, or height.

Advances in genetics (the study of heredity) and genomics (the study of genes and their function and related technology) are providing better methods for:

- Preventing diseases and abnormalities
- Diagnosing diseases
- Predicting health risks
- Personalizing treatment plans

CRITICAL COMPONENT

Genetics and Genomics

"The main difference between genomics and genetics is that genetics scrutinizes the functioning and composition of the single gene whereas genomics addresses all genes and their interrelationships in order to identify their combined influence on the growth and development of the organism" (WHO, 2012).

Dominant and Recessive Inheritance

Genes are either dominant or recessive. When a dominant and recessive gene are paired, such as a gene for brown eyes and a gene for blue eyes, the traits of the dominant gene (brown eyes) will be present. If both genes in a pair are recessive, the recessive trait will be present.

Genetic diseases and disorders are often related to a defective recessive gene and are present at birth when a person has a pair of genes with the same defect on both (Fig. 3–1). People

Autosomal Recessive-Cystic Fibrosis

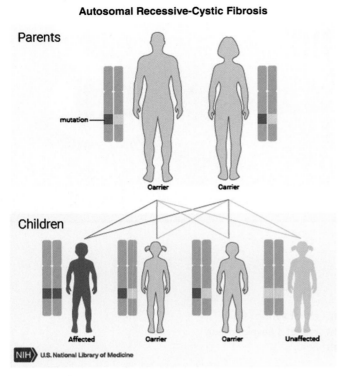

FIGURE 3–1 Two unaffected parents each carry one copy of mutation for cystic fibrosis. They have one affected child and three unaffected (two of which carry one copy of affected gene).

who have just one defective gene carry the disorder and can pass it on to a child but do not have it themselves. Examples of these autosomal-recessive disorders include cystic fibrosis, sickle cell anemia, thalassemia, and Tay-Sachs disease (Table 3–1). Autosomal-dominant disorders such as Huntington's disease (Fig. 3–2), familial hypercholesterolemia, and xeroderma pigmentation present when one or both genes in a pair carries the defect.

Sex-Linked Inheritance

Conditions can be either X-linked inheritance and Y-linked inheritance. With X-linked inheritance:

● The mutated gene is located only on the X chromosome.
● The gene can be either recessive or dominant.
● Male children who receive an X chromosome with a mutated gene present with the disorder when the Y chromosome does not carry that gene; the gene, even though it may be recessive, becomes dominant.
● Female children who have one X chromosome with a sex-linked trait disorder do not present with the trait but are carriers of the trait.
● Hemophilia is an example of an X-linked inheritance disorder (Fig. 3–3).

With Y-linked inheritance, the mutation is located only on the Y chromosome. This means the disease can be passed only from father to son.

TABLE 3–1   Genetic Diseases

DISEASE (PATTERN OF INHERITANCE)	DESCRIPTION
Sickle-cell anemia (R)	The most common genetic disease among people of African ancestry. Sickle-cell hemoglobin forms rigid crystals that distort and disrupt red blood cells; oxygen-carrying capacity of the blood is diminished.
Cystic fibrosis (R)	The most common genetic disease among people of European ancestry. Production of thick mucus clogs in the bronchial tree and pancreatic ducts. Most severe effects are chronic respiratory infections and pulmonary failure.
Tay-Sachs disease (R)	The most common genetic disease among people of Jewish ancestry. Degeneration of neurons and the nervous system results in death by the age of 2 years.
Phenylketonuria (PKU) (R)	Lack of an enzyme to metabolize the amino acid phenylalanine leads to severe mental and physical retardation. These effects may be prevented by the use of a diet (beginning at birth) that limits phenylalanine.
Huntington's disease (D)	Uncontrollable muscle contractions between the ages of 30 and 50 years, followed by loss of memory and personality. There is no treatment that can delay mental deterioration.
Hemophilia (X-linked)	Lack of factor VIII impairs chemical clotting; may be controlled with factor VIII from donated blood.
Duchenne's muscular dystrophy (X-linked)	Replacement of muscle by adipose or scar tissue, with progressive loss of muscle function; often fatal before age 20 years due to involvement of cardiac muscle.

R = recessive; D = dominant.
Scanlon & Sanders, 2015.

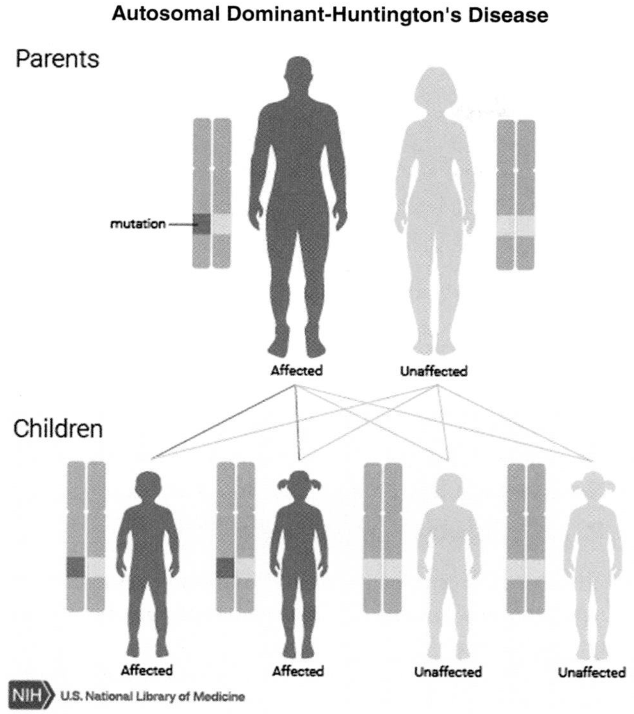

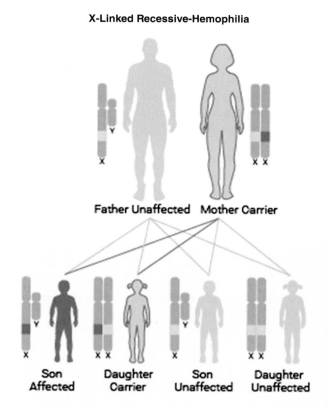

FIGURE 3-2 A man with Huntington's disease has two affected children and two unaffected children.

FIGURE 3-3 A woman who is a carrier of hemophilia has one affected son, one daughter who is a carrier and one son and one daughter who are unaffected.

Genomic Medicine

The Human Genome Project, a 13-year international, collaborative research program completed in 2003, has provided the scientific community with valuable information used in the diagnosis, treatment, and prevention of genetically linked disorders. Current genomic medicine is building upon and expanding the knowledge gained from the Human Genome Project. The National Human Genome Research Institute (NHGRI) defines *genomic medicine* as an emerging medical discipline that involves using genomic information about an individual as part of their clinical care (e.g., for diagnostic or therapeutic decision making) and the health outcomes and policy implications of that clinical use (NHGRI, 2016). Examples of genomic medicine include:

- Newborn screening for inherited, treatable genetic diseases
- Cell-free circulating DNA as a biomarker for cancer
- Pharmacogenomics to determine whether a therapy will be effective for an individual
- Development drugs that can treat genetic diseases such as ivacaftor, which treats a specific mutation for one form of cystic fibrosis (NHGRI, 2016)

Genetic Testing

Several genetic tests are selectively used in the care of childbearing families. These include:

- Carrier testing, used to identify individuals who carry one copy of a gene mutation when there is a family history of a genetic disorder. When both prospective parents are tested, the test can provide information about their risk of having a child with a genetic condition.
- Preimplantation testing, also known as preimplantation genetic diagnosis, is used to detect genetic changes in embryos created using assisted reproductive techniques. Prior to transferring an in vitro embryo into the woman's uterus, a cell from the developing fetus is removed for genetic testing.
- Prenatal testing allows for the early detection of genetic disorders such as trisomy 21, hemophilia, and Tay-Sachs disease.
- Newborn screening is used to detect genetic disorders that can be treated early in life.

Couples who have a higher risk for conceiving a child with a genetic disorder include those with:

- A maternal age older than 35
- A history of previous pregnancy resulting in a genetic disorder or newborn abnormalities
- One or both partners having a genetic disorder
- A family history of a genetic disorder

Diagnosis of genetic disorders during pregnancy allows parents to use gene therapy when available, prepare to raise a child with the specific genetic disorder, or seek genetic counseling to make the decision to continue or terminate the pregnancy.

Nursing Actions

Nursing actions for couples who elect to continue the pregnancy based on information of a genetic disorder include:

- Providing additional information about the genetic disorder.
- Referring them to support groups for parents who have children with the same genetic disorder.
- Providing a list of websites that contain accurate information about the disorder.
- Explaining that they will experience grief over the loss of the "dream child" and that this is normal.
- Encouraging them to talk openly to each other about their feelings and concerns.

Nursing actions for couples who elect to terminate the pregnancy based on information from genetic testing are as follows:

- Explaining the stages of grief they will experience.
- Informing the couple that grief is a normal process.
- Encouraging the couple to communicate with each other and share their emotions
- Referring the couple to a support group if available in their community

Nurses, especially those practicing in the obstetrical or pediatric areas, need a general understanding of genetics and the possible effects on the developing human, as they may be required to explain diagnostic procedures used in genetic testing, including purpose, findings, and possible side effects. Nurses may also need to clarify or reinforce information couples receive from their health care providers or genetic counselors. Maternal-child nurses should be able to provide information regarding:

- Genetic counseling services available in the parents' community.
- Access to genetic services.
- Procedure for referral to the different services.
- The information or services these agencies provide.

CRITICAL COMPONENT

Teratogens

The developing human is most vulnerable to the effects of teratogens during the period of organogenesis, the first 8 weeks of gestation. An example of a teratogen is toxoplasmosis.

Toxoplasma is a protozoan parasite found in cat feces and uncooked or rare beef and lamb. When an embryo is exposed to *Toxoplasma*, fetal demise, mental retardation, and blindness can result. Women who are pregnant or attempting to conceive should:

- Avoid contact with cat feces, such as through cleaning or changing a litter box.
- Avoid eating rare beef or lamb.

TERATOGENS

Birth defects can occur from genetic disorders or result from teratogen exposure. Teratogens are drugs, viruses, infections, or other exposures that have the potential to cause embryonic/fetal developmental abnormality (Table 3–2). The degree or types of malformation caused by teratogen exposure vary based on length of exposure, amount of exposure, and when it occurs during human development. Developing humans are most vulnerable to the effects of teratogens during organogenesis, which occurs during the first 8 weeks of gestation. Exposure during this time can cause gross structural defects. Exposure to teratogens after 13 weeks of gestation may cause fetal growth restriction or reduction of organ size.

ANATOMY AND PHYSIOLOGY REVIEW

Knowledge of the male and female reproductive systems is essential for the maternity nurse.

TABLE 3–2   Teratogenic Agents

AGENT	EFFECT
Drugs and Chemicals	
Alcohol	Increased risk of fetal alcohol syndrome occurring when the pregnant woman ingests six or more alcoholic drinks a day. No amount of alcohol is considered safe during pregnancy. Newborn characteristics of fetal alcohol syndrome include: • Low birth weight • Microcephaly • Mental retardation • Unusual facial features due to midfacial hypoplasia • Cardiac defects
Angiotensin-converting enzyme (ACE) inhibitors	Increased risk for: • Renal tubular dysplasia that can lead to renal failure and fetal or neonatal death • Intrauterine growth restriction

TABLE 3–2   Teratogenic Agents—cont'd

AGENT	EFFECT
Carbamazepine (anticonvulsant)	Increased risk for: • Neural tubal defects • Craniofacial defects, including cleft lip and palate • Intrauterine growth restriction
Cocaine	Increased risk for: • Heart, limbs, face, gastrointestinal tract, and genitourinary tract defects • Cerebral infarctions • Placental abnormalities
Warfarin (Coumadin)	Increased risk for: • Spontaneous abortion • Fetal demise • Fetal or newborn hemorrhage • Central nervous system abnormalities
Infections/Viruses	
Cytomegalovirus	Increased risk for: • Hydrocephaly • Microcephaly • Cerebral calcification • Mental retardation • Hearing loss
Herpes varicella (chicken pox)	Increased risk for: • Hypoplasia of hands and feet • Blindness/cataracts • Mental retardation
Rubella	Increased risk for: • Heart defects • Deafness and/or blindness • Mental retardation • Fetal demise
Syphilis	Increased risk for: • Skin, bone, and/or teeth defects • Fetal demise • Blindness and deafness
Toxoplasmosis	Increased risk for: • Fetal demise • Blindness • Mental retardation
Zika	Increased risk for: • Microcephaly • Blindness • Hearing defects • Impaired growth

American College of Obstetricians and Gynecologists (ACOG), 1997; CDC, 2017; Scanlon & Sanders, 2015.

Male

The major structures and functions of the male reproductive system are pictured in Figures 3–4 and 3–5. They include the following:

- The scrotum is a loose bag of skin and connective tissue in which the two testes are suspended. The temperature inside the scrotum is approximately 96°F, lower than body temperature. This environment facilitates the production of viable sperm (Scanlon & Sanders, 2015).
- In the fetus, the testes develop near the kidney and normally descend into the scrotum before birth. Each of the two testes is divided into lobes that contain several seminiferous tubules in which spermatogenesis takes place. Sperm travel from the seminiferous tubules and through the rete testis (a tubular network) and enter the epididymis.
- The epididymis is a coiled, tubelike structure on the posterior surface of each testis, inside which sperm complete their maturation.
- The ductus deferens, also called the vas deferens, extends from the epididymis into the abdominal cavity. In the abdominal cavity, it extends over the urinary bladder and down the posterior side of the bladder, where it joins with the ejaculatory duct.
- Two ejaculatory ducts receive sperm from the ductus deferens and secretions from the seminal vesicles. The ducts empty into the urethra.
- Located posterior to the urinary bladder, the seminal vesicles produce secretions that contain fructose, an energy source for sperm. These secretions are alkaline, which increases sperm motility.
- The prostate gland is a muscular gland located beneath the urinary bladder and surrounds the first inch of the urethra as it extends from the bladder. It secretes an alkaline fluid that further increases sperm motility.

- Bulbourethral glands, also referred to as Cowper's glands, are located below the prostate gland. They secrete an alkaline solution that coats the interior of the urethra to neutralize the acidic urine that is present.
- Located within the penis, the urethra is the final duct through which semen passes as it exits the body.
- The penis is the external male genital organ, consisting of smooth muscle, connective tissue, and blood sinuses. The penis is flaccid when blood flow to the area is minimal and becomes erect when its arteries dilate and the sinuses fill with blood.

Female

The major structures and functions of the female reproductive system, pictured in Figures 3–6 and 3–7, include the following:

- The ovaries are two oval-shaped organs, each about 4 centimeters long, located on either side of the uterus and held in place by the ovarian ligament and broad ligament. Several thousand primary follicles are present in the ovaries at birth, each containing an oocyte. The follicle cells secrete estrogen. A mature follicle is known as a graafian follicle.
- Fertilization occurs within one of the two fallopian tubes, also called oviducts. The lateral end of these tubes partially surrounds the ovary. Fringelike projections called fimbriae protrude from the lateral end to create a current that pulls the ovum into the tube. Peristaltic waves created by the fallopian tubes' smooth muscle contractions move the ovum through the tube and into the uterus, where the medial end of the tube lies (Scanlon & Sanders, 2015).
- The uterus is the site of implantation and expands during pregnancy to accommodate the developing embryo/fetus and its placenta. This organ is shaped like an upside-down pear and is about 3 inches wide, 2 inches long, and 1 inch deep. The upper portion of the uterus is known as the fundus,

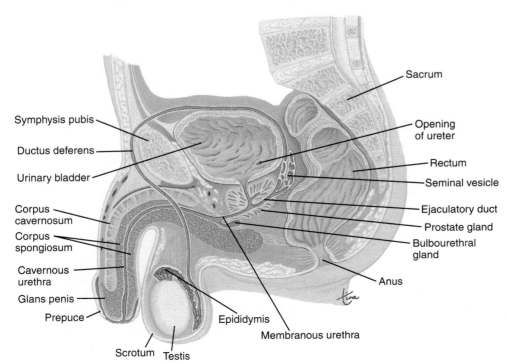

FIGURE 3–4 Male reproductive system shown in a midsagittal section through the pelvic cavity.

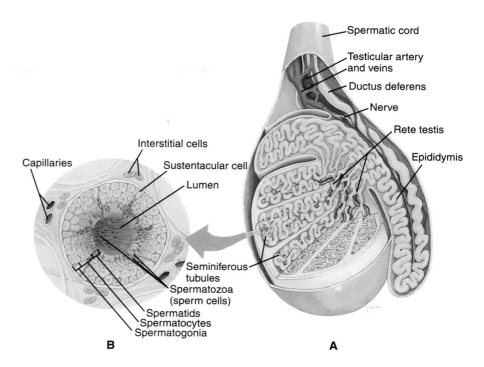

FIGURE 3-5 (*A*) Midsagittal section of the testis; the epididymis is on the posterior side of the testis. (*B*) Cross section through a somniferous tubule showing development of the sperm.

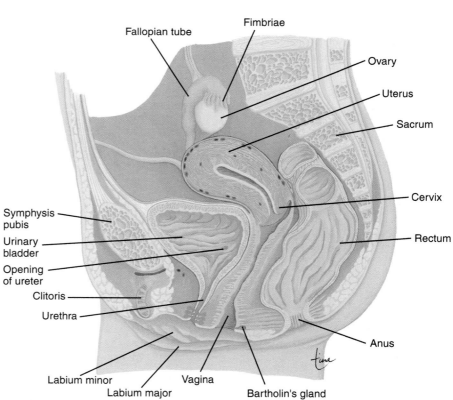

FIGURE 3-6 Female reproductive system shown in a midsagittal section through the pelvic cavity.

while the large central portion is called the body. The narrow, lower end that opens to the vagina is called the cervix. The inner lining of the uterus, called the endometrium, consists of a permanent layer (the basilar layer) and a regenerative layer (the functional layer). Each month, estrogen and progesterone stimulate the functional layer to thicken in preparation for egg implantation. If implantation occurs, the endometrium continues to thicken. If implantation does not occur, the functional layer is shed during the menstrual cycle.

● The vagina is a muscular tube approximately 4 inches long, extending from the cervix to the perineum. It has multiple functions: receiving sperm during sexual intercourse, providing exit for menstrual blood flow, and serving as the birth canal during the second stage of labor.

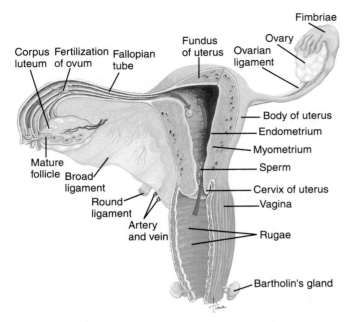

FIGURE 3-7 Female reproductive system shown in anterior view. The ovary on the left side of the illustration has been sectioned to show the developing follicles. The fallopian tube on the left side of the illustration has been sectioned to show fertilization. The uterus and vagina have been sectioned to show internal structures. Arrows indicate the movement of the ovum toward the uterus and the movement of sperm from the vagina toward the fallopian tube.

● The external genitalia, also known as the vulva, comprise the clitoris, labia majora and minora, and Bartholin's glands.
  ● The clitoris, a small mass of erectile tissue anterior to the urethral orifice, responds to sexual stimulus.
  ● The labia majora and minora are paired folds of skin that cover the urethral and vaginal openings and prevent drying of their mucous membranes.
  ● Bartholin's glands, located in the floor of the vestibule, have ducts that open onto the mucous of the vaginal orifice. Their secretions keep the mucous membranes moist and lubricate the vagina during sexual intercourse.

MENSTRUAL CYCLE

A woman's menstrual cycle is influenced by the ovarian cycle and endometrial cycle (Fig. 3–8).

Ovarian Cycle

The ovarian cycle pertains to the maturation of ova and consists of three phases:

1. The follicular phase begins the first day of menstruation and lasts 12 to 14 days. During this phase, the graafian follicle matures under the influence of two pituitary hormones: luteinizing hormone (LH) and follicle-stimulating hormone (FSH). The maturing graafian follicle produces estrogen.

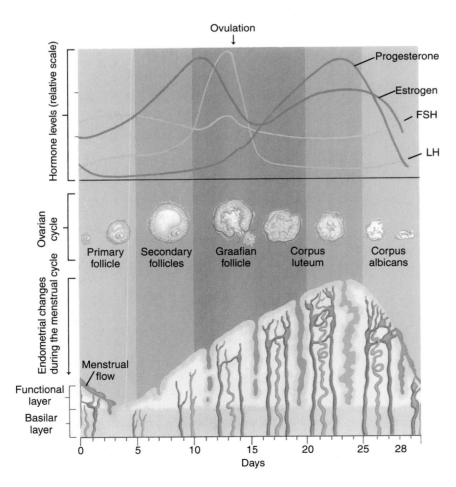

FIGURE 3-8 The menstrual cycle. The levels of the major hormones are shown in relationship to one another throughout the cycle. Changes in the ovarian follicle are depicted. The relative thickness of the endometrium is also shown.

2. The ovulatory phase begins when estrogen levels peak and ends with the release of the oocyte (egg) from the mature graafian follicle. The release of the oocyte is referred to as ovulation. LH levels surge 12 to 36 hours before ovulation. Before this surge, estrogen levels decrease and progesterone levels increase.

3. The luteal phase begins after ovulation and lasts approximately 14 days. During this phase, the cells of the empty follicle morph to form the corpus luteum, which produces high levels of progesterone and low levels of estrogen. If pregnancy occurs, the corpus luteum releases progesterone and estrogen until the placenta matures enough to assume this function. If pregnancy does not occur, the corpus luteum degenerates, resulting in a decrease in progesterone and the beginning of menstruation.

Endometrial Cycle

The endometrial cycle pertains to the changes in the endometrium of the uterus in response to the hormonal changes that occur during the ovarian cycle. This cycle consists of three phases:

1. The proliferative phase occurs following menstruation and ends with ovulation. During this phase, the endometrium prepares for implantation by becoming thicker and more vascular. These changes are in response to the increasing levels of estrogen produced by the graafian follicle.

2. The secretory phase begins after ovulation and ends with the onset of menstruation. During this phase, the endometrium continues to thicken. The primary hormone during this phase is progesterone secreted from the corpus luteum. If pregnancy occurs, the endometrium continues to develop and begins to secrete glycogen, the energy source for the blastocyst during implantation. If pregnancy does not occur, the corpus luteum begins to degrade and the endometrial tissue degenerates.

3. The menstrual phase occurs in response to hormonal changes and results in the sloughing off and expulsion of the endometrial tissue.

OOGENESIS

Oogenesis is the formation of a mature ovum (egg). This process is regulated by two primary hormones:

- Follicle-stimulating hormone (FSH): Secreted from the anterior pituitary gland, FSH stimulates growth of the ovarian follicles and stimulates the follicles to secrete estrogen.
- Estrogen: Secreted from the follicle cells, estrogen promotes the maturation of the ovum.

The process of oogenesis includes the following steps:

- FSH stimulates the growth of the ovarian follicle, which contains an oogonium (stem cell).
- Through mitosis, the oogonium within the ovary forms into two daughter cells: the primary oocyte and a new stem cell (Fig. 3–9). *Mitosis* is the process by which a cell divides and forms two genetically identical cells (daughter cells), each containing the diploid number of chromosomes.

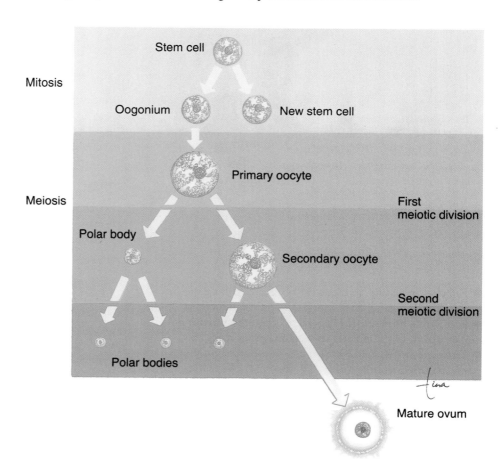

FIGURE 3–9 Oogenesis. The process of mitosis and meiosis are shown. For each primary oocyte that undergoes meiosis, only one functional ovum is formed.

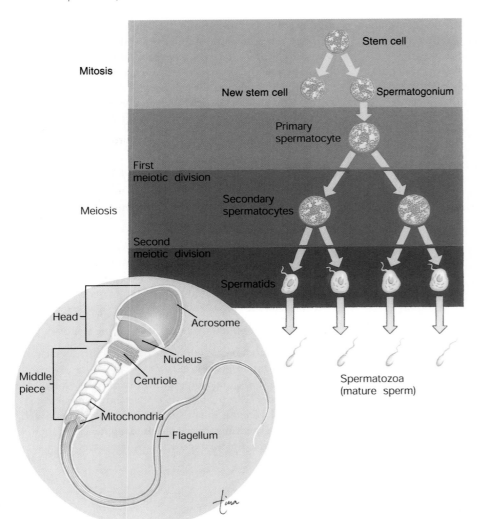

FIGURE 3–10 Spermatogenesis. The process of mitosis and meiosis are shown. For each primary spermatocyte that undergoes meiosis, four functional sperm cells are formed. The structure of the sperm cell is also shown.

- Through meiosis, the primary oocyte forms into the secondary oocyte and a polar body. The polar body forms into two polar bodies. The secondary oocyte forms into a polar body and a mature ovum. *Meiosis* is a process of two successive cell divisions that produce cells that contain half the number of chromosomes (haploid).

SPERMATOGENESIS

Spermatogenesis is the formation of mature spermatozoa (sperm), a process regulated by three primary hormones:

- Follicle-stimulating hormone (FSH): Secreted from the anterior pituitary gland, FSH stimulates sperm production.
- Luteinizing hormone (LH): Secreted from the anterior pituitary gland, LH stimulates testosterone production.
- Testosterone: Secreted by the testes, testosterone promotes the maturation of the sperm.

Through mitosis, the spermatogonium (stem cell) within the seminiferous tubules of the testes forms into two daughter cells: a new spermatogonia and a spermatogonium. The latter differentiates and is referred to as the primary spermatocyte. Through meiosis, it forms two secondary spermatocytes, each of which forms two spermatids with the haploid number of chromosomes (Fig. 3–10). Mature spermatids are called spermatozoa.

CONCEPTION

Conception, also known as fertilization, occurs when a sperm nucleus enters the nucleus of the oocyte (Fig. 3–11). Fertilization normally occurs in the outer third of the fallopian tube. The fertilized oocyte is called a zygote and contains the diploid number of chromosomes (46).

Cell Division

The single-cell zygote undergoes mitotic cell division known as cleavage. By the third day after fertilization, the zygote has morphed into a 16-cell, solid sphere called a morula. Mitosis continues; around day 5, the developing human enters the uterus and becomes a *blastocyst*. The blastocyst consists of an inner cell mass; the *embryoblast,* which will develop into the embryo; and an outer cell mass, the *trophoblast,* which assists in implantation and will become part of the placenta.

Multiple gestation refers to more than one developing embryo, such as in the case of twins. Twins can be either monozygotic or

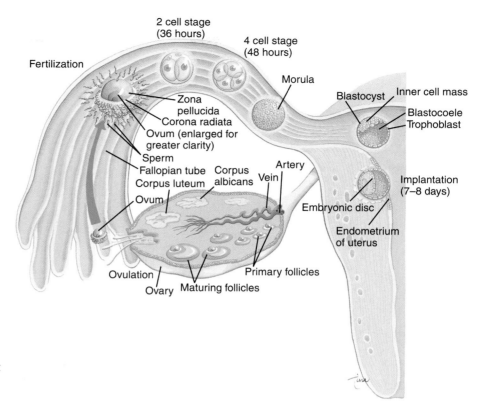

FIGURE 3–11 Ovulation, fertilization, and early embryonic development. Fertilization takes place in the fallopian tube, and the embryo reaches the blastocyst stage when it becomes implanted in the endometrium of the uterus.

dizygotic. *Monozygotic twins,* also called identical twins, result from a fertilized ovum that splits during the early stages of cell division to form two identical embryos that are genetically the same. *Dizygotic twins,* also called fraternal twins, result from two separate ova fertilized by two separate sperm; they are not genetically identical.

Implantation

Implantation, the embedding of the blastocyst into the endometrium of the uterus, begins around day 5 or 6. To prepare for implantation, progesterone stimulates the endometrium to become thicker and more vascular while enzymes secreted by the trophoblast, now referred to as the chorion, digest the surface of the endometrium. Implantation normally occurs in the upper part of the posterior wall of the uterus.

EMBRYONIC AND FETAL DEVELOPMENT

The developing human is referred to as an embryo from the time of implantation through 8 weeks of gestation.

Embryo

Organogenesis, the formation and development of body organs, occurs during this critical time of human development. Primary germ layers known as the ectoderm, mesoderm, and endoderm form the organs, tissues, and body structures of the developing human. The ectoderm is the outer germ layer, the mesoderm is the middle layer, and the endoderm is the inner layer. These primary germ layers begin to develop around day 14 (Table 3–3).

TABLE 3–3 Structures Derived From the Primary Germ Layers

LAYER	STRUCTURES DERIVED*
Ectoderm	Epidermis; hair and nail follicles; sweat glands
	Nervous system; pituitary gland; adrenal medulla
	Lens and cornea; internal ear
	Mucosa of oral and nasal cavities; salivary glands
Mesoderm	Dermis; bone and cartilage
	Skeletal muscles; cardiac muscles; most smooth muscles
	Kidneys; adrenal cortex
	Bone marrow and blood; lymphatic tissue; lining of blood vessels
Endoderm	Mucosa of esophagus, stomach, and intestines
	Epithelium of respiratory tract, including lungs
	Liver and mucosa of gallbladder
	Thyroid gland; pancreas

*These are representative lists, not all-inclusive ones. Most organs are combinations of tissues from each of the three germ layers.
Scanlon & Sanders, 2015.

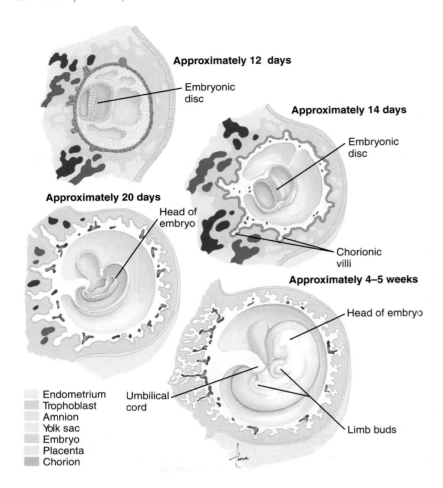

Approximately 12 days
— Embryonic disc

Approximately 14 days
Embryonic disc

Approximately 20 days
Head of embryo

Chorionic villi

Approximately 4–5 weeks
Head of embryo

Umbilical cord

Limb buds

Endometrium
Trophoblast
Amnion
Yolk sac
Embryo
Placenta
Chorion

FIGURE 3–12 Embryonic development at 12 days (after fertilization), 14 days, 20 days, and 4–5 weeks. By 5 weeks, the embryo has distinct parts but does not yet look definitely human.

The heart forms during the 3rd week of gestation and begins to beat and circulate blood during the 4th week. By the end of the 8th gestational week, the primary germ layers have transformed into a clearly defined human about 3 centimeters long with all organ systems formed (Fig. 3–12).

Fetus

The developing human is referred to as a fetus from week 9 to birth. During this stage of development, organ systems grow and mature (Table 3–4).

Fetal Circulation

The cardiovascular system begins to develop within the first few weeks after conception. The heart begins to beat during the 3rd week after conception. Fetal circulation (Fig. 3–13) has several unique features:

- High levels of oxygenated blood enter the fetal circulatory system from the placenta via the umbilical vein.
- The *ductus venosus* connects the umbilical vein to the inferior vena cava. This allows the majority of the highly oxygenated blood to enter the right atrium.
- The *foramen ovale* is an opening between the right and left atria. Blood high in oxygen is shunted to the left atrium via the foramen ovale. After delivery, the foramen ovale closes in

response to increased blood returning to the left atrium. It may take up to 3 months for full closure.
- The *ductus arteriosus* connects the pulmonary artery with the descending aorta. The majority of the oxygenated blood is shunted to the aorta via the ductus arteriosus with smaller amounts going to the lungs. After delivery, the ductus arteriosus constricts in response to the higher blood oxygen levels and prostaglandins.

PLACENTA, MEMBRANES, AMNIOTIC FLUID, AND UMBILICAL CORD

These structures provide a range of functions for the mother and developing fetus.

Placenta

- The placenta is formed from both fetal and maternal tissue (Fig. 3–14).
- The chorionic membrane that develops from the trophoblast, along with the chorionic villi, form the fetal side of the placenta. The *chorionic villi* are projections from the chorion that embed into the decidua basalis and later form the fetal blood vessels of the placenta.

TABLE 3–4 Summary of Fetal Development

GESTATIONAL WEEK	LENGTH*/WEIGHT	FETAL DEVELOPMENT/CHARACTERISTICS
12	8 cm/45 grams	Red blood cells are produced in the liver.
		Fusion of the palate is completed.
		External genitalia are developed to the point that sex of fetus can be noted with ultrasound.
		Eyelids are closed.
		Fetal heart tone can be heard by Doppler device.
16	14 cm/200 grams	Lanugo is present on head.
		Meconium is formed in the intestines.
		Teeth begin to form.
		Sucking motions are made with the mouth.
		Skin is transparent.
20	19 cm/450 grams	Lanugo covers the entire body.
		Vernix caseosa covers the body.
		Nails are formed.
		Brown fat begins to develop.
24	23 cm/820 grams	Eyes are developed. Alveoli form in the lungs and begin to produce surfactant.
		Footprints and fingerprints are forming.
		Respiratory movement can be detected.
28	27 cm/1,300 grams	Eyelids are open. Adipose tissue develops rapidly.
		The respiratory system has developed to a point where gas exchange is possible, but lungs are not fully mature.
32	30 cm/2,100 grams	Bones are fully developed. Lungs are maturing.
		Increased amounts of adipose tissue are present.
36	34 cm/2,900 grams	Lanugo begins to disappear. Labia majora and minora are equally prominent.
		Testes are in upper portion of scrotum.
40	36 cm/3,400 grams	Fetus is considered full term at 38 weeks. All organs/systems are fully developed.

*Length is measured from the crown (top of head) to the rump (buttock). This is referred to as the crown-rump length (CRL).

Sadler, 2015; Scanlon & Sanders, 2015.

- The endometrium is referred to as the decidua and consists of three layers: decidua basalis, decidua capsularis, and decidua vera. The decidua basalis, the portion directly beneath the blastocyst, forms the maternal portion of the placenta.
- The maternal side of the placenta is divided into compartments or lobes known as cotyledons.
- The placental membrane separates the maternal and fetal blood and prevents fetal blood from mixing with maternal blood, but it also allows for the exchange of gases, nutrients, and electrolytes.

Function of the Placenta

The placenta serves several critical functions for the mother and developing fetus. These include:

- Metabolic and gas exchange: In the placenta, fetal waste products and CO_2 are transferred from the fetal blood into

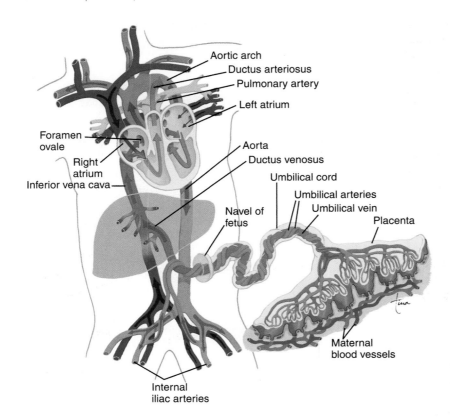

FIGURE 3–13 Fetal circulation. Fetal heart and blood vessels are shown on the left. Arrows depict direction of blood flow. The placenta and umbilical vessels are shown on the right.

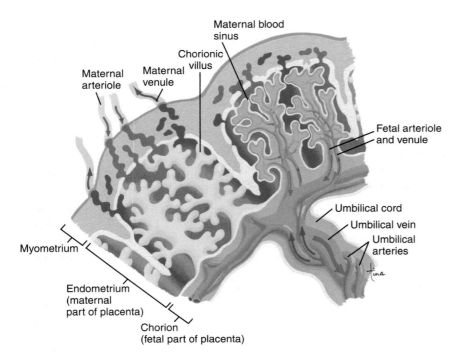

FIGURE 3–14 Placenta and umbilical cord. The fetal capillaries in the chorionic villi are within the maternal blood sinuses. Arrows indicate the direction of blood flow in the maternal and fetal vessels.

the maternal blood sinuses by diffusion. Nutrients such as glucose and amino acids and O_2 are transferred from the maternal blood sinuses to the fetal blood through the mechanisms of diffuse and active transport.

- Hormone production: The major hormones the placenta produces are progesterone; estrogen; human chorionic gonadotropin (hCG); and human placental lactogen (hPL), also known as human chorionic somatomammotropin.

  - Progesterone facilitates implantation and decreases uterine contractility.
  - Estrogen stimulates the enlargement of the breasts and uterus.

- hCG stimulates the corpus luteum so that it will continue to secrete estrogen and progesterone until the placenta is mature enough to do so. This is the hormone assessed in pregnancy tests. hCG rises rapidly during the first trimester and then rapidly declines.
- hPL promotes fetal growth by regulating available glucose and stimulates breast development in preparation for lactation.

Viruses such as rubella and cytomegalovirus can cross the placental membrane and enter the fetal system, potentially causing fetal death or defects. Drugs can also cross the placental membrane. Women should consult their health care providers before taking any medication during pregnancy. Drugs with an FDA pregnancy category of C, D, or X should be avoided during pregnancy or when attempting to conceive.

The placenta becomes fully functional between the 8th and 10th weeks of gestation. By the 9th month, it measures between 15 and 25 cm in diameter, is 3 cm thick, and weighs approximately 600 grams.

CRITICAL COMPONENT

Medications

Women who are pregnant or attempting pregnancy should consult with their health care provider before taking any prescribed or over-the-counter medications, as these can cross the placental membrane.

Embryonic Membranes

The *embryonic sac,* also called the bag of waters, is formed by the amniotic and chorionic membranes. The amniotic membrane is the inner membrane and develops from the embryoblast, while the chorionic or outer membrane develops from the trophoblast. The amniotic sac contains the embryo and amniotic fluid. Both membranes stretch to accommodate the growth of the developing fetus and subsequent increase in amniotic fluid.

Function of the Embryonic Membranes

The intact membranes help maintain a sterile environment by forming a barrier that prevents bacteria from entering the amniotic fluid through the vagina.

Amniotic Fluid

Contained within the amniotic sac (Fig. 3–15), amniotic fluid is clear and is mainly composed of water. It also contains proteins, carbohydrates, lipids, electrolytes, fetal cells, lanugo, and vernix caseosa. During the first trimester, the amniotic membrane produces amniotic fluid; during the second and third trimesters, it is produced by the fetal kidneys. The amount of amniotic fluid peaks at 800–1,000 mL around 34 weeks' gestation and decreases to 500–600 mL at term.

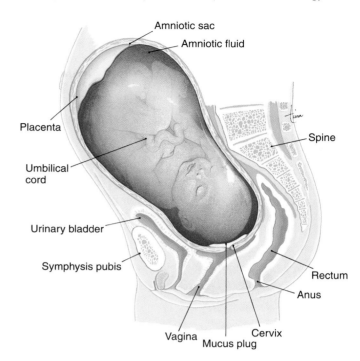

FIGURE 3–15 Fetus, placenta, umbilical cord, and amniotic fluid.

Function of Amniotic Fluid

Amniotic fluid:

- Cushions the fetus from sudden maternal movements.
- Prevents the developing human from adhering to the amniotic membranes.
- Allows freedom of fetal movement, which aids in symmetrical musculoskeletal development.
- Provides a consistent thermal environment.

Abnormalities

Problems with the amniotic fluid can cause health issues for the woman and fetus. These include:

- *Polyhydramnios* or hydramnios, which refers to excess amount of amniotic fluid (1,500–2,000 mL). Newborns of mothers who experience polyhydramnios have an increased incidence of chromosomal disorders and gastrointestinal, cardiac, and neural tube disorders.
- *Oligohydramnios,* which refers to a decreased amount of amniotic fluid (less than 500 mL at term or 50% reduction of normal amount). This is generally related to a decrease in placental function. Newborns of mothers who experienced oligohydramnios have an increased incidence of congenital renal problems.

Umbilical Cord

The umbilical cord connects the fetus to the placenta and consists of two umbilical arteries and one umbilical vein. The arteries carry deoxygenated blood while the vein carries oxygenated blood. These vessels are surrounded by Wharton's jelly, a collagenous substance that protects the vessels from compression. The umbilical cord is usually inserted in the center of the placenta and is about 55 cm long.

CRITICAL COMPONENT

Umbilical Vessels

After delivery of the newborn, assess the number of vessels in the cord. Newborns with only two vessels (one artery and one vein) have a 20% chance of having a cardiac or vascular defect. Document the number of vessels present in the newborn. Record and report abnormalities to the pediatrician or pediatric nurse practitioner.

INFERTILITY AND REPRODUCTIVE TECHNOLOGY

Infertility is defined as the inability to conceive and maintain a pregnancy after 12 months (6 months for woman older than age 35 years) of unprotected sexual intercourse. It affects 12% of women ages 15 to 44 (CDC, 2016). Infertility affects the physical, social, psychological, sexual, and economic dimensions of the couple's lives.

Causes of Infertility

A cause can be identified in approximately 80% of couples who experience infertility. Among identified causes, one-third are related to female factors alone, one-third to male factors alone, and one-third to a combination of male and female factors (CDC, 2009).

Male causative factors are classified into five categories:

1. Endocrine causes include pituitary diseases, pituitary tumors, and hypothalamic diseases that may interfere with male fertility. Low levels of LH, FSH, or testosterone can also decrease sperm production.
2. Spermatogenesis is the process in which mature functional sperm are formed. Several factors can affect the development of mature sperm. These factors are referred to as *gonadotoxins* and include:
   - Drugs (e.g., chemotherapeutics, calcium channel blockers, heroin, and alcohol)
   - Infections/viruses (e.g., prostatitis, sexually transmitted infections [STIs], and contracting mumps after puberty)
   - Systemic illness
   - Prolonged heat exposure to the testicles (e.g., use of hot tubs, wearing tight underwear, and frequent bicycle riding)
   - Pesticide exposure
   - Radiation to the pelvic region
3. Sperm antibodies are an immunological reaction against the sperm that causes a decrease in sperm motility. This is seen mainly in men who have had either a vasectomy reversal or who experienced testicular trauma.
4. Sperm transport factor includes missing or blocked structures in the male reproductive anatomy that interfere with sperm transport (e.g., vasectomy, prostatectomy, inguinal hernia, and congenital absence of the vas deferens).
5. Disorders of intercourse include erectile dysfunction (inability to achieve and/or maintain an erection), ejaculatory dysfunctions (retrograde ejaculation), anatomical abnormalities (hypospadias), and psychosocial factors that can interfere with fertility.

Female causative factors are classified into three major categories:

1. Ovulatory dysfunction includes anovulation or inconsistent ovulation. These factors have a very high success rate with appropriate treatment. Causes of ovulatory dysfunction are:
   - Hormonal imbalances
   - Hyperthyroidism and hypothyroidism
   - High prolactin levels
   - Premature ovarian failure (menopause prior to age 40)
   - Polycystic ovarian syndrome (see Chapter 19)
2. Tubal and pelvic pathology factors include damage to the fallopian tubes and uterine fibroids. Damage to the fallopian tubes is commonly related to previous pelvic inflammatory disease or endometriosis. Uterine fibroids, benign growths of the muscular wall of the uterus, can cause a narrowing of the uterine cavity and interfere with embryonic and fetal development, causing a spontaneous abortion.
3. Cervical mucus factors include infection and cervical surgeries such as cryotherapy, a medical intervention used to treat cervical dysplasia. These factors may interfere with the ability of sperm to enter or survive in the uterus.

CRITICAL COMPONENT

Risk Factors for Infertility

Women

Autoimmune disorders

Diabetes

Eating disorders or poor nutrition

Excessive alcohol use

Excessive exercising

History of cancer treated with gonadotoxic therapy or pelvic irradiation

Obesity

Older age

Sexually transmitted infections

Men

Environmental pollutants

Heavy use of alcohol, marijuana, or cocaine

Impotence

Older age

STIs

Smoking

Diagnosis of Infertility

When a couple has difficulty conceiving, both the man and the woman need to be evaluated. The woman is evaluated by her gynecologist or reproductive endocrinologist. The man is evaluated by a urologist. Common diagnostic tests to determine the underlying cause of infertility include:

- Screening for STIs.
- Laboratory tests to assess hormonal levels (thyroid-stimulating hormone [TSH], FSH, LH, anti-Müllerian hormone [AMH], and testosterone).
- Semen analysis, which entails the following:
  - The man abstains for 2 to 3 days before providing a masturbated sample of his semen.
  - Specimens are either collected at the site of testing or brought to the site within an hour of collection.
  - The semen analysis includes volume, sperm concentration, motility, morphology, white blood cell count, immunobead, and mixed agglutination reaction test.
  - Several semen analyses may be required since sperm production normally fluctuates.
- Ovulatory dysfunction analysis, which may include:
  - Basal body temperature (BBT) charting: The female partner takes her temperature each morning before rising using a basal thermometer and records her daily temperature. Ovulation has occurred if there is a rise in the temperature by 0.4°F for 3 consecutive days.
  - Ovulatory prediction kits, used more often than BBT charting.
  - Ovarian reserve testing: Used to determine size of the remaining egg reserve. On day 3 of the menstrual cycle, blood is drawn to evaluate the levels of FSH, estradiol, and AMH. The same day, a transvaginal ultrasound is performed to assess ovarian volume and antral follicle count.
  - Detecting LH surge: A rapid increase in LH 36 hours before ovulation can be tested with urine or serum. The urine test can be performed at home to assist in identifying the ideal time for intercourse when pregnancy is desired.
- Endometrial biopsy. This is performed to assess the response of the uterus to hormonal signals that occur during the cycle. The biopsy is performed at the end of the menstrual cycle in the clinical or medical office.
- Hysterosalpingogram. This is a radiological examination that provides information about the endocervical canal, uterine cavity, and fallopian tubes. Under fluoroscopic observation, dye is slowly injected through the cervical canal into the uterus. This examination can detect tubal problems such as adhesions or occlusions and uterine abnormalities such as fibroids, bicornate uterus, and uterine fistulas.
- Laparoscopy. This uses an instrument called a *laparoscope* to visualize and inspect the ovaries, fallopian tubes, and uterus for abnormalities such as endometriosis and scarring.

Treatment

Treatment depends on the cause of infertility and can range from lifestyle changes to surgery. For male infertility patients, treatment options may include:

- Hormonal therapy for endocrine factors.
- Lifestyle changes to correct abnormal sperm count, such as stress reduction, improved nutrition, smoking cessation, and elimination of drugs that have an adverse effect on fertility.
- Corticosteroids to decrease the production of sperm antibodies.
- Antibiotics to clear infections of the genitourinary tract.
- Repair of varicocele or inguinal hernia to facilitate sperm transport.
- Transurethral resection of ejaculatory ducts to treat disorders related to intercourse.

Treatments for female infertility may include:

- Treatments for anovulation, such as:
  - Lifestyle changes that include stress reduction, improved nutrition, smoking cessation, and elimination of drugs that have an adverse effect on fertility.
  - Drug therapy to stimulate ovulation: clomiphene citrate, which has a very high success rate; letrozole; injectable gonadotropins; the gonadotropin-releasing hormone [GnRH] pump; and bromocriptine.
- Surgery to open the fallopian tubes if tubal abnormalities are present.
- Removal of uterine fibroids through a surgical procedure called *myomectomy*.
- Antibiotics to treat cervical infection.

SAFE AND EFFECTIVE NURSING CARE: Understanding Medication

Clomiphene Citrate (Clomid)

- Indication: Anovulatory infertility
- Action: Stimulates release of FSH and LH, which stimulates ovulation
- Common side effects: Hot flashes, breast discomfort, headaches, insomnia, bloating, blurry vision, nausea, vaginal dryness
- Route and dose: PO; 50–200 mg/day from cycle day 3–7.
- Nursing actions:
  - Provide information on use of medication and its side effects.

Instruct woman not to drive if she is experiencing blurry vision.
Vallerand & Sanoski, 2017.

When the previously mentioned treatments are not successful, the couple is usually referred to an obstetrician who has specialized training in infertility. Additional testing is done, and

TABLE 3–5   Common Assisted Fertility Technologies

TECHNOLOGY	PROCEDURE
Artificial insemination (AI): Intracervical Intrauterine Partner's sperm Donor sperm	Sperm that has been removed from semen is deposited directly into the cervix or uterus using a plastic catheter. The sample is collected by masturbation, and the sperm are separated from the semen and prepared for insemination. Sperm can be from the partner or from a donor when the male partner does not produce sperm. Examples of fertility conditions where this procedure is used include (1) poor cervical mucus production as a result of previous surgery of the cervix, (2) anti-sperm antibodies, (3) diminished amount of sperm, and (4) diminished sperm motility.
Testicular sperm aspiration	Sperm are aspirated or extracted directly from the testicles. Sperm are then microinjected into the harvested eggs of the female partner. This is also referred to as *intra-cytoplasmic injection*. This procedure is used with men who (1) had an unsuccessful vasectomy reversal, (2) have an absence of vas deferens, or (3) have an extremely low sperm count or no sperm in their ejaculated semen.
In vitro fertilization (IVF)	IVF is a procedure in which oocytes are harvested and fertilization occurs outside the female body in a laboratory.
Zygote intrafallopian transfer (ZIFT)	In ZIFT, a zygote is placed into the fallopian tube via laparoscopy 1 day after the oocyte is retrieved from the woman and IVF is used.
Gamete intrafallopian transfer (GIFT)	In GIFT, sperm and oocytes are mixed outside the woman's body and then placed into the fallopian tube via laparoscopy. Fertilization takes place inside the fallopian tube. This procedure is used when there has been (1) a history of failed infertility treatment for anovulation, (2) unexplained infertility, and (3) low sperm count.
Embryo transfer (ET)	ET is when, through IVF, an embryo is placed in the uterine cavity via a catheter. Example of fertility condition in which this procedure is used is when the fallopian tubes are blocked.

based on the outcome, various procedures can be used to assist in fertility (Table 3–5).

Emotional Implications

Couples who are infertile experience a "roller coaster" effect during diagnosis and treatment. Each month they become excited and hopeful that they will conceive, and then the woman has a period and their excitement and hopes turn to sadness and possibly depression. Infertility can cause a crisis in the couple's lives and relationship (Sherrod, 2004). Diagnosis and treatment of infertility can cause:

- Stress, anxiety, and depression for both the female and male partner.
- Guilt for one or both partners if they blame themselves for the inability to conceive.
- Marital strain if one partner blames the other for the infertility.
- Sexual dysfunction caused by the stress of prescribed sexual activity in infertility treatment.
- Strain within the extended family, as the couple may avoid events that include children and may even isolate socially if they find it too painful to be around children.

- Lack of support network, particularly for those who do not share information about their fertility problems with family members and friends.
- Self-esteem issues, including the feeling of being "less of a man" or "less of a woman" because conception does not occur, or shame associated with the feeling of having a "defective" body.

Most couples can benefit from counseling during the time of diagnosis and treatment and after treatment ends. Ideally, counseling should start before treatment begins. Couples may have high expectations of reproductive technology and fail to recognize that treatment may not be successful. Counseling includes discussion about:

- The effects treatment may have on them as a couple, as individuals, and as a family.
- Information about different treatment methods and ethical dilemmas they may encounter
- Information about the effects, consequences, and resolution of treatment.
- The decision on when to stop treatment.
- Adoption.
- The use of surrogacy, an option for a woman with unhealthy or no eggs in which another woman is

impregnated with the partner's sperm and carries the baby on behalf of the couple.

● The use of a gestational carrier, in which a woman's own egg is fertilized by her partner's sperm and placed inside the uterus of the carrier, who agrees to carry the baby on behalf of the couple.

Evidence-Based Practice: Infertile Mother's Vulnerability to Depression

Olshansky, E. (2003). A theoretical explanation for previously infertile mothers' vulnerability to depression. *Journal of Nursing Scholarship, 35,* 263–268.

Since the 1980s, Ellen Olshansky, PhD, RN, FAAN, has researched the psychosocial effects of infertility. She synthesized the results of several grounded theory studies on the experience of infertility and summarized her theory of identity as infertility. According to her theory:

● Women who are distressed by their infertility become consumed with concerns about the infertility and often neglect their relationships with friends, spouse, or family members. This can lead to social isolation.

● Infertility becomes the focus of the couple's relationship, and other aspects of the relationship are often ignored. This can lead to a dysfunctional marriage or couple relationship.

● Career women may experience a sense of loss of self, due to the shift of focus from career to infertility. This also contributes to social isolation.

● Once pregnancy has been achieved, women often have difficulty perceiving themselves as pregnant women.

Ethical Implications

Assisted reproductive technologies (ART) are treatments that involve the surgical removal of the oocytes and combining them with sperm in a laboratory setting. These treatments include in vitro fertilization (IVF), zygote intrafallopian transfer (ZIFT), gamete intrafallopian transfer (GIFT), and embryo transfer (ET). ART has created numerous ethical dilemmas. The primary one is "surplus" embryos, those produced from hyperstimulation of the ovaries that occurs when IVF technologies are being used. Several eggs from the woman may be harvested and fertilized using IVF, but only two or three are returned to the woman's body. These surplus embryos are either frozen for future use or allowed to perish. This has raised the question of when life begins and the rights of the embryo. Other ethical questions that arise are:

● Who owns the embryos—the woman or the man?
● Who decides what will happen to the surplus embryos?
● Who has access to ART, which has substantial costs that are often not covered by health insurance providers?
● At what point should the health care provider recommend that the couple stop using ART?

● When artificial insemination with donor sperm or surrogacy is used, do you tell the child, and if so, when?
● Does the sperm donor have any rights or responsibilities regarding the child produced from his donation?

The Nurse's Role

The role of the nurse varies based on where he or she interfaces with the couple who is experiencing infertility. Nurses who work in an infertility clinic take on various roles, including counseling, teaching, supporting, and assisting in the procedures. Nurses who work in acute care, clinics, or other settings must be aware of the emotional impact infertility has on the individual and on the couple. Couples become frustrated with health care professionals who do not understand the effect of infertility on their lives (Sherrod, 2004).

CRITICAL COMPONENT

Infertility

The experience of infertility affects the individual's and the couple's emotional well-being.

Nurses' awareness of how infertility affects all aspects of the individual's and of the couple's relationship will enhance the effectiveness of the nursing care provided to these couples or individuals.

REFERENCES

American College of Obstetricians and Gynecologists (ACOG). (1997). *Teratology* (educational bulletin no. 236). Washington, DC: Author.

Centers for Disease Control and Prevention (CDC). (2009). *Infertility FAQs.* Retrieved from www.cdc.gov/reproductivehealth/infertility.

Centers for Disease Control and Prevention (CDC). (2016). *Infertility.* Retrieved from www.cdc.gov/nchs/fastats/infertility.htm.

Centers for Disease Control and Prevention (CDC). (2017). *Zika virus.* Retrieved from www.cdc.gov/zika/about/overview.html.

Genetics Home Reference. (2017). *Inheriting genetic conditions.* Retrieved from www.ghr.nlm.nih.gov.

National Human Genome Research Institute (NHGRI). (2016). *What is genomic medicine?* Retrieved from www.genome.gov/27552451/what-is-genomic-medicine/genomic-medicine.

Olshansky, E. (2003). A theoretical explanation of previously infertile mothers' vulnerability to depression. *Journal of Nursing Scholarship, 35,* 236–268.

Sader, T. (2015). *Langman's medical embryology* (13th ed.). Philadelphia, PA: Lippincott Williams & Wilkins.

Scanlon, S., & Sanders, T. (2015). *Essentials of anatomy and physiology* (7th ed.). Philadelphia, PA: F.A. Davis.

Sherrod, R. (2004). Understanding the emotional aspects of infertility: Implications for nursing practice. *Journal of Psychosocial Nursing and Mental Health Services, 42,* 40–47.

Vallerand, A., & Sanoski, C. (2017). *Davis's drug guide for nurses* (15th ed.). Philadelphia, PA: F.A. Davis.

World Health Organization (WHO). (2012). Human Genetics Programme. Retrieved from www.who.int/genomics/geneticsVSgenomics/en.

Physiological Aspects of Antepartum Care

4

Connie Miller DNP, RNC-OB, CNE, CCCE

LEARNING OUTCOMES

Upon completion of this chapter, the student will be able to:

1. Identify the major components of preconception health care.
2. Describe methods for diagnosis of pregnancy and determination of estimated date of delivery.
3. Identify the progression of anatomical and physiological changes over the course of a pregnancy.
4. Link the anatomical and physiological changes of pregnancy to signs, symptoms, and common discomforts of pregnancy.
5. Describe appropriate interventions to relieve common discomforts of pregnancy.
6. Identify the critical elements of assessment and nursing care during initial and subsequent prenatal visits.
7. Describe the elements of patient education and anticipatory guidance appropriate for each trimester of pregnancy.

Nursing Diagnosis

- Knowledge deficit related to physiological changes of pregnancy
- Knowledge deficit related to nutritional requirements during pregnancy
- Altered health maintenance related to knowledge deficit regarding self-care measures during pregnancy
- Knowledge deficit of warning signs of pregnancy
- Sleep pattern disturbance related to discomforts of late pregnancy
- Constipation related to changes in gastrointestinal tract during pregnancy
- Anxiety related to physiological changes of pregnancy
- Anxiety related to uncertain outcome of pregnancy

Nursing Outcomes

- The pregnant woman will verbalize an understanding of expected anatomical and physiological changes of pregnancy.
- The pregnant woman will report eating a diet following healthy eating practices and MyPlate guidelines with the recommended calorie intake and achieve the recommended weight gain throughout pregnancy.
- The pregnant woman will verbalize understanding of self-care needs in pregnancy such as posture/body mechanics, rest and relaxation, personal hygiene, and activity and exercise.
- The pregnant woman will verbalize an understanding of how to implement measures for relieving discomforts associated with normal physical changes. For example, she will verbalize an understanding of strategies for constipation management in pregnancy and will resume normal bowel function by using these strategies.
- The pregnant woman will verbalize understanding of warning signs of pregnancy and when to call her provider.
- The pregnant woman will verbalize understanding of strategies to accommodate sleep disturbance during pregnancy.
- The pregnant woman will verbalize strategies to reduce anxiety during pregnancy and will report experiencing a reduction in anxiety.

INTRODUCTION

The scope of this chapter is nursing care and interventions prior to conception and throughout a normal pregnancy based on an understanding of the physiological aspects of pregnancy. During pregnancy, the pregnant mother undergoes significant anatomical and physiological changes to nurture and accommodate the developing fetus (Soma-Pillay et al., 2016). These changes begin after conception and affect every organ system in the body. For most women experiencing an uncomplicated pregnancy, these changes resolve after pregnancy with minimal residual effects. It is important to understand the normal physiological changes occurring in pregnancy to help differentiate adaptations that are abnormal.

The second half of the chapter presents preconception and prenatal care. Within the continuum of reproductive health care, preconception care and prenatal care provide a platform for important health care functions, including health promotion, screening and diagnosis, and disease prevention (WHO, 2016). It has been established that by implementing timely and appropriate evidence-based practices, preconception and prenatal care can improve maternal and fetal outcomes and save lives (WHO, 2016). Crucially, it also provides the opportunity to communicate with and support women, families, and communities at a critical time in the course of a woman's life. Chapter 5 addresses the psychosocial and cultural components of the antepartum period.

Prior to pregnancy, nursing care focuses on assessment of the woman's health and potential risk factors, as well as education on health promotion and disease prevention. During pregnancy, nursing care shifts to regular assessment of the health of the pregnancy, including assessment and screening of risk factors for potential complications, education on health promotion, and disease prevention. The focus is on implementation of appropriate interventions based on risk status or actual complications and inclusion of significant others/family in care and education to promote pregnancy adaptation.

PHYSIOLOGICAL PROGRESSION OF PREGNANCY

Pregnancy results in maternal physiological adaptations involving every body system, with each change meant to protect the woman and/or the fetus and based in the maintenance of the pregnancy, the development of the fetus, and the preparation for labor and birth. To both understand a woman's experience of normal pregnancy and be effective in identifying deviations from normal, the nurse must have a basic foundation in the physiology of pregnancy.

This understanding is critical not only for risk assessment and implementation of appropriate nursing interventions to reduce risk, but also for providing effective patient education and anticipatory guidance grounded in knowledge of the normal physical changes in pregnancy and their resulting common, normal discomforts. The next sections present the changes that occur in each system, and Table 4–1 summarizes the major physiological changes and factors that influence these changes.

Reproductive System

Maternal physiological adaptations to pregnancy are most profound in the reproductive system. The uterus undergoes phenomenal growth, breasts prepare for lactation, and the vagina changes to accommodate the birthing process.

TABLE 4–1   Physiological Changes in Pregnancy

PHYSIOLOGICAL CHANGES	CLINICAL SIGNS AND SYMPTOMS
Reproductive System—Breasts	
Increased estrogen and progesterone levels: Initially produced by the corpus luteum and then by the placenta	Tenderness, feeling of fullness, and tingling sensation
	Increase in weight of breast by 400 g
Increased blood supply to breasts	Enlargement of breasts, nipples, areola, and Montgomery follicles (small glands on the areola around the nipple)
	Striae: Due to stretching of skin to accommodate enlarging breast tissue
	Prominent veins due to a twofold increase in blood flow
Increased prolactin: Produced by the anterior pituitary	Increased growth of mammary glands
	Increase in lactiferous ducts and alveolar system
	Production of colostrum, a yellow secretion rich in antibodies, begins to be produced as early as 16 weeks

TABLE 4-1   Physiological Changes in Pregnancy—cont'd

PHYSIOLOGICAL CHANGES	CLINICAL SIGNS AND SYMPTOMS
Reproductive System—Uterus, Cervix, and Vagina	
Increased levels of estrogen and progesterone	Hypertrophy of uterine wall
	Softening of vaginal muscle and connective tissue in preparation for expansion of tissue to accommodate passage of fetus through the birth canal
	Uterus contractibility increases in response to increased estrogen levels, leading to Braxton-Hicks contractions.
	Hypertrophy of cervical glands leads to formation of mucus plug, which serves as a protective barrier between uterus/fetus and vagina
	Increased vascularity and hypertrophy of vaginal and cervical glands leads to increase in leukorrhea.
	Cessation of menstrual cycle (amenorrhea) and ovulation
Enlargement and stretching of uterus to accommodate developing fetus and placenta	Increase in uterine size to 20 times that of nonpregnant uterus
	Weight of uterus increases from 70 g to 1,100 g
	Capacity increases from 10 mL to 5,000 mL—80% of that to uteroplacental
Expanded circulatory volume leads to increased vascular congestion	Blood flow to the uterus is 500–600 mL/min at term.
	Goodell's sign: Softening of the cervix
	Hegar's sign: Softening of the lower uterine segment
	Chadwick's sign: Bluish coloration of cervix, vaginal mucosa, and vulva
Acid pH of vagina	Acid environment inhibits growth of bacteria
	Acid environment allows growth of *Candida albicans*, leading to increased risk of candidiasis (yeast infection)
Cardiovascular System	
Decrease in peripheral vascular resistance	Decrease in blood pressure
Increase in blood volume by 40%–45%	Hypervolemia of pregnancy
Increase in cardiac output by 40%	Increased heart rate of 15–20 bpm
BMR increased 10%–20% by third trimester	Increased stroke volume of 25%–30%
Increase in peripheral dilation	Systolic murmurs, load and wide S1 split, load S2, obvious S3
	Increase in heart size
Increase in RBC count by 30%	Physiological anemia of pregnancy
Increase in RBC volume by 18%–33%	Hemodilution is caused by the increase in plasma volume being relatively larger than the increase in RBCs, which results in decreased hemoglobin and hematocrit values (see Appendix D for pregnancy laboratory values).
Increase in plasma volume by 50%	
Increase in WBC count	Values up to 16,000 mm^3 in the absence of infection

Continued

TABLE 4–1   Physiological Changes in Pregnancy—cont'd

PHYSIOLOGICAL CHANGES	CLINICAL SIGNS AND SYMPTOMS
Increased demand for iron in fetal development	Iron-deficiency anemia: Hemoglobin <11 g/dL and hematocrit <33%
Plasma fibrin increase of 40% Fibrinogen increase of 50% Decrease in coagulation inhibiting factors Protective of inevitable blood loss during birth	Hypercoagulability
Increased venous pressure and decreased blood flow to extremities due to compression of iliac veins and inferior vena cava	Edema of lower extremities Varicosities in legs and vulva Hemorrhoids
In supine position the enlarged uterus compresses the inferior vena cava, causing reduced blood flow back to the right atrium and a drop in cardiac output and blood pressure.	Supine hypotensive syndrome
Respiratory System Hormones of pregnancy stimulate the respiratory center and act on lung tissue to increase and enhance respiratory function. Increase of oxygen consumption by 15%–20%	Increase in tidal volume by 35%–50% Slight increase in respiratory rate Increase in inspiratory capacity Decrease in expiratory volume Slight hyperventilation Slight respiratory alkalosis
Estrogen, progesterone, and prostaglandins cause vascular engorgement and smooth muscle relaxation	Dyspnea Nasal and sinus congestion Epistaxis
Upward displacement of diaphragm by enlarging uterus Estrogen causes a relaxation of the ligaments and joints of the ribs Slight decrease in lung capacity	Shift from abdominal to thoracic breathing Chest and thorax expand to accommodate thoracic breathing and upward displacement of diaphragm
Renal System Alterations in cardiovascular system (increased cardiac output and increased blood and plasma volume) lead to increased renal blood flow of 50%–80% in first trimester and then decreases. Increased progesterone levels, which cause a relaxation of smooth muscles	Urinary frequency and incontinence and increased risk of UTI
Dilation of renal pelvis and ureters Ureters become elongated with decreased motility Decreased bladder tone with increased bladder capacity	Increased risk of UTI
Pressure of enlarging uterus on renal structures Displacement of bladder in third trimester	Urinary frequency and nocturia
Increased glomerular filtration rate	Increased urinary output

TABLE 4–1   Physiological Changes in Pregnancy—cont'd

PHYSIOLOGICAL CHANGES	CLINICAL SIGNS AND SYMPTOMS
Increased renal excretion of glucose and protein	Glucosuria and proteinuria
Decreased renal flow in third trimester	Dependent edema
Increased vascularity	Hyperemia of bladder and urethra
Gastrointestinal System	
Increased levels of hCG and altered carbohydrate metabolism	Nausea and vomiting during early pregnancy
Increased progesterone levels slow stomach emptying and relax the esophageal sphincter	Reflux of gastric contents into lower esophagus resulting in heartburn
Increased progesterone levels relax smooth muscle to slow the digestive process and movement of stool	Bloating, flatulence, and constipation
Increased progesterone levels decrease muscle tone of gallbladder and result in prolonged emptying time	Increased risk of gallstone formation and cholestasis
Changes in senses of taste and smell	Increase or decrease in appetite Nausea Pica: Abnormal; craving for and ingestion of nonfood substances such as clay or starch
Displacement of intestines by uterus	Flatulence, abdominal distention, abdominal cramping, and pelvic heaviness
Increased levels of estrogen lead to increased vascular congestion of mucosa	Gingivitis, bleeding gums, increased risk of periodontal disease
Musculoskeletal System	
Increased progesterone and relaxin levels lead to softening of joints and increased joint mobility, resulting in widening and increased mobility of the sacroiliac and symphysis pubis.	Altered gait: "Waddle" gait Facilitates birthing process Low back pain or pelvic discomfort Pelvis tilts forward, leading to shifting of center of gravity that results in change in posture and walking style, increasing lordosis. Increased risk of falls due to shift in center of gravity and change in gait and posture
Distention of abdomen related to expanding uterus, reduced abdominal tone, and increased breast size	Round ligament spasm
Increased estrogen and relaxin levels lead to increased elasticity and relaxation of ligaments.	Increased risk of joint pain and injury
Abdominal muscles stretch due to enlarging uterus	Diastasis recti
Integumentary System	
Estrogen and progesterone levels stimulate increased melanin deposition, causing light brown to dark brown pigmentation.	Linea nigra Melasma (chloasma) Increased pigmentation of nipples, areola, vulva, scars, and moles
Increased blood flow, increased BMR, progesterone-induced increase in body temperature, and vasomotor instability	Hot flashes, facial flushing, alternating sensation of hot and cold Increased perspiration

Continued

TABLE 4-1 Physiological Changes in Pregnancy—cont'd

PHYSIOLOGICAL CHANGES	CLINICAL SIGNS AND SYMPTOMS
Increased action of adrenocorticosteroids leads to cutaneous elastic tissues becoming fragile	Striae gravidarum (stretch marks) on abdomen, thighs, breast, and buttocks
Increased estrogen levels lead to color and vascular changes	Angiomas (spider nevi)
	Palmar erythema: Pinkish-red mottling over palms of hands and redness of fingers
Increased androgens lead to increase in sebaceous gland secretions	Increased oiliness of skin and increase of acne
Endocrine System	
Decreased follicle-stimulating hormone	Amenorrhea
Increased progesterone	Maintains pregnancy by relaxation of smooth muscles, leading to decreased uterine activity, which results in decreased risk of spontaneous abortions
	Decreases gastrointestinal motility and slows digestive processes
Increased estrogen	Facilitates uterine and breast development
	Facilitates increases in vascularity
	Facilitates hyperpigmentation
	Alters metabolic processes and fluid and electrolyte balance
Increased prolactin	Facilitates lactation
Increased oxytocin	Stimulates uterine contractions
	Stimulates the milk let-down or ejection reflex in response to breastfeeding
Increased hCG	Maintenance of corpus luteum until placenta becomes fully functional
Human placental lactogen/human chorionic somatomammotropin	Facilitates breast development
	Alters carbohydrate, protein, and fat metabolism
	Facilitates fetal growth by altering maternal metabolism; acts as an insulin antagonist
Hyperplasia and increased vascularity of thyroid	Enlargement of thyroid
	Heat intolerance and fatigue
Increased BMR related to fetal metabolic activity	Depletion of maternal glucose stores leads to increased risk of maternal hypoglycemia
Increased need for glucose due to developing fetus	Increased production of insulin
Increase in circulating cortisol	Increase in maternal resistance to insulin leads to increased risk of hyperglycemia
Neurological System	
	Headache
	Syncope

Blackburn, 2014; Cunningham et al., 2014; Kahn & Hoos, 2010; Mattson & Smith, 2011.

Breasts

Breast changes begin early in pregnancy and continue throughout gestation and into the postpartum period. These changes are primarily influenced by increases in hormone levels and occur in preparation for lactation (see Table 4–1).

Uterus

The uterus is described in three parts (Fig. 4–1):

● Fundus or upper portion
● Isthmus or lower segment
● Cervix, the lower narrow part, or neck; the external part of the cervix interfaces with the vagina. The cervical os is the opening of the cervix that dilates (opens) during labor to allow passage of the fetus through the vagina.

Uterine changes over the course of pregnancy are profound (see Table 4–1).

● Before pregnancy, this elastic, muscular organ is the size and shape of a small pear and weighs 40–50 g.
● During pregnancy, the uterine wall progressively thins as the uterus expands to accommodate the developing fetus.
● By mid-pregnancy, the uterine fundus reaches the level of the umbilicus abdominally.
● Toward the end of pregnancy, the enlarged uterus, containing a full-term fetus, fills the abdominal cavity and has altered the placement of the lungs and rib cage in addition to the abdominal organs (Fig. 4–2).

● Intermittent, painless, and physiological uterine contractions, referred to as *Braxton-Hicks contractions*, begin in the second trimester, but some women do not feel them until the third trimester. These contractions are irregular with no particular pattern. As the uterus enlarges, they are more noticeable.
● At term, the uterus weighs 1,100 to 1,200 g.

Vagina

The vagina is an elastic muscular canal. As pregnancy progresses, various changes take place in the vasculature and tone (see Table 4–1):

● An increase of vascularity due to the expanded circulatory needs
● An increase of vaginal discharge (leukorrhea) in response to the estrogen-induced hypertrophy of the vaginal glands
● Relaxation of the vaginal wall and perineal body, which allows stretching of tissues to accommodate the birthing process.
● Acid pH of the vagina, which inhibits growth of bacteria but allows overgrowth of *Candida albicans*. This places the pregnant woman at risk for candidiasis (yeast infection).

Ovaries

The corpus luteum, which normally degrades after ovulation when the egg is not fertilized, is maintained during the first couple months of pregnancy by high levels of human chorionic gonadotropin (hCG). At the beginning of pregnancy, the corpus

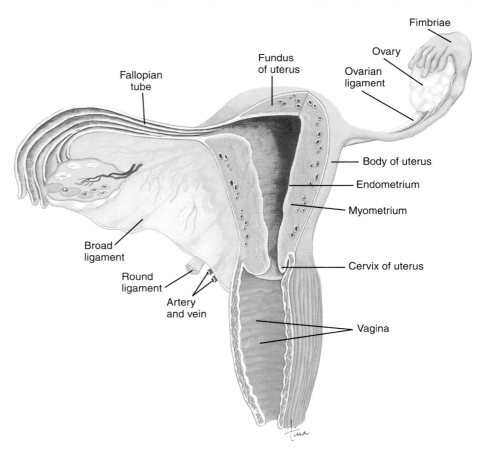

FIGURE 4-1 Reproductive system.

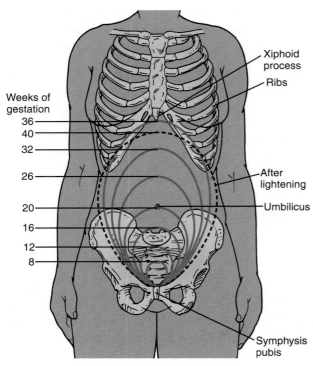

FIGURE 4–2 Uterine heights by weeks of gestation with anatomical landmarks.

luteum produces progesterone to maintain the endometrium, the thick lining of the uterus. This allows for implantation and establishment of the pregnancy. There is subsequently no shedding of the endometrium that would result in menstruation. Ovulation ceases as the hormones of pregnancy inhibit follicle maturation and release. By 6 to 7 weeks' gestation, the placenta begins producing progesterone and the corpus luteum degenerates.

Cardiovascular System

The cardiovascular system undergoes significant adaptations during pregnancy to support the maintenance and development of the fetus while also meeting maternal physiological needs during both the pregnancy and the postpartum period. Changes in the cardiovascular system in pregnancy are profound and begin early in pregnancy; by 8 weeks' gestation, the cardiac output has already increased by 20% (Soma-Pillay et al., 2016). The hemodynamic changes are also a protective mechanism for the inevitable maternal blood loss during the intrapartum period (see Table 4–1). Cardiovascular system changes include:

- Cardiac output increases 30% to 50% and peaks at 25 to 30 weeks.
- The heart rate increases 15 to 20 beats per minute (bpm).
- Stroke volume increases by 25% to 30%.
- Basal metabolic rate (BMR) increases 10% to 20% by the third trimester.
- The white blood cell (WBC) count increases, with values up to 16,000 mm³ in the absence of infection.
  - The increase is hormonally induced and similar to elevations seen in physiological stress such as exercise.

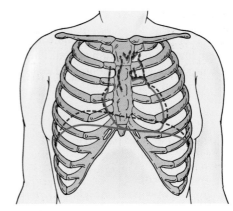

FIGURE 4–3 Dotted lines indicate displacement of heart and lungs as pregnancy progresses and uterus enlarges.

- Plasma volume increases 40% to 50% during pregnancy until reaching a peak about 32 to 34 weeks and remaining there until term.
- In response to increased oxygen requirements of pregnancy, the red blood cell (RBC) count increases 30% and RBC volume increases up to 33% with iron supplementation (up to 18% without supplementation).
  - The increase in plasma volume is relatively larger than the increase in RBCs. This hemodilution is evidenced by decreased hemoglobin and hematocrit values and is known as physiological anemia of pregnancy or pseudo anemia of pregnancy. See Appendix D for laboratory values during pregnancy.
  - Cardiac work is eased as the decrease in blood viscosity facilitates placental perfusion.
- Iron-deficiency anemia is defined as hemoglobin less than 11 g/dL and hematocrit less than 33%.
  - Maternal iron stores are insufficient to meet the demands for iron in fetal development.
- Blood volume increases by 1,500 mL or by 40% to 45% to support uteroplacental demands and maintenance of pregnancy. This is referred to as hypervolemia of pregnancy.
- The heart enlarges slightly as a result of hypervolemia and increased cardiac output.
- The heart shifts upward and laterally as the growing uterus displaces the diaphragm (Fig. 4–3).
- Hypercoagulation occurs during pregnancy to decrease the risk of postpartum hemorrhage. These changes place the woman at increased risk for thrombosis and coagulopathies.
  - Plasma fibrin increase of 40%
  - Fibrinogen increase of 50%
  - Coagulation inhibiting factors decrease
- Blood pressure decreases in the first trimester due to a decrease in peripheral vascular resistance. The blood pressure returns to normal by term.
- Supine hypotension can occur when the woman is in the supine position, as the enlarging uterus can compress the inferior vena cava.
- In most women, a systolic heart murmur or a third heart sound (gallop) may be heard by mid-pregnancy.

- Peripheral dilation is increased.
- Varicosities may develop in the legs or vulva as a result of increased venous pressure below the level of the uterus.
- Dependent edema in the lower extremities is caused by increased venous pressure from the enlarging uterus.

CRITICAL COMPONENT

Supine Hypotensive Syndrome

Supine hypotensive syndrome is a hypotensive condition resulting from a woman lying on her back in mid to late pregnancy (Fig. 4–4). In a supine position, the enlarged uterus compresses the inferior vena cava, leading to a significant drop in cardiac output and blood pressure that results in the woman feeling dizzy and faint.

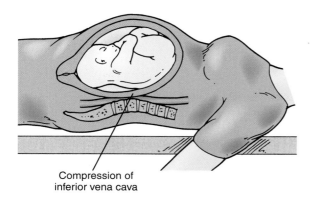

Compression of
inferior vena cava

FIGURE 4–4 Supine hypotension compression of the inferior vena cava by the gravid uterus while in the supine position reduces venous blood return to the heart, causing maternal hypotension.

Respiratory System

Throughout the course of pregnancy, the respiratory system adapts in response to physiological and anatomical demands related to fetal growth and development as well as to maternal metabolic needs (see Table 4–1). There is a significant increase in oxygen demand during normal pregnancy. This is due to a 15% increase in the metabolic rate and a 20% increased consumption of oxygen. There is a 40% to 50% increase in minute ventilation, mostly due to an increase in tidal volume, rather than in the respiratory rate (Soma-Pillay et al., 2016). Pulmonary function is not compromised in a normal pregnancy.

Physiological changes occur to accommodate the additional requirements for oxygen delivery and carbon dioxide removal in mother and fetus during pregnancy. These include the following:

- Tidal volume increases 35% to 50%
- Slight respiratory alkalosis
  - Decrease in P_{CO_2} leads to an increase in pH (more alkaline) and a decrease in bicarbonate.
  - This change promotes transport of carbon dioxide away from the fetus.

- Increases in estrogen, progesterone, and prostaglandins cause vascular engorgement and smooth muscle relaxation resulting in edema and tissue congestion, which can lead to:
  - Dyspnea.
  - Nasal and sinus congestion.
  - Epistaxis (nosebleeds).

Anatomical changes include the following:

- Diaphragm is displaced upward approximately 4 cm.
- Increase in chest circumference of 6 cm with an increase in the costal angle of greater than 90 degrees.
- Shift from abdominal to thoracic breathing as the pregnancy progresses (see Fig. 4–3).
- These anatomical changes may contribute to the physiological dyspnea that is common during pregnancy.

Renal System

The kidneys undergo change during pregnancy as they adapt to perform their basic functions of regulating fluid and electrolyte balance, eliminating metabolic waste products, and helping to regulate blood pressure (see Table 4–1). Physiological changes include the following:

- Renal plasma flow increases.
- Glomerular filtration rate (GFR) increases.
- Renal tubular reabsorption increases.
- Proteinuria and glucosuria can normally occur in small amounts related to exceeded tubal reabsorption threshold of protein and glucose due to increased volume.
  - Even though a small amount of proteinuria and glucosuria can be normal, it is important to assess and monitor for pathology.
- Shift in fluid and electrolyte balance.
  - The need for increased fluid and electrolytes results in alteration of regulating mechanisms, including the renin–angiotensin–aldosterone system and antidiuretic hormone.
- Positional variation in renal function.
  - In the supine and upright maternal position, blood pools in the lower body, causing a decrease in cardiac output, GFR, and urine output; also causing excess sodium and fluid retention.
  - A left lateral recumbent maternal position can:
    - Maximize cardiac output, renal plasma volume, and urine output.
    - Stabilize fluid and electrolyte balance.
    - Minimize dependent edema.
    - Maintain optimal blood pressure.

These changes support the increased circulatory and metabolic demands of the pregnancy because the renal system secretes both maternal and fetal waste products. Anatomical changes include the following:

- Renal pelvis dilation with increased renal plasma flow

- Ureter alterations
  - Becomes elongated, tortuous, and dilated

- Bladder alterations
  - Bladder capacity increases and bladder tone decreases; related to progesterone effect on smooth muscle of the bladder, causing relaxation and stretching.
- Urinary stasis
  - Progesterone reduces the tone of renal structures, allowing for pooling of urine.
  - Stasis promotes bacterial growth and increases the woman's risk for urinary tract infections and pyelonephritis.
- Hyperemia of bladder and urethra related to increased vascularity that results in pelvic congestion; edematous mucosa is easily traumatized.
- Most women experience urinary symptoms of frequency, urgency, and nocturia beginning early in pregnancy and continuing to varying degrees throughout the pregnancy. These symptoms are primarily a result of the systemic hormonal changes of pregnancy and may also be attributed to anatomical changes in the renal system and other body system changes during pregnancy but are not generally indicative of infection. Urinary tract infections (UTIs) are common in pregnancy and may be asymptomatic.
- Physiological changes that occur in the renal system during pregnancy predispose pregnant women to UTIs. Symptoms of a UTI include urinary frequency, dysuria, urgency, and sometimes pus or blood in the urine. Treatment includes anti-infective medication for a 7- to 10-day period. If untreated, the infection can lead to pyelonephritis or premature labor.

Gastrointestinal System

The gastrointestinal (GI) system adapts in its anatomy and physiology during pregnancy in support of maternal and fetal nutritional requirements (see Table 4–1). The adaptations are related to hormonal influences and the impact of the enlarging uterus on the GI system as pregnancy progresses (Soma-Pillay et al., 2016).

Up to 90% of pregnant women experience some degree of nausea and vomiting in pregnancy (NVP). For most affected women, the symptoms are an expected part of pregnancy and tolerated well; however, about a third of affected women experience significant distress. As the pregnancy progresses, NVP symptoms usually diminish; 60% of cases resolve by 12 weeks' gestation and 90% have symptom improvement by 16 weeks' gestation (Tan & Omar, 2011). It is important to identify women with significant NVP so they can be successfully treated.

Additional alterations in nutritional patterns commonly seen in pregnancy include:

- Increase in appetite and food intake.
- Cravings for specific foods.
  - Pica is a craving for and consumption of nonfood substances such as starch and clay. It can result in toxicity due to ingested substances or malnutrition from replacing nutritious foods with nonfood substances.
- Avoidance of specific foods.

Anatomical and physiological changes include the following:

- Uterine enlargement displaces the stomach, liver, and intestines as the pregnancy progresses.
- By the end of pregnancy, the appendix is situated high and to the right along the costal margin.
- The GI tract experiences a general relaxation and slowing of its digestive processes during pregnancy, contributing to many of the common discomforts of pregnancy such as heartburn, abdominal bloating, and constipation.
- Hemorrhoids (varicosities in the anal canal) are common in pregnancy due to increased venous pressure and are exacerbated by constipation; 30% to 40% of pregnant women experience hemorrhoidal discomfort, pruritus, and/or bleeding.
- Gallstones: Progesterone-induced relaxation of smooth muscle results in distention of gallbladder and slows emptying of bile; bile stasis and elevated levels of cholesterol contribute to formation of gallstones.
- Pruritus: Abdominal pruritus may be an early sign of cholestasis.
- Ptyalism: Increase in saliva.
- Bleeding gums and periodontal disease.
  - Increased vascularity of the gums can result in gingivitis.

Musculoskeletal System

Significant adaptation occurs in the musculoskeletal system as a result of pregnancy (see Table 4–1). Hormonal shifts are responsible for many of these changes. Mechanical factors attributable to the growing uterus also contribute to musculoskeletal adaptation. Anatomical and physiological changes include the following:

- Altered posture and center of gravity related to distention of the abdomen by the expanding uterus and reduced abdominal tone that shifts the center of gravity forward.
  - A shift in the center of gravity places the woman at higher risk for falls.
- Altered gait ("pregnant waddle"): Hormonal influences of progesterone and relaxin soften joints and increase joint mobility.
- Lordosis: Abnormal anterior curvature of the lumbar spine. The body compensates for the shift in center of gravity by developing an increased curvature of the spine.
- Joint discomfort: Hormonal influences of progesterone and relaxin soften cartilage and connective tissue, leading to joint instability.
- Round ligament spasm: Estrogen and relaxin increase elasticity and relaxation of ligaments, and abdominal distention stretches round ligaments, causing spasm and pain.
- Diastasis recti: This is the separation of the rectus abdominis muscle in the midline caused by the abdominal distention. It is a benign condition that can occur in the third trimester.

The impact of the musculoskeletal adaptations in pregnancy, which result in numerous common discomforts, can sometimes be reduced if the woman maintains a normal body weight and exercises regularly prior to and throughout her pregnancy.

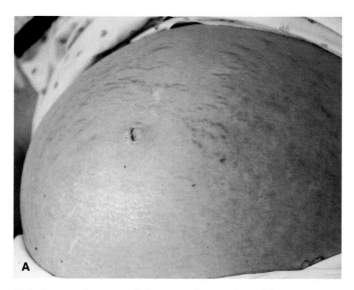

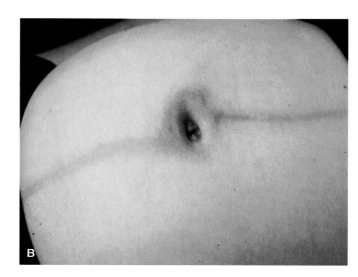

FIGURE 4-5 Pregnant abdomen with striae (**A**) and linea nigra (**B**).

Integumentary System

The integumentary system includes the skin and related structures such as hair, nails, and glands. Hormonal influences are primary factors in integumentary system adaptations during pregnancy (see Table 4–1). Anatomical and physiological changes include:

- Hyperpigmentation: Estrogen and progesterone stimulate increased melanin deposition of light brown to dark brown pigmentation.
  - Linea nigra: Darkened line in midline of abdomen (Fig. 4–5B)
  - Melasma (chloasma), also referred to as *mask of pregnancy*: This brownish pigmentation of the skin appears over the cheeks, nose, and forehead. This occurs in 50% to 70% of pregnant women and is more common in darker-skinned women. It usually occurs after the 16th week of pregnancy and is exacerbated by sun exposure.
- Striae (stretch marks): Stretching of skin due to growth of breast, hips, abdomen, and buttocks, plus the effects of estrogen, relaxin, and adrenocorticoids may result in tearing of subcutaneous connective tissue/collagen (Fig. 4–5A).
- Varicosities, spider nevi, and palmer erythema: Vascular changes related to hormonally induced increase in elasticity of vessels and increase in venous pressure from enlarged uterus.
- Hot flashes and facial flushing: Caused by increased blood supply to skin, increase in basal metabolic rate, progesterone-induced increased body temperature, and vasomotor instability.
- Oily skin and acne: Effects of increase in androgens.
- Sweating: Thermoregulation process at the level of skin increases in response to increases in thyroid activity, BMR, metabolic activity of fetus, and increased maternal body weight.

- Although none of these integumentary system adaptations is seen universally, each alteration is seen commonly, is not of pathological significance, and typically resolves or regresses significantly after pregnancy.

Endocrine System

Endocrine system adaptations are essential for maintaining the stability of both the woman and her pregnancy and for promoting fetal growth and development. Endocrine glands mediate the many metabolic process adaptations in pregnancy. General endocrine system alterations occur as a result of pregnancy, and pregnancy-specific endocrine adaptations related to the placenta develop after conception (see Table 4–1).

Physiological changes during pregnancy include significant alterations in pituitary, adrenal, thyroid, parathyroid, and pancreatic functioning. For example, the hormonal production activity and size of the thyroid gland increase during pregnancy in support of maternal and fetal physiological needs, and pancreatic activity increases during pregnancy to meet both maternal and fetal needs related to carbohydrate metabolism.

The hormones of pregnancy are responsible for most of the physiological adaptations and physical changes seen throughout the entire pregnancy. The placental hormones are initially produced by the corpus luteum of pregnancy. Once implantation occurs, the fertilized ovum and chorionic villi produce hCG.

- The high hCG level in early pregnancy maintains the corpus luteum and its production of progesterone and, to a lesser extent, estrogen until the placenta develops and takes over this function.
- After the development of a functioning placenta, the placenta produces most of the hormones of pregnancy, including estrogen, progesterone, human placental lactogen, and relaxin.

● Each of these hormones plays a role in the physiology of pregnancy, resulting in specific alterations in nearly all body systems, as described in this chapter, to support maternal physiological needs, maintenance and progression of the pregnancy, and fetal growth and development. (See Table 4–1 for details on pregnancy hormones.)

Immune System

Every aspect of the body's very complicated immune system undergoes adaptation during pregnancy to maintain a tenuous balance between preserving maternal-fetal well-being through normal immune responses and making the necessary alterations of the maternal immune system required to maintain the pregnancy. This adaptive process involves the maternal immune system becoming tolerant of the "foreign" fetal system so that the fetus is not rejected and is protected from infection. Immune function changes in pregnancy are far-reaching and beyond the scope of this chapter. This is also a relatively new body of science that is not fully understood.

SAFE AND EFFECTIVE NURSING CARE: Patient Education

Education About Pregnancy-Related Changes

- Discuss reasons for breast changes such as tenderness, enlargement, or heaviness and encourage the woman to wear a properly fitted supportive bra.
- Explain the possibility of breasts leaking colostrum.
- Educate on Braxton-Hicks contractions and contraction patterns that should be reported to the woman's health care provider.
- Discuss self-care measures to prevent yeast infections.
- Educate on the causes of supine and orthostatic hypotension and provide advice on self-care measures to prevent a hypotensive event.
- Encourage the woman to include iron-rich foods and take iron supplementation to prevent anemia.
- Instruct the woman in prevention and relief measures for dependent edema and varicosities.
- Educate and reassure the woman about normal respiratory changes and suggest symptom relief measures.
- Encourage the woman to stand, stretch, and take a deep breath periodically throughout the day.
- Educate the woman on reasons for increased frequency of urination during the first and third trimesters.
- Teach signs and symptoms of a UTI and advise her to seek prompt treatment if she experiences them.
- Encourage UTI-prevention measures such as emptying the bladder frequently, wiping front to back, washing hands before and after urination, urinating before and after intercourse, and maintaining adequate hydration with at least 8 glasses of liquid a day.

- Teach and encourage Kegel exercises and instruct the woman to wear a perineal pad if needed.
- Reassure the woman of the normalcy and self-limiting nature of nausea and vomiting of pregnancy and suggest measures to prevent and relieve it.
- Advise the woman to maintain good oral hygiene and continue routine preventive dental care.
- Encourage the woman to eat a high-fiber diet with adequate hydration and physical activity to prevent constipation and hemorrhoids.
- Instruct on preventive and relief measures for heartburn, flatulence, constipation, and hemorrhoids.
- Discuss musculoskeletal system changes during pregnancy.
- Encourage good posture and body mechanics to prevent symptoms of pain.
- Teach symptom relief measures for back or ligament pain.
- Encourage gentle abdominal strengthening exercises.
- Offer reassurance as skin pigmentation and/or other changes occur.
- Discuss normalcy of striae in pregnancy and encourage good weight control.
- Suggest maintaining skin comfort with daily bathing, lotions, oatmeal baths, nonbinding clothing.
- Advise to limit sun exposure and wear sunscreen.

PRECONCEPTION HEALTH CARE

Preconception care is a broad term that refers to the process of identifying social, behavioral, environmental, and biomedical risks to a woman's fertility and pregnancy outcome and reducing these risks through education, counseling, and appropriate intervention, when possible, before conception (Sackey, 2017). The aim is to optimize health and wellness by identifying and managing any medical, behavioral, social, environmental, or biomedical potential risks to a woman's health or fertility prior to conception in order to increase the chances of having a healthy baby (Table 4–2).

Preconception care is important because risk behaviors (e.g., smoking) and environmental exposures (e.g., Zika) can negatively affect fetal development and pregnancy outcomes. In addition, because almost half of pregnancies in the United States are unintended (Finer & Zolna, 2011), preconception care provides an opportunity to educate on risks, such as obesity, and intervene through motivational counseling or referrals to specialists as needed to reduce risks and optimize a woman's health. If pregnancy occurs, preconception care can reduce such complications as congenital disorders or fetal growth abnormalities (Sackey, 2017).

Access to Care

Various institutional, cultural, and economic barriers make it challenging for some groups of people to access the health care they need. Because perinatal nurses provide care to women

TABLE 4–2   Components of Health History and Risk Factor Assessment in Preconception Care

COMPONENT	PURPOSE AND ACTIONS
Identifying Information	
Age, gravida/para, address, race/ethnicity, religion, marital/family status, occupation, education	To determine specific risks based on sociodemographic characteristics • Provide education and anticipatory guidance. • Identify psychosocial resources and available sources of support (see Chapter 5 for detailed information on psychosocial and cultural assessment). • Refer for social services, counseling services, spiritual support.
Health Status	
Prior and present health status	To determine past and present health status • Provide education and anticipatory guidance. • Refer for additional testing/procedures. • Refer to physician specialist, counseling services, substance abuse treatment, genetic counseling, dietician, social services as indicated. • Administer rubella and/or hepatitis and flu vaccines as indicated. • Refer to cessation programs as appropriate (e.g., smoking).
Disease/Complications	
History of or current medical conditions/diseases (may include thromboembolitic blood dyscrasias, autoimmune, thyroid disorders)	To identify any components in medical history that may increase risk in the well-woman population
Surgeries (including blood transfusions)	• Initiate actions to minimize risks.
History of physical/sexual abuse	
Medication use (prescription, over the counter, complementary)	
Allergies	
Immunizations	
Family Medical	
Current health status	To determine both modifiable and nonmodifiable risk factors related to family and genetic history
Genetic	
Medical conditions/diseases	• Initiate actions to minimize risks.
Reproductive	
Menstrual	To ascertain details about menstrual cycles; past pregnancies and their outcomes; any gynecological disorders, including infertility; past or present contraceptive use; history of sexually transmitted infections; sexual orientation; past or present sexuality issues; use of safe sex practices
Obstetric	
Gynecological	
Contraceptive	
Sexual	• Assess prior pregnancy losses.

Continued

TABLE 4–2   Components of Health History and Risk Factor Assessment in Preconception Care—cont'd

COMPONENT	PURPOSE AND ACTIONS
Self-Care/Lifestyle/Safety Behaviors	To determine: • Frequency of health maintenance visits (well-woman and dental) • Bowel patterns • Sleep patterns • Stress management • Nutrition, BMI, and exercise history • Counseling on the importance of achieving a normal BMI prior to conception To identify tobacco, alcohol, and substance use/abuse, caffeine use To identify use of complementary and alternative medicine modalities To identify spiritual or religious practices To determine safety practices such as use of seat belts, sunscreen, smoke alarms, and carbon monoxide detectors, gun safety • Initiate actions to minimize risks.
Psychosocial Mental health Social	 To ascertain past and present psychological and emotional health To identify social patterns and sources of emotional and social support in family and friends • Refer to mental health providers as needed.
Cultural Beliefs/values Practices Primary language	 To identify cultural practices and beliefs/values impacting health and pregnancy • Incorporate knowledge of beliefs and practices in care. To determine need for translation • Obtain translation assistance as needed. • Provide educational materials in woman's primary language.
Environmental Home Workplace	 To identify past and current exposure to environmental or occupational hazards/toxins • Refer for environmental exposure counseling, genetic counseling when indicated.
Financial Basic needs related to food and housing Resources Health insurance	 To determine adequacy of resources to meet basic ongoing needs • Refer for social services, economic support services as indicated.

and infants, we are especially concerned with eliminating the barriers to care for these populations. Nurses are members of one of the most trusted professions and thus play an invaluable role in leading and supporting efforts to increase access to care for all women, regardless of their race, socioeconomic status, or environment. Nurses should be aware of barriers that affect access to health care and strive to reduce disparities through advocacy work with organizations such as Association of Women's Health, Obstetric and Neonatal Nurses (AWHONN); with state and federal legislators; and within their communities. Nurses can also provide support, information, and referrals to women from underserved communities (AWHONN, 2016).

Routine Physical Examination and Screening

The two primary components of a preconception health care visit are a physical examination and relevant health screening in the form of laboratory or diagnostic testing (Table 4–3).

- The physical examination includes:
  - Height and weight measurements to calculate body mass index (BMI) and assess for healthy weight.
  - Comprehensive physical examination, including breast and pelvic examination.
- Laboratory and diagnostic tests include:
  - Serum blood tests to determine blood type and Rh factor, complete blood count (CBC), cholesterol, glucose, IgG Rubella, HIV, and syphilis.
  - Urinalysis.
  - Cultures for sexually transmitted infections (STIs).
  - Papanicolaou smear (Pap smear), a screening test for cervical cancer.
  - Tuberculin skin test.
- Additional testing may be ordered based on history and physical examination findings.

Preconception Anticipatory Guidance and Education

Anticipatory guidance is the provision of information and guidance to women and their families that enables them to be knowledgeable and prepared as the process of pregnancy and childbirth unfolds. Anticipatory guidance and education in the childbearing-aged population spans topics from health maintenance, self-care, and lifestyle choices to contraception and safety behaviors. The nurse is key in providing this aspect of care (Fig. 4–6). It is imperative that a woman's age, sexual orientation, culture, religion, and additional values and beliefs are acknowledged and respected and that this information is incorporated appropriately into the nurse's teaching plan.

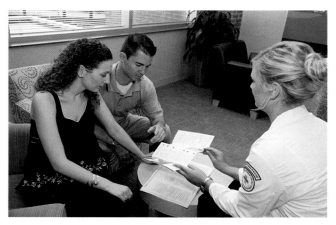

FIGURE 4–6 Nurse providing anticipatory guidance and education on self-care.

Preconception Education

The goal of preconception education is to provide a woman with information she can use to enhance her health before becoming pregnant. When a woman seeks care specifically because she is planning for a future pregnancy, more emphasis is placed on counseling and anticipatory guidance related to preparation and planning for a pregnancy.

Preconception anticipatory guidance and education topics include nutrition, vitamin supplements such as folic acid, exercise, self-care, contraception cessation, timing of conception, and modifying behaviors to reduce risks.

Nutrition

Maintaining a healthy weight is especially important for women planning a pregnancy. The BMI is a number calculated based on a person's height and weight, and represents a measure of body fat. The BMI can be used as an easy method of screening the nutritional status of women and to identify weight categories that may lead to health problems.

Currently, 36.5% of adults in the United States are obese (Ogden, Carroll, Fryar, & Flegal, 2015). The number of women in childbearing years who are overweight or obese has grown over the last three decades, and maternal obesity prior to conception has been linked to childhood obesity in their offspring, increased infant mortality, and an increased risk of fetal congenital anomalies (Bodnar et al., 2016; Meehan, Beck, Mair-Jenkins, Leonardi-Bee, & Puleston, 2014). Taking into consideration the lifelong health consequences associated with obesity, the Institute of Medicine (IOM) published guidelines in 2009 recommending that women achieve their normal BMI prior to conceiving, and this remains the current recommendation (ACOG, 2013a; IOM, 2009).

Obesity increases a woman's risk for infertility. During pregnancy, it is associated with increased perinatal morbidity and mortality from a variety of causes:

- Increased risk for antepartum complications such as hypertension, cardiac dysfunction, proteinuria, sleep apnea, nonalcoholic fatty liver disease, gestational diabetes mellitus, and preeclampsia (ACOG, 2015). Obese gravidas are 40% more likely to experience stillbirth.
- Obese pregnant women are at increased risk of cesarean delivery, failed trial of labor, endometritis, wound rupture or dehiscence, and venous thrombosis and postpartum hemorrhage (ACOG, 2015).
- Fetuses of obese gravidas are at increased risk of macrosomia and impaired growth.

CRITICAL COMPONENT

Pre-Pregnancy Weight

An overweight or obese pre-pregnancy weight increases the risk for poor maternal and neonatal outcomes and may have far-reaching implications for long-term health and development of chronic disease. At the other end of the spectrum, underweight pre-pregnancy weight and/or inadequate weight gain increases the risk for poor fetal growth and low birth weight. Women who are either significantly overweight or underweight should be counseled about potential issues with infertility and associated risks during and after pregnancy. Referral for dietary counseling and planning is recommended as needed to achieve a healthier weight before conception (ACOG, 2015; Stang & Huffman, 2016; Wilkes, 2016).

World Health Organization Body Mass Index Categories

Underweight: Less than 18.5

Normal weight: 18.5–24.9

Overweight: 25–29.9

Obesity class I: 30–34.9

Obesity class II: 35–39.9

Obesity class III: 40 or greater

World Health Organization, 2000.

Given the detrimental influence of maternal overweight and obesity on reproductive and pregnancy outcomes for the mother and child, the Academy of Nutrition and Dietetics suggests that all overweight and obese women of reproductive age receive counseling on the roles of diet and physical activity in reproductive health to ameliorate these adverse outcomes. This should be done prior to pregnancy, during pregnancy, and in the interconceptional period (Stang & Huffman, 2016).

Nutritional education for women of childbearing years should include:

● Education on diet and physical activity and their role in reproductive health.
● Advise on the importance of achieving and maintaining a healthy weight prior to conception (Meehan et al., 2014).
● Encouragement to make nutritious food choices with an emphasis on fresh fruits and vegetables, lean protein sources, low-fat or nonfat dairy foods, whole grains, and small amounts of healthy fats.
● Help in choosing appropriate foods and serving sizes (Fig. 4–7).

Prenatal Vitamins

Many women planning to conceive begin taking prenatal vitamin supplements. These contain a wide range of vitamins and minerals important for good health during pregnancy:

● Folic acid supplementation decreases risk of neural tube defects. Since 1992, the Centers for Disease Control and Prevention (CDC) has recommended daily folic acid supplementation of 0.4 mg daily for childbearing-aged women after folic acid was shown to reduce the incidence of neural tube defects (NTDs) such as spina bifida, with an expected 50% reduction in NTD incidence in the United States. The beneficial impact of folic acid supplementation is greatest between 1 month before pregnancy and through the first trimester, the period of neural tube development. Due to the large percentage of unplanned pregnancies and the fact that the neural tube

Daily Food Checklist

The checklist shows slightly more amounts of food during the 2nd and 3rd trimesters because you have changing nutritional needs. This is a general checklist. You may need more or less amounts of food.*

Food Group	1st Trimester	2nd and 3rd Trimesters	What counts as 1 cup or 1 ounce?
*Eat this amount from each group daily.**			
Fruits	2 cups	2 cups	1 cup fruit or 100% juice ½ cup dried fruit
Vegetables	2½ cups	3 cups	1 cup raw or cooked vegetables or 100% juice 2 cups raw leafy vegetables
Grains	6 ounces	8 ounces	1 slice bread 1 ounce ready-to-eat cereal ½ cup cooked pasta, rice, or cereal
Protein Foods	5½ ounces	6½ ounces	1 ounce lean meat, poultry, or seafood ¼ cup cooked beans ½ ounce nuts or 1 Tbsp peanut butter 1 egg
Dairy	3 cups	3 cups	1 cup milk 8 ounces yogurt 1½ ounces natural cheese 2 ounces processed cheese

If you are not gaining weight or gaining too slowly, you may need to eat a little more from each food group.
If you are gaining weight too fast, you may need to cut back by decreasing the amount or change the types of food you are eating.

Get a Daily Food Checklist for moms designed just for you.
Go to ChooseMyPlate.gov/Checklist.

FIGURE 4–7 USDA daily food checklist tips for pregnant moms.

closes very early in pregnancy, before many women know they are pregnant, all women of childbearing potential are recommended to take a daily supplement containing 0.4 to 0.8 mg of folic acid (Wolff, Witkop, Miller, & Syed, 2009).

- During pregnancy, women with no previous NTDs are recommended to take 0.6 mg/day. For women with a previous pregnancy affected by an NTD, 4 mg/day is recommended from 1 month before conception through the entire first trimester of pregnancy; after that, 0.4 mg/day for the remainder of the pregnancy is recommended.
- Women who have had an infant with an NTD, a medical history of pregestational diabetes, or any medical condition resulting in decreased red cell folate levels should consult their provider about recommendations for a higher dose (Goetzl, 2017).

- Calcium, magnesium, and vitamin D contribute to bone health and osteoporosis prevention throughout the life span, including during the childbearing years.
- Iron supplementation is commonly prescribed during pregnancy, although there is some controversy about the benefit of this practice as a routine recommendation.
  - A woman who is anticipating a short time between pregnancies is at risk for iron-deficiency anemia. Iron supplementation may be prescribed, and she is encouraged to include iron-rich foods in her diet in between pregnancies since she is likely to have reduced iron stores and may also be anemic from the previous recent pregnancy.
- Megadoses—doses many times the usual amount—of vitamins and minerals are not advised, as they may be toxic to the developing fetus.

Exercise

A program of regular exercise positively impacts a woman's health and may generally be continued once she has conceived. It is best to implement such a program several months in advance of conception so that when pregnancy occurs, regular exercise is already comfortable and routine. Women embarking on a new exercise regime may want to confer with their providers.

- Aerobic activity, including regular weight-bearing exercise such as walking or running, combined with stretching exercises and some type of weight work/muscle strengthening provides overall body conditioning and help with weight management, and can enhance psychological well-being.
- The weight-bearing exercise and weight/strengthening work also enhance bone health and help prevent osteoporosis.

Self-Care

Most women are pregnant for at least 1 to 2 weeks before becoming aware of their pregnancy. For this reason, it is helpful to counsel the preconception woman to decrease risk behaviors and eliminate exposure to substances that are known or suspected to be harmful during gestation as soon as she stops using contraception or begins trying to become pregnant (see Fig. 4–6). The woman should avoid:

- Illicit drugs, alcohol, tobacco (even secondhand smoke), and excessive use of caffeine.

- Medications contraindicated in pregnancy (prescription, over-the-counter, and herbal supplements).
- Environmental toxins. Exposure to some toxic substances—including lead, mercury, arsenic, cadmium, pesticides, solvents, and household chemicals—can increase the risk of miscarriage, preterm birth, and other pregnancy complications (U.S. Department of Health and Human Services, 2009).

The woman should be encouraged to:

- Use safer sex practices to prevent STIs.
- Use seat belts in a car, ensure that smoke alarms and carbon monoxide detectors are in working order, apply sunscreen when outdoors.
- Maintain adequate relaxation and sleep.
- Maintain optimal oral health and treat any periodontal disease before pregnancy, as it has been associated with adverse pregnancy outcomes, including preterm birth, low birth weight, and preeclampsia (Vamos et al., 2015).
- Discuss the use of complementary or alternative medicine modalities, such as acupuncture, herbal supplements, homeopathy, and massage, with her primary health care provider. Some of these interventions may need to be discontinued before a pregnancy for safety reasons.

Contraception Cessation

Before conception, it is ideal for a woman to have at least two or three normal menstrual periods. For all women planning a pregnancy, discontinuing contraception and tracking menstrual cycles will aid in facilitating conception and in dating the pregnancy once conception is achieved.

- Women using some form of hormonal contraception need to stop and begin using a barrier method of birth control or fertility awareness family planning techniques for the next few months before conception.
- Women using Depo-Provera for contraception need to be informed that it may take from several months up to more than a year to conceive after discontinuing injections.
- Women using an intrauterine device need to have the device removed.

Timing of Conception

Many women are interested in learning more about their menstrual cycles to gain more control over their ability to conceive.

- Preconception counseling can include basic information about the menstrual cycle, when in the cycle a woman can conceive, signs of ovulation, the life span of ovum and sperm, and how to time sexual intercourse to increase the likelihood of conception.
- Women who have used fertility awareness family planning principles are familiar with these concepts and can simply reverse the behaviors they practiced when using the method to avoid conception.

CRITICAL COMPONENT

Zika Virus Infection

The Zika virus is an infection spread primarily through infected mosquitoes (*Aedes aegypti* or *Aedes albopictus*), but it can also be sexually transmitted from a person infected by the virus, even when symptoms are not present. A pregnant woman can also spread the virus to her fetus, causing birth defects such as microcephaly, impaired growth, or visual abnormalities or hearing deficits. There is no cure for the Zika virus; symptoms, such as conjunctivitis, fever, joint or muscle pain, rash, or headache, are generally mild and can last up to a week. Currently there is no vaccine to prevent against the virus (CDC, 2017a). To avoid exposure to the virus, pregnant women should avoid travel to geographical areas known to have active mosquito transmissions of Zika, and they should protect themselves from mosquitoes, use protection throughout pregnancy against sexual transmission from a partner who may be infected, and adhere to recommendations for standard infection precautions (Lockwood, Romero, & Nielsen-Saines, 2017).

Modification of Behaviors to Reduce Risk

With each topic of conversation in preconception counseling, women gain information that helps them positively affect their overall health and reduce perinatal risk. Women can eliminate or reduce risks by modifying factors related to preexisting medical conditions, high-risk behaviors, and self-care and safety behavior deficits to improve outcomes of future pregnancies.

Nursing Actions in Preconception Care

- Provide comfort and privacy.
- Use therapeutic communication techniques.
- Obtain the health history and conduct a review of systems.
- Provide teaching about procedures.
- Assist with physical and pelvic exams and obtaining specimens.
- Provide anticipatory guidance and education related to plan of care and appropriate follow-up and assess the patient's understanding. See Table 4–3 for categories of clinical content for preconception care.
- Provide education, recommendations, and referrals to help women make appropriate behavioral, lifestyle, or medical changes based on history or physical examination.

SAFE AND EFFECTIVE NURSING CARE: Patient Education

Preconception Care and Health Care

The CDC recommendations emphasize that preconception care is not limited to a single visit to a health professional but is a process of care that is designed to meet the needs and improve the health of women during the different stages of their reproductive life. All women and men of reproductive age are candidates for preconception care. The CDC's Show Your Love is a national campaign that uses social media and a website with a variety of tips and tools, including an app, to help young adults make lifestyle choices that promote preconception health. Resources for organizations include buttons with the campaign logo to paste on Web pages, videos, checklists, and educational pamphlets to help young adults set goals and make health plans to put into action for optimal control of their preconception health and well-being (Verbiest, McClain, & Woodward, 2016).

Preconception Care for Men

As for women, preconception care for men offers an opportunity for disease prevention and health promotion. In addition, preconception care for men is an important factor in improving family planning and pregnancy outcomes for women, enhancing the reproductive health and health behaviors of men and their partners, and preparing men for fatherhood. The CDC recommends that when a couple is planning to conceive, the man should have a medical evaluation to prevent and identify disease and provide preconception education. Prior to attempting conception, management should be optimized for any high-risk behaviors or poorly controlled disease states, such as diabetes or hypertension (Verbiest et al., 2016). The CDC recommends (2017b):

- Counseling men to avoid certain risks (such as tobacco use and exposure to toxic substances).
- Counseling men to engage in healthy behaviors (such as reproductive life planning, proper nutrition, and healthy weight maintenance).

DIAGNOSIS OF PREGNANCY

The diagnostic confirmation of pregnancy is based on a combination of the presumptive, probable, and positive changes/signs of pregnancy. This information is obtained through history, physical and pelvic examinations, and laboratory and diagnostic studies.

Presumptive Signs of Pregnancy

The presumptive signs of pregnancy include all subjective signs of pregnancy (i.e., physiological changes perceived by the woman):

- Amenorrhea: Absence of menstruation
- Nausea and vomiting: Common from week 2 through 12
- Breast changes: Changes begin to appear at 2 to 3 weeks
  - Enlargement, tenderness, and tingling
  - Increased vascularity
- Fatigue: Common during the first trimester
- Urination frequency: Related to pressure of enlarging uterus on bladder; decreases as uterus moves upward and out of pelvis

- Quickening: A woman's first awareness of fetal movement; occurs around 18 to 20 weeks' gestation in primigravidas (between 14 and 16 weeks in multigravidas)

These changes could have causes outside of pregnancy and are not considered diagnostic.

Probable Signs of Pregnancy

The probable signs of pregnancy are objective signs of pregnancy and include all physiological and anatomical changes that can be perceived by the health care provider:

- Chadwick's sign: Bluish-purple coloration of the vaginal mucosa, cervix, and vulva seen at 6 to 8 weeks
- Goodell's sign: Softening of the cervix and vagina with increased leukorrheal discharge; palpated at 8 weeks
- Hegar's sign: Softening of the lower uterine segment; palpated at 6 weeks
- Uterine growth and abdominal growth
- Skin hyperpigmentation
  - Melasma (chloasma), also referred to as the *mask of pregnancy*: Brownish pigmentation over the forehead, temples, cheek, and/or upper lip
  - Linea nigra: Dark line that runs from the umbilicus to the pubis
  - Nipples and areola: Become darker; more evident in primigravidas and dark-haired women
- Ballottement: A light tap of the examining finger on the cervix causes fetus to rise in the amniotic fluid and then rebound to its original position; occurs at 16 to 18 weeks
- Positive pregnancy test results
  - Laboratory tests are based on detection of the presence of hCG in maternal urine or blood.
  - The tests are extremely accurate but not 100%. There can be both false-positive and false-negative results. Because of this, a positive pregnancy test is considered a probable rather than a positive sign of pregnancy.
  - A maternal blood pregnancy test can detect hCG levels before a missed period.
  - A urine pregnancy test is best performed using a first morning urine specimen, which has the highest concentration of hCG and becomes positive about 4 weeks after conception.
  - Home pregnancy tests are also accurate (but not 100%) and are simple to perform. These urine tests use enzymes and rely on a color change when agglutination occurs, indicating a pregnancy. The home tests can be performed at the time of a missed menstrual period or as early as 1 week before a missed period. If a negative result occurs, the instructions suggest that the test be repeated in 1 week if a menstrual period has not begun.

These changes could also have causes other than pregnancy and are not considered diagnostic. The presumptive and probable signs of pregnancy are important components of the assessment in confirming a pregnancy. Early in gestation, before any positive signs of pregnancy, a combination of presumptive and probable signs is used to make a practical diagnosis of pregnancy.

Positive Signs of Pregnancy

The positive signs of pregnancy are the objective signs of pregnancy (noted by the examiner) that can only be attributed to the fetus:

- Auscultation of the fetal heart, by 10 to 12 weeks' gestation with a Doppler
- Observation and palpation of fetal movement by the examiner after about 20 weeks' gestation
- Sonographic visualization of the fetus: Cardiac movement noted at 4 to 8 weeks

Sonographic Diagnosis of Pregnancy

Ultrasound using a vaginal probe can confirm a pregnancy slightly earlier than with the transabdominal method. With a transvaginal ultrasound, the gestational sac is visible by 4.5 to 5 weeks' gestation and fetal cardiac movement can be observed as early as 4 weeks' gestation. Ultrasound has increasingly become a routine and expected part of prenatal care. Indications for ultrasound examination of an early pregnancy for purposes of diagnosis include:

- Pelvic pain or vaginal bleeding in the first trimester
- History of repeated pregnancy loss or ectopic pregnancy (the implantation of a fertilized ovum outside the uterus)
- Uncertain menstrual history
- Discrepancy between actual size and expected size of pregnancy based on history

PREGNANCY

The antepartum (antepartal) period, also referred to as the prenatal period, begins with the first day of the last menstrual period (LMP) and ends with the onset of labor (known as the intrapartal period).

Pregnancy is also counted in terms of trimesters, each roughly 3 months in length:

- First trimester: First day of LMP through 14 completed weeks
- Second trimester: 15 weeks through 28 completed weeks
- Third trimester: 29 weeks through 40 completed weeks

Due Date Calculation

An important piece of information to share with a newly pregnant woman and her family is her "due date," or estimated date of birth. This is now more commonly known as estimated date of delivery (EDD). This date represents a best estimation as to when a full-term infant will be born. The original term used for this date was estimated date of confinement.

Calculation of the EDD is best accomplished with a known and certain LMP. If the LMP is unknown, other tools are used to determine the most accurate EDD possible:

- Physical examination to determine uterine size
- First auscultation of fetal heart rate with a Doppler and/or a fetoscope (stethoscope for auscultation of fetal heart tones)

- Date of quickening
- Ultrasound examination
- History of assisted reproduction

Naegele's Rule

Naegele's rule is the standard formula for determining an EDD based on the LMP: First day of LMP − 3 months + 7 days.

Formula for Naegele's Rule

LMP	SEPTEMBER 7
	− 3 months
	June 7
	+ 7 days
EDD	June 14

It is important to remember that the EDD as determined by Naegele's rule is only a best guess of when a baby is likely to be born. Two factors influence the accuracy of Naegele's rule:

- Regularity of a woman's menstrual cycles
- Length of a woman's menstrual cycles
  - Results may not be accurate if menstrual cycles are not regular or are greater than 28 days apart.

Most women give birth within 3 weeks before to 2 weeks after their EDD. The length of pregnancy is approximately 280 days, or 40 weeks from the first day of the LMP. In recent years, there has been conflicting or inconsistent information on the definition of a "term" pregnancy. The window for full-term gestation is between 38 and 42 weeks from the LMP; however, in 2012, a workgroup of experts met to review the definition of term gestation. Based on evidence that infant mortality is lowest for deliveries between 39 weeks 0 days and 41 weeks 6 days, the workgroup recommended that "early term" be used to refer to births between 37 weeks 0 days and 38 weeks 6 days and "late term" be used to refer to births between 41 weeks 0 days and 41 weeks 6 days (Spong, 2013).

CRITICAL COMPONENT

Classification of Deliveries From 37 Weeks of Gestation

Early term: 37 0/7 weeks through 38 6/7 weeks

Full term: 39 0/7 weeks through 40 6/7 weeks

Late term: 41 0/7 weeks through 41 6/7 weeks

Post term: 42 0/7 weeks and beyond

ACOG, 2013; Spong, 2013.

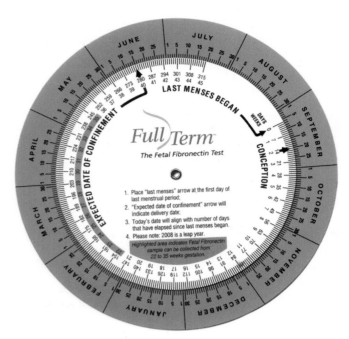

FIGURE 4–8 Gestational wheel. To use the gestational wheel, place the arrow labeled "first day of last period" from the inner circle on the date of the LMP on the outer circle. The EDD is then read as the date on the outside circle that lines up with the arrow at 40 completed weeks on the inside circle. Here the LMP is September 7 and the EDD is June 14.

BOX 4–1 | Gestational Age

What Is Gestational Age?

Gestational age refers to the number of completed weeks of fetal development, calculated from the first day of the last normal menstrual period. Embryologists date fetal age and development from the time of conception (known as *conceptual* or *embryological age*), which is usually 2 weeks less. Unless otherwise specified, all references to dating or fetal age in this textbook will be gestational ages (based on time since the last menstrual period and not time since conception).

Weeks of Gestation

Once an EDD has been determined, a pregnancy is counted in terms of weeks of gestation, beginning with the first day of the LMP and ending with 40 completed weeks (the EDD). A useful tool for quickly and easily calculating the EDD is the gestational wheel (Fig. 4–8), but it is less reliable than Naegele's rule due to variations of up to a few days between wheels. It is best to calculate a due date initially using Naegele's rule and then employ a gestational wheel to determine a woman's current gestational age (Box 4–1).

To use the gestational wheel, place the arrow labeled "first day of last period" from the inner circle on the date of the LMP on the outer circle. The EDD is then read as the date on the outside circle that lines up with the arrow at 40 completed weeks on the inside circle. With the example, the LMP is September 7 and the EDD is June 14.

Prenatal Assessment Terminology

A set of terms is used to describe obstetrical history and to define a woman's obstetrical status. An important shorthand system for explaining a woman's obstetrical history uses the terms *gravida* and *para* (G/P) in describing numbers of pregnancies and births.

- G/P is a two-digit system used to denote pregnancy and birth history.
  - Gravida refers to the total number of times a woman has been pregnant, without reference to how many fetuses there were with each pregnancy or when the pregnancy ended. It is simply how many times a woman has been pregnant, including the current pregnancy.
  - Para refers to the number of births after 20 weeks' gestation whether live births or stillbirths. There is no reference to number of fetuses delivered with this system, so twins count as one delivery, just like a singleton birth. A pregnancy that ends before the end of 20 weeks' gestation is considered an abortion, whether it is spontaneous (miscarriage) or induced (elective or therapeutic), and is not counted using the G/P system.
- GTPAL (gravida, term, preterm, abortion, living) is a more comprehensive system that provides information about each pregnancy and the pregnancy outcome. This system designates numbers of infants as follows:
  - **G** = total number of times pregnant (same as G/P system)
  - **T** = number of term infants born (between 37 and 42 weeks' gestation)
  - **P** = number of preterm infants born (between 20 and 37 weeks)
  - **A** = number of abortions (either spontaneous or induced) before 20 weeks' gestation (or less than 500 grams at birth)
  - **L** = the number of children currently living
- GTPALM may also be used, with the *M* representing pregnancies with multiple gestations.
- Nulligravida is a woman who has never been pregnant or given birth.
- Primigravida is a woman who is pregnant for the first time.
- Multigravida is a woman who is pregnant for at least the second time.

ANTEPARTAL NURSING CARE: PHYSIOLOGY-BASED NURSING ASSESSMENT AND NURSING ACTIONS

Nurse actions have significant impact on patient outcomes; the care that nurses provide to women before, during, and after birth is fundamental to the well-being of them and their newborns.

The nurse's expert knowledge confers the authority to shape the care environment and influence patient decisions. Therefore, understanding the physiological and psychosocial adaptations and changes of pregnancy improves the overall quality of health care provided to women.

Prenatal Assessment

The prenatal period is the entire period a woman is pregnant, through the birth of the baby. It is a time of transition in a family's life as they prepare for the birth of a child, affording an opportunity for positive change in all aspects of health and health maintenance behaviors. Prenatal care (PNC) is health care related to pregnancy, also referred to as antenatal care.

During ongoing interactions, the nurse places emphasis on health education and health promotion involving the woman in her care. The integrative view of health inherent in nursing care for the childbearing woman and her family contributes to a unique situation in which the antepartal patient has ready access to health information, individualized woman-centered support, and guidance to help achieve the healthiest possible pregnancy and the best possible outcome for her and her baby (Barron, 2014). The impact of this health care related to pregnancy and the possibility for positive change it engenders can extend well beyond the antepartal period into the life of the new family (WHO, 2016).

Early, adequate prenatal care has long been associated with improved pregnancy outcomes. Adequate prenatal care is a comprehensive process in which problems associated with pregnancy are identified and treated. Three basic components of adequate prenatal care have been identified: early and continuing risk assessment, health promotion, and medical and psychosocial intervention with follow-up. The aim of good prenatal care is to detect any potential problems early, prevent them if possible, and direct women to appropriate specialists or hospitals if necessary (Till, 2015).

Prenatal care reduces maternal and perinatal morbidity and mortality both directly, through detection and treatment of pregnancy-related complications, and indirectly, through the identification of women and girls at increased risk of developing complications during labor and delivery, thus ensuring referral to an appropriate level of care (WHO, 2016). PNC also provides an important opportunity to prevent and manage concurrent diseases through integrated service delivery. Additionally, prenatal care can provide reassurance of well-being to a pregnant woman and her family while providing education and information.

Prenatal nursing care and interventions also contribute to the woman's and family's ability to make informed choices about the health care of the entire family throughout the childbearing cycle, based on information provided by the nurse and integrated with the family's personal values, preferences, and beliefs. One of the *Healthy People 2020* objectives is to increase the proportion of women who receive early and adequate prenatal care from 70% to 78% (U.S. Department of Health and Human Services, 2010). Family-centered maternity care is based on a view that

TABLE 4–3   Categories of Clinical Content for Preconception Care

HEALTH PROMOTION	PERSONAL HISTORY	NUTRITION
• Family planning and reproductive life plan • Weight status • Physical activity • Nutrient intake • Folate • Substance use • STIs	• Family history • Known genetic conditions • Prior cesarean delivery • Prior miscarriage • Prior preterm birth • Prior stillbirth • Uterine anomalies	• Calcium • Dietary supplements • Essential fatty acids • Folic acid • Iodine • Iron
IMMUNIZATIONS	**INFECTIOUS DISEASES**	**MEDICAL CONDITIONS**
• Hepatitis B • HPV • Influenza • Measles, mumps, and rubella (MMR) • Tetanus, diphtheria, pertussis (Tdap) • Varicella	• Cytomegalovirus • Hepatitis C • Herpes simplex virus • HIV • Listeriosis • Malaria • STIs • Syphilis • Toxoplasmosis • Tuberculosis	• Asthma • Cardiovascular disease • Diabetes mellitus • Eating disorders • Hypertension • Lupus • Phenylketonuria (PKU) • Psychiatric conditions • Renal disease • Rheumatoid arthritis • Seizure disorders • Thrombophilia • Thyroid disease
EXPOSURES	**PSYCHOSOCIAL RISKS**	**SPECIAL POPULATIONS**
• Alcohol, tobacco, illicit substances • Environmental • Hobbies • Medications	• Access to care • Inadequate financial resources	• Disability • Immigrant and refugee populations • Survivors of cancer

pregnancy and childbirth are normal life events, a life transition that is not primarily medical but rather developmental.

● The initial prenatal visit parallels a preconception health care visit (see Tables 4–2 and 4–3). It also includes information about the health and health history of the father of the baby (i.e., age, blood type and Rh status, current health status, history of any chronic or past medical problems, genetic history, occupation, lifestyle factors impacting health, and his involvement in the woman's life and with her pregnancy).

● Early initiation of prenatal care is encouraged for optimization of maternal health and infectious disease screening (Till, 2015).

● The focus of patient education and anticipatory guidance shifts toward pregnancy-related health concerns, but the basic components of the visit and the emphasis on health maintenance and health promotion remain the same. Prenatal visits also include specific assessment of the pregnancy and fetal status. Some of these components are uniform across all prenatal visits, and others are specific to one or more trimesters of the pregnancy.

● Subsequent prenatal visits are more abbreviated than the initial visit, with nursing care and interventions focused on current pregnancy status and patient needs, always with an emphasis on patient education and anticipatory guidance (see Table 4–4 and the Clinical Pathway feature, "Content and Timing of Routine Prenatal Visits for Normal Pregnancy").

● The number of prenatal care visits in low-risk women in developed countries is 7 to 12 per pregnancy (Zolotor & Carlough, 2014). Current guidelines on the frequency of prenatal visits is monthly up to 28 weeks of gestation, then every 2 to 3 weeks between 28 and 36 weeks' gestation, and then weekly from 36 weeks' gestation until delivery (AAP/ACOG, 2012).

● The efficacy of the current model for individual prenatal care visits has been questioned as well.

TABLE 4–4 Prenatal Care: Content and Timing of Routine Prenatal Visits

	HISTORY AND PHYSICAL ASSESSMENT	LABORATORY/DIAGNOSTIC STUDIES IN NORMAL PREGNANCY (RECOMMENDED TIMING)
First Trimester		

Initial visit	Comprehensive health and risk assessment (see Table 4–1)
	
	Current pregnancy history
	
	Complete physical and pelvic examination
	
	Determine EDD
	
	Nutrition assessment, including 24-hour diet recall
	
	Psychosocial assessment (see Chapter 5)
	
	Assessment for intimate partner violence
		• Blood type and Rh factor
		• Antibody screen
		• CBC, including:
		  • Hemoglobin
		  • Hematocrit
		  • RBC count
		  • WBC count
		  • Platelet count
		• RPR, VDRL (syphilis serology)
		• HIV screen
		• Hepatitis B screen (surface antigen)
		• Genetic screening may be done between 10 0/7 weeks and 13 6/7 weeks
		• Rubella titer
		• PPD (tuberculosis screen)
		• Urinalysis
		• Urine culture and sensitivity
		• Pap smear
		• Gonorrhea and chlamydia cultures
		• Ultrasound

Return visit (4 weeks after initial visit)	Chart review Interval history Focused physical assessment: Vital signs, urine, weight, fundal height Clinical pelvimetry	
Second Trimester		
Return visits (every 4 weeks)	Chart review Interval history Nutrition follow-up Focused physical assessment: Vital signs, urine dipstick for glucose, albumin, ketones, weight, fundal height, FHR, fetal movement, Leopold maneuver, edema Pelvic exam or sterile vaginal examination if indicated Confirm established due date	• Triple screen, quad screen, or penta screen • Ultrasound • Screening for gestational diabetes at 24–28 weeks • Hemoglobin and hematocrit • Antibody screen if Rh negative • Administration of RhoGAM if Rh negative and antibody screen negative
Third Trimester		
Return visits (every 2–3 weeks until 36 weeks, then weekly until 40 weeks; typically, twice weekly after 40 weeks)	Chart review Interval history Nutrition follow-up Focused physical assessment: Vital signs, urine dipstick for glucose, albumin, ketones, weight, fundal height, FHR, fetal movement (i.e., kick counts), Leopold maneuver, edema Pelvic exam or sterile vaginal examination if indicated	Group B streptococcus screening: Vaginal and rectal swab cultures done at 35–37 weeks' gestation to determine presence of GBS bacterial colonization before the onset of labor in order to anticipate intrapartum antibiotic treatment needs Additional screening testing: • H&H if not done in second trimester • Repeat GC, chlamydia, RPR, HIV, HBsAg (if indicated and not done in late second trimester) • 1-hour glucose challenge test at 24–28 weeks

Evidence-Based Practice: CenteringPregnancy

Carter, E. B., Temming, L. A., Akin, J., Fowler, S., Macones, G. A., Colditz, G. A., & Tuuli, M. G. (2016). Group prenatal care compared with traditional prenatal care: A systematic review and meta-analysis. *Obstetrics & Gynecology, 128(3)*, 551–561.

Catling, C. J. (2017). Group versus conventional antenatal care for women. *Cochrane Database of Systematic Reviews*, (1). doi:10.1002/14651858.CD007622.pub3

Antenatal care is one of the most important health care services provided for pregnant women around the world. The generally accepted model of one-on-one prenatal care currently in use in the United States lacks a scientific basis. Because these individual prenatal visits typically last just 10 minutes, most women spend only a few hours total with their provider throughout their pregnancy. CenteringPregnancy is a group model of prenatal care delivery and is an alternative to individual prenatal care. It is designed to promote individual responsibility for health in pregnancy; provide appropriate prenatal assessment and risk screening; and provide education, social support, and a sense of community, all in a cost-effective and efficient manner.

CenteringPregnancy provides increased time in antenatal care, with women receiving between 12 and 20 hours of care in a group setting compared with an estimated 2 to 3 hours (8 to 10 visits of 15 to 20 minutes' duration) with conventional antenatal care. This likely results in increased education about pregnancy, childbirth, and early parenting, which in turn may affect perinatal outcomes. CenteringPregnancy groups typically have 5 to 12 pregnant women and meet with the provider for sessions every 2 to 4 weeks. Each session lasts 2 hours and covers topics such as promoting health through exercise, nutrition, or relaxation, all while offering social support.

Advantages of the CenteringPregnancy model of care include focus on the normalcy of pregnancy; increased time with the care provider during the pregnancy, a perceived benefit for both the care provider and the pregnant woman; efficiency for the care provider in delivering important prenatal education content; development of social connections between group members; social support for participants in managing the normal challenges of pregnancy; and validation of the woman's experience of pregnancy by a peer group (Rotundo, 2011).

A recent systematic review and meta-analysis was conducted to compare perinatal outcomes of individuals who had group prenatal care compared with individual prenatal care. Outcomes included rates of preterm birth, low birth weight, neonatal intensive care unit (NICU) admissions, and breastfeeding initiation. Four randomized control trials (RCT) and 10 observational studies were analyzed and synthesized. A decrease in low birthweight deliveries were noted in observational studies but not in the RCTs. Participating in group prenatal care did not lower preterm birth rates overall; however, a significant decrease in the risk of preterm birth was noted in African American women. Compared to individual prenatal care, no difference in rates of NICU admissions or breastfeeding mothers was found (Carter et al., 2016).

A Cochrane Review of four RCTs involving 2,450 women concluded that group antenatal care is acceptable to women and is not associated with adverse outcomes for mothers or their babies (Catling, 2017). They reported no differences between women who received group pregnancy care and those given one-to-one care in terms of important pregnancy outcomes such as preterm birth, infant birth weight, or death of the baby. Women who attended group pregnancy care rated their satisfaction as similar to women receiving individual care.

Goals of Prenatal Care

- Maintenance of maternal fetal health
- Accurate determination of gestational age
- Ongoing assessment of risk status and implementation of risk-appropriate intervention

- Build rapport with the childbearing family
- Referrals to appropriate resources

Nursing Actions

- Provide for comfort and privacy and use therapeutic communication techniques during the interview and conversation.
- Demonstrate sensitivity toward the patient related to the personal nature of the interview and conversation.
- Obtain the woman's identifying information (initial prenatal visit).
- Obtain a complete health history (initial prenatal visit) or an interval history (subsequent visits) (see Tables 4–2, 4–3, and 4–4 and the Clinical Pathway feature).
- Conduct a review of systems (initial prenatal visit).
- Obtain blood pressure, temperature, pulse, respirations, weight, height (initial prenatal visit), and BMI (initial prenatal visit).
- Assess for absence or presence of edema.
- Provide anticipatory guidance for the patient before and during the physical examination (initial prenatal visit and subsequent visits when indicated).
- Assist with physical and pelvic examination as needed (initial prenatal visit and subsequent visits when indicated).
- Assist with obtaining specimens for laboratory or diagnostic studies as ordered (initial prenatal visit and subsequent visits when indicated) and assess urine specimen for protein, glucose, and ketones.
- Provide teaching about procedures as needed (initial prenatal visit and subsequent visits when indicated).
- Provide anticipatory guidance related to the plan of care and appropriate follow-up, including how and when to contact care provider with warning signs or symptoms.
- Provide teaching appropriate for the woman, her family, and her gestational age; assess the woman's understanding of the teaching provided; and allow time for the woman to ask questions.
- Document, according to agency protocol, all findings, interventions, and education provided.
- Assess for intimate partner violence.

Cultural assessment is an important part of prenatal care. To plan culture-specific care, the nurse should assess the woman's beliefs, values, and behaviors that relate to pregnancy and childbearing. This includes information about ethnic background, religious preferences, language, communication style, common etiquette practices, and expectations of the health care system (see further discussion in Chapter 5).

First Trimester

One of the *Healthy People 2020* objectives is to increase the proportion of pregnant women who receive prenatal care beginning in the first trimester, with the target goal set at 77.9% (U.S. Department of Health and Human Services, 2010). The baseline report from the National Center for Health Statistics indicated that 70.8% of women who gave birth began prenatal care within the first 3 months of pregnancy, while 7.1% of all women received late care (beginning in the third trimester of pregnancy) or no care (Martin et al., 2010). In addition, the percentage of women with timely prenatal care declined (down 2%), and the percentage of women with late or no care increased (up 6%). Additionally, government statistics reflect a decrease in timely prenatal care and an increase in late or no prenatal care in the United States, with disparities noted among ethnic groups (i.e., Hispanics and African Americans being less timely in accessing care as compared to Euro Americans). Specifically, non-Hispanic white women (76.2%) were markedly more likely than non-Hispanic black (59.2%) and Hispanic (64.7%) mothers to begin care in the first trimester of pregnancy (Martin et al., 2010).

During the initial prenatal visit, the woman learns the frequency of follow-up visits and what to expect from her prenatal visits as the pregnancy progresses (see Table 4–4 and Clinical Pathway feature). If the patient is seen for her initial prenatal visit early in the first trimester, she may have more than one visit during that trimester. Subsequent visits are similar to those described for the second trimester. If the woman presents late for prenatal care and is in her second or third trimester at her initial prenatal visit, the nurse may need to modify typical patient education content to meet the current needs of the patient and her family.

At every prenatal care encounter, it is imperative that the nurse provides a relaxed environment for the woman and her family, one in which they feel comfortable asking questions and sharing personal details about their lives related to the health of the woman, her fetus, and the developing family.

CRITICAL COMPONENT

Intimate Partner Violence (Abuse)

Intimate partner violence (IPV) against women consists of actual or threatened physical or sexual violence and psychological and emotional abuse by a current or former partner or spouse. IVP affects women of every age, race, religion, socioeconomic status, and educational level and is the most common form of violence against women. Pregnant women are at a higher risk for IPV, especially when the pregnancy is unplanned (Martin-de-Las-Heras, Velasco, de Dios Luna, & Martin, 2015). Homicide is a leading cause of death in pregnant or recently pregnant women, and a significant portion of those homicides are committed by current or former intimate partners (Cheng, & Horon, 2010). According to the U.S. Department of Justice, Office of Violence Against Women (2012), one out of four women in the United States has experienced IPV; however, the true prevalence may be unknown due to fear of disclosure by the victim or failure on the part of the provider to screen adequately. Recent data reports the prevalence of physical violence by an intimate partner was 31.5% among women and an estimated 47.1% of women experienced at least one act of psychological aggression by an intimate partner during their lifetimes (Breiding et al., 2014). For some women, pregnancy is the only time they come into frequent contact with a health care provider. Early identification of IPV is necessary to minimize its serious physical

and mental effects, as well as its adverse health outcomes for the fetus (Bianchi, Cesario, & McFarlane, 2016). Research has documented that three simple screening questions can reliably identify abused women:

Within the last year, have you been hit, slapped, kicked, or otherwise physically hurt by someone?

Since you have been pregnant, have you been hit, slapped, kicked, or otherwise physically hurt by someone?

Within the last year, has anyone forced you to engage in sexual activities?

If a woman discloses violence, reassure her that she is not alone, that there have been others in her position before, and that help is available. Assessment for abuse during pregnancy with education, advocacy, and referral to community resources should be standard for all pregnant women during routine prenatal visits and on admission in labor. AWHONN advocates for universal screening for all pregnant women and recommends the ABCs of patient care to guide nurses caring for victims of abuse (AWHONN, 2007):

A: Alone. Reassure the woman that she is not alone, that there have been others in her position before, and that help is available.

B: Belief. Articulate your belief in the victim—that you know the abuse is not her fault and that no one deserves to be hurt or mistreated.

C: Confidentiality. Ensure the confidentiality of the information that is being provided and explain the implication of mandatory reporting laws, where applicable.

D: Documentation. Descriptive documentation with photographs, taken with the woman's permission, and a verbatim account from the patient's perspective is helpful to accurately capture and record the nature and extent of injuries.

E: Education. Education about community resources can be lifesaving. Know where you can refer a woman for help and have information about local shelters readily available. Also ask if she knows how to obtain a restraining order.

S: Safety. One of the most dangerous times for women is when they decide to leave an abusive relationship. Tell the woman to call 911 if she is in imminent danger and to consider alerting neighbors to call the police if they hear and/or see signs of conflict.

AWHONN, 2007; Bianchi, Cesario, & McFarlane, 2016; Cheng & Horon, 2010; Martin-de-Las-Heras et al., 2015; U.S. Department of Justice, 2012.

Components of Initial Prenatal Assessment

● History of current pregnancy:
   ● First day of LMP and degree of certainty about the date
   ● Regularity, frequency, and length of menstrual cycles
   ● Recent use or cessation of contraception
   ● Woman's knowledge of conception date

- Signs and symptoms of pregnancy
- Whether the pregnancy was intended
- The woman's response to being pregnant
- Obstetrical history, detail about all previous pregnancies:
  - GTPAL
  - Whether abortions, if any, were spontaneous or induced
  - Dates of pregnancies
  - Length of gestation
  - Type of birth experiences (e.g., induced or spontaneous labors, vaginal or cesarean births, use of forceps or vacuum-assist, type of pain management)
  - Complications with pregnancy, labor, or birth
  - Neonatal outcomes, including Apgar scores, birth weight, neonatal complications, feeding method, health and development since birth
  - Pregnancy loss and grieving status
- Physical and pelvic examinations:
  - The bimanual component of the pelvic examination enables the examiner to internally palpate the dimensions of the enlarging uterus. This information assists with dating the pregnancy, either confirming an LMP-based EDD or providing information in the absence of a certain LMP. When gestational age is uncertain, a decision may be made to perform an ultrasound examination of the pregnancy to determine an EDD. It is important to determine an accurate EDD as early as possible because numerous decisions related to timing of interventions and management of pregnancy are based on gestational age as determined by the EDD.
  - Clinical pelvimetry (measurement of the dimensions of the bony pelvis through palpation during an internal pelvic examination) may be performed during the initial pelvic examination; however, routine pelvimetry is not recommended (Chisholm & Levine, 2017).
- Assessment of uterine growth:
  - Uterine growth after 10 to 12 weeks' gestation is assessed by measuring the height of the fundus with the use of a centimeter measuring tape. The zero point of the tape is placed on the symphysis pubis, and the tape is then extended to the top of the fundus. The measurement should approximately equal the number of weeks pregnant. Instruct the woman to empty her bladder before the measurement because a full bladder can displace the uterus (Fig. 4–9).
  - Maternal position and examiner uniformity are variables that render this evaluation somewhat imprecise, but it is useful as a gross measure of progressive fetal growth as well as to help identify a pregnancy that is growing outside the optimal or normal range, either too large or too small for its gestational age. This serves as a screening tool for fetal growth.
- Assessment of fetal heart tones with an ultrasound Doppler in the first trimester, initially heard by 10 and 12 weeks' gestation. The normal fetal heart rate (FHR) baseline is between 110 and 160 beats per minute.
- Comprehensive laboratory and diagnostic studies:
  - Laboratory studies are ordered or obtained at the initial prenatal visit to establish baseline values for follow-up and comparison as the pregnancy progresses.

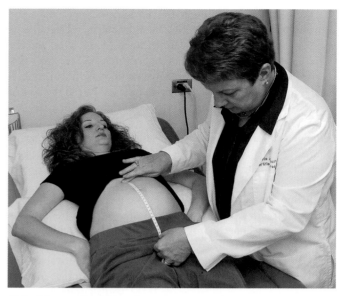

FIGURE 4–9 Fundal height measurement during prenatal visit.

- Ultrasound might be performed during the first trimester to confirm intrauterine pregnancy, viability, and gestational age.

CRITICAL COMPONENT

Warning/Danger Signs of the First Trimester

Educate pregnant women in the first trimester to contact their health care provider immediately if they experience any of the following symptoms:

- Abdominal cramping or pain indicates possible threatened abortion, UTI, or appendicitis.
- Vaginal spotting or bleeding indicates possible threatened abortion.
- Absence of fetal heart tone indicates possible missed abortion.
- Dysuria, frequency, and urgency indicate possible UTI.
- Fever or chills indicate possible infection.
- Prolonged nausea and vomiting indicate possible hyperemesis gravidarum; increased risk of dehydration.

Nutritional Assessment and Education

Approximately 40% of pregnant women in Western countries gain more than recommended during pregnancy (Gaillard, 2015). Maternal obesity during pregnancy has been linked to adverse fetal outcomes as well as childhood and adult obesity in their offspring (Gaillard, 2015). Pregnancy is a time when women are open to nutritional and lifestyle education, so it is an optimal time for needed behavioral changes in overweight and obese women (Walsh & McAuliffe, 2015; WHO, 2016). Nutrition should be discussed at all prenatal visits to reinforce the importance of appropriate weight gain, as both excessive and

BOX 4–2 | New Recommendations for Total and Rate of Weight Gain During Pregnancy, by Pre-Pregnancy BMI

The impact of pre-pregnancy weight and gestational weight gain on perinatal outcomes is significant and is directly related to infant birth weight, morbidity, and mortality. The current evidence suggests that inadequate weight gain and/or an underweight pre-pregnancy weight increases risk for poor fetal growth and low birth weight. At the other end of the spectrum, excessive weight gain and/or an overweight or obese pre-pregnancy weight increases the risk for poor maternal and neonatal outcomes and may have far-reaching implications for long-term health and development of chronic disease. Pre-pregnancy weight and BMI, as well as gestational weight gain, have increased nationally. The new recommendations for maternal weight gain in a singleton pregnancy are individualized based on pre-pregnancy BMI.

PRE- PREGNANCY BMI	TOTAL WEIGHT GAIN RECOMMENDED IN POUNDS	RATES OF WEIGHT GAIN,* 2ND AND 3RD TRIMESTER MEAN (RANGE) IN LBS/WEEK
Underweight (<18.5)	28–40	1 (1–1.3)
Normal weight (18.5–24.9)	25–35	1 (0.8–1)
	37–54 for twin pregnancies	
Overweight (25–29.9)	15–25	0.6 (0.5–0.7)
	31–50 for twin pregnancies	
Obese (≥30)	11–20	0.5 (0.4–0.6)
	25–42 for twin pregnancies	

*Calculations assume a 1.1–4.4 lb weight gain in the first trimester.

ACOG, 2013a.

inadequate weight gain in pregnancy are associated with poor perinatal outcomes.

- Discuss appetite, cravings, or food aversions.
- Obtain a 24-hour diet recall and review for obvious deficiencies.
- Based on the woman's pre-pregnancy BMI and IOM guidelines (Box 4–2):
  - Assist the woman to set weight-gain goals with a recommended weight gain of between 1 and 5 pounds during the first trimester.
  - Discuss distribution of weight gain during pregnancy (Box 4–3).
  - Encourage the woman to eat a variety of unprocessed foods from all food groups, including fresh fruits, vegetables, whole grains, lean meats or beans, and low-fat dairy products (USDA, 2017).
  - For more detailed information on nutritional needs during each trimester of pregnancy or to design a personalized daily food plan tailored to personal life circumstances, refer the patient to www.choosemyplate.gov/moms-daily-food-plan (see Fig. 4–7).
- Encourage the woman to drink 8 to 10 glasses of fluid per day and limit caffeine to 200 mg per day.
- Certain types of fish (king mackerel, orange roughy, marlin, shark, swordfish, and tilefish) should be avoided due to high levels of mercury; however, most other fish and seafood are safe as long as fully cooked. Tuna is safe but limit white (albacore) tuna to 6 ounces per week.

BOX 4–3 | Maternal Weight Gain Distribution

Baby: 7–8 lb

Placenta: 1.5 lb

Amniotic fluid: 2 lb

Breasts: 1–3 lb

Uterus: 2 lb

Increased fluid volume: 2–3 lb

Increased blood volume: 3–4 lb

Maternal fat: 6–8 lb

Macones, G., Ramin, S. M., & Barss, V. A., 2013.

- Advise on prevention of food-borne illnesses:
  - Wash hands frequently, before and after handling food. Use warm water and soap.
  - Thoroughly rinse all raw vegetables and fruits before eating.
  - Cook eggs and all meats, poultry, or fish thoroughly, and sanitize all dishes, utensils, cutting boards, or areas that contact these during food preparation.
  - Discard cooked food left out at room temperature for more than 2 hours.
  - Foods to avoid:
    - Unpasteurized juices or dairy products
    - Raw sprouts of any kind

- Unpasteurized soft cheeses like Brie, Camembert, or feta
- Refrigerated, smoked seafood
- Unheated deli meats or hot dogs
- Raw eggs
- Raw fish and shellfish
- Teas with chamomile, peppermint, licorice, or raspberry leaf
- For more detailed advice on food safety during pregnancy, visit www.fda.gov/Food/ResourcesForYou/HealthEducators/ucm081819.htm

CRITICAL COMPONENT

Initial Prenatal Labs With Rationale

Laboratory screening includes:

- Blood type and Rh factor with antibody screening to identify isoimmunization. Patients found to be Rh negative should be rescreened in the second trimester and given RhoGAM at 28 weeks and again after delivery, if the infant is Rh positive.
- Hct or Hgb blood volume in pregnancy increases more than red cell volume and hematocrit typically falls. Therefore, Hct or Hgb levels should be monitored for signs of anemia. Anemia is often caused by iron deficiency and should be treated with supplemental iron taken in addition to routine prenatal vitamins. A normal-term pregnancy requires approximately 1 g of iron, an amount not adequately supplied in the diet.
- Rubella to determine if the mother is susceptible or immune. If susceptible, she should receive vaccination postpartum.
- Varicella to determine if the mother is susceptible or immune. If susceptible, she should receive vaccination postpartum.
- Venereal disease research laboratory (VDRL) or rapid plasma regain (RPR) to check for serological evidence of syphilis so treatment can be initiated as soon as possible to avoid vertical transmission and the sequelae of congenital syphilis.
- Gonorrhea and chlamydia tests to identify and treat infection.
- Urine culture to identify and treat UTI, including asymptomatic bacteriuria, which is associated with a 25% risk of pyelonephritis if left untreated.
- Hepatitis B surface antigen to identify women whose infants need immunoprophylaxis postdelivery to minimize the risk of congenital infection and carrier status.
- HIV serology. Antiretroviral therapy during gestation and around the time of delivery can decrease the risk of vertical transmission to less than 2%. HIV-positive women should be counseled on the risks and benefits of treatment and mode of delivery.
- Women aged 21 to 29 years should have cytology screening every 3 years. Women aged 30 to 65 years should have human papillomavirus (HPV) and cytology co-screening every 5 years or cytology alone every 3 years.
- Discussion of prenatal screening for chromosome abnormalities, genetic disease, and birth defects should be performed and documented in the patient's medical record.

Topics to be addressed include:

- Prenatal screening and diagnostic tests for chromosome abnormalities—options include first trimester screening, quad screen, and integrated/sequential screening. Alpha fetal protein (AFP) alone is NOT an acceptable screening strategy for chromosome abnormalities (see Chapter 6).
- AFP for neural tube defect screening.
- Cystic fibrosis carrier screening is offered to Caucasians and discussed with other patients as they desire.
- Hemoglobin electrophoresis for patients at risk of sickle cell trait, thalassemia, or other hemoglobinopathies, including African American patients and patients of Mediterranean or Asian ancestry (sickle prep or sickle dex is inadequate because it screens only for hemoglobin S).
- Tay-Sachs, Canavan, and familial dysautonomia for patients of Eastern European Jewish ancestry.
- Tuberculosis skin test for patients at risk—for example, recent immigrants from developing countries, inmates, residents of mental institutions or group homes.

AAP/ACOG, 2012; APEC 2015.

Migrant Women

Women of reproductive age constitute a large proportion of new immigrants to the United States and are among the most vulnerable members of the population. Pregnancy can be an entry point into the health care system (HCS) for immigrant women, though they are less likely to access maternal care services than their nonimmigrant counterparts. In a systematic review, Heaman et al. (2013) reported that immigrants were more likely to receive inadequate prenatal care, initiate prenatal care late in pregnancy, and have fewer than the recommended number of prenatal appointments. A current systematic review of qualitative research indicates migrant women had pregnancy expectations strongly rooted in home beliefs, values, and practices that were supported by family, husbands, and friends. However, when women lacked support, they experienced several challenges in navigating the HCS. Furthermore, the overall experience of a woman's pregnancy is negatively affected when she believes that her health care providers (HCPs) are unsupportive, insensitive, and disrespectful to her wishes (Winn, Hetherington, & Tough, 2017). The author recommends strategies be implemented to increase cultural sensitivity within the HCS and recognize a need for awareness that immigrant women may be isolated in their new country and need additional assistance to navigate an unfamiliar system. For example, findings indicate women with support from the community and from providers were more likely to be receptive to the care and accept new practices if they understood their benefit or if the practice was supported by someone they knew. Women reported that in order to feel comfortable asking questions, it was important to feel their practices from their country of origin were respected. Understanding that a woman's expectations of pregnancy are rooted in home practices, values, and beliefs can help providers support women. Working with immigrant support groups can help identify potential cultural advisors to help new immigrants navigate the HCS (Winn, Hetherington, & Tough, 2017).

SAFE AND EFFECTIVE NURSING CARE: Patient Education

Patient education topics for women in the first trimester of pregnancy should include the following:

- General information about physical changes (see Table 4–1)
- General information about common discomforts of pregnancy
  - Relief measures for normal discomforts in early pregnancy are discussed based on patient need (Table 4–5).
- General information about fetal development: By the end of the first trimester, the fetus is 3 inches in length and weighs 1 to 2 ounces, all organ systems are present, the head is large, and the heartbeat is audible with Doppler.
- General health maintenance/health promotion information:
  - Avoid exposure to tobacco, alcohol, and recreational drugs.
  - Avoid exposure to environment hazards with teratogenic effects.
  - Obtain input from the care provider before using medications, complementary and alternative medicine, and nutritional supplements.
  - Reinforce safety behaviors (e.g., seat belt, sunscreen).
  - Recognize the need for additional rest.
  - Maintain daily hygiene.
  - Decrease the risk for UTIs and vaginal infections by wiping from front to back, wearing cotton underwear, maintaining adequate hydration, voiding after intercourse, and not douching.
  - Maintain good oral hygiene: Gentle brushing of teeth and flossing; continue routine preventative dental care.
  - Exercise 30 minutes each day: Avoid risk for trauma to abdomen, avoid overheating, and maintain adequate hydration while exercising.
  - Establish daily Kegel exercise routine to maintain pelvic floor muscle strength and decrease risk of urinary incontinence and uterine prolapse.
  - Travel is safe in low-risk pregnancy: Need to stop more frequently to stretch and walk to decrease risk of thrombophlebitis; take copy of prenatal record.
  - Use coping strategies for stress, such as relaxation exercises and meditation.
  - Communicate with partner regarding changes in sexual responses: Sexual responses/desires change throughout pregnancy. Couples need to talk openly about these changes and explore different sexual positions that accommodate the changes of pregnancy.
- Warning/danger signs that need to be reported to the care provider.

Second Trimester

Subsequent or return prenatal visits begin with a chart review from the previous visit(s) and an interval history. This history includes information about the pregnancy since the previous prenatal visit (see Table 4–4 and Clinical Pathway feature).

Components of Second-Trimester Prenatal Assessments

- Focused physical assessment
- Vital signs
  - Vital signs within normal limits; slight decrease in blood pressure toward end of second trimester
- Weight
  - Average weight gain per week depending on pre-pregnancy BMI (see Box 4–2)
- Urine dipstick for glucose, albumin, and ketones
  - Mild proteinuria and glucosuria are normal.
- FHR
  - Able to auscultate FHR with Doppler; rate 110 to 160 bpm (Fig. 4–10)
- Fetal movement
  - Assess for quickening (when the woman feels her baby move for the first time).
- Leopold's maneuvers (palpation of the abdomen) to identify the position of the fetus in utero (Chapter 8)
  - Examiner able to palpate fetal parts.
- Presence of edema
  - Slight lower-body edema is normal due to decreased venous return.
  - Upper-body edema, especially of the face, is abnormal and needs further evaluation.
- Fundal height measurement
  - Fundal height should equal weeks of gestation.
- Confirm established due date:
  - Quickening occurs around 18 weeks' gestation (usually between 18 and 20 weeks of gestation, but sometimes as early as 14 to 16 weeks of gestation in a multigravida and occasionally as late as 22 weeks of gestation in some primigravidas).
  - Ultrasound around 20 weeks' gestation to confirm EDD and scan fetal anatomy
- Laboratory and diagnostic studies:
  - Triple screen, quad screen, or penta screen blood tests at 15 to 23 weeks of gestation (Chapter 6): Screening tests for neural tube defect and trisomy 21 are not diagnostic. Amniocentesis offered if screening tests are positive.
  - Screening for gestational diabetes: 1-hour glucose challenge test recommended between 24 and 28 weeks; 3-hour glucose tolerance test (GTT) is ordered if 1-hour screen is elevated.
  - Hemoglobin and hematocrit between 28 and 32 weeks to identify anemia and the need for an iron supplement. This is the time in pregnancy when the hemoglobin and hematocrit are likely to be at their lowest, so the result provides the care provider with valuable information for management of late pregnancy.

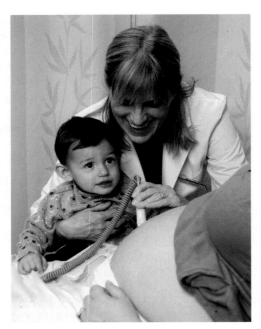

FIGURE 4–10 A nurse practitioner listening to fetal heart tone with a pregnant mom and her toddler.

- Syphilis serology if prevalent or as indicated
- Antibody screen for Rh-negative women
- All pregnant women should be offered prenatal assessment for chromosomal abnormalities by screening or diagnostic testing regardless of age or other risk factors (ACOG, 2016).
- Administer anti-D immunoglobulin (i.e., RhoGAM) to Rh-negative women with negative antibody screen results.
  - Anti-D immunoglobulin is administered at 28 weeks' gestation to help prevent isoimmunization and the resulting risk of hemolytic disease in fetuses in subsequent pregnancies.

SAFE AND EFFECTIVE NURSING CARE: Understanding Medication

Rho (D) Immune Globulin (RhoGAM)

Lab screening during an initial prenatal visit includes blood type and Rh factor with antibody screening to identify isoimmunization. Patients found to be Rh negative should be rescreened in the second trimester and given RhoGAM at 28 weeks and again after delivery if the infant is Rh positive.

- Indication: Administered to Rh-negative women prophylactically at 28 weeks' gestation to prevent isoimmunization from potential exposure to Rh-positive fetal blood during the normal course of pregnancy. Also administered with likely exposure to Rh-positive blood, such as with pregnancy loss, amniocentesis, or abdominal trauma. If the infant is Rh positive, another dose is given within 72 hours after delivery.

- Action: Prevents production of anti-Rh(D) antibodies in Rh(D)-negative women exposed to Rh(D)-positive blood. Prevention of antibody response and hemolytic diseases of the newborn (erythroblastosis fetalis) in future pregnancies of women who have conceived a Rh(D)-positive fetus.
- Adverse reactions: Pain at intramuscular (IM) site; fever
- Route/dosage: One vial standard dose (300 mcg) IM at 28 weeks' gestation. Use cautiously in patients with preexisting idiopathic thrombocytopenic purpura (ITP) anemia.

Vallerand, Sanoski, & Deglan, 2017.

CRITICAL COMPONENT

Warning/Danger Signs of the Second Trimester

- Abdominal or pelvic pain indicates possible preterm labor (PTL), UTI, pyelonephritis, or appendicitis.
- Absence of fetal movement once the woman has been feeling daily movement indicates possible fetal distress or death.
- Prolonged nausea and vomiting indicates possible hyperemesis gravidarum; at risk for dehydration.
- Fever and chills indicates possible infection.
- Dysuria, frequency, and urgency indicate possible UTI.
- Vaginal bleeding indicates possible infection, friable cervix due to pregnancy changes, placenta previa, abruptio placenta, or PTL.

SAFE AND EFFECTIVE NURSING CARE: Patient Education

Patient education topics during the second trimester should include the following:
- Information on fetal development during the second trimester
  - At 20 weeks' gestation, the fetus is 8 inches long, weighs 1 pound, and is relatively long and skinny.
- General health maintenance/health promotion topics
- Nutritional follow-up and reinforcement
  - Recommend increase in daily caloric intake by 340/kcal/day during second trimester (IOM, 2006).
  - Offer counseling and guidance on dietary intake or physical activity as needed.
- Information on physical changes during the second trimester (see Table 4–1)
- Relief measures for normal discomforts commonly experienced during the second trimester (see Table 4–5)
- Reinforce warning/danger signs that need to be reported to care provider.

- Signs and symptoms of PTL:
  - Rhythmic lower abdominal cramping or pain
  - Low backache
  - Pelvic pressure
  - Leaking of amniotic fluid
  - Increased vaginal discharge
  - Vaginal spotting or bleeding
- Signs and symptoms of hypertensive disorders:
  - Severe headache that does not respond to usual relief measures
  - Visual changes
  - Facial or generalized edema
- Information about the benefits and risks of procedures and tests with goal of enabling the woman to make informed decisions about what procedures she will choose based on her knowledge of the available options coupled with her and her family's values and beliefs.

Third Trimester

The focused assessment includes all aspects of the second trimester assessment and may also include a pelvic examination to identify cervical change, depending on weeks of gestation and maternal symptoms. Assessment of pregnancy in the third trimester becomes more frequent and involved than in previous return visits as the pregnancy advances and the fetus nears term (see Table 4–4 and the Clinical Pathway feature).

Components of Third Trimester Assessments

- Chart review
- Interval history
- Focused assessment (e.g., fundal height)
- Assessment of fetal well-being
  - Auscultation of FHR
  - Record woman's assessment of "kick counts"
    - Daily fetal movement count (kick counts) is a maternal assessment of fetal movement by counting fetal movements in a period of time to identify potentially hypoxic fetuses. Maternal perception of fetal movement was one of the earliest tests of fetal well-being and remains an essential assessment of fetal health. The pregnant woman is instructed to palpate the abdomen and track fetal movements daily by tracking fetal movements for 1 or 2 hours.
    - In the 2-hour approach recommended by the American College of Obstetricians and Gynecologists (ACOG), maternal perception of at least 10 distinct fetal movements within 2 hours is considered reassuring; once movement is achieved, counts can be discontinued for the day.

- In the 1-hour approach, the count is considered reassuring if it equals or exceeds the established baseline; in general, 4 movements in 1 hour is reassuring.
    - Define fetal movements or kick counts to include kicks, flutters, swishes, or rolls.
    - Instruct mother to keep journal or documentation of the time it takes to feel fetal movement.
    - Instruct mother to perform counts at same time every day.
    - Instruct mother to monitor time intervals it takes and to contact HCP immediately for deviations from normal (i.e., no movements or decreased movements).
  - Decreased fetal activity should be reported to the provider, as further evaluation of the fetus, such as a nonstress test or biophysical profile, is indicated.
  - Pelvic examination to identify cervical change, depending on weeks of gestation and maternal symptoms
- Leopold's maneuvers to identify the position of the fetus in utero (Chapter 8)
- Screening for Group B Streptococcus (GBS)
  - One-quarter to one-third of women are colonized with GBS in the lower gastrointestinal or urogenital tract (typically asymptomatic).
  - GBS infection in a newborn, either early onset (first week of life) or late onset (after first week of life), can be invasive and severe, with potential long-term neurological sequelae.
  - Vaginal and rectal swab cultures are done at 35 to 37 weeks' gestation to determine presence of GBS bacterial colonization before the onset of labor to anticipate intrapartum antibiotic treatment needs (Zolotor & Carlough, 2014).
- Laboratory tests and screening
  - 1-hour glucose test at 24 to 28 weeks' gestation (may have already been done in second trimester)
  - Hemaglobin and Hematocrit (H & H) (if not recently done in second trimester)
  - Repeat gonorrhea culture (GC), chlamydia, syphilis test by rapid plasma reagin (RPR) if indicated and not screened in second trimester, HIV, and hepatitis B surface antigen (HBsAg) tests as indicated
- Travel limitations may be suggested in the last month.
- Discussion of preparation for labor and birth
  - Attend childbirth classes
  - Discuss the method of labor pain management
  - Develop birth plan; list preferences for routine procedures
- Signs of impending labor
- Discussion of true versus false labor
- Instruction on when to contact the doctor or midwife
- Instructions on when to go to the birthing unit
- Discussion on parenting and infant care
  - Attend parenting classes
  - Select the method of infant feeding
  - Select the infant health care provider
  - Prepare siblings

CRITICAL COMPONENT

Warning/Danger Signs of the Third Trimester

- Abdominal or pelvic pain (PTL, UTI, pyelonephritis, appendicitis)
- Decreased or absent fetal movement (fetal hypoxia or death)
- Prolonged nausea and vomiting (dehydration, hyperemesis gravidarum)
- Fever, chills (infection)
- Dysuria, frequency, urgency (UTI)
- Vaginal bleeding (infection, friable cervix due to pregnancy changes or pathology, placenta previa, placenta abruptio, PTL)
- Signs/symptoms of PTL: Rhythmic lower abdominal cramping or pain, low backache, pelvic pressure, leaking of amniotic fluid, increased vaginal discharge
- Signs/symptoms of hypertensive disorders: Severe headache that does not respond to usual relief measures, visual changes, facial or generalized edema.

SAFE AND EFFECTIVE NURSING CARE: Patient Education

Patient education for women in the third trimester should include the following:

- Information about fetal growth during the third trimester
- At term fetus is about 17 to 20 inches in length, weighs between 6 and 8 pounds, has increased deposits of subcutaneous fat, and has established sleep and activity cycles.
- General health maintenance/health promotion topics
- Nutritional follow-up and reinforcement
  - Recommend increase in daily caloric intake by 452/kcal/day during third trimester (IOM, 2006).
  - Offer counseling and guidance on dietary intake or physical activity as needed.
- Information on physical changes during the third trimester (Table 4–4).
- Relief measures for normal discomforts commonly experienced during the third trimester (Table 4–5).
- Reinforce warning/danger signs that need to be reported to care provider.

TABLE 4–5   Self-Care/Relief Measures for Physical Changes and Common Discomforts of Pregnancy

BODY SYSTEM	PHYSICAL CHANGES AND COMMON DISCOMFORTS OF PREGNANCY (COMMON TIMING)	NURSING ACTIONS FOR PATIENT EDUCATION FOR SELF-CARE AND RELIEF MEASURES
Generalized or multisystem	Fatigue (first and third trimesters)	Reassure the woman of the normalcy of her response.
		Encourage the woman to plan for extra rest during the day and at night; focus on "work" of growing a healthy baby.
		Enlist support and assistance from friends and family.
		Encourage the woman to eat an optimal diet with adequate caloric intake and iron-rich foods and iron supplementation if anemic.
	Insomnia (throughout pregnancy)	Instruct the woman to implement sleep hygiene measures (regular bedtime, relaxing or low-key activities pre-bedtime).
		Encourage the woman to create a comfortable sleep environment (body pillow, additional pillows).
		Teach breathing exercises and relaxation techniques/measures (progressive relaxation, effleurage [a massage technique using a very light touch of the fingers in two repetitive circular patterns over the gravid abdomen], warm bath, or warm beverage before bed).
		Evaluate caffeine use.

TABLE 4–5 Self-Care/Relief Measures for Physical Changes and Common Discomforts of Pregnancy—cont'd

BODY SYSTEM	PHYSICAL CHANGES AND COMMON DISCOMFORTS OF PREGNANCY (COMMON TIMING)	NURSING ACTIONS FOR PATIENT EDUCATION FOR SELF-CARE AND RELIEF MEASURES
	Emotional lability (throughout pregnancy)	Reassure the woman of the normalcy of response.
		Encourage adequate rest and optimal nutrition.
		Encourage communication with partner/significant support people.
		Refer to pregnancy support group.
Reproductive		
Breasts	Tenderness, enlargement, upper back pain (throughout pregnancy; tenderness mostly in the first trimester)	Encourage the woman to wear a well-fitting, supportive bra.
		Instruct woman in correct use of good body mechanics.
	Leaking of colostrum from nipples (starting second trimester onward)	Reassure the woman of the normalcy.
		Recommend soft cotton breast pads if leaking is troublesome.
Uterus	Braxton-Hicks contractions (mid-pregnancy onward)	Reassure the woman that occasional contractions are normal.
		Instruct the woman to call her provider if contractions become regular and persist before 37 weeks.
		Ensure adequate fluid intake.
		Recommend a maternity girdle for uterus support.
Cervix/vagina	Increased secretions	Encourage daily bathing.
	Yeast infections (throughout pregnancy)	Recommend cotton underwear.
		Recommend wearing panty liner, changing pad frequently.
		Instruct the woman to avoid douching or using feminine hygiene sprays.
		Inform provider if discharge changes in color or is accompanied by foul odor or pruritus.
	Dyspareunia (throughout pregnancy)	Reassure the woman/couple of normalcy of response, provide information.
		Suggest alternative positions for sexual intercourse and alternative sexual activity to sexual intercourse.
Cardiovascular		
	Supine hypotension (mid-pregnancy onward)	Instruct the woman to avoid supine position from mid-pregnancy onward.
		Advise her to lie on her side and rise slowly to decrease the risk of a hypotensive event.
	Orthostatic hypotension	Advise woman to keep feet moving when standing and avoid standing for prolonged periods.
		Instruct to rise slowly from a lying position to sitting or standing to decrease the risk of a hypotensive event.

Continued

TABLE 4–5   Self-Care/Relief Measures for Physical Changes and Common Discomforts of Pregnancy—cont'd

BODY SYSTEM	PHYSICAL CHANGES AND COMMON DISCOMFORTS OF PREGNANCY (COMMON TIMING)	NURSING ACTIONS FOR PATIENT EDUCATION FOR SELF-CARE AND RELIEF MEASURES
	Anemia (throughout pregnancy; more common in late second trimester)	Encourage the woman to include iron-rich foods in daily dietary intake and take iron supplementation.
	Dependent edema lower extremities and/or vulva (late pregnancy)	Instruct the woman to: • Wear loose clothing • Use a maternity girdle (abdominal support), which may help reduce venous pressure in pelvis/lower extremities and enhance circulation • Avoid prolonged standing or sitting • Dorsiflex feet periodically when standing or sitting • Elevate legs when sitting • Position on side when lying down
	Varicosities (later pregnancy)	Instruct woman in all measures for dependent edema (see above). Suggest the woman wear support hose (put on before rising in the morning, before legs have been in dependent position). Instruct the woman to lie on her back with legs propped against a wall in an approximately 45-degree angle to spine periodically throughout the day. Instruct the woman to avoid crossing legs when sitting.
Respiratory	Hyperventilation and dyspnea (throughout pregnancy; may worsen in later pregnancy)	Reassure the woman of the normalcy of her response and provide information. Instruct the woman to slow down respiration rate and depth when hyperventilating. Encourage good posture. Instruct the woman to stand and stretch, taking a deep breath periodically throughout the day; stretch and take a deep breath periodically throughout the night. Suggest sleeping semi-sitting with additional pillows for support.
	Nasal and sinus congestion/epistaxis (throughout pregnancy)	Suggest the woman try a cool-air humidifier. Instruct the woman to avoid use of decongestants and nasal sprays and instead to use normal saline drops.
Renal	Frequency and urgency/nocturia (may be throughout pregnancy; most common in first and third trimesters)	Reassure the woman of normalcy of response. Encourage the woman to empty her bladder frequently, always wiping front to back. Stress the importance of maintaining adequate hydration, reducing fluid intake only near bedtime. Instruct her to urinate after intercourse. Teach the woman to notify her provider if there is pain or blood with urination. Encourage Kegel exercises; wear perineal pad if needed.

TABLE 4–5   Self-Care/Relief Measures for Physical Changes and Common Discomforts of Pregnancy—cont'd

BODY SYSTEM	PHYSICAL CHANGES AND COMMON DISCOMFORTS OF PREGNANCY (COMMON TIMING)	NURSING ACTIONS FOR PATIENT EDUCATION FOR SELF-CARE AND RELIEF MEASURES
Gastrointestinal		
	Nausea and/or vomiting in pregnancy (NVP) (first trimester and sometimes into the second trimester)	Reassure the woman of normalcy and self-limiting nature of response. Avoid strong odors and causative factors (e.g., spicy foods, greasy foods, large meals, stuffy rooms, hot places, or loud noises). Encourage women to experiment with alleviating factors: • Eating small, frequent meals as soon as, or before, feeling hungry • Eat at a slow pace • Eat crackers or dry toast before rising or whenever nauseous • Drink cold, clear carbonated beverages such as ginger ale, or sour beverages such as lemonade • Avoid fluid intake with meals • Eat ginger-flavored lollipops or peppermint candies • Brush teeth after eating • Wear P6 acupressure wrist bands • Take vitamins at bedtime with a snack (not in the morning) • Suggest vitamin B_6, 25 mg by mouth three times daily or ginger, 250 mg by mouth four times daily. Oral or rectal medications may be prescribed for management of troublesome symptoms. Identify, acknowledge, and support women with significant NVP to offer additional treatment options.
	Increase or sense of increase in salivation (mostly first trimester if associated with nausea)	Suggest use of gum or hard candy or use astringent mouthwash.
	Bleeding gums (throughout pregnancy)	Encourage the woman to maintain good oral hygiene (brush gently with soft toothbrush, daily flossing). Maintain optimal nutrition.
	Flatulence (throughout pregnancy)	Encourage the woman to: • Maintain regular bowel habits • Engage in regular exercise • Avoid gas-producing foods • Chew food slowly and thoroughly • Use the knee-chest position during periods of discomfort
	Heartburn (later pregnancy)	Suggest: • Small, frequent meals • Maintain good posture • Maintain adequate fluid intake but avoid fluid intake with meals • Avoid fatty or fried foods • Remain upright for 30–45 minutes after eating • Refrain from eating at least 3 hours prior to bedtime

Continued

TABLE 4–5   Self-Care/Relief Measures for Physical Changes and Common Discomforts of Pregnancy—cont'd

BODY SYSTEM	PHYSICAL CHANGES AND COMMON DISCOMFORTS OF PREGNANCY (COMMON TIMING)	NURSING ACTIONS FOR PATIENT EDUCATION FOR SELF-CARE AND RELIEF MEASURES
	Constipation (throughout pregnancy; see Concept Map feature)	Encourage the woman to: • Maintain adequate fluid intake • Engage in regular exercise such as walking • Increase fiber in diet through vegetables, fruits, and whole grains • Maintain regular bowel habits • Maintain good posture and body mechanics
	Hemorrhoids (later pregnancy)	Avoid constipation (see above). Instruct the woman to avoid bearing down with bowel movements. Instruct the woman in comfort measures (e.g., ice packs, warm baths or sitz baths, witch hazel compresses). Elevate the hips and lower extremities during rest periods throughout the day. Gently reinsert hemorrhoid into the rectum while doing Kegel exercises.
Musculoskeletal	Low back pain/joint discomfort/difficulty walking (later pregnancy)	Instruct the woman to: • Utilize proper body mechanics (e.g., stoop using knees vs. bend for lifting) • Maintain good posture • Do pelvic rock/pelvic tilt exercises • Wear supportive shoes with low heels • Apply warmth or ice to painful area • Use of maternity girdle • Use massage • Use relaxation techniques • Sleep on a firm mattress with pillows for additional support of extremities, abdomen, and back
	Diastasis recti (later pregnancy)	Instruct the woman to do gentle abdominal strengthening exercises (e.g., tiny abdominal crunches, may cross arms over abdomen to opposite sides for splinting, no sit-ups). Teach proper technique for sitting up from lying down (i.e., roll to side, lift torso up using arms until in sitting position).
	Round ligament spasm and pain (late second and third trimester)	Instruct the woman to: • Lie on side and flex knees up to abdomen • Bend toward pain • Do pelvic tilt/pelvic rock exercises • Use warm baths or compresses • Use side-lying in exaggerated Sim's position with pillows for additional support of abdomen and in between legs • Use maternity belt

TABLE 4–5   Self-Care/Relief Measures for Physical Changes and Common Discomforts of Pregnancy—cont'd

BODY SYSTEM	PHYSICAL CHANGES AND COMMON DISCOMFORTS OF PREGNANCY (COMMON TIMING)	NURSING ACTIONS FOR PATIENT EDUCATION FOR SELF-CARE AND RELIEF MEASURES
	Leg cramps (throughout pregnancy)	Instruct the woman to: • Dorsiflex foot to stretch calf muscle • Warm baths or compresses to the affected area • Change position slowly • Massage the affected area • Regular exercise and muscle conditioning
Integumentary	Striae (stretch marks) (later pregnancy)	Reassure the woman that there is no method to prevent them. Suggest maintaining skin comfort (e.g., lotions, oatmeal baths, nonbinding clothing). Encourage good weight control.
	Dry skin or pruritus (itching) (later pregnancy)	Suggestions for maintaining skin comfort: Use tepid water for baths and showers and rinse with cooler water. Avoid hot water (drying effect may increase itching). Use moisturizing soaps or body wash. Avoid exfoliating scrubs or deodorant soaps (has drying effect and may increase itching). Use of lotions, oatmeal baths, nonbinding clothing may lessen itching.
	Skin hyperpigmentation	Limit sun exposure. Wear sunscreen regularly.
	Acne	Use products developed for the face only (e.g., cleansers, sunscreen), avoid body soaps and facial scrubs (both have drying effects), body lotions/creams (clog pores); use tepid water when washing face and always follow with cold rinse to close pores before applying moisturizers (if needed) or sunscreen.
Neurological	Headaches	Maintain adequate hydration.
	Syncope	Rise slowly from sitting to standing. Instruct the woman to avoid supine position from mid-pregnancy onward. Advise her to lie on her side and rise slowly to decrease the risk of a hypotensive event.

Clinical Pathway for Prenatal Care: Content and Timing of Routine Prenatal Visits for Normal Pregnancy

Focus of Care	Initial Prenatal Visit	First Trimester	Second Trimester	Third Trimester
Frequency of prenatal visits	Initial visit	Return visit (4 weeks after initial visit) and then every 4 weeks	Return visit every 4 weeks	Return visits every 2 to 3 weeks until 36 weeks, then weekly until 40 weeks; twice weekly after 40 weeks
Assessments	Comprehensive health and risk assessment Current pregnancy • First day of LMP • Regularity, frequency, and length of menstrual cycles • Recent use or cessation of contraception • Woman's knowledge of conception date • Determine EDD • Signs and symptoms of pregnancy • Inquire whether the pregnancy was intended • Assess the woman's response to being pregnant Obstetrical history • GTPAL • Date of pregnancies • Length of gestation • Type of birth experiences • Complications with previous pregnancies • Prior pregnancy losses • Neonatal outcomes, including Apgar scores Medical history Family history Social history • Smoking • Alcohol • Substance use Sexual history and practices Complete physical assessment • Vital signs • Urine • Pelvic examination	Chart review Interval history since last visit Focused physical assessment: • Weeks gestation • Blood pressure • Urine dipstick for glucose, albumin, ketones • Weight, including cumulative weight gain or loss • Fundal height measurement • Fetal heart tones • Clinical pelvimetry	Chart review Interval history Nutrition follow-up Focused physical assessment: • Blood pressure and vital signs • Urine dipstick for glucose, albumin, ketones • Weight • Fundal height measurement • Fetal heart tones • Fetal movement—note beginning of fetal movement (quickening) • Leopold maneuver • Edema Pelvic exam or sterile vaginal examination if indicated Reevaluate pregnancy risk status	Chart review Interval history Nutrition follow-up Focused physical assessment: • Vital signs • Urine dipstick for glucose, albumin, ketones • Weight • Fundal height measurement • Leopold maneuver • Edema • Pelvic exam or sterile vaginal examination if indicated • Assessment of fetal well-being • FHR • Fetal movement (i.e., kick counts)

Clinical Pathway for Prenatal Care—cont'd

Focus of Care	Initial Prenatal Visit	First Trimester	Second Trimester	Third Trimester
	Nutrition assessment			
	• Height and weight to calculate BMI			
	• 24-hour diet recall			
	Physical activity level			
	Psychosocial and cultural assessment (see Chapter 5)			
	Depression evaluation			
	Assessment for intimate partner violence			
Laboratory and diagnostic studies	Blood type and Rh factor	Review labs	Triple screen or quad screen at 15 to 20 weeks	Group B streptococcus screening:
	Antibody screen		Ultrasound as indicated	• Vaginal and rectal swab cultures done at 35 to 37 weeks on all pregnant women
	CBC, including:		Screening for gestational diabetes with 1- hour glucose challenge test at 24 to 28 weeks	
	• Hemoglobin			Additional screening testing:
	• Hematocrit		Hemoglobin and hematocrit (see Appendix D for normal laboratory values in pregnancy)	H&H if not done recently in second trimester (see Appendix D for normal laboratory values in pregnancy)
	• RBC count			
	• WBC count			
	• Platelet count (see Appendix D for normal laboratory values in pregnancy)		Antibody screen if Rh-negative around 26 to 28 weeks	Repeat if indicated (and not done in late second trimester):
	RPR, VDRL (syphilis serology)		• Administration of RhoGAM at 28 weeks if Rh-negative and antibody-screen negative	• GC
	HIV screen			• Chlamydia
	Hepatitis B screen (surface antigen)			• RPR
	Offer genetic screening			• HIV
	Rubella titer purified protein derivative (PPD) (tuberculosis screen)			• HBsAg
	Urinalysis			1-hour glucose challenge test 24 to 28 weeks
	Urine culture and sensitivity			Ultrasound as indicated
	Pap smear			
	Gonorrhea and chlamydia cultures			
	Ultrasound			

Continued

Clinical Pathway for Prenatal Care—cont'd

Focus of Care	Initial Prenatal Visit	First Trimester	Second Trimester	Third Trimester
Prenatal education and anticipatory guidance	Provide information to the woman and her support person on the following: • Physical changes and common discomforts to expect during first trimester • Relief measures for common discomforts • Fetal development • General health maintenance/health promotion • Warning/danger signs to report to care provider • Nutrition, prenatal vitamins, and folic acid • Exercise • Self-care and modifying behaviors to reduce risks • Physiology of pregnancy • Course of care	Same as for initial visit	Provide information to the woman and her support person on the following: • Physical changes and common discomforts to expect during second trimester • Relief measures for common discomforts • Fetal development and growth during second trimester • Reinforce warning/danger signs to report to care provider • Nutritional follow-up and recommendation of increase in daily caloric intake by 340 kcal/day • Follow up on physical activity as needed • Follow up on modifiable risk patterns • Begin teaching on preparing for birth	Provide information to the woman and her support person on the following: • Physical changes and common discomforts to expect during third trimester • Relief measures for normal and common discomforts • Fetal development and growth during third trimester • Reinforce warning/danger signs to report to care provider • Nutritional follow-up and recommendation of increase in daily caloric intake by 452 kcal/day • Follow up on modifiable risk patterns Teach fetal movement kick counts Continue teaching and preparing the couple for delivery • Discussion on attending childbirth preparation classes • Teach signs of impending labor • Discuss true vs. false labor • Instruction on when to contact the care provider or go to birthing unit • Discussion on attending parenting classes • Select the method of infant feeding • Select the infant health care provider • Preparation of siblings

CONCEPT MAP |

Constipation

Altered Pattern of Elimination
- Decrease in normal frequency of defecation
- Bowel movement every 3 days
- Bloated abdominal sensation

Altered Fluid Intake Related to Occasional Nausea and Vomiting
- Reports of nausea once or twice a week
- Occasional vomiting
- Decreased oral intake

Constipation

Alteration in elimination related to physiologic and anatomic changes in pregnancy including alteration in gastrointestinal tone by relaxation of smooth muscle, increased nausea and vomiting, and displacement of small and large intestine by gravid uterus.

Decrease GI Motility Related to Effect of Prostaglandin on Smooth Muscle of Intestines
- Passage of hard and dry stool
- Increase reabsorption of water from intestines

Hemorrhoids
- Visually apparent varicosities in rectum on anal inspection
- Woman reports pain in rectum on defecation

Problem No. 1: Altered pattern of elimination
Goal: Resumption of typical bowel patterns
Outcome: Patient will resume her normal bowel patterns.

Nursing Actions

1. Assess prior bowel patterns before pregnancy, including frequency, consistency, shape, and color.
2. Auscultate bowel sounds.
3. Assess prior experiences with constipation.
4. Explore prior successful strategies for constipation.
5. Explain contributing factors to constipation in pregnancy.
6. Teach strategies for dealing with constipation, including dietary modifications, exercise, and adequate fluid intake.
7. Encourage high-fiber foods and fresh fruits and vegetables.
8. Encourage dietary experimentation to evaluate what works for her.

9. Establish regular time for bowel movement.
10. Discuss rationale for strategies.
11. Explore with the woman and discuss with the care provider use of stool softener and/or bulk laxative.
12. Encourage the patient to discuss concerns about constipation by asking open-ended questions.

Problem No. 2: Altered fluid intake related to nausea and vomiting
Goal: Normal fluid intake
Outcome: Normal fluid intake and decreased nausea and vomiting

Nursing Actions

1. Assess factors that increase nausea and vomiting.
2. Suggest small, frequent meals.

3. Decrease fluid intake with meals.

4. Avoid high-fat and spicy food.

5. Explore contributing factors to nausea in pregnancy.

6. Teach strategies for dealing with nausea in pregnancy.

7. Encourage the woman to experiment with strategies to alleviate nausea.

8. Suggest vitamin B_6 or ginger to decrease nausea.

Problem 3: Decreased gastric motility
Goal: Increased motility
Outcome: Patient has normal bowel movement.

Nursing Actions

1. Provide dietary information to increase fiber and roughage in diet.

2. Review high-fiber foods, such as pears, apples, prunes, kiwis, and dried fruits.

3. Suggest bran cereal in the morning and instruct woman to check labels for at least 4 to 5 grams of fiber per serving.

4. Discuss strategies to increase fluid intake.

5. Drink warm liquid upon rising.

6. Encourage exercise to promote peristalsis.

7. Reinforce relationship of diet, exercise, and fluid intake on constipation.

Problem 4: Discomfort with defecation because of hemorrhoids
Goal: Decreased pain with bowel movement
Outcome: Patient will have decreased pain and maintain adequate bowel function.

Nursing Actions

1. Reinforce strategies to avoid constipation.

2. Encourage the woman to not avoid defecation.

3. Instruct the woman to avoid straining on evacuation.

4. Discuss care of hemorrhoids, including witch hazel pads and hemorrhoid creams.

5. Discuss use of stool softeners.

6. Recommend that the woman support a foot on a footstool to facilitate bowel evacuation.

7. Reinforce relationship of diet, exercise, and fluid intake on constipation.

Case Study

As a nurse in an antenatal clinic, you are part of an interdisciplinary team that is caring for Margarite Sanchez during her pregnancy. Margarite is a 28-year-old G3 P1 Hispanic woman here for her first prenatal care appointment. By her LMP she is at 8 weeks' gestation. She is 5 feet, 7 inches tall and her weight today is 140 (states pre-pregnancy weight was 137, BMI = 21.5). Margarite reports some spotting 2 weeks ago that prompted her to do a home pregnancy test that was positive. The spotting has stopped. She tells you that she is very tired throughout the day and has some nausea in the morning and breast tenderness. She is happy to be pregnant but a bit surprised.

Outline the aspects of your initial assessment.

Outline for Margarite what laboratory tests are done during this first prenatal visit and rationale for the tests.

Detail the prenatal education and anticipatory guidance appropriate for the first trimester of pregnancy.

What teaching would you do for Margarite's discomforts of pregnancy?

Discuss nursing diagnosis, nursing activities, and expected outcomes related to this woman.

At 18 weeks' gestation, Margarite comes to the clinic for a prenatal visit. She states she thinks she felt her baby move for the first time last week and that the pregnancy now feels real to her. She states, "I feel great! The nausea and fatigue are gone." She is concerned she is not eating enough protein, as she has little interest in red meat but eats beans and rice at dinner. She remembers discussing with you at her first visit some screening tests for problems with the baby but now is unsure how they are done and what they are for.

Outline for Margarite nutritional needs during pregnancy, highlighting protein requirements.

Outline for Margarite the screening tests that are done in the second trimester and what they are for.

Detail the prenatal education and anticipatory guidance appropriate for the second trimester of pregnancy.

Discuss nursing diagnosis, nursing activities, and expected outcomes related to Margarite.

Margarite comes to your clinic for a prenatal visit and is now at 34 weeks' gestation. She states she feels well but has some swelling in her legs at the end of the day, a backache at the end of the day, and difficulty getting comfortable enough to fall asleep. She is also having difficulty sleeping, as she gets up to go to the bathroom two or three times a night.

She remembers from her first pregnancy some things she should be aware of that indicate a problem at the end of pregnancy but is not sure what they are.

Detail the prenatal education and anticipatory guidance appropriate for the third trimester of pregnancy.

What teaching would you do for Margarite's discomforts of pregnancy?

What warning signs would you reinforce with Margarite at this point in her pregnancy?

Discuss nursing diagnosis, nursing activities, and expected outcomes specific to Margarite.

REFERENCES

Alabama Perinatal Excellence Collaborative. (2015) APEC Guidelines for Routine Prenatal Care, guideline 1, version 7.

American Academy of Pediatrics/American College of Obstetricians and Gynecologists. (2012). *Guidelines for perinatal care* (7th ed.). Elk Grove Village, IL: American Academy of Pediatrics; Washington, DC: American College of Obstetricians and Gynecologists.

American College of Obstetricians and Gynecologists (ACOG). (2013a). ACOG Committee opinion no. 548: Weight gain during pregnancy. *Obstetrics & Gynecology, 121*(1), 210.

American College of Obstetricians and Gynecologists (ACOG). (2013b) Definition of term pregnancy. Committee Opinion No. 579. *Obstetrics & Gynecology, 122*, 1139–1140.

American College of Obstetricians and Gynecologists (ACOG). (2015). Practice bulletin no. 156: Obesity in pregnancy. *Obstetrics & Gynecology, 126*(6), e112–126.

American College of Obstetricians and Gynecologists (ACOG). (2016). Practice bulletin no. 162: Prenatal diagnostic testing for genetic disorders. *Obstetrics & Gynecology, 127*(5), e108–122.

Association of Women's Health, Obstetric and Neonatal Nurses (AWHONN). (2007). *Universal screening for domestic violence.* Washington, DC: Author.

Association of Women's Health, Obstetric and Neonatal Nurses (AWHONN). (2016). *Position Statement: Access to health care.* Washington, DC: Author.

Barron, M. (2014). Antenatal care. In K. Simpson, & P. Creehan (Eds.), *Perinatal nursing.* Philadelphia, PA: Lippincott Williams & Wilkins.

Bianchi, A. L., Cesario, S. K., & McFarlane, J. (2016). Interrupting intimate partner violence during pregnancy with an effective screening and assessment program. *Journal of Obstetric, Gynecologic & Neonatal Nursing, 45*(4), 579–591.

Blackburn, S. T. (2014). Physiologic changes of pregnancy. In K. Simpson, & P. Creehan (Eds.), *Perinatal nursing.* Philadelphia, PA: Lippincott Williams & Wilkins.

Bodnar, L. M., Siminerio, L. L., Himes, K. P., Hutcheon, J. A., Lash, T. L., Parisi, S. M., & Abrams, B. (2016). Maternal obesity and gestational weight gain are risk factors for infant death. *Obesity, 24*(2), 490–498. doi: 10.1002/oby.21335

Breiding, M., Smith, S., Basile, K. Walters, M., Chen, J., & Merrick, M. (2014). Prevalence and characteristics of sexual violence, stalking, and intimate partner violence victimization—National Intimate Partner and Sexual Violence Survey, United States, 2011. *MMWR Surveillance Summaries, 63*(8), 1–18.

Carter, E. B., Temming, L. A., Akin, J., Fowler, S., Macones, G. A., Colditz, G. A., & Tuuli, M. G. (2016). Group prenatal care compared with traditional prenatal care: A systematic review and meta-analysis. *Obstetrics & Gynecology, 128*(3), 551–561.

Catling, C. J. (2017). Group versus conventional antenatal care for women. *Cochrane Database of Systematic Reviews* (1), doi:10.1002/14651858.CD007622.pub3

Centers for Disease Control and Prevention (CDC). (1992). Recommendations for the use of folic acid to reduce the number of cases of spina bifida and other neural tube defects. *MMWR Recommendations and Reports, 41*(RR-14), 001.

Centers for Disease Control and Prevention (CDC). (2017a). *Zika virus.* Retrieved from www.cdc.gov/zika/pregnancy/index.html.

Centers for Disease Control and Prevention (CDC). (2017b). *Preconception health and health care for men.* Retrieved from www.cdc.gov/pregnancy.html.

Cheng, D., & Horon, I. L. (2010). Intimate-partner homicide among pregnant and postpartum women. *Obstetrics & Gynecology, 115*(6), 181–1186. doi: 10.1097/AOG.0b013e3181de0194

Chisholm, A., & Levine, E. M. (2017). *Routine prenatal care.* DynaMed Plus. Retrieved http://www.dynamed.com/login.aspx?direct=true&site=DynaMed&id=114252

Cunningham, F., Leveno, K., Bloom, S., Song, C., Dashe, J., Hoffman, M., . . . Sheffield, J. (2014). *William's obstetrics* (24th ed.). New York, NY: McGraw-Hill.

Finer, L. B., & Zolna M. R. (2011). Unintended pregnancy in the United States: Incidence and disparities, 2006. *Contraception, 84*(5), 478–485.

Gaillard, R. (2015). Maternal obesity during pregnancy and cardiovascular development and disease in the offspring. *European Journal of Epidemiology, 30*(11), 1141–1152.

Goetzl, L. M. (2017). *Folic acid supplementation in pregnancy.* Retrieved from www.uptodate.com/contents/folic-acid-supplementation-in-pregnancy?source=search_result&search=folic%20acid%20pregnancy&selectedTitle=5-150

Heaman, M., Bayrampour, H., Kingston, D., Blondel, B., Gissler, M., Roth, C., . . . Gagnon, A. (2013). Migrant women's utilization of prenatal care: A systematic review. *Maternal Child Health Journal, 17*, 816. doi:10.1007/s10995-012-1058-z

Institute of Medicine. (2006). *Dietary reference intakes: The essential guide to nutrient requirements.* Washington, DC: National Academies Press.

Institute of Medicine. (2009). *Weight gain during pregnancy: Reexamining the guidelines.* Washington, DC: National Academies Press.

Kahn, D. A., & Hoos, B. J. (2010). Maternal physiology during pregnancy: Introduction. In A. Decherney & L. Nathan (Eds.), *Current Diagnoses and Treatment in Obstetrics and Gynecology.* New York, NY: McGraw-Hill.

Lockwood, C. J., Romero, S. T., &Nielsen-Saines, K. (2017). *Zika virus infection: Evaluation and management of pregnant women.* Retrieved from www.uptodate.com/contents/zika-virus-infection-evaluation-and-management-of-pregnant-women?source=see_link.

Macones, G., Ramin, S. M., & Barss, V. A. (2013). *Weight gain and loss in pregnancy.* Retrieved from www.uptodate.com/contents/weight-gain-and-loss-in-pregnancy?source=see_link#H20254142.

Martin-de-Las-Heras, S., Velasco, C., de Dios Luna, J., & Martin, A. (2015). Unintended pregnancy and intimate partner violence around pregnancy in a population-based study. *Women and Birth, 28*(2), 101–105.

Martin, J. A., Hamilton, B. E., Sutton, P. D., Ventura, S. J., Mathews, T. J., Kimeyer, S., & Osterman, M. J. (2010). Births: Final data for 2007. *National Vital Statistics Reports, 58*(24).

Mattson, S., & Smith, J. (2011). *Core curriculum for maternal-newborn nursing* (4th ed.). St. Louis, MO: Elsevier.

Meehan, S., Beck, C.R., Mair-Jenkins, J., Leonardi-Bee, J., & Puleston, R. (2014). Maternal obesity and infant mortality: A meta-analysis. *Pediatrics, 133*, 863–871.

Ogden, C. L., Carroll, M. D., Fryar, C. D., & Flegal, K. M. (2015). *Prevalence of obesity among adults and youth: United States, 2011–2014.* NCHS data brief, no. 219. Retrieved from www.cdc.gov/nchs/data/databriefs/db219.pdf.

Rotundo, G. (2011). Centering pregnancy: The benefits of group prenatal care. *Nursing for Women's Health, 15*(6), 507–518.

Sackey, J. A. (2017). *The preconception office visit.* Retrieved from www.uptodate.com/contents/the-preconception-office-visit?source=search_result&search=preconception%20care&selectedTitle=1-85.

Soma-Pillay, P., Catherine, N.-P., Tolppanen, H., Mebazaa, A., Tolppanen, H., & Mebazaa, A. (2016). Physiological changes in pregnancy. *Cardiovascular Journal of Africa, 27*(2), 89–94. http://doi.org/10.5830/CVJA-2016-021.

Spong, C. Y. (2013). Defining "term" pregnancy: Recommendations from the Defining "Term" Pregnancy Workgroup. *Journal of the American Medical Association, 309*(23), 2445–2446.

Stang, J., & Huffman, L. G. (2016). Position of the Academy of Nutrition and Dietetics: Obesity, reproduction, and pregnancy outcomes. *Journal of the Academy of Nutrition and Dietetics, 116*(4), 677–691.

Stothard, K. J., Tennant, P. W., Bell, R., & Rankin, J. (2009). Maternal overweight and obesity and the risk of congenital anomalies: A systematic review and meta-analysis. *Journal of the American Medical Association, 301*(6), 636.

Tan, P. C., & Omar, S. Z. (2011). Contemporary approaches to hyperemesis during pregnancy. *Current Opinion in Obstetrics and Gynecology, 23*, 87–93.

Till, S. R. (2015). Incentives for increasing prenatal care use by women in order to improve maternal and neonatal outcomes. *Cochrane Database of Systematic Reviews, 12*, doi:10.1002/14651858.CD009916.pub2.

U.S. Department of Agriculture. (2017). *Health & nutrition information.* Retrieved from www.choosemyplate.gov/moms-pregnancy-breastfeeding.

U.S. Department of Health and Human Services. (2009). *The environment and women's health,* Office on Women's Health in the Department of Health and Human Services.

U.S. Department of Health and Human Services. (2010). *Healthy People 2020,* Office of Disease Prevention and Health Promotion Publication number 80132.

U.S. Department of Justice. (2012). *Office on violence against women.* Retrieved from www..justice.gov/archive/ovw/docs/stop-solicitation-finalversion.pdf

Vallerand, A. H., Sanoski, C. A., & Deglan, J. H. (2017). *Davis's drug guide for nurses* (15th ed.). Philadelphia, PA: F.A. Davis.

Vamos, C. A., Thompson, E. L., Avendano, M., Daley, E. M., Quinonez, R. B., & Boggess, K. (2015). Oral health promotion interventions during pregnancy: A systematic review. *Community Dentistry and Oral Epidemiology, 43*(5), 385–396.

Verbiest, S., McClain, E., & Woodward, S. (2016). Advancing preconception health in the United States: Strategies for change. *Upsala Journal of Medical Sciences, 121*(4), 222–226.

Walsh, J. M., & McAuliffe, F. M. (2015). Impact of maternal nutrition on pregnancy outcome–Does it matter what pregnant women eat? *Best Practice & Research Clinical Obstetrics & Gynaecology, 29*(1), 63–78.

Wilkes, J. (2016). AAFP Releases position paper on preconception care. *American Family Physician, 94*(6), 508.

Winn, A., Hetherington, E., & Tough, S. (2017). Systematic review of immigrant women's experiences with perinatal care in North America. *Journal of Obstetric, Gynecologic & Neonatal Nursing, 46*(5), 764–775.

Wolff, T., Witkop, C. T., Miller, T., & Syed, S. B. (2009). US Preventative Services Task Force. Folic acid supplementation for the prevention of neural tube defects: An update of the evidence for the US Preventative Services Task Force. *Annals of Internal Medicine, 150*(9), 632–639.

World Health Organization (WHO). (2000). Obesity: Preventing and managing the global epidemic. Report of a WHO consultation. Retrieved from www.who.int/nutrition/publications/obesity/WHO_TRS_894/en.

World Health Organization (WHO). (2016). *WHO recommendations on antenatal care for a positive pregnancy experience.* Retrieved from http://apps.who.int/iris/bitstream/10665/250796/1/9789241549912-eng.pdf?ua=1

Zolotor, A. J., & Carlough, M. C. (2014). Update on prenatal care. *American Family Physician, 89*(3), 199–208.

The Psycho-Social-Cultural Aspects of the Antepartum Period

5

Scout Hebinck RNC, MSN

LEARNING OUTCOMES

Upon completion of this chapter, the student will be able to:

1. Describe expected emotional changes of the pregnant woman and appropriate nursing responses to these changes.
2. Identify the major developmental tasks of pregnancy as they relate to maternal, paternal, and family adaptation.
3. Identify critical variables that influence adaptation to pregnancy, including age, parity, and social, cultural, and sexual orientation.
4. Identify nursing assessments and interventions that promote positive psycho-social-cultural adaptations for the pregnant woman and her family.
5. Analyze critical factors in preparing for birth, including choosing a provider and birth setting and creating a birth plan.
6. Identify key components of childbirth preparation education for expectant families.
7. Analyze and critique current evidence-based research in psycho-social-cultural adaptation to pregnancy.

Nursing Diagnoses

- At risk for anxiety and fear related to unknown processes of pregnancy and birth
- Deficient knowledge related to pregnancy psychosocial and emotional changes
- At risk for interrupted family processes related to role changes and developmental stressors in pregnancy
- At risk for ineffective communication related to cultural differences between family and health care providers
- Risk for increased stress and ineffective coping related to inadequate social support during pregnancy
- Risk for inadequate prenatal care related to inaccessible health care second to immigration status and sexual orientation
- Risk for ineffective coping
- Deficient knowledge related to psychosocial and emotional changes in pregnancy
- Readiness for enhanced family processes

Nursing Outcomes

The pregnant woman and her family will:

- Be able to communicate effectively with health care providers.
- Verbalize fears related to anxiety.
- Verbalize appropriate family dynamics.
- Report increasing acceptance of changes in body image.
- Seek clarification of information about pregnancy and birth.
- Demonstrate knowledge regarding expected changes of pregnancy.
- Develop a realistic birth plan and be open to possible changes.
- Exhibit acceptance of roles as parents.
- Identify appropriate support systems.
- Receive positive and effective social support.
- Express satisfaction with health care providers' sensitivity to traditional beliefs and practices of her culture or sexual orientation.

INTRODUCTION

This chapter explores the influence of culture on values and beliefs, the effects of pregnancy on the woman and on members of the immediate and extended family, and variables that influence the woman's adaptation to pregnancy. We explore topics related to patient and family empowerment, along with barriers to culturally competent care and strategies to remove those barriers. We describe how diverse cultural, ethnic, and social backgrounds function as sources of patient, family, and community values, and we explore patient-centered care with sensitivity and respect for the diversity of the human experience. Nursing actions are focused on providing autonomy and choices based on the respect for the woman's preferences, values, and needs. Health promotion, individualized care, and a family-centered approach are all crucial components of nursing care. Patient-centered care is a central concept in maternity nursing. It recognizes the patient or designee as the source of control and full partner in providing compassionate and coordinated care based on respect for patient's preferences, values, and needs.

MATERNAL ADAPTATION TO PREGNANCY

The news of pregnancy confers profound and irrevocable changes in a woman's life and the lives of those around her. With this news, the woman begins her journey toward becoming a mother. Less visible than the physical adaptations of pregnancy but just as profound are the pregnant woman's psychological adaptations and development of her identity as a mother. These are crucial aspects of the childbearing cycle. Psychological, cultural, and social variables all significantly influence this process. Psychosocial support for the pregnant woman and her family is a distinct and major nursing responsibility during the antepartum period. This chapter presents the expected emotional changes a woman and her family must navigate to achieve a positive adaptation to pregnancy. Factors influencing these changes are also described.

Successful adaptation to the maternal role requires important psychological work. Although becoming a mother has been noted to occur on a long-term continuum, the psychological groundwork is laid during the course of each woman's individual experience during pregnancy. The pregnant woman is able to use the 9 months available to her to restructure her psychological and cognitive self toward motherhood. Motherhood, an irrevocable change in a woman's life, progressively becomes part of a woman's total identity (Koniak-Griffin, Logsdon, Hines-Martin, & Turner, 2006; Mercer, 1995, 2004).

Maternal Tasks of Pregnancy

Maternal tasks of pregnancy were first identified in the psychoanalytic literature (Bibring, Dwyer, Huntington, & Valenstein, 1961), then further explored and outlined by classic maternity nurse researchers Reva Rubin, Ramona Mercer, and Regina Lederman. Rubin's research has provided a framework and core knowledge base for researchers and clinicians. She identified these significant maternal tasks women undergo during the course of pregnancy (1975, 1984):

- Ensuring a safe passage for herself and her child: the mother's knowledge and care-seeking behaviors to ensure that both she and the newborn emerge from pregnancy healthy.
- Ensuring social acceptance of the child by significant others: the woman's engagement of her family and social network in the pregnancy.
- Attaching or "binding-in" to the child: the development of maternal-fetal attachment.
- Giving of oneself to the demands of motherhood: the mother's willingness and efforts to make personal sacrifices for the child.

Building on Rubin's work, Regina Lederman (1996; Lederman & Weis, 2009) identified seven dimensions of maternal role development: acceptance of the pregnancy, identification with the motherhood role, relationship to her mother, reordering partner relationships, preparation for labor, prenatal fear of losing control in labor, and prenatal fear of losing self-esteem in labor.

Acceptance of the Pregnancy

This task focuses on the woman's adaptive responses to the changes related to pregnancy growth and development (Lederman, 1996):

- Responding to mood changes
- Responding to ambivalent feelings
- Responding to nausea, fatigue, and other physical discomforts of the early months of pregnancy
- Responding to financial concerns
- Responding to increased dependency needs

Expected findings include:

- Desire for and/or acceptance of pregnancy.
- Predominately happy feelings during pregnancy.
- Little physical discomfort or a high tolerance for the discomfort.
- Acceptance of body changes.
- Minimal ambivalent feelings and conflict regarding pregnancy by the end of her pregnancy.
- A dislike of being pregnant but a feeling of love for the unborn child.

CRITICAL COMPONENT

Ambivalent Feelings Toward Pregnancy

It is common for women to experience ambivalent feelings toward pregnancy during the first trimester. These feelings decrease as pregnancy progresses. Ambivalence that continues into the third trimester may indicate unresolved conflict. When evaluating ambivalence, it is important to assess the reason for the ambivalence and its intensity.

Identification With the Motherhood Role

Accomplishment of this task is influenced by the woman's acceptance of pregnancy and the relationship she has with her own mother. Women who have accepted their pregnancy and who have a positive relationship with their own mothers more easily accomplish this task (Lederman, 1996). Accomplishment of this task is also influenced by the woman's degree of fears about labor, such as helplessness, pain, loss of control, and loss of self-esteem (Lederman, 1996). Vivid dreams are common during pregnancy, allowing the woman to envision herself as a mother in various situations. A woman often rehearses or pictures herself in her new role in different scenarios (Rubin, 1975). The motherhood role is progressively strengthened as she attaches to the fetus. Fetal attachment influences the woman's sense of her child and her sense of being competent as a mother. Events that facilitate fetal attachment include:

- Hearing the fetal heartbeat.
- Seeing the fetus move during an ultrasound examination.
- Feeling the fetus kick or move.

Expected findings:

- Moves from viewing herself as a woman-without-child to a woman-with-child
- Anticipates changes motherhood will bring to her life
- Seeks company of other pregnant women
- Is highly motivated to assume the motherhood role
- Actively prepares for the motherhood role

Relationship to Her Mother

A woman's relationship with her mother is an important determinant of adaptation to motherhood. Unresolved mother-daughter conflicts reemerge and can confront women during pregnancy (Lederman, 1996). Four components important to the woman's relationship with her own mother are:

- Availability of the woman's mother to her in the past and in the present.
- The mother's reaction to her daughter's pregnancy.
- The mother's relationship to her daughter.
- The mother's willingness to reminisce with her daughter about her own childbirth and child-rearing experiences.

Expected findings:

- The woman's mother was available to her in the past and continues to be available during the pregnancy (Fig. 5–1).
- The woman's mother accepts the pregnancy, respects her autonomy, and acknowledges her daughter becoming a mother.
- The woman's mother relates to her daughter as an adult versus as a child.
- The woman's mother reminisces about her own childbearing and child-rearing experiences.

Reordering Partner Relationships

Pregnancy has a dramatic effect on a couple's relationship. Some couples view pregnancy and childbirth as a growth experience and an expression of deep commitment to their bond, while

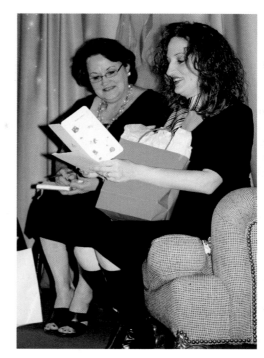

FIGURE 5–1 Pregnant woman and her mother participating in baby shower.

others view it as an added stressor to a relationship already in conflict. The partner's support during pregnancy enhances the woman's feelings of well-being and is associated with earlier and continuous prenatal care (Lederman, 1996; Lederman & Weis, 2009). A woman's partner is the fundamental and natural source of social support, favorably influencing the emotional state of pregnancy. This emotional support is manifested by caring, understanding, empathy, and generation of positive feelings in the supported person (Skurzak, 2015). There is mounting evidence that fathers and partners are influential in maternal psychological variables and smoking behavior during pregnancy (Cheng et al., 2016).

Assessment of the couple's relationship includes:

- The partner's concern for the woman's needs during pregnancy.
- The woman's concerns for her partner's needs during pregnancy.
- The varying desire for sexual activity among pregnant women.
- The effect pregnancy has on the relationship (e.g., whether it brings them closer together or causes conflict).
- The partner's adjustment to his or her new role.

Expected findings include the following:

- The partner is understanding and supportive of the woman.
- The partner is thoughtful and "pampers" the woman during pregnancy.
- The partner is involved in the pregnancy.
- The woman perceives that her partner is supportive.
- The woman is concerned about her partner's needs of making emotional adjustments to the pregnancy and new role.

- Women in relationships with established open communication about sexuality are likely to have less difficulty with changes in sexual activity.
- Couples indicate that they are growing closer to each other during pregnancy.
- The partner is happy and excited about the pregnancy and prepares for the new role.

Preparation for Labor

Preparation for labor means preparing for the physiological processes of labor as well as the psychological processes of separating from the fetus and becoming a mother to the child. Preparation for labor and birth occur through taking classes, reading, fantasizing, and dreaming about labor and birth (Lederman, 1996; Lederman & Wies, 2009). The degree of preparation for labor and birth affect the woman's level of anxiety and fear. The more prepared she feels, the lower her level of anxiety and fear.

Expected findings:

- The woman attends childbirth classes and reads books and online resources about labor and birth.
- The woman uses smartphone applications to track her pregnancy and growing fetus.
- The woman mentally rehearses (fantasizes) the labor and birthing process.
- The woman has dreams about labor and birth and works with her partner or birthing coach to develop a birth plan.
- The woman develops realistic expectations of labor and birth.
- The pregnant woman may engage in a flurry of activity known as "nesting behavior," hurrying to finish preparing for the newborn's arrival.

Prenatal Fear of Losing Control in Labor

Loss of control includes two factors (Lederman 1996; Lederman & Wies, 2009): loss of control over the body and loss of control over emotions. The degree of fear is related to:

- The woman's degree of trust with the medical and nursing staff, her partner, and other support persons.
- The woman's attitude regarding the use of medication and anesthesia for labor pain management.

Expected findings:

- The woman perceives individual attention from medical staff.
- The woman perceives that she is being treated as an adult and her questions and concerns are addressed by the medical staff.
- The woman perceives that the nursing staff is compassionate, empathetic, and available.
- The woman perceives that she is being supported by her partner and family/friends.
- The woman has realistic expectations regarding management of labor pain and these expectations are met.

Prenatal Fear of Losing Self-Esteem in Labor

Some women have fears that they will lose self-esteem in labor and "fail" during labor. When a woman feels a threat to her self-esteem, it is important to assess the following areas (Lederman & Weis, 2009):

- The source of the threat
- The response to the threat
- The intensity of the reaction to the threat

Behaviors that reflect self-esteem are:

- Tolerance of self.
- Value of self and assertiveness, and decisions about her labor process.
- Positive attitude regarding body image and appearance.

Expected findings include the ability to:

- Develop realistic expectations of self during labor and birth and have an awareness of risks and potential complications.
- Identify and respect her own feelings.
- Assert herself in acquiring information needed to make decisions.
- Recognize her own needs and limitations.
- Adjust to the unexpected and unknown.
- Recover from threats quickly.
- Verbalize fears and concerns.

As the woman prepares to experience labor, give birth, and take on the maternal role, the process of maternal adaptation to pregnancy is potentially completed. With the dominating physical discomforts of the third trimester, most women become impatient for labor to begin. There is relief and excitement about going into labor. The mother is ready and eager to deliver and hold her baby. She has prepared for her future as a mother (Rubin, 1984).

Nursing Actions

During the antepartal period, the nurse can take on a variety of roles: teacher, counselor, clinician, resource person, and role model. Nursing actions should be focused on health promotion, individualized care, and prevention of individual and family crises and are highlighted in the critical component nursing actions that facilitate adaptation to pregnancy (Lederman & Weis, 2009; Mattson & Smith, 2016).

Factors That Influence Maternal Adaptation

The ability of the woman to adapt to the maternal role is influenced by a variety of factors, including parity, maternal age, sexual orientation, single parenting, multiple gestation (twins, triples), socioeconomic factors, cultural beliefs, and history of abuse.

Multiparity

- Multigravidas may have the benefit of experience, but it should not be assumed that they need less help than a first-time mother. They know more of what to expect in terms of pain during labor, postpartum adaptation, and the many added responsibilities of motherhood, but they may need time to process and develop strategies for integrating a new member into the family.

● Pregnancy tasks may be more complex. Giving adequate attention to all of her children and supporting sibling adaptation are unique challenges faced by the multigravida. She may spend a great deal of time working out a new relationship with the first child and grieve for the loss of their special relationship. She also has to consider the financial issues associated with feeding, clothing, and providing for another child while at the same time maintaining a relationship with her partner and continuing her career, whether inside or outside the home (Jordan, 1989).

Maternal Age

Mothers who give birth at an older or younger than average age face unique circumstances and challenges.

Adolescent Mothers

Adolescence is a period of accelerated growth and change that bridges the complex transition from childhood to adulthood. The second decade of life is often a turbulent period in which adolescents experience hormonal changes, physical maturation, and, frequently, opportunities to engage in risk behaviors. The patterns of behavior they adopt may have long-term consequences for their health and quality of life. Because of the rapid physical, cognitive, and emotional developments that take place during this age period, adolescence is also a time when many health problems may first emerge. Moreover, adolescents also experience special vulnerabilities, health concerns, and barriers to accessing health care (MacKay & Duran, 2007).

Definitions of adolescence and the years encompassed vary. Adolescence is generally regarded as the period of life from puberty to maturity, the meanings of which are often debated by health professionals. Many children begin puberty by the age of 10, although there is considerable individual variation in the developmental and maturation timeline. During their teenage years, adolescents are learning financial, social, and personal independence, and they are expected to become capable of adult behaviors and responses.

Although birth rates for adolescents are decreasing and the reasons for the declines are not totally clear, evidence suggests these declines are due to more teens abstaining from sexual activity, and more teens who are sexually active using birth control than in previous years (Lindberg, Santelli, & Desai, 2016). Teen pregnancy and childbearing bring substantial social and economic costs through immediate and long-term impacts on teen parents and their children. Adolescents who have an unintended pregnancy face a number of challenges, including abandonment by their partners, increased adverse pregnancy outcomes, and inability to complete school education, which may ultimately limit their future social and economic opportunities (CDC, 2017a). For example, data indicates only about 50% of teen mothers receive a high school diploma by 22 years of age, whereas approximately 90% of women who do not give birth during adolescence graduate from high school (Perper, Peterson, & Manlove, 2010).

The major developmental task of adolescence is to form and become comfortable with a sense of self. Pregnancy presents a challenge for teenagers who must cope with the conflicting developmental tasks of pregnancy and adolescence at the same time. Achieving a maternal identity is very difficult for an adolescent who is in the throes of evolving her own identity as an adult capable of psychosocial independence from her family. Although she may achieve the maternal role, research indicates that she may function at a lower level of competence than would an older woman (Mercer, 2004).

In addition, the younger the adolescent is, the more difficulty she will have with body image changes, as well as acknowledging the pregnancy, seeking health care, and planning for the changes that pregnancy and parenting will bring. Delayed entry into prenatal care is common. There is also a higher rate of abuse among pregnant adolescents (Porter & Holness, 2011). Teten, Ball, Valle, Noonan, and Rosenbluth (2009) reviewed the prevalence rates of adolescent victimization and the prevalence of dating violence victimization for girls to be between 10% and 30% (Sutherland, 2011). Additionally, they reported that adolescent girls experiencing violence in a dating relationship were 4 to 6 times more likely than their nonabused peers to have been pregnant and 8 to 9 times more likely to have attempted suicide in the past year (Sutherland, 2011).

One contributor to a successful outcome of adolescent pregnancy is assured confidentiality with health care providers. The Association of Women's Health, Obstetric and Neonatal Nurses (AWHONN) encourages the establishment of interdisciplinary educational initiatives that will increase health care providers' competency in delivering effective and confidential adolescent health care (AWHONN, 2009).

Partner support is another important factor in maternal and infant health for adolescents. Studies show lack of partner support or poor relationships with partners during pregnancy and postpartum is associated with negative maternal behaviors, adverse emotional health, and low birth weight (Smith, Buzi, Kozinetz, Peskin, & Wiemann, 2016). In a national sample of women and girls aged 10 to 19 years who experienced pregnancy, data indicate lack of partner support was associated with adverse birth outcomes. Even after adjusting for key confounding factors, pregnancy loss and low birth weight remained lower in the group with higher partner support. Teens with partner support were less likely to have a preterm birth than those without support from the partner, although this difference was not statistically significant (Shah, Gee, & Theall, 2014). Successful adaptation to pregnancy and parenthood may greatly depend on the age of the adolescent (Fig. 5–2).

● Comprehensive and community-based health care programs for adolescents are effective in improving outcomes for the teen mother and her infant (CDC, 2017a). Examples include programs that have been implemented in schools, clinics, community agencies, or home visitation programs. Additionally, higher levels of support and higher self-esteem are associated with a more positive adaptation to mothering

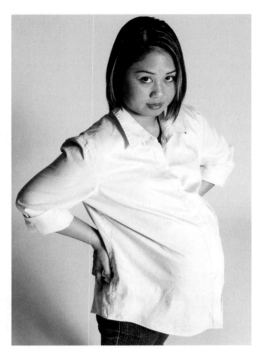

FIGURE 5–2 Pregnant adolescent.

births. In women older than 40, the risk increases for placenta previa, placenta abruptio, caesarean deliveries, preeclampsia, and gestational diabetes. In fact, 48.4% of babies born from women over the age of 40 are delivered by caesarean section (Martin, Hamilton, Osterman, Driscoll, & Mathews, 2017).

The more mature woman is better equipped psychosocially to assume the maternal role than women in younger age groups. However, she also might have increased difficulty with the changing roles in her life, experiencing heightened ambivalence. She might have difficulty balancing a career with the physical and psychological demands of pregnancy. The unpredictable nature of pregnancy, labor, and life with a newborn may challenge a woman who has developed a predictable, controlled life (Carolan, 2005; Dobrzykowski & Stern, 2003; Schardt, 2005). Older mothers are more commonly from a higher socioeconomic background and have a more extensive education. They are more likely to be established in their career, their relationships, and their lifestyles. Pregnancy is often chosen and planned. Sometimes it culminates after infertility treatments and may involve extensive use of reproductive technologies. Pregnant women in this age group are highly motivated to seek information about childbirth and parenting from books, friends, electronic resources, mommy groups, and smartphone applications.

for adolescents (Key, Gebregziabher, Marsh, & O'Rourke, 2008; Logsdon, Gagne, Hughes, Patterson, & Rakestraw, 2005; Porter & Holness, 2011; Schaffer, Jost, Pederson, & Lair, 2008).

- Early adolescence is defined as the period between ages 11 and 13 years. Adolescents in this phase of life are self-centered and oriented toward the present. Additionally, there is a greater likelihood that pregnancy at this age is a result of abuse or coercion. Moving into the maternal role is a difficult challenge for this age group. Grandmothers will play a significant role in caring for the infant as well as providing guidance to their daughter regarding mothering skills (Mercer, 1995; Pinazo-Hernandis & Tompkins, 2009).
- Middle adolescence is defined as the period between 14 and 18 years. During this time, the adolescent will be more capable of abstract thinking and understanding consequences of current behaviors.
- By age 19 to 20, as adolescents mature into late adolescence, these skills will be further developed and eventually mastered. The older pregnant adolescent is more likely to be a capable and active participant in health care decisions (DeVito, 2010).

Older Mothers

In North America, an increasing number of women have delayed childbearing until after age 35. Most women in this age group deliver at term without adverse outcomes. However, even with good prenatal care, there is an increased incidence of adverse perinatal outcomes. Chronic diseases that are more common in women over 35 may affect the pregnancy. Older mothers are also more likely to have miscarriages, fetal chromosomal abnormalities, low birth weight infants, premature births, and multiple

CRITICAL COMPONENT

Nursing Actions That Facilitate Adaptation to Pregnancy
First Trimester

- Begin psychosocial assessment at initial contact; assess woman's response to pregnancy; assess stressors in woman's life. This allows the nurse to identify issues that may require referrals and begin developing the plan of care.
- Promote pregnancy and birth as a family experience; encourage family and father or partner participation in prenatal visits; encourage questions from father and family members about the pregnancy. It is important to offer an inclusive model of care that acknowledges the needs of the family as well as the individual. Pregnancy significantly affects all family members. Meeting with family members provides additional information to the nurse and helps complete the family assessment. Positive family support is associated with positive maternal adaptation.
- Assess learning needs. This allows the nurse to provide individualized information.
- Offer anticipatory guidance regarding normal developmental stressors of pregnancy, such as ambivalence during early pregnancy, feelings of vulnerability, mood changes, and active dream/fantasy life. This allows the nurse to emphasize normalcy, health, universality, strengths, and developmental concepts, to decrease anxiety.
- Assess for increased anxieties and fear; if anxieties seem greater than normal, refer to psych care provider. Excessive anxiety, stress, and prenatal depression have a negative

impact on a woman's pregnancy and affect the physiology of the developing fetus. Specialized intervention is needed.

- Listen, validate, provide reassurance, and teach expected emotional changes. Educate partner and family members, and stress normalcy of feelings to decrease anxiety and ensure the woman feels "heard" and validated.
- If appropriate, discuss common phases through which expectant fathers progress through pregnancy. Be aware of phases of paternal adaptation when counseling parents about expected changes of pregnancy; provide anticipatory guidance regarding potential communication conflicts. This will acknowledge the partner as a significant participant in the pregnancy process and assist in improving communication and decreasing stress in the relationship.

Second Trimester

- Encourage verbalization of possible grief process during pregnancy related to body image changes, loss of old life, changing relationships with family and friends. The woman may be more anxious about body changes in the second trimester. She may begin to have fears or phobias. The nurse needs to acknowledge and validate the woman's feelings and help her work toward resolving any conflicting feelings.
- Discuss normal changes in sexual activity and provide information and acknowledge the woman's sexuality.
- Encourage "tuning in" to fetal movements; discuss fetal capacities for hearing, responding to interaction, and maternal activity. This will encourage the attachment process and help empower the woman with increased involvement in care.
- Reinforce to partner and family the importance of giving the expectant mother extra support; give specific examples of ways to help (e.g., helping her eat well, helping with heavy work, giving extra attention). This will encourage family and partner participation in the pregnancy process and promote support for the woman. A well-supported woman will likely have a more positive adaptation to pregnancy.

Third Trimester

- Encourage attendance at childbirth classes to promote knowledge and decrease fears. Childbirth education can give women the information they need to make informed decisions, such as educational information on the risks and benefits of vaginal delivery and cesarean delivery. Further, childbirth education can ensure that women from all population groups understand the relative risks and benefits of their choices, empowering them to make informed decisions regarding birthing options.
- Discuss preparations for birth, parenthood; explore expectations of labor. The woman will begin to focus more on the impending birth during the third trimester, and her learning needs will be more focused on this area. It is important to provide anticipatory information and guidance.
- Assess partner's comfort level with labor coach role and reassure as needed; stress that help in labor will be available; encourage presence of second support person if

appropriate. The woman's partner may not feel comfortable providing labor support, and it is important to discuss prior to the onset of labor so all roles can be clarified.

- Refer to appropriate educational materials on parenthood. Encourage discussions of plans, expectations with partner. Give anticipatory guidance regarding the realities of infant care, breastfeeding, and so on. This will promote communication and planning with the expectant parents, as well as a positive transition to parenthood.
- If psychosocial complications develop, plan for appropriate referrals to coordinate with social workers, nutritionist, and community agencies to ensure continuity of psychosocial assessment and provide appropriate support during the woman's pregnancy.
- Help expectant mother identify and use support systems to promote positive adaptation to pregnancy, birth, and postpartum; anticipate the need for postpartum support; and decrease the risk of postpartum depression.

(Lederman & Weis, 2009; Mattson & Smith, 2016; McCants & Greiner, 2016; Simpson & Creehan, 2014)

Lesbian Mothers

Little research has been conducted on the process of maternal adaptation to pregnancy in lesbian women. Although the developmental tasks of pregnancy are likely to be similar, the lesbian woman may face unique obstacles and challenges in today's health care environment. *Healthy People 2020* has added new objectives relating to improving the health, safety, and well-being of lesbian, gay, bisexual, and transgender individuals (HHS, 2010a).

- Lesbian women may be more likely to lack social support, particularly from their families of origin. They may be exposed to additional stress due to homophobic attitudes, particularly from the health care system. Unlike their heterosexual counterparts, the journey of lesbians to parenthood may consist of several unique steps (Wojnar & Katzenmeyer, 2014).
- Finding supportive health care providers with whom they are comfortable disclosing sexual orientation is an important need identified by lesbian women (Fig. 5–3). Heteronormative health care environments in which parents are assumed to be a man and a woman can present barriers to care for all same-sex couples. The role of the woman's partner and legal considerations of the growing family will also affect the lesbian experience of pregnancy (McManus, Hunter, & Renn, 2006; Rondahl, Bruhner, & Lindhe, 2009; Ross, 2005).
- Lesbian mothers most commonly plan their pregnancies, conceiving through donor insemination. In addition, it has been observed that many lesbian couples participate in a relatively equal division of child care. These factors can combine to help decrease the stress a lesbian mother might experience and act as protection from perinatal depression (Ross, 2005). According to Baetens and Brewayes (2001) and Wojnar (2007), many lesbian couples begin the process with negotiations about which partner will fill the role of the biological parent. The decision is usually influenced by age,

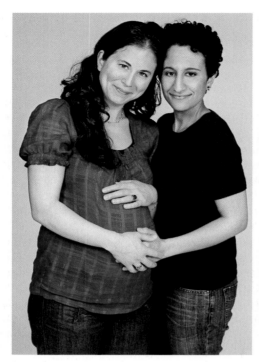

FIGURE 5–3 Lesbian pregnant couple.

desire for pregnancy, reproductive health, and security of employment (Bos, Van Balen, & Van den Boom, 2004, 2007; Renaud 2007; Wojnar & Katzenmeyer, 2014).

● Nursing assessments of lesbian women should be adapted accordingly. Nurses need to strive toward using inclusive language and avoid making assumptions about a woman's gender orientation without further information. Birth partners who are not the biological fathers experience the same fears, questions, and concerns. Birth partners need to be kept informed, supported, and included in all activities in which the mother desires their participation. To date, researchers who explored the roles of lesbian nonbiological mothers (also known as *lesbian comothers* or *social mothers*) focused on how these women sought to legitimize and formalize their roles and positions within the family (Wojnar & Katzenmeyer, 2014). Researchers have identified some similarities between lesbian nonbiological mothers and new fathers; however, they noted that lesbian nonbiological mothers did not receive the same level of societal support and recognition as fathers (Goldberg & Sayer, 2006; Wojnar & Katzenmeyer, 2014). They also reported feelings of jealousy related to perceptions of unequal ties to the children and desire to carry children themselves.

Single Parenting

The literature reports a higher degree of stress for pregnant single women, such as greater anxiety and less tangible reliable support from family and friends (Simpson & Creehan, 2014).

● Single mothers may live at or below the poverty level, facing greater financial challenges, resulting in a higher risk of

depression. With the initial news, many women must decide whether or not to proceed with the pregnancy. Single women engage in the maternal tasks of pregnancy and face more complex tasks and a variety of challenges:
  ● Telling the family may cause concern.
  ● Issues regarding legal guardianship in the event she is incapacitated must be considered.
  ● Deciding whether to put the father's name on the birth certificate.
● Some single mothers are financially stable and have well-established careers.
● The reasons surrounding the pregnancy and the presence or absence of strong support persons can significantly influence the woman's adaptation (Beeber & Canuso, 2005). Initial assessments are crucial for providing appropriate care and possible resources she may or may not need:
  ● Is the woman single by choice? Did she decide later in her life that she wanted a family unit? Or did she decide on her own she wanted to raise a baby herself?
  ● Is she a single mother by accident (e.g., death of partner following conception, separation, divorce)?
  ● Did she get pregnant by a casual acquaintance? Or a partner they are not married to and do not live with?

Multigestational Pregnancy

A multiple gestation pregnancy (twins, triples, etc.) places added psychosocial stressors on the family unit. The diagnosis shocks many expectant parents, who may need additional support and education to help them cope with the changes they face. The increased risk for adverse outcomes results in increased fears and anxieties for the pregnant woman.

● If the woman is found to be carrying more than three fetuses, the parents may receive counseling regarding selective reduction of the pregnancies to reduce the incidence of premature birth and allow the remaining fetuses to grow to term gestation.
● This situation poses an ethical dilemma and emotional strain for many parents, particularly if they have been attempting to achieve pregnancy for a lengthy time (Begley, 2000; Collopy, 2004; Damato, 2003; Maifeld, Hahn, Titler, Marita, & Mullen, 2003).

Socioeconomic Factors

The resources of the family to meet the needs for food, shelter, and health care play a crucial role in how its members respond to pregnancy. Health equity is achieved when everyone has an equal opportunity to reach his or her health potential regardless of social position or other characteristics such as race, ethnicity, gender, religion, sexual identity, or disability. Health inequities are closely linked with social determinants of health—conditions in the environments in which people are born, live, learn, work, play, worship, and age. These affect a wide range of health, functioning, and quality-of-life outcomes and risks. Certain social determinants, such as high unemployment, low education, and low income, have been associated with higher teen birth rates.

Interventions that address socioeconomic conditions like these can play a critical role in addressing disparities observed in U.S. birth rates and outcomes (CDC, 2017a).

● Financial barriers have been identified as the one of the most important factors contributing to maternal inability to receive adequate prenatal care.
● Homelessness plays a vital role in accessibility to health care, consistency in attending scheduled appointments, and receiving care after birth and beyond.
● Immigrant women face significant economic barriers. Women in this group are often marginalized, and many may work in low-income service-oriented jobs. Access to health care is often limited (Jentsch, Durham, Hundley, & Hussein, 2007; Meleis, 2003).
● The elimination of these health care disparities resulting from low income has been noted as one of the major goals of *Healthy People 2020* (HHS, 2010a).

Women Who Are Abused

Pregnancy is often a trigger for beginning or increased abuse or intimate partner violence (see Chapters 4 and 7). Abuse, whether emotional or physical, crosses all racial, ethnic, and economic lines. Abuse often gets worse during pregnancy. According to the March of Dimes, almost 1 in 6 pregnant women have been abused by a partner (March of Dimes, 2017). Pregnancy offers a unique opportunity for health care providers to recognize abuse and to intervene appropriately. Nurses must screen all pregnant women for abuse.

Military Deployment

Military deployment can significantly influence adaptation to pregnancy. Thousands of women of childbearing age are serving in the U.S. military and are being deployed. Overall, 15% of Department of Defense active-duty military personnel are women, up from 11% in 1990. In 2015, 17% of active-duty officers were female, up from their share of 12% in 1990. And 15% of enlisted personnel were female in 2015, up from 11% in 1990 (Parker, Cilluffo, & Stepler, 2017). Although women have traditionally been excluded from serving in direct combat roles in the military, they serve in positions that put them in the direct line of fire and may cause significant stress (e.g., convoy driver, patrol). Military life presents many challenging obstacles, including deployments, moves, separation from family, and possibly life as a single parent. These events can create added stressors on soon-to-be mothers (Recame, 2013).

● For women veterans, pregnancy can exacerbate mental health conditions (Mattocks et al., 2010).
● Women with deployed partners may also have more difficulty with accepting the pregnancy and experience greater conflict. Evidence shows, however, that on-base community support can have a positive effect on pregnancy acceptance for these women (Weis, Lederman, Lilly, & Schaffer, 2008; Weis & Ryan, 2012).
● The Centering Pregnancy model of care, implemented at various military treatment facilities, also shows promise for offering effective group support for military women and their spouses (Foster, Alviar, Neumeier, & Wootten, 2012).

Evidence-Based Practice: Women in the Military

Katon, J., Lewis, L., Hercinovic, S., McNab, A., Fortney, J., & Rose, S. (2017). Improving perinatal mental health care for women veterans: Description of a quality improvement program. *Maternal Child Health, 21*(8), 1598–1605.

Little is known about mental health problems or treatment among pregnant women veterans. Veterans may experience significant stress during military service that can have lingering effects. A quality improvement project was conducted in a single Veterans Administration (VA) health care system between 2012 and 2015. It included a screen for depressive symptoms (using the Edinburgh Postnatal Depression Scale three times during the perinatal period), a dedicated maternity care coordinator, an on-site clinical social worker, and an on-site OB/GYN. Information on prior mental health diagnosis was collected. The prevalence of perinatal depressive symptoms and receipt of mental health care among those with such symptoms are reported by the presence of a pre-pregnancy mental health diagnosis. Of the 199 women who used VA maternity benefits between 2012 and 2015, 56% had at least one pre-pregnancy mental health diagnosis. Compared to those without a pre-pregnancy mental health diagnosis, those with such a diagnosis were more likely to be screened for perinatal depressive symptoms at least once (61.5% vs. 46.8%). Prevalence of depressive symptoms was 46.7% among those with a pre-pregnancy mental health diagnosis and 19.2% among those without. Improving perinatal mental health care for women veterans requires a multidisciplinary approach, including on-site integrated mental health care.

Nursing Actions

● Assess adaptation to pregnancy at every prenatal visit. Early assessment and intervention may prevent or greatly reduce later problems for the pregnant woman and her family.
● Identify areas of concern, validate major issues, and make suggestions for possible changes.
● Refer to the appropriate member of the health care team and follow up.
● Establish a trusting relationship, as women may be reluctant to share information until one has been formed (e.g., questions asked at the first prenatal visit bear repeating with ongoing prenatal care).
● Assess for the need for psychotropic medications and determine if any were used in the past and were effective.
● Use psychosocial health assessment screening tools.
  ● A variety of screening tools can be used to assess adaptation to pregnancy and to identify risk factors. Psychosocial assessment reported in the literature ranges from a few questions asked by the health care provider to questionnaires and risk screening tools focusing on a specific area such as depression or abuse (Beck, 2002; Carroll et al., 2005; Midmer, Carroll, Bryanton, & Stewart, 2002; Priest, Austin, & Sullivan, 2006).
  ● The Antenatal Psychosocial Health Assessment (ALPHA) form, developed in Ontario, Canada, is a useful evidence-based prenatal tool that can identify women who would benefit from additional support and intervention (Box 5–1) (Carroll et al., 2005; Midmer et al., 2002).

BOX 5-1 | Antenatal Psychosocial Health Assessment (ALPHA)

The Antenatal Psychosocial Health Assessment is an evidence-based prenatal tool that can help providers identify women who would benefit from additional support and intervention. This tool assesses the following areas:

- Social support
- Recent stressful life events
- Couple's relationship
- Onset of prenatal care
- Plans for prenatal education
- Feelings toward pregnancy after 20 weeks
- Relationship with parents in childhood
- Self-esteem
- History or psychiatric/emotional problems
- Depression in this pregnancy
- Alcohol/drug use
- Family violence

Carroll et al., 2005.

PATERNAL ADAPTATION DURING PREGNANCY

The news of a pregnancy has a profound effect on the male partner. Men have fears, questions, and concerns regarding the pregnancy, their partner, and the transition to fatherhood. Each father brings to pregnancy a unique history of his childhood that informs his own fatherhood experience. Some relish the role and look forward to actively nurturing a child. Others may be more detached or even hostile to the idea of fatherhood.

Fathers' Participation

Changing cultural and professional attitudes have encouraged the father's participation in the birth experience. Some fathers respond well to this expectation, wishing to explore every aspect of pregnancy, childbirth, and parenting (May, 1980). Others are more task-oriented and view themselves as managers. They may direct the woman's diet and rest periods and act as coaches during childbirth but remain detached from the emotional aspects of the experience. Some are more comfortable as observers and prefer not to participate. In some cultures, pregnancy and childbirth are viewed as exclusively a woman's domain, and fathers may be removed from the experience completely. In high-risk populations, increased paternal involvement can potentially improve birth outcomes, reduce health care disparities, and increase positive maternal behaviors. Fatherhood initiatives and employment assistance are examples of programs that can promote paternal involvement

(Alio et al., 2011; Alio, Salihu, Komosky, Richman, & Marty, 2010; Misra, Caldwell, Young, & Abelson, 2010).

Effect of Pregnancy on Fathers

An expectant father may have increased concern about his partner's well-being and worry about whether they will be good parents. A current metasynthesis of research into fatherhood revealed common themes, including reports that all expectant fathers voiced some form of anxiety/worry in response to their partner's pregnancy; this was the single most powerfully shared experience. Worry appeared to be a normal cognitive process, with many men expressing worries over the health of their partner and unborn baby. Men talked about experiencing conflicting feelings in response to finding out they were going to become fathers, spanning the entire spectrum of emotions from joy to disappointment.

Men enter into the unknown realm of pregnancy with certain expectations of how they should think and feel; these expectations are imposed by oneself and by societal attitudes of male hegemony. Internal conflict arises when there seems to be a discrepancy between how men are expected to feel and how they actually feel. During the pregnancy, men can feel that their needs are neglected and their role underutilized. Unintentional stress may be caused by the way in which antenatal services are delivered and the attitudes of health professionals. Research on fathers in the second trimester revealed expectant fathers started to accept the pregnancy as real when they started to see evidence of the pregnancy in their partner's body, which was catalyzed by seeing and feeling the movements of their unborn baby. Consequently, they were able to relate to their unborn baby and pregnancy experience in a different way and started to develop an emotional attachment to their unborn baby. Toward the end stages of the pregnancy, men move away, both socially and psychologically, from their lives as non-parents and redefine themselves as fathers (Kowlessar, Fox, & Wittkowski, 2015).

- Increased emphasis on his role as provider causes a reevaluation of lifestyle and job or career status.
  - There may be anxiety about providing financial stability for his growing family.
- Changes in relationships and roles will challenge expectant fathers, creating the potential for distancing from their partners.
  - There may be a higher risk for infidelities and abuse. Abuse may begin or escalate with the news of pregnancy.
- With the focus of prenatal care on the woman and the growing fetus, the man may struggle at times to feel that he is relevant in the pregnancy (Widarsson, Kerstis, Sundquist, Engström, & Sarkadi, 2012).
- Some fathers are without models to assist them in taking on the role of active and involved parent (Genesoni & Tallandini, 2009; Hanson, Hunter, Bormann, & Sobo, 2009).
- Men may experience pregnancy-like symptoms and discomforts similar to those of their pregnant partner, such as nausea, weight gain, or abdominal pains. This is referred to as Couvade syndrome (Brennan, Ayers, Ahmed, &

Marshall-Lucette, 2007), or sympathetic pregnancy. The partner may experience minor weight gain, altered hormone levels, morning nausea, and disturbed sleep patterns.

Paternal Developmental Tasks

Paternal adaptation involves unique developmental tasks for fathers (Table 5–1). May's classic research (1982) on men identified three phases that fathers experience as the pregnancy progresses:

1. The announcement phase: Men may react to the news of pregnancy with joy, distress, or a combination of emotions, depending on whether the pregnancy is planned or unwanted.
2. The moratorium phase: During this phase, many men appear to put conscious thought of the pregnancy aside for some time, even as their partners are undergoing dramatic physical and emotional changes right before their eyes.
3. The focusing phase: This phase begins in the last trimester. Men will be actively involved in the pregnancy and their

relationship with the child. These experiences unfold concurrently but in a distinctly different manner than the pregnant woman's adaptive experience.

Nursing Actions

- Explore the man's response to news of pregnancy.
- Reassure that ambivalence is common in the early months of pregnancy.
- Reassure normalcy of pregnancy-like symptoms (Couvade syndrome).
- Encourage attendance and involvement with childbirth education (i.e., provide resources for classes, electronic resources, and smartphone applications and discuss advantages of attending classes and utilizing a father's group).
- Encourage the man to negotiate his role in labor with his partner.
- Explore his attitudes and expectations of pregnancy, childbirth, and parenting.

TABLE 5–1 Paternal Adaptation to Pregnancy

ANNOUNCEMENT PHASE

Men may react to the news of pregnancy with joy, distress, or a combination of emotions, depending on whether the pregnancy is planned or unwanted.	Occurs as the news of the pregnancy is revealed.
	It may last from a few hours to several weeks.
	It is very common at this phase for men to feel ambivalence.
	The main developmental task is to accept the biological fact of pregnancy.
	Men will begin to attempt to take on the expectant father role.

MORATORIUM PHASE

During this phase, many men appear to put conscious thought of the pregnancy aside for some time, even as their partners are undergoing dramatic physical and emotional changes right before their eyes.	This can cause potential conflict when women attempt to communicate with their partners about the pregnancy.
	Sexual adaptation will be necessary as well; men may fear hurting the fetus during intercourse.
	Feelings of rivalry may surface as the fetus grows larger and the woman becomes more preoccupied with her own thoughts of impending motherhood.
	Men's main developmental task during this phase is to accept the pregnancy. This includes accepting the changing body and emotional state of his partner, as well as accepting the reality of the fetus, especially when fetal movement is felt.

FOCUSING PHASE

The focusing phase begins in the last trimester.	Men begin to think of themselves as fathers.
Men will be actively involved in the pregnancy and their relationship with the child.	Men participate in planning for labor and delivery, and the newborn.
	Men's main developmental task is to negotiate with their partner the role they are to play in labor and to prepare for parenthood.

May, 1982.

SEXUALITY IN PREGNANCY

Physiological changes during pregnancy affect the body's hormonal milieu as well as a woman's sexual desires, responses, and practices. Sexuality in pregnancy occurs on a wide continuum of responses for women. Some women feel more beautiful and desirable with advancing pregnancy and others feel unattractive and ungainly. The sexual relationship can be significantly affected during this time. Physical, emotional, and interactional factors all play a part in the woman's and her partner's sexual response during pregnancy (Crooks & Baur, 2010). A more open discussion between clinicians and patients about sexual activity during pregnancy is relevant and may help to alleviate women's fears, close knowledge gaps, and reassure those who wish to be sexually active throughout pregnancy (Afshar, My-Lin, Mei, & Grisales, 2017).

- The desire for sexual activity varies among pregnant women. Sexual desire can vary even in the same woman at different times during the pregnancy. Typically, a woman's sexual interest and coital frequency declines in the first trimester of pregnancy, shows variable patterns in the second trimester, and decreases sharply in the third trimester (Afshar et al., 2017).
  - During the first trimester, fatigue, nausea, and breast tenderness may affect sexual desire.
  - During the second trimester, desire may increase as a result of increased sense of well-being and the pelvic congestion associated with this time in pregnancy.
  - During the third trimester, sexual interest may once again decrease as the enlarging abdomen creates feelings of awkwardness and bulk.
- Many women have some level of apprehension about sexual intercourse during pregnancy.
- Women in relationships with established open communication about sexuality are less likely to have difficulty with changes in sexual activity. For example, it may be necessary for a couple to modify intercourse positions for the pregnant woman's comfort.
  - The side-by-side, woman-above, and rear-entry positions are generally more comfortable than the man-above positions.
- Nonsexual expressions of affection are just as important.
- Common concerns related to sexual activity include:
  - Fears about hurting the fetus during intercourse or causing permanent anomalies as a result of sexual activity.
  - Fear the birth process will drastically change the woman's genitals.
- Changes in body shape and body image will influence both partners' desire for sexual expression.

Nursing Actions

- Discuss fears and concerns related to sexual activity.
- Encourage communication between partners and discuss possible changes with couples.
  - Encourage the couple to verbalize fears and to ask questions.
  - Use humor and encourage the couple to use humor to relieve anxiety or embarrassment.

- Evidence currently is insufficient to justify recommending against sexual intercourse during pregnancy. Advise pregnant women that there are no contraindications to intercourse or masturbation to orgasm provided the woman's membranes are intact, there is no vaginal bleeding, and she has no current problems or history of premature labor (Crooks & Baur, 2010).
- During prenatal visits, simply asking patients about whether they continue to be sexually active during their pregnancy may be enough to make them comfortable asking questions about their sexual health. This can open the door to review sexual positions to increase comfort for the couple with advancing pregnancy.
- Cultural influences can affect forms of sexual contact in some populations. Ethnic and religious beliefs may propagate fears about sexual intercourse, thereby leading to avoidance during pregnancy (Afshar et al., 2017). It may be important to discuss alternative forms of sexual expression.

FAMILY ADAPTATION DURING PREGNANCY

Pregnancy affects the entire family; psychosocial assessment and interventions must be considered from a family-centered perspective (Barron, 2014). The family is a basic structural unit of the community and constitutes one of society's most important institutions. It is a key target for perinatal assessment and intervention. This primary social group assumes major responsibility for the introduction and socialization of children and forms a potent network of support for its members. An understanding of the different family structures and the life cycle of the family and the related developmental tasks can assist the nurse in nursing care during pregnancy. Because of the multitude of definitions of "family" and the changing realities of the current times, there is a need for redefinition of family. One example is, "People related by marriage, birth, consanguinity or legal adoption, who share a common kitchen and financial resources on a regular basis" (Sharma, 2013, p. 308). The structure of families varies widely among and within cultures. Social scientists now commonly recognize that families exist in a variety of ways and that during their lives, children may indeed belong to several different family groups.

Changing Familial Structures

U.S. census data indicates major shifts in the configuration of families over the past several decades. A woman's family is the primary support during the childbearing years and has a direct influence on her emotional and physical health. It is essential that the nurse identify the woman's definition of family and provide care on that basis. Nurses must support all types of families (Fig. 5–4). The variety of family configurations includes (Friedman, Bowden, & Jones, 2003):

- The nuclear family: A father, mother, and child living together but apart from both sets of grandparents.
- The extended family: Three generations, including married brothers and sisters and their families.

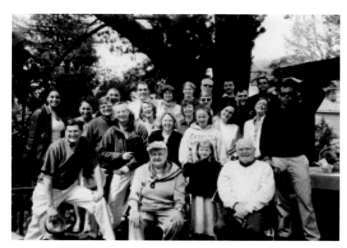

FIGURE 5–4 Multicultural family.

- Single-parent family: Divorced, never married, separated, or widowed man or woman and at least one child.
- Three-generational families: Any combination of first-, second-, and third-generation members living within a household.
- Dyad family: Couple living alone without children.
- Stepparent family: One or both spouses have been divorced or widowed and have remarried into a family with at least one child.
- Blended or reconstituted family: A combination of two families with children from one or both families and sometimes children of the newly married couple.
- Cohabiting family: An unmarried couple living together.
- Gay or lesbian family: A same-sex couple living together with or without children; children may be adopted, from previous relationships, or conceived via artificial insemination.
- Adoptive family: Single persons or couples who have at least one child who is not biologically related to them and to whom they have legally become parents.

Family theorists have identified eight stages in the life cycle of a family that provide a framework for nurses caring for childbearing families (Duvall, 1985; Friedman et al., 2003): beginning families, childbearing families, families with preschool children, families with school-aged children, families with teenagers, families launching young adults, middle-aged parents, and aging families.

Each of these stages has developmental tasks that the family needs to accomplish to successfully move to the next stage.

Developmental Tasks

The events of pregnancy and childbirth are considered a developmental (maturational) crisis in the life of a family, defined as a change associated with normal growth and development.

- All family members are significantly affected.
  - Previous life patterns may be disturbed, and there may be a sense of disorganization.

- Certain developmental tasks have been identified that a family must face and master to successfully incorporate a new member into the family unit and allow the family to be ready for further growth and development. The developmental tasks for the childbearing family are:
  - Acquiring knowledge and plans for the specific needs of pregnancy, childbirth, and early parenthood.
  - Preparing to provide for the physical care of the newborn.
  - Adapting financial patterns to meet increasing needs.
  - Realigning tasks and responsibilities.
  - Adjusting patterns of sexual expression to accommodate pregnancy.
  - Expanding communication to meet emotional needs.
  - Reorienting relationships with relatives.
  - Adapting relationships with friends and community to take account of the realities of pregnancy and the anticipated newborn.

The accomplishment of these tasks during pregnancy lays the groundwork for later adaptation required when the newborn is added to the family unit (Duvall, 1985; Friedman et al., 2003).

Nursing Actions

- Assess knowledge related to pregnancy, childbirth, and early parenting.
- Assess cultural family traditions for new family additions.
- Assess progress in developmental tasks of pregnancy.
- Explore patterns of communication related to emotional needs, responsibilities, and new roles.
- Include the entire family; assessments and interventions must be considered in a family-centered perspective.
- Provide education and guidance related to pregnancy, childbirth, and early parenting.

Sibling Adaptation

Sharing the spotlight with a new brother or sister can be a major crisis for a child. The older child often experiences a sense of loss or feels jealous at being "replaced" by the new sibling. During pregnancy, areas of change that impact siblings the most involve maternal appearance, parental behavior, and changes in the home environment such as sleeping arrangements.

- Sibling adaptation is greatly influenced by the child's age and developmental level, as well as by the attitude of the parents.
  - Children younger than 2 are usually unaware of the pregnancy and do not understand explanations about the future arrival of the newborn.
  - Children from 2 to 4 years of age may respond to the obvious changes in their mother's body but may not remember from month to month why the changes are occurring. This age group is particularly sensitive to the disruptions of the physical environment. Therefore, if the parents plan to change the sibling's sleeping arrangements to accommodate the new baby, these arrangements should be implemented well in advance of the birth. Children still sleeping in a crib should be moved to a bed at least 2 months before the baby is due.

- Children aged 4 to 5 often enjoy listening to the fetal heartbeat and may show interest in the development of the fetus. As pregnancy progresses, they may resent the changes in their mother's body that interfere with her ability to lift and hold them or engage in physical play.
- School-age children (6 to 12) are usually enthusiastic and keenly interested in the details of pregnancy and birth. They have many questions and are eager to learn. They often plan elaborate welcomes for the newborn and want to be able to help when their new sibling comes home.
- Adolescent responses to pregnancy vary according to developmental level. They may be uncomfortable with the obvious evidence of their parents' sexuality or be embarrassed by the changes in their mother's appearance. They may be fascinated and repelled by the birth process all at once. Older adolescents may be somewhat indifferent to the changes associated with pregnancy but also may respond in a more adult fashion by offering support and help.
- Expectant parents should make a special effort to prepare and include the older child as much as their developmental age allows. Preparation must be carried out at the child's level of understanding and readiness to learn (Box 5–2).
- Some children may express interest in being present at the birth. If siblings are to attend the birth, they should participate in a class that prepares them for the event. During the labor and birth, a familiar person who has no other role should be available to explain what is taking place and to comfort or remove them if the situation becomes overwhelming.

Nursing Actions

- Explore with parents' strategies for sibling preparation (see Box 5–2).
- Assess adaptation to pregnancy at every prenatal visit. Early assessment and intervention may prevent or greatly reduce later problems for the pregnant woman and her family.
- Discuss strategies to facilitate sibling adaptation based on the child's age and development.
- Facilitate discussion of the birth plan if parents want the children present during the sibling's birth and a contingency plan if the labor doesn't go as planned and additional care is needed for the child.

Grandparent Adaptation

Grandparents are often the first family members to be told about a pregnancy and must make complex adjustments to the news. When it is their first grandchild, most grandparents are delighted. A first pregnancy is also undeniable evidence that they are growing older, and some may respond negatively, indicating that they are not ready to be grandparents.

- New parents recognize that the tie to the future represented by the fetus is of special significance to grandparents.
- Grandparents provide a unique sense of family history to expectant parents that may not be available elsewhere. They can be a valuable resource and can strengthen family systems by widening the circle of support and nurturance.

BOX 5–2 | Tips for Sibling Preparation

Pregnancy

- Take the child on a prenatal visit. Let the child listen to the fetal heartbeat and feel the baby move.
- Take the child to the homes of friends who have babies to give him or her an opportunity to see firsthand what babies are like.
- Take the child on a tour of the hospital or birthing center; if available, enroll in a sibling preparation class, if age appropriate.

After the Birth

- Encourage parents to be sensitive to the changes the sibling is experiencing; jealousy and a sense of loss are normal feelings at this time.
- Plan for high-quality, uninterrupted time with the older child.
- Encourage older children to participate in care of their sibling (i.e., bringing a diaper, singing to the baby, sitting with Mom during infant feeding times).
- Teach a parent to be watchful when the older child is with the newborn; natural expressions of sibling jealousy may involve rough handling, slapping or hitting, throwing toys, and so on.
- Reassure parents that regressive behaviors in the very young child may be a normal part of sibling adjustment (i.e., return to diapers, wanting to breastfeed or take a bottle, tantrums), and with consistent attention and patience the behaviors will decrease.
- Praise the child for acting age appropriately; show the child how and where to touch the baby.
- In the hospital: Encourage sibling visitation; call older children on the phone; have visitors greet the older child before focusing on the newborn.
- Give a gift to the new sibling from the newborn; let the sibling select a gift for the baby before delivery to bring to the newborn after the birth.

- Grandparents may also be called upon for more long-term help. Teen pregnancy, parents' incarceration, substance abuse, child abuse, and death or mental illnesses of the parents are examples of situations where grandparents may have to assume the care and upbringing of the newborn. According to the U.S. Census Bureau (2010), 2.7 million grandparents were raising their grandchildren in 2010, up from 2.4 million in 2000 (Lee & Blitz, 2016).
- The demands of helping to raise a grandchild may create added stressors in their lives that grandparents may not have anticipated. Grandparent carers reported higher levels of distress in the carer role. Predictors of carer stress included severity of child behavior problems and daily hassles (Lee & Blitz, 2016).

Nursing Actions

- Assess the grandparents' response to pregnancy.
- Explore grandparents as a resource during pregnancy and early parenting.
- Involve social services, as they may assess the grandparents' financial and community resources for possible parenting.

MENTAL HEALTH DIFFICULTIES WITH PREGNANCY ADAPTATION

Women may present with psychosocial issues and concerns that are beyond the realm of the perinatal nurse. Severe and persistent mental illness (SPMI) refers to complex mood disorders that include major depressive disorder with or without psychosis; severe anxiety disorders resistant to treatment; affective psychotic disorders, including bipolar affective disorder, schizophrenia, and schizoaffective disorder; and other nonaffective subtypes of schizophrenia (McKeever, Alderman, Luff, & DeJesus, 2016). SPMIs affect 1 in 17 people and are among the leading causes of disability and impaired health-related quality of life in the United States. Caring for childbearing women with preexisting SPMI can be challenging for maternal-child health clinicians. Challenges for clinicians include early identification, accuracy of diagnoses, and appropriate management through care coordination among an interdisciplinary team that includes obstetric providers, psychiatrists, nurses, and others (McKeever et al., 2016). Nurses need to be aware of community mental health resources and be prepared to collaborate with psychiatric or mental health specialties, social services, or community agencies. Mental health issues during pregnancy can create problems for the pregnant woman across several dimensions.

- Difficulty with taking on the maternal role, making the necessary transitions to parenthood, and mourning losses associated with the time before pregnancy are all potential areas of concern.
- Prenatal depression, maternal stress, and anxiety exert biochemical influences that significantly impact the developing fetus and contribute to adverse birth outcomes that have long-term consequences (e.g., low birth weight, shorter gestational age, adverse neonatal behavioral responses) (Lederman & Weis, 2009). It is postulated that decreased utero-placental blood flow because of high maternal stress levels can affect the onset and duration of labor by interfering with mechanisms that modulate uterine contractions and impact delivery (Stadtlander, 2017).
- When assessing mood, emotional states, and anxiety, the nurse should consider these aspects: frequency, duration, intensity, and source. Screening and treatment interventions should be encouraged during the prenatal period. Early diagnosis and intervention may mitigate potential harm to the mother and child (Phua et al., 2017).
- Rates of serious mental illness (MI) during pregnancy, while low, are of concern given their association with adverse outcomes and the effects of psychotropic medication use or discontinuation during pregnancy.

Nursing Actions

- Assess adaptation to pregnancy at every prenatal visit. Early assessment and intervention may prevent or greatly reduce later problems for the pregnant woman and her family.
- Assess the woman's social support system and coping mechanisms.
- Assess the woman's mood, anxiety, and emotional state and consider frequency, duration, intensity, and source of patients' emotional response.
- Explore other mechanisms that might be helpful.
- Discuss expectations about pregnancy, childbirth, and parenting.
- Identify areas of concern, validate major issues, and make suggestions for possible changes.
- Refer to the appropriate member of the health care team and follow up with those team members for an interdisciplinary plan of care.
- Establish a trusting relationship, as women may be reluctant to share information until one has been formed (e.g., questions asked at the first prenatal visit bear repeating with ongoing prenatal care).
- Make appropriate referrals to other health professionals when needed and continue to follow up. Always act with compassion and be sure to keep each individual woman at the center of care.

PSYCHOSOCIAL ADAPTATION TO PREGNANCY COMPLICATIONS

Most of the time, pregnancy progresses with few problems and results in generally positive outcomes. However, with the diagnosis of pregnancy complications, normal concerns and anxieties of pregnancy are exacerbated. Uncertainty of fetal outcome can interfere with parental attachment.

- Response to pregnancy complications depends on:
  - Pregnancy condition.
  - Perceived threat to mother or fetus.
  - Coping skills.
  - Available support.
- Disequilibrium, feelings of powerlessness, increased anxiety and fear, and a sense of loss are all responses to the news of a pregnancy complication.
- The pregnant woman may distance herself emotionally from the fetus as she faces varying levels of uncertainty about the pregnancy, impacting attachment (Gilbert, 2010).
- Events such as antepartal hospitalization or activity restrictions may contribute to a greater incidence of depression in the pregnant woman.
- The risk of crisis for the pregnant woman and her family clearly increases due to an unpredictable or uncertain pregnancy outcome (Durham, 1998).

- How a woman and her family respond to this additional stress is crucial in determining whether a crisis will develop.
  - Having a realistic perception of the event, adequate situational support, and positive coping mechanisms help a woman maintain her equilibrium and avoid crisis.
  - Poor self-esteem, lack of confidence in the mothering role, and an inability to communicate concerns to health care providers and close unsupportive family members are all factors that increase the risk of crisis.

Research has demonstrated the physical health of mothers with a high-risk pregnancy, demographic and emotional factors, and the health condition of newborns jointly affect mental health. High-risk pregnancy is a potential risk factor for postpartum anxiety and depression and needs follow-up. High-risk pregnancies create additional health problems in both mothers and infants. Pregnant women need emotional support from both providers and family members. Counseling sessions on various aspects of pregnancy and parenthood may reduce the incidence of postpartum depression (Zadeh, Khajehei, Sharif, & Hadzic, 2012).

Nursing Actions

When caring for a pregnant woman with complications, the priority is to reestablish and maintain physiological stability. However, nurses must also be able to intervene to promote psychosocial adaptation to the news of pregnancy complications (Giurgescu, Penckofer, Maurer, & Bryant, 2006; Lederman, 2011; Mattson & Smith, 2016). The following actions can assist to reduce or limit the detrimental effects of complications on individual or family functioning:

- Provide frequent and clear explanations about the problem, planned interventions, and therapy and continue to encourage her to ask questions and/or verbalize concerns.
- Assess and encourage the use of the woman's support systems and provide systems she is unaware of that can be supportive for her.
- Support individual adaptive coping mechanisms and resource more if needed.
- Make appropriate referrals and follow up when additional assistance is needed.

SOCIAL SUPPORT DURING PREGNANCY

Social support is any support provided by a person with whom the expectant mother has a personal relationship. It involves the primary groups of most importance to the individual woman: her spouse or partner, her mother, and her close friends. Involvement of and support from the baby's partner during pregnancy is associated with improved maternal mental health and may contribute to less distressed infant temperament (Stapleton et al., 2012). Social support takes several forms; material, emotional, informational, spiritual, and comparison support have all been identified as important types of support for the pregnant woman.

- Material (instrumental) support consists of practical help such as assistance with chores, meals, and managing finances.
- Emotional support involves support that gives affection, approval, and encouragement as well as feelings of togetherness.
- Informational support consists of sharing information or helping women investigate new sources of information.
- Comparison support consists of help given by someone in a similar situation. Their shared information is useful and credible because they are experiencing or have experienced the same events in their lives.
- Spiritual support consists of creating a space for the woman to express and explore what is happening to her during pregnancy.

Social Support Research

Research from several disciplines provides evidence for the importance of social support for the pregnant woman's health, positive adaptation to pregnancy, and the prevention of pregnancy complications. It is a naturally occurring resource that can prevent health problems and complications and promote health. Receiving adequate help from others enhances self-esteem and feelings of being in control. Mothers who perceived stronger social support partners midpregnancy had lower emotional distress postpartum after controlling for their distress in early pregnancy, and their infants were reported to be less distressed in response. Partner support mediated the effects of the mothers' interpersonal security and relationship satisfaction on maternal and infant outcomes (Stapleton et al., 2012).

- Social support benefits the expectant mother the most when it matches her expectations, referred to as *perceived social support*. It is important that the woman identify and clarify her expectations and needs for support. Perceived support expectations that do not materialize for the pregnant woman can lead to increased distress and problems with adaptation to pregnancy (Ngai, Chan, & Ip, 2010).
- Pregnant women frequently need social support that differs from the support they receive. Nurses can advise the pregnant woman how best to use her existing support networks or how to expand her support network so her needs are met. Nurses have the opportunity and responsibility to help women explore potential sources of support such as childbirth education classes, electronic resources, church, work, school, or the community.
- High-risk populations, including adolescents, women with pregnancy complications, and women with low incomes, may need particular direction from nurses in obtaining adequate support (Beeber & Canuso, 2005; Logsdon et al., 2005). Involving other disciplines such as social work, psychiatry, and maternal-fetal specialists could be necessary for these populations.
- A woman's cultural background also influences the amount of social support received and who provides this support.

Women in cultures that value individualism, self-sufficiency, and independence may have more difficulty receiving social support than those from a culture that values interdependence and collectivism (Meleis, 2003).

● Recent immigrants face many challenges in obtaining needed social support. The disruption of lifelong attachments can cause anxieties and a sense of disorientation. Language barriers and socioeconomic struggles are additional stressors facing immigrant women, creating a higher risk for depression (Ganann, Sword, Thabane, Newbold, & Black, 2016). Their families, experiencing the same difficulties, may not be able to provide sufficient support. Further research is needed to examine the impact of culture on social support.

● Social support is not considered professional support, although professionals can provide supportive actions such as counseling, teaching, role modeling, or problem solving. When expectant mothers have no other means of support, some community programs employ paraprofessionals to visit them, providing education and social support. Programs that capitalize on the skills of experienced mothers living in the communities may be less expensive and more culturally sensitive than purely hospital-based programs led by teams of health care professionals. Additionally, post-delivery follow-up programs offering home-based social support may also have important benefits for socially disadvantaged mothers and children (Cannella, 2006; Dawley & Beam, 2005; Logsdon et al., 2005).

Evidence-Based Practice: Measurable Outcomes of Social Support Interventions

Hodnett, E. D., Fredericks, S., & Weston, J. (2010). Support during pregnancy for women at increased risk of low birthweight babies. *Cochrane Database of Systematic Reviews*, (6), doi:10.1002/14651858.CD000198.pub2

There is substantial evidence that social support interventions improve pregnancy outcomes on the following factors:

● Attachment to infant and improved interactions with infant
● Compliance with health care regimen
● Improved functional status
● Improved coping with changes related to pregnancy
● Increased acceptance of new role in life
● Increased incidence of breastfeeding
● Reduced physical symptoms
● Reduced loneliness
● Reduced feelings of stress or a sense of concern
● Reduced postpartum depression
● Satisfaction with intimate relationships

Pregnant women need the support of caring family members, friends, and health professionals. While programs that offer additional support during pregnancy are unlikely to prevent the pregnancy from resulting in a low birthweight or preterm baby, they may be helpful in reducing the likelihood of antenatal hospital admission and caesarean birth.

Assessing Social Support

Assessing social support is a crucial component of prenatal care. The following areas of assessment should be addressed when planning care:

● Who is available to help provide support? Who is available to provide each type of support (material, emotional, informational, comparison, and spiritual)? Is the support adequate in each category?
● With whom does the pregnant woman have the strongest relationships, and what type of support is provided by these individuals?
● Is there conflict in relationships with support providers? Is the conflict violent or has it been the source of abuse?
● Is there potential for improvement of the woman's support network? Should members who provide more stress than support be deleted and will that cause more stress? Should new members be added?
● Who are the people living with the pregnant woman?
● Who assists with household chores?
● Who assists with child care and parenting activities?
● Who does the pregnant woman turn to when problems occur or during a crisis?
● What is the woman's financial situation?

Nursing Actions

The nursing profession plays an important role in promoting patient-centered, individualized care (Wilson & Leese, 2013). Due to the strong evidence that social support improves pregnancy outcomes, the following nursing actions are recommended:

● Provide opportunities for the woman to ask for support, and rehearse with her appropriate language to use in asking for support. Encourage her to ask for support anytime.
● Invite key support providers to attend prenatal and postpartum visits.
● Facilitate supportive functioning and interactions within the family, encouraging family to ask questions and to be involved if the mother permits.
● Encourage the pregnant woman to interact with other pregnant or postpartum women she knows, and provide access if possible to Centering Pregnancy model of care.
● Suggest church, health clubs, work or school, and electronic resources as sites to meet women with similar interests and concerns.
● Provide information regarding community resources, such as mommy groups and online resources.

CHILDBEARING AND CULTURE

Childbirth is a time of transition and celebration in all cultures (Callister, 2014). Culture is a distinct way of life that characterizes a community of people. It has a significant influence on a client's

BOX 5-3 | Resources for Further Cultural Information

Alliance for Hispanic Health: www.hispanichealth.org

Arab topics: www.al-bab.com

Asian and Pacific Islander American health forum: www.apiahf.org

AT&T Language Line: www.languageline.com

Gay & Lesbian Medical Association: www.glma.org

Hmong studies Internet resource center: www.hmongstudies.com/HmongStudiesJournal

Indian Health Services: www.ihs.gov

Office of Minority Health: https://minorityhealth.hhs.gov/

Transcultural Nursing Society: www.tcns.org

perspective on health. Every culture has a set of behaviors, beliefs, and practices that profoundly influence women and their families during childbearing. Culture can influence how women think, make decisions, and act. Cultural beliefs and practices can affect the health status of pregnant women by influencing her use of health care services and her beliefs regarding her body, pregnancy, illness, and her confidence in providers and their recommendations (Barron, 2014). A culturally responsive nurse recognizes these influences and considers them carefully when planning care (Amidi-Nouri, 2011; Moore, Moos, & Callister, 2010). Box 5–3 lists resources that provide further cultural information.

● It is critical that nurses acquire the knowledge and skills to provide quality care to culturally divergent groups. Expectations of nursing practice will increasingly demand sensitivity to the cultural needs of families and competence in providing care.

● All nursing care is given within the context of many cultures: that of the patient, nurse, health care system, and the larger society. Childbirth directly involves two bodies in one; it's the only time in life when the care surrounds two (or more) humans contained in one body. The mother's body must adapt to changes associated with accommodating another life, while the baby must adapt to life outside the womb after birth (Romano, 2014).

Statistics of the U.S. Population

The U.S. Census Bureau reports one birth every 7 seconds in the United States, and a current population of 325,365,189 as of September 2017. The most recent census identifies five major groups in the United States: African American/blacks, American Indian/Alaska Native, Asian American/Pacific Islander, Hispanic/Latino, and white (U.S. Census, 2010). From a global perspective, the movement of immigrants, refugees, and diplomatic and military personnel and their families worldwide has resulted in increasingly diverse populations. Although the U.S. Census has classified these populations primarily by race, it is important to recognize that many may also identify with their country of origin, or ethnicity. Indeed, the 2010 U.S. Census has expanded its classifications in an attempt to achieve greater clarity and includes

Hispanic/Latino as a population as well as an option to select multiple races.

Culturally Sensitive Behavioral Practices

Culturally sensitive practices can be viewed from a variety of dimensions that nurses must consider when planning care (Moore et al., 2010).

● Decision making: Are decisions made by the woman alone or by others such as her partner, extended family, male elders, spiritual leaders, older adults, or possibly the oldest female relative present?

● Concept of time: Is the culture past, present, or future-oriented? This may affect the woman's understanding about the need for specific time commitments, such as prenatal care appointments.
  ● The dominant U.S. culture is future-oriented, which means people act today with expectations for future rewards. Cultures that are not future-oriented may not seek preventative care, or preconception, prenatal, or well-woman care.

● Communication: Verbal communication may be challenging due to language barriers, meanings of words in different cultures, or how willing a client is to disclose personal information.
  ● Cultures may have different practices regarding such nonverbal communication practices as eye contact, personal space, use of gestures, facial expressions, and appropriate touching. A nurse born in the United States might misinterpret a smile as agreement or understanding about something, rather than confusion about what is being explained.

● Religion: One's religious background may have a powerful influence on sexual attitudes and behaviors. It is important to appreciate that all people from one country, one neighborhood, or one faith do not share one culture or a single set of religious beliefs (Moore et al., 2010).

● Worldview: A client's understanding of how human life fits into the larger picture.
  ● How is illness explained? Examples include ancestral displeasure, body imbalance, breach of taboo, evil eye, germ theory of disease, spirit possession, or karma.

● Modesty and gender: What are the norms for interaction between men and women? What are the norms for undressing in front of someone not in your family?
  ● Some cultures accept public exposure of the human body, while in others, women are expected to cover almost all their bodies. The nurse must understand and appreciate the mores of the woman and her social group.

Common Themes for the Childbearing Family

During the prenatal period, preventing harm to the fetus and ensuring a safe and easy birth are common themes in many cultures. Common aspects influencing labor and delivery include general attitudes toward birth, preferred positions, methods of pain management, and the role of family members and the health care provider.

- The postpartum period is generally considered a time of increased vulnerability for both mothers and babies, influencing care of the new mother as well as infant care practices related to bathing, swaddling, feeding, umbilical cord care, and circumcision (Mattson & Smith, 2016).
- Pregnancy and childbirth may elicit certain customs and beliefs during pregnancy about acceptable and unacceptable practices that have implications for planning nursing care and interventions. These beliefs must be taken into consideration when assessing and promoting adaptation to pregnancy (Box 5–4).

BOX 5–4 | Examples of Cultural Prescriptions, Restrictions, and Taboos

Prescriptive Beliefs

- Remain active during pregnancy to aid the baby's circulation.
- Remain happy to bring the baby joy and good fortune.
- Drink chamomile tea to ensure an effective labor.
- Soup with ginseng root is a good general strength tonic.
- Pregnancy cravings need to be satisfied or the baby will be born with a birthmark.
- Sleep flat on your back to protect the fetus from harm.
- Attach a safety pin to an undergarment to protect the fetus from cleft lip or palate.

Restrictive Beliefs

- Do not have your picture taken because it might cause stillbirth.
- Avoid sexual intercourse during the third trimester because it will cause respiratory distress in the newborn.
- Coldness in any form may cause arthritis or other chronic illness.
- Avoid seeing an eclipse of the moon; it will result in a cleft lip or palate.
- Do not reach over your head or the cord will wrap around the baby's neck.

Taboos

- Avoid funerals and visits from widows or women who have lost children because they will bring bad fortune to the baby.
- Avoid hot and spicy foods, as they can cause overexcitement for the pregnant woman.
- An early baby shower will invite the evil eye and should be avoided.
- Avoid praising the newborn; it will call the attention of the gods to the vulnerable infant.

Adapted from Lauderdale, 2011.

BOX 5–5 | Examples of Cultural Practices/Beliefs Affecting Childbearing

- Sons are highly valued.
- Umbilical cord should be saved.
- Circumcision should be performed on the eighth day of life.
- Placenta should be buried.
- Colostrum is harmful and should be avoided.
- Technology is highly valued.
- May avoid eye contact and limit touch.
- Pregnancy requires medical attention to ensure health.
- Father's participation in labor and birth is not expected.
- The polarity of yin/yang as major life force; health requires a balance between yin (cold) and yang (heat).

Adapted from Moore, Moos, & Callister, 2010.

- Prescriptive behavior is an expected behavior of the pregnant woman during the childbearing period.
- Restrictive behavior describes activities during the childbearing period that are limited for the pregnant woman.
- Taboos are cultural restrictions believed to have serious supernatural consequences.

Cultural practices can also be classified as functional (enhances well-being), neutral (does not harm or help), or nonfunctional (potentially harmful). Nurses must be able to differentiate among these beliefs and practices, and respect functional and neutral practices even if they differ from their own beliefs (Box 5–5).

Nurses need to keep in mind that few cultural customs related to pregnancy are dangerous; although they might cause a woman to limit her activity and her exposure to some aspects of life, they are rarely harmful to herself or her fetus. When encountering nonfunctional practices, the nurse should first try to understand the meaning of the practice for the woman and her family and then work carefully to bring about change. An example of a nonfunctional practice would be the ingestion of clay during pregnancy (Lauderdale, 2011; Moore et al., 2010).

Barriers to Culturally Sensitive Care

Barriers to culturally competent care include values, beliefs, and customs as well as communication challenges (Callister, 2014). Cultural health disparities are created when nurses and other care providers fail to understand the importance of client beliefs about health and illness (Moore et al., 2010). Nurses' attitudes can create barriers to culturally competent care. Ethnocentrism, the belief that the customs and values of the dominant culture are preferred or superior in some way, creates obstacles that can make culturally sensitive care challenging to implement. Stereotyping, the assumption that everyone in a group is the same as everyone else in the group, also creates barriers. Communication barriers include not only language barriers but also lack of knowledge, fear and distrust, racism, and bias. The following factors also create barriers to care:

● Lack of diversity among health care providers. For example, white female nurses comprised 77% of the registered nurses (RNs) older than age 70; less than two-thirds of nurses younger than age 40 are white females (McMenamin, 2015).
● Strong evidence exists that the quality of health care varies as a function of race, ethnicity, and language (Amidi-Nouri, 2011; Meleis, 2003; Moore et al., 2010).
● Mainstream models of obstetric care as practiced in North America can present a strange and confusing picture to many women from different ethnic backgrounds. The predominant culture's emphasis on formal prenatal care, technology, hospital deliveries, and a bureaucratic health care system presents barriers to care for many groups.
  ● Protocols, an unfamiliar environment, and health care providers who only speak English all create barriers that confuse, intimidate, and result in inadequate access to care.
  ● Health literacy is the capacity to obtain, process, and understand basic health information and services needed to make appropriate health decisions. Approximately one-half of the adult population may lack the needed literacy skills to use the U.S. health care system. Low literacy has been linked to poor health outcomes, such as higher rates of hospitalization and less frequent use of preventive services (CDC, 2017b).
  ● These obstacles to health care significantly contribute to health care disparities, or differences in care experienced by one population compared with another population. (For further information on health care disparities, see Chapter 1.)
  ● Disparities also may occur in gender, age, economic status, religion, cultural background, disability, or sexual orientation.

Culturally Responsive Nursing Practice

Nurses have an obligation to provide patients and their families effective, understandable, and respectful care in a manner that is compatible with their cultural beliefs, practices, and preferred language. *Cultural assessment* is defined as the assessment of shared cultural beliefs, values, and customs related to health behaviors (Mattson & Smith, 2016). The goal is to gain knowledge to create an environment in which a trusting relationship with the client can be developed (see Box 5–3).

● Mandates from professional health care accrediting bodies and government agencies provide evidence of increased commitment to providing culturally appropriate health care. Examples of these directives include:
  ● The Joint Commission–mandated plan of patient care includes cultural and spiritual assessments and interventions (The Joint Commission, 2018).

● The American Association of Colleges of Nursing (AACN) has stated that nursing graduates should have the knowledge and skills to provide holistic care that addresses the needs of diverse populations. AACN has also published specific end-of-program cultural competencies for baccalaureate nursing education (AACN, 2008).
● Cultural competence is addressed explicitly in the *Healthy People 2020* focus area of health communications, stating that cultural sensitivity is necessary for effective communication with individuals and the public to stimulate systems change and to influence health behavior (U.S. DHSS, 2010a).
● The HHS office of minority health has published 14 national standards for Culturally and Linguistically Appropriate Services (CLAS standards) (U.S. DHSS, 2010a).
● Culturally sensitive nursing practice requires the nurse to maintain an open attitude and sensitivity to differences.
● Women who indicate they cannot make a decision about care or seem hesitant and uncertain may be following the culture's expectation that important decisions belong to someone other than the woman (Moore et al., 2010).

CRITICAL COMPONENT

Strategies for Nurses: Improving Culturally Responsive Care

· Maintain an open attitude.
· Recognize yourself as a part of the diversity in society and acknowledge your own belief system.
· Examine the biases and assumptions you hold about different cultures.
· Avoid preconceptions and cultural stereotyping.
· Explore and acknowledge historical and current portrayals of racial and ethnic groups in society.
· Develop an understanding of how racial or ethnic differences affect the quality of health care.
· Acknowledge the power you have to use professional privilege positively or negatively.
· Recall your commitment to "individualized care," "respect," and "professionalism."
· Identify who the client calls "family."
· Include notes on cultural preferences and family strengths and resources as part of all intake and ongoing assessments, and nursing care plans and care maps.
· Use the cultural wisdom (beliefs, values, customs, and habits) of the client to shape his or her participation in health practices and care plans.
· Seek out client-friendly teaching and assessment tools.
· Review the literature to generate a culture database.
· Read literature from other cultures and if an ethnic group is well represented in the local population, learn about that culture to provide optimal care.
· Participate in professional development/continuing education programs that address cultural competence.

- Recognize that all care is given within the context of many cultures.
- Develop linguistic skills related to your client population.
- Learn to use nonverbal communication in an appropriate way.
- Learn about the communication patterns of various cultures.
- Advocate for organizational change.
- Understand and apply the various regulatory standards (CLAS, AACN, etc.).
- Promote cultural practices that are helpful, tolerate practices that are neutral, and work to educate women to avoid practices that are potentially harmful.
- Understand and develop possible methods of support that are accepted in the culture.

Amidi-Nouri, 2011; Barron, 2014; Callister, 2014; Mojaverian & Heejung, 2013; Moore et al., 2010

Cultural practices or beliefs may not apply to all individuals, and a great deal of diversity will be found among women of any ethnic group. Educational background, family heritage, social class, economic factors, work/occupational experience, urban/rural origin, length of time in the United States (or place of migration), and a variety of individual characteristics or choices such as sexual orientation, disability, and strength of ethnic identity will all influence how women experience health and illness (Meleis, 2003).

It is also important to recognize that socioeconomic factors are often blended with culturally influenced patterns of behavior. Variations that appear to be cultural may actually reflect the socioeconomic conditions in which many minority groups live. This arises in part because some have fewer opportunities for education and upward mobility. The economic gap accentuates differences, and soon the assumption is made that observed differences are cultural in origin (May & Mahlmeister, 1994).

Cultural Assessment

When considering cultural aspects of care (Andrews & Boyle, 2011; Moore et al., 2010), the nurse caring for expectant families must answer a variety of questions to individualize care:

- What is the woman's predominant culture? To what degree does the client identify with the cultural group? Is there anything she would like to observe on her culture's traditions?
- What language does the client speak at home? What are the styles of nonverbal communication (e.g., eye contact, space orientation, touch, decision making)?
- How does the woman's culture influence her beliefs about pregnancy and childbirth? Is pregnancy considered a state of illness or health? How does the culture explain illness? Are there particular attitudes toward age at the time of pregnancy? Marriage? Who would be an acceptable father or partner? What is considered acceptable in terms of pregnancy frequency?
- Are there cultural prescriptions, restrictions, or taboos related to certain activities, dietary practices, or expressions

of emotion? What does the pregnant woman consider to be normal practice during pregnancy, birth, postpartum?
- How does the woman interpret and respond to experiences of pain? Will she want medication for pain?
- How is modesty expressed by men and women?
- Are there culturally defined expectations about male-female relationships and relationships outside the culture?
- What is the client's educational background? Does it affect her knowledge level concerning the health care–delivery system, teaching/learning, written material given, or understanding?
- How does the client relate to persons outside her cultural group? Does she prefer a caregiver with the same cultural background?
- What is the role of religious beliefs related to pregnancy and childbirth?
- How are childbearing decisions made, and who is involved in the decision-making process?
- How does the woman's predominant culture view the concept of time? (Cultures may be past, present, or future-oriented.)
- How does the woman's culture explain illness? (Examples: ancestral displeasure, germ theory, etc.)

Nursing Actions

With the increasing diverse patient population, it is imperative that nurses provide culturally sensitive care. Professionals must acknowledge belief and value systems different from their own and consider these differences when delivering care to childbearing women and their families (Callister, 2014; Leininger, 1991; Moore et al., 2010; Purnell, 2014).

- Enhance communication.
  - Greet respectfully.
  - Establish rapport.
  - Demonstrate empathy and interest.
  - Listen actively.
- Emphasize the woman's strengths; consider each woman's individuality regarding how she conforms to traditional values and norms.
- Respect functional and neutral practices.
- If proposed practices are nonfunctional, work with the woman and her support network to bring about change.
- Accommodate cultural practices as appropriate.
- Identify who the client calls "family."
- Determine who the family decision makers are and involve them in the care if mother permits.
- Provide an interpreter when necessary (Box 5–6).
- Recognize that a patient agreeing and nodding yes to the nurse's instruction or questions may not always guarantee comprehension but instead may mean confusion.
- Use nonverbal communication and visual aids in an appropriate way.
- When providing patient education, include family and elicit support from the established caretakers in the family (i.e., grandmother, aunt, etc.), and encourage questions or to verbalize concerns.
- Demonstrate how scientific and folk practices can be combined to provide optimal care.

BOX 5–6 | Working With an Interpreter

A trained medical interpreter should be used for medical interpretations. A friend or family member may not understand terms used by the health care provider. A woman may be discussing issues she wants to keep private. The interpreter can be a valuable member of the health care team.

The nurse should be alert to the client's nonverbal cues and ask the patient to repeat information that she needs to recall later.

Many nursing schools and health care institutions may prohibit nursing students from interpreting, for example, obtaining consent for a procedure, because limited knowledge about the procedure may lead the student to give inaccurate information. Phone centers can be used by phoning in and asking the operator to find the appropriate translator for the patient's language.

Adapted from Moore, Moos, & Callister, 2010.

PLANNING FOR BIRTH

Planning and preparing for childbirth requires many decisions by the woman and her family during pregnancy (i.e., choosing a provider, choosing a place of birth, planning for the birth, preparing for labor through education, and planning for labor support). These choices affect how the woman approaches her pregnancy and can contribute significantly to a positive adaptation and positive fetal outcomes.

Choosing a Provider

One of the first decisions a woman makes is to choose her care provider during pregnancy and birth. This important decision also influences where her birth will take place.

Physicians

Obstetricians and family practice physicians attend approximately 91% of births in the United States. Most physicians care for their patients in a hospital setting.

- Care often includes pharmacological and medical management of problems as well as use of technological procedures.
- They care for both low- and high-risk patients.

Midwives

The focus of midwifery care is on noninterventionist care, with an emphasis on the normalcy of the birth process.

- Midwives care for women in hospital settings, alternative birth centers, or at the family home.
- In many countries, midwives are the primary providers of care for healthy pregnant women, and physicians are consulted when medical or surgical intervention is required. In European countries, more than 75% of births are attended by midwives.

- Nurse-midwives are RNs with advanced training in care of obstetric patients. In 2014, certified nurse-midwives (CNMs) and certified midwives (CMs) attended 8% of all hospital births, an 11.1% increase since 2005. The percentage of out-of-hospital births attended by CNMs also increased 9.1% over this period, from 28.6% in 2005 to 31.4% in 2014. Both the number and percentage of CNM/CM-attended births in the United States slightly increased from 2013 to 2014 (Martin, Hamilton, Osterman, Curtin, & Mathews, 2017). The percentage of total U.S. births attended by CNMs/CMs increased from 8.2% to 8.3%, less than 10% of births in the United States, usually seeing low-risk patients. Nurse-midwives practice with physicians or independently with a contracted health care provider agency for physician backup.
- Lay midwives manage about 1% of the births in the United States and Canada, with the majority taking place in the home setting. Their training varies greatly, from being self-taught to having formal training and licensing.
- Direct-entry midwives are trained in midwifery schools or universities as a profession distinct from nursing. Increasing numbers of midwives in the United Kingdom and Ireland fall into this category.
- Given the variations in midwifery training and knowledge, pregnant women considering midwifery care may need education and information regarding the experience and credentials of the midwife providing their care to make informed decisions (Box 5–7).

Choosing a Place of Birth

Pregnant women must decide whether to give birth in a hospital setting, at a birthing center, or at home.

Hospitals

- In the United States, approximately 99% of births take place in hospital settings.
- Hospital maternity services can vary greatly, from traditional labor and delivery rooms with separate newborn and postpartum units to in-hospital birth centers.
- Labor, delivery, and recovery (LDR) rooms may be available in which the expectant mother is admitted, labors, gives birth, and spends the first 2 hours of recovery.
- In labor, delivery, recovery, postpartum (LDRP) units, the mother remains in the same room for her entire hospital stay.

Birth Centers

- Freestanding birth centers are usually built in locations separate from the hospital but may be located nearby in case transfer of the woman or newborn is needed.
- Only women at low risk for complications are included in care.
- Birth centers are usually staffed by nurse-midwives or physicians who also have privileges at the local hospital.
- They offer homelike accommodations, with emergency equipment available but stored out of view.

BOX 5–7 | Professional Position Statement: AWHONN Position Statement on Midwifery

AWHONN supports the practice of the certified nurse-midwife as a primary care provider who is prepared to independently manage most aspects of women's health care. The certified nurse-midwife's practice should include appropriate professional consultation, collaboration, and referral as indicated by the health status of the patient and applicable state and federal laws.

Background

AWHONN identifies a wide range of disparate educational requirements and certification standards in the United States that fall under the umbrella category of midwifery. The following titles are attributed to midwives without prior nursing credentials who are not graduates of American College of Nurse Midwives (ACNM)-accredited programs: direct entry, lay, licensed, or professional. Direct entry midwives cover the spectrum from the doctorally prepared European midwife to the self-taught, beginning practitioner.

The wide range of what is actually meant by the designation "midwife" can easily confuse consumers, health care institutions, and legislators. Definitions of various certification levels are:

- CNM: certified nurse-midwife (administered by ACNM)

- CM: certified midwife (administered by ACNM)

- CPM: certified professional midwife (administered by the North American Registry of Midwives). Also referred to as *direct entry, lay,* or *licensed midwife.*

- Midwives with a state license or permit (administered on a state-by-state basis). Also referred to as *direct entry, lay,* or *licensed midwife.*

- Midwives without formal credentials (no administrative oversight). Also referred to as *direct entry* or *lay midwife.*

Individual state-by-state laws govern the practice of midwifery in the United States. Certified nurse-midwives and certified midwives often practice in collaboration and consultation with other health care professionals to provide primary, gynecological, and maternity care to women in the context of the larger health care system. Certified nurse-midwives may have prescriptive privileges, admitting privileges to hospitals, and may own and/or manage freestanding practices. The scope of practice for a direct entry, or lay, midwife who is not ACC accredited is typically limited to the practice of home birth or birth center options for women but varies according to state-by-state regulations.

Association of Women's Health, Obstetric and Neonatal Nurses (AWHONN), 2000.

Home Births

- Home births are popular in European countries such as Sweden and the Netherlands, with rigorous screening policies in place to ensure that only low-risk women are having home births and are attended by trained midwives (Zielinski, Ackerson, & Kane-Low, 2015).

- In developing countries, home births may occur due to the lack of hospitals, adequate birthing facilities, and staff.

- In the United States, home births account for fewer than 1% of births. In the North American medical community, many have concluded that home birth exposes the mother and fetus to unnecessary danger. Consequently, a woman seeking a home birth may find it challenging to find a qualified health care provider willing to give prenatal care and attend the birth.

- Home births allow the expectant family to be in control of the experience, and the mother may be more relaxed than in the hospital environment. It may be less expensive, and risk of serious infection may be decreased.

- If home birth is the woman's choice, the following criteria will promote a safe home birth experience:
  - The woman must be comfortable with her decision.
  - The woman should be in good health; home birth is not for high-risk pregnancy.
  - The woman should have access to a good transportation system in case of transfer to the hospital.
  - The woman should be attended by a well-trained health care provider with adequate medical supplies and resuscitation equipment (Romano, 2010).

The Birth Plan

A birth plan is a tool by which parents can explore their childbirth options and choose those that are most important to them. A written birth plan can help women clarify their desires and expectations and communicate those desires with their care providers (Lothian, 2011).

- Birth plans typically emphasize specific requests for labor and immediate postdelivery care. Some involve expectations surrounding postpartum and newborn care as well, including breastfeeding.

- The birth plan document can be inserted into the woman's prenatal record or hospital chart as a way of communicating with care providers.

The Doula

The word *doula* comes from ancient Greek and means "woman's servant" (ICEA, 1999). A doula is an individual who provides support to women and their partners during labor, birth, and postpartum. The doula does not provide clinical care.

- Continuous support by a trained doula during labor has been associated with shorter labors, decreased need for analgesics, decreased need for medical interventions, and increased maternal satisfaction (Campbell, Lake, Falk, & Backstrand, 2006; Hodnett, Gates, Hofmeyr, & Sakala, 2011; Pascali-Bonaro & Kroeger, 2004).

- Pregnant women should be made aware of the benefits of doula care prior to coming to the hospital to deliver.

- Many hospitals have implemented doula services that are either free or fee-based.

Childbirth Education

The roots of prenatal education began in the early 1900s with classes in maternal hygiene, nutrition, and baby care taught by the American Red Cross in New York City. Childbirth education as we know it today developed as a consumer response to the increasing medical control and technological management of normal labor and birth during the 1950s and 1960s in Europe and North America. Early proponents of childbirth education such as Lamaze, Bradley, and Dick-Read focused primarily on the prevention of pain in childbirth. Methods of "natural childbirth" (Dick-Read), "psychoprophylaxis" (Lamaze), and "husband-coached childbirth" (Bradley) attained great popularity among middle-class groups.

Childbirth education has evolved since that time toward a more eclectic approach. The focus has shifted away from rigid techniques to embrace a philosophy that "affirms the normalcy of birth, acknowledges women's inherent ability to birth their babies, and explores all the ways that women find strength and comfort during labor and birth" (Lamaze International, 2009; Walker, Visger, & Rossie, 2009). The content of childbirth education classes has greatly expanded, assisting women and their families to make informed decisions about pregnancy and birth based on knowledge of their options and choices. Antenatal education programs often have a range of aims, such as to influence health behavior, build women's confidence in their ability to give birth, prepare women and their partners for childbirth, prepare for parenthood, develop social support networks, promote confident parents, and contribute to reducing perinatal morbidity and mortality. Antenatal education thus comprises a range of educational and supportive measures that help parents and prospective parents understand their own social, psychological, and physical needs during pregnancy, labor, and parenthood. From conception to childbirth, parental education is an important tool to help parents understand the milestones that are necessary for healthy social, emotional, and intellectual growth (Centers for Disease Control, 2018).

- Specialized classes are designed to meet the needs of specific groups, including classes for breastfeeding, sibling preparation, refreshers, prenatal/postpartum exercise, online childbirth preparation, and grandparents' education. Programs have been developed for adolescents, mothers expecting twins, and mothers older than 35. Nurses and childbirth educators have played an important role in the development of these innovative education programs.
- Professional organizations, including International Childbirth Education Association (ICEA), Lamaze International, and AWHONN have all published position papers that delineate expectations of basic components of prenatal education. Through the development of position papers as well as teacher training and certification programs, these organizations have ensured that childbirth educators have a sound knowledge base and specific competencies.
- The *Healthy People 2020* maternal, infant, and child health goals include an objective that commits to increasing the proportion of pregnant women who attend a formal series of prepared childbirth classes (HHS, 2010a).
- The overall goal of childbirth education is to promote the competence of expectant parents in meeting the challenges

of childbirth and early parenting. The focus is on promoting healthy pregnancy and birth outcomes, facilitating a positive transition to parenting, and decreasing anxiety around birth. Attending childbirth education (CBE) class and/or having a birth plan were associated with a vaginal delivery (Afshar et al., 2017).
- Class content typically includes the physical and emotional aspects of pregnancy, childbirth and early parenting, coping skills, and labor support techniques (Box 5–8).

BOX 5–8 | Perinatal Education: Sample Content in a Childbirth Preparation Class

Introduction

Introductions

Overview of childbirth education: Rationale and pain theory

Physical and emotional changes of pregnancy; fetal development

Nutrition, exercise, and self-care during pregnancy

Introduction to breathing and relaxation techniques

Labor

Signs of labor

Stages and phases of labor and delivery

Labor support techniques; the role of the support person in labor

Practice of breathing and relaxation techniques

Birth Plans

Labor review, incorporating labor support techniques and nonpharmacological comfort strategies

Birth options and birth plans: developing advocacy skills

Pharmacological interventions

Practice of breathing and relaxation techniques

Hospital tour

Variations in Labor

Variations of labor: back labor, prodromal labor, precipitous labor

Cesarean delivery

Medical procedures (IVs, episiotomy, assisted delivery, electronic fetal monitoring (EFM), Pitocin, epidurals)

Practice of relaxation and breathing techniques

Newborn

Review of labor; practice of relaxation and breathing techniques

Newborn care

Breastfeeding

Postpartum

Postpartum and transition to parenthood

Community resources for new parents

● Values clarification and informed decision making are emphasized, as well as the promotion of wellness behaviors and healthy birth practices. Pregnant women are encouraged to identify their own unique goals for childbirth (Green & Hotelling, 2009; Lothian, 2011).

● Class formats have evolved to meet the varied needs of expectant families and may include a traditional weekly series, one-day intensives, or online classes.

Childbirth classes remain a popular and well-established component of care during the childbearing years. However, the evidence regarding the effects of antenatal education remains inconclusive. As the body of research on childbirth and childbirth education increases and as more childbirth educators use research findings as a basis for their teaching, evidence-based practice will be enhanced.

● Nurses need to be aware of these powerful influences on the health-related decisions of childbearing women and their families. The quality of information and advice varies widely. For a list of reliable Internet resources for parent education, see Box 5–9.

● Information via technology is convenient and can be retrieved in seconds, but the results may be inaccurate, inconsistent, or poorly referenced, so trusted sources for evidence-based information should be provided by nurses.

BOX 5–9 | Internet Resources for Expectant Families

Babycenter: www.babycenter.com

Childbirth Connection: www.childbirthconnection.org

Doulas of North America: www.dona.org

Healthy Mothers, Healthy Babies Coalition: www.hmhb.org

ICEA (International Childbirth Education Association): www.icea.org

La Leche League: www.lalecheleague.org

Lamaze International: www.lamaze.org

March of Dimes: www.marchofdimes.com

American College of Nurse Midwives: www.Mymidwife.org

AWHONN Patient Education: www.Health4women.org

SAFE AND EFFECTIVE NURSING CARE: Patient Education

Mobile Phone Education: Text4Baby

Text4Baby is an innovative educational program offering perinatal education via text messages. More than 90% of American households have cell phones, the majority with text messaging capabilities. The program was developed through a collaboration of public and private partnership, including ZERO TO THREE, Voxiva, CTIA Wireless Foundation, the Department of Health and Human Services, White House Office of Science and Technology Policy, and Discovery Fit and Health. These partnerships include government agencies, corporations, academic institutions, professional associations, and nonprofit organizations. Message content was reviewed by an interdisciplinary panel of experts to ensure the information reflected evidence-based practice.

Once signed up for the service, women will receive three free SMS text messages each week timed to their due dates, throughout pregnancy until baby is 1 year old. The program provides vital health information to pregnant women and new mothers. Examples of topics include nutrition, seasonal flu prevention and treatment, mental health topics, risks of tobacco use, oral health, safe infant sleeping, and parenting. Women can sign up for the program by texting BABY to 511411 (or by texting BEBE for Spanish) (Hunt, 2015).

Evidence-Based Practice: Effectiveness of Childbirth Education

Afshar, Y., Wang, E., Mai, J., Esakoff, T., Pisarska, M., & Gregory, K. (2017). Childbirth education class and birth plans are associated with a vaginal delivery. *BIRTH, 44*(1), 29–34; Gagnon, A. J. (2011). Individual or group antenatal education for childbirth or parenthood, or both. *Cochrane Database of Systematic Reviews* (10). doi:10.1002/14651858.CD002869.pub2

Childbirth education aims to help prospective parents prepare for childbirth and parenthood. Prospective parents often look to childbirth classes or antenatal education to provide important information on issues such as decision making about and during labor, skills for labor, pain relief, infant and postnatal care, breastfeeding, and parenting skills. This antenatal education can be provided in many ways. A retrospective cross-sectional study placed women into four categories: those who attended a CBE class, those with a birth plan, those who attended a CBE class and had a birth plan, and those with neither CBE or a birth plan. In the study, 14,630 deliveries met the inclusion criteria: 31.9% of the women attended CBE, 12% had a birth plan, and 8.8 % had both. Women who attended CBE or had a birth plan were older, more likely to be nulliparous, had a lower body mass index, and were less likely to be African American. After adjusting for significant covariates, women who participated in either option or both had higher odds of a vaginal delivery. Attending CBE class and/or having a birth plan were associated with a vaginal delivery. These findings suggest that patient education and birth preparation may influence the mode of delivery. CBE and birth plans could be used as quality improvement tools to potentially decrease cesarean rates (Afshar et al., 2017). An older Cochrane review indicates there are many varied ways of providing this antenatal education, and some may be more effective than others. The review found nine trials involving 2,284 women. Interventions varied greatly, and no consistent outcomes were measured. The review of trials found a lack of high-quality evidence from trials and so the effects of antenatal education remain largely unknown. Further research is required to ensure that effective ways of helping health professionals support pregnant women and their partners in preparing for birth and parenting are investigated so that the resources used meet the needs of parents and their newborn infants. They concluded the effects of general antenatal education for childbirth or parenthood, or both, remain largely unknown. Individualized prenatal education directed toward avoidance of a repeat caesarean birth does not increase the rate of vaginal birth after caesarean section (Gagnon, 2011).

CONCEPT MAP

Maternal Adaptation to Pregnancy Complications

Frustration
* Woman expresses anger or aggression
* Withdrawal from pregnancy or partner

Fear
* Woman states she is afraid of fetal death
* Woman states she is afraid of newborn disability
* Woman is crying

Pregnancy Complication
Woman diagnosed with high-risk pregnancy

Anxiety
* Unexpected pregnancy complication
* Unanticipated interruption in normal pregnancy

Threat to Self-Esteem
* Woman feels lack of self-confidence related to pregnancy
* Woman reports feeling she has failed as a woman
* Woman feels little confidence to be a mother

Problem No. 1: Anxiety related to uncertain labor processes and fetal outcome

Goal: Decrease anxiety and possess knowledge of processes

Outcome: Verbalize fears to decrease anxiety and verbalize knowledge of processes

Nursing Actions
1. Provide time for the patient and family to express their concerns regarding fetal outcome.
2. Encourage the woman to vent apprehension, uncertainty, anger, fear, and/or worry.
3. Discuss prior pregnancy outcomes if applicable.
4. Explain pregnancy complication, management, and reason for each treatment.
5. Help the woman to obtain needed social support.
6. Refer the family to community or hospital resources such as social worker, case manager, or chaplain services as needed.
7. Provide resource information for the woman and family as issues arise.

Problem No. 2: Impaired self-esteem related to pregnancy complication

Goal: Improved self-esteem

Outcome: Patient will express improved self-esteem.

Nursing Actions
1. Encourage verbalization of feelings.
2. Practice active listening.
3. Provide emotional support.
4. Encourage the patient to participate in decision making.
5. Make needed referrals to social services and mental health specialists.

Problem 3: Anxiety related to unexpected pregnancy complication(s)

Goal: Decreased anxiety

Outcome: Patient verbalizes that she feels less anxious, verbalizes plan of care with complication(s).

Nursing Actions
1. Be calm and reassuring in interactions with patient and family.
2. Explain all information repeatedly related to complication.
3. Provide autonomy and choices.
4. Encourage patient and family to verbalize their feelings regarding diagnosis by asking open-end questions.
5. Explore past coping strategies.
6. Explore spiritual practices and beliefs with the woman.

Problem 4: Frustration related to pregnancy complication
Goal: Positive pregnancy adaptation
Outcome: Patient demonstrates adaptation to pregnancy.

Nursing Actions
1. Allow the woman to express her feelings related to loss of normal pregnancy.
2. Allow the woman to express her feelings related to not having a normal birth.
3. Allow the woman to express her feelings related to uncertainty of fetal outcome.
4. Provide choices related to management when possible.

Case Study

As a nurse in an antenatal clinic, you are part of an interdisciplinary team that is caring for Margarite Sanchez during her pregnancy. Margarite is 10 weeks pregnant and is a 28-year-old G3 P1 Hispanic woman. She began prenatal care at 8 weeks' gestation visit. She works in a day-care center. She has a 2-year-old son. José, her husband, has not accompanied her to her second prenatal appointment, as he is in his busy season as a landscaper. Margarite reports they are pleased about the pregnancy although planned to wait another year or two before attempting another pregnancy. Margarite was seen for some spotting at 6 weeks' gestation that has resolved. She tells you she has been irritable and short-tempered with her husband and son, particularly at the end of the day when she feels exhausted. She states she is relieved the spotting stopped but is not sure she feels ready to be a mother of two children. Her mother lives four blocks away, and they speak on the phone daily and see each other several times a week. She is very involved in her parish, and the women in her church study group all know she is pregnant and are all certain the baby is a girl.

Detail the aspects of your psychosocial assessment at 10 weeks' gestation.

Discuss the rationale for the assessment.

Discuss the nursing diagnosis, nursing activities, and expected outcomes related to this problem.

Discuss the importance of the pregnant woman's mother during pregnancy.

Suggest two interventions that could help to prepare Margarite's 2-year-old son during the pregnancy.

REFERENCES

Afshar, Y., My-Lin, N., Mei, J., & Grisales, T. (2017). Sexual health and function in pregnancy: Counseling about sexuality in pregnancy and postpartum offers an opportunity to allay fears and increase patient satisfaction during a unique period in a woman's life. *Contemporary OB/GYN, 62*(8), 24–30.

Afshar, Y., Wang, E., Mai, J., Esakoff, T., Pisarska, M., & Gregory, K. (2017). Childbirth education class and birth plans are associated with a vaginal delivery. *BIRTH, 44*(1), 29–34.

Alio, A., Bond, M., Padilla, Y., Heidelbaugh, J., Lu, M., & Parker, W. (2011). Addressing policy barriers to paternal involvement during pregnancy. *Maternal Child Health Journal, 15,* 425–430.

Alio, A., Salihu, H., Komosky, J., Richman, A., & Marty, P. (2010). Feto-infant health and survival: Does paternal involvement matter? *Maternal Child Health Journal, 14,* 931–937.

American Association of Colleges of Nursing. (2008). *The essentials of baccalaureate education for professional nursing practice.* Retrieved from http://aacn.nche.edu/education-resources/BaccEssentials08.pdf.

Amidi-Nouri, A. (2011). Culturally responsive nursing care. In A. Berman & S. Snyder (Eds.), *Kozier & Erb's Fundamentals of Nursing* (9th ed.). San Francisco, CA: Pearson.

Andrews, M., & Boyle, C. (2011). *Transcultural concepts in nursing care* (6th ed.). Philadelphia, PA: Lippincott Williams & Wilkins.

Association of Women's Health, Obstetric and Neonatal Nurses (AWHONN). (2000). *Policy position statement: Midwifery.* Washington, DC: Author.

Association of Women's Health, Obstetric and Neonatal Nurses (AWHONN). (2009). Confidentiality in adolescent health care. Position statement. Washington DC: Author.

Baetens, P., & Brewaeys, A. (2001). Lesbian couples requesting donor insemination: an update of the knowledge with regard to lesbian mother families, *Human Reproduction Update, 7*(5), 512–519. https://doi.org/10.1093/humupd/7.5.512

Barron, M. (2014). Antenatal care. In K. Simpson & P. Creehan (Eds.), *AWHONN perinatal nursing* (4th ed., pp. 41–70). Philadelphia, PA: Lippincott Williams & Wilkins.

Beck, C. (2002). Revision of the Postpartum Depression Predictors Inventory. *Journal of Obstetric, Gynecologic, and Neonatal Nursing, 31*(4), 394–402.

Beeber, L., & Canuso, R. (2005). Strengthening social support for the low income mother: Five critical questions and a guide for intervention. *Journal of Obstetric, Gynecologic, and Neonatal Nursing, 34*(6), 769–776.

Begley, A. (2000). Preparation for practice in the new millennium: A discussion of the moral implications of multifetal pregnancy reduction. *Nursing Ethics, 7*(2), 99–112.

Bibring, G., Dwyer, T., Huntington, D., & Valenstein, D. (1961). A study of the psychological processes in pregnancy and of the early mother-child relationships. *Psychoanalytic Study of the Child, 16*(9), 9–24.

Bos, H. M. W., Van Balen, F., & Van Den Boom, D. C. (2004). Experience of parenthood, couple relationship, social support, and child rearing goals in planned lesbian families. *Journal of Child Psychology and Psychiatry, 45,* 755–764.

Bos, H. M. W., Van Balen, F., & Van den Boom, D. C. (2007). Child adjustment and parenting in planned lesbian-parent families. *American Journal of Orthopsychiatry, 77,* 38–48.

Brennan, A., Ayers, S., Ahmed, H., & Marshall-Lucette, S. (2007). A critical review of the Couvade syndrome: The pregnant male. *Journal of Reproductive and Infant Psychology, 25*(3), 173–189.

Callister, L. (2014). Integrating cultural beliefs and practices into the care of childbearing women. In K. Simpson & P. Creehan (Eds.), *AWHONN perinatal nursing* (4th ed., pp. 41–70). Philadelphia, PA: Lippincott Williams & Wilkins.

Campbell, D., Lake, M., Falk, M., & Backstrand, J. (2006). A randomized trial of continuous support in labor by a lay doula. *Journal of Obstetric, Gynecologic, and Neonatal Nursing, 35*(4), 456–464.

Cannella, B. (2006). Mediators of the relationship between social support and positive health practices in pregnant women. *Nursing Research, 55*(6), 437–445.

Carolan, M. (2005). "Doing it properly": The experience of first time mothering over 35 years. *Health Care for Women International, 26*(9), 764–787.

Carroll, J., Reid, A., Biringer, A., Midmer, D., Glazier, R., Wilson, L., . . . Stewart, D. (2005). Effectiveness of the Antenatal Psychosocial Health Assessment

(ALPHA) form in detecting psychosocial concerns: A randomized controlled trial. *Canadian Medical Association Journal, 173*(3), 253–259.

Centers for Disease Control (CDC). (2017a). *Teen pregnancy in the United States.* Retrieved from www.cdc.gov/teenpregnancy/about/index.htm.

Centers for Disease Control (CDC). (2017b). *Lead health literacy initiative.* Retrieved from www.cdc.gov/nceh/lead/tools/leadliteracy.htm

Centers for Disease Control. (2018). *Child Development.* Retrieved from https://www.cdc.gov/ncbddd/childdevelopment/facts.html

Cheng, E. R., Rifas-Shiman, S. L., Perkins, M. E., Rich-Edwards, J. W., Gillman, M. W., Wright, R., & Taveras, E. M. (2016). The influence of antenatal partner support on pregnancy outcomes. *Journal of Women's Health, 25*(7), 672–679. doi:10.1089/jwh.2015.5462

Collopy, K. (2004). "I couldn't think that far": Infertile women's decision making about multifetal reduction. *Research in Nursing and Health, 27*(2), 75–86.

Crooks, R., & Baur, K. (2010). *Our sexuality* (11th ed.). Menlo Park, NJ: Benjamin Cummings Publishing Company.

Damato, E. (2003). Predictors of prenatal attachment in mothers of twins. *Journal of Obstetric, Gynecologic, and Neonatal Nursing, 33*(4), 436–445.

Dawley, K., & Beam, R. (2005). "My nurse taught me how to have a healthy baby and be a good mother:" Nurse home visiting with pregnant women 1888 to 2005. *Nursing Clinics of North America, 40*, 803–815.

DeVito, J. (2010). How adolescent mothers feel about becoming a parent. *Journal of Perinatal Education, 19*(2), 25–34.

Dobrzykowski, T., & Stern, P. (2003). Out of sync: A generation of first-time mothers over 30. *Health Care for Women International, 24*(3), 242–253.

Durham, R. (1998). Strategies women engage in when analyzing preterm labor at home. *Journal of Perinatology, 19*, 61–69.

Duvall, E. (1985). *Marriage and family development.* New York, NY: Harper & Row.

Foster, G., Alviar, A., Neumeier, R., & Wootten, A. (2012). A tri-service perspective on the implementation of a centering pregnancy model in the military. *Journal of Obstetric, Gynecologic, and Neonatal Nursing, 41*(2), 315–321.

Friedman, M., Bowden, V., & Jones, E. (2003). *Family nursing: Research, theory, and practice* (5th ed.). Upper Saddle River, NJ: Prentice Hall.

Gagnon, A. J. (2011). Individual or group antenatal education for childbirth or parenthood, or both. *Cochrane Database of Systematic Reviews* (10). doi:10.1002/14651858.CD002869.pub2

Ganann, R., Sword, W., Thabane, L., Newbold, B., & Black, M. (2016). Predictors of postpartum depression among immigrant women in the year after childbirth. *Journal of Women's Health, 25*(2), 155–165.

Genesoni, L., & Tallandini, M. (2009). Men's psychological transition to fatherhood: An analysis of the literature, 1989–2008. *Birth, 36*(4), 305–317.

Gilbert, E. (2010). *Manual of high risk pregnancy and delivery* (5th ed.). St. Louis, MO: C.V. Mosby.

Giurgescu, C., Penckofer, S., Maurer, M., & Bryant, F. (2006). Impact of uncertainty, social support, and prenatal coping on the psychological well-being of high risk pregnant women. *Nursing Research, 55*(5), 356–365.

Goldberg, A. E., & Sayer, A. G. (2006) Lesbian couples' relationship quality across the transition to parenthood. *Journal of Marriage and Family, 68*, 87–100.

Green, J., & Hotelling, B. A. (2009). Healthy birth practice #3: Bring a loved one, friend, or doula for continuous support. Washington, DC: Lamaze International.

Hanson, S., Hunter, L., Bormann, J., & Sobo, E. (2009). Paternal fears of childbirth: A literature review. *Journal of Perinatal Education, 18*(4), 12–20.

Hodnett, E. D., Fredericks, S., & Weston, J. (2010). Support during pregnancy for women at increased risk of low birthweight babies. *Cochrane Database of Systematic Reviews,* (6), doi:10.1002/14651858.CD000198.pub2

Hodnett, E. D., Gates, S., Hofmeyr, G., & Sakala, C. (2011). Continuous support for women during childbirth (Cochrane Review). In the *Cochrane Library,* 2.

Hunt, S. (2015). Text4Baby app. *Nursing for Women's Health, 19*(1), 77–79.

International Childbirth Education Association (ICEA). (1999). Position paper: The role and scope of the doula. *International Journal of Childbirth Education, 14*(1), 38–45.

Jentsch, B., Durham, R., Hundley, V., & Hussein, J. (2007) Creating consumer satisfaction in maternity care: The neglected needs of migrants, asylum seekers and refugees. *International Journal of Consumer Studies, 31*, 128–134.

Joint Commission (2018). The Joint Commission Standards Interpretation. Author, https://www.jointcommission.org/standards_information/jcfaq.aspx

Jordan, P. (1989). Support behaviors identified as helpful and desired by second time parents over the perinatal period. *Maternal Child Nursing Journal, 18*(2), 133–145.

Katon, J., Lewis, L., Hercinovic, S., McNab, A., Fortney, J., & Rose, S. (2017). Improving perinatal mental health care for women veterans: Description of a quality improvement program. *Maternal Child Health, 21*(8), 1598–1605.

Key, J. D., Gebregziabher, M. G., Marsh, L. D., & O'Rourke, K. M. (2008). Effectiveness of an intensive school-based intervention for teen mothers. *Journal of Adolescent Health, 42*, 394–400.

Koniak-Griffin, D., Logsdon, C., Hines-Martin, V., & Turner, C. (2006). Contemporary mothering in a diverse society. *Journal of Obstetric, Gynecologic, and Neonatal Nursing, 35*(5), 671–678.

Kowlessar, O., Fox, J. R., & Wittkowski, A. (2015). The pregnant male: A metasynthesis of first-time fathers' experiences of pregnancy. *Journal of Reproductive & Infant Psychology, 33*(2), 106–127. doi:10.1080/02646838.2014.970153.

Lamaze International. (2009). *Position paper—Lamaze for the 21st century.* Retrieved from https://www.lamazeinternational.org/p/cm/ld/fid=211.

Lauderdale, J. (2011). Transcultural perspectives in childbearing. In M. Andrews & J. Boyle (Eds.), *Transcultural concepts in nursing care* (6th ed., pp. 95–131). Philadelphia, PA: Lippincott Williams & Wilkins.

Lederman, R. (1996). *Psychosocial adaptation in pregnancy* (2nd ed.). New York, NY: Springer.

Lederman, R. (2011). Preterm birth prevention: A mandate for psychosocial assessment. *Issues in Mental Health Nursing, 32*, 163–169.

Lederman, R., & Weis, K. (2009). *Psychosocial adaptation in pregnancy: Seven dimensions of maternal role development* (3rd ed.). New York, NY: Springer.

Lee, Y., & Blitz, L. (2016). We're grand: A qualitative design and development pilot project addressing the needs and strengths of grandparents raising grandchildren. *Child & Family Social Work, 21*, 381–390.

Leininger, M. (Ed). (1991). *Culture care diversity & universality: A theory of nursing.* New York, NY: National League for Nursing Press.

Lindberg, L. D., Santelli, J. S., & Desai, S. (2016). Understanding the decline in adolescent fertility in the United States, 2007–2012. *Journal of Adolescent Health, 59*(5), 577–583.

Logsdon, C., Gagne, P., Hughes, T., Patterson, J., & Rakestraw, V. (2005). Social support during adolescent pregnancy: Piecing together a quilt. *Journal of Obstetric, Gynecologic, & Neonatal Nursing, 34*(5), 606–614.

Lothian, J. (2011). Lamaze breathing: What every pregnant woman needs to know. *Journal of Perinatal Education, 20*(2), 118–120.

MacKay, A. P., & Duran, C. (2007). Adolescent health in the United States, 2007. National Center for Health Statistics.

Maifeld, M., Hahn, S., Titler, M., Marita, G., & Mullen, M. (2003). Decision making regarding multifetal reduction. *Journal of Obstetric, Gynecologic, & Neonatal Nursing, 32*(3), 357–369.

March of Dimes. (2017). Abuse during pregnancy. Retrieved from https://www.marchofdimes.org/pregnancy/abuse-during-pregnancy.aspx

Martin, J. A., Hamilton, B. E., Osterman, M.J.K., Driscol, A. K., & Mathews, T. J. (2017). Births: Final data for 2015. National vital statistics report; vol 66, no 1. Hyattsville, MD: National Center for Health Statistics.

Mattocks, K., Skanderson, M., Goulet, J., Brandt, C., Womack, J., Krebs, E., . . . Haskell, S. (2010). Pregnancy and mental health among women veterans returning from Iraq and Afghanistan. *Journal of Women's Health, 19*(12), 2159–2166.

Mattson, S., & Smith, J. (2016). *Core curriculum for maternal newborn nursing* (4th ed.). St. Louis, MO: Elsevier Saunders.

May, K. (1980). A typology of detachment/involvement styles adopted by first time expectant fathers. *Western Journal of Nursing Research, 2*, 443–453.

May, K. (1982). Three phases of father involvement in pregnancy. *Nursing Research, 31*(6), 337–342.

May, K., & Mahlmeister, L. (1994). *Maternal & neonatal nursing, family centered care.* Philadelphia, PA: Lippincott Williams & Wilkins.

McCants, B. M., & Greiner, J. R. (2016). Prebirth education and childbirth decision making. *International Journal of Childbirth Education, 31*(1), 24–27.

McKeever, A., Alderman, S., Luff, S., & DeJesus, B. (2016). Assessment and care of childbearing women with severe and persistent mental illness. *Nursing for Women's Health, 20*(5), 484–499. doi:10.1016/j.nwh.2016.08.010

McManus, A., Hunter, L., & Renn, H. (2006). Lesbian experiences and needs during childbirth: Guidance for health care providers. *Journal of Obstetric, Gynecologic, & Neonatal Nursing, 35*(1), 13–23.

McMenamin, P. (2015). Diversity among registered nurses: Slow but steady progress. American Nurses Association.Professional Issues Panel http://www.ananurspace.org/blogs/peter-mcmenamin/2015/08/21/rn-diversity-note?ssopc=1

Meleis, A. (2003). Theoretical consideration of health care for immigrant and minority women. In P. St. Hill, J. Lipson, & A. Meleis (Eds.), *Caring for women cross culturally*. Philadelphia, PA: F.A. Davis.

Mercer, R. (1995). *Becoming a mother*. New York, NY: Springer.

Mercer, R. (2004). Becoming a mother versus maternal role attainment. *Journal of Nursing Scholarship, 36*(3), 226–233.

Midmer, D., Carroll, J., Bryanton, J., & Stewart, D. (2002). From research to application: The development of an antenatal psychosocial health assessment tool. *Canadian Journal of Public Health, 93*(4), 291–296.

Misra, D. P., Caldwell, C., Young, A. A., & Abelson, S. (2010). Do fathers matter? Paternal contributions to birth outcomes and racial disparities. *American Journal of Obstetrics and Gynecology, 202,* 99–100.

Mojaverian, T., & Heejung, K. (2013). Interpreting a helping hand: Cultural variation in the effectiveness of solicited and unsolicited social support. *Personality and Social Psychology Bulletin, 39*(1), 88–99.

Moore, M., Moos, M., & Callister, L. (2010). *Cultural competence: An essential journey for perinatal nurses*. White Plains, NY: March of Dimes Foundation.

Ngai, F., Chan, S., & Ip, W. (2010). Predictors and correlates of maternal role competence and satisfaction. *Nursing Research, 59*(3), 185–193.

Parker, K., Cilluffo, A., & Stepler, R. (2017). *6 facts about the U.S. military and its changing demographics*. PEW Research Reports. Retrieved from http://www.pewresearch.org/fact-tank/2017/04/13/6-facts-about-the-u-s-military-and-its-changing-demographics/

Pascali-Bonaro, D., & Kroeger, M. (2004). Continuous female companionship during childbirth: A crucial resource in times of stress or calm. *Journal of Midwifery & Women's Health, 49*(4), 19–27.

Perper, K., Peterson, K., & Manlove, J. (2010) Diploma attainment among teen mothers. Child trends, fact sheet publication #2010-01: Washington, DC: Child Trends.

Phua, D. Y., Kee, M.K.Z.L., Koh, D.X.P., Rifkin-Graboi, A., Daniels, M., Chen, H., . . . Meaney, M. J. (2017). Growing Up In Singapore Towards Healthy Outcomes Study Group. Positive maternal mental health during pregnancy associated with specific forms of adaptive development in early childhood: Evidence from a longitudinal study. *Developmental Psychopathology, 29*(5), 1573–1587. doi: 10.1017/S0954579417001249. PubMed PMID: 29162171.

Pinazo-Hernandis, S., & Tompkins, C. (2009). Custodial grandparents: The state of the art and the many faces of this contribution. *Journal of Intergenerational Relationships, 7*(2–3), 137–143.

Porter, L., & Holness, N. (2011). Breaking the repeat teen pregnancy cycle: How nurses can nurture resilience in at-risk teens. *Nursing for Women's Health, 15*(5), 369–381.

Priest, S., Austin, M., & Sullivan, E. (2006). Antenatal psychosocial screening for prevention of antenatal and postnatal anxiety and depression (Protocol). *Cochrane Library*, 1.

Purnell, L. (2014). *Guide to culturally competent health care* (3rd ed.). Philadelphia, PA: F.A. Davis.

Recame, M. A. (2013). Childbirth education and parental support programs within the U.S. military population. *International Journal of Childbirth Education, 28*(1), 67–70.

Renaud, M.T. (2007). We are mothers too: Childbearing experiences of lesbian families. *Journal of Obstetric, Gynecologic and Neonatal Nursing, 36*(1), 190–199.

Romano, A. (2010). Safe and healthy birth: The importance of data. *Journal of Perinatal Education, 19*(4), 52–58.

Romano, A. (2014). Why holistic care for childbirth? *International Journal Childbirth Education, 29,* 4.

Rondahl, G., Bruhner, E., & Lindhe, J. (2009). Heteronormative communication with lesbian families in antenatal care, childbirth and postnatal care. *Journal of Advanced Nursing, 65*(11), 2337–2344.

Ross, L. (2005). Perinatal mental health in lesbian mothers: A review of potential risk and protective factors. *Women & Health, 41*(3), 113–128.

Rubin, R. (1975). Maternal tasks in pregnancy. *Maternal-Child Nursing Journal, 4*(3), 143–153.

Rubin, R. (1984). *Maternal identity and the maternal experience*. New York, NY: Springer.

Schaffer, M. A., Jost, R., Pederson, B. J., & Lair, M. (2008). Pregnancy-free club: A strategy to prevent repeat adolescent pregnancy. *Public Health Nursing, 25*(4), 304–311.

Schardt, D. (2005). Delayed childbearing: Underestimated psychological implications. *International Journal of Childbirth Education, 20*(3), 34–37.

Shah, M. K., Gee, R. E., & Theall, K. P. (2014). Partner support and impact on birth outcomes among teen pregnancies in the United States. *Journal of Pediatric and Adolescent Gynecology, 27*(1), 14–19. http://doi.org/10.1016/j.jpag.2013.08.002

Sharma, R. (2013). The family and family structure classification redefined for the current times. *Journal of Family Medicine and Primary Care, 2*(4), 306–310.

Simpson, K., & Creehan, P. (Eds.). (2014). *AWHONN Perinatal Nursing* (4th ed.), Philadelphia, PA: Lippincott.

Skurzak, A. (2015). Social support for pregnant women. *Polish Journal Public Health, 125*(3), 169–172.

Smith, P., Buzi, R., Kozinetz, C., Peskin, M., & Weimann, C. (2016). Impact of a group prenatal program for pregnant adolescents on perceived partner support. *Child Adolescent Social Work, 33,* 417–428.

Stadtlander, L. (2017). Anxiety and pregnancy. *International Journal Childbirth Education, 32*(1), 32–35.

Stapleton, L., Schetter, C., Westling, E., Rini, C., Hobel, C., & Sandman, C. (2012). Perceived partner support in pregnancy predicts lower maternal and infant distress. *National Institute of Health, 26*(3), 453–463.

Sutherland, M. (2011). Implications for violence in adolescent dating experiences. *Journal of Obstetric, Gynecologic, & Neonatal Nursing, 40*(2), 225–234.

Teten, A. L., Ball, B., Valle, L. A., Noonan, R., & Rosenbluth, B. (2009). Considerations for the definition, measurement, consequences, and prevention of dating violence victimization among adolescent girls. *Journal of Women's Health, 18*(7), 923–927. doi: 10.1089/jwh.2009.1515. PubMed PMID: 19575691.

U.S. Census Bureau. (2010). *National population by race, United States, 2010*. Retrieved from https://www.census.gov/quickfacts/fact/table/US/PST045217/

U.S. Department of Health and Human Services, Health Resources and Services Administration. (2010a). *Healthy People 2020 objectives*. Retrieved from ttps://www.healthypeople.gov/2020/topics-objectives/topic/Access-to-Health-Services

U.S. Department of Health and Human Services, Health Resources and Services Administration. (2010b). *The registered nurse population: Findings from the National Sample Survey of Registered Nurses*. Washington, DC: Author.

Walker, D., Visger, J., & Rossie, D. (2009). Contemporary childbirth education models. *Journal of Midwifery and Women's Health, 54*(6), 469–476.

Weis, K., Lederman, R., Lilly, A., & Schaffer, J. (2008). The relationship of military imposed marital separations on maternal acceptance of pregnancy. *Research in Nursing & Health, 31,* 196–207.

Weis, K., & Ryan, T. (2012). Mentors offering maternal support: A support intervention for military mothers. *Journal of Obstetric, Gynecologic, and Neonatal Nursing, 42*(2), 303–314.

Widarsson, M., Kerstis, B., Sundquist, K., Engström, G., & Sarkadi, A. (2012). Support needs of expectant mothers and fathers: A qualitative study. *Journal of Perinatal Education, 21*(1), 36–44.

Wilson, C., & Leese, B. (2013) Do nurses and midwives have a role in promoting the well-being of patients during their fertility journey? *British Fertility Society, 16*(1), 2–7.

Wojnar, D. (2007). Miscarriage experiences of lesbian couples. *Journal of Midwifery and Womens Health, 52,* 479–485.

Wojnar, D., & Katzenmeyer, A. (2014) Experiences of preconception, pregnancy, and new motherhood for lesbian nonbiological mothers. *Journal of Obstetric, Gynecological & Neonatal Nursing, 43*(1), 50–59.

Zadeh, M. A., Khajehei, M., Sharif, F., & Hadzic, M. (2012). High-risk pregnancy: Effects on postpartum depression and anxiety. *British Journal of Midwifery, 20*(2), 104–113.

Zielinski, R., Ackerson, K., Kane-Low, L. (2015). Planned home birth: Benefits, risks and opportunities. *Dove Press, 7,* 361–377. https://doi.org/10.2147/IJWH.S55561

Antepartal Tests

6

Roberta F. Durham, RN, PhD

LEARNING OUTCOMES

Upon completion of this chapter, the student will be able to:

1. Define terms used in antenatal tests.
2. Identify the purpose and indication for key antenatal tests.
3. Describe the procedure, interpretation, advantages, and risks of common antenatal tests.
4. Articulate the nursing responsibilities related to key antenatal tests.
5. Identify patient teaching needs related to antenatal tests.

Nursing Diagnosis

- Deficient knowledge related to antenatal tests
- Anxiety related to antenatal tests
- Risk for disturbed maternal fetal dyad because of fetal injury or death related to invasive antenatal tests

Nursing Outcomes

- The pregnant woman and her family will understand the purpose, procedure, and results of antenatal tests.
- The pregnant woman will be able to make informed decisions about antenatal tests.
- Complications of antenatal tests will be identified promptly, and appropriate nursing interventions will be initiated.

INTRODUCTION

This chapter presents various antenatal tests offered to pregnant women, focusing on tests for at-risk and/or high-risk pregnancies. Common maternal conditions indicating need for antenatal tests are presented in Table 6–1. The purpose, indication, basic procedure, interpretation, advantages, risks, and nursing actions are outlined. Specifics on procedures are not detailed, as they may vary from institution to institution. Routine tests performed during pregnancy are presented and detailed in Chapter 4. Antenatal tests are often performed as outpatient procedures, including ultrasound, amniocentesis, and nonstress tests (NST). Antenatal tests may also be performed during an antenatal hospitalization for a high-risk pregnancy. The nurse's role and responsibility related to antenatal tests may vary based on the inpatient or outpatient setting. Nursing care may be provided before, during, and/or after a procedure.

ASSESSMENT FOR RISK FACTORS

The nurse needs to assess for factors that place the woman and/ or her fetus at risk for adverse outcomes.

- Biophysical factors originate from the mother or fetus and impact the development or function of the mother or fetus. They include genetic, nutritional, medical, and obstetric issues (see Table 6–1).
- Psychosocial factors are maternal behaviors or lifestyles that have a negative effect on the mother or fetus. Examples include smoking, caffeine use, alcohol/drug use, and psychological status.
- Sociodemographic factors are variables pertaining to the woman and her family that place the mother and the fetus at increased risk. Examples include access to prenatal care, age, parity, marital status, income, and ethnicity.

● Environmental factors are hazards in the workplace or the general environment that impact pregnancy outcomes. Various environmental substances can affect fetal development. Examples include exposure to chemicals, radiation, and pollutants.

The underlying mechanism for how some risk factors impact pregnancy outcomes is not fully understood. Many risk factors appear to have a combined or cumulative effect. Identification of risk factors for poor perinatal outcomes is essential to minimize maternal and neonatal morbidity and mortality. Risk factors are described in more detail in Chapters 7, 10, 14, and 17 as they relate specifically to pregnancy, labor, the postpartum period, and the neonate, respectively.

THE NURSE'S ROLE IN ANTEPARTAL TESTING

The nurse's role during antepartal testing varies based on the specific test. In general, it includes assessing for risk factors and providing information and emotional support and comfort to women undergoing antenatal tests. Many women having antenatal tests are at high risk for fetal and maternal complications and are anxious and vulnerable. In some instances, the nurse assists or performs the antenatal test, and in some instances this requires advanced competencies (i.e., ultrasound).

TABLE 6–1	Indications for Antepartum Fetal Surveillance: Common Maternal Conditions Indicating Need for Antenatal Tests
Maternal Conditions	Antiphospholipid syndrome
	Hemoglobinopathies
	Hypertensive disorder
	Renal disease
	Cardiac disease
	Systemic lupus erythematosus
	Insulin-treated diabetes mellitus
Pregnancy-Related Conditions	Pregnancy-induced hypertension
	Decreased fetal movement
	Hydramnios, oligohydramnios, and polyhydramnios
	Intrauterine growth restriction
	Multiple gestation with growth discrepancy or monochorionic diamniotic multiples, post-term pregnancy
	Previous unexplained fetal demise
	Isoimmunization
	Fetal anomalies

American Academy of Pediatrics and the American College of Obstetricians and Gynecologists, 2012.

CRITICAL COMPONENT

Nursing Actions Related to Antenatal Tests

Nurses are involved in antenatal testing in a variety of ways, depending on the test. Regardless of the level of involvement in antenatal testing, nurses must provide appropriate support to families and understand the variety of tests available during pregnancy, the risks and benefits of tests/procedures, the indications for tests/procedures, the interpretation of findings, the nursing care associated with the test/procedure, and the physical and psychological benefits, limitations, and implications of the test/procedure (Barron, 2014; Gilbert, 2011). Specific nursing actions for women undergoing antenatal testing include the following:

- Promote informed decisions and prevent uninformed decisions by patients.
- Assess for factors that place the woman and/or her fetus at risk for adverse outcomes.
- Establish a trusting relationship.
- Provide information regarding the test.
  - Explain how the test/procedure is performed.
  - Explain potential risks and benefits.
  - Explain what the woman can expect during the test/procedure.
  - Explain what the test measures.
  - Encourage questions.
  - Encourage and foster open communication with providers.
  - Provide online resources for further information (Box 6–1).
- Provide comfort.
  - Assist woman into a comfortable position.
  - Preserve the woman's modesty by closing doors and exposing only the portions of her body necessary for the test/procedure.
- Reassure the woman and her significant other.
  - Address concerns regarding the test/procedure such as type of discomfort or pain she may experience and effects on her and/or her unborn child.
  - If she prefers, encourage the woman's significant other to be with her during procedures.
- Provide psychological support to the woman and her significant other (Fig. 6–1).
  - Incorporate understanding of cultural and social issues.
  - Remain with the woman and her significant other during the test/procedure.
  - Assess for anxiety and provide care to reduce the level of anxiety.

- Allow client to vent feelings and frustrations with the discomfort, time-consuming demands, and limitations imposed by high-risk pregnancy and antenatal testing.
- Allow the woman to express feelings related to high-risk pregnancy.
- Encourage expression and exploration of feelings.
- Document the woman's response and the results of tests.
- Report results of tests to providers.
- Schedule appropriate follow-up.
- Reinforce information given by the woman's provider regarding the results of the tests and need for further testing, treatment, or referral.

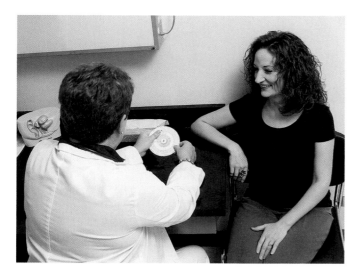

FIGURE 6–1 Nurse counseling a pregnant woman.

SCREENING AND DIAGNOSTIC TESTS

Prenatal detection of abnormalities provides an opportunity for the patient and provider to prepare and intervene. Normal test results can decrease a patients' anxiety; however, screening results are not definite. They are designed to identify those who are not affected by a disease or abnormality. Certain screening tests assess the risk that the fetus has specific common birth defects, but screening tests cannot tell whether the baby actually has a birth defect. These tests carry no risk to the fetus.

Diagnostic tests provide a yes or no answer to whether a fetus is normal or abnormal and can detect many, but not all, birth abnormalities caused by defects in a gene or chromosomes. Diagnostic testing may be done instead of screening if a couple has a family history of a birth defect, belongs to a certain ethnic group, or already has a child with a birth defect. Diagnostic tests also are available as a first choice for all pregnant women, including those who do not have risk factors. Some diagnostic tests carry risks, including a small risk of pregnancy loss.

CRITICAL COMPONENT

Antepartal Screening and Diagnostic Tests
Screening Test
A screening test is a test designed to identify those who are not affected by a disease or abnormality. Some screening tests are offered to all pregnant women, such as multiple marker screening and ultrasound. Other screening tests are reserved for high-risk pregnancies to provide information on fetal status and well-being. If the results of screening tests indicate an abnormality, further testing is indicated. Screening tests include the following:

- Amniotic fluid index (AFI)
- Biophysical profile
- Contraction stress test
- Daily fetal movement count
- Multiple marker screening: alpha-fetoprotein screening, triple marker, and quad marker
- Nonstress test (NST)
- Ultrasonography
- Nuchal translucency
- Umbilical artery Doppler flow
- Vibroacoustic stimulation

Diagnostic Tests
Prenatal diagnosis is the science of identifying structural or functional anomalies or birth defects in the fetus (Cunningham et al., 2014). Diagnostic tests help to identify a disease or provide information that aids in diagnosis. Most fetal diagnostic tests are reserved for high-risk pregnancies in which the fetus is at increased risk for developmental or physical problems.

Diagnostic tests include the following:

- Amniocentesis
- Chorionic villi sampling
- Magnetic resonance imaging
- Percutaneous umbilical blood sampling
- Ultrasonography

BIOPHYSICAL ASSESSMENT

Since the 1970s, the fetus has become more accessible with the refinement of new technology such as ultrasound. Fetal physiological parameters that can now be assessed and observed include movement, urine production, and structures and blood flow. Tests used in biophysical assessment of the fetus are ultrasonography, umbilical artery Doppler flow, and magnetic resonance imaging (MRI).

Fetal Ultrasound Imaging

Ultrasonography is the use of high-frequency sound waves to produce an image of an organ or tissue (Fig. 6–2). It is the most common diagnostic test during pregnancy (Cunningham et al., 2014).

Ultrasound use varies based on trimester (Table 6–2) and is commonly used to obtain vital information such as:

- Presence of a gestational sac.
- Gestational age.
- Fetal growth.
- Fetal anatomy and presentation when performed in the second and third trimesters.
- Placental location and possible abnormalities.
- Fetal activity.
- Number of fetuses.
- Viability.
- Amount of amniotic fluid.
- Visual assistance for some invasive procedures, such as amniocentesis.

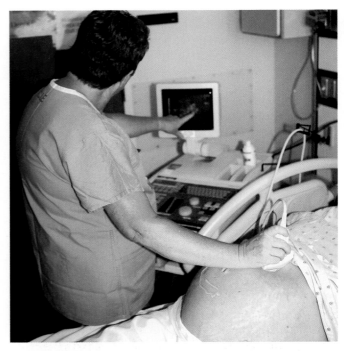

FIGURE 6–2 Nurse explains ultrasound to a pregnant woman having an ultrasound test.

TABLE 6–2   Indications for Ultrasound by Trimester of Pregnancy

FIRST TRIMESTER	SECOND TRIMESTER	THIRD TRIMESTER
Confirm intrauterine pregnancy.	Confirm the due date.	Confirm gestational age.
Confirm fetal cardiac activity.	Confirm fetal cardiac activity.	Confirm fetal viability.
Detect multiple gestation (number and size of gestational sacs).	Confirm fetal number, position, fetal size, amnionicity, and chorionicity.	Detect fetal number, position, congenital anomalies, intrauterine growth restriction (IUGR). Detect placental abruption, previa, or maturity.
Assessment of amnionicity and chorionicity of multiples.	Confirm placental location.	Detect placental position, abruption, previa, or maturity.
Visualization during chorionic villus sampling.	Confirm fetal weight and gestational age.	Assess biophysical profile.
Estimate gestational age.	Detect fetal anomalies (best after 18 weeks) or IUGR.	Assess amniotic fluid index.
Evaluate uterine structures.	Visualize for amniocentesis.	Perform Doppler flow studies.
Detect missed abortion, tubal, or ectopic pregnancy, or hydatiform mole.	Evaluate uterine and cervical structures.	Evaluate uterine and cervical structures.
Evaluate vaginal bleeding.	Evaluate vaginal bleeding.	Evaluate vaginal bleeding.
To screen for aneuploidy (nuchal translucency).	Visualize for diagnostic tests and external version.	Visualize for diagnostic tests and external version.

American Academy of Pediatrics and the American College of Obstetricians and Gynecologists, 2012; AWHONN, 2016.

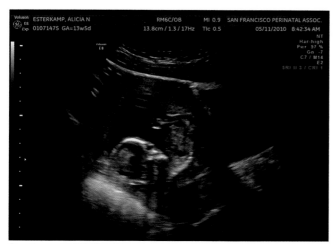

Courtesy of Allbin family

FIGURE 6–3 2D ultrasound picture.

A standard ultrasound is one that is used for evaluating fetal presentation, amniotic fluid volume, cardiac activity, placental position, gestational age measurements, fetal number, and fetal anatomy (Fig. 6–3). Other categories of ultrasound include limited obstetric ultrasound and specialized ultrasound, usually done when a standard ultrasound indicates the need for further fetal evaluation. Limited ultrasound is performed when a focused maternal/fetal ultrasound assessment is indicated by the clinical situation. It can be used to measure amniotic fluid volume, evaluate interval growth, evaluate the cervix, confirm fetal cardiac activity or fetal presentation as an adjunct to ultrasound-guided amniocentesis or external version, confirm embryonic number, measure crown-rump length, or confirm a yolk sac or uterine sac with assisted reproductive technology.

Specialized ultrasound is used for targeted or detailed anatomic examination when an anomaly is suspected based on fetal Doppler assessment, performance of biophysical profile (BPP), assessment of amniotic fluid, fetal echocardiography, or measurement of additional fetal structures (AAP & ACOG, 2012; AWHONN, 2016). Point-of-care ultrasound is ultrasound imaging performed during a patient encounter or procedure to enhance patient care (AWHONN, 2016).

Ultrasound equipment has become more portable, affordable, and efficient and thus easier to utilize at the bedside. Point-of-care sonography is brought to the patient and performed by health care providers in real time to directly correlate findings to presenting signs and symptoms. These exams are within the scope of practice for licensed registered nurses (RNs) who have the necessary knowledge, skills, and training in the specific imaging procedure to be performed. Examples in maternity nursing care where nurses may use point-of-care ultrasound are varied and include determining fetal presentation, evaluating fetal well-being (e.g., BPP), and assessing amniotic fluid volume. Performing an obstetric ultrasound primarily to produce keepsake images or to determine fetal gender without a medical indication is not recommended.

Timing

Standard ultrasounds are typically done in the first trimester to confirm pregnancy and calculate gestational age. Additional ultrasounds may be done at other times as needed. The timing and type of ultrasound performed should be such that the clinical question being asked can be answered (AAP & ACOG, 2012). A standard ultrasound performed in the second or third trimester includes evaluation of fetal presentation, quantification of amniotic fluid volume, documentation of the presence or absence of cardiac activity, placental position in relationship to the cervix, obtaining appropriate fetal biometric measurements, and determining fetal number. In addition, a fetal anatomic survey is conducted that includes imaging of specific anatomic structures (AWHONN, 2016).

Procedures

- Transvaginal ultrasound
  - Generally performed in the first trimester for earlier visualization of the fetus
  - Woman in a lithotomy position
  - Sterile covered probe/transducer inserted into the vagina
- Abdominal ultrasound
  - A full bladder is necessary to elevate the uterus out of the pelvis for better visualization when performed during the first half of pregnancy.
  - The woman is in a supine position.
  - Transmission gel and transducer are placed on the maternal abdomen.
  - The transducer is moved over the maternal abdomen to create an image of the structure being evaluated (see Fig. 6–2).

Interpretation of Results

- Postprocedure interpretation is typically done by a practitioner such as a radiologist, obstetrician, or nurse-midwife. After specialized training, nurses can perform limited obstetrical ultrasound (Box 6–2).
- Ultrasound for gestational age is determined through measurements of fetal-crown rump length, biparietal diameter, and femur length. It is most accurate when performed before 14 weeks to determine gestational age plus or minus 1 week (AAP & ACOG, 2012; Barron, 2014).
- Normal findings for the fetus are appropriate gestational age, size, viability, position, and functional capacities (see Fig. 6–3).
- Normal findings for the placenta are expected size, normal position and structure, and an adequate amniotic fluid volume.
- One screening test done by ultrasound in the first trimester is nuchal translucency. This measures the midsagittal plane with the neck of the fetus to assess the amount of fluid behind the neck (Barron, 2014). Elevated measurements are associated with trisomy 21.
- Abnormal findings should be referred for further testing and management of fetal anomalies (AAP & ACOG, 2012).

BOX 6–2 | AWHONN Ultrasound Guidelines

The Association of Women's Health, Obstetric and Neonatal Nurses (AWHONN) has developed guidelines for the didactic and clinical preparation for nurses who perform limited obstetric ultrasound. A minimum of 8 hours of didactic content is recommended in the following areas: (1) ultrasound physics and instrumentation, (2) patient education, (3) nursing accountability, (4) documentation, (5) image archiving, (6) legal and ethical issues, and (7) lines of authority and responsibility (AWHONN, 2016).

Currently there are no certification requirements for nurses performing limited ultrasound. Appropriate institutional policies, didactic and clinical education, and evaluation components are needed to ensure competence for nurses to perform limited ultrasound.

I. Obstetric first-trimester ultrasound

A. Identification of number and measurement of yolk sac(s), gestational sac(s), embryo(s), and fetus(es)

B. Identification and confirmation of early fetal cardiac activity

C. Determination of uterine versus extrauterine pregnancy

D. Use as an aid for ultrasound-guided procedures

II. Obstetric second- and third-trimester ultrasound

A. Fetal number and location

B. Fetal cardiac activity

C. Fetal position and presentation

D. Placental location

E. Amniotic fluid volume assessment

F. Biometric measurements to estimate fetal age and weight

G. Cervical length measurement

H. Use as aid for ultrasound-guided procedures

I. Modified BPP (amniotic fluid index and nonstress test)

J. Biophysical profile including: fetal tone, fetal movement, fetal breathing, amniotic fluid, and nonstress test

Association of Women's Health, Obstetric and Neonatal Nurses (AWHONN), 2016.

Advantages

- Accurate assessments of gestational age, fetal growth, and detection of fetal and placental abnormalities
- Noninvasive
- Provides information on fetal structures and status

Risks

- None, but controversy exists on the use of routine ultrasound for low-risk pregnant women, as there is no evidence it improves outcomes.

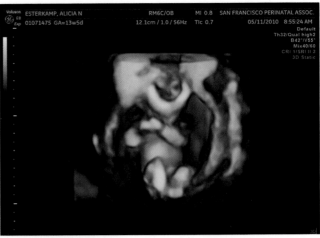

Courtesy of Allbin family

FIGURE 6–4 3D ultrasound picture.

Nursing Actions

- Explain to the woman and her family that ultrasound uses sound waves to produce an image of the baby.
- Assess for latex allergies with transvaginal ultrasound.
- For transvaginal, have patient put on gown and undress from waist down. For abdominal ultrasound, only the lower abdomen needs to be exposed.
- For transvaginal ultrasound, inform the woman that a sterile sheathed probe is inserted into the vagina. Inform her that she may feel pressure, but pain is not usually felt.
- Position patient in lithotomy for transvaginal ultrasound and supine for abdominal ultrasound.
- Provide comfort measures to the woman during the procedure, such as a pillow under her head and a warm blanket above and below her abdomen.
- Be sensitive to cultural and social as well as modesty issues.
- Provide emotional support.
- Schedule appropriate follow-up.
- Document ultrasound examination according to the institutional policy.

Three-Dimensional and Four-Dimensional Ultrasound

Three-dimensional (3D) ultrasound and four-dimensional (4D) ultrasound are advanced types of transabdominal ultrasounds that take thousands of images at once to produce a 3D or 4D image. They allow for visualization of complex facial movements and features, the branching of placental stem vessels, and connection of the umbilical vessels to the chorionic plate of the placenta (Fig. 6–4). Current recommendations are that 3D ultrasound be used only as an adjunct to conventional ultrasonography.

Purpose

- Standard determination of gestational age, fetal size, presentation, and volume of amniotic fluid

- Determination of complications such as vaginal bleeding, ventriculomegaly, hydrocephaly, and congenital brain defects
- Diagnosis of fetal malformations, uterine or pelvic abnormalities, hypoxic ischemic brain injury, and inflammatory disorders of the brain (Torgersen, 2011)

Timing

- The 3D and 4D ultrasounds are ordered as needed for further evaluation of possible fetal anomalies such as facial, cardiac, and skeletal.
- The 3D and 4D ultrasounds are most commonly requested by the patient to see a more lifelike picture of their developing baby in utero.

Procedure

- See abdominal ultrasound.

Interpretation of Results

- See abdominal ultrasound.

Advantages

- More detailed assessment of fetal structures
- 3D—presentation of placental blood flow
- Measurement of fetal organs
- 4D—allows for evaluation of brain morphology and identification of brain lesions

Risks

- Same as with standard ultrasound

Nursing Actions

- Same as with standard ultrasound

Magnetic Resonance Imaging

Magnetic resonance imaging (MRI) is a diagnostic radiological evaluation of tissue and organs from multiple planes. During pregnancy, it is used to visualize maternal and/or fetal structures for detailed imaging when screening tests indicate possible abnormalities. It is most commonly performed for suspected brain abnormality.

Purpose

- Tissue, organs, and vascular structures can be evaluated without the need to inject iodinated contrast.

Procedure

- The woman is instructed to remove all metallic objects before the test.
- The woman is placed in a supine position with left lateral tilt on the MRI table.
- The woman's abdominal area is scanned.

Interpretation

- The study is interpreted by a radiologist.

Advantages

- Provides very detailed images of fetal anatomy; particularly useful for brain abnormalities and complex abnormalities of thorax, gastrointestinal, and genitourinary systems.

Risks

- No known harmful effects

Nursing Actions

- Nurses are involved in the pre- and postprocedure.
- Explain the procedure to the woman and her family. The MRI is used to see maternal and/or fetal structures for detailed pictures.
- Address questions and concerns.

Doppler Flow Studies (Doppler Velocimetry)

Blood flow velocity measured by Doppler ultrasound reflects downstream impedance. Because more than 40% of the combined fetal ventricular output is directed to the placenta, obliteration of placental vascular channel increases afterload and leads to fetal hypoxemia. This in turn leads to dilation and redistribution of the middle cerebral artery blood flow. Ultimately, pressure rises in the ductus venosus due to afterload in the right side of the fetal heart. In this scheme, placental vascular dysfunction results in increased umbilical artery blood flow resistance, which progresses to decreased middle cerebral artery impedance followed ultimately by abnormal flow in the ductus venosus. (Cunningham et al., 2014). Three fetal vascular circuits—umbilical artery, middle cerebral artery, and ductus venosus—are currently used to determine fetal health and aid in clinical decision making for growth-restricted fetuses.

Umbilical artery Doppler flow is a noninvasive screening technique that uses advanced ultrasound technology to assess resistance to blood flow in the placenta. It evaluates the rate and volume of blood flow through the placenta and umbilical cord vessels using ultrasound. Increased resistance in the placenta, suggestive of poor function, results in reduced diastolic blood flow (Everett & Peebles, 2015). Evaluating fetal circulation and uteroplacental blood flow with Doppler flow provides critical information regarding fetal reserves and adaptation (Cypher, 2016). This assessment is commonly used in combination with other diagnostic tests to assess fetal status in intrauterine growth-restricted (IUGR) fetuses.

Purpose

- Assesses placental perfusion
- Used in combination with other diagnostic tests to assess fetal status in IUGR fetuses
- Not a useful screening tool for determining fetal compromise and therefore not recommended to the general obstetric population (AAP & ACOG, 2012)

Procedures

- The woman is assisted into a supine position.
- Transmission gel and transducer are placed on the woman's abdomen.
- Images are obtained of blood flow in the umbilical artery.

Interpretation of Results

- The directed blood flow within the umbilical arteries is calculated using the difference between systolic and diastolic flow (Everett & Peebles, 2015).
- As peripheral resistance increases, diastolic flow decreases and the systolic/diastolic increases. Reversed end-diastolic flow can be seen with severe cases of intrauterine growth restriction (AAP & ACOG, 2012).
- Umbilical artery Doppler is considered abnormal if the systolic/diastolic ratio is above the 95th percentile for gestational age, or a ratio above 3.0, or the end-diastolic flow is absent or reversed (Cunningham et al., 2014).

Advantages

- Noninvasive
- Allows for assessment of placental perfusion

Risks

- None

Nursing Actions

- Explain the procedure to the woman and her family. The Doppler test evaluates the blood flow through the placenta and umbilical cord vessels using ultrasound.
- Address questions and concerns.
- Provide comfort measures.
- Provide emotional support.
- Schedule appropriate follow-up.

Additional Doppler Studies

The middle cerebral artery (MCA) Doppler is an important indicator of fetal anemia. The role of cerebral arteries and the changes that occur in vessels in relation to the concept of "brain sparing" in potentially hypoxic fetuses is under investigation (Everett & Peebles, 2015). In the situation of chronic fetal hypoxemia or nutrient deprivation, the fetus redistributes its cardiac output to maximize oxygen and nutrient supply to the brain, described as a brain-sparing. Changes in cerebral blood flow associated with brain-sparing can be detected by Doppler sonography (Cohen, Baerts, & van Bel, 2015). However, the value of MCA Doppler in the prediction of adverse fetal outcomes has been inconsistent.

The cerebro:placental ratio is an important obstetric ultrasound tool used as a predictor of adverse pregnancy outcome. It is calculated by dividing the Doppler pulsatile indices of the MCA by the umbilical artery. The index will reflect mild increases in placental resistance with mild reductions in fetal brain vascular resistance.

The ductus venosus Doppler is Doppler velocimetry of the fetal central venous circulation that helps identify fetuses with suspected IUGR at an advanced stage of compromise. Absent or reversed flow in late diastole in the ductus venosus is associated with increased perinatal morbidity, fetal acidemia, and perinatal and neonatal mortality. The value of the Doppler velocimetry (DV) waveform is in the premature fetus with IUGR.

BIOCHEMICAL ASSESSMENT

Biochemical assessment involves biological examination and chemical determination. Procedures used to obtain biochemical specimens include chorionic villi sampling, amniocentesis, percutaneous blood sampling, and maternal assays. More than 15% of pregnancies are at sufficient risk to warrant invasive testing (Cypher, 2016).

Chorionic Villus Sampling

Chorionic villus sampling (CVS) is aspiration of a small amount of placental tissue (chorionic villi) for chromosomal, metabolic, or DNA testing. This test is used for chromosomal analysis between 10 and 12 weeks' gestation to detect fetal abnormalities caused by genetic disorders. It tests for metabolic disorders such as cystic fibrosis but does not test for neural tube defects (NTDs).

Timing

- Performed during first or second trimester, ideally at 10 to 12 weeks' gestation.

Procedure

- The woman is in a supine position or lithotomy position, depending on route of insertion.
- A catheter is inserted either transvaginally through the cervix or abdominally using a needle. With each route, ultrasonography is used to guide placement. Transabdominally, a needle is inserted through the abdomen and uterus to the placenta.
- A small biopsy of chorionic (placental) tissue is removed with aspiration.
- The villi are harvested and cultured for chromosomal analysis and processed for DNA and enzymatic analysis as indicated (Fig. 6–5).

Interpretation of Results

- Results of chromosomal studies are available within 1 week.
- Detailed information is provided on specific chromosomal abnormality detected.

Advantages

- Can be performed earlier than amniocentesis but is not recommended before 10 weeks (AAP & ACOG, 2012)
- Examination of fetal chromosomes

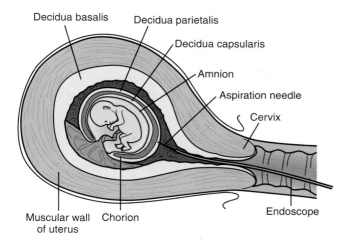

FIGURE 6–5 Chorionic villi sampling procedure.

Risks

- There is a 7% fetal loss rate due to bleeding, infection, and rupture of membranes.
- Ten percent of women experience some bleeding after the procedure.

Nursing Actions

- Review the procedure with the woman and her family. This test obtains amniotic fluid to test for fetal abnormalities caused by genetic problems.
- Instruct the woman in breathing and relaxation techniques she can use during the procedure.
- Assist the woman into the proper position.
  - Lithotomy for transvaginal aspiration
  - Supine for transabdominal aspiration
- Provide comfort measures.
- Provide emotional support.
- Recognize anxiety related to test results.
- Label specimens.
- Assess fetal and maternal well-being postprocedure. Fetal heart rate is auscultated twice in 30 minutes.
- Instruct the woman to report abdominal pain or cramping, leaking of fluid, bleeding, fever, or chills to the care provider.
- Administer RhoGAM to Rh-negative women postprocedure as per order to prevent antibody formation in Rh-negative women.

Amniocentesis

Amniocentesis is a diagnostic procedure in which a needle is inserted through the maternal abdominal wall into the uterine cavity to obtain amniotic fluid. It is commonly performed for genetic testing but can also be done for assessment of fetal lung maturity, assessment of hemolytic disease in the fetus, or intrauterine infection and therapy for polyhydramnios.

Risk factors for fetal genetic disorders include advanced maternal age (older than 35 years), history of genetic disorders,

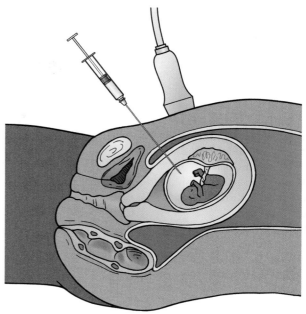

Amniocentesis:
Technique of amniocentesis is illustrated. A pocket of amniotic fluid is located by sonogram. A small amount of fluid is removed by aspiration.

FIGURE 6–6 Amniocentesis procedure.

positive screening test such as a positive alpha-fetoprotein, and known or suspected hemolytic disease in the fetus.

Timing

- Usually offered between 15 and 20 weeks for genetic testing. For other purposes, it is used as clinically indicated.

Procedure

- A detailed ultrasound is performed to take fetal measurements and locate the placenta to choose a site for needle insertion.
- A needle is inserted transabdominally into the uterine cavity using ultrasonography to guide placement (Fig. 6–6).
- Amniotic fluid is obtained.

Interpretation of Results

- Amniocentesis has an accuracy rate of 99% (AAP & ACOG, 2012; Gilbert, 2011).
- Amniotic fluid sample is sent to a lab for cell growth, and results of chromosomal studies are available within 2 weeks.
- Elevated bilirubin levels indicate fetal hemolytic disease.
- A positive culture indicates infection.
- Standards do not recommend amniocentesis be done solely to evaluate the lecithin/sphingomyelin (L/S) ratio or the presence of phosphatidyl glycerol (PG). Although amniotic fluid can be analyzed to evaluate fetal lung maturity, current practice does not recommend this. If the purpose of the test is to determine fetal lung maturity, L/S ratio, PG, and

lamellar body count (LBC), results are interpreted as follows (Cypher, 2016):

- L:S ratio greater than 2:1 indicates fetal lung maturity.
- L:S ratio less than 2:1 indicates fetal lung immaturity in increased risk of respiratory distress syndrome.
- Positive PG indicates fetal lung maturity.
- Negative PG indicates immature fetal lungs.
- An LBC of 50,000/μL or greater is highly indicative of fetal lung maturity.
- An LBC of 15,000/μL or less is highly indicative of fetal lung immaturity.
- LBC results can be hindered by the presence of meconium, vaginal bleeding, vaginal mucus, or hydramnios.

Advantages

- Examines fetal chromosomes for genetic disorders
- Direct examination of biochemical specimens

Risks

- Studies suggest a loss rate as low as 1 in 300 to 500 (AAP & ACOG, 2012).
- Trauma to the fetus or placenta
- Bleeding or leaking of amniotic fluid
- Preterm labor
- Maternal infection
- Rh sensitization from fetal blood into maternal circulation

Nursing Actions

- Review the procedure with the woman and assure her that precautions are followed during the procedure with ultrasound visualization of the fetus to avoid fetal or placental injury (Van Leeuwen & Bladh, 2015).
- Explain that in the amniocentesis procedure a needle is inserted through the abdomen into the womb to obtain amniotic fluid for testing.
- Explain that during needle aspiration, discomfort will be minimized with the use of a local anesthetic.
- Explain that a full bladder may be required for ultrasound visualization if the woman is less than 20 weeks' gestation.
- Instruct the woman in breathing and relaxation techniques she can use during the procedure.
- Provide comfort measures.
- Provide emotional support.
- Recognize anxiety related to test results.
- Prep abdomen with an antiseptic such as betadine if indicated.
- Label specimens.
- Assess fetal and maternal well-being postprocedure, monitoring and evaluating the fetal heart rate (FHR).
- Instruct the woman to report abdominal pain or cramping, leaking of fluid, bleeding, decreased fetal movement, fever, or chills to the care provider.
- Instruct woman not to lift anything heavy for 2 days.
- Administer Rho(D) immune globulin (RhoGAM) to Rh-negative women postprocedure as per order to prevent antibody formation in the Rh-negative woman.

Fetal Blood Sampling/ Percutaneous Umbilical Blood Sampling

Fetal blood sampling/percutaneous umbilical blood sampling (PUBS), or cordocentesis, is the removal of fetal blood from the umbilical cord. The blood is used to test for metabolic and hematological disorders, fetal infection, and fetal karyotyping. It can also be used for fetal therapies such as red blood cell and platelet transfusions.

Timing

- Usually used after ultrasound has detected an anomaly in the fetus
- Usually performed after 18 weeks' gestation to evaluate results of potential diagnoses and make further recommendations for medical management if necessary (Berry, Stone, Norton, Johnson, & Berghella, 2013).

Procedure

- A needle is inserted into the umbilical vein at or near placental origin and a small sample of fetal blood is aspirated (Fig. 6–7).
- Ultrasound is used to guide the needle.

Interpretation of Results

- Results are usually available within 48 hours.
- Interpretation of studies is based on the indication for the procedure.
- Biochemical testing on the blood may include a complete blood count with a differential analysis, anti-1 and anti-I cold agglutinin, ß-hCG, factors IX and VIIIC, and AFP levels (Berry, Stone, Norton, Johnson, & Berghella, 2013).

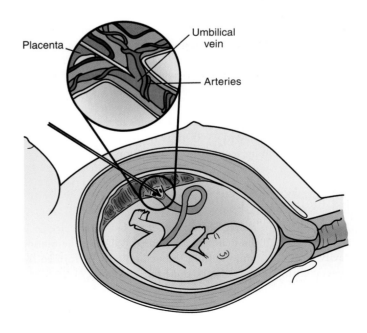

FIGURE 6–7 Percutaneous umbilical blood sampling procedure.

Advantages

● Direct examination of fetal blood sample for fetal anomalies

Risks

● Complications are similar to those for amniocentesis and include cord vessel bleeding or hematomas, maternal–fetal hemorrhage, fetal bradycardia, and risk for infection.
● The overall procedure-related fetal death rate is 1.4% but varies depending on indication (Cunningham et al., 2014).

Nursing Actions

● Nurses may be involved in the pre- and postprocedure.
● Explain the procedure to the woman and her family. During PUBS, fetal blood is removed from the umbilical cord.
● Address questions and concerns.
● Position client in a lateral or wedged position to avoid supine hypotension during fetal monitoring tests.
● Have terbutaline ready as ordered in case uterine contractions occur during procedure (Torgersen, 2011).
● Assess fetal well-being postprocedure for 1 to 2 hours via external fetal monitoring.
● Educate patient on how to count fetal movements for when she goes home (Cyper, 2016).

MATERNAL ASSAYS

Maternal assays are an increasingly common way to screen pregnant women for fetal birth defects or genetic anomalies (Allyse et al., 2015). The choice of screening tests depends on many factors, including timing of entry into prenatal care. The goal is to offer screening tests with high detection rates and low false-positive rates that provide patients with diagnostic options. Ideally, patients are seen in the first trimester and can be offered first-trimester aneuploidy screening or integrated or sequential aneuploidy screening that combines first trimester and second trimester testing (detailed in Chapter 4). The following section details a few of the maternal assays used as part of testing.

Alpha-Fetoprotein/$_1$-Fetoprotein/Maternal Serum Alpha-Fetoprotein

Alpha-fetoprotein (AFP) is a glycoprotein produced in the fetal liver, gastrointestinal tract, and yolk sac in early gestation. Assessing for the levels of AFP in the maternal blood is a screening tool for certain developmental defects in the fetus, such as fetal NTDs and ventral abdominal wall defects. Because 95% of NTDs occur in the absence of risk factors, routine screening is recommended (Cunningham et al., 2014).

Timing

● 15 to 20 weeks' gestation

Procedure

● Maternal blood is drawn and sent to the lab for analysis.

Interpretation of Results

● Increased levels are associated with defects such as NTDs, anencephaly, omphalocele, and gastroschisis.
● Decreased levels are associated with trisomy 21 (Down syndrome).
● Abnormal findings require additional testing such as amniocentesis, chorionic villus sampling, or ultrasonography to make a diagnosis.

Advantages

● 80% to 85% of all open NTDs and open abdominal wall defects and 90% of anencephalies can be detected early in pregnancy (AAP & ACOG, 2012).

Risks

● The high false-positive rate (meaning the test results indicate an abnormality in a normal fetus) can result in increased anxiety for a woman and her family as they wait for the results of additional testing. High false positives can occur with oligohydramnios, multifetal gestation, decreased maternal weight, and underestimated fetal gestational age. False low levels can also occur as a result of fetal death, increased maternal weight, and overestimated fetal gestational age (Gilbert, 2011).

Nursing Actions

● Educate the woman about the screening test. The AFP test is a maternal blood test that evaluates the levels of AFP in the maternal blood to screen for certain fetal abnormalities.
● Support the woman and her family, particularly if results are abnormal.
● Assist in scheduling diagnostic testing when results are abnormal.
● Provide information on support groups if an NTD occurs.

Multiple Marker Screen

Triple marker screening combines all three chemical markers—AFP, human chorionic gonadotropin (hCG), and estriol levels—with maternal age to detect some trisomies and NTDs. It is sometimes used as an alternative to amniocentesis. Quad screen adds inhibin-A to the triple marker screen to increase detection of trisomy 21 to 80% (Cypher, 2016).

Timing

● 15 to 16 weeks' gestation

Procedure

● Maternal blood is drawn and sent to the lab for analysis.

Interpretation

- Low levels of maternal serum alpha-fetoprotein and unconjugated estriol levels suggest an abnormality.
- hCG and inhibin-A levels are twice as high in pregnancies with trisomy 21.
- Decreased estriol levels are an indicator of NTDs.

Advantages

- 60% to 80% of cases of Down syndrome can be identified.
- 85% to 90% of open NTDs are detected.

Risks

- None

Nursing Actions

- Educate the woman about the test. This is a maternal blood test that assesses for the levels of chemicals in the maternal blood to screen for certain developmental abnormalities.
- Provide emotional support for the woman and her family.
- Assist in scheduling additional testing if needed.
- Provide information on support groups if an NTD occurs.

ANTENATAL FETAL SURVEILLANCE

The assessment of fetal status is a key component of perinatal care. A variety of methods are available for ongoing assessment of fetal well-being during pregnancy (AAP & ACOG, 2012):

- Fetal movement counting (kick counts)
- Nonstress test (NST)
- Vibroacoustic stimulation (VAS)
- Contraction stress test (CST)
- Biophysical profile (BPP)
- Amniotic fluid index (AFI)

The goal of fetal testing is to reduce the number of preventable stillbirths and to avoid unnecessary interventions. The purpose of antenatal testing is to validate fetal well-being or identify fetal hypoxemia and intervene before permanent injury or death occurs (Cypher, 2016). In most clinical situations, a normal test result indicates that intrauterine fetal death is highly unlikely in the next 7 days and is highly reassuring (AAP & ACOG, 2012). In most pregnancies, when indicated, testing begins by 32 to 34 weeks (AAP & ACOG, 2012). Antepartum testing is intended for use in pregnancies at high risk for fetal demise. Because of the risk of a high false positive potentially resulting in unnecessary delivery of a healthy baby, this testing is reserved for high-risk pregnancies. The schedule for antepartal testing for fetal surveillance may vary. For example, a recent Cochrane Review concluded there is limited evidence from randomized controlled trials to inform best practice for fetal surveillance regimens when caring for women with pregnancies affected by impaired fetal growth (Grivell, Wong, & Bhatia, 2012).

Daily Fetal Movement Count

In fetal movement counting (FMC), the pregnant woman counts fetal movements in a specified time period to identify potentially hypoxic fetuses. FMC is based on physiological principles that compromised fetuses reduce activity in response to decreased oxygenation, conserving energy. Maternal perception of fetal movement was one of the earliest and easiest tests of fetal well-being and remains an essential assessment of fetal health. Fetal activity is diminished in the compromised fetus, and cessation of fetal movement has been documented preceding fetal demise (AAP & ACOG, 2012).

Timing

- Kick counts have been proposed as a primary method of fetal surveillance for all pregnancies after 28 weeks' gestation. However, many women may begin feeling fetal movement around 16 to 20 weeks (Gilbert, 2011).

Procedure

- The pregnant woman is instructed to palpate her abdomen and track fetal movements daily for 1 to 2 hours.

Interpretation

- In the 2-hour approach, maternal perception of 10 distinct fetal movements within 2 hours is considered normal and reassuring; once movement is achieved, counts can be discontinued for the day.
- In the 1-hour approach, the count is considered reassuring if it equals or exceeds the established baseline; in general, 4 movements in 1 hour is reassuring.
- Decreased fetal movement should be reported to the provider and is an indication for further fetal assessment, such as an NST or biophysical profile (APP & ACOG, 2012).
- Fewer than four fetal movements in 2 hours should be reported to provider (Barron, 2014).

Advantages

- Done by pregnant women
- Inexpensive, reassuring, and relatively easily taught to pregnant women
- No monitoring devices are required

Risks

- None

Nursing Actions

- Teach the woman how to do kick counts and provide a means to record them. Instruct the woman to lie on her side while counting movements. Explain that maternal assessment of counting fetal movements is an important evaluation of fetal well-being.
- If fetal movement is decreased, the woman should be instructed to eat something, rest, and focus on fetal movement for 1 hour. Four movements in 1 hour is considered reassuring.

- Instruct the woman to report decreased fetal movement below normal, as this is an indication for further assessment by care providers.

Nonstress Test

The nonstress test (NST) is a screening tool that uses fetal heart rate patterns and accelerations as an indicator of fetal well-being (Fig. 6–8). The heart rate of a physiologically normal fetus with adequate oxygenation and an intact autonomic nervous system accelerates in response to movement (AWHONN, 2015). The NST records accelerations in the FHR in relation to fetal activity. It is the most widely accepted method of evaluating fetal status, particularly for high-risk pregnant women with complications such as hypertension, diabetes, multiple gestation, trauma, and/or bleeding; woman's report of lack of fetal movement; and placental abnormalities. NST is the most common method of antepartum fetal surveillance.

Procedure

- The FHR is monitored with the external FHR transducer until reactive (up to 40 minutes), while running an FHR contraction strip for interpretation.
- Monitor FHR and fetal activity for 20 to 40 minutes (placement of electronic fetal monitoring [EFM] and interpretation of EFM are described in Chapter 9).

Interpretation

- The NST is considered reactive when the FHR increases 15 beats above baseline for 15 seconds twice or more in 20 minutes (Fig. 6–9).
- In fetuses less than 32 weeks' gestation, two accelerations peaking at least 10 bpm above baseline and lasting 10 seconds in a 20-minute period is reactive (AWHONN, 2015).

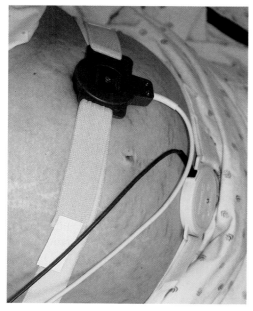

FIGURE 6–8 Monitoring for a nonstress test.

- Nonreactive NST is one without sufficient FHR accelerations in 40 minutes and should be followed up with further testing such as an ultrasound and/or biophysical profile (AAP & ACOG, 2012).
- Presence of repetitive variable decelerations that are >30 seconds requires further assessment of amniotic fluid and/or prolonged monitoring (Cunningham et al., 2014).

Advantages

- Noninvasive, easily performed, and reliable indicator of fetal well-being

Risks

- No indicated risks
- NST has a high false-positive rate of over 50% but a low false-negative rate of less than 1% (AAP & ACOG, 2012; Cypher, 2016).

Nursing Actions

- Explain the procedure to the woman and her family. The NST uses EFM to assess fetal well-being.
- Have the patient void prior to the procedure and lie in a semi-Fowler's or lateral position to avoid aortocaval compression.
- Provide comfort measures.
- Provide emotional support.
- Interpret FHR and accelerations; report results to the care provider.
- Document the date and time the test was started, the patient's name, the reason for the test, and the maternal vital signs.
- Schedule appropriate follow-up; the typical interval for testing is biweekly or weekly, depending on indication.

Vibroacoustic Stimulation

Vibroacoustic stimulation (VAS), also referred to as *fetal vibroacoustic stimulation*, is a screening tool that uses auditory stimulation (with an artificial larynx) to assess fetal well-being with EFM when NST is nonreactive. Vibroacoustic stimulation may be effective in eliciting a change in fetal behavior, fetal startle movements, and increased FHR variability. VAS is only used when the baseline rate is determined to be within normal limits. When deceleration or bradycardia is present, VAS is not an appropriate intervention (Gilbert, 2011).

Procedure

- VAS is conducted by activating an artificial larynx on the maternal abdomen near the fetal head for 1 second in conjunction with the NST. This can be repeated at 1-minute intervals up to 3 times.

Interpretation

- The NST using VAS is considered reactive when the FHR increases 15 beats above baseline for 15 seconds twice in 20 minutes.

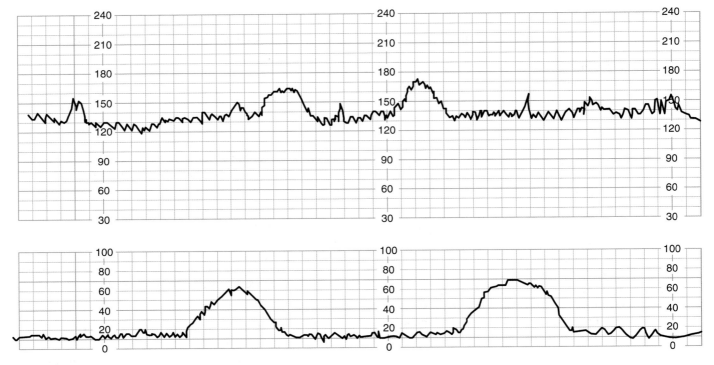

FIGURE 6–9 Fetal heart rate accelerations indicating a reactive nonstress test.

Advantages

- Using VAS to stimulate the fetus has reduced the incidence of nonreactive NSTs and reduced the time required to conduct NSTs.
- It differentiates nonreactive NSTs caused by hypoxia from those associated with fetal sleep states.
- Using the VAS decreases the incidence of faults findings of a nonreactive NST

Risks

- No adverse effects reported
- Not recommended as a routine procedure in high-risk pregnancies

Nursing Actions

- Explain the procedure to the woman and her family. The test uses a buzzer (in auditory stimulation) to assess fetal well-being.
- Position patient in a semi-Fowler's or lateral position to avoid aortocaval compression.
- Provide comfort measures.
- Provide emotional support.
- Interpret FHR and accelerations and conduct VAS appropriately. Report results to physician or midwife and document.
- Schedule appropriate follow-up.

Contraction Stress Test

The contraction stress test (CST), formerly known as an *oxytocin challenge test*, is a screening tool to assess the ability of the fetus to maintain a normal FHR in response to uterine contractions in women with a nonreactive NST at term gestation. The purpose of the CST is to identify a fetus that is at risk for compromise through observation of the fetal response to intermittent reduction in utero placental blood flow associated with stimulated uterine contractions (UCs) (AAP & ACOG, 2012; Treanor, 2015).

Procedure

- Monitor FHR and fetal activity for 20 minutes.
- If no spontaneous UCs, contractions can be initiated in some women by having them brush the nipples for 10 minutes or with IV oxytocin.

Interpretation

- The CST is considered negative or normal when there are no significant variable decelerations or no late decelerations in a 10-minute strip with three UCs in more than 40 seconds, assessed with moderate variability.
- The CST is positive when there are late decelerations of FHR with 50% of UCs.
- A positive result has been associated with an increased rate of fetal death, fetal growth restriction, lower 5-minute Apgar scores, cesarean section, and the need for neonatal resuscitation due to neonatal depression (AAP & ACOG, 2012). This requires further testing such as BPP.
- The CST is equivocal or suspicious when there are intermittent late or significant variable decelerations, and further testing may be done or the test repeated in 24 hours.

Advantages

- Negative CSTs are associated with good fetal outcomes.

Risks

- CST has a high false-positive rate, which can result in unnecessary intervention.
- Cannot be used with women who have a contraindication for uterine activity (conditions with an increased risk for preterm labor, bleeding, or uterine rupture).

Nursing Actions

- Explain the procedure to the woman and her family. The CST stimulates contractions to evaluate fetal reaction to the stress of contractions.
- Have patient void before testing.
- Position patient in a semi-Fowler's position.
- Monitor vitals before and every 15 minutes during the test.
- Provide comfort measures.
- Provide emotional support.
- Correctly interpret FHR and contractions.
- Safely administer oxytocin (i.e., avoid uterine tachysystole). Uterine tachysystole is defined as more than five uterine contractions in 10 minutes, fewer than 60 seconds between contractions, or a contraction greater than 90 seconds with a late deceleration occurring (Gilbert, 2011).
- Recognize adverse effects of oxytocin.
- Schedule appropriate follow-up.

Amniotic Fluid Index

The AFI is a screening tool that measures the volume of amniotic fluid with ultrasound to assess fetal well-being and placental function. The amniotic fluid level is based on fetal urine production, which is the predominate source of amniotic fluid and is directly dependent on renal perfusion (Cypher, 2016). In prolonged fetal hypoxemia, blood is shunted away from fetal kidneys to other vital organs. Persistent decreased blood flow to the fetal kidneys results in reduction of amniotic fluid production and oligohydramnios. In conjunction with NST, AFI is a strong indicator of fetal status, as it is accurate in detecting fetal hypoxia.

Procedure

- Ultrasound measurement of pockets of amniotic fluid in four quadrants of the uterine cavity via ultrasound.

Interpretation of Results

- Average measurement in pregnancy is 8 cm to 24 cm (Cunningham et al., 2014).
- Abnormal AFI is below 5 cm. An AFI less than 5 cm is indicative of oligohydramnios, associated with increased prenatal mortality and a need for close maternal and fetal monitoring.
- Represented graphically: decreased uteroplacental perfusion → decreased fetal renal blood flow → decreased urine production → oligohydramnios
- An AFI above 24 cm is polyhydramnios, which may indicate fetal malformation such as NTDs, obstruction of fetal gastrointestinal tract, or fetal hydrops.

Advantages

- AFI reflects placental function and perfusion to the fetus as well as overall fetal condition.

Risks

- None

Nursing Actions

- Explain the procedure to the woman and her family. This test uses ultrasound to measure the amount of amniotic fluid to assess fetal well-being and how well the placenta is working.
- Provide comfort measures.
- Provide emotional support.
- Schedule appropriate follow-up.
- Special training in obstetric ultrasound is required for evaluation of amniotic fluid volume (see Box 6–2).

Biophysical Profile

The BPP is an ultrasound assessment of fetal status along with an NST. The BPP was first introduced as an intrauterine Apgar score in response to high proportion of false-positive NSTs and CSTs. It utilizes real-time ultrasound with EFM to assess five biological variables: FHR reactivity, fetal movement, tone, breathing, and amniotic fluid volume. If fetal oxygen consumption is reduced, the immediate fetal response is reduction of activity regulated by the CNS. The BPP provides improved prognostic information because physiological parameters associated with chronic and acute hypoxia are evaluated. It is indicated in pregnancies involving increased risk of fetal hypoxia and placental insufficiency, such as maternal diabetes and hypertension. Some controversy exists related to this test, as a Cochrane Review concluded that available evidence from randomized clinical trials provides no support for the use of BPP as a test of fetal well-being in high-risk pregnancies (Grivell, Wong, & Bhatia, 2012).

Procedure

- BPP consists of an NST with the addition of 30 minutes of ultrasound observation for five indicators: FHR reactivity, fetal breathing movements, fetal movement, fetal tone, and measurement of amniotic fluid.
  - NST reactive
  - Fetal breathing movements: One or more episodes of rhythmic breathing movements of 30 seconds or movement within 30 minutes is expected.
  - Fetal movement: Three or more discrete body or limb movements in 30 minutes are expected.
  - Fetal tone: One or more fetal extremity extensions with return to fetal flexion or opening and closing of the hand is expected within 30 minutes.
  - Amniotic fluid volume: A pocket of amniotic fluid that measures at least 2 cm in two planes perpendicular to each other is expected.

TABLE 6–3   Biophysical Profile Scoring

FETAL BIOPHYSICAL PROFILES	SCORE 2	SCORE 0
Movement	At least three episodes of trunk or limb movement	Less than three episodes of trunk or limb movement
Tone	At least one episode of active extension with return to flexion of the fetal limb or trunk; opening and closing of the hand is deemed normal tone	Absent movement or slow extension/flexion
Breathing movement	At least one breathing episode lasting a minimum of 30 seconds	Absent breathing movement or less than 30 seconds of sustained breathing movement
Amniotic fluid	At least one pocket of amniotic fluid that measures at least 2 cm in two perpendicular planes	Absent pockets of amniotic fluid that measures at least 2 cm in two perpendicular planes
Nonstress test (NST)	Reactive	Nonreactive

Cypher, 2016.

Interpretation

● A score of 2 (present) or 0 (absent) is assigned to each of the five components.
● A total score of 8/10 is reassuring.
● A score of 6/10 is equivocal and may indicate the need for repeat testing in 12 to 24 hours of delivery, depending on gestational age.
● A score of 4/10 is nonreassuring and warrants further evaluation and consideration of delivery (AAP & ACOG, 2012).
● A score of 2/10 or less prompts immediate delivery.
● Fetal activity decreases or stops to reduce energy and oxygen consumption as fetal hypoxemia worsens. Decreased activity occurs in reverse order of normal development.
● Fetal activities that appear earliest in pregnancy (tone and movement) are usually the last to cease, and activities that are the last to develop are usually the first to be diminished (FHR variability) (Table 6–3).

Advantages

● Lower false-positive rate compared to other tests

Risks

● None

Nursing Actions

● Explain the procedure to the woman and her family. The BPP is an ultrasound evaluation of fetal status and involves observation of various fetal reflex activities.
● Provide comfort measures.
● Provide emotional support.
● Special training in obstetric ultrasound is required for interpretation of ultrasound components of the test (see Box 6–2).

● Schedule appropriate follow-up; the typical interval for testing is 1 week but for specific pregnancy complications, it may be biweekly.

Modified Biophysical Profile

The modified BPP combines an NST as an indicator of short-term fetal well-being and AFI as an indicator of long-term placental function to evaluate fetal well-being. It is indicated in high-risk pregnancy related to maternal conditions or pregnancy-related conditions (see Table 6–1).

Procedure

● A modified BPP combines the use of an NST with an AFI.

Interpretation

● A modified BPP is considered normal when the NST is reactive and the AFI is greater than 5 cm. An AFI less than or equal to 5 is indicative of oligohydramnios. Oligohydramnios is associated with increased perinatal mortality, and decreased amniotic fluid may reflect acute or chronic fetal asphyxia (Treanor, 2015). Amniotic fluid volume changes more slowly over time as the fetus preferentially shunts cardiac output to the heart and brain while decreasing renal perfusion and thus fetal urine output, thereby decreasing the volume of amniotic fluid.

Advantages

● Less time to complete
● NST and AFI considered most predictive of perinatal outcomes.

Risks

● None

Nursing Actions

● Explain the procedure to the woman and her family. A modified BPP is an NST and measurement of the amount of amniotic fluid.
● Provide comfort measures.
● Provide emotional support.
● Special training in ultrasound is required for interpretation of amniotic fluid volume (see Box 6–2).
● Schedule appropriate follow-up; the typical interval for testing is 1 week, but for specific pregnancy complications it may be biweekly.

REFERENCES

Allyse, M., Minear, M. A., Berson, E., Sridhar, S., Rote, M., Hung, A., & Chandrasekharan, S. (2015). Non-invasive prenatal testing: a review of international implementation and challenges. *International Journal of Women's Health, 7,* 113–126. http://doi.org/10.2147/IJWH.S67124

American Academy of Pediatrics and the American College of Obstetricians and Gynecologists. (2012). *Guidelines for perinatal care* (7th ed.). Elk Grove Village, IL: Author.

Association of Women's Health, Obstetric and Neonatal Nurses (AWHONN). (2015). *Fetal heart rate monitoring: Principles and practice* (5th ed.). Washington, DC: Author.

Association of Women's Health, Obstetric and Neonatal Nurses (AWHONN). (2016). *Ultrasound examinations performed by nurses in obstetric gynecologic and reproductive medicine settings: Clinical competencies and education guide* (4th ed.). Washington, DC: Author.

Barron, M. Antenatal tests. In K. Simpson, P. Creehan, & Association of Women's Health, Obstetrics and Neonatal Nursing. (2014). *Perinatal nursing.* Philadelphia, PA: Lippincott.

Berry, S. M., Stone, J., Norton, M.E., Johnson, D., & Berghella, V. (2013). Fetal blood sampling. *Society for Maternal-Fetal Medicine, 209*(3), 170–180.

Cohen, E., Baerts, W., & van Bel, F. (2015). Brain-sparing in intrauterine growth restriction: Considerations for the neonatologist. *Neonatology, 108,* 269–276.

Cunningham, F., Leveno, K., Bloom, S., Spong, C., Dashe, J., Hoffman, B., . . . Sheffield, J. (2014). *Williams obstetrics* (24rd ed.). New York, NY: McGraw-Hill.

Cypher, R. (2016). Antepartal fetal surveillance and prenatal diagnosis. In S. Mattson & J. Smith (Eds.), *Core curriculum for maternal-newborn nursing* (5th ed., pp. 135–158). St Louis, MO: Elsevier.

Everett, T., & Peebles, D. (2015) Antenatal tests of fetal wellbeing. *Seminars in Fetal and Neonatal Medicine, 20*(3), 138–143.

Gilbert, E. (2011). *Manual of high risk pregnancy and delivery* (6th ed.). St. Louis, MO: C. V. Mosby.

Grivell, R., Wong, L., & Bhatia, V. (2012). Regimens of fetal surveillance for impaired fetal growth. *Cochrane Database of Systematic Reviews, 13*(6), CD007113. doi:10.1002/14651858.CD007113.pub3.

Torgerson, K.L. (2011). Antepartal fetal surveillance. In S. Mattson & J. Smith (Eds.), *Core curriculum for maternal-newborn nursing* (4th ed., pp. 161–2000). St. Louis, MO: Elsevier Sanders.

Treanor, C. (2015). Antenatal fetal assessment and testing. In *Fetal heart rate monitoring: Principles and practice* (5th ed.). Washington, DC: Author.

Van Leeuwen, A., & Bladh, M. (2015). *Davis's comprehensive handbook of laboratory and diagnostic tests with nursing implications.* Philadelphia, PA: F.A. Davis.

High-Risk Antepartum Nursing Care

7

Roberta F. Durham RN, PhD
Megan E. Levy RN, BSN
Rachael Miller RN, BSN

LEARNING OUTCOMES

Upon completion of this chapter, the student will be able to:

1. Describe the primary complications of pregnancy and related nursing and medical care.
2. Delineate clinical features indicative of pregnancy complications and tests to predict, screen for, diagnose, and manage high-risk conditions.
3. Identify potential antenatal complications for the woman, the fetus, and the newborn.
4. Formulate a plan of care that includes the physical, emotional, and psychosocial needs of women diagnosed with pregnancy complications.
5. Describe the key aspects of teaching for women with antenatal complications.
6. Demonstrate understanding of knowledge related to preexisting medical complications of pregnancy and related management.

Nursing Diagnosis

- Ineffective childbearing process
- Risk for disturbed maternal fetal dyad
- Risk of maternal injury related to pregnancy complications
- Risk for ineffective family coping related to high-risk pregnancy
- Risk of maternal injury related to preexisting medical conditions
- Disturbance in self-esteem or self-identity related to high-risk pregnancy
- Risk of maternal stress related to pregnancy complications
- Interrupted family process
- Powerlessness related to uncertain pregnancy outcome
- Risk of fetal injury related to complications of pregnancy
- Caregiver role strain

Nursing Outcomes

- The woman is able to maintain a healthy pregnancy.
- The woman will understand warning signs and management of pregnancy complications.
- Family exhibits a pattern of management of adaptive tasks by family involved with the pregnancy challenges.
- The woman and her family will receive adequate support related to high-risk pregnancy and disruption in family functioning.
- The woman will verbalize acceptance and understanding of pregnancy complication and management of pregnancy complications.
- Family exhibits a pattern of family function that supports the well-being of the family.
- The woman reports a perception that her actions do significantly impact outcomes and participates in decisions related to management of pregnancy complications.
- The woman will give birth to a healthy infant without complications.
- Woman reports she is able to fulfill responsibilities to her family.

INTRODUCTION

This chapter presents information on key complications and high-risk conditions that can occur during pregnancy and on preexisting medical conditions that have the potential to be exacerbated by pregnancy. An overview of each complication is presented, including underlying pathophysiology, risk factors, risks posed to the woman and fetus, and typical medical management and nursing actions.

The nature of perinatal nursing is unpredictable, and pregnancy complications can arise abruptly, resulting in rapid deterioration of maternal and fetal status. It is imperative that nurses understand the underlying physiological mechanisms of pregnancy, the impact of complications on maternal and fetal well-being, and current interventions to optimize maternal and fetal outcomes. Pregnancy complications can have profound effects on the physical, emotional, and psychosocial health of women and their newborns both during and beyond pregnancy, ultimately increasing future health risks for women and their children. Nurses have a significant collaborative and direct role in the care of women with pregnancy complications. Nurses can optimize outcomes for women and newborns by providing safe care during the perinatal period and act as advocates for women and families during the difficult perinatal period. They are the members of the health care team who are most present with mothers and newborns, and they can provide the ongoing surveillance needed for women with complicated and challenging high-risk pregnancies (Phillips & Boyd, 2016).

GESTATIONAL COMPLICATIONS

Although most pregnant women experience normal pregnancy, various complications can develop during pregnancy that affect maternal and fetal well-being. When women experience pregnancy these complications, astute assessment, rapid intervention, and a collaborative team approach are essential to optimize maternal and neonatal outcomes. In this section, complications related to pregnancy are presented along with the physiological and pathological basis for the most common complications of pregnancy. Nursing care and appropriate management are discussed.

Risk Assessment

A high-risk pregnancy is one of greater risk to the mother or her fetus than an uncomplicated pregnancy. Pregnancy places additional physical and emotional stress on a woman's body. Health problems that occur before a woman becomes pregnant or during pregnancy may also increase the likelihood for a high-risk pregnancy (National Institute of Child Health and Human Development [NICHHD], 2013). The goal of risk assessment is to identify pregnant women at risk for developing complications and promote risk-appropriate care that will enhance maternal and fetal outcomes. These factors include

BOX 7-1 | Common Risk Factors

A high-risk pregnancy is one that threatens the health or life of the mother or her fetus. For most women, early and regular prenatal care promotes a healthy pregnancy and delivery without complications. But some women are at an increased risk for complications even before they get pregnant for a variety of reasons.

Risk factors for a high-risk pregnancy can include:

- Existing health conditions, such as high blood pressure, diabetes, or being HIV-positive
- A history of prior pregnancy complications
- Complications that arise during pregnancy, such as gestational diabetes or preeclampsia
- Being overweight or obese
- Carrying more than one fetus (twins and higher-order multiples)
- Being ≤ 18
- Advanced maternal age increases the risk because of pre-existing health problems and increased risk of pre-eclampsia and diabetes

demographic, medical, obstetric, sociocultural, lifestyle, and environmental risks.

Risk assessment tools have poor predictive value but can be helpful in distinguishing between women at high and low risk for complications. No cause-and-effect relationship between risk factors and poor outcomes has been established. For example, up to one-third of women who develop complications may not have identifiable risk factors. Additionally, the underlying causes of some complications, such as preterm labor and intrauterine growth restriction, are not fully understood. Racial and ethnic disparities exist for multiple adverse obstetric outcomes and do not appear to be explained by differences in patient characteristics (Grobman et al., 2015). The prevalence of preterm birth, fetal growth restriction, fetal demise, maternal mortality, and inadequate receipt of prenatal care all vary by maternal race/ethnicity. These disparities have their roots in maternal health behaviors, genetics, the physical and social environments, and access to and quality of health care (Bryant, Worjoloh, Caughey, & Washington, 2010). Common risk factors are presented in Box 7-1. Specific risk factors are discussed related to each complication presented.

CRITICAL COMPONENT

Nursing Activities to Promote Adaptation to Pregnancy Complications

Pregnancy complications represent a threat to both the woman and fetus's health and to the emotional well-being of the family. Assessment of emotional status and coping of the entire family is necessary to provide comprehensive care. Implementing an individualized plan of care will facilitate the family's transition during an often unexpected and frightening experience (Gilbert, 2011). Responses to high-risk pregnancy can include:

• Stress and anxiety about the maternal illness and its effect on the fetus, and the disruption to their home- and work-related activities.
• Threats to self-esteem; the woman may feel she has somehow failed as a woman and/or is failing as a mother. Self-blaming commonly occurs for real or imagined wrongdoing.
• Disappointment and frustration often occurs when goals of having a healthy pregnancy, a normal birth, and a healthy baby are impeded by a pregnancy complication.
• Conflict can occur when competing and opposing goals are presented during a high-risk pregnancy.
• Crisis occurs when the woman and her family are threatened by a pregnancy complication and an uncertain outcome.

Some general nursing actions include the following:

• Provide time for the woman and family to express their concerns and feelings, which may include apprehension, fear, anger, disappointment, and frustration. Talking can help them identify, analyze, and understand their experience and fears. Practice active listening.
• Provide information repeatedly with patient and significant other(s) to facilitate a realistic appraisal of events. That includes explaining high-risk conditions, procedures, diagnostic tests, and treatment plans in layman's terms, providing ongoing updates, and clarifying misconceptions. Discussing the underlying causes of a complication with the woman may help to alleviate feelings of self-blaming and guilt.
• Facilitate referrals related to the condition, which may include social services and chaplain services to enhance family coping and provide resources.
• Encourage the woman and her family to participate in decision making and express preferences to enhance autonomy and patient-centered care.
• If patient is hospitalized, have flexible guidelines for the family to minimize separation.
• Be a skilled communicator; take emotional "temperature" in the room and convey accurate assessment of psychological state of the patient and family.
• Be a witness to events, which can help during debriefing and with patient processing in high-risk situations.

Preterm Labor and Birth

Preterm labor (PTL) is defined as regular contractions of the uterus resulting in changes in the cervix before 37 weeks of gestation. Preterm birth (PTB) is defined as birth between 20 ⁶⁄₇ weeks of gestation and 36 ⁶⁄₇ weeks of gestation. The preterm birth rate, which declined from 2007 to 2014, increased slightly to 9.63% in 2015 (compared with 9.57% in 2014). Increases in preterm births were seen among non-Hispanic black and Hispanic women (PeriStats, 2017).

PTB is the leading cause of neonatal mortality and the most common reason for antenatal hospitalization (American College of Obstetricians and Gynecologists [ACOG], 2016a). In the United States, approximately 12% of all live births occur before term, and PTL preceded approximately 50% of these preterm births. Although the causes of PTL are not well understood, the burden of PTB is clear—preterm births account for approximately 70% of neonatal deaths and 36% of infant deaths as well as 25% to 50% of cases of long-term neurologic impairment in children. Average expenditures for premature/low birthweight (LBW) infants were more than 10 times as high as uncomplicated newborns (March of Dimes, 2015). A 2006 report from the Institute of Medicine estimated the annual cost of preterm birth in the United States to be $26.2 billion or more than $51,000 per premature infant.

Identifying women who will give birth preterm is an inexact science. According to the Institute of Medicine (2007), PTB is a complex cluster of problems with overlapping factors of influence. Its causes may include individual behavioral and psychosocial factors, neighborhood characteristics, environmental exposures, medical conditions, infertility treatments, biological factors, and genetics. Many of these factors occur in combination, particularly in those who are socioeconomically disadvantaged or who are members of racial and ethnic minority groups. Approximately three-quarters of all preterm births occur spontaneously, and the remainder result from medical intervention (ACOG, 2012b). Most preterm births are a result of spontaneous PTL; however, between 20% and 25% of preterm births are intentional, necessary, and indicated for problems such as hypertension, preeclampsia, hemorrhage, and intrauterine growth restriction (IUGR) where early delivery would improve either maternal or fetal status. There are three main situations in which preterm labor and premature birth may occur (NICHD, 2017).

● Spontaneous preterm labor and birth refers to unintentional, unplanned delivery before the 37th week of pregnancy. This type of preterm birth can result from several causes, such as infection or inflammation, although the cause of spontaneous preterm labor and delivery is usually unknown. A history of delivering preterm is one of the strongest predictors for subsequent preterm births.
● Medically indicated preterm birth is when the health care provider recommends preterm delivery in the existence of a serious medical condition such as preeclampsia. In these cases, health care providers often take steps to keep the baby in the womb as long as possible to allow for additional growth and development, while also monitoring the mother and fetus for health issues. Providers also use additional interventions, such as steroids, to help improve outcomes for the baby.
● Non-medically indicated (elective) preterm delivery. Some late-preterm births result from inducing labor or having a cesarean delivery in the absence of a medical reason to do so, even though this practice is not recommended. Research indicates that even babies born at 37 or 38 weeks of pregnancy are at higher risk for poor health outcomes than babies born at 39 weeks of pregnancy or later. Therefore, unless there are

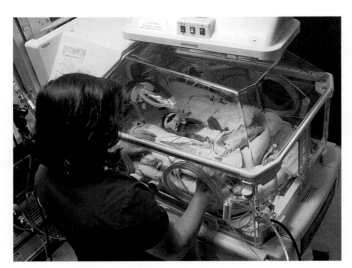

FIGURE 7–1 Premature infant in the NICU.

medical problems, health care providers should wait until at least 39 weeks of pregnancy to induce labor or perform a cesarean delivery to prevent possible health problems.

The discussion in this section focuses on spontaneous preterm labor.

A preterm/premature infant is born after 20 weeks and before 37 weeks (36 ⁶/₇ weeks) of gestation (Fig. 7–1). More specific classifications of prematurity include (PeriStats, 2017):

● Late preterm infant: An infant born between 34 and 37 weeks of gestation (34 ⁰/₇–36 ⁶/₇ weeks)
● Very preterm infant: An infant born before 32 completed weeks of gestation
● Viability: The threshold for viability is at 25 and rarely, fewer completed weeks gestation (ACOG, 2016c)
● Periviability: Approximately 0.5% of all births occur before the third trimester of pregnancy, and these very early deliveries result in the majority of neonatal deaths and more than 40% of infant deaths. *Periviable birth* is delivery occurring from 20 ⁰/₇ weeks to 25 ⁶/₇ weeks of gestation (ACOG, 2017b)

Long-term sequelae for preterm infants include cerebral palsy, hearing and vision impairment, and chronic lung disease. Long-term costs include not only health care costs but also special education costs for learning problems, costs of developmental services, and health care costs for long-term sequelae associated with prematurity. Survival rates for extremely preterm or extremely low-birth-weight (LBW) newborns born at the threshold of viability (25 or fewer completed weeks of gestation) has certainly improved in the last three decades, largely as the result of a greater use of assisted ventilation in the delivery room and surfactant therapy and increased use of antenatal and neonatal corticosteroids. However, this improvement in survival has not been associated with an equal improvement in morbidity. The incidence of chronic lung disease, sepsis, and poor growth remains high and may even have increased. There is concern that the treatment of extremely preterm and extremely LBW newborns may result in unforeseen effects into adulthood, and that the neurodevelopmental outcome

and cognitive function of extremely preterm and extremely LBW infants may be suboptimal (ACOG 2002; ACOG 2016c; ACOG 2017b). The goals of *Healthy People 2020* and the March of Dimes are to reduce the preterm birth rate from 12.2% to 11.4% (March of Dimes, 2015).

Increases in preterm birth rates from 2014 to 2015 were seen for infants born to non-Hispanic black (from 13.23%–13.41%) and Hispanic (9.03%–9.14%) women; the rate for non-Hispanic white women was essentially stable at 8.88% in 2015, compared with 8.91% for 2014. Rates had declined for each group since 2007, however, down 10% for non-Hispanic white (from 9.90% in 2007), 9% for non-Hispanic black (14.71%), and 2% for Hispanic (9.35%) infants. During 2011 to 2013 (average) in the United States, preterm birth rates were highest for black infants (16.5%), followed by Native Americans (13.4%), Hispanics (11.5%), whites (10.3%) and Asians (10.1%) (March of Dimes, 2015) During 2011 to 2013 (average) in the United States, preterm birth rates were highest for women ages 40 and older (16.5%), followed by women younger than age 20 (13.3%), ages 30 to 39 (11.6%) and ages 20 to 29 (11.0%) (March of Dimes, 2015).

Pathophysiological Pathways of Preterm Labor

The causes of preterm labor and premature birth are numerous, complex, and only partly understood. Medical, psychosocial, and biological factors may all play a role in preterm labor and birth (NICHD, 2017). Spontaneous PTB may be characterized by a syndrome composed of several components including uterine (PTL), chorioamnionic-decidual (premature rupture of membranes), and cervical (cervical insufficiency) (Owen & Harger, 2007). Yet the specific causes of spontaneous preterm labor and delivery are largely unknown.

Preterm labor is characterized as a series of complex interactions of factors. No single factor acts alone, but multiple factors interact to initiate a cascade of events that result in preterm labor and birth (Reedy, 2014). The pathways to preterm birth are thought to be multicausal, and related to various contributing factors (Iams, 2007; March of Dimes, 2006a). There are many pathways from risk factors to the terminal cascade of events resulting in labor. PTL likely occurs when local uterine factors prematurely stimulate this cascade or when suppressive factors that inhibit the cascade and maintain uterine quiescence are withdrawn prematurely. The four major factors leading to preterm labor are excessive uterine stretch or distension, decidual hemorrhage, intrauterine infection, and maternal or fetal stress. Uteroplacental vascular insufficiency, exaggerated inflammatory response, hormonal factors, cervical insufficiency, and genetic predisposition also play a role (Fig. 7–2), including:

● Excessive uterine stretch or distention
  ● Prostaglandins can be produced, stimulating the uterus to contract when overdistended from multiple gestation, polyhydramnios, or uterine abnormalities.
● Decidual activation
  ● From hemorrhage
  ● From fetal-decidual paracrine system
  ● From upper genital tract infection

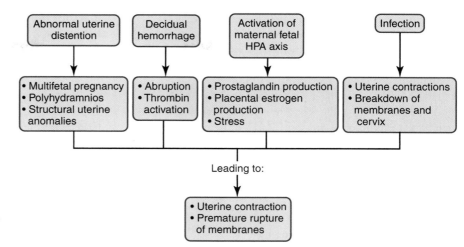

FIGURE 7-2 Pathophysiological pathways for preterm labor.

- Premature activation of the normal physiological initiators of labor, activation of the maternal-fetal hypothalamic–pituitary adrenal (HPA) axis.
- Inflammation and infection in the decidua, fetal membranes, and amniotic fluid are associated with preterm birth.

Inflammatory cytokines or bacterial endotoxins can stimulate prostaglandin release resulting in cervical ripening, contractions, and weakening and rupture of membranes.

Stress and psychosocial factors are also hypothesized to contribute to a stress response that results in uterine contractions (UCs). Studies of chronic and catastrophic stress exposures are suggestive of an association between stress and preterm birth. The search for a biological explanation for the pathways through which stress might affect preterm birth risk has led to extensive literature on the role of corticotropin-releasing hormone (CRH) as a potential mediator of this relationship. While some studies have shown higher levels of CRH in women destined to have a preterm birth, these findings have not been consistent. It remains likely, however, that neuroendocrine pathways underlie the relationship between acute and chronic stressors on PTB and low birth weight risk (Grobman et al., 2015). Because we do not know what triggers normal labor at term, it is difficult to know what causes PTL. Extensive research has been conducted over the past three decades to predict which women are at risk to deliver preterm so that intensive interventions can be implemented to prevent prematurity.

Risk Factors for Preterm Labor and Birth

Despite its use for decades, risk factor assessment alone has a limited utility for identifying who will deliver preterm (March of Dimes, 2011). Fifty percent of women who deliver preterm have no risk factors. Seventy percent of women who are at risk for preterm delivery deliver at term. Research indicates a complex interplay of multiple risk factors is responsible for preterm deliveries (PeriStats, 2017).

A host of behavioral, psychosocial, socio-demographic, and medical/pregnancy conditions, and biological factors are associated with risk for preterm birth (March of Dimes, 2018). The most consistently identified risk factors include a history of

preterm birth; for example, the additive risk associated with multiple prior preterm births is especially evident when early preterm births are considered. Women with one prior preterm delivery before 35 weeks have a 16% recurrence risk, those with two early preterm deliveries have a 41% risk, and those with three prior preterm deliveries have a 67% risk of subsequent preterm birth before 35 weeks (U.S. Department of Health and Human Services [DHHS], 2008; NIH).

The three most common risk factors for preterm birth are (Reedy, 2014):

- Prior preterm birth (single most important factor reoccurrence rates of up to 40%)
- Multiple gestation (50% of twins delivered preterm, ≥90% higher multiples delivered preterm)
- Uterine/cervical abnormalities, diethylstilbestrol (DES) exposure

Other risk factors include (ACOG, 2016a; Goldstein, 2007):

- Fetal anomalies
- History of second trimester loss, incompetent cervix or cervical insufficiency
- IVF pregnancy
- Hydramnios or oligohydramnios
- Infection, especially genitourinary infections and periodontal disease
- Premature rupture of membranes
- Short pregnancy interval (less than 9 months)
- Pregnancy associated problems such as hypertension, diabetes, and vaginal bleeding
- Chronic health problems such as hypertension, diabetes, or clotting disorders
- Inadequate nutrition, low BMI, low pre-pregnancy weight, or poor weight gain
- Age younger than 17 or older than 35 years old
- Late or no prenatal care
- Obesity, high BMI, or excessive weight gain
- Working long hours, long periods of standing
- Ancestry and ethnicity
  - Preterm birth rates are highest for African American infants (13.3% vs. 9.6%). In the United States, the preterm

birth rate among black women is 48% higher than the rate among all other women (March of Dimes, 2018).

- Maternal unmarried status is associated with an increased risk of preterm birth as well as low birth weight and small for gestational age (Shah, Zao, & Ali, 2011).
- Preterm birth is more likely in the presence of intimate partner violence (IPV), mental health issues, substance abuse, and other psychosocial stressors (March of Dimes, 2018).
  - Maternal exposure to domestic violence is associated with significantly increased risk of LBW and PTB. Inadequate prenatal care, higher incidences of high-risk behaviors, direct physical trauma, stress, and neglect are postulated mechanisms (Shah & Shah, 2010).
- Lack of social support
- Smoking, alcohol, and illicit drug use
- Lower education and socioeconomic status, poverty

Most preterm births (75%) are a result of spontaneous preterm labor (40%) and/or preterm premature rupture of membrane (PPROM) (35%) and related diagnoses (Creasy, Resnik, & Iams, 2004; Iams, 2007; Owen & Harger, 2007). However, more than 20% of preterm births are clinically indicated for complications (medically indicated preterm birth).

Prediction and Detection of Preterm Labor

Early detection of pregnant women who will give birth prematurely has been extensively researched since the 1970s with few definitive findings. No screening methods have been found to be consistently effective. Tests for preterm birth prediction include biomarkers for decidual-membrane separation, such as fetal fibronectin; proteomics to identify inflammatory activity; and genomics for susceptibility for preterm birth. Since 1998, cervical length, bacterial vaginosis, and the presence of fetal fibronectin in cervicovaginal fluid have been identified as factors most strongly linked to risk of spontaneous preterm births (March of Dimes, 2011).

Two methods thought to hold promise in predicting preterm delivery in first-time pregnancies identified only a small proportion of cases and do not appear suitable for widespread screening, according to a large study by a National Institutes of Health research network. The researchers found no benefit to combining the results of the two tests. They concluded that, alone and together, the methods did not identify enough preterm births to support routine screening of first-time pregnancies (Esplin et al., 2017).

- Transvaginal cervical ultrasonography
  - In symptomatic women, a cervical length of >30 mm reliably excludes preterm labor.
  - A cervical length of <20 mm has strong positive predictive value.
- Fetal fibronectin has a low positive predictive value but a high negative predictive value, thereby making it a useful test to predict those women who will NOT deliver preterm.

Risks for the Woman Related to Preterm Labor and Birth

- Complications related to treatment with tocolytics such as cardiac arrhythmias, pulmonary edema, and even congestive heart failure

Risks for the Fetus and Newborn Related to Preterm Labor and Birth

- Complications of prematurity and long-term sequelae associated with prematurity (see Chapter 17)

Assessment Findings

Criteria for the diagnosis of preterm labor have varied, and there is not universal agreement on criteria. Signs or symptoms a woman may experience include:

- Change in type of vaginal discharge (watery, mucus, or bloody)
- Increase in amount of discharge
- Pelvic or lower abdominal pressure
- Constant low, dull backache
- Mild abdominal cramps, with or without diarrhea
- Regular or frequent contractions or uterine tightening, often painless
- Possible ruptured membranes

CRITICAL COMPONENT

Diagnosis of Preterm Labor

Preterm birth is defined as birth between 20 $^{0}/_{7}$ weeks of gestation and 36 $^{6}/_{7}$ weeks of gestation. The diagnosis of preterm labor generally is based on clinical criteria of regular uterine contractions accompanied by a change in cervical dilation, effacement, or both, or initial presentation with regular contractions and cervical dilation of at least 2 cm (ACOG, 2016a). Less than 10% of women with the clinical diagnosis of preterm labor actually give birth within 7 days of presentation. It is important to recognize that preterm labor with intact membranes is not the only cause of preterm birth; numerous preterm births are preceded by either rupture of membranes or other medical problems necessitating delivery.

Medical Management

Historically, nonpharmacologic treatments to prevent preterm births in women with preterm labor have included bed rest, abstention from intercourse and orgasm, and hydration. These approaches are no longer recommended as evidence for their effectiveness is lacking and adverse effects have been reported (ACOG, 2016a). Management now focuses on delaying delivery for 48 to 72 hours to administer antenatal steroids and allow time to facilitate fetal lung maturity. Medical management includes the following measures.

- Tocolytic drugs are medications used to suppress uterine contractions in preterm labor. The evidence supports the use of first-line tocolytic treatment with beta-adrenergic agonist therapy, calcium channel blockers, or NSAIDs for short-term prolongation of pregnancy (up to 48 hours) to allow for the administration of antenatal steroids (ACOG, 2016a). These agents have drawbacks and potential serious adverse effects (Table 7–1). A review of evidence on tocolytic

TABLE 7–1   Common Tocolytic Agents

AGENT OR CLASS	MATERNAL SIDE EFFECTS	FETAL OR NEWBORN ADVERSE EFFECTS	CONTRAINDICATIONS	NURSING CARE
Calcium channel blockers Ex: Nifedipine (Procardia)	Dizziness, flushing, and hypotension; suppression of heart rate, contractility, and left ventricular systolic pressure when used with magnesium sulfate; and elevation of hepatic enzymes	No known adverse effects	Hypotension and preload-dependent cardiac lesions, such as aortic insufficiency	Assess for side effects including hypotension, dizziness, headache, nausea, palpitations, flushing, and edema. Assist woman when getting up from bed and when ambulating. Assess pulse and blood pressure before and after administration. Monitor hepatic enzymes (LFTs).
Nonsteroidal anti-inflammatory drugs Ex: Indomethacin	Nausea, esophageal reflux, gastritis, and emesis	Premature closure of fetal ductus arteriosus, interventricular hemorrhage, oligohydraminos, necrotizing enterocolitis in preterm newborns, and patent ductus arteriosus in newborn	Platelet dysfunction of bleeding disorder, hepatic dysfunction, gastrointestinal ulcerative disease, hepatitis, renal dysfunction, and asthma (in women with hypersensitivity to aspirin)	Assess for gastrointestinal upset. Assess level and characteristics of pain.
Beta-adrenergic receptor agonists Ex: Terbutaline, Ritodrine	Tachycardia, arrhythmias, palpitations, shortness of breath, chest discomfort, pulmonary edema, hyperglycemia, hypokalemia, hypotension, and tremor	Fetal tachycardia, alterations in fetal glucose metabolism	Tachycardia-sensitive maternal cardiac disease and poorly controlled diabetes mellitus, maternal hyperthyroidism, and seizure disorders	Monitor heart rate, blood pressure, and respiratory rate. Strict I&O for fluid overload. Assess blood glucose levels. Evaluate patient for anxiety and tremors. Use cautiously when administering to an asthma patient and monitor for respiratory distress.
Magnesium sulfate Use of magnesium sulfate as a tocolytic for short-term prolongation of pregnancy (up to 48 hours) to allow for the administration of antenatal corticosteroids in pregnant women who are at risk of preterm delivery	Causes lethargy, drowsiness, flushing, diaphoresis, nausea, vomiting, headache, pulmonary edema, loss of deep tendon reflexes, respiratory depression, hypotension, and cardiac arrest; suppresses heart rate, contractility and left ventricular systolic pressure when used with calcium channel blockers; and produces neuromuscular blockade when used with calcium-channel blockers	Neonatal depression fetal and neonatal bone demineralization	Myasthenia gravis	Assess deep tendon reflexes and for clonus. Assess respiratory status, including rate, rhythm, and depth. Monitor serum magnesium levels. Keep calcium gluconate available for use as an antidote. Monitor strict intake and output.

ACOG, 2016a; Reedy, 2014.

therapy revealed a small improvement in pregnancy prolongation and that extended use has little or no value (Dodd, Crowther, Dare, & Middleton, 2006; Han, Crowther, and Moore, 2010). Interventions to reduce the likelihood of delivery should be reserved for women with preterm labor at a gestational age at which a delay in delivery will provide benefit to the newborn. Because tocolytic therapy generally is effective for up to 48 hours, current recommendations indicate only women with fetuses that would benefit from a 48-hour delay in delivery should receive tocolytic treatment (ACOG, 2016a). Tocolytic therapy is typically administered between 24 to 34 weeks' gestation.

● Women with preterm contractions without cervical change, especially those with a cervical dilation of less than 2 cm, generally should not be treated with tocolytics.
● Maintenance therapy with tocolytics is ineffective for preventing preterm birth and improving neonatal outcomes and is not recommended for this purpose (ACOG, 2016a).

● Antibiotics should not be used to prolong gestation or improve neonatal outcomes in women with preterm labor and intact membranes. This recommendation is distinct from recommendations for antibiotic use for preterm premature rupture of membranes and group B streptococci carrier status (ACOG, 2016a).

● Progesterone supplementation may be useful to prevent preterm birth for women with a history of spontaneous preterm birth (ACOG, 2008; Dodd, Jones, Flenady, Cincotta, & Crowther, 2013). Data suggest that progesterone may be important in maintaining uterine quiescence in the latter half of pregnancy by limiting the production of stimulatory prostaglandins and inhibiting the expression of contraction- associated protein genes within the myometrium (Norwitz & Caughey, 2011). The use of progesterone is associated with benefits in infant health following administration in women at increased risk of preterm birth due either to a prior preterm birth or where a short cervix has been identified on ultrasound examination. Use of 17-alpha-hydroxyprogesterone-caproate at 250 mg/week beginning at 16 weeks to 36 weeks of gestation, is considered safe. It is not recommended for prophylactic use in multiple gestation.

● Neonatal neuroprophylaxis with intravenous magnesium sulfate administration is recommended to reduce microcapillary brain hemorrhage in premature birth of the neonate. Accumulated available evidence suggests that magnesium sulfate reduces the severity and risk of cerebral palsy in surviving infants if administered when birth is anticipated before 32 weeks of gestation (ACOG, 2010a; ACOG, 2016a).

● Corticosteroid therapy with antenatal steroids is currently recommended to women at risk of preterm birth. A single course of corticosteroids is recommended for pregnant women between 24 weeks and 34 weeks of gestation who are at risk of delivery within 7 days (ACOG, 2016a). Betamethasone is one antenatal steroid given to women to accelerate fetal lung maturity, thereby decreasing the severity of respiratory distress syndrome and other complications of prematurity in the neonate. Treatment with antenatal corticosteroids

reduces the risk of neonatal respiratory distress syndrome, cerebroventricular hemorrhage, necrotizing enterocolitis, and infectious morbidity in the neonate when used between 24 and 34 weeks' gestation (Roberts, Brown, Medley, & Dalziel, 2017).

If UCs decrease to fewer than five per hour, women are often transferred to less acute antenatal units for further observation for several days. If they remain stable, they may be discharged to home undelivered. Discharge instructions typically include self-monitoring of uterine activity, and signs and symptoms of preterm labor. Maintenance tocolytic therapy has no demonstrated benefit (Cunningham et al., 2014).

Contraindications

Contraindications to treating preterm labor include:

● Intrauterine fetal demise
● Lethal fetal anomaly
● Nonreassuring fetal status
● Severe preeclampsia or eclampsia
● Maternal bleeding with hemodynamic instability
● Chorioamnionitis
● Preterm premature rupture of membranes in the absence of maternal infection (tocolytics may be considered for the purposes of maternal transport, steroid administration, or both)
● Maternal contraindications to tocolysis (agent-specific)
  ● Active hemorrhage
  ● Severe maternal disease
  ● Fetal compromise
  ● Chorioamnionitis
  ● Fetal death
  ● Previable gestation and PPROM

Tocolysis is generally contraindicated when the maternal and fetal risks of prolonging pregnancy or the risks associated with these drugs are greater than the risks associated with preterm birth. Contraindications to tocolysis for preterm labor include severe preeclampsia, placental abruption, intrauterine infection, pulmonary hypertension, maternal hemodynamic instability, intrauterine fetal demise, lethal congenital or chromosomal abnormalities, fetal maturity, and fetal compromise (ACOG, 2016a).

SAFE AND EFFECTIVE NURSING CARE: Understanding Medication

Medication Antenatal Corticosteroids

The most beneficial intervention for improvement of neonatal outcomes among patients who give birth preterm is the administration of antenatal corticosteroids. A single course of corticosteroids is recommended for pregnant women between 24 weeks and 34 weeks of gestation who are at risk of delivery within 7 days. A Cochrane meta-analysis concluded neonates whose mothers receive antenatal corticosteroids have significantly lower severity, frequency, or both of respiratory distress syndrome, intracranial hemorrhage, necrotizing enterocolitis and death (Roberts et al., 2017).

- Indication: Given to women at 24 and 34 weeks' gestation with signs of preterm labor or at risk to deliver preterm in the next 7 days
- Action: Stimulate the production of more mature surfactant in the fetal lungs to prevent respiratory distress syndrome in premature infants
- Adverse reactions: Will raise blood sugar and may require temporary insulin coverage to maintain euglycemia in diabetic women
- Route and dose: Betamethasone 12 mg IM every 24 hours × 2 doses or Dexamethasone four 6-mg doses IM every 12 hours

A single repeat course of antenatal corticosteroids may be considered in women who are less than 34 weeks of gestation, who are at risk of preterm delivery within the next 7 days, and whose prior course of antenatal corticosteroids was administered more than 14 days previously. Rescue course corticosteroids could be provided as early as 7 days from the prior dose, if indicated by the clinical situation (ACOG, 2016a).

Nursing Actions

Nurses can provide expertise in directing patient care, stabilizing the woman and fetus, counseling, coordinating care, and providing patient teaching (Grey, 2006; March of Dimes, 2006b). Immediate care, including assessment and stabilization, occurs in labor and delivery. If uterine activity decreases, generally to fewer than 5 UCs/hr, with no further cervical change, women are often moved to a less intensive care setting than a labor and delivery unit. Once moved to an antenatal high-risk unit, they are often observed for several days and, if stable, discharged to home undelivered.

Immediate care:

- Review the prenatal record for risk factors and establish gestational age through history and ultrasound (ultrasound early in pregnancy is more reliable for gestational age).
- Assess the woman and fetus for signs and symptoms of:
  - Vaginal and urinary infection
  - Rupture of membranes
  - Sterile speculum exam to assess for ferning of amniotic fluid
  - Vaginal bleeding or vaginal discharge
  - Dehydration
- Assess fetal heart rate (FHR) and uterine contractions.
  - Report fetal tachycardia or increased uterine contractions to the health care provider.
- Obtain vaginal and urine cultures as per orders.
- Obtain fFN as per orders.
  - This should be obtained before the sterile vaginal exam. Contraindicated if rupture of membranes (ROM), bleeding, sexual intercourse, or prior collection in the last 24 hours.

- Maintain strict input and output (I&O) while on tocolytics and provide oral or IV hydration.
- May restrict total intake to 3,000 mL/24 hr if on tocolytics.
- Administer tocolytic agents as per protocol.
  - Monitor for adverse reactions (see Table 7–1).
- Administer antenatal steroids per orders.
- Position the patient on her side to increase uteroplacental perfusion and decrease pressure on the maternal inferior vena cava.
- Assess vital signs per protocol for tocolytic administered.
  - Report to the provider blood pressure greater than 140/90 mm Hg or less than 90/50 mm Hg; heart rate greater than 120; temperature greater than 100.4°F (38°C).
- Auscultate lungs for evidence of pulmonary edema.
- Assess cervical status with a sterile vaginal exam unless contraindicated by ROM or bleeding (may be done by the health care provider to minimize multiple exams); cervical ultrasound may be done (cervical length of less than 30 mm may be clinically significant).
- Notify the care provider of findings.

Continuing care once the woman is stable includes the following measures.

- Provide emotional support to the woman by providing opportunities to discuss her feelings. Women often feel guilt that they caused the preterm labor, are concerned for the infant's health, and have anxiety and sadness over loss of "normal" newborn and normal pregnancy labor and delivery.
- Facilitate a clear understanding of the treatment plan and the woman and family's involvement in clinical decision making.
- Facilitate consultations with the neonatal staff regarding neonatal survival rates, the anticipated care of the newborn, treatments, complications, and possible long-term disabilities. The family may be taken on a tour of NICU.
- Monitor the woman's response to treatment including FHR baseline and variability and uterine contractions, maternal vital signs, woman's response while on tocolytics, increase in vaginal discharge, or ROM.
- Assessment of women on tocolytics is based on tocolytic used and is detailed in Table 7–1, but generally includes monitoring of blood pressure and pulse and auscultation of lungs for pulmonary edema. Watch for:
  - Shortness of breath, chest tightness or discomfort, cough, oxygen saturation less than 95%, increased respiratory and heart rates
  - Changes in behavior such as apprehension, anxiety, or restlessness
- Encourage a side-lying position to enhance placental perfusion.
- Evaluate laboratory reports such as urine and cervical cultures.
  - White blood cell (WBC) counts are elevated in women who have received corticosteroids; therefore, elevated WBCs are not indicative of infection.

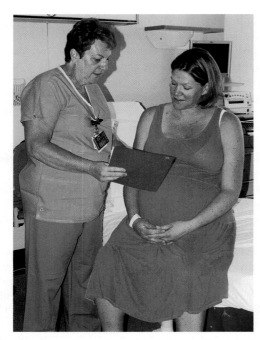

FIGURE 7–3 Nurse doing discharge teaching with high-risk pregnant woman in the hospital.

- Provide ongoing reassurance and explanations to the woman and her family.
- Explain the purpose and side effects of the medication.
- Set short-term goals such as completion of a gestational week or milestones.
- Facilitate family interactions and visiting by having flexible visiting policies.
- Assist the family in participating in plan of care.
- Some women enjoy keeping a journal to help them deal with boredom and isolation (Reedy, 2014).
- Provide referral information about online support groups.
- Discuss the emotional and behavioral responses they can expect from other children based on developmental age of children.

Discharge Plan

Approximately 30% of preterm labor spontaneously resolves and 50% of patients hospitalized for preterm labor give birth at term (ACOG, 2016a). Interventions to reduce the likelihood of delivery should be reserved for women with preterm labor at a gestational age at which a delay in delivery would improve neonatal outcomes. All plans should be decided in consideration with the woman's and family's strengths, needs, and goals in mind and should be made with their participation (Durham, 1998; Maloni, 1998) (Fig. 7–3). Discharge teaching should include a review of warning signs and how and when to call the provider (Box 7–2).

Programs have demonstrated some improvement in outcomes with nurse phone or home care follow-up (Gilbert, 2011). Typically, women treated for preterm labor are sent home without follow-up at home except for weekly prenatal visits.

Preterm Premature Rupture of Membranes/Chorioamnionitis

Premature rupture of membranes (PROM) is rupture of membranes before the onset of labor. Membrane rupture before labor and before 37 weeks of gestation is referred to as preterm PROM. Management is influenced by gestational age and the presence of complicating factors such as clinical infection, abruptio placentae, labor, or nonreassuring fetal status. Preterm premature rupture of membranes (PPROM) is rupture of membranes with a premature gestation (<37 weeks). It occurs in about 3% of pregnancies yet is responsible for about 30% of all preterm births. Premature rupture of membranes is defined as rupture of the chorioamniotic membranes before the onset of labor but at term. Adding to the confusion is prolonged rupture of membranes, which is greater than 24 hours (PROM). This section focuses on those women that have rupture of membranes preterm (PPROM) because it accounts for approximately one-third of premature births. Once the membranes rupture preterm, most women go into labor within a week. The term latency refers to the time from membrane rupture to delivery. Previable PROM is rupture of membranes (ROM) before 23 to 24 weeks, preterm PROM remote from term is from 24 to 32 weeks' gestation, and preterm PROM near term is 31 to 36 weeks' gestation (Jazayeri, 2016).

Spontaneous PPROM occurs in the absence of medical intervention and is usually secondary to ascending infection. Iatrogenic PPROM occurs after medical intervention has occurred and may be secondary to invasive fetal testing such as chorionic villus sampling, amniocentesis, or fetoscopy. PPROM contributes to about one third of preterm (before 37 weeks) births. Spontaneous premature rupture of membranes is a multifactorial but choriodecidual infection and inflammation appears to be an important factor, especially with preterm PROM at earlier gestations (ACOG, 2016b). Bacterial infections are thought to weaken the membranes leading to rupture, but in most cases the cause is unknown. It has also been postulated that stress and strain on the membranes from uterine activity causes the membranes to become less elastic and more prone to rupture with repeated strain. Other factors that play a role in tissue degradation and immune modulation, such as altered levels of hormones (including relaxin) and micronutrients (including vitamin C), may be important in PPROM (Crowley, Grivell, and Dodd, 2016). Preterm PROM often occurs in the absence of recognized risk factors or an obvious cause (ACOG, 2016b).

The optimal approach to clinical assessment and treatment of women with term and preterm PROM remains controversial. Management hinges on knowledge of gestational age and evaluation of the relative risks of delivery versus the risks of expectant management (e.g, infection, abruptio placentae, and umbilical cord accident). Current management of preterm PROM (PPROM) involves either initiating birth soon after preterm PROM or alternatively, adopting a "wait and see" approach (expectant management). It is unclear which strategy is most beneficial for mothers and their babies. However, a recent Cochrane Review of evidence reveals no difference in the incidence of neonatal sepsis between women who were delivered immediately or were managed expectantly in PPROM prior to 37 weeks' gestation. In pregnancies complicated by preterm premature rupture of the membranes a policy of expectant management with careful observation is associated with better outcomes for the mother and baby (Bond et al, 2017). Regardless of obstetric management or clinical presentation, birth within 1 week of membrane rupture occurs in at least one half of patients with preterm PROM (ACOG, 2016b). Women presenting with PROM before neonatal viability should be counseled regarding the risks and benefits of expectant management versus immediate delivery. Counseling should include a realistic appraisal of neonatal outcomes. Immediate delivery should be offered.

Risk Factors for Preterm PROM

- Previous preterm PROM or preterm delivery
- Bleeding during pregnancy
- Short cervical length
- Hydramnios
- Multiple gestation (up to 15% in twins, up to 20% in triplets)
- Sexually transmitted infections (STIs)
- Low body mass index
- Low socioeconomic status
- Cigarette smoking and illicit drug use

Risks for the Woman

- Maternal infection (i.e., chorioamnionitis, endometritis)
- Abruptio placenta and retained placenta
- Increased rates of cesarean birth

Risks for the Fetus and Newborn

- Fetal or neonatal sepsis
  - The earlier the fetal gestation at ROM, the greater the risk for infection.
  - The membranes serve as a protective barrier that separates the sterile fetus and fluid from the bacteria-laden vaginal canal.
- Preterm delivery and complications of prematurity including respiratory distress, sepsis, intraventricular hemorrhage, necrotizing enterocolitis, and an increased risk of neurodevelopmental impairment
- Hypoxia or asphyxia because of umbilical cord compression or umbilical cord accidents due to decreased fluid and ROM
- Fetal deformities if preterm PROM before 26 weeks' gestation

Assessment Findings

- Confirmed premature gestational age by prenatal history and ultrasound
- Confirmed rupture of membranes with speculum exam and positive ferning test
- Oligohydramnios on ultrasound may be seen but is not diagnostic

Medical Management

The risk of perinatal complications changes drastically with gestational age at membrane rupture, so a gestational age-based approach is appropriate for medical management (ACOG, 2016b). Medical treatment is aimed at balancing the risks of prematurity and the risks of infections. Unless near-term gestation premature PROM, management is aimed at prolonging gestation for the woman who is not in labor, not infected, and not experiencing fetal compromise. Evaluation of gestational age, fetal presentation, and fetal well-being must be determined. Conservative management refers to treatment directed at continuing the pregnancy. Gestational age is a primary consideration when considering delivery versus expectant management. Nonreassuring fetal status, clinical chorioamnionitis, and significant abruptio placentae are clear indications for delivery. Otherwise, gestational age is a primary factor when considering delivery versus expectant management. According to ACOG (2016b), guidelines for management include:

- Patients with PROM before 34 % weeks of gestation should be managed expectantly if no maternal or fetal contraindications exist.
- To reduce maternal and neonatal infections and gestational-age dependent morbidity, a 7-day course of therapy with a combination of intravenous ampicillin and erythromycin followed by oral amoxicillin and erythromycin is recommended during expectant management of women with preterm PROM who are less than 34 % weeks of gestation.
- Women with preterm PROM and a viable fetus who are candidates for intrapartum GBS prophylaxis should receive intrapartum GBS prophylaxis to prevent vertical transmission regardless of earlier treatments.
- A single course of corticosteroids is recommended for pregnant women between 24 % weeks and 34 % weeks of gestation, and may be considered for pregnant women as early as 23 % weeks of gestation who are at risk of preterm delivery within 7 days. Antenatal corticosteroids have been shown to reduce the risk of neonatal respiratory distress, intraventricular hemorrhage (bleeding within the ventricles of the baby's brain), and neonatal death in the preterm neonate.
- Women with preterm PROM before 32 % weeks of gestation who are thought to be at risk of imminent delivery should

be considered candidates for fetal neuroprotective treatment with magnesium sulfate. Delivery is recommended when preterm PROM occurs at or beyond 34 weeks of gestation.

- Numerous sealing techniques have been employed which aim to restore a physical barrier against infection and encourage the reaccumulation of amniotic fluid. Routine use of sealants is currently not recommended due to a lack of sufficient evidence to support the safety and effectiveness of such interventions (Crowley et al., 2016).
- For women with PROM at 37 % weeks gestation or more, if spontaneous labor does not occur near the time of presentation in those who do not have contraindications to labor, labor should be induced.
- At 34 % weeks or greater gestation, delivery is recommended for all women with ruptured membranes.
- Digital cervical examinations should be avoided in patients with PROM unless they are in active labor or imminent delivery is anticipated.
- In the setting of ruptured membranes with active labor, therapeutic tocolysis has not been shown to prolong latency or improve neonatal outcomes. Therefore, therapeutic tocolysis is not recommended.
- Monitor for infection, abrutio placenta, and fetal compromise, as they are all indications for delivery.
- The outpatient management of preterm PROM with a viable fetus has not been sufficiently studied to establish safety and therefore is not recommended. Most women presenting with preterm prelabor rupture of membranes (PPROM) will require hospital management. The most recent Cochrane Review concluded there is insufficient evidence on the safety of home versus hospital management to make recommendations for clinical practice (El Senoun, Dowswell, Mousa, 2014).

Nursing Actions

- Assess FHR and uterine contractions.
- Assess for signs of infection including:
  - Maternal and/or fetal tachycardia
  - Maternal fever 100.4°F (38°C) or greater
  - Uterine tenderness
  - Malodorous fluid or vaginal discharge
- Monitor for labor and for fetal compromise.
- Provide antenatal testing including non-stress tests (NSTs) and biophysical profiles (BPPs).

Evidence-Based Practice: Cochrane Review on Social Support During At-Risk Pregnancy

Hodnett, E. (2010). Support during pregnancy for women at increased risk of low birth-weight babies. *Cochrane Database of Systematic Reviews*, 6. Accessed November 23, 2012.

Programs offering additional support during pregnancy were not effective in reducing the number of babies born too early and babies with low birth weights. Babies born to mothers in socially disadvantaged situations are more likely to be small and to have health problems. Programs providing emotional support, practical assistance, and advice have been offered in addition to usual care.

Randomized trials of additional support during at-risk pregnancy by either a professional (social worker, midwife, or nurse) or specially trained layperson, compared to routine care. They defined additional support as some form of emotional support (e.g., counseling, reassurance, sympathetic listening), information, and/or advice, either in home visits or during clinic appointments, and could include tangible assistance (e.g., transportation to clinic appointments, assistance with care of other children at home).

The review of 17 randomized controlled trials involving 12,264 women found that women who received additional support during pregnancy were less likely to be admitted to the hospital for pregnancy complications and to have a cesarean birth. However, the additional support did not reduce the likelihood of giving birth too early or that the baby was smaller than expected.

Authors' Conclusions
Pregnant women need the support of caring family members, friends, and health professionals. While programs which offer additional support during pregnancy are unlikely to prevent the pregnancy from resulting in a low birth weight or preterm baby, they may be helpful in reducing the likelihood of antenatal hospital admission and caesarean birth.

Cervical Insufficiency

The term cervical insufficiency is used to describe the inability of the uterine cervix to retain a pregnancy in the absence of the signs and symptoms of clinical contractions, or labor, or both in the second trimester (ACOG, 2014a). Controversy exists in the medical literature pertaining to issues of pathophysiology, screening, diagnosis, and management of cervical insufficiency. The diagnosis of cervical insufficiency is challenging because of a lack of objective findings and clear diagnostic criteria. Diagnosis is based on a history of painless cervical dilation after the first trimester with subsequent expulsion of the pregnancy in the second trimester, typically before 24 weeks of gestation, without contractions or labor and in the absence of other clear pathology such as bleeding, infection, or ruptured membranes (ACOG, 2014a).

The pathophysiology of cervical insufficiency is still poorly understood. It is associated with previous cervical trauma such as cervical dilation and curettage or cauterization, and abnormal cervical development from genetics or diethylstilbestrol (DES) exposure in utero, cervical lacerations, and/or local or systemic hormonal effects. Various diagnostic tests in the nonpregnant woman have been suggested to confirm the presence of cervical insufficiency, but none have been validated in rigorous scientific studies and they should not be used to diagnose cervical insufficiency (ACOG, 2014a).

Risks to the Woman

- Repeated second trimester or early third trimester births
- Reported complications of cerclage include rupture of membranes, chorioamnionitis, cervical lacerations, and suture displacement

Risk to the Fetus and Newborn

- Preterm birth and consequences of prematurity

Assessment Findings

● Although patients usually are asymptomatic, some may report nonspecific symptoms, such as backache, uterine contractions, vaginal spotting, pelvic pressure, or mucoid vaginal discharge.
● Shortened cervical length or funneling of the cervix, although use of ultrasound to diagnose cervical incompetence is not currently recommended (Cunningham et al., 2014).

Medical Management

Certain nonsurgical approaches, including activity restriction, bed rest, and pelvic rest, have not been proved to be effective for the treatment of cervical insufficiency and their use is not recommended (ACOG, 2014a). Vaginal pessary has been used, but evidence is limited for potential benefit of pessary placement and has only been studied in select high-risk patients. Surgical treatment of incompetent cervix is cerclage, a type of purse-string suture placed cervically to reinforce a weak cervix (Fig. 7–4). The standard transvaginal cerclage methods currently used include modifications of the McDonald and Shirodkar techniques.

Indications for Cervical Cerclage in Women With Singleton Pregnancies

● History of one or more second-trimester pregnancy losses related to painless cervical dilation and in the absence of labor or abruptio placentae
● Prior cerclage due to painless cervical dilation in the second trimester
● Painless cervical dilation in the second trimester
● Current singleton pregnancy, prior spontaneous preterm birth at less than 34 weeks of gestation, and short cervical length (less than 25 mm) before 24 weeks of gestation

A history-indicated cerclage (also known as prophylactic cerclage) is based on classic historic features of cervical insufficiency noted above. History-indicated cerclage can be considered in a patient with a history of unexplained second-trimester delivery in the absence of labor or abruptio placentae. History indicated cerclages typically are placed at approximately 13 to 14 weeks of gestation.

Women who present with advanced cervical dilation in the absence of labor have historically been candidates for examination-indicated cerclage, also called an emergency or rescue cerclage. Women with a current singleton pregnancy, prior spontaneous preterm birth at less than 34 weeks of gestation, and short cervical length (less than 25 mm) before 24 weeks of gestation may benefit from cerclage placement and evidence suggests that cerclage placement is associated with significant decreases in preterm birth outcomes and improved neonatal outcomes. Cerclage placement in women without a prior spontaneous preterm birth and a cervical length less than 25 mm detected between 16 weeks and 24 weeks of gestation has not been associated with a significant reduction in preterm birth. Cerclage may increase the risk of preterm birth in women with a twin pregnancy and an ultrasonographically detected cervical length less than 25 mm and is not recommended (ACOG, 2014a).

● Most patients at risk of cervical insufficiency can be safely monitored with serial transvaginal ultrasound examinations in the second trimester, beginning at 16 weeks and end at 24 weeks of gestation.
● Obtain transcervical ultrasound to evaluate cervix for cervical length; funneling may be done but is not diagnostic.
● Perform cervical cultures for chlamydia, gonorrhea, and other cervical infections.
  ● Prophylactic cerclage may be placed in women with a history of unexplained recurrent painless dilation and second trimester birth, generally between 12 and 16 weeks of gestation.
  ● Rescue cerclage is placed after the cervix has dilated with no perceived contractions, up to about 24 weeks of gestation (Cunningham et al., 2014).
● Administer antibiotics or tocolytics, but this has not been demonstrated to be effective and is controversial in perioperative period (Owen & Harger, 2007).
● A firm recommendation on whether a cerclage should be removed after premature PROM cannot be made, and either removal or retention is reasonable.
● If cervical change, painful contractions, or vaginal bleeding progress, cerclage removal is recommended. Cerclage is removed if infection occurs, or labor develops.

Postoperative Nursing Actions

● Monitor for uterine activity with palpation.
● Monitor for vaginal bleeding and leaking of fluid/rupture of membranes.
● Monitor for infection.
  ● Maternal fever
  ● Uterine tenderness
● Discharge teaching may include teaching patient to:
  ● Monitor for signs and symptoms of uterine activity, rupture of membranes, bleeding, infection.
  ● Modify activity and pelvic rest for a week.
  ● Transvaginal McDonald cerclage removal is recommended at 36 to 37 weeks of gestation.

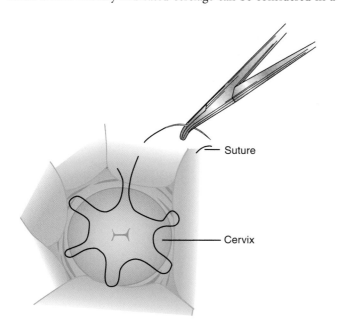

Suture

Cervix

FIGURE 7–4 Cerclage.

Multiple Gestation

Multiple gestation pregnancies are those with more than one fetus. They result from either the fertilization of one zygote that subsequently divides (monozygotic) or the fertilization of multiple ova. The twin birth rate declined in 2015 to 33.5 per 1,000 total births; the 2014 twinning rate (33.9) was an all-time high. The triplet and higher-order multiple birth rate dropped 9% from 2014 to 2015 and is down 46% since the 1998 peak (Martin, Hamilton, Osterman, Driscoll, & Mathews, 2017). Recent declines in triplet and higher order multiple (HOM) birth rates have been linked to changes in ART procedures. The increased incidence in multifetal gestations has been attributed to two main factors: 1) a shift toward an older maternal age at conception, when multifetal gestations are more likely to occur naturally, and 2) an increased use of assisted reproductive technology (ART), which is more likely to result in a multifetal gestation. Approximately one-third of twins are monozygotic (from one egg) and two-thirds are dizygotic (from two eggs) (Fig. 7–5A & B).

- Monozygotic twins are from one zygote that divides in the first week of gestation. They are genetically identical and similar in appearance and always have the same gender.
- Dizygotic twins result from fertilization of two eggs and may be the same or differing genders. If the fetuses are of differing gender, they are dizygotic and therefore dichorionic.
- Either of these processes can be involved in the development of higher order multiples.

The rate of twin specific complications varies in relation to zygocity and chorionicity. There are two principal placental types, monochorionic (one chorion) and dichorionic (two chorions). Dizygotic twins are always dichorionic/diamniotic and may be the same or different genders. Among monozygotic twins 30% dichorionic/diamniotic and have separate placentas and amniotic sacs. About 70% are monochorionic/diamniotic with a single placenta with two amniotic sacs. There are increased rates of perinatal mortality and neurological injury in monochorionic, diamniotic twins compared with dichorionic pairs (Fig. 7–5A). Only 1% of monozygotic twins are monoamniotic that share the same amniotic sac. Because they share the same sac, monoamniotic twins have a fetal mortality rate of 50% to 60% due to entangling of umbilical cords (Creasy et al., 2004) (Fig. 7–5B). Because monozygotic twins are from a single fertilized ovum, they are always the same gender. Conjoined twins may result from an aberration in the twinning process ascribed to incomplete splitting of an embryo into two separate twins (Cunningham et al., 2014). Although multiple gestations are only about 3% of births in the United States, they contribute disproportionately to maternal, fetal, and neonatal morbidity and mortality. Risks for both the fetus and the woman increase with increased number of fetuses. Compared with women with twins, women with triplets or higher order multiples (HOM) are at even higher risk of pregnancy related morbidities and mortality (Bowers, 2014).

Twin pregnancy is associated with higher rates of almost every potential complication of pregnancy. The most serious risk is spontaneous preterm delivery, which plays a major role in the increased perinatal mortality and short-term and long-term

morbidity observed in these infants. Higher rates of fetal growth restriction and congenital anomalies also contribute to adverse outcome in twin births. In addition, monochorionic twins are at risk for complications unique to these pregnancies, such as twin-twin transfusion syndrome (TTTS), which can be lethal or associated with serious morbidity (ACOG, 2014c).

Risks for the Woman

Twin pregnancy is associated with higher rates of almost every potential complication of pregnancy

- Hypertensive disorders and preeclampsia, which tend to develop earlier and be more severe, are related to enlarged placenta.
- Gestational diabetes often occurs due to physiological changes related to supporting multiple fetuses.
- Antepartum hemorrhage, abruptio placenta, placenta previa
- Anemia related to dilutional anemia
- Peripartum cardiomyopathy, pulmonary edema, and pulmonary embolism
- Intrahepatic cholestasis
- Acute fatty liver
- Cesarean birth

Risks for the Fetus and Newborn

- Increase in fetal morbidity and mortality due to sharing uterine space and placental circulation
  - Increased perinatal mortality (threefold higher than in singleton pregnancy)
  - Intrauterine fetal death of one fetus after 20 weeks' gestation increases the risks to the surviving fetus(es).
- Delivery before term is the major reason for increased morbidity and mortality in twins. Rate of preterm delivery is 50% higher in twins and at least 90% higher in triplets and higher order multiples. As the number of fetuses increases, the duration of gestation decreases.
- Increase of low birth weight neonates (20% higher than singleton)
- Monochorionic twins have a shared fetoplacental circulation, which puts them at risk for specific serious pregnancy complications, such as twin-twin transfusion syndrome and twin anemia-polycythemia sequence. These complications increase the risk for neurologic morbidity and perinatal mortality in monochorionic twins compared with dichorionic twins. In addition to the complications associated with monochorionic twinning, monoamniotic twins also are at risk for cord entanglement and conjoined twins.
- Increase of intrauterine growth restriction (IUGR) and discordant growth (weight of one fetus differs significantly from the others, usually ≥25%) related to placental insufficiency.
  - Discordant growth and twin-to-twin transfusions from sharing a placenta occurs.
  - Vascular anastomosis between twins can occur with monochorionic twin placentas. Most of these vascular communications are hemodynamically balanced and do not impact fetal development and perfusion.

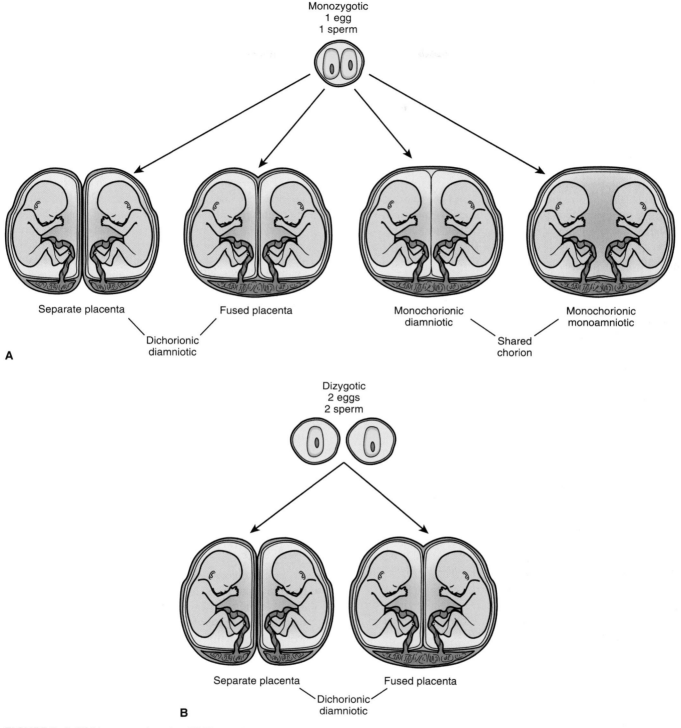

FIGURE 7–5 (**A**) Monozygotic twins. (**B**) Dizygotic twins.

- In twin-to-twin transfusion syndrome, blood is transfused from donor twin to recipient twin. Twin-to-twin transfusion is due to an imbalance in blood flow through the vasculature of the placenta because of arteriovenous anastomosis in the placenta. This results in overperfusion of one twin and can result in circulatory overload and heart failure and underperfusion and anemia of the co-twin.

- Increase of congenital, chromosomal, and genetic defects, in particular structural defects, with monozygotic twins.

Assessment Findings

Ultrasound examination is the only safe and reliable method for definitive diagnosis of twin gestation. Early ultrasound assessment also provides accurate estimation of gestational age, which is important in all pregnancies, but particularly important in management of twin pregnancies because of the higher risks for preterm delivery and growth restriction. In addition, chronionicity and amnionicity can be determined by ultrasound examination.

Nearly every maternal system is affected by the physiological changes that occur in multiple gestations. These changes are greater in multiple pregnancies than in singleton pregnancies (Bowers, 2014).

- Elevation of human chorionic gonadotropin (hCG) may contribute to increased nausea and vomiting gonadotropin (hCG) and alpha-fetoprotein.
- Fundal height and size greater than dates and palpation of excessive number of fetal parts during Leopold's maneuver
- Maternal blood volume expansion is greater than 50% to 60%, an additional 500 cc rather than 40% to 50% with singleton gestation.
- Increased cardiac output by 20% and increased stroke volume.
- Uterine growth is substantially greater, and uterine content may be up to 10 L and weigh in excess of 20 pounds. This can cause increased lower back and ligament pains and increase susceptibility to supine hypotension. Increased uterine size displaces lungs and can result in increased dyspnea and shortness of breath. Increased uterine distension increases risk of PTL and PPROM.
- Increased plasma volume 50% to 100% (results in dilutional anemia)
- Increased iron-deficiency anemia
- Increased dermatosis

Antepartal Medical Management

A woman pregnant with multiple fetuses needs ongoing, frequent surveillance of the pregnancy because of the increased rates of complications, including:

- Ultrasound for discordant fetal growth and IUGR, as well as placental sites, dividing membranes, congenital anomalies, and gender(s)
- Genetic testing for anomalies
- Monitor for preterm labor and prevent preterm birth
  - Corticosteroids for fetal lung maturity are effective in reducing respiratory distress syndrome (RDS) and other complications of prematurity.
- Monitor for maternal anemia.
- Fetal surveillance including NST, BPP
- Monitor for hypertension and preeclampsia.
- Monitor for hydramnios.
- Monitor for antepartal hemorrhage.
- Monitor for intrauterine fetal demise.
- Nutritional consult
- Consultation with perinatologist if complications occur

Interventions, such as prophylactic cerclage, prophylactic tocolytics, prophylactic pessary, routine hospitalization, and bed rest have not been proved to decrease neonatal morbidity or mortality and therefore should not be used in women with multifetal gestations (ACOG, 2014c; da Silva Lopes, 2017).

Intrapartum Medical Management

Many complications of labor and birth are encountered more often in multiple gestation deliveries, including preterm labor, uterine contractile dysfunction, abnormal presentation, umbilical cord prolapse, abruption, and postpartum hemorrhage. The best method by which to deliver pregnancies in which only the presenting twin is cephalic remains controversial. Evidence supports a vaginal trial of labor in late preterm and term twins. Routes of delivery for preterm twins lighter than 1500 g remains unclear, with compelling data for both planned cesarean and planned vaginal delivery. No data support planned cesarean for birthweight discordance alone. Risks of trial of labor after cesarean (TOLAC) for women with twins appear similar to risks for women with singletons, particularly for those who successfully undergo vaginal birth after cesarean (VBAC). For each of the clinical scenarios above, however, two major factors remain constant: (1) obstetricians need to be prepared for and skilled in breech extraction of the second twin; and (2) individualized patient counseling regarding mode of delivery is important when offering a vaginal trial of labor to women with a twin gestation (ACOG, 2014c; Christopher, Robinson, & Peaceman, 2011). Further discussion of multiple birth is in Chapter 10.

Preparation for birth of multiples includes:

- Type and crossmatch blood immediately available
- Ultrasound to confirm placental location and fetal positions
- Continuous electronic fetal monitoring (EFM) of all fetuses
- Cesarean birth access should be immediately available, including anesthesia, obstetricians, circulating nurse, and scrub personnel.
- Agents for hemorrhagic management available, including medications and blood products
- The neonatal team available should be sufficient for all infants.
- Triplets and higher multiples are delivered by cesarean birth.

Nursing Actions

- Assess for the following possible complications:
  - Uterine contractions as preterm labor can be more difficult to identify in women pregnant with multiple gestations because of more discomfort, stretching, and pressure with multiple fetuses, and overdistention of the uterus results in more uterine irritability (Gilbert, 2011).
  - Hypertension or preeclampsia
  - Antepartal hemorrhage
- Conduct antepartal surveillance including NST, amniotic fluid index (AFI), and BPP.
- Provide information to the woman and her family regarding signs and symptoms of preterm labor, preeclampsia, and other possible complications related to multiple gestations.
- Facilitate nutritional consult. The woman has an increased need for iron, calcium, and magnesium to support growth of multiple fetuses.
- Parents expecting multiples have unique educational needs due to the high-risk pregnancy and unknowns of parenting multiple infants (Bowers, 2014).

- Provide emotional support to the woman and family. The woman and her family often experience an increase of stress related to fear of pregnancy loss, high-risk pregnancy, and potential complications during pregnancy and delivery, and anxiety related to caring for more than one infant.
- Explain plan for PNC and antenatal testing and follow-up related to multiple gestation.
- Assess woman's and her partner's response to twin diagnosis and adaptation to multiple gestation
  - Acknowledge feeling of distress and fear toward pregnancy.
  - Provide family with information on multiple and support groups.
- Provide psychological support appropriate to family's response.
- Discuss the plan of care for delivery. Cesarean birth is often recommended for multiples.
- Facilitate referrals such as perinatologist, neonatologist, and social worker.

Hyperemesis Gravidarum

Hyperemesis gravidarum is vomiting during pregnancy that is so severe it leads to dehydration, electrolyte and acid-base imbalance, starvation ketosis, and weight loss. The condition is defined as uncontrolled vomiting requiring hospitalization, severe dehydration, muscle wasting, electrolyte imbalance, ketonuria, and weight loss of more than 5% of body weight. Most of these patients also have hyponatremia, hypokalemia, and a low serum urea level (Wegrzyniak, Repke, & Ural, 2012). Ptyalism is also a typical symptom of hyperemesis. The symptoms of this disorder usually peak at 9 weeks of gestation and subside by approximately 20 weeks of gestation. Approximately 1% to 5% of patients with hyperemesis must be hospitalized. Women who experienced hyperemesis in their first pregnancy have a high risk for recurrence. Hyperemesis appears to be related to rapidly rising serum levels of pregnancy related hormones such as chorionic gonadotropin (hCG), progesterone, and estrogen levels. An association has been noted with *H. pylori,* but evidence is inconclusive (ACOG, 2004b). Other factors may include a psychological component related to ambivalence about the pregnancy, but this is controversial. Regardless of the cause, a woman experiencing hyperemesis presents in the clinical situation severely dehydrated and physically and emotionally debilitated, sometimes in need of hospitalization to manage profound and prolonged nausea and vomiting (ACOG, 2015a; Gilbert, 2011; Queenan, Hobbins, & Spong, 2005). Hospital admission is appropriate for those with persistent vomiting after rehydration and intravenous antiemetic therapy, as well as women who present with abnormal electrolyte levels and acid-base balance (ACOG, 2015c).

Assessment Findings

- Vomiting that may be prolonged, frequent, and severe
- Weight loss, acetonuria, and ketosis
- Signs and symptoms of dehydration including:
  - Lightheadedness, dizziness, faintness, tachycardia, or inability to keep food/fluids down for more than 12 hours

- Dry mucous membranes
- Poor skin turgor
- Malaise
- Low blood pressure

Medical Management

Most patients respond to intravenous hydration and a short period of gut rest, followed by reintroduction of oral intake and pharmacologic therapy (ACOG, 2015c).

- Treatment of nausea and vomiting of pregnancy with vitamin B_6 or vitamin B_6 plus doxylamine is safe and effective and should be considered first-line pharmacotherapy (ACOG, 2015c; Matthews, Dowswell, Haas, Doyle, & O'Mathúna, 2010).
- Intravenous hydration should be used for the patient who cannot tolerate oral liquids for a prolonged period or if clinical signs of dehydration are present. Correction of ketosis and vitamin deficiency should be strongly considered. Dextrose and vitamins, especially thiamine, should be included in the therapy when prolonged vomiting is present.
- In refractory cases of nausea and vomiting of pregnancy, the following medications have been shown to be safe and efficacious in pregnancy: antihistamine H_1 receptor blockers, phenothiazines, and benzamides (ACOG, 2015c).
- Laboratory studies to monitor kidney and liver function
- Correction of ketosis and vitamin deficiency should be strongly considered. Dextrose and vitamins, especially thiamine, should be included in the therapy when prolonged vomiting is present.

Nursing Actions

- Assess factors that contribute to nausea and vomiting.
- Reduce or eliminate factors that contribute to nausea and vomiting, such as triggers including stuffy rooms and odors.
- Treatment of nausea and vomiting of pregnancy with ginger has shown beneficial effects and can be considered as a nonpharmacological option.
- In refractory cases of nausea and vomiting of pregnancy, use antiemetics as ordered.
- Early treatment of nausea and vomiting of pregnancy is recommended to prevent progression to hyperemesis gravidarum.
- Provide emotional support. These patients and their families often need emotional support to help deal with stress and anxiety about the maternal illness and its effect on the fetus, and the disruption to their home- and work-related activities
- Provide comfort measures such as good oral hygiene.
- Administer IV hydration with vitamins and electrolytes as per orders.
- Check weight daily.
- Monitor I&O and specific gravity of urine to monitor hydration. Fluids should be consumed at least 30 minutes before or after solid food to minimize the effect of a full stomach.
- Assess nausea and vomiting.
- Monitor laboratory values for fluid and electrolyte imbalances.

- Ensure that the woman remains NPO until vomiting is controlled, then slowly advance the diet as tolerated.
- Facilitate nutritional and dietary consult.
- Taking prenatal vitamins before bed with a snack, instead of in the morning or on an empty stomach, may also be helpful. Pyridoxine Vitamin B6 can improve nausea.
- Determine the woman's food preferences and provide them.
- Minimizing fluid intake with meals can decrease nausea and vomiting.
- Explore complementary therapies to manage hyperemesis, such as traditional Chinese medicine, hypnotherapy, and acupuncture (see Chapter 4). In a recent Cochrane Review on nausea and vomiting in pregnancy, 27 trials, with 4041 women, were reviewed covering many interventions, including acupressure, acustimulation, acupuncture, ginger, vitamin B6, and several antiemetic drugs (Matthews et al., 2010). Evidence regarding the effectiveness of P6 acupressure, auricular (ear) acupressure, and acustimulation of the P6 point was limited. Acupuncture (P6 or traditional) showed no significant benefit to women in pregnancy. The use of ginger products may be helpful to women, but the evidence of effectiveness was limited and not consistent. There was only limited evidence from trials to support the use of pharmacological agents including vitamin B6, and anti-emetic drugs to relieve mild or moderate nausea and vomiting.

Intrahepatic Cholestasis of Pregnancy

Intrahepatic cholestasis of pregnancy (ICP), also known as obstetric cholestasis, is the most common pregnancy-specific liver disease. It is a reversible type of hormonally influenced cholestasis and frequently develops in late pregnancy in individuals who are genetically predisposed. ICP is characterized by generalized itching, often commencing with pruritus of the palms of the hands and soles of the feet, with no other skin manifestations. It most often presents in the late second or early third trimester of pregnancy and approximately 1% of pregnancies in the United States are affected by this condition.

ICP has no clear etiology and is believed to be a multifactorial disorder with environmental, hormonal, and genetic contributions. The diagnosis is based on physical examination and laboratory findings, but, in general, ICP is a diagnosis of exclusion. The incidence is 0.3-0.5% among the general population with up to 15% incidence in Latin American countries. Incidence also increased among those with hepatitis C infection (6-16%). Risk factors and associations include multiple gestation, chronic hepatitis C, and prior history or family history of intrahepatic cholestasis. Affected individuals have a defect involving the excretion of bile salts, which leads to increased serum bile acids. These are deposited within the skin, causing intense pruritus.

ICP is associated with an increased risk of preterm delivery, meconium passage, intrapartum fetal heart rate abnormalities, and fetal death as intrauterine fetal death (IUFD) incidence is most often less than 5% in reports (Society for Maternal Fetal Medicine, 2017). The risk of complications for the fetus is associated with the serum level of maternal serum bile acids, and women

with more severe cholestasis are at greater risk (Williamson & Geenes, 2014). The etiology of intrahepatic cholestasis of pregnancy is complex and appears to relate to the cholestatic effect of reproductive hormones in genetically susceptible women.

Assessment Findings

- The presenting feature of intrahepatic cholestasis of pregnancy is pruritus in most cases. This typically occurs in the third trimester, with up to 80% of women presenting after 30 weeks of gestation. Pruritus is defined as an unpleasant sensation of the skin that provokes the desire to scratch. It is often the only symptom associated with ICP and may be so severe that it disturbs sleep. The pruritus typically affects the palms of the hands and the soles of the feet but may occur anywhere. It is often worse at night and gradually worsens as the pregnancy advances.
- Lab evidence of cholestasis includes elevated bile acids (>10 umol/L). Up to 60% of patients will have elevated transaminases and 20% of patients will have increased direct bilirubin levels (Society for Maternal Fetal Medicine, 2017).
- Signs and symptoms of ICP may include systemic symptoms of cholestasis, such as dark urine and pale stools. Some women also may become clinically jaundiced, but this is rare.
- Lab evidence of cholestasis includes elevated bile acids (>10 umol/L). Up to 60% of patients will have elevated transaminases and 20% of patients will have increased direct bilirubin levels (Society for Maternal Fetal Medicine, 2017).

Medical Management

- There are no preventative therapies or interventions available.
- Upon diagnosis of intrahepatic cholestasis, prenatal intervention for treatment of symptoms of cholestasis is indicated. Ursodeoxycholic acid (UDCA) has been most effective for treatment of pruritis. The starting dose of UDCA is 300 mg twice daily and can be increased to 600 mg twice daily when pruritis persists after a week of therapy. UDCA also decreases bile acids and transaminase levels though this has not been demonstrated to improve fetal outcomes. S-Adenosylmethionine can be used with UDCA for a synergistic reduction in bile acid and transaminase levels. Antihistamines, corticosteroids, or cholestyramine can be used for pruritis but are not superior to UDCA (Society for Maternal Fetal Medicine, 2017).
- Antihistamines are usually ineffective at relieving severe pruritus in women with ICP.
- Risk of fetal complications is increased in women whose serum bile acid level exceeds 40 micromoles/L and may be further increased if the woman has other coexistent pregnancy complications such as gestational diabetes or preeclampsia.
- Antepartum fetal monitoring is recommended in the antenatal management of intrahepatic cholestasis. However, the type, duration, or frequency of testing has not been identified. The mechanisms of fetal death are not understood. Most fetal demises occur late in gestation and may occur in the presence of previously reassuring fetal testing (Society for Maternal Fetal Medicine, 2017).

- While an evidence-based recommendation is not available for the timing of delivery when cholestasis of pregnancy is encountered, most management strategies would advocate delivery between 37–38 weeks.
- ICP is associated with an increased risk of intrapartum and postpartum hemorrhage (Phillips & Boyd, 2015)
- Current consensus favors twice-weekly nonstress testing with or without Doppler testing and induction at 37 weeks.

Nursing Actions

- Monitor laboratory values and liver function.
- Some women may find that aqueous cream with 2% menthol relieves their pruritus, but it has no effect on the biochemical abnormalities associated with intrahepatic cholestasis of pregnancy.
- Mild itching can often be relieved with topical antipruritics and by keeping the skin well-moisturized. Emollient lotions and primrose oil may provide some relief. Increasing water intake may help keep skin hydrated and aid in excretion of toxic wastes from the body. Evaluate excoriated skin areas for possible skin infections (Phillips & Boyd, 2015).
- Resolution of pruritis usually occurs within days of delivery.
- All women with ICP should have their liver function and serum bile acids checked 6 to 8 weeks postnatally to ensure resolution.
- Explore complementary therapies to manage pruritis such as herbal remedies like milk thistle, guar gum, dandelion root, and activated charcoal; however, there is no evidence to support the use of herbal medicines or dietary supplements in the treatment of ICP.

DIABETES MELLITUS

Diabetes mellitus is an epidemic in the United States that affects 29.1 million people (CDC, 2014) and complicates more than 200,000 pregnancies each year (American Diabetes Association [ADA], 2014). There is a direct correlation between the obesity epidemic and the increased rate of diabetes and associated health risks. About 47% of gestational diabetes cases were attributed to being overweight, obese, and/or extremely obese (AWHONN, 2016). Though obesity predisposes women to developing diabetes, especially in pregnancy, not all women who are overweight or obese will become diabetic.

Diabetes is a complex disorder with various pathological mechanisms involved in the secretion and absorption of insulin, which results in hyperglycemia and end organ damage. It is associated with long-term harm and resulting dysfunction of the eyes, kidneys, heart, and blood vessels. Diabetes in all forms is the most common metabolic disease of pregnancy (ACOG, 2013b).

- Type 1 diabetes is a result of autoimmunity of beta cells of the pancreas resulting in absolute insulin deficiency and is managed with insulin. About 5%-10% of patients diagnosed with diabetes are type I (ADA, 2014).
- Type 2 diabetes is characterized by insulin resistance and inadequate insulin production. This is the most prevalent

form of diabetes and is linked to increased rates of obesity and sedentary lifestyle. It is managed primarily with diet and exercise; the addition of oral antihyperglycemic or insulin may be indicated if hyperglycemia continues. For optimum control, many women who have type 2 diabetes require insulin during pregnancy (AWHONN, 2016).

Diabetes in Pregnancy

Women with diabetes in pregnancy can be divided into two groups: pregestational diabetes and gestational diabetics (GDM). For many of pregnancy complications, particularly diabetes, medical management is continually under investigation and recommendations for treatment are changing. This chapter provides a general discussion of diabetes in pregnancy and then considers pregestational diabetes, followed by a discussion of gestational diabetes. Many of the same principles apply in the approach to both conditions.

- Pregestational diabetes is categorized as either type 1 or type 2 diabetes.
- Gestational diabetes mellitus (GDM) is glucose intolerance that does not present prior to pregnancy.

Some of the normal physiological changes in pregnancy present challenges for managing diabetes in pregnancy. The physiological changes that accompany pregnancy produce a state of insulin resistance. To spare glucose for the developing fetus, the placenta produces several hormones that antagonize insulin:

- Human placental lactogen
- Progesterone
- Growth hormone
- Corticotropin-releasing hormone

These hormones shift the primary energy sources to ketones and free fatty acids.

Most pregnant women maintain a normal glucose level in pregnancy despite increasing insulin resistance by producing increased insulin. Whether preexisting or gestational diabetes, the risk of the perinatal morbidity and mortality for the woman and neonate are significant.

For pregestational or gestational diabetes, the treatment goals are the same and management strategies are similar:

- Maintain euglycemia control.
- Minimize complications.
- Prevent prematurity.

Overall, diabetes in pregnancy is a complex health problem that requires a multidisciplinary approach to facilitate a healthy outcome for both the woman and her baby. Care for women with diabetes should begin before conception and for GDM at the time of diagnosis. The goal of preconception care is to maintain the lowest possible glycosylated hemoglobin (HbA$_1$C) without episodes of hypoglycemia (AWHONN, 2016).

- Assessment and education regarding current diabetes self-management skills
- Exploration of strategies to improve adherence to treatment regimen

- Involvement of the woman and her family in the treatment regimen (essential in improving adherence to treatment regimen)
- Establishment of mutual goals for glycemic controls and self-monitoring

Pregestational Diabetes

Pregestational diabetes is used to describe the blood glucose (BG) levels that are found to be above the normal range but below the cutoff for diagnosing overt or clinical diabetes in the nonpregnant woman (AWHONN, 2016) Though woman may not meet the criteria for clinical diabetes, many have the components of metabolic syndrome which include central adiposity (waste circumference >35 in women), dyslipidemia, hyperglycemia, and hypertension. It is also common to see women with polycystic ovarian syndrome. It is unlikely that women diagnosed with pregestational diabetes will have improvement of their hyperglycemia once pregnant. Due to the increase of insulin resistance, women would benefit from early diagnosis and management of glucose levels (AWHONN, 2016)

Pregestational diabetics have a fivefold increase in the incidence of major fetal anomalies of the heart and central nervous system (CNS). The precise mechanism for teratogenesis in diabetic women is not well-understood but is believed to be related to hyperglycemia and deficiencies in membrane lipids and prostaglandin pathways. The quality of diabetic control throughout pregnancy is key in the prevention of major complications of diabetes and the associated risks for diabetes during pregnancy (AWHONN, 2016).

Risks for the Woman

- Diabetic ketoacidosis (DKA, 1%), especially in second trimester
- Hypertensive disorders and preeclampsia
- Metabolic disturbances related to hyperemesis, nausea, and vomiting of pregnancy
- Preterm labor (25% risk)
- Spontaneous abortion (≥30% risk)
- Polyhydramnios/oligohydramnios: Polyhydramnios related to fetal anomalies and fetal hyperglycemia (20% risk). Oligohydramnios related to decreased placental perfusion.
- Cesarean delivery
- Labor disturbances related to increased fetal size and shoulder dystocia (AWHONN, 2016)
- Exacerbation of chronic diabetes-related conditions such as heart disease, retinopathy, nephropathy, and neuropathy
- Infection related to hyperglycemia (80% risk): urinary tract infection, chorioamnionitis, and postpartum endometritis
- Induction of labor
- Postpartum hemorrhage and subsequent anemia (AWHONN, 2016)

Risks for the Fetus and Newborn

- Congenital defects including cardiac, skeletal, neurological, genitourinary, and gastrointestinal related to maternal hyperglycemia during organogenesis (first 6 to 8 weeks of pregnancy)
- Growth disturbances, macrosomia related to fetal hyperinsulinemia
- Hypoglycemia related to fetal hyperinsulinemia
- Hypocalcemia and hypomagnesemia
- Intrauterine growth restriction related to maternal vasculopathy and decreased maternal perfusion
- Asphyxia related to fetal hyperglycemia and hyperinsulinemia
- Respiratory distress syndrome related to delayed fetal lung maturity
- Polycythemia (hematocrit <65%) related to increased fetal erythropoietin
- Hyperbilirubinemia related to polycythemia and red blood cell breakdown
- Prematurity because of maternal complications
- Cardiomyopathy related to maternal hyperglycemia
- Birth injury related to macrosomia
- Stillbirth in poorly controlled maternal diabetes, especially after 36 weeks' gestation

Long-Term Risks to the Neonate

- Development of metabolic syndrome, prediabetes, and type II diabetes
- Impaired intellectual and psychomotor development
- Exposure to hyperglycemia in utero has been shown to affect epigenesist and is thought to change the expression of genes. As a result, it can contribute to increased risk for chronic illness later in life.

Preconception Assessment and Findings

- Classification of hyperglycemia based on abnormal blood glucose levels (HbA1c) and frequency in self-testing
- Presence of vascular and/or nerve dysfunction or involvement and treatment
- Evaluation of diet and proper calorie intake based on BMI
- Medication regimen evaluation and adjustment as necessary
- Evaluation of signs of metabolic syndrome and/or polycystic ovarian syndrome
- Evaluation of BMI

Self-Management

Comprehensive self-management of diabetes is complex yet essential for successful pregnancy outcomes. Measures include:

- Self-monitoring of blood glucose (SMBG) by checking blood glucose levels 4 to 8 times per day (before and after meals and at bedtime) in pregnancy. This is the most important parameter for determining metabolic control. Table 7–2 indicates glycemic goals for pregnancy.
- Self-monitoring of urine ketone. Women should test the first void specimen for ketones when blood glucose level is greater than 200 mg/dL, during maternal illness, and/or when glucose control is altered. Moderate to large amounts of ketones are an indication of inadequate food intake and should be reported to care provider.

TABLE 7–2 Normal Pregnancy Blood Glucose Values and Targeted Blood Glucose Values for Pregnant Women With Diabetes

NORMAL PREGNANCY BG VALUES		TARGET BG FOR PREGNANT WOMEN WITH DIABETES
Fasting	70.9 ± 7.8 mg/dl	≤ 95 mg/dl
Premeal		≤ 100 mg/dl
1 hour after meals	108.9 ± 12.9 mg/dl	≤ 140 mg/dl
2 hours after meals	99.3 ± 10 mg/dl	≤ 120 mg/dl
Mean	88 ± 10 mg/dl	100 mg/dl
A1C	4.5%–5.2%	< 6%

AWHONN, 2016.

- Record keeping of blood glucose levels, food intake, insulin, and activity needs to be maintained for appropriate management of treatment regimen.
- Exercise is beneficial for glycemic control and overall well-being. Generally, exercise three times a week for at least 20 minutes is recommended, but some contraindications such as hypertension and preeclampsia do exist.
- Review signs and symptoms of maternal hypoglycemia for the prevention and management of hypoglycemic episodes. Patients should always carry a source of fast-acting carbohydrate with them, such as hard candy or fruit juice.

Medical Management

Preconception care for women with pregestational diabetes is key to decrease risks to the woman and her fetus for a successful pregnancy. Achieving euglycemic control for 1 to 2 months is recommended, with recommended HbA$_1$C less than 7%. Pregnancies complicated by preexisting diabetes are managed by a multidisciplinary team including a perinatologist, diabetes nurse educator, and dietitian. Screening at diagnosis of pregnancy may include kidney, heart, thyroid function, and ophthalmic exams. Additional fetal diagnostic testing typically includes regular ultrasound examinations, intensive prenatal care schedule, and antenatal testing. The insulin needs of type 1 diabetic women increase such that by the end of pregnancy, insulin needs may be two to three times that of pre-pregnancy levels and may require three or four injections per day of Humulin insulin.

Medical Nutritional Therapy

Medical nutritional therapy (MNT) is a cornerstone of diabetes management for all pregnant women and the goal is to provide adequate nutrition, prevent diabetic ketoacidosis, and promote euglycemia. MNT needs to be individualized and continually adjusted based on blood glucose values and insulin regimen and the woman's lifestyle. A registered dietitian should meet with the woman regularly to assess and reevaluate her nutritional needs. The Institute of Medicine recommends a calorie intake

minimum of 1800 kcals/day for all pregnant women, including those who are overweight and obese. The nutritional calorie value should be broken down to an intake of 40% carbohydrates, 20% protein, and 30% to 40% fat. However, all diet plans should be individualized and set by a registered dietitian and certified diabetes educator (AWHONN, 2016).

Risks of Complications During Delivery

Timing of delivery is a tremendous challenge in pregnancies complicated by diabetes. At term, the risk of stillbirth increases, as does the risk of macrosomia. However, intervention may place the woman at risk for prolonged labor and operative delivery. Thus, care providers must determine which pregnancies should be allowed to go into spontaneous labor and which are in need of labor induction. Most guidelines state that diabetes in pregnancy is not an automatic indication for scheduled cesarean delivery (Cunningham et al., 2014).

Complicating the issue of when and how to deliver is the fact that infants of diabetic women (IDM) have delayed pulmonary lung maturity and are at risk for respiratory distress syndrome (RDS) and transient tachypnea of the newborn (TTN). Excess maternal glucose levels result in excess insulin production by the fetus in utero, which is known to result in delayed surfactant production, interfering with fetal lung maturity (AWHONN, 2016).

The following are general recommendations for intrapartal care:

- Evaluate fetal lung maturity by checking if amniotic fluid is positive for phosphatidylglycerol, to try to avert RDS in the newborn who is less than 38 weeks' gestation. The lecithin/sphingomyelin (L/S) ratio is not a specific indicator for fetal lung maturity in diabetic women.
- Maintain maternal plasma glucose levels at 70 to 110 mg/dL during labor.
- Administer intravenous insulin when necessary to achieve desired glucose levels.

Nursing Actions

Nurses play a key role in educating women on the importance of strict glycemic control and adopting a healthy lifestyle (AWHONN, 2016). For pregnant women with type 1 diabetes, this means learning about the effects pregnancy has on the management of diabetes and the adjustments required to the prior diabetic management regimen. The pregnancy represents new stressors and challenges for diabetic women and their families. Women may feel vulnerable and anxious about their health and that of their fetus.

● Provide information on:
    ● Physiological changes in pregnancy and the impact on diabetes
    ● Changes in insulin requirements during pregnancy with advancing gestation
● Assist the woman in arranging for dietary counseling with a dietitian.
● Dietary counseling should include the woman's preferences and pregnancy requirements along with assessment of calorie intake and dietary pattern through 24-hour dietary recall and importance of timing of medication if necessary.
● Review self-monitoring of blood glucose, urine ketones, signs and symptoms of hyper- and hypoglycemic episode, dietary intake, and activity.
● Emphasize the importance of record keeping of dietary intake, urine ketones, glucose levels, and activity.
● Instruct the woman to bring records to prenatal appointments to be reviewed by the primary health care provider.
● Review signs, symptoms, and treatment of hyperglycemia based on the individualized treatment plan.
● Review signs, symptoms, and treatment of hypoglycemia (blood glucose <70 mg/dL) including:
    ● Diaphoresis; tachycardia; shakiness; cold, clammy skin; blurred vision; extreme fatigue; mental confusion and irritability; somnolence; and pallor (Daley, 2014)
    ● Ingest 10 to 15 g of carbohydrate for blood glucose of 60 mg/dL to raise blood glucose by 30 to 40 mg/dL in 30 minutes
● Review signs and symptoms of diabetic ketoacidosis, including:
    ● Abdominal pain, nausea and vomiting, polyuria, polydipsia, fruity breath, leg cramps, altered mental status, and rapid respirations (Daley, 2014)
● Care for women admitted to the hospital in diabetic ketoacidosis during pregnancy should be provided by nurses with experience in intensive care and obstetrics. The goals of care include fluid resuscitation, restoration of electrolyte balance, reduction of hyperglycemia, and treatment of underlying cause such as infection (AWHONN, 2016)
● Provide information on when and how to call the care provider:
    ● Glucose levels greater than 200 mg/dL, moderate ketones in urine, persistent nausea and vomiting, decreased fetal movement, and other indicators based on individualized plan of care (Daley, 2014)

● Provide information on management of nausea, vomiting, and illness:
    ● The glucose level should be checked every 1 to 2 hours, urine ketones checked every 4 hours; insulin should still be given with vomiting (Daley, 2014)
● Provide an expected plan of prenatal care, antenatal tests, and fetal surveillance.
● Provide an expected plan for labor and delivery.
● Assist the woman in arranging to meet with a diabetic nurse educator:
    ● Ideally, women are referred to a diabetic nurse educator to help them to learn self-care management of diabetes and to facilitate regulation of diabetes in pregnancy.
● Emphasize that changes in the management plan may be necessary every few weeks due to the physiological changes of pregnancy.
● Arrange for antenatal testing:
● Antenatal testing generally starts at 28 weeks' gestation and includes NST and BPP.

Gestational Diabetes Mellitus

Gestational diabetes mellitus (GDM) and pregestational diabetes have very similar predisposing factors; both are characterized by elevated blood sugar levels that do not meet criteria for clinical diabetes diagnosis. GDM is defined by ACOG as a carbohydrate intolerance leading to hyperglycemia that is first discovered in pregnancy. It accounts for about 90% of diabetic pregnancies (ACOG, 2013b). This definition applies whether the GDM is controlled only with diet and exercise or with insulin as well. When medical nutrition therapy is inadequate to control glucose in GDM, insulin is required. Approximately 7% of pregnancies are complicated by GDM; however, the prevalence may range from 1% to 14% depending on the population and diagnostic tests performed. Increased prevalence is found in Hispanic, African American, Native American, and Asian and Pacific Islander populations (ADA, 2014).

The metabolic changes that occur during pregnancy lower glucose tolerance and as a result, blood glucose levels rise and more insulin is produced. However, as the pregnancy develops, insulin demand increases. For most pregnant women, this is a normal physiological process. Pregnant women who have continued hyperglycemia are diagnosed with gestational diabetes. Insulin resistance during pregnancy stems from a variety of factors, including alterations in growth hormone and cortisol secretion (insulin antagonists), human placental lactogen secretion (which is produced by the placenta and affects fatty acids and glucose metabolism, promotes lipolysis, and decreases glucose uptake), and insulinase secretion (which is produced by the placenta and facilitates metabolism of insulin). In addition, estrogen and progesterone contribute to a disruption of the glucose insulin balance. Increased maternal adipose deposition, decreased exercise, and increased caloric intake also contribute to this state of relative glucose intolerance (AWHONN, 2016)

Two main contributors to insulin resistance are:

● Increased maternal adiposity
● Insulin desensitizing hormones produced by the placenta

The placenta produces human chorionic somatomammotropin (HCS), cortisol, estrogen, and progesterone. HCS stimulates pancreatic secretion of insulin in the fetus and reduces peripheral uptake of glucose. It has been proposed that as the placenta increases in size with increasing gestation, so does the production of these hormones, leading to a progressive insulin-resistant state. Women with deficient insulin secretory capacity develop GDM. Because maternal insulin does not cross the placenta, the fetus is exposed to maternal hyperglycemia and in response produces more insulin, which promotes growth and subsequent macrosomia.

The American Association of Obstetricians and Gynecologists recommends routine screening for all pregnant women at 24 to 28 weeks of gestation, with a two-step screening method for diagnosis. This two-step method was developed based on studies that showed that women with GDM have a 30% to 50% chance of developing type II diabetes within 20 years after pregnancy. The first step in the two-step process is a non-fasting 1-hour 50-g oral glucose tolerance test (a positive test is a result of 135 mg/dL to140 mg/dL). Women who test positive move on to the second step, a 3-hour glucose tolerance test performed on a separate day after 8 to 12 hours of fasting. The 3-hour test is done after the woman ingests a 100-g glucose load; plasma glucose levels are drawn at 1, 2, and 3 hours post glucose load. If two or more glucose levels are above these thresholds, a diagnosis of GDM is made: fasting ≥95 mg/dL, 1-hour ≥180 mg/dL, 2-hour ≥155 mg/dL, and 3-hour ≥140 mg/dL (ACOG, 2013b). Less stringent criteria have been proposed and may be used by some institutions or providers.

Risk Factors for GDM

- No known risk factors are identified in 50% of patients with GDM.
- History of fetal macrosomia
- Strong family history of diabetes
- Obesity

Risks for the Woman

- Hypoglycemia and DKA
- Preeclampsia
- Cesarean birth
- Development of non-gestational diabetes

Risks for the Fetus and Newborn

Risks for newborns born to GDM are similar to the risks for newborns born to pregestational diabetic women, except GDM newborns are not at risk for congenital anomalies.

- Macrosomia
  - Macrosomia places the fetus at risk for birth injuries such as brachial plexus injury.
- Intrauterine growth restriction
- Hypoglycemia during the first few hours post-birth
- Hyperbilirubinemia
- Shoulder dystocia
- Respiratory distress syndrome
- Birth trauma
- The magnitude of fetal–neonatal complications is proportional to the severity of maternal hyperglycemia.

Assessment Findings

- Abnormal glucose screening results between 24 to 28 weeks of gestation

Medical Management

- GDM may be managed by care providers with consultation and referral as appropriate.
- For most women with GDM, the condition is controlled with a well-balanced diet and exercise.
- Up to 40% of women with GDM may need to be managed with insulin.
- Oral hypoglycemic agents may be used, but there is not agreement on their recommended use during pregnancy.
- Cesarean birth is recommended for estimated fetal weight >4,500 g.
- Women with GDM need to be monitored for type 2 diabetes after the birth.

Nursing Actions

- The cornerstone of management of GDM is glycemic control. For women diagnosed during pregnancy with GDM, this means learning many complex skills and management strategies to maintain a healthy pregnancy.
- The goal of therapy is to maintain euglycemia throughout pregnancy.
- Teach the woman to test glucose four times a day, one fasting and three postprandial checks/day (suggested glucose control is to maintain fasting glucose less than 95 mg/dL before meals, and between 120 to 135 mg/dL after meals) (Hoffert Gilmartin, Ural, & Repke, 2008) (Fig. 7–6 and Table 7–2).

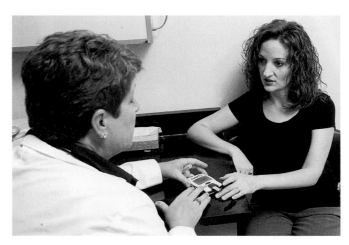

FIGURE 7–6 Blood glucose levels need to be checked regularly for any woman who has diabetes at any time during pregnancy.

- Provide information on effects of elevated glucose on developing fetus and rationale for managing euglycemic glucose levels.
- Encourage active participation in management and decision making.
- Teach the woman to monitor fasting ketonuria levels in the morning.
- Teach proper self-administration of insulin (site selection, insulin onset, peak, duration, administration). For the gestational diabetic, consider that it may be the first insulin administration time related to the pregnancy. Unlike for women with preexisting diabetes, this can create a tremendous change in lifestyle. Successful self-administration of insulin requires patience, support and encouragement, and reassurance by the nurse educator (AWHONN, 2016).
- Teach the woman signs and symptoms and treatment for hypoglycemia, hyperglycemia, and diabetic ketoacidosis outlined above.
- Reinforce diet management. This calorie distribution will help 75% to 80% of GDM women become normoglycemic.
- Reinforce plan of care related to self-management and fetal surveillance.
- Exercise has been shown to improve glycemic control. The mechanism of this improvement is mostly secondary to increasing tissue sensitivity to insulin. Walking 10 to 15 minutes after a meal is beneficial and can be managed by most pregnant women. Exercising three or more times a week for at least 15 to 30 minutes duration is recommended.

CRITICAL COMPONENT

Key Concepts in Diabetes Management

- Pregnancy outcomes are greatly improved among women who have strict blood glucose control.
- Fetal risk and infant morbidity are relative to the level of glycemic control during pregnancy.
- Euglycemia during preconception period time reduces the risk that a woman with diabetes will spontaneously miscarry or have an infant with congenital defect.
- Risk for gestational diabetes should be performed early in pregnancy.
- A history of gestational diabetes mellitus increased the risk for development of overt type 2 diabetes in women (AWHONN, 2016).

HYPERTENSION IN PREGNANCY

Hypertension is identified as systolic pressure 140 mm Hg or greater or diastolic pressure 90 mm Hg or greater. Hypertensive disorders of pregnancy are the most common complication of pregnancy, affecting 10 percent of pregnant women, and are the second leading cause of maternal death and a significant contributor to neonatal morbidity and mortality. Hypertension is directly responsible for 17.6% of maternal deaths in the United States and has increased more than 50% since 1990 (Task Force on Hypertension in Pregnancy, 2013). Hypertensive disorders are classified into four categories:

- Preeclampsia is a multisystem hypertensive disease unique to pregnancy, with hypertension accompanied by proteinuria after the 20th week of gestation. Eclampsia is the onset of convulsions or seizures that cannot be attributed to other causes in a woman with preeclampsia.
- Chronic hypertension with superimposed preeclampsia includes the following scenarios:
  - Women with hypertension only in early gestation who develop proteinuria after 20 weeks of gestation.
  - Women with hypertension and proteinuria before 20 weeks who develop a sudden exacerbation of hypertension, suddenly manifest other signs and symptoms such as an increase in liver enzymes, present with thrombocytopenia, manifest with symptoms of right upper quadrant pain and severe headaches, develop pulmonary edema or congestion, develop renal insufficiency, or have sudden substantial sustained increases in protein excretion.
- Gestational hypertension: Systolic BP ≥140/90 for the first time after 20 weeks, without other signs and systemic finding of preeclampsia.
- Chronic hypertension: Hypertension (BP ≥140/90) before conception. High blood pressure known to predate conception or detected before 20 weeks of gestation (Task Force on Hypertension, 2013).

Preeclampsia/Eclampsia

Preeclampsia is a hypertensive, multisystem disorder of pregnancy whose etiology remains unknown. The rate of preeclampsia in the United States has increased 25% in the last two decades and is a leading cause of maternal and infant illness and death (ACOG, 2013c). Currently, ACOG defines preeclampsia as new-onset hypertension after 20 weeks' gestation with two blood pressure readings at least 140 mm Hg systolic and/or at least 90 mm Hg diastolic taken at least 4 hours apart. In addition, a woman will have proteinuria greater than 300 mg in 24 hours (protein/creatinine ratio ≥ 0.3 mg/dl) or new-onset systemic disease. Preeclampsia is best described as a pregnancy-specific syndrome of reduced organ perfusion secondary to vasospasm and endothelial activation (Cunningham et al., 2014). Three diagnostic considerations have emerged in recent literature. First, is that it is widely accepted that there are different presentations of the disease depending on the timing of symptom onset. Second, proteinuria is no longer an inclusion criterion for diagnosis of preeclampsia (ACOG, 2013c; Task Force on Hypertension in Pregnancy, 2013). Third, a diagnosis of mild preeclampsia is no longer appropriate based on clinical presentation, because this designation undermines the potential for disease progression. Early-onset preeclampsia is defined as onset of symptoms before 34 weeks' gestation and is associated with more severe disease. Women with early-onset preeclampsia often have abnormal uterine artery Doppler waveforms and IUGR and are more likely to experience adverse perinatal outcomes, including preterm birth. It is proposed that poor placentation is a key factor in early-onset

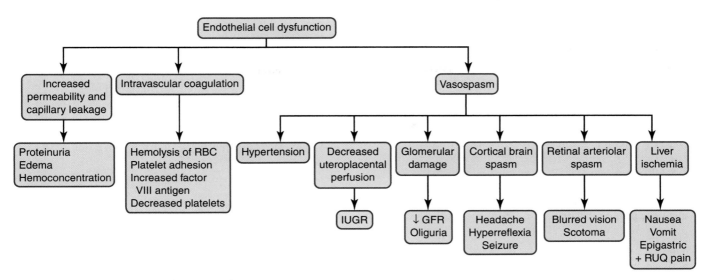

FIGURE 7-7 Pathophysiological changes of preeclampsia.

disease. Women with late-onset disease (onset of symptoms after 34 weeks) frequently have more favorable maternal and fetal outcomes. This disease subset is thought to be triggered by abnormal immune response. New-onset postpartum preeclampsia appears to have yet a different clinical presentation, complicating the diagnosis.

Although management is evidence-based, preventative measures/screening tools are lacking, and treatment remains symptomatic. Delivery is no longer considered the cure. Preeclampsia is a disease of pregnancy accompanied by underlying systemic pathology that can have severe maternal and fetal impact.

- The incidence of preeclampsia complicating pregnancy is 5-11% (Cunningham et al., 2014).
- Despite extensive research, there is no consensus as to the cause of preeclampsia.
- ACOG currently recommends prophylaxis with aspirin for women with a history of preeclampsia and preterm birth, or with two or more prior pregnancies complicated by preeclampsia (Task Force on Hypertension in Pregnancy, 2013).

Pathophysiology of Preeclampsia

To understand the pathophysiological mechanisms of preeclampsia, it is important to review the normal physiological changes of pregnancy. Normal pregnancy is a vasodilated state in which peripheral vascular resistance decreases 25%. Within the first weeks, the woman's blood pressure falls, largely due to a general relaxation of muscles within the blood vessels. Diastolic blood pressure drops 10 mm Hg at mid-pregnancy and gradually returns to pre-pregnant levels at term. There is a 50% rise in total blood volume by the end of the second trimester, and cardiac output increases 30% to 50%. Increased renal blood flow leads to an increased glomerular filtration rate. Because preeclampsia is a syndrome of reduced organ perfusion secondary to vasospasm and endothelial activation, the physiological changes that predispose women to preeclampsia also affect other organs/systems such as the hepatic system, renal system, coagulation system, central nervous system, eyes, fluid and electrolytes, and pulmonary system (Fig. 7–7).

Disease pathways for preeclampsia are thought to involve immune system malfunction, ischemia, oxidative stress, inflammatory response, thrombosis, and endothelial dysfunction. Although signs and symptoms of preeclampsia are not evident until later in pregnancy, the pathologic process most likely begins shortly after conception. It is theorized that this process involves two distinct stages: placental abnormalities and clinical manifestation of maternal disease. Fetal morbidity and mortality are consequences of impaired or incomplete placentation. Establishment of intervillous uteroplacental circulation begins at 8 to 10 weeks gestation and involves invasion of trophoblasts into the uterine vasculature. This remodeling of the uterine vasculature involves replacement of the smooth muscle layer of the spiral arteries, resulting in large capacity, dilated vessels with the low resistance necessary to increase placental circulation, and oxygenation to the fetus. Incomplete transformation of the spiral arteries occurs with preeclampsia. Cytotrophoblasts invade the decidua of the spiral arteries but not the myometrial portion of the artery, and this shallow invasion leads to narrow vessels with high resistance and poor placental perfusion.

An additional pathophysiologic vascular alteration occurring with preeclampsia is acute atherosis. Atherosis increases the likelihood of placental pathology, including hypoperfusion and placental infarcts. These pathologic processes may lead to placental hypoxia and ultimately fetal compromise, including IUGR, fetal heart rate decelerations, acidemia, potential developmental deficits, or fetal death (Phillips & Boyd, 2016). The placenta is evident as the root cause of preeclampsia (ACOG, 2013c).

The second stage of preeclampsia is maternal systemic disease and onset of clinical signs and symptoms. It is proposed that suboptimal placental perfusion triggers an inflammatory response, resulting in the release of pro-inflammatory cytokines, serum soluble Flt-1, and soluble endoglin into maternal circulation. Other inflammatory factors are C-reactive protein and interleukin-6.

This process causes a cascading effect of endothelial damage, vasospasm, altered hemostasis, and activation of the coagulation system. Critical maternal organs affected are the brain, liver, kidneys, and vascular system. Preeclampsia is now known to have a genetic link involving inflammatory signal processing.

● In preeclampsia, there is an increase in microvascular fat deposition within the liver, which is proposed as one cause of epigastric pain. Liver damage may be mild or may progress to HELLP syndrome (Hemolysis, Elevated Liver enzymes, and Low Platelets). Hepatic involvement can lead to periportal hemorrhagic necrosis in the liver that may cause a subcapsular hematoma, potentially resulting in right upper quadrant pain or epigastric pain. This may signal worsening preeclampsia (NHBPEP, 2000).

● In 70% of preeclamptic patients, glomerular endothelial damage, fibrin deposition, and resulting ischemia reduce renal plasma flow and glomerular filtration rate (NHBPEP, 2000). Protein is excreted in the urine. Uric acid, creatinine, and calcium clearance are decreased and oliguria develops as the condition worsens. Oliguria is a sign of severe preeclampsia and kidney damage.

● The coagulation system is activated in preeclampsia and thrombocytopenia occurs, possibly due to increased platelet aggregation and deposition at sites of endothelial damage, activating the clotting cascade. A platelet count below 100,000 cells/mm³ is an indication of severe preeclampsia (NHBPEP, 2000).

● Endothelial damage to the brain results in fibrin deposition, edema, and cerebral hemorrhage, which may lead to hyper-reflexia and severe headaches and can progress to eclampsia (NHBPEP, 2000).

● Retinal arterial spasms may cause blurring or double vision, photophobia, or scotoma (NHBPEP, 2000).

● The leakage of serum protein into extracellular spaces and into urine, by way of damaged capillary walls, results in decreased serum albumin and tissue edema (NHBPEP, 2000).

● Pulmonary edema is most commonly caused by volume overload related to left ventricular failure as the result of extremely high vascular resistance (Cunningham et al., 2014).

CRITICAL COMPONENT

Preeclampsia: Signs, Symptoms, and Severe Features

Preeclampsia is defined as new-onset hypertension after 20 weeks gestation with two blood pressure readings at least 140 mm Hg systolic and/or at least 90 mm Hg diastolic taken at least 4 hours apart. In addition, a woman will have proteinuria greater than 300 mg in 24 hours (protein/creatinine ratio ≥ 0.3 mg/dl) or new-onset systemic disease including thrombocytopenia (platelet count < 100,000 μl), impaired liver function (hepatic transaminase levels elevated twice above normal values and/or persistent right upper quadrant or epigastric abdominal pain), creatinine level indicative of renal insufficiency (>1.1 dl), new-onset cerebral/visual symptoms such as persistent headache, or visual disturbances (Task Force on Hypertension in Pregnancy, 2013).

Severe features of preeclampsia consist of one or more of the following signs or symptoms. Symptoms that preeclampsia has progressed to the severe stage of the disease include:

- Blood pressure ≥160/110 mm Hg. Two readings taken 4 hours apart with the woman on bed rest. Women with blood pressures in this range have an increased risk of stroke.
- Visual problems (blurred or double vision, blind spots, flashes of light or squiggly lines, loss of vision), persistent headache
- Pulmonary edema, new shortness of breath (due to fluid in the lungs)
- Abnormal liver function test and may see pain in the mid- or right-epigastrium (similar to heartburn)
- Abnormal kidney tests (e.g., serum creatinine >1.1 mg/dL)
- Low platelet count (<100,000)
- Liver abnormalities (detected by blood tests)
- HELLP syndrome

ACOG, 2017a; Task Force on Hypertension in Pregnancy, 2013)

Risk Factors for Preeclampsia/Eclampsia

● Nulliparity
● Age younger than 20 or older than 35 years
● Obesity
● Multiple gestation
● Family history of preeclampsia
● Chronic hypertension, kidney disease, lupus, or diabetes prior to pregnancy
● Previous preeclampsia or eclampsia
● Gestational diabetes

Risks for the Woman

● Cerebral edema/hemorrhage/stroke
● Disseminated intravascular coagulation (DIC)
● Pulmonary edema
● Congestive heart failure
● Maternal sequelae resulting from organ damage include renal failure, HELLP syndrome (hemolysis, elevated liver enzymes, and low platelets), thrombocytopenia and disseminated intravascular coagulation, pulmonary edema, and eclampsia (seizures), hepatic failure
● Abruptio placenta
● Women with a history of preeclampsia have a 1.5 to 2 times higher risk of developing heart disease later in life.

Risks for the Fetus and Newborn

● Fetal/neonatal morbidity and mortality are consequences of intrauterine growth restriction (IUGR), prematurity, and placental abruption.
● Fetal intolerance to labor because of decrease placental perfusion
● Stillbirth

In addition, we now know that the intrauterine environment associated with IUGR programs the fetus for adult disease later

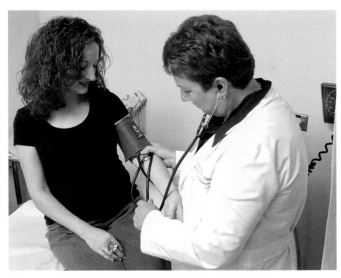

FIGURE 7–8 Take the woman's blood pressure while she is seated and with her arm at heart level.

in life. Newborns with IUGR are at increased risk for metabolic and cardiovascular diseases as adults, including type 2 diabetes, obesity, metabolic syndrome, and hypertension.

Assessment Findings

Accurate assessment is essential so that early recognition of worsening disease will allow for timely intervention that may improve maternal and neonatal outcome.

● Elevated blood pressure: Hypertension with systolic pressure 140 mm Hg or greater and diastolic pressure 90 mm Hg or greater. Blood pressure should be measured with the woman at rest. The proper cuff size is one whose bladder circles at least 80% of the upper arm. A mercury sphygmomanometer is most accurate. The arm should be supported at the level of the heart (see Fig. 7–8).
● Proteinuria is no longer a diagnostic criterion. According to the new ACOG guidelines, the diagnosis of preeclampsia no longer requires the detection of high levels of protein in the urine (proteinuria). Evidence shows organ problems with the kidneys and livers can occur without signs of protein, and that the amount of protein in the urine does not predict how severely the disease will progress.
● Lab values may indicate elevations in liver function tests, diminished kidney function, and altered coagulopathies.
● Evidence tells us that preeclampsia is a dynamic process. Diagnosing a woman's condition as "mild preeclampsia" is not helpful because it is a progressive disease, progressing at different rates in different women. Appropriate care requires frequent re-evaluation for severe features of the disease and appropriate actions outlined in the new guidelines.

Medical Management

Management for preeclampsia is expectant or expedient birth, depending on the severity of disease, gestational age, and fetal status. Women with early-onset preeclampsia (<34 weeks

gestation) will need corticosteroids to facilitate fetal lung maturity and may require magnesium sulfate.

Once diagnosed, the woman and fetus should be monitored weekly for indications of worsening condition, as preeclampsia is a progressive disease. However, women can also present with abrupt onset of the disease. Indications of worsening preeclampsia are treated with hospitalization and evaluation. Antihypertensive drugs are used to control elevated blood pressure. Delivery is indicated in severe preeclampsia, even before term, to protect the woman and fetus from severe sequelae. Care in labor and delivery includes use of magnesium sulfate to prevent seizures.

The primary goal in preeclampsia is to control the woman's blood pressure and prevent seizure activity and cerebral hemorrhage. Induced birth is indicated for women at less than 34 weeks' gestation with severe features of preeclampsia or for unstable maternal/fetal status at any gestation. Medical management includes the following measures.

● Magnesium sulfate, a central nervous system depressant, has been proven to help reduce seizure activity without documentation of long-term adverse effects to the woman and fetus.
● Antihypertensive medications are used to control blood pressure (see Table 7–3).
● Outpatient management for women with mild preeclampsia is an option if the woman can adhere to activity restriction, frequent office visits, blood pressure monitoring, and antenatal testing.
● Induced birth is indicated for women at less than 34 weeks' gestation with severe features of preeclampsia or for unstable maternal/fetal status at any gestation (Cluver, 2017).
● For hypertensive disorders as a group, planned early delivery appears to be better for the mother after 34 weeks' gestation. However, it is unclear whether planned early delivery increases risks for the baby, especially at earlier gestations, and more research is needed to guide practice according to a recent Cochrane Review (Cluver, 2017).

Nursing Actions

● Accurate assessment is essential because early recognition of worsening disease allows for timely intervention and may improve maternal and neonatal outcome.
● Blood pressure should be measured with the woman seated and her arm at heart level, using an appropriate sized cuff (Fig. 7–8). Placing the woman in a left lateral recumbent position is no longer recommended to evaluate blood pressure, as it gives an inaccurately low blood pressure reading (Cunningham et al., 2014; NHBPEP, 2000).
● Administer antihypertensive as per orders (generally for blood pressure >160/110 mm Hg) (see Table 7–3).
● Administer magnesium sulfate as per orders.
● Assess for CNS changes including headache, visual changes, deep tendon reflexes (DTRs), and clonus (Box 7–3 and Fig. 7–9).
● Auscultate lung sounds for clarity and monitor the respiratory rate.
● Assess for signs and symptoms of pulmonary edema such as:
  ● Shortness of breath, chest tightness or discomfort, cough, oxygen saturation less than 95%, increased respiratory and heart rates

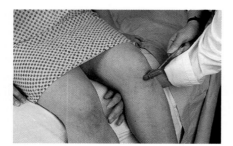

FIGURE 7–9 Assessing DTRs.

BOX 7–3 | Assessment Of Deep Tendon Reflexes

PHYSICAL ASSESSMENT	GRADE
None elicited	0
Sluggish or dull	1
Active, normal	2
Brisk	3
Brisk with transient or sustained clonus	4
(see Fig. 7–9)	

- Changes in behavior, such as apprehension, anxiety, or restlessness
- Assess for epigastric pain or right upper quadrant pain indicating liver involvement.
- Assess weight daily and assess for edema to assess for fluid retention.
- Check urine for proteinuria (may include 24-hour urine collection) and specific gravity.
- Evaluate laboratory values including:
  - Elevations in serum creatinine >1.1 mg/dL
  - Hematocrit levels >35
  - Low platelet count <100,000/mm^3
  - Elevated liver enzymes AST and ALT > 2X the upper limit of normal (Poole, 2014)

- Perform antenatal fetal testing and fetal heart rate monitoring (NST and BPP).
- Check intake of adequate calories and protein.
- Maintain accurate I&O to evaluate kidney function. Total fluid intake may be restricted to 2,000 mL/24 hr.
- Provide a quiet environment to decrease CNS stimulation.
- Maintain bed rest in the lateral recumbent position.
- Provide information to the woman and her family. Education is key in helping with the understanding of the disease process and the plan of care.
- Report deterioration in maternal or fetal status to provider.

TABLE 7–3 Preeclampsia/Eclampsia Medications

DRUG NAME OR CLASS	ADMINISTRATION AND USE	CONTRAINDICATIONS
Magnesium sulfate	IV access: Load 4–6 grams 10% magnesium sulfate in 100 mL solution over 20 minutes. Maintenance dose: 1–2 grams/hour. No IV access: 10 grams of 50% solution IM (5 grams in each buttock)	Pulmonary edema, renal failure, myasthenia gravis
Antihypertensive medications	For SBP ≥160 or DBP ≥110 Labetalol: (20 mg, 40 mg, 80 IV over 2 minutes, escalating doses, repeat q 10 min). Maximum cumulative dose should not exceed 220 mg in 24 hours. Hydralazine: (5–10 mg IV over 2 minutes, repeat q 20 min until target BP reached). Maximum cumulative IV-administered dose should not exceed 25 mg in 24 hours. *If persistent seizures, consider anticonvulsant medications and additional workup.	Labetalol: Avoid in asthma or heart failure, can cause neonatal bradycardia
Anticonvulsant medications	For recurrent seizures or when magnesium sulfate is contraindicated. Lorazepam (Ativan): 2–4 mg IV x1, may repeat once after 10–15 min Diazepam (Valium): 5–10 mg IV q 5–10 min to maximum dose 30 mg	

ACOG, 2017a.

SAFE AND EFFECTIVE NURSING CARE: Understanding Medication

Intravenous Administration of Magnesium Sulfate

Magnesium sulfate is indicated for women with severe features of preeclampsia. Although the exact method of action in seizure prophylaxis is not clearly understood, therapeutic levels of the drug will result in cerebral vasodilation, thereby reducing ischemia caused by vasospasm. Magnesium sulfate also slows neuromuscular conduction, depresses the vasomotor center, and decreases central nervous system irritability (Poole, 2014). Continuous intravenous administration:

- Loading dose: 4–6 g diluted in 100 mL of IV fluid administered over 15–20 minutes
- Continuous infusion: 2 g/hr in 100 mL of IV fluid for maintenance
- Laboratory evaluation: Measure serum magnesium level at 4–6 hours, after onset of treatment. Dosage should be adjusted to maintain a therapeutic level of 4 to 8 mg/dl.
- Duration: Intravenous infusion should continue for 24 hours post-delivery.
- The antidote for magnesium toxicity is calcium gluconate or calcium chloride 5–10 mEq given IV slowly over 5–10 minutes.

CRITICAL COMPONENT

Care of the Woman on Magnesium Sulfate

Potential Side Effects	Nursing Actions
Maternal: Nausea Flushing Diaphoresis Blurred vision Lethargy Hypocalcemia Depressed reflexes Respiratory depression-arrest Cardiac dysrhythmias Decreased platelet aggregation Circulatory collapse	Assess vital signs before beginning infusion and every 5–15 minutes during loading dose, then every 30–60 minutes until the patient stabilizes. Frequency is then determined by the patient status. Assess DTRs every 2 hours. Deep tendon reflexes can be elicited by striking the tendon of a partially stretched muscle briskly, using the flat or pointed surface of the reflex hammer (Poole, 2014). Patellar, or knee-jerk, reflexes may be unreliable in women who have had regional anesthesia, and brachial reflexes should be used. Reflexes are graded on a scale of 0 to +4, with 0 being an absent reflex and +4 being a hyperactive reflex.

Potential Side Effects	Nursing Actions
	Clonus is associated with central nervous system excitability and can be elicited by dorsiflexing the foot against the nurse's hand and then releasing it suddenly. Beats of clonus occur when the foot taps against the examiner's hand instead of returning to normal position. Monitor strict intake and output. Patients with oliguria or renal disease are at risk for toxic levels of magnesium. Monitor serum magnesium levels (therapeutic level is 5–7 mg/dL). Monitor for signs and symptoms of magnesium toxicity: • Decreased reflexes could be a sign of pending respiratory depression. • Loss of DTRs • Respiratory depression: respiratory rate <14 breaths/min • Oliguria, urine output <30 mL/hr • Shortness of breath or chest pain • EKG changes • If toxicity is suspected, discontinue the infusion and notify the health care provider. Respiration difficulty and cardiac arrest can occur with magnesium levels above 12 mEq/L. • Keep calcium gluconate immediately available (1g IV). • Maintain seizure precautions and keep resuscitation equipment nearby. • Patients receiving IV labetalol for blood pressure control should have cardiac monitoring. • Maintain continuous fetal heart rate monitoring. Report abnormal findings including: Urine output < 30 ml/hour Respiratory rate < 12 breaths/minute

Continued

Potential Side Effects	Nursing Actions
	SpO$_2$ < 95% Persistent hypotension Absent deep tendon reflexes Altered maternal levels of consciousness Abnormal laboratory test values
Fetal/neonatal: Fetal heart rate decreased variability Respiratory depression Hypotonia Decreased suck reflex Signs and symptoms of magnesium toxicity	Monitor FHR. Alert the neonatal team before delivery of use of magnesium sulfate in labor.

CRITICAL COMPONENT

Emergent Therapy for Acute-Onset, Severe Hypertension During Pregnancy and the Postpartum Period

Pregnant women or women in the postpartum period with acute-onset, severe systolic hypertension; severe diastolic hypertension; or both require urgent antihypertensive therapy. Acute-onset, severe systolic (greater than or equal to 160 mm Hg) hypertension; severe diastolic (greater than or equal to 110 mm Hg) hypertension; or both can occur during the prenatal, intrapartum, or postpartum periods. The goal is not to normalize BP, but to achieve a range of 140–150/90–100 mm Hg to prevent repeated, prolonged exposure to severe systolic hypertension, with subsequent loss of cerebral vasculature autoregulation. In the event of a hypertensive crisis, with prolonged uncontrolled hypertension, maternal stabilization should occur before delivery, even in urgent circumstances. Treatment with first-line agents should be expeditious and occur as soon as possible within 30–60 minutes of confirmed severe hypertension to reduce the risk of maternal stroke.

Intravenous (IV) labetalol and hydralazine have long been considered first-line medications for the management of acute-onset, severe hypertension in pregnant women and women in the postpartum period. Immediate release oral nifedipine also may be considered as a first-line therapy, particularly when IV access is not available.

It is important to note differences in recommended dosage intervals between these options, which reflect differences in their pharmacokinetics. Protocols should be followed for maternal monitoring of blood pressure every 5 to 15 minutes. None of the recommended drugs require cardiac monitoring.

Although all three medications are appropriately used for the treatment of hypertensive emergencies in pregnancy, each agent can be associated with adverse effects. Parenteral hydralazine may increase the risk of maternal hypotension (systolic BP, 90 mm Hg or less). Parenteral labetalol may cause neonatal bradycardia and should be avoided in women with asthma, heart disease, or congestive heart failure. Nifedipine has been associated with an increase in maternal heart rate, and with overshoot hypotension.

ACOG, 2017a.

Fetal Assessment

Preeclampsia exposes the fetus to an adverse intrauterine environment. Hypoperfusion of the placenta can result in chronic hypoxia, IUGR, asphyxia, and fetal death. Antenatal fetal surveillance is used to detect compromised fetal status in the hope of preventing asphyxia and stillbirth. Fetal well-being is evaluated by the following measures.

- Fetal movement is a critical component of nursing assessment, and a woman's report of decreased fetal movement should always be investigated.
- Biophysical profile can be used to screen for acute or chronic fetal hypoxia by examining five fetal parameters most affected by hypoxia. These include the nonstress test, fetal movement, fetal breathing, fetal tone, and amniotic fluid index (see Chapter 6). A normal score is 8 (without nonstress test) to 10 (with reactive nonstress test); a score of 4 or less is considered abnormal and indicative of fetal compromise.
- Oligohydramnios is associated with an increased risk of perinatal morbidity and mortality, and therefore this finding is especially concerning. Because amniotic fluid is comprised mostly of fetal urine, low fluid volume would indicate a lack of renal perfusion.
- Evaluation and decision making regarding fetal IUGR is facilitated by umbilical artery Doppler velocimetry testing. This measures hemodynamic changes in the fetal/placental circulation unit. The S/D ratio is most commonly measured, and the value should decline as a normal pregnancy progresses, reflecting increased blood flow to the fetus due to decreased placental resistance. However, when pregnancy is complicated by preeclampsia, atherosis of the placental vessels results in an increase in placental resistance. An elevated S/D ratio (>3 to 4) is seen with fetal growth restriction before clinical signs of fetal distress and possibly even before an abnormal biophysical profile. The blood flow through the umbilical arteries should be forward. If this flow, called the end diastolic flow, is an absent or reversed-end diastolic flow, this is indicative of fetal compromise and placental dysfunction and warrants increased surveillance and assessment for birth.

Eclampsia

Eclampsia is the occurrence of seizure activity in the presence of preeclampsia. Eclampsia can occur ante-, intra-, or postpartum;

about 50% of cases occur antepartum. Eclampsia is thought to be triggered by one or more of the following:

- Cerebral vasospasm
- Cerebral hemorrhage
- Cerebral ischemia
- Cerebral edema

Warning signs of potential eclampsia include:

- Severe persistent headaches
- Epigastric pain
- Nausea and vomiting
- Hyperreflexia with clonus
- Restlessness

Care during a seizure includes (Box 7–4):

- Remaining with the patient.
- Calling for help.
- Providing for patient safety by assessing airway and breathing.
  - Lower the head of the bed and turn the woman's head to one side.
  - Anticipate the need for suctioning to decrease the risk of aspiration.
  - Aspiration is the leading cause of maternal mortality (Poole, 2014).
- Preventing maternal injury.
  - If possible, a padded tongue blade should be inserted to prevent tongue injury (a tongue blade is still recommended by guidelines but not typically used in clinical practice).
  - Keep side rails up and padded, if possible.
- Recording the time, length, and type of seizure activity.
- Notifying the physician.

After the seizure, the nurse should:

- Rapidly assess maternal and fetal status.
- Assess airway; suction if needed.
- Administer supplemental oxygen: 10 L/min via mask.
- Ensure IV access.
- Administer magnesium sulfate per orders.
- Provide a quiet environment.

HELLP Syndrome

HELLP syndrome (Hemolysis, Elevated Liver enzymes, and Low Platelets) is the acronym used to designate the variant changes in laboratory values that can occur as a complication of severe preeclampsia.

- Hemolysis is a result of red blood cell destruction as the cells travel through constricted vessels.
- Elevated liver enzymes result from decreased blood flow and damage to the liver.
- Low platelets result from platelets aggregating at the site of damaged vascular endothelium causing platelet consumption and thrombocytopenia (Cunningham et al., 2014; Sibai, 2004).

BOX 7–4 | Eclampsia Protocol

Assessment Findings

Confirm findings again within 10 minutes after calling the physician.

- SBP <90 mmHg or >160 mmHg; DBP >100 mmHg (***Not applicable for SBP <90 when 30 minutes or less post epidural and anesthesiologist present.)
- Heart rate <50 bpm or >120 bpm
- Respiratory rate < 10 bpm or >30 bpm
- Oxygen saturation <95%
- Oliguria <35 mL/hr × 2 hours
- Maternal agitation, confusion, or unresponsiveness
- Blurred vision
- Proteinuria
- Non-remitting headache or shortness of breath in a hypertensive patient

Diagnostic/Lab Tests to Consider

- Pulse oximeter
- CBC, CMP
- Urinalysis
- Type and screen or type and cross match if bleeding
- Magnesium level
- EKG
- CT angiogram or perfusion scan in patients with acute chest pain
- CXR if patient is short of breath, particularly if pre-eclamptic
- Echocardiogram

Eclampsia Nursing Interventions

- Call for assistance and notify primary physician.
- Designate team leader, checklist reader/recorder, and primary RN.
- Ensure side rails are up and padded.
- Protect airway and improve oxygenation; administer supplemental oxygen (100% non-rebreather face mask); ensure suction and bag-mask ventilation are available; maternal pulse oximetry.
- Place in lateral decubitis position.
- Monitor and record description, characteristics, and duration of seizure activity, if present.
- Continuous fetal monitoring
- Establish and maintain IV access; draw preeclampsia labs.
- Administer magnesium sulfate.
- Administer antihypertensive therapy.
- Develop delivery plan, if appropriate.
- Update and communicate with patient, family, and obstetric team.

Continued

BOX 7–4 | Eclampsia Protocol—cont'd

Provider Notification

- RN will notify attending OB of patient's status and request a bedside evaluation, and the OB physician will evaluate the patient within 10 minutes.
- The in-house OB will also be notified and will provide a bedside evaluation if the attending OB is unavailable.
- If the in-house OB is not immediately available, they will receive a verbal report and determine if further action is necessary.
- The OB will decide the planned frequency of monitoring and re-evaluation, as well as criteria for immediate physician notification, and any necessary diagnostic therapeutic interventions.
- A "huddle" will take place and members, including the OB, primary RN, charge RN, and anesthesiologist, will discuss the management plan.
- If condition persists or worsens after interventions, consider calling a Rapid Response.

ACOG, 2017a; Council on Patient Safety in Women's Health Care, 2017.

Women with severe preeclampsia have an increased risk (7% to 24%) of developing HELLP syndrome. HELLP may develop in women who do not present with the cardinal signs of severe preeclampsia. HELLP may appear at any time during the pregnancy in 70% of cases, and in the immediate postpartum period for 30% of cases (Queenan et al., 2005). The only definitive treatment is delivery. However, some women may experience worsening HELLP syndrome over the first 48-hour postpartum period. Women with only some of the laboratory changes are diagnosed with partial HELLP syndrome.

CRITICAL COMPONENT

Laboratory Values Indicative of HELLP Syndrome

Platelets	<100,000/mm^3
Liver enzymes (AST, ALT)	Elevated AST: > 2 X upper limit of normal Elevated ALT: >2 X upper limit of normal
Bilirubin (indirect)	Elevated: >1.2 mg/dL
LDH	Elevated: >600 units/L

Risks for the Woman

- Abruptio placenta
- Renal failure
- Liver hematoma and possible rupture
- Death

Risks for the Fetus and Newborn

- Preterm birth
- Death

Assessment Findings

- The woman may present with a complaint of general malaise, nausea, and right upper gastric pain.
- The woman may have unexplained bruising, mucosal bleeding, petechiae, and bleeding from injection and IV sites.
- Assessment findings are related to alternations in laboratory tests associated with changes in liver function and platelets.

Medical Management

The only definitive cure for HELLP syndrome is immediate delivery of the fetus and placenta. Resolution of disease is generally in 48 hours postpartum. Medical management may include replacement of platelets and is the same as those for the women with severe preeclampsia (Poole, 2014).

Nursing Actions

- Perform a thorough assessment of the woman related to the diagnosis of preeclampsia.
- Evaluate laboratory tests.
- Notify the physician immediately if HELLP syndrome is suspected or lab values deteriorate.
- Administer platelets as per orders.
- Assessment and management are the same for the women diagnosed with HELLP syndrome as for the women with severe preeclampsia.
- Provide the woman and the family with information regarding HELLP and its treatment.
- Provide emotional support to the woman and her family, as the woman and family are at risk for increased levels of anxiety related to diagnosis (Mattson & Smith, 2011).

PLACENTAL ABNORMALITIES AND HEMORRHAGIC COMPLICATIONS

Major blood loss during pregnancy is a significant contributor to both maternal and fetal morbidity and mortality. Hemorrhage predisposes a woman to hypovolemia, anemia, infection, and premature birth. Significant maternal blood loss can cause decreased perfusion and oxygen to the fetus, resulting in progressive deterioration of fetal status and even death (Burke-Sosa, 2014). Placental abnormalities and hemorrhagic complications of pregnancy are presented in this section.

The major causes of antepartum hemorrhage are placenta previa and placental abruption. The basic principles of immediate care of women with either type of antepartum hemorrhage include assessment of maternal and fetal condition, prompt maternal resuscitation if required, and consideration of early delivery if there is evidence of fetal distress and if the baby is mature enough to be potentially capable of survival. Up to 15% of maternal cardiac output, and up to 1000 mL/min flows through the placental bed at term; unresolved bleeding can result in maternal exsanguination in 8 to 10 minutes (Burke-Sosa, 2014).

Placental disorders such as placenta previa, placenta accreta, and vasa previa are all associated with vaginal bleeding in the second half of pregnancy. They are also important causes of serious fetal and maternal morbidity and even mortality. Moreover, the rates of previa and accreta are increasing, probably because of increasing rates of cesarean delivery, maternal age, and assisted reproductive technology. The routine use of obstetric ultrasonography as well as improving ultrasonographic technology allows for the antenatal diagnosis of these conditions. In turn, antenatal diagnosis facilitates optimal obstetric management (Silver, 2015).

For the fetus, significant blood loss can result in negative alterations in maternal hemodynamic status and decreased oxygen. When bleeding decreases the blood flow to the placenta, maternal fetal gas exchange is reduced and the fetus is at risk for progressive deterioration including hypoxemia, hypoxia, asphyxia, and death (Burke-Sosa, 2014). The risk is directly related to the amount and duration of blood loss.

CRITICAL COMPONENT

Vaginal Bleeding

A sterile vaginal exam is contraindicated in all pregnant women with extensive vaginal bleeding until the source of bleeding is identified. If a vaginal exam is performed with a placenta previa torrential, vaginal bleeding could occur related to dislodging of the placenta from maternal tissues. Maternal blood loss results in decreased oxygen-carrying capacity, which directly impacts oxygen delivery to maternal organs and placental blood flow, thus decreasing oxygen to the fetus. Therefore, the management of placenta previa and all placental abnormalities is dependent on maternal and fetal status.

Placenta Previa

The incidence of placenta previa is estimated to be 1 in 200 pregnancies at term and varies throughout the world (Cunningham et al., 2014). Placenta previa occurs when the placenta attaches to the lower uterine segment of the uterus, near or over the internal cervical os instead of in the body or fundus of the uterus (Fig. 7–10). The cause is unknown (Silver, 2015). Women with placenta previa have an approximately 10-fold increased risk of antepartum vaginal bleeding. The mechanism of bleeding is uncertain but appears to be attributable to separation of the placenta from the underlying decidua, resulting from contractions, cervical effacement, cervical dilation, and/or advancing gestational age (Silver, 2015). Hemorrhage is especially likely to occur during the third trimester with development of the lower uterine segment and when uterine contractions dilate the cervix, thereby applying shearing forces to the placental attachment to the lower segment, or when separation is provoked by vaginal examination. Placenta previa is most often diagnosed before the onset of bleeding when ultrasound is performed for other indications (Burke-Sosa, 2014).

In the past, previas were characterized as complete, partial, and marginal depending on how much of the internal endocervical os was covered by the placenta. However, the use of transvaginal ultrasonography allows for precise localization of the placental edge and the cervical os. Accordingly, the nomenclature has been modified to eliminate the terms "partial" and "marginal." Instead, all placentas overlying the os (to any degree) are termed previas and those near to but not overlying the os are termed low-lying (Silver, 2015).

Risk Factors for Placenta Previa

- Endometrial scarring
  - Previous placenta previa
  - Prior cesarean birth
  - Abortion involving suction curettage
  - Multiparity or short pregnancy interval
- Impeded endometrial vascularization
  - Advanced maternal age (>35 years)
  - Diabetes or hypertension
  - Cigarette smoking
  - Uterine anomalies/fibroids/endometritis

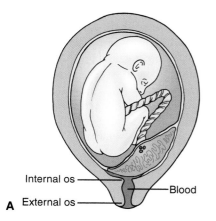
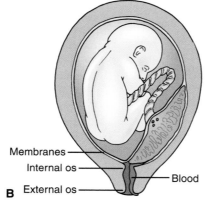
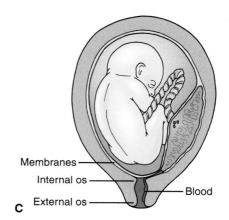

FIGURE 7–10 Placenta previa. (**A**) Previa (**B**) Previa. (**C**) Low-lying placenta

● Increased placental mass
  ● Large placenta
  ● Multiple gestation

Risks for the Woman

● Hemorrhagic and hypovolemic shock related to excessive blood loss necessitating blood transfusion, hysterectomy, maternal intensive care unit admission.
● Because of the large volume of maternal blood flow to the uteroplacental unit at term, unresolved bleeding can result in maternal exsanguinations in 10 minutes.
● Potential Rh sensitization as Rh-negative women can become sensitized during any antepartum bleeding episode.
● Other risks from hemorrhage include septicemia, thrombophlebitis, and even maternal death.

Risks for the Fetus and Newborn

● Disruption of uteroplacental blood flow can result in progressive deterioration of fetal status, and the degree of fetal compromise is related to the volume of maternal blood loss (Burke-Sosa, 2014).
● Blood loss, hypoxia, anoxia, and death (<10%) related to maternal hemorrhage may occur.
● Fetal anemia may develop due to maternal blood loss.
● Neonatal morbidity and mortality is related primarily to prematurity (Silver, 2015).

Assessment Findings

● The "classic" presentation used to be painless vaginal bleeding in the third trimester. Bleeding may be associated with abdominal pain, contractions, or both.
● Hemodynamic changes can be associated with blood loss.
● Fetal heart rate changes are associated with maternal blood loss.
● Bleeding usually occurs near the end of the second trimester or in the third trimester of pregnancy, and initial bleeding episodes may be slight.
● The first episode of bleeding is rarely life-threatening or a cause of hypovolemic shock.
● Ultrasound confirms placental location at the cervix and transvaginal ultrasonography also improves the accuracy of the diagnosis in the third trimester. Many placenta previas noted at mid-pregnancy during routine screening ultrasounds will no longer be present by the time of delivery. The relationship between the cervix and the placenta changes over time with the placenta typically "moving away" from the cervix. Accordingly, only approximately 10% to 20% of previas at 20 weeks of gestation will remain previas in the late third trimester.
● Maternal findings may also include fear and anxiety.
● A vaginal exam is contraindicated.

Emergency Medical Management

● Cesarean delivery is necessary when either maternal or fetal status is compromised as a result of extensive hemorrhage.
● Cesarean birth is necessary in practically all women with placenta previa because the placenta is at the cervix, and labor

and cervical dilation results in placental hemorrhage (Silver, 2015).
● Vaginal delivery may be attempted with a low-lying placenta if one can proceed with an emergency cesarean birth if needed.
● Placenta previa may be associated with placenta accreta, placenta increta, or placenta percreta.
● There is an increased risk of postpartum hemorrhage in the setting of previa, even without accreta, and blood is transfused as needed.

Medical Management After Stabilization

When the maternal and fetal status is stable and bleeding is minimal (<250 mL), prolonging the pregnancy and delaying delivery may be possible. This expectant management or conservative management is performed when the fetus is premature to allow for fetal lungs to mature. The benefits of a planned delivery under optimal circumstances and before labor or bleeding must be weighed against the risks of prematurity. This typically includes close observation and hospitalization. If the woman and fetus remain stable and bleeding stops, discharging the woman home may be a consideration. The mainstay of antepartum care is "expectant management." Most women with asymptomatic previa (no bleeding or contractions) are managed as outpatient. A Cochrane Review of clinical trials revealed little evidence of any clear advantage or disadvantage to a policy of home versus hospital care (Neilson, 2009). Although often prescribed, the benefits of bed rest, pelvic rest, or reduced activity remain unproven (Silver, 2015).

Nursing Actions

Nursing actions are related to maternal fetal status and the amount of vaginal bleeding and include the following.

● Perform the initial assessment:
  ● Evaluation of color, character, and amount of vaginal bleeding and weigh the amount
  ● Arrangement for ultrasound to determine placental location
  ● Determination of fetal well-being, gestational age, and fetal lung maturity
  ● Assessment of vital signs for increased pulse and respiratory rate and falling blood pressure every 5 to 15 minutes if active bleeding. The woman can have up to a 40% maternal blood loss before exhibiting hemorrhagic hemodynamic changes in the blood pressure and pulse.
● Notify the physician of any of the following:
  ● Onset or increase in vaginal bleeding
  ● Blood pressure less than 90/60 mm Hg; pulse less than 60 or more than 120 bpm
  ● Respirations less than 14 or more than 26 breaths/min
  ● Temperature greater than 100.4°F (38°C)
  ● Urine output less than 30 mL/hr
  ● Saturated oxygen less than 95%
  ● Decreased level of consciousness
  ● Onset or increase in uterine activity
  ● Category II or III FHR pattern

- Assess abdominal pain, uterine tenderness, irritability, and contractions.
- Initiate bed rest with bathroom privileges.
- Establish and maintain IV access with large-bore IV in case blood replacement therapy is needed.
- Administer oxygen at 8 to 10 L/min per mask.
- Ensure availability of hold clot and blood components.
- Assess FHR and uterine activity and facilitate antenatal testing as ordered.
- Give corticosteroids to accelerate fetal lung maturity, if indicated.
- Monitor lab values including CBC, platelets, and clotting studies.
- Inform the patient and family of maternal and fetal status, and reassure the patient and her family. Explain interventions and reasons they are being performed.
- Anticipate a cesarean birth if patient is unstable.
- If undelivered and mother is RH negative, administer RhoGAM.

Placental Abruption

Placental abruption, also referred to as abruptio placentae, is bleeding at the decidual-placental interface that causes partial or complete placental detachment prior to delivery of the fetus. The diagnosis is typically reserved for pregnancies over 20 weeks of gestation. Placental abruption is initiated by hemorrhage into the decidual basalis. A hematoma forms, leading to destruction of the placenta adjacent to it. In some instances, spiral arterioles that nourish the decidua and supply blood to the placenta rupture. Bleeding into the decidua basalis results in hemorrhage and placental separation (Fig. 7–11).

Although several risk factors are known, the etiopathogenesis of placental abruption is multifactorial and not well understood. The separation may be partial or total and can be classified as grade 1 (mild), 2 (moderate), or 3 (severe) (Gilbert, 2011). Bleeding with placental abruption is almost always maternal. This is a uniquely dangerous condition for the woman and fetus because of its potentially serious complications. Placental abruption complicates approximately 1 percent of pregnancies, with two-thirds classified as severe due to accompanying maternal, fetal, and neonatal morbidity.

A majority of placental abruption cases appear to have long-standing chronic etiology (Elsasser et al., 2010). The major clinical findings are vaginal bleeding and abdominal pain, often accompanied by hypertonic uterine contractions, uterine tenderness, and a nonreassuring fetal heart rate (FHR) pattern (Elsasser, Ananth, Prasad, & Vintzileos, 2010). Clinical diagnosis for abruption should include one or more of the following: retroplacental bleeding or clot, sonographic visualization of abruption, or painful vaginal bleeding accompanied by nonreassuring fetal status or uterine hypertonicity (Elsasser et al., 2010). Maternal and fetal status determines the management of the pregnancy. A concealed hemorrhage occurs in about 10% of abruptions. This results in uterine tenderness and abdominal pain. The fetal response to abruptio placenta depends on the volume of blood loss and the extent of uteroplacental insufficiency. Management depends on maternal and fetal status and gestational age. About half of abruptions occurred before 37 weeks of gestation and 14 percent occurred before 32 weeks (Tikkanen, 2011).

Risk Factors

- Previous abruption increases risk up to 15%
- Hypertensive disorders, prior cesarean section, maternal age, multiple gestation, preterm premature rupture of membranes, uterine anomalies/fibroids
- Abdominal trauma
- Cocaine, methamphetamine use, and/or cigarette smoking
- Thrombophilia

Risks for the Woman

- Maternal risks include obstetric hemorrhage, need for blood transfusions, emergency hysterectomy, disseminated intravascular coagulopathy, and renal failure.
- Maternal death is rare but seven times higher than the overall maternal mortality rate.

Three grades of abruption placentae

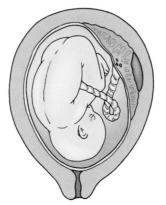 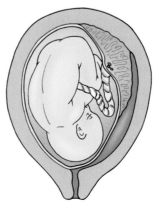 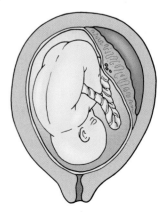

FIGURE 7–11 Three grades of abruptio placentae.

Mid Grade
(< 15% placenta separates
with concealed hemorrhage)

Moderate Grade 2
(Up to 50% placenta separates
with apparent hemorrhage)

Severe Grade 3
(> 50% placenta separates
with concealed hemorrhage)

Risks for the Fetus and Newborn

● Perinatal consequences include low birthweight, preterm delivery, asphyxia, stillbirth, and perinatal death.
● In developed countries, approximately 10% of all preterm births and 10% to 20% of all perinatal deaths are caused by placental abruption.

Assessment Findings

● Vaginal bleeding is present in up to 80% of women with abruption. Maternal assessment findings with active bleeding include:
  ● Hypovolemic shock, hypotension, oliguria, thready pulse, shallow/irregular respirations, pallor, cold, clammy skin, and anxiety
  ● Vaginal bleeding (but can be concealed hemorrhage)
  ● Severe abdominal pain and tense abdomen or continuous, dull back pain
  ● Uterine contractions/tenderness/hypertonus/increasing uterine distention
  ● Nausea and vomiting
  ● Decreased renal output
  ● Remember, during pregnancy signs of shock are usually not until 25% to 30% of maternal blood loss has occurred.
  ● Kleihauer–Betke test in maternal blood may be positive and indicate the presence of fetal red blood cells.
● Fetal assessment findings include:
  ● Tachycardia
  ● Bradycardia
  ● Category II or III FHR patterns including: loss or variability of FHR, late decelerations, decreasing baseline
  ● Maternal findings may also include fear and anxiety.

Emergency Medical Management

If abruption results in unstable or deteriorating maternal or fetal status, delivery by cesarean is indicated. Treatment includes:

● Monitoring maternal volume status and coagulation status
● Correcting coagulation defects
● Restoring blood loss
● Assessing fetal status
● Expediting delivery as indicated

Medical Management After Stabilization

If the maternal status is stable and the fetus is immature, then expectant management would include:

● Hospitalization and close monitoring of maternal and fetal status including signs and symptoms of abruption such as bleeding, uterine activity or hypertonus, and abdominal pain, and monitoring maternal laboratory and coagulation studies.
● Corticosteroids may be given to accelerate fetal lung maturity and tocolysis may be considered.

Nursing Actions

● Close monitoring of maternal and fetal status including signs and symptoms of abruption such as vaginal bleeding, uterine pain, activity or hypertonus, abdominal pain and monitoring maternal laboratory and coagulation studies.
● Palpate the uterus for contractions/tenderness/hypertonus/increasing uterine distension.
● Monitor maternal cardiovascular status for hypotension and tachycardia.
● Establish and maintain IV access with a large-bore needle.
● Administer oxygen at 8 to 10 L/min by mask.
● Assess FHR for baseline changes, variability, and periodic changes indicative of an abnormal FHR.
● Provide emotional support to the woman and her family, reassure the patient and her family, and provide information to the woman and her family regarding treatment plan and status of their infant.
● Measure and estimate blood loss.
● Anticipate a cesarean birth if patient or fetus is unstable.
● If undelivered and mother is RH negative, administer RhoGAM.

Placenta Accreta

Placenta accreta is a general term used to describe the clinical condition when part of the placenta, or the entire placenta, invades and is inseparable from the uterine wall. When the chorionic villi invade only the myometrium, the term placenta increta is appropriate; whereas placenta percreta describes invasion through the myometrium and serosa, and occasionally into adjacent organs, such as the bladder. Clinically, placenta accreta becomes problematic during delivery when the placenta does not completely separate from the uterus and is followed by massive obstetric hemorrhage, leading to disseminated intravascular coagulopathy; the need for hysterectomy; surgical injury to the ureters, bladder, bowel, or neurovascular structures; adult respiratory distress syndrome; acute transfusion reaction; electrolyte imbalance; and renal failure. The average blood loss at delivery in women with placenta accreta is 3,000 to 5,000 mL (ACOG, 2012b). As many as 90% of patients with placenta accreta require blood transfusion, and 40% require more than 10 units of packed red blood cells. Maternal mortality with placenta accreta has been reported to be as high as 7%. Maternal death may occur despite optimal planning, transfusion management, and surgical care (ACOG, 2012b). The incidence of placenta accreta has increased and seems to parallel the increasing cesarean delivery rate. Placenta accreta can be diagnosed by ultrasound prenatally but typically is diagnosed after delivery when the placenta is retained. If the placenta does not separate readily, rapid surgical intervention is needed.

● Placenta accreta: Invasion of the trophoblast is beyond the normal boundary (80% of cases).
● Placenta increta: Invasion of the trophoblast extends into uterine myometrium (15% of cases).
● Placenta percreta: Invasion of the trophoblast extends into the uterine musculature and can adhere to other pelvic organs (5% of cases).

One of the most important modifiers of clinical outcome is prenatal diagnosis of accreta. Several studies confirm decreased hemorrhage and other maternal complications in cases diagnosed antenatally rather than intrapartum. Prenatal diagnosis allows for optimal management, which typically includes planned cesarean hysterectomy before the onset of labor or bleeding. Diagnosing placenta accreta before delivery allows for multidisciplinary planning in an attempt to minimize potential maternal or neonatal morbidity and mortality. The diagnosis is usually established by ultrasonography and occasionally supplemented by magnetic resonance imaging (MRI).

Risk Factors for Placenta Accreta

- Women at greatest risk of placenta accreta are those who have myometrial damage caused by a previous cesarean delivery with either anterior or posterior placenta previa overlying the uterine scar.
- The risk of placenta accreta was 3%, 11%, 40%, 61%, and 67% for the first, second, third, fourth, and fifth or greater repeat cesarean deliveries, respectively (Silver et al., 2006).
- Placenta previa without previous uterine surgery is associated with a 1% to 5% risk of placenta accreta.
- Advanced maternal age
- Multiparity
- Any condition resulting in myometrial tissue damage followed by a secondary collagen repair

Risks for the Woman

- Hemorrhagic and hypovolemic shock related to excessive blood loss. Maternal morbidity is common and 25% to 50% of patients are admitted to an intensive care unit.
- Increased risk of infection, thromboembolism, pyelonephritis, pneumonia, adult respiratory distress syndrome, and renal failure.
- Surgical complications also are common, owing to the frequent need for hysterectomy.

Risks for the Fetus and Newborn

- The average gestational age of delivery of accretas is typically 34 to 36 weeks of gestation, usually resulting from medically indicated preterm birth.
- At term, a placenta accreta typically does not present a risk to the fetus or neonate, but presents a problem in management after delivery.

Assessment Findings

- The mainstay of antenatal diagnosis is obstetric ultrasonography.
- Maternal assessment findings at delivery include:
  - Hypovolemic shock
  - Hypotension
  - Oliguria
  - Thready pulse
  - Shallow/irregular respirations
  - Pallor
  - Cold, clammy skin
  - Anxiety

Medical Management

The timing of delivery in cases of suspected placenta accreta must be individualized (ACOG, 2012b). This decision should be made jointly with the patient, obstetrician, and neonatologist. Patient counseling should include discussion of the potential need for hysterectomy, the risks of profuse hemorrhage, and possible maternal death. Generally, the recommended management of suspected placenta accreta is planned preterm cesarean hysterectomy with the placenta left in situ as removal of the placenta is associated with significant hemorrhagic morbidity. However, this approach might not be considered first-line treatment for women who have a strong desire for future fertility. Therefore, surgical management of placenta accreta may be individualized (ACOG, 2012b).

Nursing Actions

- Monitor lab values including CBC and clotting studies.
- Provide emotional support to the woman and her family.
- Provide information to the woman and her family regarding treatment plan and timing of birth.

Abortion

Abortion is the spontaneous or elective termination of pregnancy before 20 weeks' gestation. Abortions are referred to as induced, elective, therapeutic, and spontaneous. Induced abortion is the medical or surgical termination of pregnancy before fetal viability. Elective abortion is termination of pregnancy before fetal viability at the request of the woman but not for reasons of impaired health of the mother or fetal disease. According to the most recent national estimates, 18% of all pregnancies in the United States end in abortion. Compared with 2012, the total number, rate, and ratio of reported abortions for 2013 decreased 5%. Additionally, from 2004 to 2013, the number, rate, and ratio of reported abortions decreased 20%, 21%, and 17%, respectively.

Termination of pregnancy is done transcervically through dilation of the cervix, then evacuation of the uterus mechanically by curettage, scraping of the contents, or vacuum. Legally induced abortions have an extremely low complication rate. Medical abortion, which involves the use of medications rather than a surgical procedure to induce an abortion, is an option for women who wish to terminate a first-trimester pregnancy (ACOG, 2014b). Early medical abortion with medications such as mifepristone and misoprostol can be highly effective. In 2013, the majority (66.0%) of abortions were performed by ≤8 weeks' gestation, and nearly all (91.6%) were performed by ≤13 weeks' gestation. Few abortions were performed between 14 and 20 weeks' gestation (7.1%) or at ≥21 weeks' gestation (1.3%). From 2004 to 2013, the percentage of all abortions performed at ≤13 weeks' gestation remained consistently high (≥91.5%) and among those performed at ≤13 weeks' gestation, the percentage performed at ≤6 weeks' gestation increased 16%. Most recent data indicate that most abortions (70%) were performed by curettage at ≤13 weeks' gestation and over 20% were performed by early medical abortion (a nonsurgical abortion at ≤8 weeks' gestation) (Jatlaoui et al.,

2016). Women in their twenties accounted for the majority of abortions in 2013 and throughout the period of analysis.

Therapeutic abortion is termination of pregnancy for serious maternal medical indications or serious fetal anomalies. This section focuses on spontaneous abortion as it is associated with hemorrhage. An abortion is defined as legal if it was performed by a licensed clinician within the limits of state law. An abortion is defined as illegal if it was performed by any person other than a licensed clinician.

Nearly all abortions are a result of unintended pregnancy. Multiple factors influence the incidence of abortion, including access to health care services, including contraception; the availability of abortion providers; state regulations, such as mandatory waiting periods or parental involvement laws, and legal restrictions on abortion providers; increasing acceptance of nonmarital childbearing; shifts in the racial/ethnic composition of the U.S. population; and changes in the economy and the resulting impact on fertility preferences and use of contraception (Jatlaoui et al., 2016). However, because unintended pregnancy precedes nearly all abortions, efforts to reduce the incidence of abortion need to focus on helping women, men, and couples avoid unwanted pregnancies.

Early Pregnancy Loss

Spontaneous abortion is defined as a nonviable, intrauterine pregnancy with either an empty gestational sac or a gestational sac containing an embryo or fetus without fetal heart activity within the first 12 ⁶/₇ weeks of gestation. In the first trimester, the terms miscarriage, spontaneous abortion, and early pregnancy loss are used interchangeably.

Hemorrhage in the decidua basalis followed by necrosis of the tissue usually accompanies abortion. Approximately 10% of pregnancies end in spontaneous abortion. Most (80%) occur in the first 12 weeks of gestation and are termed early abortion, and more than half of those are a result of chromosomal abnormalities (ACOG, 2015b). Early pregnancy losses typically are related to an abnormality of the zygote, embryo, fetus, or at times the placenta. Late pregnancy losses are between 12 and 20 weeks' gestation.

Risk Factors for Early Pregnancy Loss

- Increased parity
- Increased maternal and paternal age
- Endocrine abnormalities such as diabetes or luteal phase defects
- Drug use or environmental toxins
- Immunological factors such as autoimmune diseases
- Infections
- Systemic disorders
- Genetic factors
- Uterine or cervical abnormalities

Assessment Findings for Early Pregnancy Loss

- Uterine bleeding first, then cramping abdominal pain in a few hours to several days later
- Ultrasound confirms diagnosis. Early pregnancy loss can be diagnosed with certainty in a woman with an ultrasound-

documented intrauterine pregnancy who subsequently presents with reported significant vaginal bleeding and an empty uterus on ultrasound examination.
- In other instances, the diagnosis of early pregnancy loss is not as clear. Depending on the specific clinical circumstances and how much diagnostic certainty the patient desires, a single serum β-hCG test or ultrasound examination may not be sufficient to confirm the diagnosis of early pregnancy loss.

Medical Management for Early Pregnancy Loss

Accepted treatment options for medical management include expectant management, medical treatment, or surgical evacuation depending on classification and signs and symptoms. In patients for whom medical management of early pregnancy loss is indicated, initial treatment using 800 micrograms of vaginal misoprostol generally is recommended, with a repeat dose as needed.

Accepted treatment options for early pregnancy loss include expectant management, medical treatment, or surgical evacuation. In women without medical complications or symptoms requiring urgent surgical evacuation, treatment plans can safely accommodate patient treatment preferences.

Women who are Rh(D) negative and unsensitized should receive 50 micrograms of Rh(D)-immune globulin immediately after surgical management of early pregnancy loss or within 72 hours of the diagnosis of early pregnancy loss with planned medical management or expectant management in the first trimester.

There are no effective interventions to prevent early pregnancy loss. As with expectant management of early pregnancy loss, women opting for medical treatment should be counseled on what to expect while they pass pregnancy tissue, provided information on when to call regarding bleeding, and given prescriptions for pain medications. Counseling should emphasize that the woman is likely to have bleeding that is heavier than menses (and potentially accompanied by severe cramping). The woman should understand how much bleeding is considered too much. An easy reference for the patient to use is the soaking of two maxi pads per hour for 2 consecutive hours. The patient should be advised to call her obstetrician-gynecologist or other gynecologic provider if she experiences this level of bleeding. As with expectant management, it also is important to counsel patients that surgery may be needed if medical management does not achieve complete expulsion.

Patients undergoing expectant management may experience moderate-to-heavy bleeding and cramping. Educational materials instructing the patient on when and who to call for excessive bleeding and prescriptions for pain medications should be provided.

Nursing Actions Related to Care After Early Pregnancy Loss

- Monitor vital signs per protocol and PRN.
- Monitor bleeding.
- Review labs.
- Give RhoGAM if indicated.
- Follow agency guidelines and facilitate and support the family's decisions about disposition of the products of conception.

● Assess significance of loss to woman and family (Gilbert, 2011).
  ● Acknowledge feeling of sadness, distress, or relief toward pregnancy loss.
  ● Give parents' choices and opportunities for decision making.
  ● Provide family with information on miscarriage, pregnancy loss, and support groups.
● Provide psychological support appropriate to family's response.
● Provide resources to patient and family to educate them about the psychological effects of pregnancy loss.
● Connect patient/family with aftercare, as needed.
● Schedule post-discharge follow-up meeting with patient, as needed.
● Discharge teaching related to self-care and warning signs, including:
  ● Teach pericare.
  ● Pelvic rest includes no tampons, douching, or sexual intercourse for several weeks.
  ● Teach patient to monitor for excessive bleeding and signs and symptoms of infection such as fever and uterine tenderness or foul-smelling discharge.
  ● Teach about diet high in iron and protein for tissue repair and red blood cell replacement.
  ● Review plan for follow-up with care provider.
    ○ Follow-up typically includes confirmation of complete expulsion by ultrasound examination, but serial serum β-hCG measurement may be used instead in settings where ultrasonography is unavailable. Patient-reported symptoms also should be considered when determining whether complete expulsion has occurred.

Ectopic Pregnancy

An ectopic pregnancy (EP) occurs when a fertilized egg grows outside the uterus as a result of the blastocyst implanting somewhere other than the endometrial lining of the uterus (Fig. 7–12). The embryo or fetus in an ectopic pregnancy is absent or stunted, and this is a nonviable pregnancy. Most ectopic pregnancies occur in the fallopian tube (95%), but the fertilized ovum can also implant in the ovary, cervix, or abdominal cavity (5%). Because most ectopic pregnancies are tubal, the focus of this section is on tubal ectopic pregnancy. In a tubal pregnancy, the tube lacks a submucosal layer, and the fertilized ovum burrows through the epithelium of the tubal wall, tapping into the blood vessels; however, the tubal environment cannot support the rapidly proliferating trophoblast.

As the pregnancy grows, it can cause the tube to rupture (burst). If this occurs, it can cause major internal bleeding. This can be life-threatening and must be treated with surgery. The incidence of tubal pregnancy is increasing and not always reported, but is estimated at 1% to 2% (Panelli, Phillips, & Brady, 2015). Hemorrhage from ectopic pregnancy is still the leading cause of pregnancy-related maternal death in the first trimester and accounts for 4% to 10% of all pregnancy-related deaths, despite improved diagnostic methods leading to earlier detection and treatment. Women with tubal pregnancy have diverse clinical symptoms that largely depend on whether there is a rupture.

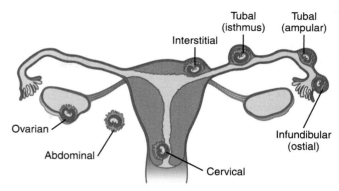

FIGURE 7–12 Sites for ectopic pregnancy.

Risk Factors for Ectopic Pregnancy

Up to 50% of women diagnosed with EPs have no identifiable risk factors; however, a number of risk factors have been associated with EP. Prior EP is a strong risk factor for recurrent EP, with a recurrence rate of 5% to 25%, or up to 10 times the risk in the general population (Panelli et al., 2015). Women who have abnormal fallopian tubes are at higher risk of ectopic pregnancy. Abnormal tubes may be present in women who have had the following conditions:

● Pelvic inflammatory disease (an infection of the uterus, fallopian tubes, and nearby pelvic structures)
● Previous ectopic pregnancy
● Infertility
● Pelvic or abdominal surgery
● Endometriosis
● Sexually transmitted diseases
● Prior tubal surgery (such as tubal sterilization)

Other factors that increase a woman's risk of ectopic pregnancy include the following:

● Cigarette smoking
● Exposure to the drug diethylstilbestrol (DES) during her mother's pregnancy
● Increased age

Risks for the Woman

● Hemorrhage related to rupture of fallopian tube
● Decreased fertility related to removal of fallopian tube

Assessment Findings

Most women now present prior to tubal rupture, and with advances in diagnosis and imaging, the outcomes have dramatically improved. Common findings are:

● Pelvic or abdominal pain
● Light or heavy bleeding that is not at the time of your normal menstrual period (abnormal vaginal bleeding)
● Abdominal or pelvic pain, which can be sudden and sharp and ache without relief or seem to come and go. It may occur on only one side.

- Blood from the ruptured tube can build up under the diaphragm, causing shoulder pain.
- Weakness, dizziness, or fainting caused by blood loss.
- Vital signs become unstable, indicating hypovolemia if hemorrhage is significant.

Medical Management

- Diagnosis generally is made with clinical signs, physical symptoms, serial human chorionic gonadotropin (hCG) levels, transvaginal ultrasonography, and serum progesterone levels.
- Early diagnosis allows for surgical or medical management of unruptured ectopic pregnancy. Treatment in stable patients is often medical, though patients meeting certain clinical criteria or with EPs outside the fallopian tube may require differing and/or more invasive treatment, including excision by laparoscopy or, less commonly, laparotomy.
- If the pregnancy is small and the tube is not ruptured, in some cases the pregnancy can be removed through a small cut made in the tube using laparoscopy. In this procedure, a slender, light-transmitting telescope is inserted through a small opening in your abdomen in a hospital with general anesthesia. A larger incision in the abdomen may be needed if the pregnancy is large or the blood loss is a concern. Some or all of the tube may need to be removed.
- If the pregnancy is small and has not ruptured the tube, sometimes drugs can be used instead of surgery to treat ectopic pregnancy. Medication stops the growth of the pregnancy and permits the body to absorb it over time, allowing the woman to keep her fallopian tube. Non-surgical medical management of ectopic pregnancy may be indicated in an unruptured and hemodynamically stable woman (ACOG, 2008a). Methotrexate, a folic acid antagonist and type of chemotherapy agent, will cause dissolution of the ectopic mass. For patients who are medically unstable or experiencing life-threatening hemorrhage, immediate surgical treatment is indicated.

Nursing Actions

- Ensure stabilization of cardiovascular status.
- Offer explanations and reassurance related to the plan of care.
- Assess response to diagnosis related to anxiety, fear, guilt.
- Provide support related to the pregnancy loss.
- Explain plan for follow-up care, which is determined by treatment plan, surgical or medical.
- Give RhoGAM if indicated.
- Assess significance of loss to woman and family (Gilbert, 2011):
  - Acknowledge feeling of sadness, distress, or relief toward pregnancy loss.
  - Give parents' choices and opportunities for decision making.
  - Provide family with information on pregnancy loss and support groups.
- Provide psychological support appropriate to family's response.

- Discharge teaching related to self-care and warning signs including:
  - Teach patient to monitor for severe abdominal pain, excessive bleeding, and signs and symptoms of infection such as fever.
  - Teach about diet high in iron if woman experiences a high estimated blood loss (EBL).
  - Review plan for follow-up with care provider.
  - Teach patient appropriate pain management.
  - Teach patient signs and symptoms that need to be reported, such as severe abdominal pain, fever, bleeding.
- Special considerations for teaching women treated with methotrexate (ACOG, 2008a):
  - Because methotrexate affects rapidly dividing tissues, gastrointestinal side effects, such as nausea, vomiting, and stomatitis, are the most common. Therefore, women treated with methotrexate should be advised not to use alcohol and nonsteroidal anti-inflammatory drugs (NSAIDs).
  - It is not unusual for women treated with methotrexate to experience abdominal pain 2 to 3 days after administration, presumably from the cytotoxic effect of the drug on the trophoblast tissue, causing tubal abortion.

Gestational Trophoblastic Disease

The term gestational trophoblastic disease refers to a spectrum of placental related tumors. Gestational trophoblastic disease (GTD) is a group of rare diseases in which abnormal trophoblast cells grow inside the uterus after conception (Cunningham et al., 2014). GTD is categorized into molar and nonmolar tumors. Gestational trophoblastic neoplasia (GTN) is a type of gestational trophoblastic disease (GTD) that is almost always malignant. Nonmolar tumors are grouped as gestational trophoblastic neoplasia or malignant gestational trophoblastic disease (ACOG, 2004a). As an example, one of the nonmalignant tumors will be described.

A hydatidiform mole is a benign proliferating growth of the trophoblast in which the chorionic villi develop into edematous, cystic, vascular transparent vesicles that hang in grapelike clusters without a viable fetus (Fig. 7–13). A hydatidiform mole develops in 1 to 2 of 1,000 pregnancies in the United States (Cunningham

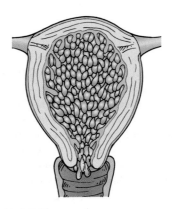

FIGURE 7–13 Hydatidiform mole.

et al., 2014). Most hydatidiform moles are benign, but they sometimes become cancerous. Having one or more of the following risk factors increases the risk that a hydatidiform mole will become cancer. This is a nonviable pregnancy. In a normal pregnancy, the trophoblast cells develop into the placenta and have chorionic villi that form the endometrium. With a hydatidiform mole pregnancy, there is a proliferation of the placenta and trophoblastic cells, which absorb fluid from the maternal blood. Fluid accumulates into the chorionic villi and vesicles form out of the chorionic villi (see Fig. 7–13). The erythroblastic tissue of the complete hydatidiform mole never develops into a fetus. The erythroblastic tissue of a partial hydatidiform mole may include some fetal tissue, but this is always abnormal and never matures.

Risk Factors

- Maternal age younger than 20 or older than 35 years
- Previous molar pregnancy

Risks for the Woman

- Increased risk of choriocarcinoma

Assessment Findings

In addition to vaginal bleeding and uterine enlargement, other presenting symptoms or signs may include:

- Pelvic pain or sensation of pressure
- Anemia
- Hyperemesis gravidarum
- Hyperthyroidism (secondary to the homology between the beta-subunits of hCG and thyroid-stimulating hormone (TSH), which causes hCG to have weak TSH-like activity)
- Preeclampsia early in pregnancy
- Amenorrhea
- Nausea and vomiting
- Abnormal uterine bleeding ranges from spotting to profuse hemorrhage
- Enlarged uterus
- Abdominal cramping and expulsion of vesicles

Diagnosis of Medical Management

- The routine use of ultrasound in early pregnancy can diagnose molar pregnancy much earlier than before.
- hCG and transvaginal ultrasound

Medical Management

- Immediate evacuation of mole with aspiration/suction D&C
- After molar evacuation, all patients should be monitored with serial hCG determinations to diagnose and treat malignant sequelae promptly. Oral contraceptives have been demonstrated to be safe and effective during post treatment monitoring based on randomized controlled trials.
- Women with nonmetastatic gestational trophoblastic disease should be treated with single-agent chemotherapy (ACOG, 2004a).

- Follow-up of hCG levels should be obtained for at least 6 months to detect trophoblastic neoplasia. After hCG levels fall to normal for 6 months, pregnancy can be considered.
- Women with metastatic gestational trophoblastic disease should be referred to specialists with experience treating this disease.

Nursing Actions for Post Evacuation of Mole

- Monitor for signs and symptoms of hemorrhage such as abnormal VS, abdominal pain, vaginal bleeding.
- Assess uterus.
- Offer explanations and reassurance related to the plan of care.
- Offer emotional support related to pregnancy loss.
- Assess response to diagnosis and treatment plan related to anxiety, fear, guilt.
- Provide support related to the pregnancy loss.
- Explain plan for follow-up care related to serial hCG.
- Give RhoGAM if indicated.
- Assess significance of loss to woman and family (Gilbert, 2011).
  - Acknowledge feeling of sadness, distress, or relief toward pregnancy loss.
  - Give parents' choices and opportunities for decision making.
  - Provide family with information on pregnancy loss and support groups.
- Provide psychological support appropriate to family's response.
- Offer resources to patient and family to educate about the psychological effects of pregnancy loss.
- Schedule post-discharge follow-up meeting with patient, as needed.
- Discharge teaching related to self-care and warning signs including (Cunningham et al., 2014; Genovese, 2016):
  - Teach patient to monitor for severe abdominal pain, excessive bleeding, and signs and symptoms of infection such as fever.
  - Review plan for follow-up with care provider and encourage adherence to follow-up regime.
  - Teach patient appropriate pain management.
  - Discuss contraception options and reason to prevent pregnancy for one year.
- Emphasize importance of medical follow-up with regular HCG levels because of the risk of malignant trophoblastic disease and choriocarcinoma.
- Prophylactic chemotherapy is not routinely recommended (ACOG, 2004a).

CRITICAL COMPONENT

Psychosocial Consideration Related to Pregnancy Complications

A woman with pregnancy complication often requires increased surveillance during pregnancy and may require hospitalization. This can result in additional stress for herself, her partner, and her family (Durham, 1998). Hospitalization may involve not only loss of normal routine, but loss of control. Women with high-risk pregnancies may undergo unplanned cesarean birth and/or disruption of birth plans. High-risk pregnancies can result in financial hardship from loss of work hours and increased cost of medical care. Research has found that hospitalized antepartum women reported high levels of physical, emotional, familial, and financial hardship, and a feeling of uncertainty associated with hospitalization (Cowswell, Middleton, & Weeks, 2009). Women may have fear of death or loss of their fetus. After a pregnancy with unplanned outcomes, a woman may experience anxiety related to future pregnancies. It is common for women with high-risk pregnancies to deliver newborns that require tertiary care in the NICU. Mothers may also experience separation from their newborns because of transport of the newborn. Some women report feeling powerless because of this separation. Maternal separation also represents a barrier for women desiring to breastfeed their newborns. These women will require lactation support. Successful breastfeeding for a duration of 6 to 12 months may decrease the risk of future health concerns for the mother and her newborn (Phillips & Boyd, 2016).

INFECTIONS

Infections are a common complication of pregnancy. Intrauterine or perinatally transmitted infections can have severe and debilitating effects on the mother, her sex partner, and the fetus. Infections can be acquired by the fetus transplacentally, such as with HIV; may ascend the birth canal; or can be acquired though contact at the time of a vaginal birth, such as herpes. The impact of infection on pregnancy depends on the infectious organism involved. A thorough history for mother and sex partner should be taken to determine risk of sexually transmitted disease and counseled on perinatal testing recommendations for screening and treatment.

Some infectious agents, such as trichomoniasis and vaginosis, are easily treated and affect only the mother. Other infections, such as rubella and syphilis, can actively infect the fetus during pregnancy. The recommendations to screen pregnant women are thus based on the disease severity and sequelae of prevalence in population, state laws requirements, and the associated costs (CDC, 2015a). In the following section, infections such as HIV, gonorrhea, chlamydia, syphilis, hepatitis B, HPV, HSV, TORCH infections, UTI/pyelonephritis, and GBS are reviewed, highlighting maternal and fetal effects, treatment, and nursing implications (CDC, 2015a).

Human Immunodeficiency Virus (HIV/AIDS)

Human immunodeficiency virus (HIV) is a chronic illness caused by the retrovirus of the lentivirus family that has an affinity for the T-lymphocytes, macrophages, and monocytes. HIV/AIDS is a virus passed from one person to another through blood and sexual contact. There is an increased risk for HIV/AIDS among female adults and adolescents <25 years of age (CDC, 2015c). In 2011 there were about 8,100 females living with classified stage 3 (AIDS) (CDC, 2015a; CDC, 2015b).

Transmission of HIV/AIDS happens through sexual contact without condoms, a high number of partners, presence of genital sores, and presence of other sexually transmitted diseases. It is also transmitted by exposure to blood, blood products, or by-products such as blood transfusion, needle sharing, and accidental inoculation via occupational exposure (CDC, 2015b). Transmission of HIV perinatally happens through transplacental, intrapartal, and breast milk exposure. Before the use of antiviral therapy in pregnancy, the risk of infection for a neonate to an HIV seropositive mother was approximately 25%, ranging from 13% to 39%. However, today most pregnant women who have HIV are on a regular antiretroviral drug regimen, decreasing their HIV viral load to undetectable. As a result, the rate of maternal-child transmission has decreased (CDC, 2015b).

Factors Associated With Increased Perinatal Transmission

- Mother with AIDS
- Preterm delivery
- Decreased maternal CD4 count
- High maternal viral load
- Chorioamnionitis
- Blood exposure due to episiotomy, vaginal laceration, and forceps delivery

Risks to Fetus and Newborn

- Risk of transmission is 20% to 25% without the use of antiretroviral drugs but can be as low as 2% with appropriate antepartal drug treatment.
- Preterm delivery
- Preterm PROM
- IUGR

Assessment Findings

- Physical findings include fever, fatigue, vomiting, diarrhea, weight loss, generalized lymphadenopathy, cognitive changes, neurological disorder, PID, TORCH infections, oral gingivitis, vaginitis, and opportunistic infection.
- Psychosocial findings include anxiety, fear, lack of social support, stress, depression, denial, emotional instability, financial instability, and lack of resources.

Medical Management

- Perform routine screening starting at first perinatal visit. CD4 counts should be tested at first antenatal visit and every three months during pregnancy. HIV RNA should be tested between 36 and 38 weeks' of gestation to determine safest method of delivery (Panel on Treatment of Pregnant Women with HIV Infection and Prevention of Perinatal Transmission, 2018).
- Treatment of at least three antiretroviral drugs

Nursing Actions in Antepartal Period

- Provide education and counseling on plan of care.
- Provide education and counseling on potential consequences of pregnancy on HIV disease progress, risk for transmission, and consequences for neonate.
- Education to facilitate health promotion
  - Adequate sleep
  - Adequate diet as protein deficiency can depress immunity; adequate zinc and vitamin A for cell growth
  - Avoidance of infection
- Provide emotional support.
- If the woman is diagnosed with HIV during pregnancy, she needs extensive and ongoing education and counseling on plan of care and management.

Nursing Actions in Intrapartal Period

- Avoid using instruments during birth.
- Leave fetal membranes intact.
- Avoid fetal scalp electrode.
- Avoid episiotomy and assisted vaginal delivery.
- Provide and reinforce education.
- Provide emotional support.

Sexually Transmitted Infections/ Diseases (STI/STD)

Sexually transmitted infections (STIs), sometimes referred to as sexually transmitted diseases (STDs) remain a major public health challenge in the United States. The Centers for Disease Control and Prevention (CDC, 2015a) estimates that 20 million new infections occur every year, almost half of them among young people age 15 to 24 years. STIs affect women of every socioeconomic and educational level, age, race, and ethnicity. The two most common reported infections in the United States are chlamydia and gonorrhea, which primarily affect women ages 15 to 24 (CDC, 2015a). Women also receive routine testing for syphilis, hepatitis B, HIV, and human papillomavirus (HPV) during prenatal care. Though not routinely tested, if the woman has a history of herpes simplex virus (HSV) or reports new onset signs and symptoms, further testing is recommended.

In addition to the physical and psychological consequences, the costs of treating STIs are estimated at more than $16 billion annually (CDC, 2015a). Table 7–4 provides a summary of fetal and maternal effects and management of STIs/STDs. Women who are pregnant can become infected with the same STIs as women who are not pregnant. Pregnancy does not provide protection for the woman or the baby, and consequences of an STI can be serious in pregnancy, even life-threatening for the woman and her baby. Intrauterine or perinatal transmitted STIs can have severely debilitating effects on women, their partners, and their fetuses. All women should be screened for STIs during their first prenatal visit.

Prevention and control of STDs is the best way to reduce and eliminate potential harm. Five strategies used to promote prevention include (CDC, 2015a):

- Accurate risk assessment and education and counseling of persons at risk on ways to avoid STDs through changes in sexual behaviors and use of recommended prevention services

- Pre-exposure vaccination of persons at risk for vaccine-preventable STDs
- Identification of asymptomatically infected persons and persons with symptoms associated with STDs
- Effective diagnosis, treatment, counseling, and follow up of infected persons; and evaluation, treatment, and counseling of sex partners of persons who are infected with an STD

Risks for the Woman

- STIs can cause pelvic inflammatory disease (Table 7–4).
- Pelvic inflammatory disease (PID) can lead to infertility, chronic hepatitis, and cervical and other cancers.
- STIs during pregnancy can lead to PTL, PROM, and uterine infection.
- Table 7–4 summarizes information on maternal effects and management of STIs (CDC, 2015b).

Risks for the Fetus

- STIs can pass to the fetus by crossing the placenta; some can be transmitted to the baby during delivery as the baby passes through the birth canal (see Table 7–3).
- Harmful effects to babies include preterm birth, low birth weight, neonatal sepsis, and neurological damage.

Assessment Findings

- Many STIs in women are "silent" without signs and symptoms, making routine screening for STIs during the first prenatal visit an important part of routine prenatal care.
- Physical findings include low-grade temperature, poor personal hygiene, genital warts, purulent urethral or cervical discharge, friable cervix, genital lesions, tender uterus, pain on motion of cervix, inguinal adenopathy, and rash on palms and soles of feet.
- Positive STI cultures and test results

Medical Management

- Provide routine screening of STIs and HIV at first prenatal visit.
- Treat bacterial STIs with antibiotics.
- Prescribe antiviral medications for viral STIs to reduce symptoms.

Nursing Actions

- Provide information on STIs.
- Provide emotional support.
- Instruct the woman on correct administration of medications and other treatments and importance of completing treatment.
- Instruct the patient on the warning signs of complication (fever, increased pain, bleeding).
- Provide information on the importance of abstaining from intercourse until the patient and her partner are free of infection.
- Provide the partner with treatment as indicated.

TABLE 7–4   Summary of Fetal and Maternal Effects and Management of STIs/STDs

INFECTION	MATERNAL EFFECTS	FETAL EFFECTS	MANAGEMENT	NURSING ISSUES
Chlamydia *Chlamydia Trachomatis*	Three-fourths of women have no symptoms, so it is known as a "silent" disease; may have burning on urination or abnormal vaginal discharge.	Contact at delivery may cause conjunctivitis and/or premature birth. The efficacy of ophthalmia neonatorum prophylaxis is unclear.	During pregnancy, treatment with oral antibiotics such as amoxicillin, azithromycin, erythromycin	Can lead to pelvic inflammatory disease (PID). Treat all infected partners. Retest in 3 weeks.
Gonorrhea *Neisseria Gonorrhoeae*	Most women have no symptoms but may have burning on urination, increased purulent yellow-green vaginal discharge, or bleeding between periods. Rectal infection can cause anal itching, discharge, and bleeding. Can lead to PID.	Contact at birth. Ophthalmia neonatorum may cause sepsis and/or blindness. To prevent gonococcal ophthalmia neonatorum, a prophylactic antibiotic ointment should be instilled into the eyes of all newborns.	During pregnancy, treatment with antibiotics such as cephalosporin	Can lead to PID. Complete treatment.
Group B Streptococcus *Streptococcus Agalactiae* (GBS)	Women are typically asymptomatic carriers. Symptoms can include abnormal vaginal discharge, urinary tract infections, chorioamnionitis.	Transmission rates are low, 1%–2%, but infection can result in invasive GBS with permanent neurological sequelae.	If GBS-positive at 35–37 weeks of gestation or GBS status unknown, treat with antibiotics in labor to prevent neonatal transmission; penicillin or ampicillin IV	GBS-positive women receive intrapartum antibiotic prophylaxis.
Hepatitis B (HBV)	50% asymptomatic; may have low-grade fever, anorexia, nausea and vomiting, fatigue, rashes. Chronic infection can lead to cirrhosis of the liver and liver cancer.	90% of infected infants have chronic infection. Cirrhosis of the liver Liver cancer	Serial testing for viral load can be completed. No specific treatment is available.	HBsAg-positive pregnant women should be reported to the state or local health department for timely and appropriate prophylaxis for their infants. Immunoprophylaxis of all newborns born to HBsAg-positive women. HBIG to neonate at delivery and hepatitis B vaccination series initiated.
Hepatitis CRNA Virus (HCV)	80% of persons infected have no symptoms. Can lead to chronic liver disease, cirrhosis, and liver cancer.	Exposure transplacentally. Estimated 2%–7% transmission rate. Little research on treatment of children.	Ribavirin and interferon, but are contraindicated in pregnancy	Breastfeeding is not contraindicated.
Human Papillomavirus (HPV) Thirty or more types infect the genital area.	The majority of HPV infections are asymptomatic but can cause genital warts. Genital warts are flat, papular, or pedunculated growths on the genital mucosa.	Route of transmission unclear. Can cause respiratory papillomatosis.	Testing for HPD is done with routine PAP smear. If warts are present, they may be removed during pregnancy. Treatment reduces but does not eliminate HPV infection.	The presence of genital warts is not an indication for cesarean delivery.

TABLE 7–4	Summary of Fetal and Maternal Effects and Management of STIs/STDs—cont'd			
INFECTION	**MATERNAL EFFECTS**	**FETAL EFFECTS**	**MANAGEMENT**	**NURSING ISSUES**
Syphilis *Treponema Pallidum*	Ulcer or chancre, then maculopapular rash advancing to CNS and multiorgan damage.	Transplacental transmission. Congenital syphilis may cause preterm birth, physical deformity, neurological complications, stillbirth, and/or neonatal death.	Penicillin	
Trichomonas *Trichomonas Vaginalis*	Malodorous yellow-green vaginal discharge and vulvar irritation. Can lead to premature rupture of membrane and preterm labor.	Preterm delivery and low birth weight. Respiratory and genital infection.	Metronidazole	
Candidiasis *Candida Albicans**	Results from a disturbance in vaginal flora. Pruritus, vaginal soreness, dyspareunia, abnormal vaginal discharge with a yeasty odor		Topical azole therapies	
Bacterial Vaginosis†	50% of women are asymptomatic. A fishy odor and/or vaginal discharge. Can result in preterm labor and/or premature rupture of membranes.	Premature rupture of membranes, chorioamnionitis, and/or preterm birth	Metronidazole or clindamycin	
Human Immunodeficiency Virus (HIV/AIDS)	May be asymptomatic for years. HIV weakens the immune system. It may manifest as mononucleosis-like symptoms such as fever, fatigue, sore throat, and lymphadenopathy.	Early antiretroviral treatment has been shown to be effective in reducing maternal–fetal transmissions. Placental transmission but <2% transmission with maternal treatment with antiretroviral medications. 15%–25% transmission to fetus without maternal treatment. Antibody screening is not reliable during infancy because maternally produced IgG antibodies to HIV are present for up to 18 months.	Antiviral	Cesarean birth may be considered. Breastfeeding is contraindicated. Case management follow-up for both the woman and her baby.

CDC, 2015a & c.

*Not an STI.

† A polymicrobial clinical syndrome

TORCH Infections

TORCH is an acronym that stands for Toxoplasmosis, Other (hepatitis B), Rubella, and Cytomegalovirus and Herpes simplex virus. TORCH infections are unique in their pathogenesis and have potentially devastating effects on the fetus (Table 7–5). Each disease can cross the placenta and may adversely affect the developing fetus. These teratogenic effects of each disease vary depending on the developmental stage and gestational time of exposure (CDC, 2015a).

Cytomegalovirus (CMV) is the most common cause of congenital infection, and the risk of vertical transmission to the fetus in pregnancy is 30% to 40%. CMV has been identified to cause CNS deficits such as mental retardation, cerebral palsy, seizures, chorioretinitis, and neurosensory hearing loss when transferred to the fetus. Women who develop a CMV infection in the first trimester are more likely to deliver fetuses with neurosensory birth deficits and CNS sequelae than women infected in the second or third trimester. In cases where maternal CMV infection is suspected, it is important to evaluate the risk to the fetus of being infected and/or symptomatically affected by CMV to provide appropriate counseling and guidance to parents (Carlson, Norwitz, & Stiller, 2010).

Risk Factors

The risk status for these infections varies based on route of transmission. Some are sexually transmitted diseases, such as herpes; others have various routes of transmission to woman (CDC, 2015b).

Risk for the Woman

- Depends on the infectious agent (CDC, 2015b; see Table 7–5)

Risks for the Fetus

- The usual route of transmission to the fetus is transplacentally (see Table 7–5).
- Infections acquired in utero can result in intrauterine growth restriction, prematurity, chronic postnatal infection, and even death.

Assessment Findings

- Maternal assessment findings vary with the organism (see Table 7–5).

Medical Management

- Medical management varies based on the organism, trimester of exposure, and clinical evidence of neonatal sequelae (see Table 7–5).

Nursing Actions

- Nursing considerations vary with the organism (see Table 7–5).
- Provide emotional support.
- Instruct woman on treatment plan.

Urinary Tract Infection and Pyelonephritis

Urinary tract infections (UTI) are the most common bacterial infections during pregnancy. They are associated with risk to both mother and fetus and can contribute to preterm labor and birth, cause low birth weight, lead to pyelonephritis and overall increase the risk of perinatal mortality. Pregnant women can be both symptomatic and asymptomatic. Those with symptomatic UTI are treated prophylactically throughout their pregnancy with oral antibiotics (Johnson & Wolfe, 2014).

Assessment and Findings

- Infections can develop from the ascending colonization of preexisting vaginal, perineal and fecal flora.
- Maternal physiological and anatomical factors can predispose women to ascending infections. Urinary retention due to an enlarging uterus and urinary stasis due to hormonal changes can also contribute to UTIs.
- History of UTI before in pregnancy or childhood.
- Increased risk of UTI related to advanced maternal age, low socioeconomic status, underlining chronic illnesses such as preeclampsia, sickle cell trait, diabetes, and hypertension.
- Associated with poor hygiene, frequent intercourse, recent catheterization, and abdominal trauma or pelvic surgery
- Symptoms include frequency, dysuria, hematuria, fever, chills, malaise, nocturia, malodorous urine, flank pain or tenderness, nausea, vomiting, diarrhea, and low abdominal tenderness or pain.
- Diagnostic testing of urine. Positive result associated with more than 100,000 colonies /mL of bacteria in the urine from a clean catch midstream sample.
- *E. Coli* account for 80% to 90% of UTIs.

Medical Management

- All pregnant women should have a urine culture completed at first prenatal appointment.
- Obtain follow-up cultures and surveillance for recurrent UTI.

Nursing Actions

- Provide education and support of prevention and signs and symptoms of UTI.
- Instruct patient on the use and importance of completion of antibiotic treatment with possible prophylactic treatment throughout pregnancy.
- Instruct patient on the early labor precautions and to report them immediately.
- Provide information related to proper hygiene and wiping, prompt void, and adequate daily hydration.

Group Beta Streptococcus (GBS)

Group B Streptococcus (GBS) colonizes the female genital tract and rectum. It has been known to cause UTI, pyelonephritis, chorioamnionitis, preterm labor, vaginal discharge, postpartum

TABLE 7–5 Torch Infections

INFECTION	MATERNAL EFFECTS	FETAL EFFECTS	PREVENTION AND MANAGEMENT	NURSING ISSUES
Toxoplasmosis *Toxoplasma Gondii* Single-celled protozoan parasite Transplacental transmission	Most infections are asymptomatic but may cause fatigue, muscle pains, pneumonitis, myocarditis, and lymphadenopathy.	Severity varies with gestational age and congenital infection. Can lead to spontaneous abortion, low birth weight, hepatosplenomegaly, icterous, anemia, chorioretinitis, and/or neurological disease. Incidence of congenital infection is low.	Avoid eating raw meat and contact with cat feces. Treatment with sulfadiazine or pyrimethamine after the first trimester	Teach women to avoid raw meat and cat feces. Almost 50% of adults have an antibody to this organism.
Other infections hepatitis B Direct contact with blood or body fluid from infected person	30%–50% of infected women are asymptomatic. Symptoms include low-grade fever, nausea, anorexia, jaundice, hepatomegaly, preterm labor, and preterm delivery.	Infants have a 90% chance of becoming chronically infected, HBV carrier, and a 25% risk of developing significant liver disease.	Infant receives HBIG and hepatitis vaccine at delivery.	Universal screening recommended in pregnancy. HBV can be given in pregnancy.
Rubella (German measles) Nasopharyngeal secretions Transplacental	Erythematous maculopapular rash, lymph node enlargement, slight fever, headache, malaise	Overall risk of congenital rubella syndrome is 20% for primary maternal infection in the first trimester and 50% if the woman is infected in the first 4 weeks of gestation. Anomalies include deafness, eye defects, CNS anomalies, and severe cardiac malformations.	Primary approach to rubella infection is immunization. If the woman is pregnant and not immune, she should not receive the vaccine until the postpartum period.	If the woman is not immune, she should not receive the vaccine until the postpartum period and be counseled to not become pregnant for 3 months.
Cytomegalovirus (CMV) Virus of herpes group Transmitted by droplet contact and transplacentally	Most infections are asymptomatic, but 15% of adults may have mononucleosis-like syndrome.	Infection to fetus is most likely with primary maternal infection and timing of infection with first- and second-trimester exposure. May result in low birth weight, IUGR, hearing impairment microcephaly, and CNS abnormalities.	No treatment is available.	
Herpes Simplex Virus (HSV) Chronic lifelong viral infection Contact at delivery and ascending infection	Painful genital lesions. Lesions may be on external or internal genitalia.	Transmission rate of 30%–50% among women who acquire genital herpes near time of delivery and is low (<1%) among women with recurrent genital herpes. Mortality of 50%–60% if neonatal exposure to active primary lesion is related to neurological complications of massive infection sepsis and neurological complications.	No cure available. Acyclovir to suppress outbreak of lesions.	Most common viral STI. Protect the neonate from exposure with cesarean delivery if active lesion.

Source: *CDC, 2015a & c.*

endometritis, post cesarean section wound infection, and in rare instances endocarditis (American Academy of Pediatrics [AAP] and the American College of Obstetricians and Gynecologists [ACOG], 2012).

Maternal and Neonatal Risks

- Premature labor
- Maternal intrapartum fever for prolonged rupture of membranes >12 hours
- Neonatal prematurity
- Transmission rate from mother to infant at birth is 50% to 75%
- On rare occasions, ultrasound has shown evidence of fetal hydrops and has been associated with fetal death.
- Prevalence of neonatal GBS is 0.5 per 1000 births.
- Approximately 30% to 50% of pregnant women are carriers of GBS.

Assessment and Findings

- Common cause of sepsis, meningitis, and pneumonia
- Positive test for GBS in current pregnancy or previous pregnancy. CDC recommends routine cultures of vagina and rectum between 35 and 37 weeks' gestation.

Medical Management

- Treatment of positive test results with ampicillin or penicillin during labor
- Review of previous history of GBS

Nursing Management

- Provide instruction on the importance of GBS antibiotic therapy during pregnancy.
- Assess for signs and symptoms of fever or sepsis during prenatal care through delivery.

TRAUMA DURING PREGNANCY

Trauma is the leading cause of maternal death during pregnancy and is more likely to cause maternal death than any other complication of pregnancy. The most common cause of maternal death by trauma is abdominal injury (resulting in hemorrhagic shock) and head injury. Motor vehicle accidents and domestic violence/intimate partner violence are the predominant causes of reported trauma during pregnancy (Mendez-Figueroa, Dahlke, Vrees, & Rouse, 2013). Injury to the pregnant woman can result from blunt or penetrating trauma. The most common cause of blunt injury is motor vehicle accidents. The most common cause of penetrating trauma is from gunshot wounds. The mechanisms of maternal and fetal injury, gestational age of the fetus, and secondary complications determine the maternal-fetal response to trauma. Maternal outcome in trauma corresponds to the severity of the injury.

Fetal outcome depends on injury and maternal physiological response (Van Otterloo, 2016).

It is essential to keep in mind that at term, 15% of maternal cardiac output, 750 mL to 1000 mL/min, flows through the placental bed; unresolved bleeding can lead to maternal exsanguination in 8 to 10 minutes (Burke-Sosa, 2014).

A wide array of complications has been associated with obstetric trauma, including maternal injury, death, shock, hemorrhage, intrauterine fetal demise, abruptio placenta, and uterine rupture; therefore, timely and efficient evaluation is critical to ensure maternal-fetal well-being. That typically includes history and physical examination, lab work, assessment of fetal heart rate and uterine activity, ultrasound, and radiologic studies (Mirza, Devine, & Gaddipati, 2010). Goals of management of the pregnant patient suffering trauma focuses on prevention of hypoxemia, acidosis, hypotension, and hyperventilation to stabilize the mother and avoid fetal hypoxia (Callahan, 2016).

Pregnancy causes both anatomic and physiological changes that impact the woman's response to traumatic injury. For example, increased plasma volume by 50% and increased red blood cell volume of 30% can mask hemorrhage. Any condition that results in maternal hypotension, such as hemorrhage or hypovolemia, results in vasoconstriction of the uterine arteries and shunting of blood to vital organs. The shunting of blood from the uteroplacental unit maintains maternal blood pressure at the expense of perfusion to the fetus. The pregnant woman has decreased oxygen reserves and decreased blood buffering capacity, which leaves the pregnant trauma patient vulnerable to hypoxemia and less able to compensate when acidemia occurs (Baldisseri, 2016; Maharaj, 2007). Two catastrophic events can occur during pregnancy after blunt trauma to the abdomen:

- Placental abruption
- Uterine rupture

Extensive discussion of management and care during trauma in pregnancy is beyond the scope of this chapter, but key elements of stabilization of the woman and the fetus and assessments are briefly reviewed. Treatment priorities for injured pregnant women typically are directed as they would be for nonpregnant women. Some important considerations related to pregnancy are presented in the following section.

Assessment Findings

Assessment findings are based on injury. Initial maternal evaluation is the systematic evaluation performed according to the standard Advanced Trauma Life Support (ATLS) protocols. Initial maternal evaluation and resuscitation takes precedence over fetal evaluation. Early recognition of maternal compromise and rapid resuscitation reduces maternal mortality, which in turn reduces fetal mortality.

- Physiological changes in pregnancy might delay the usual vital sign changes of hypovolemia; blood loss of up to 1,500 mL can occur without a change in maternal vital sign changes.
- Uterine contractions more frequently than every 10 minutes may be an indication of placental abruption (Cunningham et al., 2014).

● Fetal well-being reflects maternal and fetal status, and conversely fetal heart rate changes may indicate maternal deterioration such as hypoxia.

Medical Management

Treatment priorities and medical management for the pregnant trauma patient are the same as for the non-pregnant woman in the initial evaluation. Admission and continuous fetal monitoring for 24 to 48 hours after stabilization, particularly for abdominal injuries because of the increased incidence of placental abruption, is recommended.

● Pregnant women greater than 20 weeks should be monitored for a minimum of four hours for uterine activity. The Kleinhauer-Betke test should be performed on all pregnant women who sustain major trauma.
● Consider obstetrical ultrasound.

Nursing Actions

● Treatment priorities for injured pregnant women typically are directed as they would be for non-pregnant women.
● Initial actions in trauma care are focused on maternal stabilization (Callahan, 2016).
● Evaluate uterine activity and fetal status.
● All women of childbearing age should be screened for intimate partner violence.
● To improve the effectiveness of CPR, clinicians should perform left lateral uterine displacement by tilting the whole maternal body 25 to 30 degrees.

PREGESTATIONAL COMPLICATIONS

Women who enter pregnancy with a preexisting disease or chronic medical condition are at increased risk for complication and are considered high risk. These high-risk pregnancies require extensive surveillance and collaboration of multiple disciplines to achieve an optimal pregnancy outcome. Women often experience fear and anxiety for their health and that of the fetus regarding the impact of the chronic disease on the pregnancy outcome. Any preexisting medical disease can complicate the pregnancy or be exacerbated during pregnancy. Increasing numbers of women with chronic diseases are achieving pregnancy. Nursing care is focused on decreasing complications and providing support and education to patients and families to facilitate their participation in their health care during pregnancy.

Women and their families should participate in decision making and the plan of care to optimize outcomes for both the woman and the fetus. Maternal safety is the prime consideration in all pregnancies. The major preexisting medical complications that impact pregnancy are discussed in this chapter, although all of the possible preexisting medical conditions impacting pregnancy are beyond the scope of this chapter. When caring for women who have preexisting diseases, textbooks on high-risk pregnancy management and perinatal journals are the best sources of information.

CRITICAL COMPONENT

The Importance of Patient-Centered Pregnancy Care

Women experiencing pregnancy complications are especially physiologically, psychologically, emotionally, and spiritually vulnerable. Nurses are in a unique position to explore a woman's needs and advocate for the woman's participation in management of pregnancy complications. It is essential to recognize the patient or designee as the source of control and full partner in providing compassionate and coordinated care based on respect for the patient's preferences, values, and needs.

Some suggestions to foster respect for a woman's preferences, values, and needs include:

• Elicit patient values, preferences, and expressed needs as part of clinical interview, implementation of care plan, and evaluation of care.
• Communicate patient values, preferences, and expressed needs to other members of the health care team.
• Value the patient's expertise with her own health and symptoms.
• Respect patient and family preferences for degree of active engagement in care process.

Cardiovascular Disorders

Pregnancy complicated by cardiovascular disease is potentially dangerous to maternal and fetal well-being and is the leading non-obstetric cause of maternal mortality (Yancy, 2016). The incidence of cardiac disease among pregnant women ranges from 0.5% to 4% and varies in form and severity (Gaddipati & Troiano, 2013). Cardiac disease during pregnancy may be categorized as congenital, acquired, or ischemic. The spectrum and severity of heart disease observed in reproductive-age women is changing. Today, congenital heart disease accounts for more than half of cardiac disease in pregnancy, and ischemic heart disease is on the rise as a result of obesity, hypertension, diabetes, and delayed childbearing (Arafeh, 2014). Some of the normal cardiac changes during pregnancy can exacerbate cardiac disease during pregnancy, including:

● Increase in total blood volume 30% to 50%
● Increase in cardiac output that peaks at 28 to 32 weeks of gestation
● Plasma volume expansion by 45%
● Increase in RBC by 20%
● Increased cardiac output by 40%
● Increased heart rate by 15%
● Decreased diastolic blood pressure by 10 to 15 mm Hg at 24 to 32 weeks (Arafeh, 2014)

- Heart slightly enlarges and displaces upward and to the left anatomically.
- The weight of the gravid uterus can lie on the inferior vena cava, causing compression and hypotension and decreasing cardiac output.
- Increased estrogen leads to vasodilatation, which lowers peripheral resistance and increases cardiac output.
- Autonomic nervous system influences are more prominent on blood pressure.

Marked hemodynamic changes in pregnancy can have a profound effect on the pregnant woman with cardiac disease and may result in exceeding the functional capacity of the diseased heart (Arafeh, 2014; Cunningham et al., 2014; Yancy, 2016), resulting in:

- Pulmonary hypertension
- Pulmonary edema
- Congestive heart failure
- Maternal or fetal death

Extensive discussion of specific cardiac disorders and their management is beyond the scope of this text. Reference to texts that deal with management of high-risk pregnancy, particularly during labor and delivery, is indicated when caring for women with underlying heart disease, but general principles are presented. The management of cardiac disease is related to the cardiac disorder that is present and the impact it has on cardiac function responsible for specific symptoms.

Risks for the Woman

- Maternal mortality with cardiac disorders ranges from 1% to 50% based on cardiac disorder.
- Maternal effects include severe pulmonary edema, systemic emboli, and congestive heart failure.

Risks for the Fetus and Newborn

- Fetal effects are a result of decreased systemic circulation and/or decreased oxygenation.
- If maternal circulation is compromised because of decreased cardiac function, uterine blood flow is reduced, which can result in intrauterine growth restriction. Fetal oxygenation is impaired when maternal oxygenation is impaired.
- Fetal hypoxia can result in permanent CNS damage depending on length and severity of decreased oxygenation.
- If the woman has congenital heart disease, there is an increased incidence of fetal congenital cardiac anomalies (Yancy, 2016).
- Neonatal death secondary to maternal cardiac disease ranges from 3% to 50%.

Assessment Findings

- Diagnosis of cardiac disease is based on symptoms and diagnostic tests, which may include ECG, echocardiogram, and lab tests.
- The usual signs of deteriorating cardiac function include:
  - Dyspnea, severe enough to limit usual activity
  - Progressive orthopnea

- Paroxysmal nocturnal dyspnea
- Syncope during or after exertion
- Palpitations
- Chest pain with or without activity
- Arrhythmias
- Fatigue
- Cyanosis
- Thromboembolitic changes
- Fluid retention

Medical Management

Medical management varies based on cardiac disease and should include collaboration between obstetricians, maternal fetal medicine specialists, cardiologists, anesthesiologists, and other specialists as needed. Discuss with the woman estimations of maternal and fetal mortality, potential chronic morbidity, and interventions to minimize risk during pregnancy and delivery.

- Obtain laboratory test to evaluate renal function and profusion (electrolytes, serum creatinine, proteins, and uric acid).
- Invasive hemodynamic monitoring using pulmonary artery catheters, peripheral arterial catheters, or central venous pressure monitors may be necessary.
- Drug therapy is dependent on cardiac lesion.
- Vaginal delivery is recommended for most patients with cardiac disease.
- Preterm delivery may be indicated for deteriorating maternal or fetal status.

Nursing Actions

- Nursing measures are directed toward prevention of complications and early identification of deteriorating cardiac status.
- Review the woman's history related to cardiovascular disorder, including previous therapies or surgery, current medications, and current functional classification of cardiac disease.
- Conduct a cardiovascular assessment (Gaddipati & Troiano, 2013) that includes:
  - Auscultation of heart, lungs, and breath sounds
  - LOC, BP, HR, capillary refill check
  - Evaluation of respiratory rate and rhythm
  - Evaluation of cardiac rate and rhythm
  - Body weight and weight gain
  - Assessment of skin color, temperature, and turgor
  - Identification of pathological edema
- Additional noninvasive assessment may include:
  - O_2 saturation via pulse oximeter
  - Arrhythmia assessment with 12-lead EKG
  - Electrocardiogram
  - Urinary output
  - Electronic fetal monitoring
- Review laboratory results related to renal function and perfusion.
  - Electrolytes, blood urea nitrogen (BUN), serum creatinine, proteins, uric acid
- Determine the patient's and family's understanding of the effect of her cardiac disease on her pregnancy.

- Provide information to the woman and her family regarding status of woman and fetus and plan of care.
  - Antepartal testing including NSTs, BPPs, and ultrasounds
  - New medications may include anticoagulation therapy; therefore, women need to learn to give self-injections.
- Provide emotional support to the woman and her family.
- Refer patient to high-risk pregnancy support groups.
- Monitor for signs and symptoms of thromboembolism and infection.
- Review diet and activity guidelines.
- Discuss the importance of regular medical follow-up with multidisciplinary team.
- Facilitate home health and other referrals PRN.

Hematological Disorders

Pregnancy results in intravascular volume expansion, with the increase in plasma volume larger than the rise in erythrocyte volume, resulting in hemodilution of pregnancy that results in a drop in the hemoglobin and hematocrit. During pregnancy, there is an increased potential for thrombosis resulting from increased levels of coagulation factors and decreased fibrinolysis, venous dilation, and obstruction of the venous system by the gravid uterus. Thromboembolic diseases occurring most frequently in pregnancy include deep vein thrombosis and pulmonary embolism; both are addressed in this chapter.

Iron-Deficiency Anemia

Anemia complicates 15% to 60% of all pregnancies (Yancy, 2016), and 75% of those anemias are a result of iron deficiency related to a diet low in iron content and insufficient iron stores. Pregnancy results in an intravascular volume expansion with the increase in plasma volume larger than the rise in RBCs, resulting in the hemodilution of pregnancy; the net result is a physiological drop in hemoglobin and hematocrit values. Iron deficiency anemia during pregnancy is the consequence primarily of expansion of plasma volume without normal expansion of maternal hemoglobin mass. During pregnancy, the two main causes of iron-deficiency anemia are iron deficiency and acute blood loss (Cunningham et al., 2014). Anemia is present if the hemoglobin drops below 11 g/dL in the first and third trimesters and below 10 g/dL in the second trimester (Yancy, 2016). Discussion of acquired and inherited anemias and hemoglobinopathies are beyond the scope of this chapter.

Risk Factors

- History of poor nutritional status or eating disorder
- Close spacing of pregnancies
- Multiple gestation
- Excessive bleeding
- Adolescence

Risks for the Woman

- Fatigue
- Reduced tolerance to activity

Risks for the Newborn

- Preterm birth
- Intrauterine growth restriction

Assessment Findings

- Pallor
- Fatigue, weakness, and malaise
- Reduced exercise tolerance and dyspnea
- Anorexia and/or pica
- Edema
- Hemoglobin below 10 to 11 g/dL
- Hematocrit below 30%
- Serum ferritin levels below 10 to 15 mg/L (Cunningham et al., 2014)

Medical Management

- Iron supplementation with at least 200 mg daily of elemental iron compounds, such as ferrous sulfate, fumarate, or gluconate (Cunningham et al., 2014)

Nursing Actions

- Refer the woman to a dietitian for nutritional counseling and reinforce dietary interventions.
- Advise that taking iron supplementation at bedtime and on an empty stomach may increase absorption and decrease gastrointestinal upset.
- Discuss strategies to deal with constipation PRN.
- Assess fatigue and develop interventions and a plan of care to deal with fatigue.
- Monitor hemoglobin and hematocrit levels throughout pregnancy.

Pulmonary Disorders

Normal physiological changes of pregnancy can cause a woman with a history of compromised respiratory function to decompensate. Pulmonary disease has become more prevalent in women of childbearing age. Pulmonary diseases, such as pneumonia or tocolytic-induced pulmonary edema, can develop during pregnancy whereas other conditions such as asthma preexist. It is important to remember that some of the normal respiratory changes during pregnancy can exacerbate respiratory disease during pregnancy. Alteration in the immune system and mechanical and anatomical changes have a cumulative effect to decrease tolerance to hypoxia and acute changes in pulmonary function (Gilbert, 2011; McMurtry-Baird & Kennedy, 2014). These include the following:

- Increased progesterone during pregnancy results in maternal hyperventilation and increased tidal volume.
- Changes in configuration of the thorax with advancing pregnancy decrease residual capacity and volume while oxygen consumption increases.
- Increased estrogen levels result in mucosal edema, hypersecretion, and capillary congestion.
- Respiratory physiology in normal pregnancy tends toward respiratory alkalosis.

Respiratory emergencies, such as pulmonary embolism and amniotic fluid embolism (anaphylactoid syndrome), are discussed in other sections of the chapter. Asthma is presented as an exemplar of the impact of pregnancy on a preexisting pulmonary disorder.

Asthma

Asthma is the most common form of lung disease that can impact pregnancy and complicates about 8% of pregnancies. Asthma is a chronic syndrome characterized by varying levels of airway obstruction, bronchial hyperresponsiveness, and bronchial edema. Severe and poorly controlled asthma may be associated with increased prematurity, need for cesarean delivery, preeclampsia, growth restriction, and maternal morbidity and mortality (AAP & ACOG, 2012).

Diagnosis and management goals of asthma during pregnancy are the same as for nonpregnant women. People with asthma have airways that are hyperresponsive to allergens, viruses, air pollutants, exercise, and cold air. This hyperresponsiveness is manifested by bronchospasm, mucosal edema, and mucus plugging the airways. Goals of therapy include (Yancy, 2016):

- Optimal control of asthma and maintaining adequate oxygenation of the fetus by preventing hypoxic episodes in the mother
- Maintaining normal pulmonary function
- Managing exacerbations aggressively
- Frequently assessing medication needs and response
- Identifying, avoiding, and controlling asthma triggers to protect the pulmonary system from irritants and allergen exposure
- Relief of bronchospasm
- Resolution of airway inflammation to reduce airway hyper-responsiveness
- Improvement of pulmonary function

Risks for the Woman

- Pregnancy has varying effects on asthma, with about one-third of pregnant women becoming worse, one-third improving, and one-third remaining the same (Yancy, 2016). If symptoms worsen, they tend to do so between 17 to 24 weeks' gestation.
- With aggressive management of asthma, pregnancy outcomes can be the same as for nonasthmatic pregnant women.
- Uncontrolled asthma increases the risk of preeclampsia, hypertension, and hyperemesis gravidarum.

Risks for the Fetus and Newborn

- Hypoxia to the fetus is a major complication.
- Preterm birth
- Low birth weight
- Fetal-growth restriction

Assessment Findings

- Signs and symptoms of asthma:
  - Cough (productive or nonproductive)
  - Wheezing
  - Tightness in chest
  - Shortness of breath
  - Increased respiratory rate (>20 breaths/min)
- Signs and symptoms of hypoxia:
  - Cyanosis
  - Lethargy
  - Agitation or confusion

- Intercostal retractions
- Respiratory rate >30 breaths/min

Medical Management

Asthma should be aggressively treated during pregnancy, as the benefits of asthma control far outweigh the risks of medication use. During pregnancy, monthly evaluation of pulmonary function and asthma history are conducted. Serial ultrasound for fetal growth and antepartal fetal testing is done for moderately or severely asthmatic women.

Medications commonly used for asthma management are considered safe during pregnancy and include bronchodilators, anti-inflammatory agents such as inhaled steroids, oral corticosteroids, allergy injections, and antihistamines. Corticosteroids should be given early to all patients with severe acute asthma (Cunningham et al., 2014).

Nursing Actions

- Take a detailed history and assessment of respiratory status, including pulmonary function tests (PFTs) and blood gases (ABGs). Pulmonary function testing should be routine in the management of chronic and acute asthma (Cunningham et al., 2014).
- Assess for signs and symptoms including cough, wheezing, chest tightness, and sputum production.
- Care for women with acute asthma exacerbations includes:
  - Oxygen administration to maintain Pao_2 greater than 95%
  - Ongoing maternal pulse oximeter
  - Baseline arterial blood gases as per orders
  - Baseline pulmonary function tests performed to gather baseline data as per orders
  - Beta-agonist inhalation therapy as ordered
- Monitor maternal oxygen saturation (should be at 95% to oxygenate the fetus).
- Assess fetal well-being and for signs of fetal hypoxia.
- Evaluate pulmonary function test results and laboratory tests (i.e., arterial blood gases).
- Explain the plan of care and goals.
- Teach the woman to avoid allergens and triggers.
- Teach the woman to monitor pulmonary function daily and her normal parameters.
- Teach the woman the role of medications, correct use of medications, and adverse effects of medications.
- Teach the woman to recognize signs and symptoms of worsening asthma and provide a treatment plan to manage exacerbations appropriately.
- Discuss warning signs and symptoms to report to the provider, such as dyspnea, shortness of breath, chest tightness, or exacerbations of signs and symptoms beyond the woman's baseline asthma status (Yancy, 2016).

Chronic Kidney Disease

Chronic kidney disease can be classified into the following broad categories: GN (primary and secondary); interstitial nephropathy, chronic pyelonephritis (including malformations, reflux nephropathy, and residual scars of previous pyelonephritis), diabetic nephropathy, polycystic kidney disease, isolated persistent urinary anomalies, recurrent stone disease, acute pyelonephritis occurring during pregnancy, kidney transplantation, persistent urinary anomalies, and renal function impairment (Piccoli et al., 2010). Pregnancy results in important alterations in acid-base, electrolyte, and renal function due to pregnancy-associated physiologic changes in renal and systemic hemodynamics.

Understanding these changes is essential when evaluating pregnant women with renal disease. Kidney size increases by about 1 to 1.5 cm, primarily in the collecting system. Dilatation of the ureters and pelvis occurs and is presumed to be secondary to the smooth muscle–relaxing effect of progesterone. Kidney size increases by about 1 to 1.5 cm, primarily in the collecting system. Dilatation of the ureters and pelvis occurs and is presumed to be secondary to the smooth muscle–relaxing effect of progesterone.

Assessment Findings

- Abnormal kidney function tests, including creatinine, BUN, uric acid, electrolytes, 24-hour urine protein
- Maternal consequences of chronic kidney disease include hypertension, proteinuria, edema, fatigue, lethargy, headache, anemia

Medical Management

Pregnant patients with kidney disease are often under the care of a maternal-fetal specialist who has advanced training in high-risk obstetrics. These patients receive frequent obstetric follow-up that includes careful blood pressure monitoring, renal function testing, and 24-hour urine protein collections. Consultation with a nephrologist often occurs, particularly for patients with more advanced disease and those with progressive renal failure.

Almost all patients with significant renal disease and/or hypertension in late pregnancy, or when the likelihood of fetal viability is very high, are delivered and managed as non-gravid patients. If progressive renal failure occurs either in early pregnancy or before fetal viability can be assured, however, dialysis may need to be considered. A discussion of dialysis is beyond the scope of this chapter. Anemia should be treated with erythropoietin and careful attention to iron therapy. Nutritional support that allows weight gains of 0.3 to 0.5 kg/wk should be maintained in the second and third trimesters.

Nursing Actions

- Monitor labs for renal function, anemia, and preeclampsia.
- Provide follow-up and reinforcement of nutritional support that allows weight gains of 0.3 to 0.5 kg/wk which should be maintained in the second and third trimesters.
- Monitor for signs and symptoms of preeclampsia.
- Provide comfort measures based on symptoms.
- Explain procedures and plan of care.

Gastrointestinal Disorders

A pregnant woman that presents with gastrointestinal disorders needs a work up as with any non-pregnant individual.

Cholelithiasis

Cholelithiasis is the presence of gallstones in the gallbladder. The incidence of cholelithiasis in pregnant women is 3.5% (Tran,

Ahn, & Reau, 2016). Cholelithiasis is common in pregnancy because increased estrogen levels cause cholesterol supersaturation and increased gallstone formation. Cholecystitis is the second most common surgical condition in pregnancy. Decreased muscle tone allows gallbladder distension and thickening of the bile and prolongs emptying time during pregnancy, increasing the risk of cholelithiasis. Additionally, cholesterol and biliary sludge are thought to be major factors in stone formation, and biliary sludge may increase during pregnancy (Cunningham et al., 2014). Symptomatic cholecystitis was previously managed conservatively, but more recent data suggests high rates of recurrent symptoms (40%–90%), increased rates of hospitalizations, preterm labor, and deliveries, and spontaneous abortions when intervention is deferred. Early surgical intervention with laparoscopic cholecystectomy after ERCP is now preferred.

Assessment Findings

- Colicky abdominal pain presents in the right upper quadrant; anorexia, nausea, and vomiting; fever.
- Gallstones are present on an ultrasound scan.

Medical Management

Cholelithiasis was typically treated with conservative management such as IV fluids, bowel rest, nasogastric suctioning, diet, and antibiotics. Increasingly, it is managed by surgical intervention with laparoscopic cholecystectomies (Cunningham et al., 2014). If gallbladder disease is nonacute, surgical intervention may be delayed until the postpartum period.

Nursing Actions

- Manage pain, administering pain medication as needed.
- Manage nausea and vomiting, minimizing environmental factors that cause nausea and vomiting such as odors.
- Administer antiemetics as needed.
- Provide comfort measures based on symptoms.
- Explain procedures and plan of care including dietary restrictions.

Liver Disease

A pregnant patient presenting with abnormal liver tests should undergo standard workup as with any non-pregnant individual.

Acute Fatty Liver of Pregnancy

Acute fatty liver of pregnancy (AFLP) is a rare disorder characterized by the onset of abdominal pain and jaundice, typically occurring after week 34 of gestation. The pathogenesis involves microvesicular fatty infiltration of hepatocytes, which may be related to defective mitochondrial beta-oxidation of fatty acid (Tran, Ahn, & Reau, 2016). The diagnosis is established via the clinical presentation and laboratory studies. Hyperbilirubinemia is the predominant laboratory abnormality, with mild elevations of aspartate aminotransferase (AST) and alanine aminotransferase (ALT) levels also occurring. Severe cases may result in hypoglycemia, coagulation abnormalities, and even fulminant hepatic failure. Most women with this disorder have acute kidney injury but only a small percentage require dialysis. The median gestation age at the time of identification is 36 weeks. Risk factors include twin pregnancies and low body mass index.

While most patients recover completely, fulminant hepatic failure requires liver transplantation. Women with AFLP should be delivered promptly; expectant management is not appropriate. A pregnant patient presenting with abnormal liver tests should undergo standard workup as with any non-pregnant individual.

Assessment Findings

- Presenting symptoms are non-specific: nausea, vomiting, and abdominal pain. Concomitant preeclampsia is present in roughly half of the affected women. Striking aminotransferase elevations and hyperbilirubinemia are typical. Hepatic failure can manifest with signs of hepatic dysfunction such as encephalopathy, coagulopathy, and hypoglycemia. Renal dysfunction and pancreatitis are common (Tran, Ahn, & Reau, 2016).
- Computed tomography may show a hypodense fatty liver compared with the spleen. Ultrasound imaging may demonstrate homogeneous fatty infiltrate without focal infiltrates.

Medical Management

Women with AFLP should be delivered promptly; expectant management is not appropriate (Tran, Ahn, & Reau, 2016). While most patients recover completely, hepatic failure requires liver transplantation.

Nursing Actions

- Manage pain, administering pain medication as needed.
- Children of mothers affected by AFLP should be monitored carefully for manifestations of deficiency of long-chain 3-hydroxyacyl-coenzyme A dehydrogenase, including hypoketotic hypoglycemia and fatty liver.
- Provide comfort measures based on symptoms.

Venous Thromboembolic Disease

Venous thromboembolism (VTE) is a blood clot that starts in a vein. It is the third leading vascular diagnosis after heart attack and stroke, affecting about 300,000 to 600,000 Americans each year. There are two types of VTE: deep vein thrombosis (DVT) is a clot in a deep vein, usually in the leg, but sometimes in the arm or other veins. Pulmonary embolism (PE) occurs when a DVT clot breaks free from a vein wall, travels to the lungs, and blocks some or all the blood supply. Blood clots in the thigh are more likely to break off and travel to the lungs than blood clots in the lower leg or other parts of the body.

Thromboembolism is a blood clot that can potentially block blood flow and damage the organs, a leading cause of maternal morbidity and mortality in the United States. The risk of venous thrombosis and pulmonary embolism in otherwise healthy women is considered highest during pregnancy and postpartum (Cunningham et al., 2014). Pregnancy is a hypercoagulable state with increased fibrin generation, increased coagulation factors, and decreased fibrinolytic activity. Venous stasis in the lower extremities, increased blood volume, and compression of the inferior vena cava and pelvic veins with advancing gestation all combine to increase risk five times over non-pregnant women. About 80% of thromboembolic events during pregnancy are venous, with pulmonary embolism and other VTE responsible for 1.1 deaths per 100,000 deliveries, or 9% of all maternal deaths in the United States (Bates, Middeldorp, Rodger, James, & Greer, 2016).

Physiologic and anatomic changes during pregnancy increase the risk for thromboembolism. Hypercoagulability, increased venous stasis, decreased venous outflow, uterine compression of the inferior vena cava and pelvic veins, reduced mobility, and changes in levels of coagulation factors normally regulating hemostasis all result in an increased thrombogenic state. Risk for deep vein thrombosis during pregnancy is greatest in the left lower extremity. About half of the cases of venous thromboembolism during pregnancy are associated with a common risk factor for thrombophilia. Acquired and/or inherited thrombophilia are associated with severe preeclampsia, abruption, intrauterine growth restriction (IUGR), intrauterine fetal demise (IUFD), preterm birth, and recurrent miscarriage. Thrombophilia can be an inheritable hypercoagulable condition caused by mutations in clotting mechanisms. The most common acquired thrombophilia during pregnancy is antiphospholipid antibody syndrome (APLA). These antibodies are a result of antigenic changes in endothelial and platelet membranes which promote thrombosis. Other risk factors for VTE unrelated to pregnancy include a personal history of VTE, thrombophilia, obesity, hypertension, and smoking (ACOG, 2011b). Medical conditions such as diabetes, heart disease, hypertension, renal disease, sickle-cell disease, smoking, or serious infections increase the risk of complications in pregnancy (American Academy of Pediatrics [AAP] and the American College of Obstetricians and Gynecologists [ACOG], 2012).

Assessment Findings

- Classic signs of DVT are dependent edema, abrupt unilateral leg pain, erythema, low-grade fever, and positive Homan's sign (i.e., pain with dorsiflexion of foot).
- A PE may present with shortness of breath, tachypnea, tachycardia, dyspnea, pleural chest pain, fever, and anxiety.

Medical Management

Objective tests for DVT include Doppler ultrasound, magnetic resonance venography, and pulsed Doppler study. Chest X-ray, CT, and electrocardiography are used to diagnose PE. ACOG recommends preventive treatment with anticoagulant medication for women who have had an acute VTE during pregnancy, a history of thrombosis, or those at significant risk for VTE during pregnancy and postpartum, such as women with high-risk acquired or inherited thrombophilias. Women with a history of thrombosis should be evaluated for underlying causes to determine whether anticoagulation medication is appropriate during pregnancy. Most women who take anticoagulation medications before pregnancy will need to continue during pregnancy and postpartum. Treatment goals include prevention of further clot propagation, prevention of PE, and prevention of further venous thromboembolism.

- Anticoagulation therapy is required for women experiencing a DVT during pregnancy with heparin compounds titrated to achieve an aPTT of 1.5 to 2.5 times control values.

Intravenous anticoagulation should be maintained for at least 5 to 7 days, after which treatment is converted to subcutaneous heparin (Cunningham et al., 2014).

- Early reviews concluded that low-molecular-weight heparins (LMWH) are safe and effective for use throughout pregnancy. The American College of Obstetrics and Gynecologists (ACOG) concluded that risks associated with LMWH use were rare and that no cause-and-effect relationship has been established between LMWH and congenital anomalies or maternal hemorrhage (Cunningham et al., 2014).
- Treatment of PE is to stabilize a woman with a life-threatening PE and transfer to ICU. Thromboembolitic therapy and catheter or surgical embolectomy may be done.

Nursing Actions

- Begin ambulation after symptoms dissipate (Cunningham et al., 2014).
- Administer elastic stockings.
- Manage pain, administering pain medication as needed.
- Teach woman how to administer heparin SQ to her abdomen.
- Instruct woman to report side effects such as bleeding gums, nosebleeds, easy bruising, or excessive trauma at injection sites.

Evidence-Based Practice: Venous Thromboembolism Bundle

D'Alton, M., Friedman, A., Smiley, R., Montgomery, D., Paidas, M., D'Oria, R., … Clark, S. (2016). National Partnership for Maternal Safety: Consensus Bundle on Venous Thromboembolism. *Journal of Obstetric, Gynecologic & Neonatal Nursing, 45*(5), 706–717.

Obstetric venous thromboembolism is a leading cause of severe maternal morbidity and mortality. Maternal death from thromboembolism is amenable to prevention, and thromboprophylaxis is the most readily implementable means of systematically reducing the maternal death rate. Observational data support the benefit of risk-factor-based prophylaxis in reducing obstetric thromboembolism. This bundle, developed by a multidisciplinary working group and published by the National Partnership for Maternal Safety under the guidance of the Council on Patient Safety in Women's Health Care, supports routine thromboembolism risk assessment for obstetric patients, with appropriate use of pharmacologic and mechanical thromboprophylaxis. Safety bundles outline critical clinical practices that should be implemented in every maternity unit. The bundle is divided into four domains: The *Readiness* domain, which supports establishment of risk-assessment strategies throughout pregnancy. Risk assessment should occur at four time points in pregnancy: (a) during the first prenatal visit, (b) during all antepartum admissions, (c) immediately postpartum during a hospitalization for childbirth, and (d) on discharge home after a birth. The *Recognition* domain, which reviews clinical recommendations from major existing guidelines for patients recognized to be at increased risk for thromboembolism. The *Response* domain, which outlines specific recommendations for prophylaxis for at-risk patients from the NPMS working group; and the *Reporting and Systems Learning* domain, which includes recommendations for quality assurance and surveillance.

Maternal Obesity

Maternal obesity, defined by a BMI of ≥30, has long been recognized as a risk factor in pregnancy. Currently, one in five women is at risk for being obese at the beginning of pregnancy (American Academy of Pediatrics [AAP] and the American College of Obstetricians and Gynecologists [ACOG], 2012). Being overweight or obese during pregnancy is associated with many adverse outcomes, including miscarriage, impaired glucose tolerance, and sleep apnea (Opray, Grivell, Deussen, & Dodd, 2015). Obesity during pregnancy increases the risk of morbidity and mortality for both the mother and baby and is a well-established risk factor for the development of comorbid conditions such as preeclampsia, gestational and type 2 diabetes, and thrombosis (ACOG, 2015d). Many of the systemic physiological alterations that occur during pregnancy may be altered when the pregnant woman is obese. For example:

- The typical increase in cardiac output associated with pregnancy is compounded when a woman is obese and is influenced by the degree and duration of obesity. Cardiac output increases by 30 to 50 mL/min for every 100 g of fat deposited. Blood volume is increased as well. A degree of cardiac hypertrophy is normal during pregnancy, but obesity exaggerates the hypertrophy and contributes to myocardial dilation.
- Although obese women can experience more frequent episodes of obstructive sleep apnea (OSA) than women with normal BMI, pregnancy may exert a protective effect on OSA occurrence.
- Pregnant women are more prone to gastric reflux, given associated hormonal and anatomic changes. The incidence of hiatus hernia is greater in obese patients, and abdominal pressure and intragastric volume are increased.
- Pregnancy is a hypercoagulable state, and obesity further increases the risk of thrombosis by promoting venous stasis, increasing blood viscosity, and promoting activation of the coagulation cascade.
- A large panniculus, a thick layer of adipose tissue in the abdominal area sometimes called a fatty apron, may contribute to uterine compression and exaggerate the vena cava syndrome to which pregnant women are susceptible.

Risks for the Woman

- Preeclampsia
- Deep vein thrombosis
- Urinary tract infections
- Gestational diabetes
- Preterm birth
- Cesarean delivery
- Operative and post-operative complications
  - Prolonged operating times
  - Excessive blood loss
  - Wound infection
  - Thromboembolism
  - Endometritis

Risks for the Fetus/Newborn

- Congenital anomalies, including cardiac and neural tube defects
- Growth abnormalities and facial clefting

- Macrosomia
- Miscarriage
- Stillbirth

Assessment Findings

- BMI of ≥30 kg/m². Body mass index calculated at the first prenatal visit should be used to provide diet and exercise counseling guided by IOM recommendations for gestational weight gain during pregnancy (ACOG, 2015d).

Medical Management

- Provide specific information on maternal risks of obesity in pregnancy.
- Early pregnancy screening for glucose intolerance (gestational diabetes or overt diabetes) should be based on risk factors, including maternal BMI of 30 or greater, known impaired glucose metabolism, or previous gestational diabetes (ACOG, 2015d).
- Provide specific information on the increased risk for an infant with a neural tube defect and for a stillborn infant.
- These risks require heightened and ongoing evaluation of the pregnant woman and fetus.

Nursing Actions

- Measure and record height and weight of woman and calculate BMI.
- Reinforce information on maternal and fetal risks associated with obesity.
- Provide teaching on signs and symptoms of preeclampsia, diabetes, sleep apnea, and vena cava syndrome.
- Ensure woman understands plan of care for increased and ongoing evaluation of pregnancy.
- Because pregnancy presents an ideal time during which to initiate simple healthy behaviors, such as walking and proper diet that can be maintained after birth, offer suggestions and encouragement for lifestyle changes.
- Obese women who have even small weight reductions before pregnancy may have improved pregnancy outcomes. Interpregnancy weight loss in obese women may decrease the risk of a large-for-gestational-age neonate in a subsequent pregnancy (ACOG, 2015d).
- Provide referrals to dietitian for nutritional counseling and reinforce guidelines for diet and weight gain. Recommended weight gain in obese women is 11 to 20 pounds (Cunningham et al., 2014).
- Use caution when shifting the panniculus to assess for fetal heart sounds or when providing personal hygiene, as the redistributed weight may alter maternal hemodynamics and increase the risk of vena cava compression.
- Encouraging the woman to sleep in a sitting position may help, as effects of obesity on the respiratory system are decreased in this position.
- Making appropriate environmental changes to accommodate the larger patient, such as assuring that patient beds, examining tables, and chairs can support at least 400 pounds.

Thyroid Disorders

Thyroid disorders are common in young women and thus managed frequently in pregnancy. There is an intimate relationship between maternal and fetal thyroid function, which makes identifying thyroid disorders an important aspect of antenatal assessment and care. Care of thyroid disorders during pregnancy is essential to both the mother and baby because maternal TSH-receptor-blocking antibodies can cross the placenta and cause fetal thyroid dysfunction. However, identifying thyroid disorders in pregnancy can be difficult because many of the signs and symptoms can mirror those of pregnancy itself (Cunningham et al., 2014).

Hyperthyroidism

Hyperthyroidism or symptomatic thyrotoxicosis is caused by hyperfunctioning of the thyroid gland in which it produces excessive amounts of thyroid hormone. Grave's disease is responsible for 90% to 95% of hyperthyroidism cases in pregnant women (Van Otterloo, 2016). Compared with controlled maternal hyperthyroidism, inadequately treated maternal hyperthyroidism is associated with a greater risk of preterm delivery, severe preeclampsia, and heart failure with an increase in medically indicated preterm deliveries, low birth weight infants, and possible fetal loss.

Assessment Findings

- Tachycardia
- Failure to gain weight or weight loss
- Nervousness, tremors
- Frequent stools
- Excessive sweating
- Heat intolerance
- Insomnia
- Palpitations
- Hypertension
- Markedly depressed TSH levels
- Elevated serum free T4 (fT4) and total triiodothyronine (TT3) levels

Medical Management

- Medication must be used cautiously, as many antithyroid drugs can cause birth defects and fetal thyroid problems (Van Otterloo, 2016).
- Thionamide drugs: Propylthiouracil (PTU) approved for use during pregnancy (Cunningham et al., 2014).
- Use of Iodine 131 for treatment of Grave's disease after the first trimester can result in destruction of the fetal thyroid gland; therefore, it is contraindicated during pregnancy (American Academy of Pediatrics [AAP] and the American College of Obstetricians and Gynecologists [ACOG], 2012).
- Monitor fetal growth and development through ultrasound testing and fundal height measurement.
- Assess thyroid hormone levels (TSH and thyroxine) periodically throughout pregnancy and adjust medication dosage accordingly.
- Monitor hepatic enzymes.
- Monitor WBC for leukopenia.

Nursing Actions

- Provide teaching on signs and symptoms of hyperthyroidism and treatment plan, including daily medication and side effects.
- Educate woman and family on the plan of care for increased and ongoing evaluation of pregnancy, including frequent monitoring of thyroid levels to ensure that the lowest possible amount of antithyroid medication is administered for control of patient's symptoms while minimizing fetal exposure to antithyroid medications (Van Otterloo, 2016).
- Provide nutritional counseling to meet additional calorie requirements.
- Discuss information regarding fetal status and potential maternal and fetal complications associated with hyperthyroidism in pregnancy.

Hypothyroidism

Hypothyroidism is caused by inadequate thyroid hormone production and is associated with elevated TSH levels and decreased FT4 levels.

Assessment Findings

- Fatigue
- Constipation
- Muscle cramps
- Weight gain
- Cold intolerance
- Hair loss
- Dry skin
- Clinical or overt hypothyroidism is characterized by abnormally high TSH levels and abnormally low thyroxine levels.
- Subclinical hypothyroidism is defined by an elevated serum TSH level and normal serum thyroxine.

Medical Management

- Levothyroxine (Synthroid) 1 to 2 µg/kg/day or approximately 100 µg/day, adjusted by 25 to 50 µg increments until TSH levels become normal (Cunningham et al., 2014).
- Surveillance of TSH and thyroxine levels measured at 4-6 week intervals
- If replacement therapy is inadequate or not instituted during pregnancy, there is high risk of fetal mortality and morbidity.

Nursing Actions

- Reinforce information on maternal and fetal risks associated with hypothyroidism.
- Provide teaching on signs and symptoms of hypothyroidism and treatment plan, including daily medication.
- Ensure the woman and family understand the plan of care for increased and ongoing evaluation of pregnancy.

Systemic Lupus Erythematosus

Systemic lupus erythematosus is a heterogenous autoimmune disease characterized by immune system abnormalities, including overactive B lymphocytes. These overactive lymphocytes result in tissue and cellular damage and immunosuppression. Almost 90 percent of lupus cases are in women, and the disease is encountered relatively frequently in pregnancy (Cunningham et al., 2014). SLE increases the risk of spontaneous abortion, intrauterine fetal death, preeclampsia, intrauterine growth retardation, and preterm birth. Prognosis for both mother and child is best when SLE is quiescent for at least 6 months before the pregnancy and when the mother's underlying renal function is stable and normal or near normal (Khurana, 2017). Lupus nephritis can get worse during pregnancy. In general, pregnancy does not cause flares of SLE.

Assessment Findings

- Malaise
- Fever
- Weight loss
- Arthritis
- Rash
- Pleuro-pericarditis
- Photosensitivity
- Anemia
- Cognitive dysfunction

Medical Management

- There is no cure for SLE; thus, lupus management consists primarily of monitoring maternal clinical and laboratory conditions as well as fetal well-being (Cunningham et al., 2014).
- Low-dose aspirin throughout pregnancy
- Monitor for complication of pregnancy such as spontaneous abortion, intrauterine fetal death, preeclampsia, intrauterine growth retardation, and preterm birth.
- Corticosteroids during acute flare-ups
- Methylprednisolone

Nursing Actions

- Monitor and identify flare-ups.
- Provide teaching on signs and symptoms of SLE and disease process, as well as treatment plan throughout pregnancy.
- Ensure woman and family understand the plan of care for increased and ongoing evaluation during pregnancy.
- Reinforce a low-salt diet is recommended in pregnancy to prevent weight increase and hypertension. Calcium and vitamin D supplementation may be advised to prevent osteoporosis.
- Reinforce adherence to an exercise program may help prevent bone loss and depression. Strenuous activity is best avoided when patients have flare-ups.

SUBSTANCE USE

Alcohol abuse and other substance use disorders are major, often underdiagnosed health problems for women, regardless of age, race, ethnicity, and socioeconomic status, and have resulting high costs for individuals and society (ACOG, 2015a). Substance use disorder is commonly defined as pathologic pattern of behaviors related to the use of any of 10 separate classes of substances, including alcohol and licit and illicit substances.

BOX 7–5 | Substances That Are Commonly Misused or Abused

Alcohol (ethanol)

Cannabinoids (marijuana and hashish)

Club drugs (methylenedioxymethamphetamine [MDMA], flunitrazepam, and gamma-hydroxybutyrate [GHB])

Dissociative drugs (ketamine, phencyclidine [PCP] and analogs, *Salvia divinorum*, and dextromethorphan)

Hallucinogens (lysergic acid diethylamide [LSD], mescaline, and psilocybin)

Opioids (heroin and opium)

Other compounds (anabolic steroids and inhalants)

Prescription medications (central nervous system depressants, stimulants, and opioid pain relievers)

Stimulants (cocaine, amphetamine, and methamphetamine)

Tobacco

National Institute on Drug Abuse, 2013.

BOX 7–6 | Nursing Interventions With Substance-Using Patients

The nurse caring for a pregnant woman who abuses substances should take the following measures.

- Advocate for intervention and treatment referral for those patients with positive screening results (Box 7–8).
- Provide health education about the risks to the fetus of substance use during pregnancy and facilitate early diagnosis and appropriate intervention and referral.
- Maintain a nonjudgmental and nonpunitive attitude; remember addiction is a disease.
  - It has been proposed that government policies can be viewed as either "facilitative" or "adversarial." Facilitative policies improve women's access to prenatal care, food, shelter, and treatment. Adversarial policies propose that women who fail to seek treatment are liable to criminal prosecution and may diminish utilization of prenatal care and support services, such as housing, education and job training, financial support services, parenting education, legal services, and aftercare.
- Nurses have a responsibility to treat their patients with substance use disorder with dignity and respect and to try to establish a therapeutic alliance with these patients.
- Encourage prenatal visits and ongoing assessmemt for pregnancy complications and provide information on fetal growth and development.
- Provide specific suggestions to decrease smoking, alcohol intake and substance use.
- Provide written information of resources at appropriate educational level.
- Nurses should familiarize themselves with resources available through their local hospital and community to appropriately and effectively discuss treatment options for patients.
- Nurses should be aware of strategies for safe and effective pain management in women with long-term opioid exposure, which results in tolerance and hyperalgesia.
- Nurses should communicate the unique needs of pregnant women and position themselves as advocates for the benefit of timely and ongoing treatment that will improve perinatal and neonatal outcomes rather than focus on their criminalization.

Alcohol, cigarette, and illicit drug use during pregnancy can cause poor pregnancy and birth outcomes including low birth weight, developmental disabilities, preterm birth, and infant mortality (March of Dimes, 2013). The first 8 weeks of pregnancy are the most critical in terms of embryonic development, and substances ingested in that period can have a teratogenic effect (Sullivan, 2016). Recent reports show that nearly 5.9% of pregnant women use illicit drugs (Substance Abuse and Mental Health Services Administration [SAMHSA], 2013), 15.3% of pregnant women use tobacco, and for pregnant women in the first trimester, binge or heavy drinking of alcohol is as high as 11.9% (Hudak, Tan, & Committee on Drugs and Committee on Fetus and Newborn, 2014) .The findings in this report suggest that many U.S. women, particularly those in the third trimester, are getting the message and abstaining from substance use. Still, a sizeable proportion of women in the first trimester of pregnancy were past-month users of alcohol, cigarettes, or marijuana, and one in seven women used cigarettes in the second or third trimester (Box 7–5). In addition, many women resume use of these substances after childbirth, and that resumption appears to be rapid given the higher rates for mothers of infants younger than 3 months old compared with pregnant women in the second or third trimesters. Effective interventions for women to further reduce substance use during pregnancy and to prevent postpartum resumption of use could improve the overall health and well-being of mothers and infants (Box 7–6).

Polydrug abuse among pregnant women with substances such as alcohol and tobacco with marijuana or cocaine has become very common (March of Dimes, 2011). In these cases, it can be difficult to determine which complications are associated with which substance. For example, recent research shows that smoking tobacco or marijuana, taking prescription pain relievers, or using illegal drugs during pregnancy is associated with double or even triple the risk

of stillbirth. Specifically, for tobacco use there is a 1.8 to 2.8 times greater risk of stillbirth, with the highest risk found among the heaviest smokers. Marijuana use carries a 2.3 times greater risk of stillbirth; evidence of any stimulant, marijuana, or prescription pain reliever use has a 2.2 times greater risk of stillbirth; and passive exposure to tobacco carries a 2.1 times greater risk of stillbirth (National Institute of Child Health and Human Development, 2013).

Risks of specific complications vary based on substance used; however, general risks resulting from substance abuse for both the woman and fetus/newborn are presented. Pregnant women using illicit substances often fear legal consequences and may avoid seeking prenatal care. A nonjudgmental and factual approach with attention toward reducing risks offers the best approach for these complex pregnancies. Chemically dependent pregnant women may engage in other risky behaviors. A holistic, comprehensive approach to care that deals not only with the prenatal aspects of care, but also with the complex social and psychological contributing factors, is needed. The Association of Women's Health, Obstetric and Neonatal Nurses (AWHONN) opposes laws and other reporting requirements that result in incarceration or other punitive legal actions against women because of a substance abuse disorder in pregnancy (AWHONN, 2015). Box 7-6 reviews nursing interventions with substance using patients.

Smoking/Tobacco Use

Smoking is one of the most important modifiable causes of poor pregnancy outcomes in the United States, and is associated with maternal, fetal, and infant morbidity and mortality (ACOG, 2017c). Smoking has been linked to doubling a woman's risk of having a low birth weight baby, slowing fetal growth, and increasing the risk of preterm delivery, spontaneous abortion, and stillbirth. Compared to babies of nonsmokers, babies whose mothers smoked during pregnancy are up to three times more likely to die from sudden infant death syndrome (SIDS). Furthermore, smoking during pregnancy doubles a woman's risk of experiencing placenta previa and placenta abruption, both of which can cause heavy bleeding that adversely affect mother and baby. An estimated 5% to 8% of preterm deliveries, 13% to 19% of term deliveries of infants with low birth weight, 23% to 34% cases of SIDS, and 5% to 7% of preterm-related infant deaths can be attributed to prenatal maternal smoking (ACOG, 2017c). The risks of smoking during pregnancy extend beyond pregnancy-related complications. Children born to mothers who smoke during pregnancy are at an increased risk of asthma, infantile colic, and childhood obesity.

Nearly 16% of women smoke during their pregnancies. Statistics show that 910 infant deaths occur because of smoking during pregnancy and an estimated $350 million dollars are spent each year in healthcare due to the effects of smoking while pregnant (National Institute on Drug Abuse, 2013). Although quitting smoking before 15 weeks of gestation yields the greatest benefits for the pregnant woman and fetus, quitting at any point can be beneficial. There is conflicting evidence as to whether nicotine replacement therapy increases abstinence rates in pregnant smokers.

The physiological effects of smoking are a result of transient intrauterine hypoxemia and are dose-dependent. The more the woman smokes, the greater the risk. Cigarette smoke contains many chemicals, particularly nicotine and carbon monoxide, that cause adverse pregnancy outcomes such as low birth weight and prematurity. Nicotine reduces uterine blood flow and carbon monoxide binds to hemoglobin, reducing the oxygen-carrying capacity of the blood which increases the risk of fetal morbidity and mortality.

Assessment & Findings

● Gather a history of prior tobacco use, current use, quantity of use daily, and exposure to other family members that smoke.

● Physical findings include a cough, congestion and smell of tobacco in the air or on their clothing.
● Psychosocial findings include denial, anxiety, depression, anger, and guilt.
● An ultrasound can be performed as a diagnostic test to detect intrauterine fetal growth (IUGR).

Medical Management

● Provide education with smoking cessation education and information around smoking and its health hazards to the woman and fetus (American Cancer Society, 2015).

Nursing Management

Health care professionals have a responsibility to routinely screen patients for tobacco use, to implement or support evidence-based smoking cessation strategies, and to refer patients to smoking cessation programs and resources. Nurses have the expertise in health promotion, disease prevention, women's health issues, and holistic care to provide the continuity of care necessary during and after pregnancy to support and monitor a woman's efforts to quit smoking (AWHONN, 2010). Additionally, AWHONN supports educational programs at the federal, state, and local levels that increase public awareness of the health risks for women and their babies related to smoking during pregnancy, increasing smoking bans, and taxation of cigarettes. Although quitting smoking before 15 weeks of gestation yields the greatest benefits for the pregnant woman and fetus, quitting at any point can be beneficial (ACOG, 2017c). Nurses should:

● Assess patients smoking habits and timing.
● Support patient in decreasing smoking intake.
● Provide and help patient identify alternative coping mechanisms instead of smoking. Examples are having a nutritious snack, walking to relieve stress, relaxation as a substitute.
● Refer patient to appropriate programs for stress reduction and smoking cessation support (Sullivan, 2016) (Box 7–7).

Alcohol

Alcohol consumption during pregnancy is a major health problem, and prenatal exposure to alcohol remains the leading known preventable cause of birth defects in the United States (Mattson & Smith, 2011). Among pregnant women, 1 in 10 reported any alcohol use and 1 in 33 reported binge drinking in the past 30 days (CDC, 2014).

Among pregnant women, the highest prevalence of alcohol use was among those who were 35 to 44 years, college graduates, and not married (Tan et al., 2015). Because a safe level of alcohol intake during pregnancy cannot be determined, both the U.S. Surgeon General and the March of Dimes Foundation recommend that pregnant women not consume any alcohol. White women were more likely than Hispanic women to have consumed alcohol in the past month regardless of their pregnancy status. Generally, higher education status and higher family income were associated with higher rates of alcohol use among all women of childbearing age regardless of their pregnancy status. Among women aged 18 to 44, those with a college education were nearly twice as likely

> ## BOX 7-7 | Patient Referrals for Information and Support on Quitting Substance Use During Pregnancy
>
> Alcoholics Anonymous
>
> www.aa.org
>
> Narcotics Anonymous
>
> www.na.org
>
> Smoking Cessation
>
> www.ahrq.gov/consumer/tobacco/quits.htm
>
> www. helppregnantsmokersquit.org/quit/toll_free.asp.
>
> www.cancer.org
>
> www.marchofdimes.org

as their counterparts with less than a high school education to have used alcohol in the past month in each pregnancy status category. Similarly, women age 15 to 44 with annual family incomes of $75,000 or higher had the highest rates of alcohol use in the prior month compared with those with lower family incomes in all three pregnancy status categories (USDHHS, Substance Abuse and Mental Health Services Administration, 2008).

Other data from the CDC reports 10.2% of pregnant women (about 1 in 10) drink during pregnancy, and 1.9% of pregnant women (about 1 in 50) reported binge drinking in the past 30 days. The National Institute on Alcohol Abuse and Alcoholism defines at-risk alcohol use for healthy women as more than three drinks per occasion or more than seven drinks per week and any amount of drinking for women who are pregnant or at risk of pregnancy. Binge drinking is defined as more than four drinks per occasion. Almost 50% of binge drinking occurs among otherwise moderate drinkers. Heavy alcohol use is binge drinking on 5 or more days in the past month. Moderate drinking is defined as one drink per day. Alcohol use disorder (AUD) is a medical condition that doctors diagnose when a patient's drinking causes distress or harm. When evaluating a patient's drinking habits, it is important to verify the description of "a drink" to determine the actual amount of alcohol consumed.

Pregnant women age 15 to 17 years may need alcohol prevention services tailored for their age group, as nearly 16% of them used alcohol in the past month. Pregnant women in this age group consumed an average of 24 drinks in the past month (i.e., they drank on an average of six days during the past month and an average of about four drinks on the days that they drank).

Alcohol is a teratogen. Fetal alcohol spectrum disorder (FASD) is the most severe result of prenatal drinking, affecting 40,000 newborns in the U.S. annually. Recent reports from specific U.S. sites report the prevalence of FAS to be 2 to 7 cases per 1,000, and the prevalence of Fetal Alcohol Spectrum Disorders (FASD) to be as high as 20 to 50 cases per 1,000 (March of Dimes, 2013). When a pregnant woman drinks, alcohol passes swiftly to the fetus through the placenta. Because alcohol is processed more slowly in the fetus's liver, the alcohol level can be even higher and can remain elevated longer. Drinking alcohol during pregnancy can result in a wide range of physical and mental birth defects. The term "fetal alcohol spectrum disorder" (FASD) is used to describe the many problems associated with alcohol exposure prior to birth. Fetal alcohol syndrome is associated with abnormalities, growth defects, and facial dysmorphia. However, for every child born with fetal alcohol syndrome, many more are born with neurobehavioral defects caused by prenatal alcohol exposure. Alcohol-related birth defects include growth deformities, facial abnormalities, central nervous system impairment, behavioral disorders, and impaired intellectual development.

Alcohol can affect a fetus at any stage of pregnancy, and the cognitive defects and behavioral problems that result from prenatal alcohol exposure are lifelong. In early pregnancy during organogenesis and perhaps before the patient's recognition of pregnancy, the fetus may be particularly vulnerable to maternal binge or heavy alcohol use. Alcohol-related birth defects are completely preventable. Even moderate alcohol consumption during pregnancy may alter psychomotor development, contribute to cognitive defects, and produce emotional and behavioral problems in children, although patient denial and underreporting make it difficult to quantify these effects. There is evidence of varying susceptibility to alcohol's effect on the developing fetus. Although alcohol consumption may have negative consequences for any pregnant woman, the effects of alcohol may be more potent in mothers who are older, in poor health, or who also smoke or use drugs. Chapter 17 provides additional information on FASDs. The consensus is that no level of drinking alcohol is considered safe in pregnancy.

Assessment & Findings

- Five criteria for determining risk for FAS including drinking during pregnancy, cluster of birth defects, facial abnormalities, brain damage, and fetal growth restriction.
- History of prenatal care from a nonjudgmental perspective
- Screening with the Four P's of pregnancy (Chasnoff, Wells, McGourty, & Bailey, 2007) includes the following questions:
  - Have you ever used drugs or alcohol during pregnancy?
  - Have you had a problem with drugs or alcohol in the past?
  - Does your partner have a problem with drugs or alcohol?
  - Do you consider one of your parents to be an addict or alcoholic? (Chasnoff, Wells, McGourty, & Bailey, 2007)
- Risk factors include history of substance abuse, current or recent drug use, previous child with FAS, smoking, multiple sex partners, recent abuse, and mental health problems.
- Physical findings: Poor nutrition or hygiene, tremors, edema, agitated, memory loss, and hepatomegaly
- Psychological findings: Depression, fear, anxiety, lack of family support, denial, hostility, anger, unplanned pregnancy, and low self-esteem
- Diagnostic studies: Blood alcohol level, STI testing, and serial sonogram

Medical Management

- Inpatient or outpatient treatment for alcohol or other drugs
- Provide written information of resources at appropriate educational level
- Case management and increasing prenatal visits

Nursing Management

- Health education on the effects of alcohol and potential dangers
- Referral to community support and resources (see Box 7–7)
- Assessment for risk factors and physical/psychological affects

Illicit Drugs

An average of 5.9% of pregnant women use illicit drugs such as marijuana, cocaine, amphetamines, heroin, and Ecstasy (SAMHSA, 2013). The effect of the drug on placental function and fetal development depends on its nature. For example, cocaine causes vasoconstriction that can impact the placenta and uterus, resulting in placental abruption or preterm birth (Sullivan, 2016). Women who use illicit drugs are counseled to stop, except for heroin users, for whom methadone treatment is recommended to prevent stillbirth.

Cocaine

Cocaine abuse and addiction is a complex problem which involves physiological changes in the brain as well as psychosocial and environmental factors. Biologically, cocaine blocks the reuptake of catecholamines at the nerve terminal, which increases circulating catecholamines in the blood and leads to vasoconstriction. Cardiovascular and neurological complications such as hypertension, tachycardia, uterine contractions, myocardial infarction, dysrhythmias, subarachnoid hemorrhage, thrombocytopenia, seizures, and even sudden death have been described among patients who abuse cocaine. Stimulants such as cocaine, crank, and crystal meth are correlated to the abnormal neurobehavioral affects in the neonate as a result of direct exposure instead of association of withdrawal symptoms (Hudak et al., 2014). Acute use of cocaine during the third trimester can result in preterm labor, a greater incidence of PROM, abruptio placentae, precipitous delivery, increased risk for meconium staining, and premature and low birth weight infants (Forray, 2016).

Opioid Use

The prevalence of opioid use disorder in the United States continues to rise and is a public health crisis. It is thus increasingly important for providers to be educated on opioid prescribing and that patients have access to accurate information and appropriate treatment (ACOG, 2012b). Opioid abuse in pregnancy includes the use of heroin and the misuse of prescription opioid analgesic medications.

In addition to the use of screening tools, certain signs and symptoms may suggest a substance use disorder in a pregnant woman. Pregnant women with opioid addiction often seek prenatal care late in pregnancy; exhibit poor adherence to their appointments; experience poor weight gain; or exhibit sedation, intoxication, withdrawal, or erratic behavior. Opioid-assisted therapy during pregnancy can prevent complications of illicit opioid use and narcotic withdrawal, encourage prenatal care and drug treatment, reduce criminal activity, and avoid risks of associating with a drug culture. Comprehensive opioid-assisted therapy that includes prenatal care reduces the risk of obstetric complications.

Methadone maintenance, as prescribed and dispensed daily by a registered substance abuse treatment program, is part of a comprehensive package of prenatal care, chemical dependency counseling, family therapy, nutritional education, and other medical and psychosocial services as indicated for pregnant women with opioid dependence (ACOG, 2012b).

Heroin abuse during pregnancy is linked to adverse consequences for both mother and fetus. Hazards of heroin to the fetus are believed to be directly related to the physiological dependence effect on the fetus and the maternal lifestyle associated with heroin use. Opioids such as heroin, morphine, and methadone are central nervous system depressants that can cross the placenta and blood brain barrier, potentially causing withdrawal signs in the neonate (Hudak et al., 2014). The primary effects of heroin include analgesia, sedation, feeling of well-being, and euphoria. Women who use heroin during pregnancy typically do not seek early prenatal care for fear of detection of heroin use and are at an increased risk to exposure to serious infections such as STDs, hepatitis, and HIV. The neonatal effects of prenatal heroin exposure include withdrawal symptoms, increased incidence of meconium aspiration at birth, increased incidence of sepsis, IUGR, and neurodevelopmental behavioral problems (Sullivan, 2016).

Marijuana

Marijuana is the most commonly used illicit drug (National Institute of Drug Abuse, 2013) and the second most common drug used overall after alcohol. About one in 25 women in the U.S. reports using marijuana while pregnant (Ko, Farr, Tong, Creanga, & Callaghan, 2015). Marijuana use causes tachycardia and low blood pressure, which can result in orthostatic hypotension. Research has shown that neonates born to mothers who used marijuana during pregnancy can have an altered response to visual stimuli, increased tremulousness, and even a high-pitched cry that may indicate a problem with neurological development and developmental problems (Mark, Desai, & Terplan, 2016; Sullivan, 2016).

Risks for the Woman Using Substances During Pregnancy

- Preterm labor
- PPROM
- Poor weight gain and nutritional status
- Placental abnormalities (placenta previa, abruptio placentae)

Risks for the Fetus and Newborn

- Fetal effects may include CNS abnormalities and intrauterine growth restriction, small for gestational age, low birth weight, prematurity, and stillbirth.
- Effects of maternal substance use on the fetus differ based on the drug the woman has taken. The effect on the neonate are detailed in Chapter 17.
- Neonatal withdrawal syndrome (symptoms are dependent on drug used during pregnancy) (see Chapter 17)
- Sudden infant death syndrome (SIDS)

Assessment Findings in Women Using Substances During Pregnancy

A variety of screening tools have been proposed, and screening for smoking, alcohol use, and illicit drugs is recommended to start at the first prenatal visit. Universal screening of all pregnant women is recommended in a supportive and nonjudgmental manner (Gilbert, 2011). One simple screening tool includes asking the following four questions for a yes or no response, described as Ewing's 4 P's (Taylor, Zaichkin, & Bailey, 2002).

- Have you ever used alcohol or drugs during this pregnancy?
- Have you had a problem with drugs or alcohol in the past?
- Does your partner have a problem with drugs or alcohol?
- Do you consider one of your parents to have a problem with drugs or alcohol?

A yes answer to any of these questions should trigger further evaluation of habits. Additionally, a toxicology screen of a urine sample can be attained to evaluate for certain drug use.

Medical Management

- Screen for substance use in pregnancy with all pregnant women (ACOG, 2012a).
- Refer to multispecialty clinics.
- Refer to drug treatment programs.
- Screen for domestic violence.
- Conduct frequent urine toxicology tests.
- Use targeted ultrasound to rule out congenital anomalies.
- Provide patient education.
- Conduct antepartal testing.

Nursing Actions for the Woman Using Substances During Pregnancy

Women are more receptive to treatment and lifestyle changes during pregnancy; therefore, pregnancy may be a window of opportunity for chemically dependent women to enter treatment. To facilitate this, nurses must be armed with the knowledge and information necessary to screen and identify women who abuse substances during pregnancy. Because of the substantial costs and repercussions of drug use during pregnancy for newborns, women, and society, it is essential to devise methods of intervention that decrease this risky behavior. Many women who need substance abuse treatment may not receive it due to lack of money or child care, fear of losing custody of their children, or other barriers. For successful recovery, women often need a continuum of care for an extended period, including comprehensive inpatient or outpatient treatment for alcohol and other drugs, case management for coordination of prenatal care, counseling, and other mental health treatment (see Box 7–7). Nursing actions include the following.

- Provide health education about the risks to the fetus of substance use during pregnancy and facilitate early diagnosis and appropriate intervention and referral.
- Laws governing drug screening during pregnancy vary from state to state. Nurses must be aware of laws and local guidelines for toxicology screening of pregnant women and treatment options and availability of programs, as many treatment programs will not accept pregnant women.
- Counsel women who test positive for drug or alcohol use and those who smoke during pregnancy to stop and supply referrals to assist with cessation and refer to local treatment centers for pregnant women (Box 7–7).
- Maintain a nonjudgmental and nonpunitive attitude; remember that addiction is a disease.
- Nurses should remain up to date with current treatment approaches and strategies to addiction management in pregnancy (see Box 7–8).

It has been proposed that government policies can be viewed as either "facilitative" or "adversarial." Facilitative policies improve women's access to prenatal care, food, shelter, and treatment. Adversarial policies propose that women who fail to seek treatment are liable to criminal prosecution and may diminish utilization of prenatal care and support services, such as housing, education and job training, financial support services, parenting education, legal services, and aftercare. Research shows that residential substance abuse treatment designed specifically for pregnant women and women with children can have substantial benefits in terms of recovery, pregnancy outcomes, parenting skills, and women's ability to maintain or regain custody of their children.

BOX 7–8 | Resources for Further Information on Substance Abuse Treatment for Health Professionals

Resources for Further Information

Alcoholics Anonymous (AA)

check your local phone book for listings in your area

Internet address: http://www.aa.org

National Council on Alcoholism and Drug Dependence, Inc. (NCADD)

217 Broadway, Suite 712

New York, NY 10007

Phone: (212) 269–7797; Fax: (212) 269–7510

HOPE LINE: (800) NCA–CALL (24-hour Affiliate referral)

Email: national@ncadd.org

Internet address: http://www.ncadd.org

National Institute on Alcohol Abuse and Alcoholism

5635 Fishers Lane

Bethesda, MD 20892–9304

(301) 443–3860; Fax: (301) 480–1726

Internet address: http://www.niaaa.nih.gov

National Organization on Fetal Alcohol Syndrome

900 17th Street, NW, Suite 910

Washington, DC 20006

(800) 66–NOFAS; Fax: (202) 466–6456

Internet address: http://www.nofas.org

March of Dimes

https://www.marchofdimes.org/

Substance Abuse and Mental Health Services Administration (SAMHSA)

Treatment Facility Locator

(800) 662–HELP

Internet address: http://www.findtreatment.samhsa.gov

CONCEPT MAP

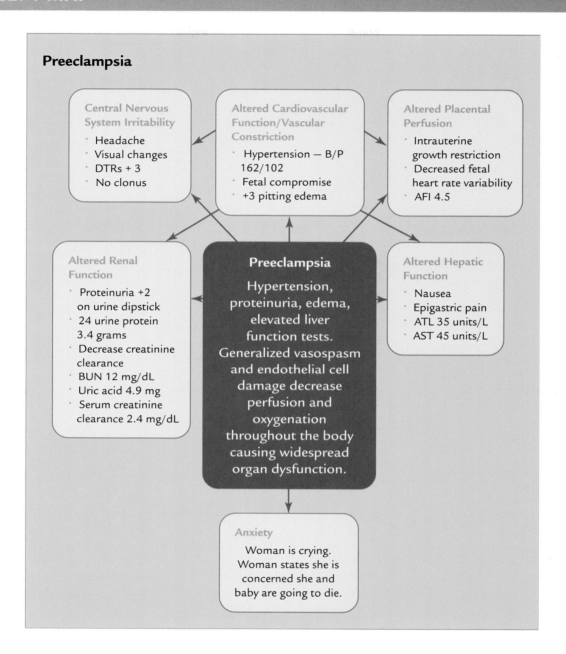

Preeclampsia

Central Nervous System Irritability
- Headache
- Visual changes
- DTRs + 3
- No clonus

Altered Cardiovascular Function/Vascular Constriction
- Hypertension — B/P 162/102
- Fetal compromise
- +3 pitting edema

Altered Placental Perfusion
- Intrauterine growth restriction
- Decreased fetal heart rate variability
- AFI 4.5

Altered Renal Function
- Proteinuria +2 on urine dipstick
- 24 urine protein 3.4 grams
- Decrease creatinine clearance
- BUN 12 mg/dL
- Uric acid 4.9 mg
- Serum creatinine clearance 2.4 mg/dL

Preeclampsia
Hypertension, proteinuria, edema, elevated liver function tests. Generalized vasospasm and endothelial cell damage decrease perfusion and oxygenation throughout the body causing widespread organ dysfunction.

Altered Hepatic Function
- Nausea
- Epigastric pain
- ATL 35 units/L
- AST 45 units/L

Anxiety
Woman is crying. Woman states she is concerned she and baby are going to die.

Problem No. 1: Central nervous system irritability
Goal: Prevent seizures and cerebral edema.
Outcome: Patient will remain seizure free and not develop neurological sequelae.

Nursing Actions
1. Monitor CNS changes including headache, dizziness, blurred vision, and scotoma.
2. Maintain seizure precautions.
3. If treated with magnesium sulfate, see Critical Component: Care of the Woman on Magnesium Sulfate.
4. Restrict fluids to total of 125 mL/hr or as ordered.
5. Monitor I&O.
6. Assess DTRs.
7. Maintain bed rest in the lateral position.
8. Provide an environment that is conducive to decreased stimulation, such as low lights, decreased noise, and uninterrupted rest periods.
9. Teach the patient relaxation techniques.

Problem No. 2: Altered cardiovascular function/vasoconstriction
Goal: Normal blood pressure
Outcome: Blood pressure within acceptable limits, below 140/90 mm Hg

Continued

Nursing Actions

1. Monitor BP every hour or more frequently if elevated.
2. Administer antihypertensive medication as ordered related to hypertensive parameters.
3. Assess edema.
4. Assess lungs for pulmonary edema.
5. Maintain bed rest in the left lateral position.

Problem 3: Anxiety related to harm for self and fetus
Goal: Decreased anxiety.
Outcome: Patient verbalizes that she feels less anxious.

Nursing Actions

1. Be calm and reassuring in interactions with the patient and her family.
2. Explain all procedures.
3. Explain results of test and procedures.
4. Teach patient relaxation and breathing techniques.
5. Encourage the patient and family to verbalize their feelings regarding recent hemorrhage by asking open-ended questions.

Problem 4: Altered renal function
Goal: Maintain adequate renal function.
Outcome: The patient will maintain adequate renal function.

Nursing Actions

1. Monitor and maintain strict I&O.
2. Report urine output <30 mL/hr.
3. Check urine protein and specific gravity.
4. Evaluate kidney function tests.
5. Report changes in urine output or worsening kidney function laboratory values to the care provider.
6. Assess edema.

Problem 5: Altered hepatic function
Goal: Maintain adequate hepatic function.
Outcome: The patient will maintain adequate hepatic function.

Nursing Actions

1. Assess epigastric pain, right upper quadrant pain, nausea, and vomiting.
2. Interpret laboratory tests related to liver function (AST, LDH).
3. Report changes in liver function tests to the care provider.

Problem No. 6: Altered placental perfusion
Goal: Maintain fetal oxygenation.
Outcome: Assessments of fetal status remain within normal limits.

Nursing Actions

1. Assess FHR baseline, variability, and for Category II or III FHR patterns.
2. Provide interventions for intrauterine resuscitation of fetus (IV fluid, O_2, lateral position).
3. Report any abnormal FHR patterns to the care provider.
4. Facilitate antenatal testing.
5. Instruct the woman in daily kick counts.

Case Study

As the nurse, you evaluate Mallory Polk in triage in the labor and delivery unit. She presented in the triage unit at 8 p.m. at 32 weeks' gestation with complaints of a persistent low, dull backache; increased vaginal discharge; and pelvic pressure in her vagina for two days with some vaginal spotting this evening when she went to the bathroom. She attributed the discomforts of backache and pulling to working long hours for the past week in arbitration on a "big case," as she is a partner in a large law firm. Mallory is a 42-year-old single African American woman. She is accompanied by her sister Alison, who is visiting for the week from out of state. When placed on the monitor, Mallory is having contractions every 5 to 7 minutes that she reports as "menstrual cramping." The FHR is in the 150s baseline with accelerations to 170s with moderate variability. A review of her prenatal record reveals she is a G2 P0 and the pregnancy is a result of in vitro fertilization. She has received regular prenatal visits. She does not smoke or drink alcohol. Her prenatal laboratory results are as follows:

- Blood type A+
- RPR NR
- GBS negative
- Hgb 12.4
- Hct 32.1
- Hepatitis negative

Prenatal Care Summary

Mallory began prenatal care at 10 weeks' gestation and receives regular prenatal care. She conceives after three attempts at in vitro fertilization. She has no prior medical complications and has experienced a normal pregnancy. Her first pregnancy was terminated at 6 weeks of gestation. She is allergic to shellfish and is allergic to sulfa drugs. An ultrasound at 12 weeks confirms a gestational age of 32 weeks.

Detail the aspects of your initial assessment and what you would report to her physician.

Within 40 minutes of arrival, you phone her physician, who is completing a delivery, and report your assessment findings. The physician comes to the unit in 10 minutes to evaluate Mallory. Based on her assessment, she orders an IV lactated Ringer's 300-mL bolus, a CBC, and urinalysis clean catch; does a fetal fibronectin; and does a sterile vaginal exam that reveals her cervix is 2 cm dilated/75% effaced/0 station. Her physician orders a 4-g magnesium sulfate bolus over 30 minutes, then 2 g per hour. Betamethasone is to be given 12 mg now and to be repeated in 24 hours. An ultrasound is ordered for fetal size and position. Her physician discusses the plan of care for treatment of preterm labor with Mallory and answers her questions, and Mallory agrees to the plan to attempt to stop the contractions and delay delivery.

What are your immediate priorities in nursing care for Mallory? Discuss the rationale for the priorities.

State nursing diagnosis, expected outcome, and interventions related to this problem.

List Mallory's risk factors for preterm labor.

What teaching would you include?

Within 10 minutes of starting the magnesium sulfate bolus, she reports feeling hot and flushed and feels burning at the IV site. After the magnesium sulfate bolus is complete, you start the magnesium sulfate infusion at 2 g per hour. At midnight, her contractions slow down to every 15 minutes or 4 to 5 contractions/hour. The FHR baseline is 140s with minimal variability and periodic accelerations. An ultrasound reveals the fetus is vertex, estimated fetal weight (EFW) is 1,560 g, and fetal fibronectin is positive.

What are the assessments for a woman treated for preterm labor on magnesium sulfate?

Discuss the rationale for the assessments.

What teaching would you include in the nursing action plan?

At 7 a.m. when you sign off, Mallory is sleeping intermittently. Her contractions are 23 per hour and the FHR is normal. Mallory is very concerned about giving birth to a premature baby. She is concerned that a baby will not survive at this gestation and states, "I have always wanted to be a mother and was so happy when I was finally ready to have a baby and conceived with IVF." She is worried about not being able to return to work over the next few days and weeks, as she has many active cases pending over the next few weeks. She states that she is not ready for the baby to come and has not set up the crib or finished the nursery. She feels guilty that she did not come to the hospital sooner and considered the backache as just part of pregnancy discomforts. Before you leave, you have requested Mallory be seen that day by the neonatal clinical specialist to review status and care for neonates born prematurely and to have Mallory's sister tour the NICU.

Detail the aspects of your psychosocial assessment for a woman with a high-risk pregnancy.

Discuss the rationale for the assessment.

Discuss nursing diagnosis, nursing actions, and expected outcomes related to this psychosocial assessment.

The next night, you come onto your shift at 7 p.m. and care for Mallory again. She remains on the magnesium sulfate and appears to be tolerating the medication. Her magnesium level is 5.6 mEq/L. She still feels warm and somewhat lethargic with sore muscles from being in bed all day. She is due for her second dose of betamethasone. Her I&O for the past 24 hours are: I: 2,500 mL; O: 2,300 mL. The plan is to stop the magnesium sulfate and transfer her to the antenatal unit in the morning and observe her for a day or so.

Detail the aspects of your ongoing assessment for a woman treated with magnesium sulfate and diagnosed with preterm labor.

Discuss the rationale for the assessment.

At 3:20 p.m. she reports feeling a gush of fluid from her vagina after a strong contraction. Between her legs is a large amount of clear fluid. The FHR is baseline 140s with minimal variability and accelerations. Mallory appears frightened and anxious. She is crying and her sister is at her side holding her hand and reassuring her.

What are your immediate priorities in nursing care for Mallory?

Discuss the rationale for the priorities.

Within 45 minutes, her physician comes in to see Mallory and does an SVE. She is 5 cm, 90% effaced, and +1 station, and an ultrasound reveals the fetus is vertex. The physician recommends they turn off the magnesium sulfate and anticipate a vaginal birth because of the advanced preterm labor. Mallory agrees with the plan.

REFERENCES

American Academy of Pediatrics (AAP) and the American College of Obstetricians and Gynecologists (ACOG). (2012). *Guidelines for perinatal care* (7th Ed.). Elk Grove Village, IL: Authors.

American Cancer Society. (2015). Smoking while you are pregnant or breastfeeding. Retrieved from https://www.cancer.org/cancer/cancer-causes/tobacco-and-cancer/smoking-while-you-are-pregnant-or-breastfeeding.html

American College of Obstetricians and Gynecologists (ACOG). (2002). Perinatal care at the threshold of viability. ACOG Practice Bulletin No. 38. *International Journal of Gynecology & Obstetrics, 79*(2), 181–188.

American College of Obstetricians and Gynecologists (ACOG). (2004a). Diagnosis and treatment of gestational trophoblastic disease. ACOG Practice Bulletin No. 53.

American College of Obstetricians and Gynecologists (ACOG). (2004b). Nausea and vomiting of pregnancy. ACOG Practice Bulletin No. 52.

American College of Obstetricians and Gynecologists (ACOG). (2008a). Medical management of ectopic pregnancy. ACOG Practice Bulletin No. 94. *Obstetrics & Gynecology, 111*(6), 1479–1485.

American College of Obstetricians and Gynecologists (ACOG). (2010). Committee Opinion No. 445: Magnesium sulfate before antepartal preterm birth for neuroprotection. *Obstetric & Gynecology,* 669–671.

American College of Obstetricians and Gynecologists (ACOG). (2012a). Committee Opinion No. 524: Opioid use, dependency, and addiction in pregnancy. *Obstetrics & Gynecology, 119*(5), 1070–1076.

American College of Obstetricians and Gynecologists (ACOG). (2012b). Committee Opinion No. 529: Placenta accreta. *Obstetrics & Gynecology,* 120, 207–211.

American College of Obstetricians and Gynecologists (ACOG). (2013a). Committee Opinion No. 560: Medically indicated later preterm and early term deliveries. *Obstetrics & Gynecology,* 121(4), 908–910.

American College of Obstetricians and Gynecologists (ACOG). (2013). Gestational diabetes mellitus. ACOG Practice Bulletin No. 137. *Obstetrics & Gynecology,* 122(2 Pt 1), 406–416.

American College of Obstetricians and Gynecologists (ACOG). (2013c). Hypertension in pregnancy Practice Guideline WQ 244. Retrieved from https://www.acog.org/Clinical-Guidance-and-Publications/Task-Force-and-Work-Group-Reports/Hypertension-in-Pregnancy

American College of Obstetricians and Gynecologists (ACOG). (2014a). Cerclage for the management of cervical insufficiency. ACOG Practice Bulletin No. 142. *Obstetrics & Gynecology,* 123, 372–379.

American College of Obstetricians and Gynecologists (ACOG). (2014b). Medical management of first-trimester abortion. Practice Bulletin No. 143. *Obstetrics & Gynecology,* 123(3), 676–692.

American College of Obstetricians and Gynecologists (ACOG). (2014c). Multifetal gestations: Twin, triplet, and higher-order multifetal pregnancies. ACOG Practice Bulletin No. 144. *Obstetrics & Gynecology,* 123(5), 1118–1132.

American College of Obstetrics and Gynecologists (ACOG). (2015a). Committee Opinion No. 633: Alcohol abuse and other substance use disorders: Ethical issues in obstetric and gynecologic practice. *Obstetrics & Gynecology,* 125(6),1529–1537.

American College of Obstetricians and Gynecologists (ACOG). (2015b). Early pregnancy loss. ACOG Practice Bulletin No. 150. *Obstetrics & Gynecology,* 2015; 125:1258–1267.

American College of Obstetricians and Gynecologists (ACOG). (2015c). Nausea and vomiting of pregnancy. ACOG Practice Bulletin No. 153. *Obstetrics & Gynecology,* 126(3), e12–24.

American College of Obstetricians and Gynecologists (ACOG). (2015d). Obesity in pregnancy. ACOG Practice Bulletin No. 150. VOL. 126, NO. 6,

American College of Obstetricians and Gynecologists (ACOG). (2016a) Management of preterm labor. ACOG Practice Bulletin No. 171. *Obstetrics & Gynecology,* 128, e155–164.

American College of Obstetricians and Gynecologists (ACOG). (2016b). Premature rupture of membranes. Practice Bulletin No. 172. *Obstetrics & Gynecology,128*, e165–77.

American College of Obstetricians and Gynecologists (ACOG). (2017a). Committee Opinion No. 692: Emergent therapy for acute-onset, severe hypertension during pregnancy and the postpartum period.*Obstetrics & Gynecology,129*, e90–95.

American College of Obstetricians and Gynecologists (ACOG). (2017b). Periviable birth. Obstetric Care Consensus No. 4. *Obstetrics & Gynecology,130*, e187–189.

American College of Obstetricians and Gynecologists (ACOG). (2017c). Smoking Cessation During Pregnancy Committee Opinion No. 741. *Obstetrics & Gynecology, 130*, e200–204.

American Diabetes Association (ADA). (2014). Diagnosis and classification of diabetes mellitus. *Diabetes Care, 37*(1), 81–91.

Arafeh, J. (2014). Cardiac disease in pregnancy. In K. Simpson & P. Creehan (Eds.), *Perinatal nursing* (4th ed.). Philadelphia, PA: Lippincott, Williams & Wilkins.

Association of Women's Health, Obstetric and Neonatal Nurses (AWHONN). (2010). Smoking and women's health position statement. *Journal of Obstetric, Gynecologic, & Neonatal Nursing, 39*, 611–613.

Association of Women's Health, Obstetric and Neonatal Nurses (AWHONN). (2015). Criminalization of pregnant women with substance use disorders position statement 2015. *Journal of Obstetric, Gynecologic, & Neonatal Nursing, 44*, 155–157. doi: 10.1111/1552-6909.1253

Association of Women's Health, Obstetric and Neonatal Nurses (AWHONN). (2016). The nursing care of the woman with diabetes in pregnancy evidence-based clinical practice guideline. Evidence-Based Clinical Practice Guideline Development Team. Association of Women's Health, Obstetric and Neonatal Nurses, Washington D.C.

Baldisseri, M. (2016). *Shock and pregnancy.* Retrieved from https://www.uptodate.com/contents/shock in pregnancy

Bates, S. M., Middeldorp, S., Rodger, M., James, A. H., & Greer, I. (2016). Guidance for the treatment and prevention of obstetric-associated venous thromboembolism. *Journal of Thrombosis and Thrombolysis, 41*, 92–128. http://doi.org/10.1007/s11239-015-1309-0

Bond, D., Middleton, P., Levett, K., van der Ham, D., Crowther, C., Buchanan, S., & Morris J. (2017). Planned early birth versus expectant management for women with preterm prelabour rupture of membranes prior to 37 weeks' gestation for improving pregnancy outcome. *Cochrane Database of Systematic Reviews, 3*. CD004735. doi: 10.1002/14651858.CD004735.pub4.

Bowers, N. (2014). Multiple gestation. In K. Simpson & P. Creehan (Eds). *Perinatal nursing* (4th ed.). Philadelphia, PA: Lippincott, Williams & Wilkins.

Bryant, A., Worjoloh, A., Caughey, A., & Washington. A. (2010). Racial/ethnic disparities in obstetric outcomes and care: Prevalence and determinants. *American Journal of Obstetrics & Gynecology,202*(4), 335–343.

Burke-Sosa, M. (2014). Bleeding in pregnancy. In K. Simpson & P. Creehan (Eds.), *Perinatal nursing* (4th ed.). Philadelphia, PA: Lippincott, Williams & Wilkins.

Callahan, L. (2016). Management of non-obstetrical surgery and trauma in pregnancy. In S. Mattson & J. E. Smith (Eds.), *Core curriculum for maternal-newborn nursing* (5th ed.). St. Louis, MO: Elsevier.

Carlson, A., Norwitz, E. R., & Stiller, R. J. (2010). Cytomegalovirus infection in pregnancy: Should all women be screened? *Reviews in Obstetrics & Gynecology, 3*(4), 172–179.

Centers for Disease Control and Prevention (CDC). (2014). *Fetal alcohol spectrum disorder (FASDs): Facts about FASDs.* Retrieved from www.cdc.gov/ncbddd/fasd/facts.html.

Centers for Disease Control and Prevention (CDC). (2015a). Fact sheet. Reported STDS in the United States 2015 National Data for chlamydia, gonorrhea and syphilis. https://www.cdc.gov/nchhstp/newsroom/docs/factsheets/std-trends-508.pdf

Centers for Disease Control (CDC). (2015b). Morbidity and Mortality Weekly Report. Sexually transmitted disease treatment guidelines. *Recommendations and Reports, 64*(3).

Centers for Disease Control and Prevention (CDC). (2015c). Sexually transmitted disease surveillance. Atlanta, GA: U.S. Department of Health & Human Services.

Chasnoff, I. J., Wells, A, McGourty, R. F., & Bailey, L. K. (2007). Validation of the 4P's Plus© Screen for Substance Use in Pregnancy. *Journal of Perinatology, 27*, 744–748.

Christopher, D., Robinson, B., & Peaceman, A. (2011). An evidence-based approach to determining route of delivery for twin gestations. *Reviews in Obstetrics & Gynecology, 4*(3–4), 109–116.

Cluver, C. (2017). Planned early delivery versus expectant management for hypertensive disorders from 34 weeks gestation to term. *Cochrane Database of Systematic Reviews, 1*. doi:10.1002/14651858.CD009273.pub2

Council on Patient Safety in Women's Health Care. (2017). Hypertension safety bundle: Severe hypertension in pregnancy. Retrieved from http://safehealthcareforeverywoman.org/patient-safety-bundles/severe-hypertension-in-pregnancy/

Cowswell, T., Middleton, P., & Weeks, A. (2009) Antenatal day care units versus hospital admission for women with complicated pregnancy. *Cochrane Database of Systematic Reviews,4*. CD001803. doi: 10.1002/14651858.CD001803.pub2.

Creasy, R., Resnik, R., & Iams, J. (Eds.). (2004). *Maternal-fetal medicine* (5th ed.). Philadelphia, PA: W. B. Saunders.

Crowley A., Grivell R., & Dodd J. (2016). Sealing procedures for preterm prelabour rupture of membranes. *Cochrane Database of Systematic Reviews, 7*. CD010218. doi: 10.1002/14651858.CD010218.pub2.

Cunningham, E., Leveno, K., Bloom, S., Spong, C., Dashe, J., Hoffman, B., . . . Sheffield, J. (2014). *Williams obstetrics* (24th ed.). New York, NY: McGraw-Hill.

Daley, J. (2014). Diabetes in pregnancy. In K. Simpson & P. Creehan. *Perinatal nursing* (4th ed.). Philadelphia, PA: Lippincott, Williams & Wilkins.

D'Alton, M., Friedman, A., Smiley, R., Montgomery, D., Paidas, M., D'Oria, R., . . . Clark, S. (2016). National Partnership for Maternal Safety: Consensus Bundle on Venous Thromboembolism. *Journal of Obstetric, Gynecologic & Neonatal Nursing, 45*(5), 706–717.

da Silva Lopes, K. (2017). Bed rest with and without hospitalization in multiple pregnancy for improving perinatal outcomes. *Cochrane Database of Systematic Reviews, 4*. doi:10.1002/14651858.CD012031.pub2

Dodd, J., Crowther, C., Dare, M., & Middleton, P. (2006) Oral betamimetics for maintenance therapy after threatened preterm labour. *Cochrane Database of Systematic Reviews, 1*. CD003927. doi: 10.1002/ 14651858.CD003927.pub2.

Dodd, J., Jones, L., Flenady, V., Cincotta, R., & Crowther, C. (2013). Prenatal administration of progesterone for preventing preterm birth in women considered to be at risk of preterm birth. *Cochrane Database of Systematic Reviews, 7*. CD004947. doi: 10.1002/14651858.CD004947.pub3

Durham, R. (1998). Strategies women engage in when managing preterm labor at home. *Journal of Perinatology,18*, 61–64.

Elsasser, D., Ananth, C., Prasad, V., Vintzileos, A., &New Jersey-Placental Abruption Study Investigators. (2010). Diagnosis of placental abruption: relationship between clinical and histopathological findings. *European Journal of Obstetrics, Gynecology, and Reproductive Biology, 148*(2), 125. http://doi.org/10.1016/j.ejogrb.2009.10.005

El Senoun, G., Dowswell, T., & Mousa, H. (2014). Planned home versus hospital care for preterm prelabour rupture of the membranes (PPROM) prior to 37 weeks' gestation. *Cochrane Database Systematic Reviews,14*(4):CD008053. doi:10.1002/14651858.CD008053.pub2. Review.

Esplin, M. S., Elovitz, M. A., Iams, J. D., Parker, C. B., Wapner, R. J., Grobman, W. A., . . . Reddy, U. M. (2017). Predictive accuracy of serial transvaginal cervical lengths and quantitative vaginal fetal fibronectin levels for spontaneous preterm birth among nulliparous women. *Journal of the American Medical Association,317*(10), 1047–1056. doi: 10.1001/jama.2017.1373. PubMed PMID: 28291893.

Forray, A. (2016). Substance use during pregnancy. *F1000Research, 5*, F1000 Faculty Rev–887. http://doi.org/10.12688/f1000research.7645.1

Gaddipati, S., & Troiano, N. (2013). Cardiac disorders in pregnancy. In N. Troiano, C. Harvey, & B. Chez (Eds.), *High risk & critical care obstetrics* (3rd ed.). Philadelphia, PA: Wolters Kluwer/Lippincott Williams & Wilkins.

Genovese, S. K. (2016). Hemorrhagic disorders. In S. Mattson & J. E. Smith (Eds.), *Core curriculum for maternal-newborn nursing* (5th ed.). St. Louis, MO: Elsevier.

Gilbert, E., (2011). *Manual of high risk pregnancy and delivery* (5th ed.). St. Louis, MO: C. V. Mosby.

Goldstein, R. (2007). Management of preterm labor. In J. Queenan (Ed.), *High risk pregnancy.* American College of Obstetricians and Gynecologists. Wiley Blackwell

Grey, B. (2006). A ticking uterus. *Lifelines,10*, 380–389.

Grobman, W. A., Bailit, J. L., Rice, M. M., Wapner, R. J., Reddy, U. M., Varner, M.W., . . . VanDorsten, J. P. (2015). Eunice Kennedy Shriver National Institute of Child Health and Human Development (NICHD) Maternal-Fetal Medicine Units (MFMU) Network. Racial and ethnic disparities in maternal morbidity and obstetric care. *Obstetrics & Gynecology, 125*(6), 1460–1467. doi: 10.1097/AOG.0000000000000735.

Han, S., Crowther, C., & Moore, V. (2010). Magnesium maintenance therapy for preventing preterm birth after threatened preterm labour. *Cochrane Database of Systematic Reviews, 7*. CD000940. doi: 10.1002/14651858.CD000940.

Hodnett, E. (2010). Support during pregnancy for women at increased risk of low birthweight babies. *Cochrane Database of Systematic Reviews, 6.*

Hoffert Gilmartin, A., Ural, S., & Repke, J. (2008). Gestational diabetes mellitus review. *Obstetrics & Gynecology, 1*(3),129–134.

Hudak, M. L., Tan, R. C. & Committee on Drugs and Committee on Fetus and Newborn. (2014). Neonatal drug withdrawal. *Pediatrics,133*(5), 937–938.

Iams, J. (2007). Predication and early detection of preterm labor. In J. Queenan (Ed.), *High risk pregnancy.* Washington D.C.: American College of Obstetricians and Gynecologists.

Institute of Medicine (US) (2007). Committee on Understanding Premature Birth and Assuring Healthy Outcomes, Behrman, R. E., Butler, A. S. (Eds.), *Preterm birth: Causes, consequences, and prevention.* Washington, DC: National Academies Press (US). Available from: https://www.ncbi.nlm.nih.gov/books/NBK11362/ doi: 10.17226/11622

Institute of Medicine. (2007). *Preterm birth: causes, consequences, and prevention.* Washington, DC: National Academy Press.

Jatlaoui, T., Ewing, A., Mandel, M., Simmons, K., Suchdev, D., Jamieson, D., & Pazol, K. (2016). Abortion surveillance—United States, 2013. *MMWR Surveillance Summary,65*(12), 1–44. doi: http://dx.doi.org/10.15585/mmwr.ss6512al.

Jazayeri, A. (2016). Premature rupture of membranes. Retrieved from https://emedicine.medscape.com/article/261137-overview

Johnson, E., & Wolfe Jr., J. S. (2014). Urinary tract infections in pregnancy. Retrieved from https://emedicine.medscape.com/article/452604-overview

Khurana, R. (2017). Systemic lupus erythematosus and pregnancy. Retrieved from https://emedicine.medscape.com/article/335055-overview

Ko, J. Y., Farr, S. L., Tong, V. T., Creanga, A. A., & Callaghan, W. M. (2015). Prevalence and patterns of marijuana use among pregnant and nonpregnant women of reproductive age. *American Journal of Obstetrics & Gynecology,213*(2), 201.e1–201.e10

Maharaj, D. (2007). Intrapartum fetal resuscitation: A review. *Internet Journal of Gynecology and Obstetrics,9*(2).

Maloni, J. A. (1998). *Antepartum bedrest: Case studies, research & nursing care.* Washington, DC: Association of Women's Health, Obstetric and Neonatal Nurses.

March of Dimes. (2006a). Compendium on preterm birth: Employing systems-based practice for patient care. Produced in cooperation with American Academy of Pediatrics, the American College of Obstetricians and Gynecologists & Association of Women's Health, Obstetric and Neonatal Nurses.

March of Dimes. (2006b). Compendium on preterm birth: Epidemiology and biology of preterm birth. Produced in cooperation with American Academy of Pediatrics, The American College of Obstetricians and Gynecologists & Association of Women's Health, Obstetric and Neonatal Nurses.

March of Dimes. (2011). Healthy Babies are worth the wait: Preventing preterm births through community-based interventions: Implementation manual. https://www.marchofdimes.org/prematurity-campaign-progress-report-2012.pdf

March of Dimes. (2013). *Quick facts: Smoking/alcohol/drugs.* Retrieved from www.marchofdimes.org/Peristats/ViewTopic.aspx?reg=99&top=9&lev=0&slev=1

March of Dimes. (2015). *Perinatal data snapshots: United States: Maternal and infant health overview.* Retrieved from www.marchofdimes.com.

March of Dimes. (2018). Preterm labor and preterm bith: Are you at risk? Retrieved from www.marchofdimes.org/complications/preterm-labor-and-premature-birth-are-you-at-risk.aspx

Mark, K., Desai, A., & Terplan, M. (2016). Marijuana use and pregnancy: Prevalence, associated characteristics, and birth outcomes. *Archives Women's Mental Health, 19*(1), 105–111.

Martin, J. A., Hamilton, B. E., Osterman, M. J. K., Driscoll, A. K. Matthews, T. K. (2017). Births: Final data for 2015. *National Vital Statistics Report,66*(1).

Matthews, A., Dowswell, T., Haas, D. M., Doyle, M., & O'Mathúna, D. (2010). Interventions for nausea and vomiting in early pregnancy. *Cochrane Database of Systematic Reviews,9*. CD007575. doi: 10.1002/14651858.CD007575.pub2.

Mattson, S., & Smith, J. E. (Eds.). (2011). *Core curriculum for maternal-newborn nursing* (4th ed.). St. Louis, MO: Elsevier Saunders.

McMurtry-Baird, S., & Kennedy, B. (2014). Pulmonary complications in pregnancy. In K. Simpson & P. Creehan (Eds.), *Perinatal nursing* (4th ed.). Philadelphia, PA: Lippincott, Williams & Wilkins.

Mendez-Figueroa, H., Dahlke, J. D., Vrees, R. A., & Rouse, D. J. (2013) Trauma in pregnancy: an updated systematic review. *American Journal of Obstetrics & Gynecology, 209,* 1.

National High Blood Pressure Education Program (NHBPEP). (2000). Working group report on high blood pressure in pregnancy (NHBPEP Publication No. 00-3029). Washington, DC: National Heart Lung and Blood Institute.

National Institute of Child Health and Human Development (NICHHD). (2013). Tobacco, drug use in pregnancy can double risk of stillbirth. NIH network study documents elevated risk associated with marijuana, other substances [news release]. Bethesda, MD: National Institute of Child Health and Human Development.

National Institute of Child Health and Human Development (2017). Preterm labor and birth. Bethesda, MD: Eunice Kennedy Shriver National Institute of Child Health and Human Development; January 31, 2017.

National Institute on Drug Abuse. (2013). *Commonly abused drugs.* Retrieved from https://www.drugabuse.gov/.

Neilson, J. (2009). Interventions for suspected placenta previa. *Cochrane Database of Systematic Reviews, 1.* doi:10.1002/14651858.CD001998

Norwitz, E., & Caughey, A. (2011). Progesterone supplementation and the prevention of preterm birth.*Reviews in Obstetrics & Gynecology,4*(2), 60–72.

Opray, N., Grivell, R., Deussen, A., & Dodd, J. (2015). Directed preconception health programs and interventions for improving pregnancy outcomes for women who are overweight or obese. *Cochrane Database of Systematic Reviews,7.* CD010932. doi:10.1002/14651858.CD010932.pub2.

Owen, J., & Harger, J. (2007). Cerclage and cervical incompetency. In J. Queenan (Ed.), *High risk pregnancy.* Washington, DC:The American College of Obstetricians and Gynecologists.

Panel on Treatment of Pregnant Women with HIV Infection and Prevention of Perinatal Transmission. (2018) Recommendations for Use of Antiretroviral Drugs in Transmission in the United States. Available at http://aidsinfo.nih.gov/contentfiles/lvguidelines/ PerinatalGL.pdf. Accessed 5-2-2918

Panelli, D. Phillips, C. & Brady. P. (2015). Incidence, diagnosis and management of tubal and nontubal ectopic pregnancies: A review. *Fertility Research and Practice,1,* 15.

PeriStats. (2017). National Center for Health Statistics, final natality data. Retrieved from www.marchofdimes.com/peristats.

Phillips, C., & Boyd, M. (2015). Intrahepatic cholestasis of pregnancy. *Nursing for Women's Health, 19*(1), 46–57.

Phillips, C., & Boyd, M. (2016). Assessment, management, and health implications of early-onset preeclampsia. *Nursing For Women's Health,20*(4), 402–414.

Piccoli, G. B., Attini, R., Vasario, E., Conijn, A., Biolcati, M., D'Amico, F., . . . Todros, T. (2010). Pregnancy and chronic kidney disease: A challenge in all CKD stages.*Clinical Journal of the American Society of Nephrology,5*(5), 844–855.

Poole, J. (2014). Hypertension disorders in pregnancy. In K. Simpson & P. Creehan (Eds.), *Perinatal nursing* (4th ed.). Philadelphia, PA: Lippincott, Williams & Wilkins.

Queenan, J., Hobbins, J., & Spong, C. (2005). *Protocols in high risk pregnancies.* Malden, MA: Blackwell.

Reedy, N. (2014). Preterm labor and birth. In K. Simpson & P. Creehan (Eds.), *Perinatal nursing* (4th ed.). Philadelphia, PA: Lippincott, Williams & Wilkins.

Roberts, D., Brown, J., Medley, N., & Dalziel, S. R. (2017). Antenatal corticosteroids for accelerating fetal lung maturation for women at risk of preterm birth. *Cochrane Database of Systematic Reviews, 3.* CD004454. doi: 10.1002/14651858 .CD004454.pub3.

Shah, P., & Shah, J. (2010). Maternal exposure to domestic violence and pregnancy and birth outcomes: A systematic review and meta-analyses. *Journal of Women's Health,19*(11), 2017–2031. doi:10.1089/jwh.2010.2051

Shah, P., Zao, J., & Ali, S. (2011). Maternal marital status and birth outcomes: A systematic review and meta-analyses. *Maternal & Child Health Journal,15*(7), 1097–1109. doi:10.1007/s10995-010-0654-z

Sibai, B. (2004). Diagnosis, controversies, and management of the syndrome of hemolysis, elevated liver enzymes, and low platelet count [High Risk Pregnancy Series: An expert's view]. *Obstetrics & Gynecology, 103,* 981–991.

Silver, R. (2015). Abnormal placentation: Placenta previa, vasa previa, and placenta accreta. *Obstetrics & Gynecology, 26*(3), 654–668.

Silver, R. M., Landon, M. B., Rouse, D. J., Leveno, K. J., Spong, C. Y., Thom, E. A., . . . Mercer, B. M. (2006). Maternal morbidity associated with multiple repeat cesarean deliveries. National Institute of Child Health and Human Development Maternal-Fetal Medicine Units Network. *Obstetrics & Gynecology,107,* 1226–1232.

Society for Maternal Fetal Medicine. (2017). Understanding intrahepatic cholestasis of pregnancy. Retrieved from http://www.mfmsm.com/understanding-intrahepatic-cholestasis-of-pregnancy-patient-guide-page.html?products_id=292&cPath=149

Substance Abuse and Mental Health Services Administration (SAMHSA). (2013). Results from the 2012 National Survey on Drug Use and Health: Mental health findings. Retrieved from https://www.samhsa.gov/data/sites/default/files/NSDUHresults2012/NSDUHresults2012.pdf

Sullivan, C. (2016). Substance abuse in pregnancy. In S. Mattson & J. E. Smith (Eds.), *Core curriculum for maternal-newborn nursing* (5th ed.). St. Louis, MO: Elsevier.

Tan, C., Denny, C., Cheal, N., Sniezek, J., Kanny, D., & CDC. (2015). Alcohol use and binge drinking among women of childbearing age—United States, 2011–2013. *MMWR Morbidity and Mortality Weekly Report, 64*(37), 1042–1046.

Task Force on Hypertension in Pregnancy and American College of Obstetricians and Gynecologists. (2013). Hypertension in pregnancy. Retrieved from https://www.acog.org/Clinical-Guidance-and-Publications/Task-Force-and-Work-Group-Reports/Hypertension-in-Pregnancy

Taylor, P., Zaichkin, J., & Bailey, D. (2002). *Substance abuse during pregnancy: Guidelines for screening.* Retrieved from http://contentmanager.med.uvm.edu/docs/default-source/vchip-documents/vchip_screening_for_preg_subabuse.pdf?sfvrsn=2

Tikkanen, M. (2011). Placental abruption: Epidemiology, risk factors and consequences. *Acta Obstetricia et Gynecologica Scandinavica, 90,* 140.

Tran, T., Ahn, J., & Reau, N. (2016). ACG clinical guideline: Liver disease and pregnancy. *American Journal of Gastroenterology,2.* doi: 10.1038/ajg.2015.430

U.S. Department of Health and Human Services, Substance Abuse and Mental Health Administration. (2008). Results from the 2007 National Survey on Drug Use and Health: National Findings, Office of Applied Studies, DHHS, publication no. SMA 08-4343. Rockville, MD: Author.

U.S. Department of Health and Human Services. (2018). Recommendations for the Use of Antiretroviral Drugs in Pregnant Women with HIV Infection and Interventions to Reduce Perinatal HIV Transmission in the United States. Rockville, MD: Author. Retrieved from https://aidsinfo.nih.gov/guidelined

Van Otterloo, L. (2016). Trauma in pregnancy. In S. Mattson & J. E. Smith (Eds.), *Core curriculum for maternal-newborn nursing* (5th ed.). St. Louis, MO: Elsevier.

Wegrzyniak, L., Repke, J., & Ural, S. (2012). Treatment of hyperemesis gravidarum. *Obstetrics & Gynecology, 5*(2). 78–84. doi: 10.3909/riog0176

Williamson, C., & Geenes, V. (2014). Intrahepatic cholestasis of pregnancy. *Obstetrics & Gynecology, 124,* 120–133. doi: 10.1097/AOG.0000000000000346

Yancy, M. (2016). Other medical complications. In S. Mattson & J. E. Smith (Eds.), *Core curriculum for maternal-newborn nursing* (5th ed.). St. Louis, MO: Elsevier.

The Intrapartal Period

Intrapartum Assessment and Interventions

Sylvia A Fischer RN, MSN, CNM, FNP-C

LEARNING OUTCOMES

Upon completion of this chapter, the student will be able to:
1. Describe the four stages of labor and the related nursing and medical care.
2. Demonstrate understanding of supportive care of the laboring woman.
3. Identify the five Ps of labor.
4. Describe the mechanism of spontaneous vaginal delivery and related nursing care.

Nursing Diagnoses

- Deficient knowledge of labor process
- Pain related to the labor and delivery process
- Fear related to unknowns of labor; threat of potential harm to self or fetus
- Risk of ineffective maternal/fetal perfusion related to perfusion in labor
- Risk of infection related to vaginal exams after rupture of membranes

Learning Outcomes

- The woman will understand the process and interventions related to labor.
- The woman will have decreased pain.
- The woman will have decreased fear during labor.
- The woman's vital signs and fetal heart rate remain stable.
- The woman will be free of infection.

INTRODUCTION

The intrapartum period begins with the onset of regular uterine contractions (UCs) and lasts until the expulsion of the placenta. The process by which this normally occurs is called labor. Childbirth is the period from the conclusion of the pregnancy to the start of the infant's extrauterine life. This chapter discusses the intrapartum/childbirth process, including the factors affecting labor and delivery, progression of labor and delivery, and the nursing care involved.

LABOR TRIGGERS

The question of when and how labor begins has been studied for years. The exact cause of the onset of labor is not completely understood, although there are several theories. Generally, it is proposed

that labor is triggered by both maternal and fetal factors that may be caused by an inflammatory process (Reyes-Lagos, Echeverria-Arjonilla, Pelia-Castillo, Montiel-Castro, & Pacheco-Lopez, 2014), a genetic component, and/or biomarkers in cervicovaginal fluid (Heng, Liong, Rice, DiQuinzio, & Georgioi, 2015). Unfortunately, even with substantial research, there is no concrete evidence of how labor initiates or what mechanisms are triggered at the time of labor. There is some evidence that the myometrium is stimulated by prostaglandins and oxytocin (biochemical factors) and becomes active. This initiates more contractions that become synchronized and softening of the cervix, which was previously protective (Simpson & O'Brien-Abel, 2014) (Fig. 8–1).

Maternal Factors

- Uterine muscles are stretched to the threshold point, leading to release of prostaglandins and oxytocin that stimulate contractions.

219

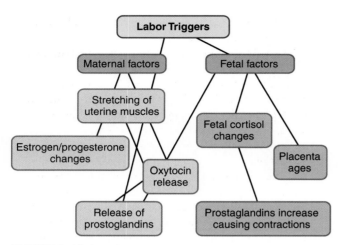

FIGURE 8–1 Labor triggers.

- Increased pressure on the cervix stimulates the nerve plexus, causing release of oxytocin by the maternal pituitary gland, which then stimulates contractions.
- Estrogen increases, stimulating the uterine response.
- Progesterone, which has a quieting effect on the uterus, is withdrawn, allowing estrogen to stimulate contractions.
- Oxytocin stimulates myometrial contractions. Oxytocin and prostaglandin work together to inhibit calcium binding in muscle cells, raising intracellular calcium levels and activating contractions.
- The oxytocin level surges from stretching of the cervix.

Fetal Factors

- As the placenta ages, it begins to deteriorate, triggering initiation of contractions.
- Prostaglandin synthesis by the fetal membranes and the decidua stimulates contractions.
- Fetal cortisol, produced by fetal adrenal glands, rises and acts on the placenta to reduce progesterone that quiets the uterus and increases prostaglandin that stimulates the uterus to contract.

SIGNS OF IMPENDING LABOR

A few weeks before labor, changes occur that indicate the woman's body is preparing for the onset of labor. These changes are also referred to as premonitory signs of labor.

- Lightening: This refers to the descent of the fetus into the true pelvis approximately 2 weeks before term in first-time pregnancies. The woman may feel she can breathe more easily but often experiences urinary frequency at this stage from increased bladder pressure. In subsequent pregnancies, this may not occur until labor begins.
- Braxton-Hicks: These contractions are irregular UCs that do not result in cervical change and are associated with "false labor." Braxton-Hicks contractions are usually not painful, don't happen at regular intervals, don't get closer together, may stop with a change in activity or position, and do not feel stronger over time. These contractions begin to coordinate the many muscle layers of the uterus to perform when true labor begins. True labor is characterized by regular uterine contractions that result in progressive dilation and effacement of the cervix and fetal descent into the pelvis (Simpson & OBrien-Abel, 2014).
- Cervical changes. The cervix ripens, becomes soft, and may become partially effaced and begin to dilate. The woman may lose her mucous plug or have a change in discharge.
- Nesting. Some women experience a burst of energy or feel the need to put everything in order, which is sometimes referred to as nesting.
- Less commonly, some women experience a 1- to 3-pound weight loss and others experience diarrhea, nausea, or indigestion preceding labor.
- The woman may experience low backache and sacroiliac discomfort due in part to the relaxation of the pelvic joints.
- The woman may experience a brownish or blood-tinged cervical mucus discharge referred to as bloody show.

FACTORS AFFECTING LABOR

Labor is defined by UCs that bring about effacement and dilation of the cervix. Factors that have been traditionally identified as the essential components in the outcome of labor and delivery include the 5 "P's":

- Powers (the contractions)
- Passage (the pelvis and birth canal)
- Passenger (the fetus)
- Psyche (the response of the woman)
- Position (maternal postures and physical positions to facilitate labor)

Powers

Powers refers to the involuntary UCs of labor and the voluntary pushing or bearing-down powers that combine to propel and deliver the fetus and placenta from the uterus (see Chapter 9 for assessment of UCs). Research shows that myometrial and decidual oxytocin receptors fluctuate during pregnancy. By the third trimester, the myometrial receptors increase by more than 300%, while uterine sensitivity of oxytocin also increases (Riemer & Heymann, 1998). Though no theory has been proven correct, studies support that pacemaker cells in the uterus send signals to other cells (Sultatos, 1997) and that the posterior lobe of the pituitary gland secretes oxytocin to stimulate contractions (Fuchs, Husslein, & Fuchs, 1991; Simpson & O'Brien-Abel, 2014).

Uterine Contractions

- The uterine muscle, known as the myometrium, contracts and shortens during the first stage of labor. Synchronizing of

these muscles focuses on the uterus & adnexa, partially due to the cervical dilation and lower uterine segment thinning (Shnol, Paul, & Belfer, 2014).
- The upper segment composes two-thirds of the uterus and contracts to push the fetus down.
- The lower segment composes the lower third of the uterus and the cervix and is less active, allowing the cervix to become thinner and pulled upward.
- Uterine contractions are responsible for the dilation (opening) and effacement (thinning) of the cervix in the first stage of labor.
- Uterine contractions are rhythmic and intermittent.
- Each contraction has a resting phase or uterine relaxation period that allows the woman and uterine muscle a pause for rest. This pause allows blood flow to the uterus and placenta that was temporarily reduced during the contraction phase. It is during this pause that much of the fetal exchange of oxygen, nutrients, and waste products occurs in the placenta. With every contraction, 500 mL of blood leaves the utero–placental unit and moves back into maternal circulation thus ridding the utero-placental unit of waste and bringing in a replenished oxygen supply.
- Uterine contractions are described in the following ways (Fig. 8–2):
  - Frequency: Time from beginning of one contraction to the beginning of another. It is recorded in minutes (e.g., occurring every 3 to 4 minutes).
  - Duration: Time from the beginning of a contraction to the end of the contraction. It is recorded in seconds (e.g., each contraction lasts 45 to 50 seconds).
  - Intensity: Strength of the contraction. It is evaluated with palpation using the fingertips on maternal abdomen and is described as:
    - Mild: The uterine wall is easily indented during contraction.
    - Moderate: The uterine wall is resistant to indentation during a contraction.
    - Strong: The uterine wall cannot be indented during a contraction.
- There are three phases of a contraction (see Fig. 8–2):
  - Increment phase: Ascending or buildup of the contraction that begins in the fundus and spreads throughout the uterus; the longest part of the contraction.
  - Acme phase: Peak of intensity but the shortest part of the contraction.
  - Decrement phase: Descending or relaxation of the uterine muscle.
- Contractions facilitate cervical changes (Fig. 8–3A, B, C).
  - Dilation and effacement occurs during the first stage of labor when UCs push the presenting part of the fetus toward the cervix, causing it to open and thin out as the musculofibrous tissue of the cervix is drawn upwards (see Fig. 8–3B).
  - Dilation is the enlargement or opening of the cervical os.
    - The cervix dilates from closed (or <1 cm diameter) to 10 cm diameter (see Fig. 8–3C).
    - When the cervix reaches 10 cm dilation, it is considered fully or completely dilated and can no longer be palpated on vaginal examination.
  - Effacement is the shortening and thinning of the cervix (Fig. 8–3A, B, C).
    - Before the onset of labor, the cervix is 2 to 3 cm long and approximately 1 cm thick (Fig. 8–3A).
    - The degree of effacement is measured in percentage and goes from 0% to 100%.
  - Effacement often precedes dilation in a first-time pregnancy. Effacement and dilation progression of the cervix occurs together in subsequent pregnancies.

Bearing-down powers occur once the cervix is fully dilated (10 cm), and the woman feels the urge to push; she will involuntarily bear down. The urge to push is triggered by the Ferguson reflex, activated

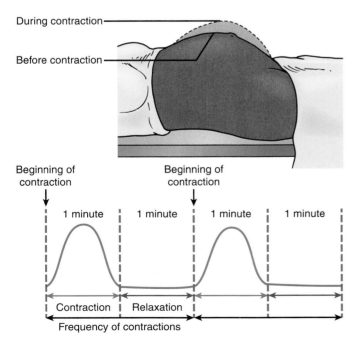

During contraction

Before contraction

Beginning of contraction

Beginning of contraction

1 minute | 1 minute | 1 minute | 1 minute

Contraction | Relaxation

Frequency of contractions

FIGURE 8–2 Frequency and duration of a contraction.

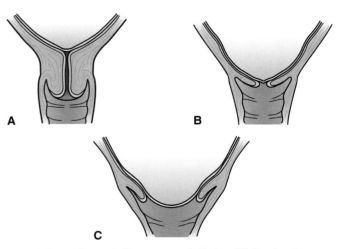

FIGURE 8–3 Cervical effacement and dilation. (*A*) Cervix prior to labor is closed and not effaced. (*B*) Cervix in latent phase of labor is effaced and starting to dilate. (*C*) Cervix in labor is effaced and dilating.

when the presenting part stretches the pelvic floor muscles. Stretch receptors are activated, releasing oxytocin and stimulating contractions (Simpson & O'Brien-Abel, 2014). The bearing-down powers are enhanced when the woman contracts her abdominal muscles and pushes. Multiple studies in the last 20 years have shown significant evidence that maternal fatigue is less and the abnormal FHR tracings associated with closed glottis sustained pushing are decreased when the woman pushes, with no significant increase of the second stage of labor. (Simpson & O'Brien-Abel, 2014). Studies done in the late 1990s and early 2000s demonstrated less injury to the pelvic floor and perineal injuries with pushing (Simpson & O'Brien-Abel, 2014). A review of nine randomized control trials (RCT) done by de Tayrac and Letouzey (2016) demonstrated that spontaneous pushing had no adverse fetal effects, higher maternal satisfaction, and no significant change in labor duration. Interventions in the second stage of labor should be realized independently with consideration of the situation at hand. It is important to consider the duration of pushing, parity, epidural analgesia, adequacy of pushing efforts, maternal and fetal status and progress, as well as the woman's preferences (Kopas, 2014).

Evidence-Based Practice: Labor Down or Bear Down

Osbourne, K., & Hanson, L. (2014). Labor down or bear down: A strategy to translate second stage labor evidence to perinatal practice. *Journal of Perinatal & Neonatal Nursing, 28*(2), 117–126.

Mother-initiated, spontaneous pushing in the second stage of labor begins at the time the woman feels the urge to push. Spontaneous pushing is defined as a mother's response to a natural urge to push or a bearing-down effort that comes and goes several times during each contraction. It does not involve timed breath holding or counting to 10 (Association of Women's Health, Obstetric and Neonatal Nurses [AWHONN], 2014c). Scientific evidence supports spontaneous physiologic approaches to a second stage labor management. However, most women in the U.S. receive instructions from care providers to use prolonged Valsalva bearing-down efforts as soon as the cervix is completely dilated. Delaying bearing-down efforts during the second stage of labor until the woman feels the urge to push results in optimal use of maternal energy, has no detrimental maternal or fetal effects, and results in improved fetal oxygenation. Though most commonly used with woman who receive epidural anesthesia, laboring down is just one component of physiologic second stage labor care that can be used to achieve optimal maternal and neonatal outcomes.

Active-directive pushing: Women historically have been put in the lithotomy position and given instructions to take a deep breath, hold it, and bear down with a closed glottis for at least 10 seconds, at least three times during one contraction as soon as they were complete, regardless of whether they felt the urge to push.

Physiologic second-stage labor care (laboring down): Encourage the women to wait until she feels an urge to push to initiate spontaneous bearing-down efforts. Support them in bearing down in response to natural urges. This passive descent is followed by an active urge to bear down.

Evidence-based practice: Waiting to push based on the woman's physical and emotional readiness has been recommended for decades (Caldeyro-Barcia, 1979; Osborn & Hanson, 2014; Roberts & Wooley, 1996). Having women labor upright in comfortable positions and not in the lithotomy position or on their backs has shown improved fetal oxygenation and APGAR scores.

The authors hope to translate the scientific evidence to clinical practice by providing tools and strategies to implement EBP second-stage labor care that encourage physiologic pushing to enhance EBP in the second stage.

Passage

The passage includes the bony pelvis and the soft tissues of the cervix, pelvic floor, vagina, and introitus (external opening to the vagina). Although all these anatomical areas play a role in the birth, the maternal pelvis is the greatest determinate in the vaginal delivery of the fetus. The assessment of the size and shape of the pelvis is important. Assessment of the pelvis is performed manually through palpation with a vaginal exam by the care provider during pregnancy.

Pelvis

- Types of bony pelvis (Fig. 8–4):
  - Gynecoid (most common type and found in about 50% of women)
  - Android
  - Anthropoid
  - Platypelloid (least common type and found in about 3% of women)
- The anatomical structure of the pelvis includes the ileum, the ischium, pubis, sacrum, and coccyx (Fig. 8–5).
- The bony pelvis is divided into:
  - False pelvis, which is the shallow upper section of the pelvis.
  - True pelvis, which is the lower part of the pelvis and consists of three planes, the inlet, the midpelvis, and the outlet. The measurement of these three planes defines the obstetric capacity of the pelvis.
- The pelvic joints include the symphysis pubis, the right and the left sacroiliac joints, and the sacrococcygeal joints.
- The actions of the hormones estrogen and relaxin during pregnancy soften cartilage and increase elasticity of the ligaments, allowing room for the fetal head.
- Station refers to the relationship of the ischial spines to the presenting part of the fetus and assists in assessing for fetal descent during labor (Fig. 8–6). Station 0 is the narrowest diameter the fetus must pass through during a vaginal birth.

Soft Tissue

- The soft tissue of the cervix effaces and dilates, allowing the descending fetus into the vagina.
- The soft tissue of the pelvic floor muscles helps the fetus in an anterior rotation as it passes through the birth canal.
- The soft tissue of the vagina expands to allow passage of the fetus.

Passenger

The passenger is the fetus. The fetus and its relationship to the passageway are the major factors in the birthing process. The relationship between the fetus and the passageway is affected by the fetal skull, fetal attitude, fetal lie, fetal presentation, fetal

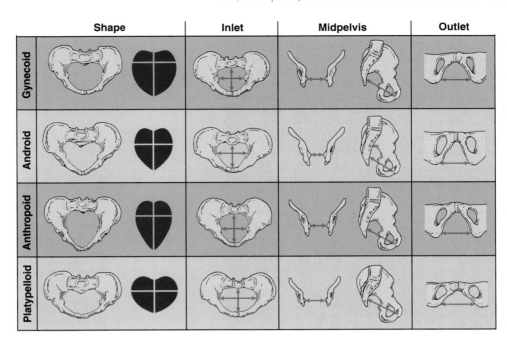

	Shape		Inlet	Midpelvis		Outlet
Gynecoid						
Android						
Anthropoid						
Platypelloid						

FIGURE 8–4 Pelvic types: gynecoid, android, anthropoid, and platypeloid.

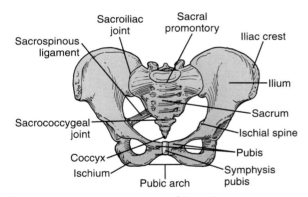

FIGURE 8–5 Anatomical structures of the pelvis.

position, and fetal size. At the onset of labor, the position of the fetus with respect to the birth canal is critical (Cunningham et al., 2014). In general, in the United States, when a fetus is in a position other than cephalic (head first), a cesarean delivery is considered. Size of the fetus alone is less significant in the birthing process than the relationship among fetal size, position, and pelvic dimensions (Mattson & Smith, 2011).

Fetal Skull

- The fetal head usually accounts for the largest portion of the fetus to come through the birth canal.
- Bones and membranous spaces help the skull to mold during labor and birth.
- Molding is the ability of the fetal head to change shape to accommodate/fit through the maternal pelvis (Fig. 8–7).
- The fetal skull is composed of two parietal bones, two temporal bones, the frontal bone, and the occipital bone (Fig. 8–8A).
  - The biparietal diameter (BPD), 9.25 cm, is the largest transverse measurement and an important indicator of head size (see Fig. 8–8B).

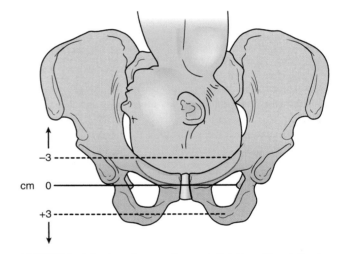

FIGURE 8–6 Station of presenting part: Fetal head in relation to ischial spines.

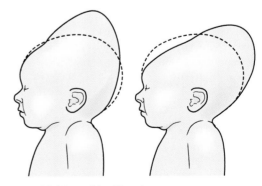

FIGURE 8–7 Molding of fetal head.

- The membranous space between the bones (sutures) and the fontanels (intersections of these sutures) allows the skull bones to overlap and mold to fit through the birth canal (see Fig. 8–8A&B).

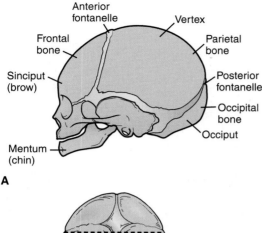

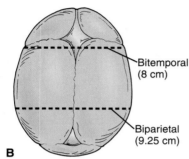

FIGURE 8–8 Bones of the fetal skull. (*A*) Bones of fetal skull (side view) (*B*) Diameter of fetal skull.

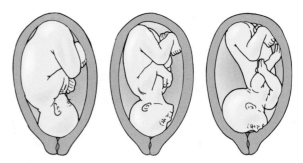

FIGURE 8–9 Fetal attitude or posture (flexed).

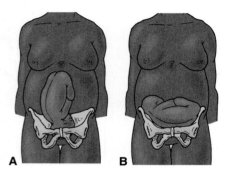

FIGURE 8–10 Fetal lie. (*A*) Longitudinal lie. (*B*) Transverse lie.

- Sutures are used to identify the positioning of the fetal head during a vaginal exam. By identifying the anterior fontanel in relationship to the woman's pelvis, the examiner can determine the position of the head and the degree of rotation that has occurred.

Fetal Attitude or Posture

Fetal attitude or posture is the relationship of fetal parts to one another, noted by the flexion or extension of the fetal joints (Fig. 8–9).

- At term, the fetus's back becomes convex and the head flexed such that the chin is against the chest. This results in a rounded appearance with the chin flexed forward on the chest, arms crossed over the thorax, the thighs flexed on the abdomen, and the legs flexed at the knees.
- With proper fetal attitude, the head is in complete flexion in a vertex presentation and passes more easily through the true pelvis.

Fetal Lie

Fetal lie refers to the long axis (spine) of the fetus in relationship to the long axis (spine) of the woman.

- The two primary lies are longitudinal and transverse (Fig. 8–10 A&B).
  - In the longitudinal lie, the long axes of the fetus and the mother are parallel (most common).
  - In the transverse lie, the long axis of the fetus is perpendicular to the long axis of the mother.
- A fetus cannot be delivered vaginally in the transverse lie.

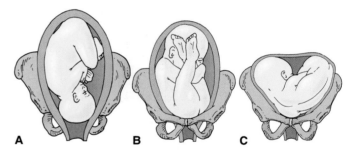

FIGURE 8–11 Fetal presentation. (*A*) Cephalic. (*B*) Breech. (*C*) Shoulder.

Presentation

Fetal presentation is determined by the part or pole of the fetus that first enters the pelvic inlet. There are three main presentations (Fig. 8–11):

- Cephalic (head first) (Fig. 8–11A)
- Breech (pelvis first) (Fig. 8–11B)
- Shoulder (shoulder first) (Fig. 8–11C)

Presenting Part

The presenting part is the specific fetal structure lying nearest to the cervix. It is determined by the attitude or posture of the fetus. Each presenting part has an identified denominator or reference point used to describe the fetal position in the pelvis.

- Cephalic presentations: The presenting part is the head (Fig. 8–12).
  - This accounts for 95% of all births (Mattson & Smith, 2011).

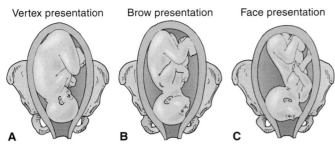

FIGURE 8–12 Cephalic presentation, (*A*) Vertex. (*B*) Brow. (*C*) Face.

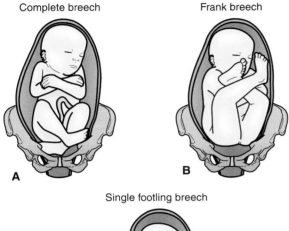

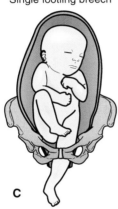

FIGURE 8–13 Breech presentation. (*A*) Complete. (*B*) Frank. (*C*) Footling.

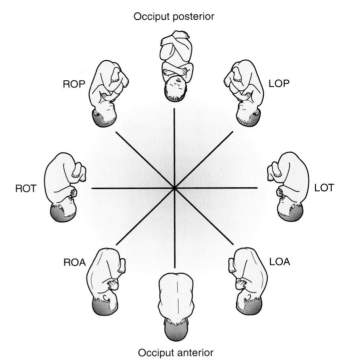

FIGURE 8–14 Variety of fetal positions with vertex presentation.

- The degree of flexion or extension of the head and neck further classifies cephalic presentations.
  - Vertex presentation indicates that the head is sharply flexed and the chin is touching the thorax. The denominator is the occiput.
  - Frontum or brow presentation indicates partial extension of the neck with the brow as the presenting part. The denominator is the frontum.
  - Face presentation indicates that the neck is sharply extended and the back of the head (occiput) is arching to the fetal back. The denominator is the mentum-chin.
- Breech presentations: The presenting part is the buttock and/or feet (Fig. 8–13).
  - Breech presentations are further classified as follows:
    - Complete breech: Complete flexion of the thighs and the legs extending over the anterior surfaces of the body (Fig. 8–13A)

- Frank breech: Complete flexion of thighs and legs (Fig. 8–13B)
- Footling breech: Extension of one or both thighs and legs so that one or both feet are presenting (Fig. 8–13C)
- Transverse presentation: The presenting part is usually the shoulder (see Fig. 8–10B).
  - This usually is associated with a transverse lie.
- Compound presentation: The fetus assumes a unique posture usually with the arm or hand presenting alongside the presenting part.

Fetal Position

The fetal position is the relation of the denominator or reference point to the maternal pelvis (Fig. 8–14).

- There are six positions for each presentation: right anterior, right transverse, right posterior, left anterior, left transverse, and left posterior.
- The occiput is the specific fetal structure for a cephalic presentation (see Fig. 8–11A).
- The sacrum is the specific fetal structure for a breech presentation (see Fig. 8–11B).
- The acromion is the specific fetal structure for a shoulder presentation (see Fig. 8–11C).
- The mentum is the specific fetal structure for the face presentation (see Fig. 8–12C).
- Position is designated by a three-letter abbreviation (Fig. 8–14):
  - First letter: Designates location of presenting part to the left (L) or right (R) of the woman's pelvis

- Second letter: Designates the specific fetal part presenting: occiput (O), sacrum (S), mentum (M), and shoulder (A)
- Third letter: Designates the relationship of the presenting fetal part to the woman's pelvis such as anterior (A), posterior (P), or transverse (T)

Psyche

Nursing care of the woman during the intrapartum period addresses not only the physical aspect of care but also the psychosocial aspect, ideally resulting in woman's wellness and satisfaction. Mental and physical preparation for childbirth helps the woman manage labor and promotes a sense of security and safety. A woman's experience and satisfaction during the labor and birthing process can be enhanced by coordination of collaborative goals between the woman and health care personnel in the plan of care. This influences her self-esteem, self-confidence, relationship to others, and general view of life. During her pregnancy, the woman should confer with her provider about pregnancy-related changes and what to expect in labor. By looking at how she handles pain, stress, anxiety, and what her preferences are, she can then make a plan of action to maintain control and autonomy when in labor. Encourage the woman to identify comforting items (such as pictures, music, visualization techniques, a favorite gown, and support people) to provide solace in the hospital environment (Simkin, Hanson, & Ancheta, 2017).

Factors that influence the woman's coping mechanism include her culture, expectations, a strong support system, and type of support during labor.

Culture

Culture influences the woman's reaction to labor expectations and how she interacts with others. The nurse must be culturally aware and sensitive to the needs and practices of the individual by integrating the woman's cultural and religious values, beliefs, and practices to provide a mutually acceptable plan of care. When the woman feels actively involved in creating a plan of care that integrates her cultural and/or religious values, beliefs, and practices, she will feel safer and more in control.

Culture and Birth Traditions

Nurses are practicing in an increasingly multicultural society with diverse cultural rituals, beliefs and practices surrounding women's health issues, including menstruation, pregnancy and childbirth. Increased cultural competence among health care providers can often reduce barriers to optimal care. Culturally sensitive communication is open, respectful, and nonjudgmental, and acknowledges that the nurse is willing to learn (Dean, 2010).

Giving birth is a pivotal life event, and the meaning of birth and parenthood is culturally defined (Moore, Moos, & Callister, 2010). Culture influences all aspects of a woman's response to labor and impacts factors such as:

- Who is with the woman in labor, their role, and who participates in decision making
- Preferences for use of pharmacological and non-pharmacological pain management in labor

- Who the woman wants to care for her in relation to gender and modesty
- Response to labor

The nurse must consider these factors to help women formulate their concerns, priorities, and decisions during childbirth.

Behaviors in birth are complex and personal. It is important for nurses to have a general understanding of birth practices of the cultural groups prevalent in the area where they work (Dean, 2010). Nurses are becoming more culturally aware through education and on-the-job training and finding it essential to recognize and examine their own traditions, beliefs, and prejudices so they can provide appropriate care and support to women and their families. According to the U.S. Department of Health and Human Services, Office of Minority Health. (2016), culturally competent care is more than a nicety; it is essential in the delivery of quality and safe care to childbearing women and their families. Strategies for providing culturally sensitive care are presented in Chapter 5. By identifying the patient's beliefs and being sensitive to her experiences of the health care system, nurses can provide individualized care to the women and her support system and give helpful information and guidance when differences are encountered.

SAFE AND EFFECTIVE NURSING CARE: Cultural Competence

Strategies for Nurses: Improving Culturally Responsive Care in Labor & Birth

Ethnicity, race, and religion may influence a woman's values, practices, and preferences during labor and birth. A flexible approach to care is required to meet the individualized needs of the woman during labor and birth. Nurses should be knowledgeable of the customs and beliefs of the specific cultural groups receiving care (AWHONN, 2011a). Providing individually focused, culturally sensitive care may enhance the likelihood of a positive birth experience. This may include the following measures:

- Learn the traditions of the cultural groups you often care for and the specific preferences of each woman and her family.
- Recognize there are subcultures within cultures.
- Listen to the woman and her support persons and help them find meaningful and acceptable support activities.
- Identify who the client calls "family."
- Expectations for the role of the woman's partner regarding support behaviors during labor and birth may vary greatly from one culture to the next.
- Use the beliefs, values, customs, and expectations of the woman to shape her plan of care for labor and birth.
- Include notes on cultural preferences and family strengths and resources as part of all intake and ongoing assessments and nursing care plans.

- Instead of focusing on technology, look beyond the routine and appreciate the needs of each woman.
- Develop linguistic skills related to your patient population.
- Learn to use nonverbal communication in an appropriate way.
- Learn about the communication patterns of various cultures.
- Recognize and acknowledge your own belief system while maintaining an open attitude.
- Examine the biases and assumptions you hold about different cultures.
- Avoid preconceptions and cultural stereotyping.
- Recognize all care is given within the context of many cultures.
- Advocate for organizational change that is flexible to cultural variations.

Amidi-Nouri, 2011; AWHONN, 2011a; Callister, 2014; Moore, Moos, & Callister, 2010; Simpson & O'Brien-Abel, 2014.

Expectations

- Expectations for the birth experience are related to how childbirth is viewed by the woman (e.g., as a natural process or as a stressful or threatening experience). The nurse should review the woman's expectations to help alleviate fear and to help set realistic goals.
- Unrealistic expectations can cause an increase in maternal anxiety.
- Past experiences and complications of pregnancy, labor, and birth strongly influence women's expectations of labor and response to labor.
- Women who have experienced a negative previous birthing experience are at risk for increased anxiety; women who experienced a positive previous birthing experience have lower anxiety levels.
- Women who are recent immigrants may have had very different birth experiences in other countries, and that influences their expectations, hopes, and fears.
- Current pregnancy experience with difficulty conceiving, an unplanned pregnancy, or a high-risk pregnancy may increase a woman's anxiety and fears.

CRITICAL COMPONENT

Nursing Support of Laboring Women

AWHONN asserts that continuously available labor support from a registered nurse (RN) is a critical component to achieve improved birth outcomes. The RN assesses, develops, implements, and evaluates an individualized plan of care based on each woman's physical, psychological and socio-cultural needs, including the woman's desires for and expectations of the laboring process. Labor care and labor support are powerful nursing functions and it is incumbent on health care facilities to provide an environment that encourages the unique patient-RN relationship during childbirth. For women in labor, continuous support can result in the following:

- Shorter labor
- Decreased use of analgesia/anesthesia
- Decreased operative vaginal births or cesarean births
- Decreased need for oxytocin/uterotonics
- Increased likelihood of breastfeeding
- Increased satisfaction with the childbirth experience (AWHONN, 2011a)

Labor is a dynamic event in a woman's life during which she needs adequate emotional and physical support and comfort. Non-pharmacologic methods of supporting and comforting women in labor have been shown to be therapeutic and to impact on women's experiences and birth outcomes (AWHONN, 2014c).

A recent Cochrane Review concluded that continuous support during labor may improve outcomes for women and infants, including increased spontaneous vaginal birth, shorter duration of labor, and decreased caesarean birth, instrumental vaginal birth, use of any analgesia, use of regional analgesia, low five-minute Apgar score, and negative feelings about childbirth experiences (Bohren, Hofmeyr, Sakala, Fukuzawa, & Cuthbert, 2017). The number of women who have access to non-pharmacologic labor support interventions provided or supervised by an RN is currently unknown, but has been demonstrated to impact birth outcomes (Zielinski, Gilbert Brody, & Low, 2016).

Support System

The woman's perception of being able to maintain control during labor and delivery is an important contributing factor to a positive and favorable evaluation of childbirth. This includes control of pain perception, control over emotions and actions, and being able to influence decisions while being an active participant (Mackey, 1995). Studies have shown that with a support person, be it a family member, friend, doula, or professional such as a nurse, the patient experiences decreased anxiety and feels more in control. This results in fewer interventions, a significantly lower level of pain, and enhanced overall maternal satisfaction (Bohren et al., 2017; Kobayashi et al., 2017).

Nursing care of women in early or latent labor should incorporate the following types of support and interventions:

- Encourage her to do normal, distracting activities and rest as needed.
- Provide emotional support, including continuous presence, reassurance, and praise.
- Provide information about labor progress and advice regarding coping techniques.
- Offer comfort measures (e.g., comforting touch, massage, warm baths/showers, promoting adequate fluid intake and output).
- Serve as an advocate, including assisting the woman in articulating her wishes to others.

A woman's feeling of empowerment during labor is due in part to a trustful relationship with the professionals and the partners.

Feeling empowered results in an increased ability to feel control, strength of the body, satisfaction, and reassurance, and a better ability to manage pain. Inadequate support from the professionals could lead to a negative birth experience where women feel abandoned, immobilized, and not prioritized by the professionals.

CRITICAL COMPONENT

Supportive Care for Adolescents in Labor

Adolescents may have a very different view of labor and birth as they struggle with self-identity and self-esteem. It can pose a challenge for providers and nurses to work with adolescents to promote a positive birthing experience, and they must understand adolescent development, expectations, and needs to do so. According to Sauls (2010), four themes became apparent based on feedback of over 180 adolescents in three tertiary centers during their postpartum interviews:

- Respectful nurse caring: During interactions, be kind and friendly and make her feel welcome. Include her in decision making, informing her of her options related to her care.
- Assistance with pain control: Assist her with pain management options with explanations of both pharmacological and non-pharmacological choices. Assess often her ability to manage her pain.
- Nursing support of the adolescent's support person: Pay attention to her support person's emotional and physical needs. Encourage them as they work through labor, including them in explanations and plan of care discussions.
- Childbirth guidance: Orient her and her support system to hospital facilities and to the birthing process, anticipating questions and explaining procedures. Answer questions truthfully and in an age-appropriate manner.

Nurses should establish environments in which adolescents' rights are protected (AWHONN, 2010). Pregnant adolescents often require special care and attention during the second stage of labor. The young adolescent has fewer coping mechanisms, less experience to draw on, incomplete cognitive development, fewer problem-solving capabilities, and an ego identity that is more easily threatened by the stress and discomfort of labor. Interventions that support the normal physiologic processes of the second stage of labor should be age- and developmentally appropriate for adolescents (AWHONN, 2010).

AWHONN, 2010; Sauls, 2010.

Adoptive Parents

For women relinquishing their newborn to adoptive parents, the birth plan must consider issues surrounding labor support, who will be with the birth mother, and the extent of the adoptive parents' involvement in the labor and after birth. When preparing the birth plan, birth mothers should be asked if they want the prospective adoptive parents to be present for the birth, whether in the waiting room or in the labor room itself, or whether they prefer the adoptive parents remain at home during labor and birth.

Commonly, birth mothers decide to have some time alone at the hospital. This gives them a chance to feel settled in the decision and make peace before placement. Supporting the wishes of the birth mother is the priority and duty of the nurse caring for the laboring woman. The experience of birth and the moments after belong to the birth mother, and nurses must allow the birth family to have their time. When the adoptive parents will have contact with the newborn is the birth mother's decision in most situations.

Because society views the relinquishment of an infant as a voluntary choice, there may be no acknowledgment that a loss has occurred, and thus no expectation for the birth mother to go through a grief process with subsequent adjustment. Relinquishing mothers value and need someone who will support them and their interests at this vulnerable point in their lives. The attitudes of the health care provider can affect how much control the relinquishing mother has over the adoption process (Clutter, 2014). Nurses involved with women at the time of relinquishment can be of significant help in the resolution of grief. A comprehensive review of older research indicated that birth mothers did not receive acknowledgment of their loss from health professionals involved in their care (Askren & Bloom, 1999). Simple recognition of the loss and its significance will go a long way toward assisting with resolution. With recognition comes the need for a structure in place to assist the woman as she attempts to deal with her loss. Postpartum telephone calls and/or support groups may be beneficial in this area. Referrals for long-term counseling may be needed (Clutter, 2014).

Gestational Surrogacy

The practice of gestational surrogacy involves a woman known as a gestational carrier who agrees to bear a genetically unrelated child with the help of assisted reproductive technologies for an individual or couple who intend(s) to be the legal and rearing parent(s), referred to as the intended parent(s) (American College of Obstetricians and Gynecologists [ACOG], 2016). Gestational surrogacy is an increasingly common form of family building that can allow individuals or a couple to become parents despite circumstances in which carrying a pregnancy is biologically impossible or medically contraindicated. Nurses may become involved in gestational surrogacy through caring for the gestational carrier or for the intended parent(s). Although gestational surrogacy increases options for family building, this treatment also involves ethical, medical, psychosocial, and legal complexities that must be considered to minimize risks of adverse outcomes for the gestational carrier, intended parent(s), and resulting children (ACOG, 2016).

Generally, the surrogate accepts responsibility to maintain the pregnancy and perform conventional measures for fetal growth until the child is born (Tavakkoli, 2017). In surrogacy, families have a business agreement surrounding the pregnancy and birth, so multiple families are involved in the hospital stay. Although inconsistently reported due to a lack of regulation, surrogacy for human reproduction appears to be on the increase in the United States (Armour, 2012). State laws surrounding these arrangements vary and are evolving, and clear policies and procedures that outline the legal processes are needed (Schafer, 2014).

Nurses are integral for a smooth process of care and to promote satisfaction for the surrogate and intended parents. Surrogacy arrangements surrounding the birth are typically detailed as part of a surrogacy contract. However, regulation and standards are changing and current knowledge of relevant hospital and legal standards is essential to provide care for surrogate families (Dunk, 2016). Everyone involved in surrogacy may need early and ongoing support, education, care options, and counseling (Dunk, 2016). Remember the gestational surrogate is the patient and is always the nurses' primary concern. When the adoptive parents have contact with the newborn is the decision of the birth mother in most situations.

Labor Support

Since the mid-20th century, most women have given birth in a hospital rather than at home, even in poorer, low resource countries. Access to continuous care and support during labor has become the exception rather than the routine in the hospital setting. Concerns about the consequent dehumanization of women's birth experiences have resulted in demands for a return to continuous, one-to-one support by women for women during labor (Fig. 8–15).

Two complementary theoretical explanations have been offered for the effects of labor support on childbirth outcomes (Bohren et al., 2017). Both explanations hypothesize that labor support enhances labor physiology and woman's feelings of control and competence.

- First theory: During labor, women may be uniquely vulnerable to unfamiliar environmental influences; current obstetric care frequently subjects women to institutional routines, high rates of intervention, unfamiliar personnel, and lack of privacy, resulting in stress (Lederman, Lederman, Work, & McCann, 1978).
  - These conditions may have an adverse effect on the progress of labor and on the development of feelings of competence and confidence; this may in turn impair adjustment to parenthood and establishment of breastfeeding and increase the risk of depression.
  - This response may, to some extent, be buffered by the provision of support and companionship during labor.
- Second theory describes two pathways: enhanced passage of the fetus through the pelvis and soft tissues, and decreased stress response (Hodnett, 2002).
  - Enhanced feto-pelvic relationships may be accomplished by encouraging mobility and effective use of gravity, supporting women to assume their preferred positions, and recommending specific positions for specific situations.
  - Studies of the relationships among fear and anxiety, the stress response, and pregnancy complications have shown that anxiety during labor is associated with high levels of the stress hormone epinephrine in the blood, which may lead to abnormal fetal heart rate (FHR) patterns in labor, decreased uterine contractility, a longer active labor phase with regular well-established contractions, and low Apgar scores (Lederman, 1986).

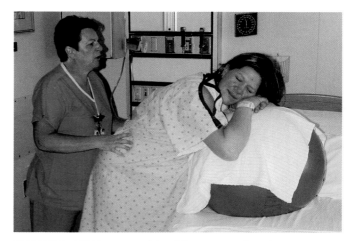

FIGURE 8–15 Woman receiving labor support from her nurse.

- Emotional support, information and advice, comfort measures, and advocacy may reduce anxiety and fear and associated adverse effects during labor.
  - Anxiety (a sense of uneasiness in response to a vague unspecific threat) can interfere with labor and increase nausea and crying, as well as interfering with the ability to focus. Emotional factors can contribute to the experience of increased pain due to high levels of anxiety (Shnol et al., 2014).
  - Fear (a painful, uneasy feeling in response to an identifiable threat) can be fear related to the unknown, fear of injury to self and fetus, or fear of pain. Fear can decrease UCs and enhance the perception of pain. Procedures and an unfamiliar environment can result in a sense of loss of control and feeling of helplessness. Women in labor can feel abandoned (Mattson & Smith, 2011). Preexisting expectations and fear itself elicits a request for c-section, predisposing the woman to higher levels of pain (Shnol et al., 2014).
  - Nurses can help and support women to be actively involved in their own care by allowing time for discussion, listening to worries and concerns, and offering information to help women gain increased self-determination in the context of care (Nordgren & Fridlund, 2001).
  - Psychosocial factors may also influence a woman's ability to cope and anxiety levels. If she has poor coping skills and high anxiety, she may experience increased pain. Positive expectations on the part of the woman correlate to better pain relief and labor responses (Shnol et al., 2014).

Position

Discussion of the influence on labor includes a fifth "P," maternal position during labor and birth. The woman's position affects both anatomical and physiological adaptations to labor (Fig. 8–16). Position is now more accurately referred to as freedom of movement during labor, allowing the woman to labor in the position she finds most comfortable. Registered nurses

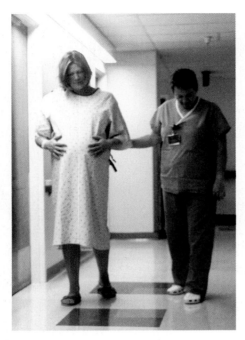

FIGURE 8–16 Woman walking in labor with her nurse.

are integral to this process: they suggest alternatives and support the woman in choosing positions that are most conducive to her individualized needs and tailored to her current stage and phase of labor. Walking, moving, and changing positions are all important options to facilitate freedom of movement. Resting places other than beds, such as rocking chairs and birthing balls, may be suggested. RNs provide advice, support, and encouragement to women to empower them to take advantage of the full range of options during labor. Women should have unlimited access to positions that are restful and comfortable for them. Registered nurses should be knowledgeable about positioning techniques for women with epidural analgesia, and they play a key role in supporting position changes that facilitate the birth process, promote maternal comfort, and maintain patient safety.

- Freedom of movement should be an option for women since it is known to enhance the ability of some women to cope with the pain of labor (AWHONN, 2014c). Using a variety of positions makes it easier for the woman to work with her body and with the fetus as the fetus moves through the pelvis (AWHONN, 2014c). During the first stage of labor, an upright position (walking, sitting, kneeling, or squatting) and/or a lateral position is encouraged (Fig. 8–17A).
  - These positions are used to decrease the compression of the maternal descending aorta and ascending vena cava that could result in a compromised cardiac output. Compression of these vessels can lead to supine hypotension, resulting in decreased placental perfusion (Simpson & O'Brien-Abel, 2014)
  - The upright position has shown benefits of aiding in the descent of the infant and more effective contractions that result in shorter labor as well as decreasing the need

for pain medication, oxytocin, and mechanical-assisted deliveries. Being in an upright, squatting, or side-lying position also demonstrated less severe lacerations or need for episiotomies (Gupta, Sood, Hofmeyr, & Vogel, 2017; Simpson & O'Brien-Abel, 2014).
  - Frequent position changes are associated with a reduction of fatigue, an increase of comfort, and improved circulation to both mother and fetus.
- Maternal position in the second stage of labor can impact the natural urge to push. Upright positions provide the advantage of gravity to help the mother move the fetus through the pelvis, and gravity-neutral positions may be more relaxing. Upright positions include standing, kneeling, and squatting. Gravity-neutral positions include side-lying and hands-knees (AWHONN, 2014d).
  - During the second stage of labor, the upright position has been shown to increase the pelvic outlet and better aligns the fetus with the pelvic inlet (Fig. 8–17B) (Simkin, Hanson, & Ancheta, 2017).
- The position most used in births in the United States is the lithotomy position, which allows for provider visualization and control during the delivery process.

ONSET OF LABOR

As the woman comes closer to term pregnancy, the uterus becomes more sensitive to oxytocin and the contractions increase in frequency and intensity. This can be an anxious time for the woman and family in determining if she needs to proceed to the birthing center. An understanding of true versus false labor can help to alleviate some of these fears.

True Labor Versus False Labor

True labor contractions occur at regular intervals and increase in frequency, duration, and intensity (Fig. 8–18).
- True labor contractions bring about changes in cervical effacement and dilation.
- False labor is characterized by irregular contractions with little or no cervical change.

Assessment of Rupture of the Membranes (ROM)

Spontaneous rupture of the membranes (SROM) may occur before the onset of labor but typically occurs during labor. Once the membranes have ruptured, the protective barrier to infection is lost, and ideally the woman should deliver within 24 hours to reduce the risk of infection to herself and her fetus.

Assessing the Status of Membranes

Different techniques may be used to confirm rupture of membranes (ROM):

- A speculum exam may be done to assess for fluid in the vaginal vault (pooling).

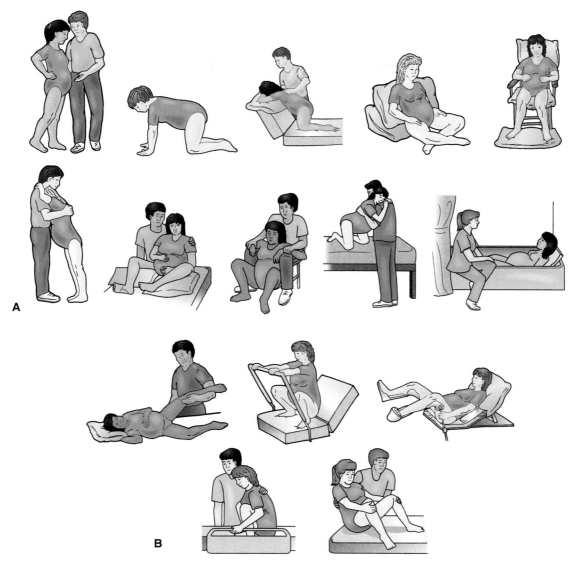

FIGURE 8–17 (**A**) Positions for labor. (**B**) Positions for pushing.

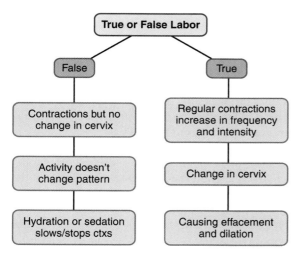

FIGURE 8–18 True vs. false labor.

● Ferning: During a sterile speculum exam, a sample of fluid in the upper vaginal area is obtained, placed on a slide, and assessed for "ferning pattern" under a microscope (Fig. 8–19A). A ferning pattern confirms ROM.

● AmniSure testing kit: The AmniSure ROM Test is a rapid, non-invasive monoclonal immunoassay that detects PAMG-1, an amniotic protein that appears in vaginal secretions if ROM has occurred. This aids clinicians with the diagnosis of ROM in pregnant women with signs and symptoms suggestive of the condition. According to published data it is ~99% accurate.

● Nitrazine paper: The paper turns blue when in contact with amniotic fluid. Can be dipped in the vaginal fluid or fluid-soaked Q-tip can be rolled over the paper (Fig. 8–19B). This method is no longer common.

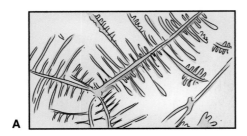

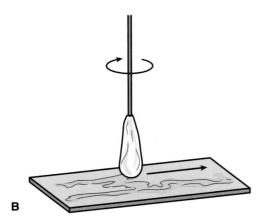

FIGURE 8–19 Assessment of rupture of membranes (**A**) Ferning pattern of dried amniotic fluid seen under microscope. (**B**) Placing fluid on nitrizine paper with Q-tip. (reordered)

Nursing Actions

- Assess the FHR.
  - There is an increased risk of umbilical cord prolapse with ROM.
  - There is a higher risk of umbilical cord prolapse when the presenting part is not engaged.
- Assess the amniotic fluid for color, amount, and odor.
  - Normal amniotic fluid is clear or cloudy with a normal odor that is similar to that of ocean water or the loam of a forest floor.
  - Fluid can be meconium-stained; this must be reported to the care provider as it may indicate fetal compromise in utero.
- Document the date and time of SROM, characteristic of fluid, and FHR.

Guidelines for Going to the Birthing Facility

By law, all pregnant women have access to medical care regardless of their ability to pay (Box 8-1). By discussing when to go to the birthing facility with the pregnancy care provider before labor happens, women will have less anxiety and be more prepared when labor begins. This decision depends on on each woman's past pregnancy history, location of the birth center, and risk status of the pregnancy. A general rule of thumb for first-time pregnancy with no risk factors is to wait until contractions are 5 minutes apart, last 60 seconds, and are regular

BOX 8–1 | Emergency Medical Treatment and Active Labor Act

The Emergency Medical Treatment and Active Labor Act (EMTALA) is a federal regulation enacted to ensure treatment for a woman seeking care in an emergency or if she thinks she is in labor, regardless of her ability to pay. Nurses who work in the labor and delivery unit(s) of the hospital need to be familiar with EMTALA regulations (Angelini & Mahlmeister, 2005). In general, the criteria for admission to the hospital for labor are cervical dilation to 3 to 4 cm and/or ruptured membranes (Cunningham et al., 2014).

for at least an hour. The woman should go to the birthing center immediately when:

- The membrane ruptures, or water breaks.
- She is experiencing intense pain.
- Bloody show increases.

MECHANISM OF LABOR

The positional changes in the presenting part required to navigate the birth canal constitute the mechanism of labor. These mechanisms are cardinal movements of labor (Fig. 8–20).

- Engagement: When the greatest diameter of the fetal head passes through the pelvic inlet; can occur late in pregnancy or early in labor (see Fig. 8–20A).
- Descent: Movement of the fetus through the birth canal during the first and second stages of labor (see Fig. 8–20A).
- Flexion: When the chin of the fetus moves toward the fetal chest; occurs when the descending head meets resistance from maternal tissues; results in the smallest fetal diameter to the maternal pelvic dimensions; normally occurs early in labor (see Fig. 8–20A).
- Internal rotation: When the rotation of the fetal head aligns the long axis of the fetal head with the long axis of the maternal pelvis; occurs mainly during the second stage of labor (see Fig. 8–20B).
- Extension: Facilitated by resistance of the pelvic floor that causes the presenting part to pivot beneath the pubic symphysis and the head to be delivered; occurs during the second stage of labor (see Fig. 8–20C).
- External rotation/restitution: During this movement, the sagittal suture moves to a transverse diameter and the shoulders align in the anteroposterior diameter. The sagittal suture maintains alignment with the fetal trunk as the trunk navigates through the pelvis (see Fig. 8–20D). Head and shoulders rotate to move under the symphysis pubis.
- Expulsion: The anterior shoulder usually comes first followed by the remainder of the body (see Fig. 8–20E).

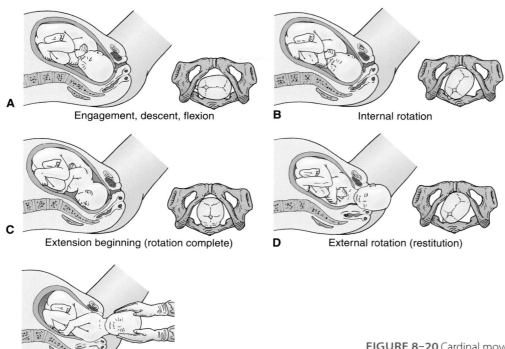

A   Engagement, descent, flexion

B   Internal rotation

C   Extension beginning (rotation complete)

D   External rotation (restitution)

E   Expulsion

FIGURE 8–20 Cardinal movements of labor. (**A**) Engagement, descent, and flexion. (**B**) Internal rotation. (**C**) Extension. (**D**) External rotation. (**E**) Expulsion.

STAGES OF LABOR AND CHILDBIRTH

Labor or parturition is the process in which the fetus, placenta, and membranes are expelled through the uterus. The care of women and families during labor and delivery requires astute and ongoing assessments of the bio-psycho-social adaptation of the woman and fetus. Because childbirth is a natural process, care should move forward on a continuum from noninvasive to least invasive intervention and from non-pharmacological to pharmacological interventions according to the desires of the woman and assessment of health care providers based on individual clinical situations (Simpson & O'Brien-Abel, 2014).

In the United States, 98.8% of all infants were delivered in hospitals. Out-of-hospital deliveries represented only 1.5% of births. Doctors delivered 92.1% of births and certified nursemidwives (CNMs) delivered 8.1% (Martin, Hamilton, Osterman, Driscoll, & Mathews, 2017). Because most babies are delivered in the hospital by physicians, nurses in the intrapartal setting have a key role in providing comprehensive and individualized care for women and their families. To provide this care, nurses must understand the process of labor, birth, and postpartum. By understanding the stages and phases of labor, the nurse can facilitate, assist, and provide care for the woman, the fetus, and her support systems (see Concept Map).

CRITICAL COMPONENT

Care Practices That Support and Promote Normal Physiologic Birth

A normal physiologic labor and birth is powered by the innate human capacity of the woman and fetus. This birth is more likely to be safe and healthy because there is no unnecessary intervention that disrupts normal physiologic processes. Supporting the normal physiologic processes of labor and birth, even in the presence of such complications, has the potential to enhance best outcomes for the mother and infant (Zielinski et al., 2016).

The World Health Organization and Lamaze International identified six birth practices that support and promote normal physiologic birth:

1. Labor begins on its own: Support the normal physiologic process.
2. Freedom of movement throughout labor: Allow women to move around and adapt positions of their choosing.
3. Continuous labor support from family, friends, doulas, or nursing staff.
4. Minimize interventions to allow healthy labor progress.
5. Spontaneous pushing in non-supine positions.
6. NO separation of mother and baby.

American College of Nurse Midwives, 2013; Romano & Lothian, 2008.

TABLE 8–1   Stages and Phases of Labor

STAGES	1ST			2ND	3RD	4TH Immediate Postpartum
Phases	Latent	Active	Transition	Expulsive	Placenta	
Length	Primip: average 6–12 hours Multip: average 6 hours	Average length of phase range is 1–6 hours Primip: 2 hours from 6 cm to complete Multip: 1.5 hours from 6 cm to complete	Average length of phase range is 1–2 hours, but up to 4 can be normal Primip: 1–2 hours Multip: 0.5–2 hours	Primip: average 2–4 hours Multip: average less than 1 hour	1–20 minutes	First 2–4 hours after delivery
Cervix	Effacing; dilating to 4 cm Now active labor is defined as 6 cm	Effacing; dilating to 7 cm Now active labor is defined as ≥6 cm	Effacing; dilating to 10 cm Now active labor is defined as 6 cm and there is little discussion of transition	Fully dilated (10 cm) and effaced	Closing	Closing
Uterine Contractions	Frequency: 5–15 min Duration: 10–30 sec Intensity: mild	Frequency: 3–5 min Duration: 30–45 sec Intensity: mod/ strong	Frequency: 1–2 min Duration: 40–60 sec Intensity: strong	Frequency: 1–2 min Duration: 50–90 sec Intensity: less painful, expulsive	Less painful contractions	Cramping
Show	None or some	Increasing	Heavy	Heavy		
Membranes	Usually intact	Intact or ruptured	Usually ruptured	Ruptured		
Station	Primip: 0 Multip: –2 0	Primip: 0 – +2 Multip: 0 – +2	Primip: 0 – +2 Multip: 0 – +2	Primip: progress to +4 Multip: progress to +4		
Biological Response	Cramps, backache Excited, anxious, happy, relief, curious, quiet or talkative, needs information and reassurance	May become restless, have labored respiration and tendency to hyperventilate Increasing fears, increasing anxieties, serious, feels threatened May be more serious and inwardly focused	Leg cramps, nausea, vomiting, hiccups, belches, perspiration on forehead and upper lip, a pulling or stretching sensation deep in pelvis Panic, emotional, irritable response to external environment stimuli	Intra-abdominal pressure is exerted (bearing down), urge to push, perineum bulges and flattens, perineal burning and stretching Desires to sleep between contractions, amnesic between contractions	Uterus rises and becomes globular shape, gush or flood as placenta separates, umbilical cord lengthens, cramping May want to sleep, proud, happy, relief, may or may not display emotions	Postpartum chills, hunger, thirst, drowsy, moderate to heavy lochia, usually painless uterine contractions

TABLE 8-1 Stages and Phases of Labor—cont'd

STAGES	1ST			2ND	3RD	4TH
Phases	Latent	Active	Transition	Expulsive	Placenta	Immediate Postpartum
Personal System	Thoughts centered on self, labor, and baby	Needs human presence	Becomes limited, losing control, thoughts are on self, uncooperative, amnesic between contractions, dependent	Slow to react, focus on delivery	Relieved	
Maternal Biological System	1. B/P, pulse, resp. temp q 1–2 hour 2. Begin Friedman graph 3. Assess cervical changes by SVE 4. Assess FHR and UC's 30 minutes or per protocol 5. Ascertain presence of bloody show and ROM 6. Encourage relaxation 7. Clear liquids or intake per protocol 8. Encourage void q 2 hours 9. Position of comfort	1. B/P, pulse, resp. temp q 1–2 hour 2. Friedman graph 3. Assess cervical changes by SVE PRN 4. Assess FHR and UCs q 15–30 minutes or per protocol 5. Assess vaginal secretions and for ROM 6. Relaxing environment 7. Clear liquids or intake per protocol 8. Encourage void q 2 hours 9. Side or semi-Fowlers position 10. Wet washcloth, mouth care, perineal care, clean dry linen	1. B/P, pulse, resp. temp. q 1 hour 2. Friedman graph 3. SVE to assess cervix, fetal position 4. Assess FHR and UCs q 15 minutes or per protocol 5. Assess vaginal secretions and for ROM 6. Relaxing environment 7. Clear liquids or intake per protocol 8. Check bladder distention 9. Encourage slow breathing 10. Relieve muscle leg cramps 11. Multip—prepare for delivery at 8 cm	1. B/P, pulse, resp. q 1 hour 2. SVE to assess position, station and progress 3. Assess FHR & UC q 5–15 min or per protocol 4. Assess patient readiness and urge to push 5. Prepare primip for delivery at 10 cm 6. Assist in comfortable position for pushing, encourage upright positions 7. Use squatting bars and birthing balls 8. Teach and utilize open glottis pushing 9. Support and facilitate patient's spontaneous pushing efforts 10. Encourage to rest between contractions 11. Ice chips or intake per protocol	1. B/P, pulse, resp. q 15 minutes 2. Assess for bleeding 3. Assess for placental detachment 4. Encourage relaxation 5. Ice chips or intake per protocol	1. VS q 15 min × 1 hour the q 30 minutes 2. Assess fundus, lochia q 15 minutes × 1 hour, then 30 minutes 3. Inspect perineum q 15 min × 1 hour, then q 30 minutes 4. Check for bladder distention 5. Position of comfort 6. Diet and fluid as tolerated

Continued

TABLE 8–1   Stages and Phases of Labor—cont'd

STAGES	1ST			2ND	3RD	4TH Immediate
Phases	Latent	Active	Transition	Expulsive	Placenta	Postpartum
Pain	1. Initiate non-pharmacological pain management strategies 2. Assist in diversional activities 3. Encourage control breathing 4. Position changes and ambulation 5. Use non-pharmacological pain management strategies	1. Relaxation and controlled breathing 2. Back rub 3. Pharmacological pain management 4. Position changes and ambulation 5. Use non-pharmacological pain management strategies	1. Relaxation and controlled breathing 2. Palpate contractions lightly 3. Pharmacological pain management 4. Position changes 5. Use non-pharmacological pain management strategies	1. Support leg, chest, arms, and back 2. Positioning 3. Pharmacological pain management 4. Relaxation breathing between contractions 5. Assist with breathing and pushing 6. Use nonpharmacological pain management strategies	1. Relaxation breathing 2. Positioning 3. Use non-pharmacological pain management strategies	1. Positioning 2. Analgesics 3. Use non-pharmacological pain management strategies
Fetal Biological System	1. Assess FHR q 30 minutes or per protocol 2. Leopold's maneuver for fetal position 3. SVE exam of patient 4. Position patient off of back	1. Assess FHR q 15–30 minutes or per protocol 2. Position patient off of back	1. Assess FHR q 15 minutes or per protocol 2. Position patient off of back	1. Assess FHR after each contraction 2. Observe perineum for crowning	1. Assess condition of newborn at birth 2. Apgar scores 1 min and 5 minutes 3. Maintain airway 4. Maintain body heat 5. Facilitate early contact with parents 6. Baby I.D.	1. V.S. q 15 minutes × 1 hr, then q 30 minutes 2. Facilitate skin to skin contact with parents 3. Initiate breast feeding 4. Give routine meds 5. Maintain thermoregulation 6. Initial assessment
Social System	1. Patient's identification of support person(s) 2. Assist support person(s) in his/her role 3. Include support person(s) in patient teaching and care 4. Encourage support person(s) to remain with patient	1. Assist support person(s) with comfort measures and positions of comfort for patient 2. Assist support person in relaxation breathing exercises 3. Encourage support person(s) to remain with patient 4. Assist support person in focusing on patient labor	1. Assist support person with relaxation breathing 2. Assist support person identifying changes and tension and keeping patient relaxed 3. Reassurance	1. Prepare support person(s) for delivery—scrubs, mask, cap, shoe covers 2. Assist support person(s) with relaxations breathing 3. Assist support person in supporting patient during contractions and pushing	1. Reassurance 2. Praise 3. Early contact with baby 4. Explain procedures	1. Support person(s) to remain with patient and baby 2. Explain procedures, education

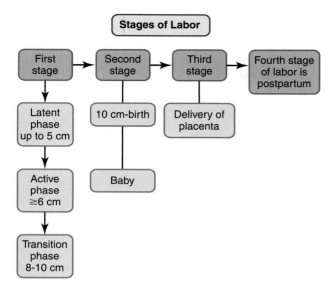

FIGURE 8-21 Stages of labor.

Labor and birth is divided into four stages (Table 8–1, Fig. 8–21):

● The first stage begins with onset of labor and ends with complete cervical dilation.
● The second stage begins with complete dilation of cervix and ends with delivery of the baby.
● The third stage begins after delivery of the baby and ends with delivery of the placenta.
● The fourth stage begins after delivery of the placenta and is completed 4 hours later; it is the immediate postpartum period (see Fig. 8–21).

Evidence-Based Practice: Early Admission vs. Active Labor Admission

Cheyne, H., Hundley, V., Dowding, D., Bland, J., Martin, M. P., & Greer, I. (2008). Effects of algorithm for diagnosis of active labour: Cluster randomized trial. *British Medical Journal, 337*, a2396.

According to data from more than 11,000 births indicates that admitting at <4cm dilated places woman at risk for increased medical interventions, epidurals, oxytocin augmentation, and cesarean sections. Early admission resulted in 84% epidural rate compared to 71% of late admissions of nulliparous women. NICU admissions and maternal breastfeeding difficulties also increased. Early admission may increase the chances of cesarean section for nulliparous woman in early labor. ACOG (2014) currently considers cervical dilation of 6 cm as the threshold for the active phase of labor. Women who are admitted to labor and delivery during the latent phase of labor are more likely to be diagnosed with slow labor progress. The diagnosis of active labor has important clinical and resource implications for the care of women in labor. Admission of women who are not in active labor is a considerable problem, leading to higher levels of medical intervention, than for those admitted in active labor.

First Stage

The first stage of labor is defined as the progression of cervical changes. This stage is divided into three phases: latent phase,

active phase, and transition. Characteristics of the first stage of labor are as follows:

● It begins with onset of true labor and ends with complete cervical dilation (10 cm) and complete effacement (100%).
● Stage 1 is the longest stage, typically lasting 12 hours for primigravidas and 8 hours for multigravidas.
● There are normally tremendous variations in lengths of labor (Cunningham et al., 2014).
● The bag of waters or fetal membranes usually ruptures during this stage.
● The woman's cardiac output increases.
● The woman's pulse may increase.
● Gastrointestinal motility decreases, which leads to increase in gastric emptying time (Mattson & Smith, 2011).
● The woman experiences pain associated with UCs that result in the dilation and effacement of the cervix.
● The first stage has three phases: the latent, active, and transition phases (see Table 8–1).

Assessment

Assessment during all phases of the first stage of labor includes:

● Maternal vital signs
● The woman's response to labor and pain
● FHR and UCs
● Cervical changes
● Fetal position and descent in the pelvis

Nursing Actions

Nursing actions during all phases of the first stage of labor are related to:

● Diet and hydration
    ● Once admitted to the hospital, medical orders typically limit oral intake to clear liquids.
    ● The WHO recommends women dictate their oral intake of carbohydrates to decrease maternal ketosis (Sharts-Hopko, 2010). ACOG endorses clear liquids during labor (2014).
    ● Evidence suggests there is no reason to restrict oral intake in labor although unrestricted intake in the hospital setting is rare (Singata, Tranmer, & Gyte, 2013; Tranmer, Hodnett, Hannah, & Stevens, 2005).
● Activity and rest
    ● Encouraging frequent position changes and upright positions assists labor progression, facilitates fetal descent, and decreases pain perception.
● Elimination
    ● Frequent emptying of bowel and bladder assists in comfort of the mother, provides more pelvic room as baby descends, and decreases pressure and injury to the urethra and bowel.
● Comfort
    ● Providing comfort measures and therapies facilitates labor progress, decreases pain perception, and supports maternal coping mechanisms to manage the labor process.
● Support and family involvement
    ● Shown to provide emotional and physical support to the laboring mother, decreasing stress, and possibly facilitating labor progress.

- Education
  - Providing education and information about labor, procedures, and hospital policies will decrease maternal and family anxiety and fear. Empowers the women to make informed decisions.
- Safety
  - Providing a safe, friendly environment will enhance the birthing experience.
- Documentation of labor admission and progression (Figs. 8–22 and 8–23)

Evidence-Based Practice: Oral Intake in Labor

Singata, M., Tranmer, J., & Gyte, G. M. L. (2013). Restricting oral fluid and food intake during labour. *Cochrane Database of Systematic Reviews, 8.* doi:10.1002/14651858.CD003930.pub3.

In some cultures, food and drinks are consumed during labor for nourishment and comfort to help meet the demands of giving birth. Restricting fluids and foods during labor is common practice across many birth settings, with women only allowed sips of water or ice chips. Restriction of oral intake may be unpleasant for some women and may adversely influence their experience of labor. A current Cochrane Review of five research studies involving 3,130 women concluded no benefit or harm to unrestricted oral intake in labor. The authors concluded that since evidence shows no benefit or harms, there is no justification for the restriction of fluids and food in labor for women at low risk of complications (Singata et al., 2013). Nurses can engage in revision of policies to reflect current evidence and support patients' autonomy in labor.

Latent Phase

The latent phase is the early and slower part of labor. The average length of this phase is 6 hours for primigravida from admission to the hospital and similar for multigravida. However there is a large range in normal length for this phase and it may normally take many hours to reach the active phase of labor. Women in this phase are usually both excited and apprehensive about the start of labor. They are talkative and able to relax with the contractions. Many women choose to stay home during this phase, although some are admitted to the birth center. Indications for admittance are cervical change/ROM or fetal intolerance of labor. Most can go home to a more relaxed setting at this stage and return to the birth center when labor progresses. Awaiting admission until active labor decreases the need for medical interventions and facilitates fetal descent and labor support of the family to the patient. However, a recent Cochrane Review concluded additional assessment and enhanced support in early labor compared to traditional care showed that these enhanced interventions may reduce the use of epidural, prevent the need to augment labor with oxytocin, and increase maternal satisfaction (Kobayashi et al., 2017).

Characteristics of this phase are:

- Cervical dilation from 0 to 4 cm with effacement from 0% to 40%.
- Mild intensity contractions occur every 5 to 10 minutes, lasting 30 to 45 seconds. Women often describe them as feeling like strong menstrual cramps.

Medical Interventions

- Laboratory tests, which may include complete blood count (CBC), urinalysis, and possible drug screening.
- Order IV or saline lock.
- Order intermittent fetal monitoring or continuous fetal and uterine monitoring.

CRITICAL COMPONENT

Nonpharmacological Strategies for Nurses and Comfort Measures in Labor

Labor support is a repertoire of techniques used to help women with the process of childbirth (Wood & Carr, 2003). Providing support and comfort is one of the primary activities of nurses and includes:

Emotional Support
- Sustaining physical presence, eye contact
- Verbal encouragement, reassurance, and praise
- Listening to woman and family
- Distraction

Physical Support
- Comfort measures such as ice chips, fluids, food, and pain medications
- Hygiene including mouth care, pericare, and changing soiled linens
- Assistance with position changes and ambulation
- Reassuring touch, massage
- Application of heat and cold
- Hydrotherapy in shower and tub. Hydrotherapy is safe and effective as a complementary pain management therapy (Stark & Miller, 2009).
- Calm environment (dim lighting, quiet, music, minimize interruptions)

Informational Support
- Provide information on the progress of labor.
- Explain all procedures.
- Communicate in lay language so the woman and her family understand.
- Offer advice.
- Use interpreters as needed.

Advocacy
- Support decisions made by the woman and her family.
- Ensure respect for the woman's decisions.
- Manage the environment, which includes visitors.
- Translate the woman's wishes to others.
- Offer advice.

Support of the Partner and Family
- Offer support and praise.
- Role model therapeutic behaviors.
- Assist the partner with food and rest.
- Provide breaks if desired or needed.

Burke, 2014; Wood & Carr, 2003.

Labor and Delivery Admission Record

PT. NAME: _____ AGE: _____ CARE PROVIDER: _____

ADMIT DATE/TIME: _____

EDC	LMP	Weeks of Gestation	Gravida	Para	Term	Preterm	Spontaneous Abortion	Elective Abortion	Living	Stillborn	C-Section	VBAC

T	P	R	BP	Height	Weight	Pre-Pregnant weight	Weight Gain	How Admitted		Accompanied By	

Date/Time Care Provider Notified	Date/Time Seen By Care Provider	Reason for Admission

Onset of Labor	Contraction Frequency (Min)

Dilatation (cm)   **Effacement (%)**   **Station**

Contraction Duration (Sec)   **Contraction Quality**
None   Mild   Moderate   Strong

Pelvic Exam By:

Pain Level Assessment: *Pain scale 0–10*

Admission Membranes: Intact   Ruptured   Bulging   Unknown

Fern: N/A   Negative   Positive   Equivocal

AROM/SROM (Date/Time):

Amniotic Fluid:

Amount: None   N/A   Copious   Large   Moderate   Small   Scant
Color: N/A   Clear   Bloody   Meconium   Heavy   Light   Particulate
Odor: None   N/A   Normal   Foul
Amniotic Fluid Comments:

Vaginal Bleeding: None   Normal   Frank bleeding

Describe Vaginal Bleeding:

Mental Status: Alert   Anxious   Confused

Feeding Preference: Breast   Bottle   Breast/bottle   Undecided

Support Person: None   Husband   Partner   Other

Support Person(s) Name:

Anesthesia Plans: None Local Epidural Spinal General Pudendal
                     Paracervical
Anesthesia Plans Other:

Anesthesia Class: Yes   No   Yes, Previous Pregnancy

Attended Prenatal Class: Yes   No   Yes, Previous Pregnancy

Labor Teaching Initiated: Yes   No   N/A
   Fetal Well-being   Yes   No   N/A
   Labor Progress   Yes   No   N/A
   Pain Relief Measures Yes   No   N/A
   Other

Nutritional screen:
[ ] N/A
[ ] History of Diabetes/Gestational Diabetes
[ ] History of Eating Disorder
[ ] Multiple Pregnancy
[ ] Special Diet/Vegetarian Diet
[ ] Pt. is 18 Years Old or Younger
[ ] Failure to Gain at Least 1/2 lb. per
    Wks. of Gestation
[ ] Food Allergies
[ ] Other _____

Describe Last Solid Intake (Include Date/Time):

Describe Last Fluid Intake (Include Date/Time):

In-Pt. Dietary Referral Entered in Computer: Yes No N/A	In-Pt. Dietary Referral Entered in Computer: Yes No N/A

Medication Allergy: Yes   No
Medication Allergy Detail:

Food Allergies: Yes   No
Food Allergy detail:

Latex Allergy: Yes   No
Describe Latex Reaction:

Allergy Sticker on Chart: Yes N/A	Allergy Band on Patient: Yes N/A

Prenatal Vitamins This Pregnancy: Yes No	Anticoagulants This Pregnancy: Yes No	Describe:

For current prescription/over the counter medications taken during pregnancy see Home Medication Order Sheet.

Prescription/over the counter medications previously taken during pregnancy:

Addressograph

(continued on next page)

FIGURE 8–22 Labor and delivery admission sheet.

Labor and Delivery Admission Record (continued)

PT. NAME: _____

GBS Yes Results: Negative Results Positive Date: **Tested:** No Unknown	**Drug Use:** Denies Yes *If Yes, Describe:* **Drug Use Comments:**

Blood
Type/Rh: Rhogam   This
                      Pregnancy: N/A   Yes   No   No Record
	Contact Lenses: Yes No Soft Hard Lenses Lenses
	                            Lenses Lenses In Out

Rubella: Immune Non-immune Unknown	**HBsAg:** Negative Positive Unknown	**RPR:** Non-Reactive Reactive Unknown	**Glasses:** Yes No **Dentures:** Yes No **Body Piercing:** Yes No **Body Piercing** **Location/Removed:**

Hemoglobin = _____ g/dl Initials: _____ Reference Range: 11–14 g/dl (pregnancy) **HIV:** Non-Reactive Reactive	**Support System After Birth:** Family Friends Community None **If None, Social Service Referral Entered In** **Computer:** Yes No N/A

Heart Disease: Yes No **Hypertension:** Yes No	**History of** Denies Emotional Physical Sexual *If Other,* **Abuse:** Other _____ *Describe*
MVP: Yes No **Diabetes:** Yes No	**Social Service Referral** **Entered in Computer:** Yes No N/A
Asthma: Yes No **DVT:** Yes No	

Blood Transfusion: Yes No **Blood Transfusion Reason/Yr:**	**Special Needs:** None Spiritual Cultural Emotional *If Other,* Other _____ Hearing/vision impaired: Yes No *Describe*

Sexually Denies Chlamydia Syphilis Gonorrhea **Transmitted** HIV HPV/Genital Warts Herpes **Diseases:** Other _____	**Social Service** **Pastoral Service** **Referral Entered** **Referral Entered** **in Computer:** Yes No N/A **in Computer:** Yes No N/A

Exposure to Infectious Denies Measles Mumps HIV/AIDS **Disease This Pregnancy:** Chicken Pox TB Hepatitis Other	**Interpreter needed?** Yes No Primary language: _____
	Psychosocial Comments:

Cervical Denies D & C LEEP Cervical biopsy **Procedures:** Laser Cryo/Cautery Other _____	**Room Orientation:** EFM Bed Phone Call Light Visitors Computer

History of Major **Illness or Surgery:**	**Does the Patient Have an Advance Directive?**

Patient History Detail:	**If No Copy on Chart, Remind Pt.**
	    If Yes, is Yes **to Have Family Member Bring** **Referral** Yes
	Yes **Copy in** **Copy AND Send Advance** **Entered in**
	     Chart? No **Directive Referral to Pastoral** **Computer:** No
	                         Services

Past Pregnancy   None   PIH   Cystitis   Pyelitis   Preterm Labor
Complications: Preterm Birth   Anemia   Rh Sensitization
                 Positive GBS   Other _____
 	
Comments:
	If No, Does Pt. Yes **If Yes, Was** Yes **Referral** Yes
	      Want Additional **Referral Sent** **Entered in**
	No **Information or** **to Pastoral** **Computer:** No
	      Assistance? No **Care?** No

Complications None PIH Cystitis Preterm Labor **Current** Anemia Rh sensitization **Pregnancy:** Placental abnormalities _____ **Comments:** Other _____	**Disposition** Sent Home Kept with Pt. Valuables in Security Office **of Valuables:** Pt. Encouraged to Take Valuables Home Other _____

Fetal Assessments None Non-Stress Test OCT **Done This Pregnancy:** CVS BPP US Amnio	**Valuables Comments:**

Previous Labor Durations:	**Pt. Wants Other Physician or Family Notified:** Yes No
Sibling History:	**Other Physician/Family Notified:**

Family N/A Adopted Heart Disease HTN Diabetes Cancer **History:** Bleeding Disorder Other _____ **Family History** **Comments:**	

Smoke Denies <5 per day 5–10 per day **Use/Frequency:** >10 per day >20 per day	**Alcohol** Denies Occasional 3–5 Drinks/Week 6 or More Drinks/Week **Use:**

Morse Fall Scale Score:
[ ] < 45, low fall risk; initiate appropriate interventions
[ ] > 50, high fall risk; initiate appropriate interventions
[ ] ≥ 4 medications associated with increased fall risk;
     high fall risk; initiate appropriate interventions

Initiate Care Plan if:
[ ] Anticipated physiological fall risk
[ ] Unanticipated physiological fall risk
[ ] Accidental fall risk

Immunization History
Vaccines: Influenza   Yes   No   Date _____
          Pneumonia   Yes   No   Date _____
          Tetanus   Yes   No   Date _____
          PPD   Yes   No   Date _____

Nursing _____ **Assessment** _____ **Summary:** _____	Requests cord blood banking: Y N Cord blood banking type: ☐ NA ☐ St. Louis Cord Blood Bank ☐ Private cord blood bank

Addressograph

FIGURE 8–22 cont'd

		DATE:				KEY
		TIME:				**Variability**
Cervix	Dilation					Ab = Absent (undetectable)
	Effacement					Min = Minimal (>0 out ≤5 bpm)
	Station					Mod = Moderate (6–25 bpm)
						Mar = Marked (>25 bpm)
Fetal Heart	Baseline Rate					**Accelerations**
	Variability					+ = Present and appropriate for gestational age
	Accelerations					∅ = Absent
	Decelerations					**Decelerations**
	STIM/pH					E = Early
	Monitor Mode					L = Late
						V = Variable
Uterine Activity	Frequency					P = Prolonged
	Duration					**Stim/pH**
	Intensity					+ = Acceleration in response to stimulation
	Resting Tone					∅ = No response to stimulation
	Monitor Mode					Record number for scalp pH
	Oxytocin milliunits/min					**Monitor mode**
						A = Auscultation/Palpation
	Pain					E = External u/s or toco
	Coping					FSE - Fetal spiral electrode
	Maternal Position					IUPC = Intrauterine pressure catheter
	O2/LPM/Mask					**Frequency of uterine activity**
	IV					∅ = None
						Irreg = Irregular
	Nurse Initials					**Intensity of uterine activity**

Patient Name: Physician/CNM:

Narrative notes:

KEY (continued):
Intensity of uterine activity
M = Mild
Mod = Moderate
Str = Strong
By IUPC = mm Hg
Resting tone
R = Relaxed
By IUCP = mm Hg
Coping
W = Well
S = Support provided
For pain use 0–10 scale
Maternal position
A = Ambulatory
U = Upright
SF = Semi-Fowler's
RL = Right lateral
LL = Left lateral
MS = Modified Sims'

FIGURE 8–23 Key labor documentation example.

Nursing Actions (see Clinical Pathway and Concept Map)

● Admit to the labor unit and orient the woman, her partner, and family to the labor room.

● The review of the prenatal record will give information from pregnancy onset to the present. The prenatal record should include all lab tests and ultrasounds (for estimated date of delivery (EDD) and placental location) as well as any prior obstetrical history (pregnancy, births, abortions, and living children). A review of allergies and medications, trends in vital signs and weight gain, chronic conditions, or pregnancy-related complications will also be a part of the record. Biochemical and infectious disease laboratory test results; for example, Group B streptococcus (GBS) status, are also included.

● Complete labor and delivery admission record (Fig. 8–22).

● Review childbirth plan and discuss the woman's expectations.

  ● Woman may present with a birth plan: Some providers and childbirth educators encourage the family to think about how they "see" the labor and birth process. It is a wish list that allows the woman to express her wishes and preferences and communicate with care providers during her prenatal appointments. This discussion should include hospital policies and medical interventions. Review this plan with the woman during the admission process and clarify what you can and cannot provide. This will facilitate open communication and show respect for her expectations.

- Teach and reinforce relaxation and breathing techniques.
  - Support what they have been practicing or teach techniques as needed to decrease pain and anxiety.
- Obtain laboratory tests as per orders.
  - Provides information on patient status and health.
- Start IV or insert saline lock, if ordered.
  - Provides access for fluids and or medications if needed.
- Review the woman's report of onset of labor.
- Assess and record the following (see Fig. 8–22 and Clinical Pathway and Concept Map):
  - Maternal vital signs
  - FHR
  - Uterine contractions
  - Cervical dilation and effacement; and fetal presentation, position, and station by performing a sterile vaginal examination (SVE) (Fig. 8–24, Box 8–2).
  - Status of membranes
  - Amniotic fluid for color, amount, consistency, and odor
  - Vaginal bleeding or bloody show for amount and characteristics of vaginal discharge
  - Fetal position with Leopold maneuver (Fig. 8–25, Box 8–3)
  - Deep tendon reflexes
  - Signs of edema
  - Heart and lung sounds
  - Emotional status
  - Pain and discomfort
- Review laboratory results, note blood Rh status hematocrit and hemoglobin and dipstick urine for glucose and protein or send urine specimen to the lab for analysis.
- Review GBS status, if GBS positive intrapartum IV antibiotic prophylaxis is given.
  - Group B streptococci (GBS), also known as Streptococcus agalactiae, can cause perinatal morbidity and mortality. Between 10% and 30% of pregnant women are colonized with GBS in the vagina or rectum. Implementation of national guidelines for intrapartum antibiotic prophylaxis since the 1990s has resulted in an approximate 80% reduction in the incidence of early-onset neonatal sepsis due to GBS. Vertical transmission of GBS during labor or delivery may result in invasive infection in the newborn during the first week of life. Penicillin remains the drug of choice, with ampicillin as an alternative (ACOG, 2011a).

BOX 8–2 | Sterile Vaginal Exam

Intrapartal Sterile Vaginal Exam

To perform a vaginal exam, the labia are separated with a sterile gloved hand. Fingers are lubricated with a water-soluble lubricant. The first and second fingers are inserted into the introitus; the cervix is located and the following parameters are assessed (Fig. 8–24):

- Cervical dilation: This measurement estimates the dilation of the cervical opening by sweeping the examining finger from the margin of the cervical opening on one side to that on the other.
- Cervical effacement: This measurement estimates the shortening of the cervix from 2 cm to paper-thin measured by palpation of cervical length with the fingertips. The degree of cervical effacement is expressed in terms of the length of the cervical canal compared to that of an unaffected cervix. When it is reduced by one-half (1 cm), it is 50% effaced. When the cervix is thinned out completely, it is 100% effaced.
- Position of cervix: Relationship of the cervical os to the fetal head and is characterized as posterior, midposition, or anterior.
- Station: Level of the presenting part in the birth canal in relationship to the ischial spines. Station is 0 when the presenting part is at the ischial spines or engaged in the pelvis.
- Presentation: Cephalic (head first), breech (pelvis first), shoulder (shoulder first)
- Fetal position: Locate presenting part and specific fetal structure to determine fetal position in relation to the maternal pelvis.

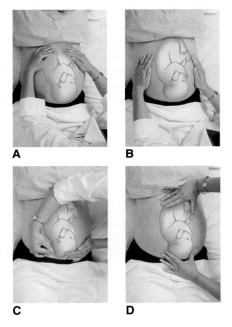

A **B**

C **D**

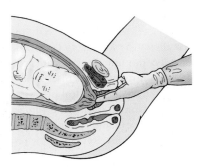

FIGURE 8–24 Sterile vaginal exam.

FIGURE 8–25 Leopold's maneuver.

BOX 8–3 | Leopold's Maneuvers

The purpose of Leopold's maneuvers is to inspect and palpate the maternal abdomen to determine fetal position, station, and size (Fig. 8–25).

- The first maneuver is to determine what part of the fetus is located in the fundus of the uterus.
- The second maneuver is to determine location of the fetal back.
- The third maneuver is to determine the presenting part.
- The fourth maneuver is to determine the location of the cephalic prominence.

Mattson & Smith, 2011.

- Intrapartum GBS prophylaxis (CDC, 2010) is indicated:
  - Previous infant with invasive GBS disease
  - GBS bacteria during any trimester of current pregnancy
  - Positive GBS vaginal-rectal screening culture in late gestation during current pregnancy
  - Unknown GBS status at onset of labor with <37 weeks gestation, or ROM >18 hours, or temperature > 100.4°F or >38.0°C
- Document allergies, history of illness, and last food intake.
- Encourage fluid intake; food may or may not be restricted.
- Provide comfort measures.
- Encourage the woman to walk as much as possible by:
  - Explaining the importance of walking in facilitating labor progression and fetal descent and rotation and in making UCs more efficient
  - Walking with the woman, which can provide a comforting and reassuring presence and distraction
- Assess cultural needs and incorporate beliefs in the nursing care and delivery plan.
- Establish a therapeutic relationship through active listening and providing labor support (Box 8–4).
- Incorporate understanding of the couple's maturity level, educational level, and previous experience into nursing care.
- Review the labor plan with the woman and her partner.
- Inquire about concerns and questions the woman and/or her partner have concerning the labor and birth process.
- Provide clear explanations and updates on progress.
- These nursing actions will provide information to the nurse to facilitate teaching moments, decrease patient anxiety, and support the plan of care.

CRITICAL COMPONENT

Teamwork and Collaboration: Leading Health Care Organizations Issue Recommendations for Quality Patient Care in Labor and Delivery

Although the infant mortality rate in the United States declined in 2010, the U.S. rate remains higher than in most European nations. In addition, U.S. health care providers have seen an increase in pregnancy complications. These trends, along with the recognition that collaboration among physicians, midwives, and nurses is essential to positive health outcomes, prompted professional organizations from the nation's leading obstetrics, family medicine, and pediatric organizations to develop joint recommendations. This "Call to Action" includes recommendations for health care providers and administrators:

- Ensure that patient-centered care and patient safety are organizational priorities that guide decisions for policies and practices.
- Foster a culture of openness by promoting the active communication of good outcomes and opportunities for improvement.
- Develop forums to facilitate communication and track issues of concern.
- Provide resources for clinicians to be trained in the principles of teamwork, safety, and shared decision making.
- Develop methods to systematically track and evaluate care processes and outcomes.
- Facilitate cross-departmental sharing of resources and expertise.
- Ensure that quality obstetric care is a priority that guides individual and team decisions.
- Identify and communicate safety concerns and work together to mitigate potential safety risks.
- Disseminate and use the best available evidence, including individual and hospital-level data, to guide practice patterns.

The joint call to action underscores the collective belief among health care providers that ongoing collaboration is a key element to improving health care outcomes. By providing interprofessional collaboration and care management for families in labor, the overall experience can promote optimal patient care, satisfaction, and maternal and fetal outcomes (AWHONN, 2011).

Active Phase

In the active phase of labor, now defined as ≥6 cm, the median duration from 6 cm to complete cervical dialation is 2 hours in primiparous women and 1.5 hours in multiparous women. Average length of phase range is 1 to 6 hours. Data indicates that after 6 cm, labor accelerates much faster in mulitparous than primiparous. Women in this phase may have decreased energy and experience fatigue. They become more serious and turn attention to internal sensations. As labor progresses, most women turn inward. Characteristics of this phase include the following:

- The consortium on safe labor reviewed more than 19,000 births and determined that nulliparous and parous woman dilate at a similar rate between 4-6 cm, much slower than Friedman (1955) determined in the 1950s: "6 is the new 4" (Zhang et al., 2010). The older standard was cervical dilation progression *from* 4 cm to 7 cm with effacement of 40% to 80%.
- Fetal descent continues.

- Contractions become more intense, occurring every 2 to 5 minutes with duration of 45 to 60 seconds.
- Discomfort increases; this is typically when the woman comes to the birth center or hospital if she has not done so already.

BOX 8–4 | Standard Of Practice. AWHONN Position Statement: Nursing Support Of Laboring Women

The Association of Women's Health, Obstetric and Neonatal Nurses (AWHONN) asserts that continuously available labor support from a registered nurse (RN) is a critical component to achieve improved birth outcomes. The RN assesses, develops, implements and evaluates an individualized plan of care based on each woman's physical, psychological and socio-cultural needs, including the woman's desires for and expectations of the laboring process. Labor care and labor support are powerful nursing functions, and it is incumbent on health care facilities to provide an environment that encourages the unique patient---RN relationship during childbirth (AWHONN, 2011a). The support provided by the RN should include the following:

- Assessment and management of the physiological and psychological processes of labor
- Facilitation of normal physiologic processes, such as the women's desire for movement in labor
- Provision of emotional support and physical comfort measures, informational support, and advocacy
- Evaluation of fetal well-being during labor
- Instruction regarding the labor process
- Patient advocacy and collaboration among members of the health care team
- Role modeling to facilitate family participation during labor and birth
- Direct collaboration with other members of the health care team to coordinate patient care

AWHONN, 2011a.

CRITICAL COMPONENT

Redefining Active Labor

ACOG currently defines the active phase of labor as cervical dilation of 6 cm as the threshold for the active phase of most women in labor. Thus, before 6 cm of dilation is achieved, standards of active phase progress should not be applied (ACOG, 2014). Recently, several professional organizations have come out in support of physiologic birth practices and the reduction in the number of unnecessary interventions during birth (ACOG, 2014; AWHONN, 2014b), increasing recognition of the benefits of physiologic birth and the risks of medical interventions

during labor and birth and increasing focus on avoiding unnecessary interventions during labor. Although interventions are sometimes necessary and not always detrimental, they can lead to interruption in normal physiologic labor and may result in further interventions that do not improve health outcomes (Zielinski et al., 2016). Redefining active labor to 6 cm dilation can assist in identifying when delays in labor are appropriately identified based on this new classification and avoid the use of interventions guiding the latent phase of labor before labor is well-established.

Medical Interventions

- Rupture membranes if not previously ruptured, if indicated.
- Evaluate fetal status by fetal monitoring as indicated, either intermittent or continuous.
- Perform internal monitoring with application of internal fetal electrode and/or uterine transducer, if necessary.
- Pain assessment: Order pain medication or epidural anesthesia.
- Evaluate progression in labor.

Nursing Actions (see Clinical Pathway and Concept Map)

- Monitor FHR and contractions every 15 to 30 minutes.
- Monitor maternal vital signs every 2 hours; every 1 hour if ROM.
- Perform intrapartal vaginal exam as needed to assess cervical changes and fetal descent (see Box 8–2).
- Assess pain (location and degree).
- Administer analgesia as per orders and desire of woman.
- Evaluate effectiveness of epidural or other pain medication.
- Monitor intake and output (I&O), hydration status, and for nausea and vomiting.
- Offer oral fluids as per orders (ice chips, popsicles, carbohydrate liquids, and water). Encourage the woman to listen to her body regarding hydration and nausea and allow her to decide when she has had enough intake.
- Offer clear explanations and updates of progress.
- Promote comfort measures.
- Assist with elimination (bladder distension can hinder fetal descent).
- Encourage breathing and relaxation methods (see Box 8–4).
  - Review and reinforce relaxation techniques.
  - Maintain eye contact and physical proximity to the woman.
  - Develop a rhythm and breathing style to deal with each contraction.
  - Use a direct and gentle voice and have a calm and confident manner.
  - Use touch or massage if acceptable to the woman.
- Interdisciplinary collaboration management of labor assists in communicating the woman's progress and status with other care providers.
- Incorporate the support person in care of patient by:
  - Role modeling supportive behaviors
  - Offering support and praise

- Explain procedures before initiating, asking permission from the patient.
- Assess the environment for adjustments to be made; typically decrease stimulation with dim lighting and decrease noise and interruptions.
- Provide reassurance, updates on progress, and positive reinforcement.

Transition Phase

The transition phase was traditionally defined as dilation from 8 to 10 cm. Current discussions of management of labor now use active labor as 6 cm to complete dilation. The transition phase is being phased out and is often subsumed under active labor. In transition, women are easily discouraged and irritable, and may be overwhelmed and panicky. They often feel and act out of control. Characteristics of this phase are:

- Cervical dilation from 8 to 10 cm with complete (100%) effacement
- Intense contractions every 1 to 2 minutes lasting 60 to 90 seconds
- Exhaustion and increased difficulty concentrating
- Increase of bloody show
- Nausea and vomiting
- Backache: Woman complains of back pressure, hand goes over hip, rubbing and pressing on area.
- Trembling
- Diaphoresis, especially upper lip and facial area
- May have a strong urge to bear down or push, more vocal with primal noises and facial expressions.

Medical Interventions

- Perform amniotomy (AROM) if not previously done.
- Assess fetal position and cervix.
- Prepare for delivery.

Nursing Actions (see Clinical Pathway and Concept Map)

- Assess FHR and UCs every 15 minutes.
- Provide calming support and reassurance, speaking slowly in low, soothing tone, giving short and clear directs such as: "You are in control;" "It is normal to feel so much pressure as the baby moves down;" "You are doing a great job working with your contractions."
  - Woman who are given encouragement and empowered to follow their body will have less anxiety and fear of the process and will perform with more control and conviction.
- Encourage the woman to breathe during contractions and rest between contractions by staying with patient and breathing with her (see Box 8–4). Assist with breathing and relaxation methods by demonstrating breathing through demonstration and reinforcement.
  - Providing support and encouragement will assist in decreasing fear and anxiety.
- Assess I&O and assist with toileting as needed.
  - Bladder distension may hinder fetal descent, cause bladder trauma and discomfort.

- Promote comfort measures.
- Attend to the woman's hygiene needs, such as mopping her brow and face, providing pericare, and changing chux.
  - Providing comfort and hygiene measures shows attention to and respect for the patient's personal needs.
- Prepare the room and couple for delivery.
  - Familiarize the woman and support people with usual routine and keep them informed of what to expect.
  - Open the delivery tray.
  - Turn on the infant radiant warmer.
- Use brief explanations, as the woman's focus is narrowed.
- Remain in the room with the woman and family.
- Provide encouragement and reassurance to the woman and her support person(s).
  - Keep them apprised of labor progress, such as changes in cervical dilation.
  - Compliment them on their effective breathing and relaxation techniques.

Second Stage

The woman enters the second stage of labor when cervical dilation is complete (10 cm) (see Table 8–1). This stage ends with the birth of the baby (Fig. 8–26). Women in the second stage may have a burst of energy, be more focused, and feel like they can actively participate in facilitating birth with active pushing efforts. Phases of the second stage of labor are as follows:

- Latent or resting phase is characterized by a period of rest and relative calm. The urge to bear down is usually not well-established, particularly for women with regional analgesia/anesthesia. The fetus can passively descend in the pelvis during this time without maternal expulsive efforts.
- Descent or active phase is characterized by increasing intensity of uterine contractions and strong urges to bear down with the activation of Ferguson's reflex. During this phase, bearing-down efforts are most effective for promoting birth.
- Physiologic processes of the second stage of labor are the normal bodily function by which the fetus traverses the pelvic outlet and is expelled from the uterus through the force of strong uterine contractions, voluntary and involuntary bearing down, and stretching of the soft tissues of the female reproductive tract. The process involves numerous hemodynamic changes that may affect the reproductive, cardiac, respiratory, gastrointestinal, and renal systems. Changes in maternal physiology during the second stage of labor may also be influenced by maternal position and energy level, pain, and hydration.

Characteristics of this stage include the following:

- Average length is 1 to 2+ hours for primigravida and less than 1 hour for multigravida, although a second stage of several hours may still be normal if there is progress.
- Woman may feel an intense urge to push or bear down when the baby reaches the pelvic floor.
  - Studies have shown that bearing down in the second stage is less tiring and more effective when started after the woman has the urge to do so rather than before.

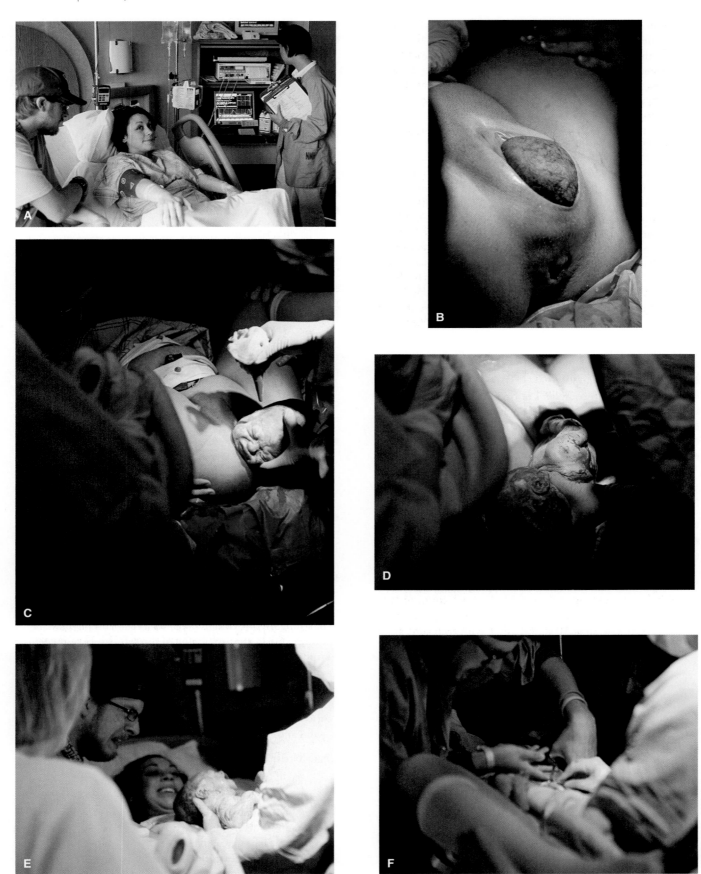

FIGURE 8–26 Vaginal birth sequence. (*A*) Pushing in an upright position allows the use of gravity to promote fetal descent. (*B*) Crowning. (*C*) Birth of the head. (*D*) Birth of the shoulders. (*E*) The infant is shown to the new parents. (*F*) The baby's father cuts the umbilical cord.

Nulliparous women with epidurals who delayed their efforts until feeling the urge to push (Ferguson's reflex) had 27% shorter pushing time. This decreased maternal fatigue, provided increased maternal satisfaction in the birth experience, and allowed women to fully participate in postpartum activities (Gillesby et al., 2010; Osbourne & Hanson, 2014).

- Contractions are intense, occurring every 2 minutes and lasting 60 to 90 seconds.
- Bloody show increases.
- The perineum flattens and the rectum and vagina bulge.

Although it was once thought that limiting the second stage of labor to 2 hours was essential to decrease the risks of fetal morbidity and mortality, we now know that waiting more than 2 hours for the fetus to descend spontaneously is usually safe for the fetus. As long as the fetal heart rate (FHR) is reassuring and evidence shows fetal descent, waiting a reasonable time for spontaneous birth usually poses no risk to the fetus. Current data suggest a prolonged second stage beyond 4 hours may increase maternal risk of operative vaginal birth and perineal trauma (AWHONN, 2008).

Pushing

Preferred pushing techniques vary in practice. Although women who use spontaneous pushing techniques may have a slightly longer second stage, the benefits of such pushing are well-documented. However, some nurses, midwives, and physicians continue to instruct patients to "take a deep breath, hold it, and push." Pushing techniques (AWHONN, 2008) include the following:

- Closed glottis (involuntary) refers to spontaneous pushing against a closed glottis (Valsalva) in response to the descent of the fetal presenting part on the perineum.
- Closed glottis (voluntary), also referred to as the Valsalva technique, involves a voluntary directed strenuous bearing-down effort against a closed glottis for at least 10 seconds. The woman is instructed to take a deep breath and hold it for as long as she can (during each count of 10) using the entire contraction. This method usually involves two to three pushes of 10 seconds each with each contraction (Roberts & Woolley, 1996).
- Directed pushing refers to instructions from care providers to the woman concerning how to push and often includes directions to "hold your breath" (closed glottis or Valsalva technique) to a count of 10 or more seconds. Instructions also may be given concerning positioning during pushing; often a supine or semi-Fowler's position is advised rather than encouraging the woman to choose her own position of comfort.
- Nondirected pushing refers to care providers encouraging the woman to choose whatever method she feels is effective to push her baby out, including choosing the position during pushing, deciding whether to hold her breath during pushing efforts, and determining the duration of each pushing effort.
- Open glottis refers to spontaneous, involuntary bearing-down accompanying the forces of the uterine contraction and is usually characterized by expiratory grunting or vocalizations. The spontaneous method usually involves three to four pushes of 6 to 8 seconds with each contraction (Simpson & O'Brien-Abel, 2014).

To maximize pushing efforts, the nurse should assess the woman's knowledge of pushing techniques, expectations for pushing, presence of Ferguson's reflex, intensity of uterine contractions, readiness to push, and the fetal presentation, position, and station. With adequate information, the woman can actively participate in the decision to start pushing. When pushing begins, women should be encouraged to push for 6 to 8 seconds, followed by a slight exhale, and repeat this pattern for three to four pushes per contraction or as tolerated by the woman and her fetus.

Perineal Stretching

Measures proposed to enhance perineal stretching and decrease perineal trauma include the application of warm compresses, gentle perineal massage and stretching, and perineal massage with warm oil during the second stage of labor. No evidence from any randomized clinical trial published to date confirms that use of warm compresses or second-stage perineal massage with or without oil decreases the need for episiotomy or the risk of perineal trauma (AWHONN, 2008).

Evidence-Based Practice: AWHONN Evidence-Based Clinical Practice Guideline: Nursing Management of Second Stage of Labor

AWHONN clinical practice recommendations for management of pushing include the following:

- Assess the woman's knowledge of pushing techniques, expectations for pushing, presence of Ferguson's reflex (urge to bear down), and readiness to push as well as the fetal presentation, position, and station.
- Pushing techniques may vary. Pushing efforts may be directed or nondirected, but nondirected pushing is preferable. Women should be permitted to choose whether to hold their breath while pushing (closed- vs. open-glottis pushing).
- When pushing begins, women should be encouraged to push for 6 to 8 seconds, followed by a slight exhale, and repeat this pattern for three to four pushes per contraction or as tolerated by the woman and her fetus.
- Woman can be encouraged to bear down and hold it as long as she can or "do whatever comes naturally" when conditions are physiologically appropriate for active pushing.
- Whenever possible, discourage the traditional practice of breath holding for 10 seconds with each contraction. Closed glottis pushing, also referred to as the Valsalva technique, involves a voluntary or directed strenuous bearing-down effort against a closed glottis for at least 10 seconds. This method usually involves two to three pushes of 10 seconds each during a contraction.
- Provide birthing aids such as birthing balls, squat bars, birthing stools, and cushions to support the woman and the pelvis.
- Evaluate the effectiveness of pushing efforts and descent of the presenting part.
- Support and facilitate the woman's spontaneous pushing efforts.

Continued

- Evaluate the effectiveness of upright or other positions on fetal descent, rotation, and maternal-fetal condition.
- Upright positioning for the second stage of labor refers to the patient's position sitting with the head of the bed at a 45-degree angle or greater, squatting, kneeling, or standing during the second stage of labor. A woman may use birthing aids such as birthing balls and squatting bars to help maintain her position. Benefits of upright positioning include possible increase of pelvic diameter by 30%, shortened duration of second stage, decreased pain, and decreased perineal trauma.
- A recent Cochrane Review suggests several possible benefits for upright posture in women without epidural anesthesia, such as a reduction in the duration of second stage of labor and reduction in episiotomy rates and assisted deliveries. However, there is an increased risk of blood loss greater than 500 mL and there may be an increased risk of second degree tears (Gupta et al., 2017).
- Ferguson's reflex is a physiological response of the woman, activated when the presenting part of the fetus is at least at +1 station; it is usually accompanied by spontaneous bearing-down efforts. Pushing efforts may be delayed until the Ferguson reflex is present.
- Delayed pushing is waiting for fetal descent and or initiation of Ferguson's reflex before pushing begins in the second stage of labor. Delayed pushing is also referred to as "laboring down," "passive descent," and "rest and descend."
- Delayed pushing may also be appropriate for women with epidural anesthesia/analgesia who do not feel the urge to push.

AWHONN, 2008.

Medical Interventions

- Prepare for delivery.
- Provide reassurance to the woman while she pushes and brings baby down through the birth canal.
- Support fetal head and maternal perineum to avoid performing episiotomy (Box 8–5).
- Assist the woman in birthing her child.

Nursing Actions (see Clinical Pathway)

- Instruct the woman to bear down with the urge to push.
  - More progress is made and fewer traumas are noted to mother and fetus with spontaneous pushing efforts.
- Monitor for fetal response to pushing; check FHR every 5 to 15 minutes or after each contraction.
  - Assess fetal heart rate response to pushing efforts.
- Explain the need for vaginal examinations and the pressure and/or pain sensations anticipated. Negotiate when exams will be performed whenever possible. Perform vaginal examinations only as needed, share findings with the woman and her partner, and acknowledge and apologize for the discomfort caused during these procedures
- Provide comfort measures and allow woman to be in position of comfort.
- Provide reassurance, empathy, and encouragement to the woman by methods such as acknowledging the stress and

BOX 8–5 | Episiotomy and Lacerations

Episiotomy is an incision in the perineum to provide more space for the presenting part at delivery (see Fig. 8–27). Routine use of episiotomy at delivery is no longer typical.

A median or midline episiotomy is at the midline and tends to heal more quickly with less discomfort. A mediolateral episiotomy is cut at a 45-degree angle to the left or right and may be used for a large infant. It tends to heal more slowly, causes greater blood loss, and is more painful. Lacerations are tears in the perineum that may occur at delivery (see Fig. 8–28).

- Lacerations can occur in the cervix, vagina, and/or the perineum (see Fig. 8–30A).
- A first-degree laceration involves the perineal skin and vaginal mucous membrane (see Fig. 8–30B).
- A second-degree laceration involves skin, mucous membrane, and fascia of the perineal body (see Fig. 8–30C).
- A third-degree laceration involves skin, mucous membrane, and muscle of the perineal body and extends to the rectal sphincter (see Fig. 8–30D).
- A fourth-degree laceration extends into the rectal mucosa and exposes the lumen of the rectum (see Fig. 8–30E).

work of labor, acknowledging unpleasant sensations, and encouraging woman's spontaneous pushing efforts.
- Attend to perineal hygiene as needed, as the woman may pass stool with pushing.
  - Provides a cleaner pathway.
- Validate and explain the physical sensations experienced by the woman during the second stage of labor. Give praise and encouragement of progress made.
- Encourage rest between contractions by breathing with the patient and therapeutic touch.
  - Decreases fatigue and hypoxia in fetus by providing increased oxygenation.
- Review and reinforce pushing technique by:
  - Maintaining eye contact.
  - Developing a rhythm and pushing style to deal with each contraction that maximizes the woman's urge to push.
  - Using direct, simple, and focused communication, avoiding unnecessary conversation.
- Advocate on the woman's behalf for her desires of the delivery plan. Facilitate collaboration or negotiation among other caregivers on behalf of the woman to support care decisions and preferences whenever possible.
- Evaluate the father's, partner's, or labor coach's knowledge of physical, emotional, and psychosocial support needed during labor and augment as needed to meet the individual woman's need.
- Assist the support person and partner.
  - Role model supportive behaviors.
  - Offer support, praise, and encouragement.
  - Assist with food and rest and provide breaks.

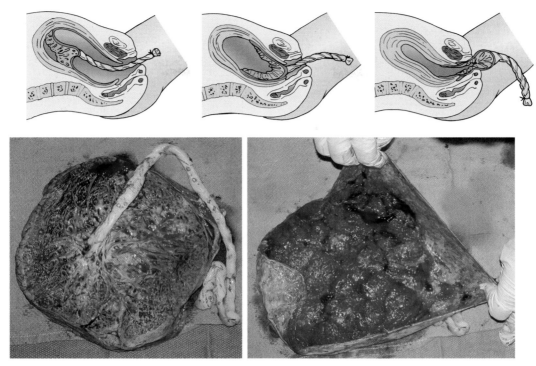

FIGURE 8–27 (*A*) Delivery of the placenta. (*B*) Delivered placenta (fetal side). (*C*) Inside of placenta (maternal side).

Third Stage

The third stage of labor begins immediately after the delivery of the fetus and involves separation and expulsion of the placenta and membranes (see Table 8–1). As the infant is born, the uterus spontaneously contracts around its diminishing contents. This sudden decrease in uterine size is accompanied by a decrease around placental implantation. This results in the decidual layer separating from the uterine wall. Placental separation typically occurs within a few minutes to less than a half hour after delivery. Once the placenta separates from the wall of the uterus, the uterus continues to contract until the placenta is expelled (Fig. 8–27). This process typically takes 1 to 20 minutes post-delivery of the baby and occurs spontaneously. Signs that signify the impending delivery of the placenta include:

● Upward rising of the uterus into a ball shape
● Lengthening of the umbilical cord at the introitus
● Sudden gush of blood from the vagina

Active management of the third stage of labor (AMTSL) includes uterotonic drugs (oxytocin is the gold standard), controlled cord traction, and fundal massage (AWHONN, 2015). These interventions decrease postpartum hemorrhage (PPH) and cause uterine contractions and placenta expulsion (AWHONN, 2014a). The placenta, membranes, and cord are examined by the care provider for completeness and anomalies.

CRITICAL COMPONENT

Quantification of Blood Loss After Birth

Normal blood loss for a vaginal birth is approximately 500 ml within 24 hours. Visual estimation of blood loss (EBL) is common practice in obstetrics; however, the inaccuracy of EBL has been well-established and blood loss can be underestimated by up to 50% (AWHONN, 2014b). AWHONN recommends that cumulative blood loss be formally measured or quantified after every birth. Inaccurate measurement of postpartum blood loss has the following implications:

• Underestimation can lead to delay in delivering lifesaving hemorrhage interventions.
• Overestimation can lead to costly, invasive, and unnecessary treatments such as blood transfusions that expose women to unnecessary risks.

Direct measurement of blood loss can be accomplished by two complementary approaches. The easiest to initiate is to collect blood in calibrated, under-buttocks drapes for vaginal birth.

The second approach is to weigh blood-soaked items and clots. These items can be collected in a single bag and weighed using a gravimetric method. By using this method, the weight of dry pads is subtracted from the total weight to obtain an estimate of blood loss. Weigh all blood-soaked materials and clots to determine cumulative volume (AWHONN, 2014c; Main et al., 2015).

SAFE AND EFFECTIVE NURSING CARE:
Understanding Medication

Uterotonics

The use of uterotonics for the prevention of PPH during the third stage of labor is recommended for all births (WHO, 2012). Oxytocin is the recommended uterotonic drug for the prevention of PPH. Oxytocin should be used for management of third stage of labor for all births (AWHONN, 2014a).

Oxytocin (Pitocin)

- Classification: hormone/oxytocic
- Route: Oxytocin should be administered only by the intramuscular (IM) or intravenous (IV) route, not by IV push. As a high-alert medication, IV oxytocin pre-mixed bags should be:
  - Infused via an IV infusion pump to control oxytocin administration
  - Prominently and clearly labeled with bright-colored labeling
  - Stored separately to prevent a 1000 milliliter IV bag with oxytocin being mistaken for a plain 1000 milliliter bag used for IV fluid resuscitation bolus
- Administer IV oxytocin by providing a bolus dose followed by a total minimum infusion time of 4 hours after birth, or per hospital policy. For women at high risk for a postpartum hemorrhage, continuation beyond 4 hours is recommended. Rate and duration should be titrated according to uterine tone and bleeding.
- Common dosing is oxytocin 20 units in 1-liter normal saline (NS) or lactated Ringer's (LR) solution with an initial bolus rate 1000 ml/hour bolus for 30 minutes (equals 10 units) followed by a maintenance rate 125 ml/hour over 3.5 hours (equals remaining 10 units).
- Give oxytocin 10 units IM in women without IV access.
- Actions: Stimulates uterine smooth muscle that produces intermittent contractions. Has vasopressor and antidiuretic properties.
- Indications: Control of PP (postpartum) bleeding after placental expulsion.

Methylergonovine (Methergine)

- Classification: Oxytocic/ergot alkaloids
- Route/Dosage: PO 200–400 mcg (0.4–0.6 mg) every 6 to12 hours for 2 to 7 days. IM 200 mcg (0.2 mg) every 2 to 4 hours up to 5 doses. IV (for emergencies only) same dosage as IM.
- Actions: Directly stimulates smooth and vascular smooth muscles causing sustained uterine contractions.
- Indications: Prevent or treat PP hemorrhage/uterine atony/subinvolution. Contraindicated in hypertensive patients.

Carboprost—Tromethamine (Hemabate)

- Classification: Prostaglandin
- Route/Dosage: IM 250 mcg injected into a large muscle or the uterus.
- Actions: Contraction of uterine muscle
- Indications: Uterine atony

Misoprostol (Cytotec)

- Classification: antiulcer/prostaglandins
- Route/Dosage: PO/Rectally 200-1,000 mcg
- Actions: Acts as a prostaglandin analogue causes uterine contractions.
- Indications: To control PP hemorrhage. This medication is used off-label and is not yet approved by the FDA for this use.

AWHONN, 2014a; Vallerand, Sanoski, & Deglin, 2017.

Medical Interventions

- At delivery, the neonate is often placed skin-to-skin on mother's chest.
- Await delivery of the placenta, typically within 20 minutes of delivery.
- If the third stage of labor lasts more than 30 minutes, IV/IM oxytocin (10 IU) may be used to manage the retained placenta. If the placenta is retained and bleeding occurs, the manual removal of the placenta should be expedited. Whenever the manual removal of the placenta is undertaken, a single dose of prophylactic antibiotics is recommended (WHO, 2012).
- Inspect the placenta after delivery: Intact, three-vessel cord, cord attachment to placenta.
- Order pain medications and uterotonics if necessary.

Nursing Actions (see Clinical Pathway and Concept Map)

- Administer uterotonic per protocol after delivery of the placenta.
- Assess maternal vital signs every 15 minutes.
- Encourage the woman to breathe with contractions and relax between contractions.
- Encourage mother-baby interactions by providing immediate newborn contact, if the newborn is stable.
- Administer pain medications as per order.
- Complete documentation of the delivery (Fig. 8–28).
  - Documentation of delivery includes labor summary, delivery summary for mother and baby, infant information, infant resuscitation, and documentation of personnel in attendance.
- Explain all forthcoming procedures.
- Stay with the woman and her family.

Fourth Stage

The fourth stage begins after delivery of the placenta and typically ends within 4 hours or with the stabilization of the mother. After the placenta delivers, the primary mechanism by which hemostasis is achieved at the placental site is vasoconstriction produced by a well-contracted myometrium. During this stage, the nurse is caring for both the woman and her newborn child (see Table 8–1). This stage also begins the

Delivery/Newborn Record

LABOR SUMMARY

Time   Date

Regular contractions began: _____ _____
Time of Oxytocin start: _____ _____
BOW ruptured: _____ _____
(best estimate) 4cm: _____ _____
10cm: _____ _____

Labor description:
- [ ] spontaneous
- [ ] augmented, oxytocin
- [ ] induced, oxytocin
- [ ] AROM for induction
- [ ] no labor

- [ ] Cervical ripening agent _____
- [ ] IUPC
- [ ] Amino infusion

Previous C/S: [ ] No   VBAC   [ ] No
             [ ] Yes attempted: [ ] Yes

Amniotic fluid rupture:
- [ ] Spontaneous
- [ ] Artificial

Color:
- [ ] Clear
- [ ] Light mec. (stain)
- [ ] Medium mec.
- [ ] Thick mec.
- [ ] Cloudy
- [ ] Bloody

Fetal monitoring in labor:
- [ ] Auscultation only
- [ ] External monitor
- [ ] Internal monitor
- [ ] Both
- [ ] IFM site

Analgesics: before delivery
drug   dose   time
_____ _____ _____
_____ _____ _____

Labor analgesia:
- [ ] none   [ ] epidural
- [ ] narcotic   [ ] both
- [ ] _____ cervical dil@epid

Steroids for lung maturity: Date _____ Time _____ Date _____ Time _____
Antibiotic started: (prior to birth): [ ] <4 hrs [ ] ≥4 hrs [ ] >24 hrs
Why: [ ] GBS ⊕ Pending / Preterm   # Doses before birth _____
      [ ] Cardiac prophylaxis
      [ ] Fever / Chorioamnionitis
      [ ] Other: _____
Peak maternal temp [ ] <99.5 [ ] 99.5–101.9 [ ] ≥102

GROUP B STREP SCREEN	APGAR SCORE		Cord around neck X
Universal Risk Factors		1 min	5 min	
[ ] Previous GBS infected infant				
[ ] ⊕ urine cx for GBS in current pregnancy	Heart Rate			
Culture Based	Respiratory Effort			Umbilical Vessel Number:
[ ] negative				
[ ] positive	Muscle Tone			
[ ] not available	Reflex Irritability			
Risk Based (Intrapartum)				
[ ] No risk factors	Color			[ ] Voided in DR
[ ] < 37 weeks				
[ ] ROM ≥ 18 hours	TOTAL			[ ] Stool in DR
[ ] Maternal temp ≥ 100.4				

DELIVERY–MOTHER

Method of Delivery:
- [ ] Vertex, Vaginal
- [ ] Breech, Vaginal
- [ ] Cesarean Section
- [ ] Vacuum
- [ ] Forceps

Episiotomy/Laceration:
- [ ] None
- [ ] Median
- [ ] Mediolateral
- [ ] Laceration
- [ ] Repaired

PLACENTA:
- [ ] Spontaneous
- [ ] Assist
- [ ] Manual
Abnormalities:

Medications at Delivery:
drug   dose   time
Pitocin   IV IM   units
_____ _____ _____

PEDIATRICIAN:

DELIVERY SUMMARY

Baby [____] **of a** [____] **gestation**
      Birth Order   Plurality

                    Time   Date
DELIVERY: _____ _____
PLACENTA: _____ _____
C/S start time: _____ _____
Uterine incis. time: _____ _____
C/S finish time: _____ _____

INFANT   (circle)   Boy   Girl

Weight _____ lb _____ gm
Length _____ in _____ cm
Head circ _____ in _____ cm

Delivery Outcomes:
- [ ] live birth admitted for regular care
- [ ] live birth admitted to trans. nursery
- [ ] live birth admitted to NICU
- [ ] neonatal death in delivery room
- [ ] fetal death before admission
- [ ] fetal death after admission

Feeding:
- [ ] Breast
- [ ] Bottle

Gest. Age @ Delivery
_____

I.D. BAND #: [_____]
Bands Checked by:
_____ RN _____ RN

Cord Blood to Lab: [ ] Yes [ ] No
Cord Gases Sent: [ ] Yes [ ] No
Specimen to Lab: [ ] Type _____
Culture to Lab: [ ] Type _____

RESUSCITATION

Check ALL that apply:
- [ ] suction
- [ ] oxygen
- [ ] mask vent
- [ ] intubation for resuscitation
- [ ] chest compression
- [ ] medications
- [ ] volume

Respirations: [ ] Spontaneous
[ ] Delayed _____ min
[ ] Narcan Given
Time: _____
Dose: _____
Route: _____
By whom: _____

For Meconium Babies:
- [ ] Not intubated
- [ ] Intubated – ∅ Below Cords
- [ ] Intubated – Meconium noted

Note: _____
_____
_____
_____

Newborn attended by _____ RN/MD
[ ] Newborn admitted time: _____ am/pm
MR # _____   Pat # _____
Pediatrician notified of delivery: K # _____
   Name _____ MD
   Date _____ Time _____ am/pm
   Via _____ by _____

DELIVERING PHYSICIAN/CNM:	APN/NICU STAFF AT DELIVERY:	ANESTHESIOLOGIST:
ASSIST MD/CNM:	OB/RN AT DELIVERY:	RN SIGNATURE DATE/TIME:

Patient's Data/Addressograph

FIGURE 8–28 Documentation of delivery.

CRITICAL COMPONENT

Newborn-Family Attachment: The Golden Hour

An important goal during the fourth stage is the newborn-family attachment. This is promoted by allowing early contact with the newborn and encouragement of eye contact and touch. The baby is placed skin-to-skin on the mother and covered with a warm blanket. Positive maternal bonding behaviors include making eye contact, touching and talking to the baby, smiling and cuddling the newborn, and similar actions. This is often the best time to institute breastfeeding. The newborn may remain in the labor and delivery room with the family for the immediate recovery period.

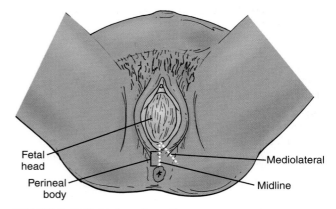

FIGURE 8–29 Episiotomy lacerations.

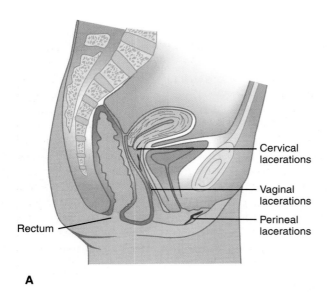

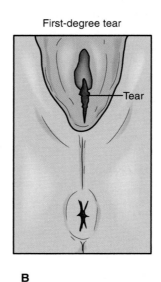

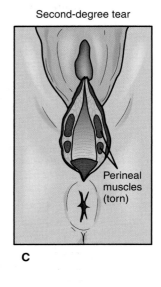

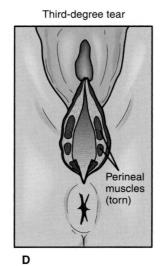

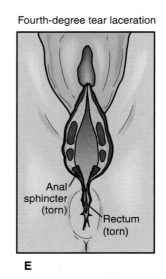

FIGURE 8–30 (*A*) Potential locations of lacerations. (*B*) First-degree tear. (*C*) Second-degree tear. (*D*) Third-degree tear. (*E*) Fourth-degree tear.

postpartum period (see Chapter 12 for a discussion of postpartum period).

Medical Interventions

- Repair the episiotomy or laceration (see Box 8–5) (Figs. 8–29 and 8–30).
- Inspect the placenta.
- Assess the fundus for firmness.
- Order uterotonics.
- Order pain medications, if necessary.

Nursing Actions (see Clinical Pathway and Concept Map)

- Explain all procedures.
- Assess the uterus for position, tone, and location, intervening with fundal massage as necessary.
- Assess lochia for color, amount, and clots. May weigh initial blood loss on scale to estimate EBL (1 gm = 1 cc) to provide for a more accurate evaluation of blood loss (AWHONN, 2014c).
- Administer medications as per orders.
- Assist the care provider with repair of lacerations and/or episiotomy.
- Assess maternal vital signs every 15 minutes.
- Monitor perineum for unusual swelling or hematoma formation.
- Apply ice packs to the perineum.
- Monitor for bladder distention.
  - *Assist the woman to the bathroom and measure void.*
- Assess for return of full motor-sensory function if epidural or spinal anesthesia is used.
- Assess pain and medicate as per orders.
- Stay with the mother and family.
- Offer congratulations and reassurance on a job well done to the woman and family.
- Explore with the family any requests they have for keeping the placenta. Some cultures consider the placenta part of the woman's body and there are a variety of rituals associated with disposal of the placenta. Efforts should be made to accommodate those requests (Callister, 2014).
- Encourage mother-baby interaction by:
  - Providing immediate newborn contact
  - Assisting with early breastfeeding, if desired
  - Pointing out the newborn's quiet, alert state
- Monitor newborn status, including temperature, heart and respiratory rates, skin color, adequacy of peripheral circulation, type of respiration, level of consciousness, and tone and activity every 30 minutes.
- Provide an opportunity for the support person to interact with newborn (Fig. 8–31).

THE NEWBORN

Newborn transition and initial care typically occur in the labor and delivery room. Initial assessments can be safely done with the infant skin-to-skin on the mother's abdomen after delivery,

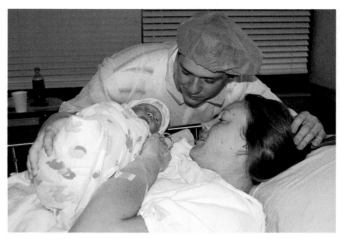

Courtesy of Chapman family

FIGURE 8–31 Newly delivered baby in the delivery room with family.

if the infant is stable. Researchers demonstrated that newborns have better outcomes, including stable temperature, heart rate, respiratory rate, and glucose levels, when they transition to extrauterine life and establish immediate skin-to-skin contact with their mothers (AWHONN, 2014d; 2016).

Apgar scores should be obtained at 1 minute and 5 minutes after birth. If the 5-minute Apgar score is less than 7, additional scores should be assigned every 5 minutes up to 20 minutes. Temperature, heart and respiratory rates, skin color, adequacy of peripheral circulation, type of respiration, level of consciousness, tone, and activity should be monitored and recorded at least every 30 minutes until the newborn's condition has remained stable for at least 2 hours. The Apgar score is a rapid assessment of five physiological signs that indicate the physiological status of the newborn and includes (Table 8–2):

- Heart rate based on auscultation
- Respiratory rate based on observed movement of chest
- Muscle tone based on degree of flexion and movement of extremities
- Reflex irritability based on response to tactile stimulation
- Color based on observation

Each component is given a score of 0, 1, or 2. An Apgar score of:

- 0 to 3 indicates severe distress
- 4 to 6 indicates moderate difficulty with transition to extrauterine life
- 7 to 10 indicates stable status.

The Apgar score is not used to determine the need for resuscitation, nor is it predictive of long-term neurological outcome of the neonate (American Academy of Pediatrics [AAP] and American College of Obstetrics and Gynecology [ACOG], 2006). Rather it is a rapid, objective, convenient shorthand for reporting the status of the newborn and the response to resuscitation immediately after birth.

At every delivery, one person should be solely responsible for assessment of the neonate response to the birth and have the

TABLE 8–2   Neonatal Apgar Score

SCORE			
Sign	0	1	2
RESPIRATORY EFFORT	Absent	Slow, irregular	Good cry
HEART RATE	Absent	Slow, below 100 bpm	Above 100 bpm
MUSCLE TONE	Flaccid	Some flexion of extremities	Active motion
REFLEX ACTIVITY	None	Grimace	Vigorous cry
COLOR	Pale, blue	Body pink, blue extremities	Completely pink

capacity to initiate resuscitation of the neonate if needed. Only 1% of neonates need extensive resuscitation at birth (American Academy of Pediatrics [AAP] and the American College of Obstetricians and Gynecologists [ACOG], 2012). The initial steps of resuscitation are to provide warmth by placing the baby under a radiant heat source, positioning the head in a "sniffing" position to open the airway, clearing the airway if necessary with a bulb syringe or suction catheter, drying the baby, and stimulating breathing. Further discussion of neonatal resuscitation is beyond the scope of this book except to mention optimal management of oxygen during neonatal resuscitation becomes particularly important because of the evidence that either insufficient or excessive oxygenation can be harmful to the newborn infant. A comprehensive discussion of the newborn's transition to extrauterine life, physical assessment, and routine procedures are presented in Chapter 15.

AWHONN (2014d) is currently focused on initiatives to increase the percentage of healthy, term newborns of stable mothers who receive uninterrupted skin-to-skin contact for at least 60 minutes. All routine procedures and assessments should be performed while the newborn is skin-to-skin with the mother. Procedures that require separation of the mother and infant, such as bathing and weighing, should be delayed until after the initial period of skin-to-skin contact. Skin-to-skin contact is described as holding the unclothed, diapered newborn on the mother's or caretaker's bare chest, usually in an upright position (Moore, Moos, & Callister, 2010). Skin-to-skin contact is also referred to as kangaroo care. The following recommendations for full-term, healthy newborns represent the consensus of the AWHONN Power of Touch Scientific Advisory Panel (AWHONN, 2016).

- All stable infants greater than 37 weeks and 0 days gestation born by vaginal or cesarean birth should be placed in immediate skin-to-skin contact for at least the first hour of life or until the first breastfeeding is completed.
- All mothers of stable infants greater than 37 weeks and 0 days gestation should be offered the option of skin-to-skin contact during painful neonatal procedures, such as vaccinations and blood sampling, whenever possible.
- All parents of healthy infants greater than 37 weeks and 0 days gestation should be encouraged to have frequent, uninterrupted skin-to-skin contact with their newborns while in the hospital and after discharge.

- Uninterrupted skin-to-skin contact should be encouraged for at least the first hour of life after birth and until the first breastfeeding is completed as long as the mother and newborn remain stable. If desired, skin-to-skin contact can be extended to the first two to three hours of life if the mother and infant remain stable. Routine care practices should ideally be delayed until the initial skin-to-skin session is completed.

One of the first procedures after birth is newborn identification. Perinatal nurses must be meticulous when recording the identification band number and birth and newborn information and applying identification bands to mothers and newborns. Institutional policies for newborn identification and newborn safety may vary.

Three medications are routinely administered to newborns:

- Erythromycin ointment is administered to the eyes as prophylaxis to prevent gonococcal and Chlamydia infections.
- Vitamin K is administered via intramuscular injection to prevent hemorrhagic disease caused by vitamin K deficiency.
- Hepatitis B virus vaccine is recommended for all newborns (American Academy of Pediatrics Committee on Infected Diseases, 2009).

Newborn care is discussed in Chapter 15.

Overview of Neonatal Resuscitation

Newly born infants who do not require resuscitation can generally be identified by a rapid assessment of the following three characteristics:

- Term gestation?
- Crying or breathing?
- Good muscle tone?

If the answer to all three of these questions is "yes," the baby does not need resuscitation and should not be separated from the mother. The baby should be dried, placed skin-to-skin with the mother, and covered with dry linen to maintain temperature. Observation of breathing, activity, and color should be ongoing (Weiner, Zaichkin, & Kattwinkel, 2016).

The initial steps of resuscitation are to provide warmth by placing the baby under a radiant heat source, positioning the head in a "sniffing" position to open the airway, clearing the airway if necessary with a bulb syringe or suction catheter, drying the baby, and stimulating breathing.

If the answer to any of the above assessment questions is "no," the infant should receive an initial assessment and one or more of the following four categories of action in sequence:

Initial Assessment: Determine if newborn can remain with the mother or should be moved to a radiant warmer for further evaluation and care.

A. **Airway** Perform initial steps to open the airway (reposition, open mouth, clear secretions if necessary).

B. **Breathing** Newborns with apnea or bradycardia may need positive-pressure ventilation, and newborns with labored breathing or low-oxygen saturation may need continuous positive airway pressure (CPAP) or oxygen therapy.

C. **Circulation** If the newborn has severe and persistent bradycardia despite assisted ventilation, perform chest compressions coordinated with PPV.

D. **Drug** If assisted ventilation and coordinated compressions are unsuccessful and severe bradycardia persists, administer epinephrine and continue with PPV and chest compressions.

The sequence algorithm for neonatal resuscitation is available at http://eccguidelines.heart.org/wp-content/uploads/2015/10/Neonatal-Resuscitation-Algorithm.pdf

MANAGEMENT OF PAIN AND DISCOMFORT DURING LABOR AND DELIVERY

Pain in childbirth is a universal experience and considered a normal occurrence. Most pain in labor results from normal physiologic events (Burke, 2014). Pain associated with labor has been described as one of the most intensely painful experiences possible. Labor pain differs from other conditions in which pain is experienced in several ways.

Understanding the cause and characteristics of pain in the labor and delivery setting helps the nurse develop a plan of care for the woman in each stage of the labor process. Labor pain is acute pain and presents in many ways. During the first stages of labor pain is caused by uterine muscle hypoxia, accumulation of lactic acid in the muscles, lower uterine and cervical stretching, traction on pelvic organs, and pressure on the bony pelvis. The size and position of the fetus can also demonstrate pain in the pelvis, rectal and adnexae and cause discomfort as well as lumbosacral plexus. During the second stage, pain is caused by pelvic muscle distention and pressure on the perineum, cervix, urethra, and rectum. Back pain during labor is thought to be caused by pressure of the fetal occiput on the maternal spine and pelvis.

Factors influencing pain response include both the physical and psychosocial:

- Rate of cervical dilation and strength of contractions.
- Size and position of fetus impacts length of labor.

- Sleep deprivation and exhaustion from long labor increases pain perception.
- Culture of the woman influences her response to labor and pain. Pain behaviors are culturally bound.
- The woman's labor support system can affect her anxiety level and perception of pain.
- Previous birth experiences may increase or decrease anxiety.
- Childbirth preparation may decrease anxiety and decrease pain.
- The woman's expectations influence her satisfaction with her birth experience.

Pain in childbirth is transmitted from the periphery of the body along nerve pathways to the brain. This pain is attributable to:

- Uterine contractions resulting in uterine pain from a decrease in blood supply to the uterus.
- Increased pressure and stretching of the pelvic structures resulting in the pulling and expansion of ligaments, muscle, and peritoneum.
- Cervical dilation and stretching resulting in the stimulation of the nerve ganglia.

Pain Response and Culture

It is well-established that pain is a highly complex phenomenon that involves biological, psychological, and social variables, and that is especially true of women's experiences of pain in labor. Cultural differences have been identified in women's experiences of pain in labor. Patients' culturally-based responses to pain are often divided into two categories: stoic and emotive (Carteret, 2011). Stoic patients are less expressive of their pain and tend to "grin and bear it." They may tend to withdraw. Emotive patients are more likely to verbalize their expressions of pain. Whether a patient is stoic or emotive may reflect his or her cultural background. If we use such broad generalizations to help understand human behavior, however, we must always keep in mind that while culture is a framework that directs human behavior, not everyone in every culture conforms to a set of expected behaviors or beliefs. Rigid use of generalizations leads to cultural stereotyping which in turn can lead to serious inaccuracies. Any individual's experience of pain will manifest itself in emotional and behavioral responses particular to his or her culture, personal history, and unique perceptions (Callister, 2014).

Communication with patients can be improved and patient care enhanced when we make efforts to bridge the divide between cultures and the beliefs and practices that make up patients' value systems (ACOG, 2011b). Through careful listening and probing nurses can uncover what is really happening with each patient's pain. Sometimes pain measurement tools that rely on numbers or any kind of linear format, such as a row of faces, may not work well across cultures (Carteret, 2011).

Gate Control Theory of Pain

The gate control theory of pain can be applied to the process of labor and birth (Fig. 8–32). This theory states that sensation

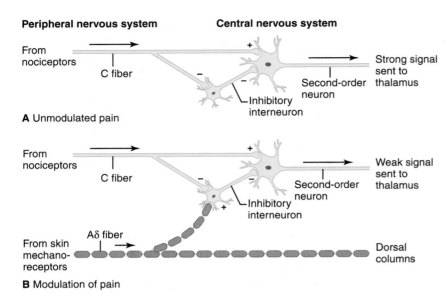

Peripheral nervous system   **Central nervous system**

A Unmodulated pain

B Modulation of pain

FIGURE 8–32 Gate control theory of pain modulation. (**A**) Normally C-fibers carrying slow pain signals block inhibitory interneurons and transmit their signals across the synapse unimpeded. (**B**) A-delta fibers carrying pleasurable signals from touch excite inhibitory interneurons, which then block the transmission of slow pain signals (+ equals transmission, – equals no transmission).

of pain is transmitted from the periphery of the body along ascending nerve pathways to the brain. Because of the limited number of sensations that can travel along these pathways at any given time, an alternate activity can replace travel of the pain sensation, thus closing the gate control at the spinal cord and reducing pain impulses traveling to the brain. Based on this premise, the application of pressure to certain areas of the body, the cutaneous stimulation such as effleurage (gentle stroking of the abdomen) or the use of heat or cold, can have a direct effect on closing the gate, which then limits the transmission of pain. A similar gating mechanism can be found in the descending nerve fibers from the hypothalamus and cerebral cortex. Strategies such as breathing, focusing, and visual and auditory stimulation may affect whether pain impulses reach the level of conscious awareness.

Non-Pharmacological Management of Labor Discomfort

Non-pharmacological management of labor discomfort includes preparation by the woman for childbirth, cutaneous stimulation, thermal stimulation, mental stimulation, and the presence of a support person(s). It is essential that nurses have a repertoire of strategies to help patients manage discomfort and pain during labor. A willingness to try a variety of strategies, adapt those that are effective, and modify and abandon those that are ineffective is an important aspect of care. Usually, no one strategy works for very long in labor, making flexibility and adaptability key qualities for labor nurses.

- Childbirth preparation methods: Education and explanation of birth process is offered through classes to the woman and her support person before the delivery time. In these classes, the woman and her partner learn about pregnancy, the labor process, the painful aspects of labor, and methods to help relieve the discomforts of pregnancy and childbirth.

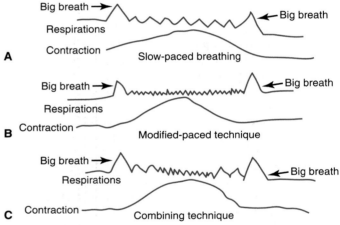

A   Slow-paced breathing

B   Modified-paced technique

C   Combining technique

FIGURE 8–33 Space breathing technique graph. (**A**) Slow-paced breathing is with big breath at beginning and end of contraction; the typical rate is fewer than 10 breaths per minute (**B**) Modified-paced breathing is with a big breath at the beginning and end of the contraction and rapid shallow breaths that are comfortable for the woman at a rate of about twice normal respirations. (**C**) Combining technique. Big breath at the beginning and end of the contraction with more rapid and shallow breathing at the peak of the contraction.

- Relaxation and breathing techniques: Varied breathing patterns that promote relaxation and avoidance of pushing before complete cervical dilation. Most childbirth preparation methods teach some form of relaxation and breathing techniques (Fig. 8–33). Most women are taught to take a deep breath at the beginning of the contraction to signal the onset of the contraction and then to breathe slowly during the contraction. As labor pain increases, the woman may need to breathe in a more rapid and shallow manner. On occasion, a woman will experience hyperventilation from this type of breathing. Symptoms are related to respiratory alkalosis and include tingling of the fingers or circumoral numbness, lightheadedness, or dizziness. This undesirable side effect can be eliminated by having the woman breathe into a bag or cupped hands. This causes her to rebreathe carbon dioxide and reverses the respiratory alkalosis. Discuss with the woman and her support team how they plan on managing labor. This will stimulate conversation, facilitate a plan of care to assist them in pain management, and give an opportunity to teach and or support them as needed.

- Effleurage is cutaneous stimulation by lightly stroking the abdomen in rhythm with breathing during contractions. Another form of cutaneous stimulation is back massage and/or counter pressure to the sacral area by another. Counter pressure is exerted to the sacral area with the heel of the hand or fist to relieve the sensation of intense pain in the back caused by internal pressure of the fetal head. This increased internal pressure by the fetal head is often associated with the posterior position of the fetus during labor. As labor advances, women may not want to be touched.

- Thermal stimulation: Application of warmth or cold, such as use of warm showers or ice packs. The use of hydrotherapy via whirlpools, warm baths, or showers is very effective and promotes relaxation and comfort. This may reduce the woman's anxiety and promote well-being, causing a reduction in catecholamine production that interferes with uterine contractility. Application of cold may release musculoskeletal pain, and the numbing effect of cold may decrease the sensation of pain.

- Mental stimulation: Focal points, imagery, and music help the woman to concentrate on something outside her body. This helps her to focus away from the pain. With imagery, the woman is encouraged to picture a relaxing scene.

- Support person(s): Significant other(s) and/or a doula provide emotional support and physical comfort and aids in a beneficial form of care. Research has shown that support early in labor significantly relieves pain, improves outcomes, decreases interventions and complication rates, enhancing overall maternal satisfaction (Simkin & O'Hara, 2002). A doula can also be used as a support for women during pregnancy through postpartum. Doulas are unique in that they are trained to provide support, promote comfort, and instill confidence to the laboring woman. Doulas are trained through many organizations and paid by the family that hires them. Doulas do not perform clinical tasks and do not have direct communication responsibility to care providers (Burke, 2014). Some studies have shown that women who used a doula had shorter labors, less use of analgesia, fewer instrument deliveries, and fewer C-sections (Hodnett, 2002).

Complementary Therapy

Many therapies have been used to promote relaxation and decrease the perception of pain while providing a complement to decrease the use of pharmacological interventions (Burke, 2014; Zwelling, Johnson, & Allen, 2006).

- Aromatherapy: Essential oils can be inhaled through vaporizers or used in a carrier oil or lotion with massage to promote relaxation and decrease the perception of pain. A few drops placed in a bath can be an adjunct to hydrotherapy. Lavender and jasmine oils promote relaxation and decrease pain perception, while peppermint may decrease feelings of nausea.

- Massage: Multiple studies have shown massage to decrease pain and promote relaxation, which in turn promotes labor progress. A quiet, soothing voice encouraging the woman to imagine a safe place can assist in relaxation. This used in conjunction with aromatherapy has proven to enhance relaxation in laboring women, allowing women to have better control of labor.

- Birthing ball: This ball (65-cm) originated in physical therapy programs but has been used successfully in the labor suite. It facilitates an upright position, opens the pelvis, and allows the woman to roll or bounce as she deems necessary to manage her contractions and pain.

- Hydrotherapy: Water has been used in many areas of medicine for many years to promote relaxation and pain control. The use of a shower or large tub is ideal for releasing endorphins, decreasing muscle tension, and promoting circulation. The use of hydrotherapy with ruptured membranes (ROM) has shown no increase of infections. The many benefits of hydrotherapy include less medication needs, less anesthesia, faster labors, facilitation of fetal positions (which decreases the number of instrumental deliveries), fewer episiotomies, decrease in blood pressure and edema, promotion of diuresis, and increased satisfaction in the birthing experience. Data indicates hydrotherapy is a safe nonpharmacologic measure (AWHONN, 2008).

- Self-hypnosis: Use of self-hypnosis during labor and birth has been investigated and studies suggest it can reduce labor pain and requests for parenteral analgesia and regional analgesia/anesthesia during labor (AWHONN, 2008). The use of self-hypnosis as a method to decrease pain during labor has not been widespread in North America.

- Music therapy: Music calms the spirit and decreases stress and distress by diverting attention from the pain receptors and promoting relaxation.

- Acupuncture: This traditional Chinese therapy improves energy flow, reduces pain and anxiety, and helps labor progress (Simpkin, Hanson, & Ancheta, 2017).

- Sterile water injections: SQ injection of .5 ml of sterile water gives about 60-90 minutes of lower back pain relief (Simpkin, Hanson, & Ancheta, 2017).

These complementary therapies are used in some form today either alone or in combination in all birthing venues from home births to stand-alone birth centers to hospital suites. They can assist the woman and her support team by providing comfort, empowering the birth experience as the woman sees it, and promoting a safe non-invasive birth.

Most classes teach a variety of strategies to manage labor pain. Specific methods include:

- Dick-Read method: Advocates birth without fear by education and environmental control and relaxation.

● Lamaze: Promotes psychoprophylaxis with conditioning and breathing.
● Bradley: This is husband-coached childbirth and support focused on working with and managing the pain rather than being distracted from it.

CRITICAL COMPONENT

Non-Pharmacological Approaches

Non-pharmacologic labor support includes physical and emotional nursing interventions that support a woman in labor to enhance her physical comfort, confidence in her ability to give birth, and sense of being cared for and being safe. A registered nurse or other members of the care team with licenses must supervise non-licensed individuals performing labor support interventions. Individuals must have evidence-based knowledge concerning how to perform and customize non-pharmacologic labor support interventions. Non-pharmacologic labor support is discussed earlier in the chapter and a summary of nursing interventions include the following:

• Stay in the room with the woman.
• Encourage the woman to labor in positions of her choice, e.g., walk or use a balance ball.
• Interventions and strategies can include:
  • Guided imagery and therapeutic breathing
  • Touch therapy, such as a back rub, leg massage, or counter pressure
  • Hydrotherapy in a tub or shower
  • Application of warm or cool compresses to various parts of the woman's body
  • Aromatherapy
  • Provide emotional support: Verbally encourage, reassure, and praise the woman and provide easy to understand information about how labor is progressing and how she and her baby are doing;
  • Support the woman's nutritional needs
  • Advocate for the woman by helping her articulate her wishes to others.

AWHONN, 2014a; Hodnett, Gates, Hofmeyr, & Sakala, 2012.

Pharmacological Management of Labor Discomfort

Pain management for childbirth is a primary concern for obstetric nurses, midwives, and physicians. The advancement of obstetric anesthesia practice has had an important impact on the role of perinatal nurses. The perinatal nurse is an integral member of the health care team who works collaboratively with the obstetric and anesthesia health care providers to address women's needs for pain management during labor and birth. As the need for a wide variety of pain management options has emerged, researchers have focused on enhancing the efficacy and safety of various forms of obstetric analgesia and anesthesia, including neuraxial, or regional, analgesia for childbirth (AWHONN, 2011b).

Pharmacological management of discomfort and pain requires the nurse to assess the woman's preferences for pain management throughout labor. The decision to use pain medication in labor should be made by the woman in collaboration with her physician or midwife. The unique circumstances of every labor influence the experience and perception of pain (Burke, 2014).

● Assessment of pain is an essential part of nursing care.
  ● Assessment of labor pain should include intensity, location, pattern, and degree of distress for the woman, as well as using pain scale with numerical self-report using a scale of 1 to 10.
● The use of medication in the relief of pain during labor falls into two major categories: Analgesia (Table 8–3) and anesthesia (Table 8–4).
● Basic principles when using analgesia include:
  ● Labor should be established.
  ● Medication should provide relief to the woman with minimal risk to the baby.
  ● Neonatal depression may occur if medication is given within an hour before delivery.
  ● Women with a history of drug abuse may have a lessened effect from pain medication and require higher doses.
● Basic principles for anesthesia include:
  ● Local anesthesia is used at the time of delivery for episiotomy and repair.
  ● Regional anesthesia is used during labor and at delivery.
  ● Regional anesthesia includes the pudendal block, epidural block, and spinal block.
  ● Regional or general anesthesia is used for cesarean deliveries. (Chapter 11 addresses care of cesarean birth women.)

Parenteral Opioids

The use of opioids in labor is common. Advantages include availability, ease of administration, and cost. Depending on the dose, route of administration, and stage of labor parenteral analgesia does not illuminate pain but causes a blunting effect, leading to a decrease in sensation of pain and inducing somnolence (Burke, 2014). Opioids cross the placenta and can cause neonatal respiratory depression.

Nitrous Oxide Analgesia

A new interest in self-administered nitrous oxide for labor analgesia has emerged in recent years in the United States. It has been used widely in Europe for decades with favorable results (Stewart & Collins, 2012). A recent published review concludes nitrous oxide analgesia is safe for mothers, neonates, and those who care for women during childbirth (Rooks, 2011). In the context of obstetric analgesia, "nitrous oxide" usually refers to a half-and-half combination of oxygen and nitrous oxide gas, called by the trade name "Nitronox." It is self-administered by the laboring woman using a mouth tube or face mask when she determines that she needs it, about a minute before she anticipates the onset of a strong contraction until the pain eases. Its use can be started and stopped at any point during labor according to the woman's needs and preferences. It takes effect in about

TABLE 8–3   Analgesic Medications in Labor

MEDICATION	CLASS	SIDE EFFECTS	NURSE INTERVENTION
Morphine sulfate	Opioid	Respiratory depression	Cautious use in 2nd stage.
Butorphanol 2–4 mg IM 0.5–2 mg IV	Opioid agonist–antagonist	Respiratory depression	Check maternal history for drug abuse. Do not give to drug dependent woman due to possible precipitation of sudden withdrawal response in woman and baby.
Nalbuphine (Nubain) 10 mg IM or IV	Opioid agonist crosses the placenta and enters breast milk	Respiratory depression and may temporarily affect fetal heart rate and cause bradycardia (ACOG 2019)	Monitor for side effect such as bradycardia in fetus and respiratory depression
Sublimaze (Fentanyl) 50–100 mcg IM 25–50 mcg IM May be used in conjunction with regional anesthesia	Short acting opioid agonist Crosses the placenta rapidly Synthetic opioid	FHR changes Hypotension Maternal/fetal/neonatal CNS depression Respiratory depression	Monitor for side effects such as sedation, nausea, vomiting, itching. Monitor respiratory rate and effort.

Vallerand, Sanoski, & Deglin, 2017 Davis's Drug Guide for nurses, 15th ed. FA Davis; American College of Obstetricians and Gynecologists (ACOG). ACOG practice bulletin no. 209:obstetric analgesia and anesthesia. Obstet Gynecol.2019.

TABLE 8–4   Anesthesia in Labor and Delivery

TYPE OF ANESTHESIA	TIME GIVEN AND EFFECTS	ADVERSE EFFECTS	NURSING IMPLICATIONS
LOCAL: Anesthetic injected into perineum at episiotomy site	Second stage of labor, immediately before delivery Anesthetizes local tissue for episiotomy and repair	Risk of a hematoma Risk of infection	Monitor for: Return of sensation to area Increased swelling at site of injection
REGIONAL: **Pudendal Block:** Anesthetic injected in the pudendal nerve (close to the ischial spines) via needle guide known as "trumpet"	Second stage of labor, prior to time of delivery Anesthetizes vulva, lower vagina and part of perineum for episiotomy and use of low forceps	Risk of local anesthetic toxicity Risk of a hematoma Risk of infection	Monitor for: Return of sensation to area Increased swelling Signs and symptoms of infection Urinary retention
Epidural Block: Anesthetic injected in the epidural space: Located outside the dura mater between the dura and spinal canal via an epidural catheter	First stage and/or second stage of labor Can be used for both vaginal and cesarean births Has the potential of 100% blockage of pain Can be used with opioids such as Sublimaze to allow walking during first stage of labor and effective pushing in second stage of labor	Most common complication is hypotension Other side effects include nausea, vomiting, pruritis, respiratory depression, alterations in FHR	**Pre-anesthesia care** Obtain consent. Check lab values—especially for bleeding or clotting abnormalities, platelet count. IV fluid bolus with normal saline or lactated Ringer's Ensure emergency equipment is available. Do time-out procedure verification

Continued

TABLE 8–4   Anesthesia in Labor and Delivery—cont'd

TYPE OF ANESTHESIA	TIME GIVEN AND EFFECTS	ADVERSE EFFECTS	NURSING IMPLICATIONS
			Post-procedure care
			Monitor maternal vital signs and FHR every 5 min initially and after every re-bolus then every 15 minutes and manage hypotension or alterations in FHR.
			Urinary retention is common and catheterization may be needed.
			Assess pain and level of sensation and motor loss.
			Position woman as needed (on side to prevent inferior vena cava syndrome).
			Assess for itching, nausea and vomiting, and headache and administer meds PRN.
			When catheter discontinued, note intact tip when removed.
Spinal Block: Anesthetic injected in the sub-arachnoid space	Second stage of labor or in use for cesarean section Rapid acting with 100% blockage of sensation and motor functioning. Can last up to 3 hours.	Adverse effects are similar to the epidural with the addition of a spinal head-ache. A blood patch often provides relief.	Interventions are same as for epidural. Monitor site for leakage of spinal fluid or formation of hematoma. Observe for headache.
GENERAL ANESTHESIA: Use of IV injection and/ or inhalation of anesthetic agents that render the woman unconscious.	Used mainly in emergency cesarean birth	Risk for fetal depression Risk for uterine relaxation Risk for maternal vomiting and aspiration	Obtain consent. Ensure woman is NPO. IV with large-bore needle. Place indwelling urinary catheter. Administer medications to decrease gastric acidity as ordered such as ant-acids: Bicitra or Proton pump inhibitor: Protonix. Place wedge to hip to prevent vena cava syndrome. Assist with supportive care of newborn.

AWHONN, 2011b; Pitter & Preston, 2001; Spratto & Woods, 2006.

50 seconds after the first breath and the effect is transient—essentially gone when no longer needed. It is simple to administer and does not interfere with the release and function of endogenous oxytocin, and has no adverse effects on the normal physiology and progress of labor. This analgesia may be of help for women who want to have an unmedicated birth but may need help at some point during labor and want to use a method that is under their control (Rooks, 2007; AWHONN, 2011b).

Epidural Anesthesia

Epidural anesthesia is one of the most common forms of pain relief during labor in the United States. In a recent report, 61% of women who had a singleton birth in a vaginal delivery in 2008 received epidural or spinal anesthesia (Osterman & Martin, 2011). Epidural anesthesia involves the placement of a very small catheter and injection of local anesthesia and or analgesia between the fourth and fifth vertebrae into the epidural space. A combined spinal epidural analgesia (CSE) involves the injection of local anesthetic and/or analgesic into the subarachnoid space. Some patients may be able to ambulate with this type of anesthesia, so it's sometimes called a "walking epidural." Because of the widespread use of epidural anesthesia in labor, AWHONN has generated evidence-based practice guidelines for care of pregnant women receiving regional anesthesia/analgesia (AWHONN, 2011b).

- Three of every five women undergoing labor in the United States use this method each year and the rate of epidural use in labor appears to be increasing (Osterman & Martin, 2011). Some research shows that epidural analgesia is associated with a lower rate of spontaneous vaginal delivery, a higher rate of instrumental (e.g., vacuum suction and/or forceps) vaginal delivery, longer labors, and increased incidence of intrapartum fevers and/or suspected sepsis (Buckley, 2005; Osterman & Martin, 2011). A review of the evidence has concluded that research about the effects of regional anesthesia/analgesia on the progress of labor may not be significant (AWHONN, 2011b; Simpson & O'Brien-Abel, 2014).
- Elevations in maternal temperature associated with regional anesthesia have been reported and may not be clinically significant. They may be associated with decreased maternal hyperventilation, reduced perspiration, and altered thermoregulatory transmission.
- A wide variety of medications and dosing regimens are used for regional analgesia/anesthesia. Nurses are responsible for knowing general information about classification of these medications, their actions, potential side effects, and complications (AWHONN, 2011b).

CRITICAL COMPONENT

Epidural Anesthesia

Epidural labor analgesia involves the placement of a catheter and injection of a local anesthetic or analgesic agent or both into the epidural space, typically in the lumbar region. Partial loss of sensation may occur.

- Nurses monitor but do not manage the care of women receiving epidural anesthesia.
- Catheter dosing of intermittent and continuous infusion of regional analgesia/anesthesia is outside the scope of registered nursing.
- Only qualified, licensed anesthesia providers should perform insertion, injection, and/or manage rate changes of a continuous infusion (AWHONN, 2011b).
- Responsibilities of nurses caring for women receiving regional anesthesia/analgesia are assessment, monitoring, and interventions to minimize complications.
- After the stabilization of the patient after regional anesthesia, the nurse monitors the woman's vital signs, mobility, level of consciousness, and perception of pain, as well as fetal status.

Nursing Actions Before the Epidural

Nursing actions are based on AWHONN (2011b) guidelines (see Table 8–4)

- Assess woman's level of pain.
- Determine the woman's and her family's knowledge and concerns about epidural anesthesia.
- Provide information about options for anesthesia/analgesia.
- Notify obstetrical and anesthesia care providers when the woman requests epidural anesthesia.
- Assess and document baseline blood pressure, pulse, respiratory rate, and temperature.
- Assess FHR to confirm a normal FHR pattern; if indeterminate or abnormal, report to the physician or midwife.
- Encourage the patient to void before initiation of epidural anesthesia.
- If ordered, administer an IV bolus as ordered to decrease incidence of hypotension.
- Obtain platelet count, blood type, and screen.
- Conduct a pre-procedure verification process per facility policy.
- Conduct time-out. The time-out involves the immediate members of the procedure team: the anesthesia provider and the nurse. During the time-out, the team members agree and verify the correct patient identity, the correct site and the procedure to be done (Joint Commission on Accreditation of Healthcare Organizations, 2017).

Nursing Actions During Administration of Epidural Anesthesia

- Assist the anesthesia provider, anesthesiologist, or nurse anesthetist (CRNA) with placement of the epidural, including placement of patient in the lateral position with head flexed toward chest, or sitting position with head flexed on chest, elbows on knees and feet supported on stool (AWHONN, 2011b; Simpson & O'Brien-Abel, 2014) (Figs. 8–34 and 8–35).

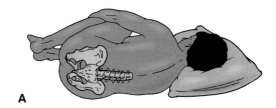

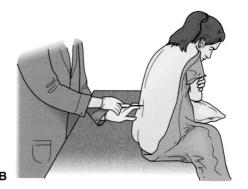

FIGURE 8–34 Lateral (*A*) and sitting (*B*) positions for placement of spinal and epidural block.

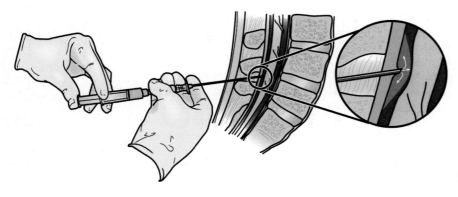

FIGURE 8–35 Technique for epidural block.

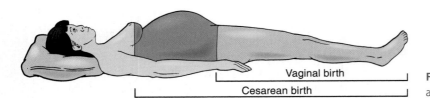

Vaginal birth
Cesarean birth

FIGURE 8–36 Levels of anesthesia necessary for vaginal and cesarean births.

Nursing Actions After Epidural Administration

● Monitor vital signs according to agency protocols, generally every 5 to 15 minutes. Assess for hypotension and respiratory distress.
  ● Up to 40% of women may experience hypotension. Difficulty breathing may indicate the catheter is in the subarachnoid space.
  ● Hypotension is defined as systolic blood pressure less than 100 mm Hg or a 20% decrease in blood pressure from preanesthesia levels. Notify the anesthesia provider if the patient becomes hypotensive.
● Assess FHR every 5 to 15 minutes.
● Facilitate lateral or upright positioning with uterine displacement.
  ● Helps to avoid supine hypotension
● Assess for effectiveness of the epidural and the woman's pain levels and description of pain.
  ● Notify the anesthesia provider of inadequate pain relief.
● Assess for sedation if opioid medication is administered with local anesthesia.
  ● Drowsiness can occur in up to 50% of women who receive combination local/opioid analgesia.
● Assess the level of motor blockade according to agency criteria.
  ● If the patient receives an epidural that allows ambulation: Before ambulation, the nurse assesses somatosensory status, motor strength, and ability to ambulate.
● Monitor for pruritis.
  ● Up to 90% of women who receive opioids in epidurals have itching. Medicate as indicated.
● Monitor for nausea and vomiting.
  ● Up to 50% of women experience this and may be treated with antiemetics.

● Assess for post-procedural headache.
  ● Occurs in up to 3% of women related to leakage of spinal fluid with inadvertent puncture. If this occurs, it should be reported to the anesthesia provider.
● Assess the woman for urinary retention.
  ● This occurs in some women who receive epidural anesthesia because of decreased motor function. Catheterization is typically necessary.
● Assess the partner's or support person's response to epidural pain relief and answer questions.
● Monitor uterine contractions as uterine activity may slow for up to 60 minutes after epidural placement. This may be a side effect of the neuroaxial block and usually no treatment is needed. Some providers will initiate oxytocin augmentation to stimulate contractions.
● Monitor for signs and symptoms of intravascular injection including: This normally occurs during placement and is monitored by a test dose being given by the anesthesiologist.
  ● Maternal tachycardia or bradycardia
  ● Hypertension
  ● Dizziness
  ● Tinnitus (ringing in the ears)
  ● Metallic taste in the mouth
  ● Loss of consciousness

If intravascular injection occurs, the anesthesia care provider should be immediately notified and care includes administering oxygen, fluids, and medication as ordered. Initiating CPR may be necessary.

● A higher level of anesthesia is necessary for a cesarean birth than for labor (Fig. 8–36).

Evidence-Based Practice: Expectant Fathers and Labor Epidurals

Chapman, L. (2000). Expectant fathers and labor epidurals. *Maternal Child Nursing, 25,* 133–138.

A qualitative research study using grounded theory methodology was conducted to describe and explain the expectant father's experience during labor and birth when epidural anesthesia/analgesia is used for labor pain management. Based on the research data a theory, "cruising through labor," was developed. The epidural labor process is different from non-epidural labor and is comprised of six phases:

- Holding out
- Surrendering
- Waiting
- Getting
- Cruising
- Pushing

Expectant fathers explained that before the epidural they felt like they were "losing" their partner as the increasing pain caused the woman to focus inward and away from interaction with those in the labor room. The expectant fathers explained that they felt a loss of connection with their partner and a loss of control. They felt that the pain of labor overtook their partner and was all-encompassing. The men further explained that they felt helpless, frustrated, and a sense of losing her to the pain of labor.

The men explained that the labor nurse played a significant role in supporting them during this time. The major supportive behaviors by the nurse were:

- Remaining in the labor room
- Explaining what was happening to their partner
- Including the men in the care of their partner

Expectant fathers reported that once the epidural was administered and the woman experienced relief from labor pain, they saw a dramatic change in their partner's behavior. They often stated, "She's back," that she was comfortable and able to interact with those around her. One man stated, "She wasn't in pain. Her color was back. Her pain was gone. She wasn't throwing up. She was back. She was comfortable."

Men further explained that the effects of the epidural in decreasing the degree of labor pain allowed the men to shift their focus from labor pain management to enjoying the labor and birthing experience (Figs. 8–37 and 8–38).

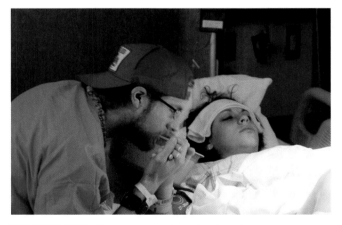

FIGURE 8–37 Partners experiencing labor together.

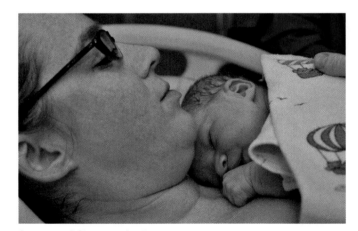

Courtesy of Chapman family

FIGURE 8–38 A new family.

Clinical Pathway for Intrapartal Maternal and Fetal Assessment

	Active Labor	Second Stage Labor (Active Pushing)	Third Stage of Labor (Delivery of Placenta)	Fourth Stage of Labor (Immediate Postpartum)
Maternal Vital Signs	P, R, BP every hour; temp every 2 hours unless ROM then every hour	P, R, BP every hour; temp every 2 hours unless ROM then every hour	P, R, BP every 15 minutes	P, R, BP every 15 minutes
FHR	Every 15–30 minutes*	Assessment every 5–15 minutes*	NA	Initiate neonatal transition care
Uterine Activity	Every 15–30 minutes**	Assessment every 5–15 minutes**	NA	NA
				Fundal and lochia checks every 15 minutes
Pain Status	Every 30 minutes and PRN	Assessment every 15 minutes	Assessment every 15 minutes	Assessment every 15 minutes
Response to Labor	Every 30 minutes and PRN	Assessment every 15 minutes	Assessment every 15 minutes	
Comfort Measures	Every 30 minutes and PRN	Assessment every 15 minutes and PRN	Assessment every 15 minutes and PRN	Assessment every 15 minutes and PRN
Maternal Position	Every 30 minutes and PRN	Change every 30 minutes and PRN		
Vaginal Exam/Fetal Station/Progress in Descent	As needed	As needed, at least every 30 minutes	NA	NA
Intake and Output	Every 8 hours	Assess bladder distension		Assess bladder distension

P, pulse; R, respirations; BP, blood pressure; FHR, fetal heart rate.

*FHR characteristics include baseline rate, variability, and presence or absence of accelerations and periodic or episodic decelerations.

**Uterine activity included contraction frequency, duration, intensity, and uterine resting tone.
AWHONN2008.

CONCEPT MAP

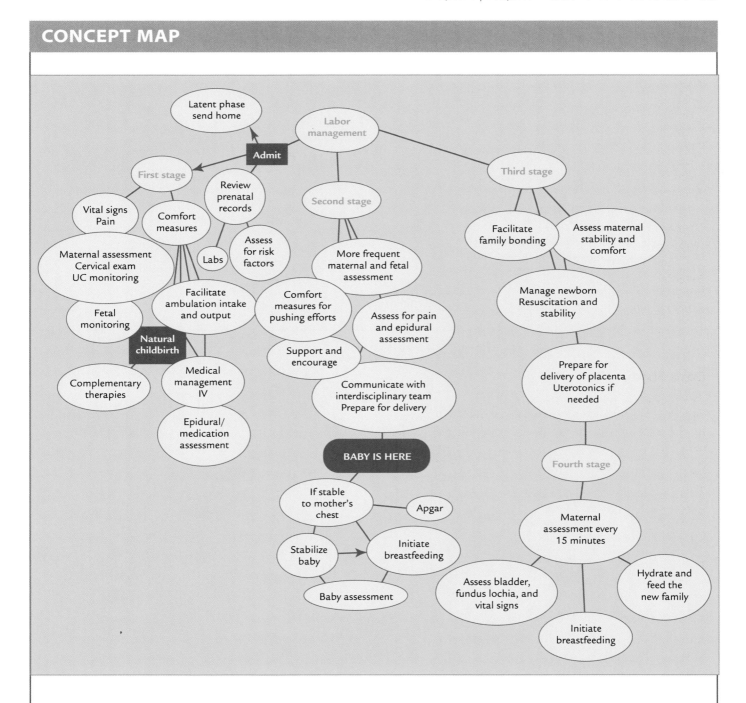

For Labor and Birth

First Stage of Labor

Goal: Safe delivery for mother and baby

Outcome: Safe delivery for mother and baby

Nursing Actions

1. Perform admission procedures and orient patient to setting.
2. Review prenatal records.
3. Assess FHR and uterine activity.
4. Assess maternal vital signs and pain.
5. Assist with ambulation and maternal position changes.
6. Provide comfort measures.

7. Discuss pain management options.
8. Administer pain meds PRN.
9. Monitor I&O and provide oral and/or IV hydration as indicated.
10. Provide ongoing assessment of labor progress.
11. Request an immediate bedside evaluation by a physician or CNM.

Second Stage of Labor

Goal: Safe delivery for mother and baby

Outcome: Safe delivery for mother and baby

Continued

Nursing Actions
1. Perform more frequent maternal and fetal assessment.
2. Review prenatal records.
3. Assess FHR and uterine activity.
4. Assess maternal vital signs and pain.
5. Encourage open glottis pushing efforts.
6. Provide comfort measures for pushing efforts.
7. Provide ongoing assessment and encouragement of labor progress.
8. Communicate with interdisciplinary team.
9. Prepare for delivery.

Third Stage of Labor
Goal: Safe delivery of placenta and transition for baby
Outcome: Safe delivery of placenta and transition for baby
Nursing Actions
1. Facilitate family bonding.
2. Assess maternal vital signs and pain.

3. Assess maternal stability.
4. Prepare for delivery of placenta and need for uterotonics.

Fourth Stage of Labor
Goal: Safe recovery of mom and baby
Outcome: Safe recovery of mom and baby
Nursing Actions
1. Facilitate family bonding.
2. Assess maternal vital signs and pain.
3. Assess maternal stability, fundus, lochia, bladder, perineum.
4. Provide comfort measures and pain meds.
5. Initiate breastfeeding.
6. Provide food and fluids for patient when stable.

Case Study

As the nurse, you admit Margarite Sanchez to the labor and delivery unit. She arrived in the triage unit at midnight in early labor. She presented with uterine contractions that were 5 minutes apart for 3 hours. Patient is a 28-year-old G3 P1 Hispanic woman. She is 39 weeks' gestation. José, her husband, has accompanied her to the unit. Two years ago, she had a normal spontaneous vaginal delivery NSVD after an 18-hour labor for a baby girl, Sonya, who was 7 lbs., 3 oz.

Margarite's cervix is now 4 cm/80%/0 station and fetal position is left occiput anterior (LOA).

Prenatal Labs
Blood type O+
RPR NR
GBS negative
Hepatitis B negative
Hgb
Hct
Vital signs: Blood pressure 110/60; pulse 84 bpm; respiratory rate 18; temperature 98.6°F (37°C).

Began prenatal care at 10 weeks of gestation and received regular prenatal care. She gained 22 pounds during pregnancy, and her current weight is 164 lbs. She is 5 feet, 4 inches tall. She has no prior medical complications and has experienced a normal pregnancy. Her first pregnancy ended in miscarriage at 8 weeks' gestation. She has no allergies to food or medication. She does not have a birth plan and states, "I just hope for a normal delivery and a healthy baby."

Detail the aspects of your initial assessment.

EFM reveals a FHR pattern that is normal, category I, with a FHR baseline of 140s moderate variability with accelerations to 160s for 20 seconds. She is uncomfortable with contractions and rates her pain at 5. She requests ambulation, as she feels more comfortable with walking.

At 0120 she has SROM for a large amount of clear amniotic fluid. FHR is baseline 130s with moderate variability, and accelerations and contractions are every 3 minutes and feel moderate to palpation. Her SVE reveals her cervix is 6 cm/90/0 station. She is very uncomfortable with contractions but does not want pain medication at this time. José appears anxious and at a loss for how to help his wife.

What are your immediate priorities in nursing care for Margarite and José Sanchez?
Discuss the rationale for the priorities.
What teaching would you include?
State nursing diagnosis, expected outcome, and interventions related to managing her labor pain.
What are appropriate interventions to manage her labor pain non-pharmacologically?

At 2 a.m. Margarite is increasingly uncomfortable with contractions and cries out that she can no longer take the pain. Her cervical exam is 6/100/0. She requests pain medication and is given a dose of Nubain at 0215 for pain relief in active labor. José asks how much longer the labor will be and when the baby will be born.

Detail the aspects of your ongoing assessment.
What are your current priorities in nursing care for Margarite Sanchez?
Discuss the rationale for the priorities.
Further teaching would include the following:
State nursing diagnosis, expected outcome, and interventions related to this problem.

At 0410 Margarite is very uncomfortable with contractions and cries out that she feels more pressure. She vomits a small amount of bile-colored fluid, and is perspiring and breathing hard with contractions. Her cervical exam is 8/100%/0. She requests pain medication and is given a dose of Nubian (nalbuphine hydrochloride) at 0440 for pain relief in transition.

What are appropriate interventions?

At 0630 Margarite reports an urge to bear down and push with contractions, is very uncomfortable with contractions, and cries out that she feels more pressure. Her sterile vaginal exam (SVE) reveals she is 10 cm/100% and +1 station. She has a strong urge to push with contractions that are every 2 minutes and strong to palpation. The fetal heart rate is 130 with moderate variability, and the FHR drops to 90 bpm for 40 seconds with pushing efforts.

What are your immediate priorities in nursing care for Margarite Sanchez? Discuss the rationale for the priorities.
What does the FHR indicate?
Teaching would include the following:
State nursing diagnosis, expected outcome, and interventions related to managing her labor pain.

Margarite continues to bear down, using open glottis pushing with contractions, and the fetal head is descending with contractions. The fetal heart rate is 130 with moderate variability and the FHR drops to 90 bpm for 40 seconds with pushing efforts. At 7:30 a.m. Margarite is increasingly unfocused with contractions and states, "I can't push . . . call my doctor to get the baby out!" José is at her side, holding her hand and encouraging her pushing efforts.

What are your immediate priorities in nursing care for Margarite Sanchez? Discuss the rationale for the priorities.

At 0815 Margarite continues to bear down with contractions and the fetal head is descending with contractions. The FHR is 130 with moderate variability and the FHR drops to 90 bpm for 40 seconds with pushing efforts. Margarite is focused with contractions. The fetal head is starting to crown with pushing efforts.

What are your immediate priorities in nursing care for Margarite Sanchez? Discuss the rationale for the priorities.

Her doctor comes into the labor and delivery room and she delivers a baby boy at 0839, with a second-degree perineal laceration. Her son weighs 3,800 g and 1- and 5-minute Apgar scores are 8 and 9.

Both Margarite and José begin to cry when their son is born, and José holds his son and hugs his wife. The placenta is delivered apparently intact at 0845. Both Margarite and her son are stable, and you initiate immediate postpartum and transition care for the mother and baby.

REFERENCES

American Academy of Pediatrics Committee on Infectious Diseases. (2009). Red Book: 2009 Report of the Committee on Infectious Diseases (28th ed.). Elk Grove Village, IL: Author.

American Academy of Pediatrics (AAP) and the American College of Obstetricians and Gynecologists (ACOG). (2012). *Guidelines for perinatal care* (7th Ed.). Elk Grove, IL: Authors.

American College of Nurse Midwives. (2013). Supporting healthy and normal physiologic childbirth: A consensus statement by ACNM, MANA, and NACPM. *Journal of Perinatal Education, 22*(1), 14–18. doi.org/10.1891/1058-1243.22.1.14

American College of Obstetricians and Gynecologists (ACOG). (2011a). Committee Opinion No. 485: Prevention of early-onset group B streptococcal disease in newborns. *Obstetrics & Gynecology, 117.*

American College of Obstetricians and Gynecologists (ACOG). (2011b). Committee Opinion No. 493: Cultural sensitivity and awareness in the delivery of health care. *Obstetrics & Gynecology, 117,* 1258–1261.

American College of Obstetricians and Gynecologists (ACOG). (2014). Safe prevention of the primary cesarean delivery. Obstetric Care Consensus No. 1. *Obstetrics & Gynecology, 123,* 693–711.

American College of Obstetricians and Gynecologists (ACOG). (2016). Committee Opinion No. 660: Family building through gestational surrogacy. *Obstetrics & Gynecology, 127*(3), e97–e103. doi:10.1097/AOG.0000000000001352

Amidi-Nouri, A. (2011). Culturally responsive nursing care. In A. Berman & S. Snyder (Eds.), *Kozier & Erb's fundamentals of nursing* (9th ed.). San Francisco, CA: Pearson.

Angelini, D., & Mahlmeister, L. (2005). Liability in triage: Management of EMTALA regulations and common obstetric risks. *Journal of Midwifery & Women's Health, 50*(6), 472–478.

Armour, K. (2012). An overview of surrogacy around the world: Trends, questions and ethical issues. *Nursing for Women's Health, 16*(3), 231–236.

Askren, H., & Bloom, K. (1999). Postadoptive reactions of the relinquishing mother: A review. *Journal of Obstetric, Gynecologic & Neonatal Nursing, 28*(4), 395–400.

Association of Women's Health, Obstetric and Neonatal Nurses (AWHONN). (2008). *Nursing care and management of the 2nd stage of labor* (2nd ed.). Washington, DC: Author.

Association of Women's Health, Obstetric and Neonatal Nurses (AWHONN). (2010). Confidentiality in adolescent health care. *Journal of Obstetric, Gynecologic, & Neonatal Nursing, 39,* 127–128.

Association of Women's Health, Obstetric and Neonatal Nurses (AWHONN). (2011a). Nursing support of laboring women. *Journal of Obstetric, Gynecologic, & Neonatal Nursing, 40,* 665–666. doi10.1111/j1552-6909.2011.01288.x

Association of Women's Health, Obstetric and Neonatal Nurses (AWHONN). (2011b). *Nursing care of the woman receiving analgesia/anesthesia in labor* (2nd ed.). Washington, DC: Author.

Association of Women's Health, Obstetric and Neonatal Nurses (AWHONN). (2014a). Guidelines for oxytocin administration after birth. *Journal of Obstetric, Gynecologic, & Neonatal Nursing, 44,* 161–164. doi:10.1111/1552-6909.12528

Association of Women's Health, Obstetric and Neonatal Nurses (AWHONN). (2014b). Non medically indicated induction and augmentation of labor. *Journal of Obstetric, Gynecologic, & Neonatal Nursing, 43*(5), 678–681.

Association of Women's Health, Obstetric and Neonatal Nurses (AWHONN). (2014c). Quantification of blood loss. Practice Brief No. 1. *Journal of Obstetric, Gynecologic, & Neonatal Nursing, 44,* 158–160. doi:10.1111/1552-6909. 12519 C 2014

Association of Women's Health, Obstetric and Neonatal Nurses (AWHONN). (2014d). *Women's health and perinatal nursing care quality refined draft.* Author. Retrieved from https://www.awhonn.org/page/NursingQualityMeasures specifications: For testing of feasibility, validity and reliability.

Association of Women's Health, Obstetric and Neonatal Nurses (AWHONN). (2016). Immediate and sustained skin-to-skin contact for the healthy term newborn after birth: Practice Brief No. 5. *Journal of Obstetric, Gynecologic, & Neonatal Nursing, 45*(6).

Bohren, M. A., Hofmeyr, G. J., Sakala, C., Fukuzawa, R. K., & Cuthbert, A. (2017). Continuous support for women during childbirth. *Cochrane Database of Systematic Reviews, 7.* doi:10.1002/14651858.CD003766.pub6

Buckley, L. (2005). *Evidence-based care sheet: Epidural analgesia in labor & childbirth.* Glendale, CA: Cinahl Information Systems.

Burke, C. (2014). Pain in labor: Nonpharmacologic and pharmacologic management. In K. Simpson & P. Creehan (Eds.). *AWHONN Perinatal nursing* (4th ed.). Philadelphia, PA: Lippincott.

Caldeyro-Barcia, R. (1979). The influence of maternal position on time of spontaneous rupture of the membranes, progress of labor, and fetal head compression. *Birth, 6*(1), 7–15. https://doi.org/10.1111/j.1523-536X.1979.tb01297.x

Callister, L. C. (2014). Integrating cultural beliefs and practices when caring for childbearing women. In K. Simpson & P. Creehan (Eds.), *AWHONN Perinatal nursing* (4th ed.). Philadelphia, PA: Lippincott.

Carteret, M. (2011). Cultural aspect of pain management. In *Dimension of culture: Cross cultural communications for health care professionals*. Retrieved from http://www.dimensionsofculture.com/2010/11/cultural-aspects-of-pain-management/

Centers for Disease Control and Prevention (CDC). (2010). Prevention of perinatal group B streptococcal disease. *Morbidity and Mortality Weekly Report, 59*.

Chapman, L. (2000). Expectant fathers and labor epidurals. *Maternal Child Nursing, 25*, 133–138.

Cheyne, H., Hundley, V., Dowding, D., Bland, J., Martin, M. P., & Greer, I. (2008). Effects of algorithm for diagnosis of active labour: Cluster randomized trial. *British Medical Journal, 337*, a2396.

Clutter, L. B. (2014). Adult birth mothers who made open infant adoption placements after adolescent unplanned pregnancy. *Journal of Obstetric, Gynecologic, & Neonatal Nursing, 43*(2), 190–199.

Cunningham, E., Leveno, K., Bloom, S., Spong, C., Dashe, J., Hoffman, B., . . . Sheffield, J. (2014). *Williams obstetrics* (24th ed.). New York, NY: McGraw-Hill.

Dean, R. A. K. (2010). Cultural competence. *Nursing for Women's Health, 14*, 50–59. doi:10.1111/j.1751-486X.2010.01507.x

de Tayrac, R., Letouzey, V. (2016). Methods of pushing during vaginal delivery and pelvic floor and perineal outcomes: A review. *Current Opinion Obstetrics and Gynecology, 28*(6), 470–476. doi:10.1097/GCO.00000000000000325

Dunk, R. (2016). Assisting families during surrogacy. *Journal of Obstetric, Gynecologic, & Neonatal Nursing, 45*(3), S33.

Friedman, E.A. (1955). Primigravid labor: a graphicostatistical analysis. *Obstetrics and Gynecology, 6*, 567–589.

Fuchs, A. R., Husslein, P., & Fuchs, F. (1991). Oxytocin secretion and human parturition: Pulse frequency and duration increase during spontaneous labor in women. *American Journal of Obstetrics and Gynecology, 164*, 1515–1523.

Gillesby, E., Burns, S., Dempsey, A., Kirby, S., Mogensen, K., Naylor, K., . . . Whelan, B. (2010). Comparison of delayed versus immediate pushing during second stage of labor for nulliparous women with epidural anesthesia. *Journal of Obstetrics, Gynecologic, & Neonatal Nursing, 39*(6), 635–644. doi:10.1111/j.1552-6909.2010.01195.x.

Goer, H., & Romano, A. (2016). *Optimal care in childbirth: The case for a physiologic approach*. Seattle, WA: Classic Day Publishing.

Gupta, J. K., Sood, A., Hofmeyr, G. J., & Vogel, J. P. (2017). Position in the second stage of labour for women without epidural anesthesia. *Cochrane Database of Systematic Reviews, 5*. doi:10.1002/14651858.CD002006.pub4

Heng, Y., Liong, S., Rice, G., DiQuinzio, M., & Georgiou, H. (2015). Human cervicovaginal fluid biomarkers to predict term and preterm labor. *Frontiers in Physiology, 6*, 151. doi:10.3389/fphys.2015.00151

Hodnett, E. (2002). Pain and women's satisfaction with the experience of childbirth: A systemic review. *American Journal of Obstetrics and Gynecology, 186*(5), S160–S172.

Hodnett, E. D., Gates, S., Hofmeyr, G. J., & Sakala, C. (2012). Continuous support for women during childbirth. *Cochrane Database of Systematic Reviews, 10*. CD003766.

Joint Commission on Accreditation of Healthcare Organizations. (2017). Glossary. In *Comprehensive accreditation manual for hospitals*. Oakbrook Terrace, IL: Author.

Kobayashi, S., Hanada, N., Matsuzaki, M., Takehara, K., Ota, E., Sasaki, H., Nagata, C., & Mori, R. (2017). Assessment and support during early labour for improving birth outcomes. *Cochrane Database of Systematic Reviews 2017, 4*. Art. No.: CD011516. DOI: 10.1002/14651858.CD011516.pub2

Kopas, M. (2014). A review of evidence-based practices for management of the second stage of labor. *Journal of Midwifery & Women's Health, 59*(3). doi:10.1111/jmwh.12199

Lederman, R. (1986). Maternal anxiety in pregnancy: Relationship to health status. *Annual Review of Nursing Research, 2*, 27–61.

Lederman, R. P., Lederman, E., Work, B. A., & McCann, D. S. (1978). The relationship of maternal anxiety, plasma catecholamines, and plasma cortisol to progress in labor. *American Journal of Obstetrics and Gynecology, 132*(5), 495–500.

Mackey, M. C. (1995). Women's evaluation of their childbirth performance. *Maternal-Child Nursing Journal, 23*(2), 57–72.

Main, E. K., Goffman, D., Scavone, B. M., Low, L. K., Bingham, D. Fontaine, P. L., . . . Levy, B. S. (2015). National partnership for maternal safety: Consensus bundle on obstetric hemorrhage. *Journal of Obstetrics, Gynecologic, & Neonatal Nursing, 44*, 462–470. doi:10.1111/1552-6909.1272

Martin, J. A., Hamilton, B. E., Osterman, M., Driscoll, A. K., & Mathews, T. E. (2017). Births: final data for 2015. *National Vital Statistics Reports, 66*(1).

Mattson, S., & Smith, J. E. (2011). *Core curriculum for maternal-newborn nursing* (4th ed.). St. Louis, MO: Elsevier Saunders.

Moore, M., Moos, M., & Callister, L. (2010). *Cultural competence: An essential journey for perinatal nurses*. White Plains NY: March of Dimes Foundation.

Nordgren, S., & Fridlund, B. (2001). Patients' perceptions of self-determination as expressed in the context of care. *Journal of Advanced Nursing, 35*(1), 117–125.

Oguz Orhan, E., Dilbaz, B., Akasakal, S., Altinbas, S., & Erkaya, S. (2014). Prospective randomized trial of oxytocin administration for active management of the third stage of labor. *International Journal of Gynecology and Obstetrics, 127*(2), 175–179.

Osbourne, K., & Hanson, L. (2014). Labor down or bear down: A strategy to translate second stage labor evidence to perinatal practice. *Journal of Perinatal & Neonatal Nursing, 28*(2).

Osterman, M. J. K., & Martin, J. A. (2011). Epidural and spinal anesthesia use during labor: 27-state reporting area, 2008. *National Vital Statistics Reports, 59*(5).

Pitter, C., & Preston, R. (2001). Modern pharmacologic methods in labor analgesia. *International Journal of Childbirth Education, 16*(2), 15–19.

Reyes-Lagos, J., Echeverria-Arjonilla, J., Pelia-Castillo, M., Montiel-Castro, A., & Pacheco-Lopez, G. (2014). Physiological, immunological and evolutionary perspectives of labor as an inflammatory process. *Advances in Neuroimmune Biology, 5*, 75–89. doi:10.3233/NIB-140085

Riemer, K. R., & Heymann, M. A. (1998). Regulation of uterine smooth muscle function during gestation. *Pediatric Research, 44*, 615–627. doi:10.1203/00006450-199811000-00001

Roberts, J., & Woolley, D. (1996). A second look at the second stage of labor. *Journal of Obstetrics, Gynecology and Neonatal Nursing, 25*(5), 415–423.

Romano, A., & Lothian, J. (2008). Promoting, protecting & supporting normal birth: A look at the evidence. *Journal of Obstetrics, Gynecologic, & Neonatal Nursing, 37*, 94–105.

Rooks, J. (2007). Guest editorial. Nitrous oxide for pain in labor—why not in the United States? *Birth: Issues in Perinatal Care, 34*(1), 3–5.

Rooks, J. P. (2011). Safety and risks of nitrous oxide labor analgesia: A review. *Journal of Midwifery & Women's Health, 56*(6), 557–565. doi:10.1111/j.1542-2011.2011.00122.x.

Sauls, D. J. (2010). Promoting a positive childbirth experience for adolescents. *Journal of Obstetric, Gynecologic, & Neonatal Nursing, 39*, 703–712.

Schafer, D. (2014). Gestational carrier delivery: What do I do now? *Journal of Obstetric, Gynecologic, & Neonatal Nursing, 43*, S94.

Sharts-Hopko, N. (2010). Oral intake during labor: A review of the evidence. *Maternal Child Nursing, 35*(4), 197–203.

Shnol, H., Paul, N., & Belfer, I. (2014) Labor pain mechanisms. *International Anesthesiology Clinics, 52*(3), 1–17.

Simkin, P., Hanson, L., & Ancheta, R. (2017). *The labor progress handbook: Early intervention to prevent and treat dystocia* (4th ed.). Hoboken, NJ: Wiley-Blackwell.

Simpson, K., & O'Brien-Abel, N., (2014). Labor and birth. In K. Simpson & P. Creehan (Eds.), *AWHONN Perinatal Nursing* (4th ed.). Philadelphia, PA: Lippincott.

Simkin, P., & O'Hara, M. (2002). Nonpharmacologic relief of pain during labor: Systemic reviews of five methods. *American Journal of Obstetrics & Gynecology, 186*(5), S131–S159.

Singata, M., Tranmer, J., & Gyte, G. M. L. (2013). Restricting oral fluid and food intake during labour. *Cochrane Database of Systematic Reviews, 8*. doi:10.1002/14651858.CD003930.pub3.

Spratto, G., & Woods, A. (2006). *2006 PDR nurse's drug handbook*. Clifton Park, NY: Delmar.

Stark, M., & Miller, M. (2009). Barriers to the use of hydrotherapy in labor. *Journal of Obstetric, Gynecologic, & Neonatal Nursing, 38*(6), 667–675. doi:10.1111/j.1552-6909.2009.01065.x.

Stewart, L., & Collins, M. (2012). Nitrous oxide as labor analgesia. *Nursing for Women's Health, 16*(5), 398–409. doi:10.1111/j.1751-486X.2012.01763.x.

Sultatos, L. G. (1997). Mechanisms of drugs that affect uterine motility. *Journal of Nurse-Midwifery, 42*, 367–370. doi:10.1016/S0091-2182(97)60134-2

Tavakkoli, S. N. (2017). Personhood and moral status of the embryo: Its effect on validity of surrogacy contract revocation according to Shia Jurisprudence

Perspective. *International Journal of Fertility & Sterility, 11*(3), 226–233. doi:10.22074/ijfs.2017.4970

Tranmer, J. E., Hodnett, E. D., Hannah, M. E., & Stevens, B. J. (2005). The effect of unrestricted oral carbohydrate intake on labor progress. *Journal of Obstetric, Gynecologic, & Neonatal Nursing, 34,* 319–328. doi:10.1177/0884217505276155

U.S. Department of Health and Human Services, Office of Minority Health. (2016). National Standards for Culturally and Linguistically Appropriate Services in Health and Health Care: Compendium of State-Sponsored National CLAS Standards Implementation Activities. Washington, DC: U.S. Department of Health and Human Services.

Vallerand, A., Sanoski, C., & Deglin, J. (2017). *Davis's drug guide for nurses* (15th ed.). Philadelphia, PA: F.A. Davis.

Weiner, G. M., Zaichkin, J., Kattwinkel, J. (Eds.). (2016). *Textbook of neonatal resuscitation* (7th ed.). Elk Grove Village, IL: American Academy of Pediatrics and American Heart Association.

Wood, S., & Carr, K. (2003). *The art and science of labor support.* White Plains, NY: March of Dimes.

World Health Organization (WHO). (2012). *WHO recommendations for the prevention and treatment of postpartum haemorrhage.* Retrieved from www.who.int/reproductivehealth/publications/maternal_perinatal_health/9789241548502/en/index.html.

Zhang, J., Landy, H. J., Branch, D. W., Burkman, R., Haberman, S., Gregory, K. D., . . . Reddy, U. M. (2010). Contemporary patterns of spontaneous labor with normal neonatal outcomes. *Obstetrics and Gynecology, 116*(6), 1281–1287. http://doi.org/10.1097/AOG.0b013e3181fdef6e

Zielinski, R. E., Gilbert Brody, M., & Low, L. K. (2016). The value of the maternity care team in the promotion of physiologic birth. *Journal of Obstetric, Gynecologic, & Neonatal Nursing, 45*(2), 276–284.

Zwelling, E., Johnson, K., & Allen, J. (2006). How to implement complementary therapies for laboring women. *Maternal Child Nursing, 31*(6), 364–370.

Fetal Heart Rate Assessment

9

Janice Stinson, RNC, PhD

LEARNING OUTCOMES

Upon completion of this chapter, the student will be able to:

1. Define terms used in electronic fetal monitoring (EFM).
2. Identify the modes of fetal heart rate assessment: auscultation, palpation, EFM.
3. Describe the components of fetal heart rate (FHR) and uterine contraction (UC) patterns essential to interpretation of monitor strips.
4. Articulate the physiology of FHR patterns.
5. Distinguish between Category I, II, and III fetal heart rate patterns and appropriate nursing actions based on these interpretations.

Nursing Diagnoses

- Risk for disturbed maternal fetal dyad
- Deficient knowledge of EFM assessment and interventions
- Impaired fetal oxygenation and perfusion related to impaired uteroplacental perfusion
- Risk of fetal injury related to respiratory or metabolic acidemia

Nursing Outcomes

- The pregnant woman and family will verbalize basic understanding of fetal monitoring.
- Intrauterine resuscitation strategies will be initiated for Category II or III EFM patterns.

INTRODUCTION

This chapter introduces basic electronic fetal monitoring (EFM) concepts. Fetal heart rate (FHR) assessment began almost 200 years ago when Swiss surgeon Francois-Isaac Mayor (1818) and nobleman Vicomte de Kergaradec (1821) reported the presence of fetal heart sounds via auscultation (hearing sounds via ear-to-abdomen, Picard horn, or stethoscope) (Freeman, Garite, & Nageotte, 2003). Electronic monitors that could continually record indirect abdominal phono and fetal electrocardiography (ECG) were developed in the 1950s (Edward H. Hon in the United States, Roberto Caldeyro Barcia in Uruguay, and Konrad Hammacher in Germany). Hon compared heart rate and patterns of FHR changes with labor variables and neonatal outcomes. FHR assessment transitioned from an auditory skill to visual assessment of data and continues to be the primary method for intrapartum fetal surveillance despite concerns regarding its efficacy and ability to improve neonatal outcomes (Freeman, 2002; Tucker, Miller, & Miller, 2009) (Box 9–1).

The goal of fetal monitoring is to interpret and continually assess fetal oxygenation (Lyndon & Ali, 2015) and prevent significant fetal acidemia while minimizing unnecessary intervention and promoting a satisfying family-centered birth experience (Lyndon, O'Brien-Abel, & Simpson, 2015). EFM is a technique for fetal assessment based on the fact that the FHR reflects fetal oxygenation (Lyndon et al., 2015). Current practice indicates that EFM is used for virtually all women during labor in the United States. While it is essential in the assessment of maternal and fetal well-being in antepartal and intrapartal settings, keep in mind that other evidence-based options such as intermittent auscultation are appropriate for laboring women (True & Bailey, 2016).

BOX 9–1 | Principles of Fetal Monitoring

Overall Goals

- Support maternal coping and labor progress
- Maximize uterine blood flow
- Maximize umbilical blood flow
- Maximize oxygenation
- Maintain appropriate uterine activity

Nursing Actions

- Review plans/expectations with woman and her family
- Maintain calm environment
- Stay at the bedside as much as possible
- Monitor only at the level needed for this patient
- Frequent position changes; upright positioning
- Judicious use of technology
- Avoid:
  - Unnecessary interventions
  - Tachysystole
  - Supine position
  - Coached pushing
  - Valsalva pushing

BOX 9–2 | AWHONN Fetal Heart Monitoring Clinical Position Statement

The Association of Women's Health, Obstetric and Neonatal Nurses (AWHONN) asserts that care by registered nurses (RNs) skilled in fetal heart monitoring (FHM) techniques, including auscultation and electronic fetal monitoring (EFM), is essential to maternal and fetal well-being during antepartum care, labor, and birth. EFM requires advanced assessment and clinical judgment. It is within the nurse's scope of practice to implement customary interventions in response to FHM data and clinical assessment. Interprofessional policies should support the RN in making decisions regarding fetal monitoring practice, intervening independently when appropriate to maternal and/or fetal condition.

A woman's preferences and clinical presentation should guide selection of FHM techniques with consideration given to use of the least invasive methods. In general, the least invasive method of monitoring is preferred to promote physiological labor and birth. Labor is dynamic; therefore, consideration of maternal preferences and identification of risk factors should occur upon admission to the birth setting and be ongoing throughout labor.

AWHONN, 2015.

Nurses are expected to independently assess, interpret, and intervene based on interpretations of EFM patterns. Assessments and interactions with monitored women and their families are individualized to provide information and explanation and reduce anxiety (Box 9-2). Clear and accurate communication with care providers and the perinatal team is essential for optimizing perinatal outcomes.

CRITICAL COMPONENT

Teamwork and Collaboration

Teamwork and collaboration means to function effectively within nursing and interprofessional teams, fostering open communication, mutual respect, and shared decision making to achieve quality patient care. Communication and collaboration are particularly essential in EFM. In 2004, the Joint Commission published Sentinel Event Alert Issue #30, Preventing Infant Death and Injury During Delivery. The Joint Commission analyzed 47 cases of perinatal death or permanent disability and found that 72% of root causes identified were related to communication issues among health care providers. The Joint Commission recommended the use of consistent fetal heart monitoring terminology among perinatal-care providers as one strategy to improve communication. Some suggestions to foster your development in this area include:

- Following communication practices that minimize risks associated with EFM communication among providers.
- Appreciating the importance of intra- and interprofessional collaboration to improve patient outcomes.
- Integrating the contributions of others who play a role in helping patient and her family achieve a healthy birth.
- Respecting the centrality of the patient/family as core members of any health care team.
- Acknowledging your own potential to contribute to effective team functioning in this critical setting.

TERMINOLOGY RELATED TO FETAL ASSESSMENT

Definitions used in this chapter are from the National Institute of Child Health and Human Development (NICHD) Research Planning Workshop (1997) and the 2008 NICHD Workshop Report on Electronic Fetal Monitoring: Update on Definitions, Interpretations and Research Guidelines publications (American College of Obstetrics and Gynecologists [ACOG], 2010; Macones, Hankins, Spong, Hauth, & Moore, 2008). There is a current movement to standardize language for FHR interpretations. It is critical for labor units to select one set of definitions for FHR patterns for all types of professional communications (AWHONN, 2015; Simpson, 2004b) (Table 9–1 and Box 9–3). Clinicians should be familiar with these definitions and use them consistently in clinical practice.

MODES OR TYPES OF FETAL AND UTERINE MONITORING

Types of fetal and uterine monitoring include the following.

Auscultation

Auscultation refers to the use of the fetoscope or Doppler to listen to the FHR without the use of a paper recorder (Feinstein,

TABLE 9-1   Terminology Related to Fetal Heart Rate Assessment

TERMINOLOGY	DEFINITION
Baseline FHR	FHR rounded to increments of 5 bpm during a 10-minute window. There must be at least 2 minutes of identifiable baseline segments (not necessarily contiguous). Does not include accelerations or decelerations or periods of marked variability (amplitude >25 bpm). • Periodic: changes in baseline of FHR occur in relation to UCs. • Episodic: changes in baseline of FHR occur independent of UCs. • Recurrent: changes in baseline of FHR occur in greater or equal to 50% of the contractions in a 20-minute period. • Intermittent: changes in baseline of FHR in less than 50% of the contractions in a 20-minute period.
Baseline variability	Fluctuations in the baseline FHR that are irregular in amplitude and frequency. The fluctuations are visually quantified as the amplitude of the peak to trough in bpm. It is determined in a 10-minute window, excluding accelerations and decelerations. It reflects the interaction between the fetal sympathetic and parasympathetic nervous system. • Absent: Amplitude range is undetectable. • Minimal: Amplitude range is visually detectable ≤5 bpm. • Moderate: Amplitude from peak to trough is 6 bpm to 25 bpm. • Marked: Amplitude range >25 bpm.
Indeterminant FHR	FHR that does not meet the criteria of baseline FHR.
Accelerations	Visually apparent, abrupt increase in FHR above the baseline. The peak of the acceleration is ≥15 bpm over the baseline FHR for ≥15 seconds and <2 minutes. • Before 32 weeks' gestation, acceleration is ≥10 beats over the baseline FHR for ≥10 seconds. Prolonged accelerations are ≥2 minutes but ≤10 minutes.
Deceleration	Transitory decrease in the FHR from the baseline. • Early deceleration is a visually apparent gradual decrease in FHR from baseline to nadir (lowest point of the deceleration) taking more than 30 seconds. The nadir occurs at the same time as the peak of the UC. Onset, nadir, and recovery match the onset, peak, and end of the UC. It's always periodic. • Variable deceleration is a visually apparent abrupt decrease in the FHR from baseline to nadir taking less than 30 seconds. The decrease in FHR is greater or equal to 15 bpm and less than 2 minutes in duration. It can be periodic or intermittent. • Late deceleration is a visually apparent gradual decrease of FHR from baseline to nadir taking more than 30 seconds. Nadir occurs at the peak of the UC. Onset, nadir, and recovery after the respective onset, peak, and end of the UC. Always periodic. • Prolonged deceleration is a visually apparent abrupt or gradual decrease in FHR below baseline that is ≥15 bpm lasting ≥2 minutes but ≤10 minutes. It can be periodic or intermittent.
Variation in baseline	Sinusoidal pattern: visually apparent smooth sine wave like undulating pattern in FHR baseline with a cycle frequency of 3-5/minutes that persists for ≥20 minutes. Benign sinusoidal patterns contain accelerations that last less than 20 minutes. A sinusoidal appearing FHR pattern can occur following maternal administration of some opioids (butorphanol and fentanyl). This undulating FHR pattern is of short duration and is also referred to as pseudosinusoidal or medication-induced sinusoidal (Lyndon, O'Brien-Abel, & Simpson, 2015).
Tachycardia	• Baseline FHR of >160 bpm lasting 10 minutes or longer.
Bradycardia	• Baseline FHR of <110 bpm lasting for 10 minutes or longer.
Normal FHR	• Category I (see Critical Component: Three-Tier FHR Interpretation System) reflects absence of metabolic acidemia at the time the EFM pattern is observed (AWHONN, 2015), and reflects favorable physiological response to maternal-fetal environment.
Abnormal FHR	• Category II and III (see Critical Component: Three-Tier FHR Interpretation System) reflects unfavorable physiological response to maternal fetal environment.

ACOG, 2010; Lyndon & Ali, 2015; Macones et al., 2008.

BOX 9–3 | Common Abbreviations for Electronic Fetal Monitoring

BPM	BEATS PER MINUTE
ED	Early deceleration
EFM	Electronic fetal monitoring
FHR	Fetal heart rate
FSE	Fetal scalp electrode
IA	Intermittent auscultation
IUPC	Intrauterine pressure catheter
LD	Late deceleration
MVU	Montevideo units
PD	Prolonged deceleration
TOCO	Tocodynamometer
VAS	Vibroacoustic stimulation
UC	Uterine contractions
US	Ultrasound
VD	Variable deceleration
VE	Vaginal examination

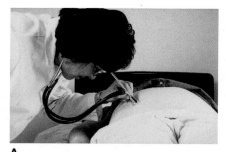

A

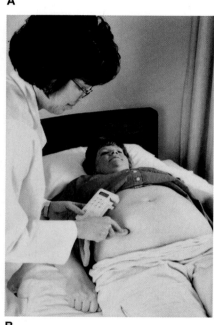

B

FIGURE 9–1 Auscultation of fetal heart rate. (*A*) Fetoscope. (*B*) Doppler ultrasound stethoscope.

Sprague, & Trepanier, 2008) (Fig. 9–1A&B). Auscultation with a fetoscope allows the practitioner to hear the sounds associated with the opening and closing of ventricular valves via bone conduction. A Doppler, by contrast, uses sound waves that are deflected from fetal heart movements similar to that used on an EFM external ultrasound transducer. This ultrasound device then converts information into a sound that represents cardiac events.

A paper recorder provides additional information on a tracing for clinician assessment, such as determining the difference between the categories in the three-tiered FHR interpretation system. This is because auscultation limits assessment data to FHR baseline, rhythm, and changes from baseline. Auscultation cannot detect certain types of decelerations and variability that can be detected by a combination of a paper recorder and ultrasound technology (part of electric monitoring).

A recent Cochrane Review evaluated using a handheld Doppler and intermittent EFM in labor was associated with an increase in caesarean sections due to fetal distress. There was no clear difference in neonatal outcomes, but long-term outcomes for the infants were not reported. The authors of this Cochrane Review reported a range in the quality of the evidence and noted that uncertainty remains regarding the use of intermittent auscultation (IA) and intermittent FHR in labor (Martis, Emilia, Nurdiati, & Brown, 2017). Research evidence supports the use of structured intermittent auscultation (SIA) as a method of fetal surveillance during labor for low-risk pregnancies (Feinstein et al., 2008; Lyndon & Ali, 2015; True & Bailey, 2016). An updated position statement from ACOG supports intermittent auscultation in low risk pregnancy in labor (ACOG, 2017).

Normal findings of SIA include normal baseline between 110 and160 beats per minute (bpm) and regular rhythm; presence of

BOX 9–4 | Guidelines and Procedure for Auscultation

1. Explain the procedure to the woman and her family.
2. Palpate the maternal abdomen to determine fetal position (Leopold's maneuvers).
3. Place the Doppler over the area of maximum intensity of fetal heart tones, generally over the fetal back.
4. Palpate maternal radial artery to differentiate maternal heart rate from FHR.
5. Determine relationship between uterine contractions (UCs) and FHR by palpating for UCs during period of FHR auscultation.
6. Count FHR between contractions for at least 30 to 60 seconds to determine the baseline rate.
7. Determine differences between baseline FHR and fetal response to contractions by counting FHR after a UC using multiple consecutive 6- to 10-second intervals for 30 to 60 seconds (protocols may differ based on location).

Killion, 2015.

FHR increases from baseline, and the absence of FHR decreases from baseline. To identify the baseline rate, the FHR should be auscultated and counted between contractions when the fetus is not moving for at least 30 to 60 seconds. Once the baseline is established, the FHR is then auscultated and counted while palpating maternal pulse for 15 to 60 seconds between contractions (Killion, 2015) (see Box 9–4). Successful implementation of SIA can be achieved by considering the following guidelines:

- Presence of nurses and providers experienced in auscultation and recognition of auditory changes in FHR
- Institutional policy developed to address the technique and frequency of assessment
- Clinical interventions (e.g., change to EFM) when concerning findings are present
- Nurse to laboring women ratio of 1:1
- User-friendly documentation tools for recording SIA findings
- Ready availability of auscultation devices
- Culture embracing the normalcy of childbirth and minimization of unnecessary interventions (True & Bailey, 2016)

In summary, fetoscope and Doppler obtain information differently but are both appropriate in certain auscultation clinical situations.

Palpation of Contractions

When the uterus contracts, the musculature becomes firm and tense and can be palpated with the fingertips by the nurse. The frequency, duration, tone, and intensity of contractions can be assessed by palpation (AWHONN, 2015; Lyndon et al., 2015). This is a subjective assessment and can be biased by the fat distribution around the pregnant woman's uterus.

- Palpation of uterine contractions is done by the nurse placing her fingertips on the fundus of the uterus and assessing the degree of tension as the contractions occur.
- The intensity of contractions is measured at the peak of the contraction and is rated as:
  - Mild or 1+ feels like the tip of the nose (easily indented)
  - Moderate or 2+ feels like the chin (can slightly indent)
  - Strong or 3+ feels like the forehead (cannot indent uterus)
- The resting tone is measured between contractions and listed as either soft or firm uterine tone.
- Palpation is a subjective assessment and can be biased by the fat distribution on the pregnant woman's abdomen.

External Electronic Fetal and Uterine Monitoring

External electronic fetal and uterine monitoring uses an ultrasound device to detect FHR and a pressure device to assess uterine activity, which is attached to a paper recorder (Fig. 9–2 and Box 9–5).

- The FHR is measured via an ultrasound transducer, an external monitor.
  - External EFM detects FHR baseline, variability, accelerations, and decelerations.

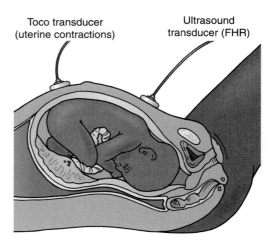

FIGURE 9–2 External monitoring showing placement of the ultrasound and tocodynamometer.

BOX 9–5 | Guidelines for Placement of an External Electronic Fetal Monitor

Explain the procedure to the woman and her family. For example: "The monitor records your baby's heart rate and uterine contractions, and it tells us the baby's response to uterine contractions. We place two monitors on your abdomen and secure them with belts. You can move around in bed and we will adjust the monitors."

FHR

Use Leopold's maneuvers to locate fetal back.

Apply ultrasound gel to FHR ultrasound transducer and place it on the woman's abdomen at the location of the fetus's back and move the transducer until clear signal and FHR is heard. Secure with monitor belt.

UCS

Place the uterine activity sensor (tocodynamometer) in the fundal area where the contraction feels strongest to palpation. Secure the monitor with a belt.

- External heart rate monitors receive waveforms from the fetal heart interpreted by the computer in the fetal monitor to produce audible sound and visual tracing to reflect the FHR.
- Fetal monitors average three consecutive beat-to-beat intervals and then assign the FHR (Killion, 2015). Although autocorrelation now minimizes doubling and halving of the FHR (erroneous readings), this can still occur. Therefore, providers are instructed to take precautions against misinterpretations by verification of FHR via monitoring of maternal heart rate via palpating the maternal radial pulse and maternal pulse oximetry (Killion, 2015).
- Today, many EFMs allow the monitoring of both the FHR and the maternal heart rate (MHR) via sensors within the tocodynamometer (TOCO), both appearing on the printout paper. MHR usually is significantly lower than the FHR and tends to increase as labor progresses and during contractions and pushing efforts.

- Location of the FHR via EFM changes in maternal position and as the fetus descends during labor, especially in the second stage (AWHONN, 2015; Lyndon et al., 2015).
- Erratic FHR recordings or gaps on a paper recorder may be caused by inadequate conduction of ultrasound signal, displacement of the transducer (may be picking up maternal heart rate), fetal or maternal movement, inadequate ultrasound gel, or fetal arrhythmia (may need to auscultate to verify).
- Contractions are measured via TOCO, also an external uterine monitor.
  - The relative frequency and duration of uterine contractions (UCs) and relative resting tone, which is the tone of the uterus between contractions, can be measured by this method.
  - External contraction monitor, TOCO, is a strain gauge that detects skin tightness or contour changes resulting from UCs. It should be placed via palpation at the uterine fundus, during maximum uterine contraction intensity, ideally at a smooth part of the uterus where no fetal small parts are felt. Appropriate placement of the TOCO may change during labor. Also, it may be more difficult to monitor tightening of the skin with increased fat distribution around the maternal abdomen.
  - External uterine monitors cannot measure pressure/intensity of contractions.
  - Pressure/intensity of the contraction must be estimated by palpation of contractions.
  - Contractions not recording on a paper recorder may occur when the transducer is placed away from strongest area of contraction or when resting tone is not dialed to 10 to 20 mm Hg when the uterus is relaxed.

Internal Electronic Fetal and Uterine Monitoring

Internal electronic fetal monitoring uses a fetal scalp electrode (FSE)/internal scalp electrode applied to the presenting part of the fetus to directly detect FHR. Internal electronic uterine monitoring involves an intrauterine pressure catheter (IUPC) placed in the uterine cavity to directly measure uterine contractions (Fig. 9–3 and Box 9–6). Membranes must be ruptured for both methods (AWHONN, 2015).

The decisions to insert an FSE are based on the need for continuous FHR tracing when troubleshooting methods do not alter quality of tracing. A nurse or care provider certified to attach this should be aware of relative contraindications to direct methods of monitoring. These include chorioamnionitis, active maternal genital herpes, HIV, positive group B streptococcus testing (Coviden, 2012), and conditions that preclude vaginal exams (e.g., placenta previa and undiagnosed vaginal bleeding).

The contraction and resting tone intensity is a combination of pressure from myometrial muscle contraction and intrauterine hydrostatic pressure (pressure exerted from amniotic fluid above the catheter). Therefore, positioning of the patient-measuring IUPC pressures in left, right, supine, and lateral will prevent

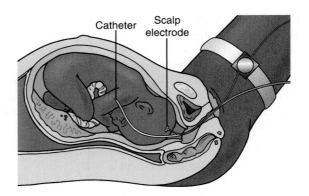

FIGURE 9–3 Internal monitoring, showing placement of the fetal scalp electrode and intrauterine pressure catheter.

BOX 9–6 | Guidelines for Placement of an Internal Electronic Fetal Monitor

Explain the procedure to the woman and her family. For example: "The internal fetal scalp electrode allows us to directly monitor your baby's heart rate. It is clipped on the baby's scalp during a vaginal exam and the monitor is attached to your leg. You can still move around and go to the bathroom.

"The intrauterine pressure catheter tells us exactly how strong your contractions are. It is a direct measurement of the pressure of your contractions. It is placed in your uterus during a vaginal exam."

FHR

Placement of the FSE requires skills and techniques of vaginal examination and EFM. There are risks, limitations, and contraindications, such as abnormal presentation, placenta previa, or preexisting infections such as herpes, HIV, or Group B streptococcus.

For placement of FSE, a vaginal exam is performed and the guide tube with the electrode is advanced and attached to the presenting part of the fetus. The membranes must be ruptured for placement and cervix dilated to 2 cm.

UCS

Placement of an IUPC is an invasive procedure where the nurse should have knowledge and understanding of indications and contraindications and risks of internal monitoring. For placement of the IUPC, the manufacturer directions are reviewed as there are several types of IUPC with different set-up guidelines. The IUPC and the guide tube are inserted in the vagina with a vaginal exam, and the catheter is advanced through the cervix into the amniotic cavity. The membranes must be ruptured for placement and cervix dilated to 2 cm.

Killion, 2015

---

possible erroneous conclusions about induction or augmentation management.

- FHR is measured via FSE.
- Internal EFM detects FHR baseline, variability, accelerations, decelerations, and limited information on some types of arrhythmias.
- It is attached to the presenting part of the fetus by the nurse or care provider.

IUPC monitoring is initiated based on the clinical need for additional uterine activity information. It may be used when external monitoring is inadequate due to maternal obesity or lack of progress in labor when quantitative analysis of uterine activity is needed for clinical decision making. In addition, an IUPC may be inserted to treat a worsening Category II tracing (e.g., recurrent variable decelerations with nadir greater than 60 mm Hg from baseline) via amnioinfusion. IUPCs provide an objective measure of the frequency, duration, and intensity of contractions (as opposed to palpation, which is subjective) and resting tone, both expressed in mm Hg.

- Contractions are measured via IUPC.
  - IUPC provides an objective measure of the pressure of contractions, expressed as mm Hg.
  - IUPC monitoring can detect actual frequency, duration, and strength of UCs and resting tone in mm Hg.
  - Uterine contraction intensity is measured using an IUPC = Peak pressure minus the baseline pressure in mm Hg.
  - Contraction intensity varies during labor, from 30 mm Hg in early spontaneous labor to 70 mm Hg in transition to 70 to 90 mm Hg in the second stage.
  - Peak pressure is the maximum uterine pressure during a contraction measured with an IUPC.
  - Resting tone or baseline pressure is the uterine pressure between contractions and should be about 5 to 20 mm Hg.
  - The contraction and resting tone intensity is a combination of pressure from myometrial muscle contraction as well as intrauterine hydrostatic pressure (pressure exerted from amniotic fluid above the catheter). Therefore, positioning of the patient—measuring IUPC pressures in left, right, supine, and lateral—will prevent possible erroneous conclusions about induction or augmentation management (AWHONN, 2015).
  - Uterine contractions may also be quantified via Montevideo units (MVUs) measured by the peak pressure for each contraction in a 10-minute period. ACOG has recommended at least 200 MVUs every 10 minutes for 2 hours as adequate uterine contraction intensity for normal progress of labor (Cunningham et al., 2014).
  - An IUPC can be used to perform an amnioinfusion.
  - The IUPC is inserted by the care provider. Some institutions may have protocols for nurses to insert IUPCs; nurses need to check hospital policy on IUPC insertion.

Telemetry

Telemetry is a type of continuous EFM that involves connecting the patient to a radio frequency transmitter that allows her to walk and take a bath without having to be connected to the monitor via cables. Nurses can oversee the fetal and uterine information as if the patient were connected directly to the monitor (Tucker et al., 2009). It can be used in all phases of labor.

Monitor Paper Used for the Electronic Fetal Monitor

Monitor paper is used for EFM (Fig. 9–4). At a paper speed of 3 cm per minute (standard for the United States), each dark

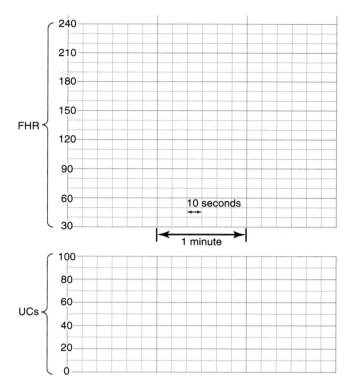

FIGURE 9–4 Monitor paper indicating timing on grid.

vertical line represents 1 minute and each lighter vertical line represents 10 seconds.

The FHR is recorded on the top grid of the paper in bpm while uterine contractions are recorded on the lower grid in mm Hg with IUPC and relative height for TOCO. Some EFM systems allow for maternal pulse to be recorded on the top grid of the paper. Maternal pulse can be obtained via a blood pressure cuff or pulse oximetry; some TOCOs now have sensors that can detect maternal pulse. Clinicians may need this additional information to distinguish between maternal and fetal heart rate. Both external and internal fetal monitors may inadvertently pick up maternal rate, which is especially critical if the fetus is not tolerating labor or has died (Lyndon & Ali, 2015).

AWHONN STANDARDS FOR FREQUENCY OF ASSESSMENT OF FHR

Frequency of FHR assessment is based on assessment of risk status, stage of labor, and ongoing clinical assessment (AWHONN, 2015; Lyndon et al., 2015).

- Intermittent auscultation (IA) (Box 9–7): Absent risk factors:
  - Every 1 hour in latent phase
  - Every 5 to 30 minutes in active and transition phases
- Intermittent EFM
  - Latent and active phase of first stage for low-risk labors (Category I), need EFM for 10 to 30 minutes every 1 to 2.5 hours, with particular attention to noting baseline,

variability, and accelerations and decelerations for 30 seconds before, during, and after a UC.

- Need continuous EFM during second stage
- Continuous EFM
  - Continuous fetal monitoring requiring external or internal monitoring became a part of routine maternal care during the 1970s.
  - By 2002, 85% of live births (3.4 million out of 4 million) were monitored by continuous monitoring.
  - This method of monitoring led to an increase in cesarean and instrumental (vacuum, forceps) vaginal births.
  - A decrease in neonatal seizures is the sole benefit of this method of perinatal management (Alfirevic, Devane, Gyete, & Cuthbert, 2017).
  - It is considered necessary if risk factors are present (Box 9–8).
- With risk factors, women should be monitored every 30 minutes during the latent phase, every 15 minutes during the active phase, and every 5 minutes during the second stage.
  - Thick meconium upon rupture of membranes
  - Rupture of membranes (greater than 24 hours at term)
  - Maternal fever
  - Vaginal bleeding in labor
  - Intrauterine infection/chorioamnionitis
  - Previous cesarean section
  - Abnormal vital signs
  - Fetal conditions (anomalies, anemia, intrauterine growth restriction, multiple gestation, breech presentation, prematurity, isoimmunization)

- Fetal intolerance of labor (as evidenced by late decelerations, variable decelerations, nadir below 60 bpm)
- Decreased fetal activity
- Maternal conditions (e.g., hypertensive disorders, diabetes, cholestasis, preexisting diseases, morbid obesity, labor dystocia)
- Use of uterine stimulants (misoprostol, dinoprostone, oxytocin)
- Epidural, other maternal analgesic interventions
- Preterm labor (less than 37 weeks)
- Post-term pregnancy (greater than 42 weeks)
- Category II or III upon admission to labor and delivery unit
- The frequency of assessment increases:
  - When indeterminate Category II or abnormal Category III FHR characteristics are heard
  - Before and after rupture of membranes or administration of medication
- When indeterminate or abnormal characteristics are heard, electronic FHR monitoring is used to:
  - Clarify pattern interpretation.
  - Assess baseline variability.
  - Further assess fetal status.

It is common practice for all women to have a baseline EFM tracing of at least 20 minutes at the time they are first evaluated in labor. Routine continuous FHR monitoring remains controversial. Nurses may use a decision tree to manage fetal assessment.

BOX 9–7 | Assessment and Documentation Recommendations of Fetal Status During Labor With Intermittent Auscultation

	LATENT PHASE (<4 CM)	LATENT PHASE (4–5 CM)	ACTIVE PHASE (≥6 CM)	SECOND STAGE (PASSIVE FETAL DESCENT)	SECOND STAGE (ACTIVE PUSHING)
Low-risk without oxytocin	At least hourly	Every 15–30 minutes	Every 15–30 minutes	Every 15 minutes	Every 5–15 minutes

*Assessment frequency should also be determined by maternal-fetal condition and may need to be done more frequently depending on the clinical situation.

Macones et al., 2008.

BOX 9–8 | Electronic Fetal Heart Monitoring Assessment Recommendations for Fetal Status During Labor

	LATENT PHASE (<4CM)	LATENT PHASE (4-5 CM)	ACTIVE PHASE (≥6 CM)	SECOND STAGE (PASSIVE FETAL DESCENT)	SECOND STAGE (ACTIVE PUSHING)
Low-risk without oxytocin	At least hourly	Every 30 minutes	Every 30 minutes	Every 15 minutes	Every 15 minutes
With oxytocin or risk factors	Every 15 minutes with oxytocin, every 30 minutes without	Every 15 minutes	Every 15 minutes	Every 15 minutes	Every 15 minutes

*Assessment frequency should also be determined by maternal-fetal condition and may need to be done more frequently depending on the clinical situation.

Macones et al., 2008.

Evidence-Based Practice: Electronic Fetal Heart Rate Monitoring for Fetal Assessment During Labor

Alfirevic, Z., Devane, D., Gyte, G. M. L., & Cuthbert, A. (2017). Continuous cardiotocography (CTG) as a form of electronic fetal monitoring (EFM) for fetal assessment during labour. *Cochrane Database of Systematic Reviews, 2*. Art. No.: CD006066. DOI: 10.1002/14651858. CD006066.pub3.

Electronic fetal monitoring, also referred to as *cardiotocography,* records changes in the FHR and their temporal relationship to uterine contractions. The aim of EFM is to identify babies who may be short of oxygen (hypoxic) to guide additional assessments of fetal well-being and determine if the baby needs to be delivered by caesarean section or instrumental vaginal birth.

A systematic review of randomized and quasi-randomized controlled trials was conducted to evaluate the effectiveness and safety of continuous cardiotocography when used as a method to monitor fetal well-being during labor.

This review included 13 trials involving over 37,000 women. One trial (4,044 women) compared continuous CTG with intermittent CTG; all other trials compared continuous CTG with intermittent auscultation. Compared with intermittent auscultation, continuous cardiotocography showed no significant improvement in overall perinatal death rate (risk ratio [RR] 0.86, 95% confidence interval [CI] 0.59 to 1.23) but was associated with halving neonatal seizure rates (RR 0.50, 95% CI 0.31 to 0.80). There was no difference in cerebral palsy rates (RR 1.75, 95% CI 0.84 to 3.63). There was an increase in caesarean sections associated with continuous CTG (RR 1.63, 95% CI 1.29 to 2.07). Women were also more likely to have instrumental vaginal births (RR 1.15, 95% CI 1.01 to 1.33). There was no difference in the incidence of cord blood acidosis (RR 0.92, 95% CI 0.27 to 3.11) or use of any pharmacological analgesia (RR 0.98, 95% CI 0.88 to 1.09).

Compared with intermittent CTG, continuous CTG made no difference to caesarean section rates (RR 1.29, 95% CI 0.84 to 1.97) or instrumental births (RR 1.16, 95% CI 0.92 to 1.46). Less cord blood acidosis was observed in women who had intermittent CTG; however, this result could have been due to chance (RR 1.43, 95% CI 0.95 to 2.14).

Overall, methodological quality of the studies reviewed was mixed. The authors concluded that EFM during labor is associated with reduced rates of neonatal seizures, but no clear differences in cerebral palsy, infant mortality, or other standard measures of neonatal well-being. However, continuous CTG was associated with an increase in caesarean sections and operative vaginal births. The authors believe the real challenge is how best to convey this uncertainty to women to enable them to make an informed choice without compromising the normality of labor.

INFLUENCES ON FETAL HEART RATE

An understanding of FHR physiology aids in the interpretation of FHR patterns. The FHR responds to multiple physiological factors. The following sections review the influences of these factors on the FHR.

Uteroplacental Unit

At term, about 10% to 15% of maternal cardiac output (600 cc to 750 cc) perfuses the uterus per minute. Oxygenated blood from the mother is delivered to the intervillous space in the placenta via the uterine arteries. Maternal-fetal exchange of oxygen, carbon dioxide, nutrients, waste products, and water occurs in the intervillous space across the membranes that separate fetal and maternal circulations. Oxygen and carbon dioxide diffuse across the membranes rapidly and efficiently (Menihan & Kopel, 2008).

- Effective transfer of oxygen and carbon dioxide between fetal and maternal blood streams is dependent on:
  - Adequate uterine blood flow.
  - Sufficient placental area.
  - Unconstricted umbilical cord.
- Appropriate oxygenation to the fetus depends on:
  - Adequate oxygenation of the mother.
  - Adequate blood flow to the placenta.
  - Adequate uteroplacental circulation.
  - Adequate umbilical circulation.
  - The fetus's own innate ability to initiate compensatory mechanisms to regulate the FHR.
- Additional factors in the fetal environment that influence fetal oxygenation include:
  - Uteroplacental function.
  - Uterine activity.
  - Umbilical cord issues.
  - Maternal physiological function.

A basic understanding of the extrinsic influence on FHR, such as normal physiological changes in pregnancy, uterine and placental blood flow, and umbilical blood flow, improves the nurse's ability to assess FHR patterns (Lyndon & Ali, 2015). The influences related to labor are discussed in Chapter 10.

Autonomic Nervous System

The autonomic nervous system is divided into the parasympathetic and sympathetic nervous systems.

Parasympathetic Nervous System

- Parasympathetic stimulation decreases the FHR.
- The parasympathetic nervous system is primarily mediated by the vagus nerve innervating the sinoatrial and atrioventricular nodes in the heart.
- Vagus nerve stimulation slows FHR and helps maintain variability.
  - Variability in FHR develops at 28 to 30 weeks' gestation.

Sympathetic Nervous System

- Sympathetic nervous system (SNS) stimulation increases the FHR.
- Nerves are distributed widely in the fetal heart, and stimulation increases the strength of the fetal heart contraction.
- SNS is responsible for FHR variability.
- Action occurs through release of norepinephrine.
- Stimulation of SNS increases FHR.
- SNS may be stimulated during hypoxemia.

Baroreceptors

- Baroreceptors are stretch receptors in the aortic arch and the carotid arch that detect pressure changes.

- They provide a protective homeostatic mechanism for regulating heart rate by stimulating a vagal response and decreasing FHR, fetal blood pressure, and cardiac output.

Central Nervous System (CNS)

- The CNS is the integrative center responsible for variations in FHR and baseline variability related to fetal activity.
- The CNS regulates and coordinates autonomic activities, mediates cardiac and vasomotor reflexes, and responds to fetal movement.

Chemoreceptors

- Chemoreceptors are located in the aortic arch and the CNS.
- They respond to changes in fetal O_2 and CO_2 and pH levels. Decreased O_2 and increased CO_2 cause peripheral chemoreceptors to stimulate the vagal nerve and slow the heart rate, and central chemoreceptors respond to an increased heart rate and increased blood pressure.

Hormonal Regulation

- The fetus responds to a decrease in O_2 or uteroplacental blood flow by releasing hormones that maximize blood flow to vital organs, such as the heart, brain, and adrenals.
- Epinephrine, norepinephrine, catecholamines, and vasopressin facilitate hemodynamic changes in response to changes in fetal oxygenation. Fetal hypoxia causes a release of epinephrine and norepinephrine that increases FHR and blood pressure. Vasopressin increases blood pressure in response to hypoxia.
- Renin–angiotensin secreted by the kidneys produces vasoconstriction in response to hypovolemia.

FETAL RESERVES

Placental reserve describes the reserve oxygen available to the fetus to withstand the transient changes in blood flow and oxygen during labor (Lyndon & Ali, 2015). In a healthy maternal-fetal unit, the placenta provides oxygen and nutrients beyond the baseline needs of the fetus.

- When oxygen is decreased, blood flow is deferred to vital fetal organs to compensate.
- When placental reserves of oxygen are depleted, the fetus may not be able to adapt to or tolerate decreased oxygen that occurs during a labor contraction.
- Fetal adaptation to the stresses of labor occurs through homeostatic mechanisms.
  - Prolonged or repeated hypoxemia may deplete reserves, resulting in decompensation.
  - Interpretation of FHR data requires the ability to differentiate three types of fetal responses:
    - Nonhypoxic reflex responses such as FHR accelerations
    - Compensatory responses to hypoxemia, such as variable decelerations
    - Impending decompensation responses such as late decelerations (Lyndon & Ali, 2015)

Umbilical Cord Blood Acid-Base Analysis After Delivery

Umbilical cord blood acid base acidosis analysis can be a useful, objective way to quantify fetal acid-base balance at birth and may be critical in evaluating whether a poor neonatal outcome is due to a hypoxic event before or during labor. An understanding of respiratory and metabolic acidosis and acidemia and associated clinical applications is required to interpret the findings (AWHONN, 2015).

Although maternal and fetal components of oxygen transport are similar, some features of oxygen transport are unique to the fetus. Fetal oxygen transport is directly dependent on the maternal transport system. The fetus has lower oxygen tension (30%) than the adult (100%). Fetuses have higher oxygen affinity (due to different fetal hemoglobin) than adults. The amount of oxygen transported to the fetus may be affected by the sufficiency of blood flow to the uterus and placenta, the integrity of the placenta, and the blood flow through the umbilical cord.

Normally, the fetus can maintain normal aerobic metabolism even though there are transient decreases in blood flow to the uterus. However, when available oxygen in the intervillous space falls below 50% of normal levels, a sequential process occurs:

1. Redistribution of blood to vital organs (heart, brain, and adrenal glands). In scenarios where oxygen is altered chronically, fetal growth will decelerate and lead to intrauterine growth restriction (IUGR).
2. Fetal myocardium will change in oxygen consumption, leading to changes in FHR, such as FHR variability.
3. Fetus will convert from aerobic to anaerobic metabolism.

In fetal heart muscle cells, normal cellular metabolism utilizes glucose and oxygen for aerobic metabolism. Carbon dioxide and water are the waste products that need to be taken away from the muscle cell by the fetal blood flow and increase of hydrogen ions in the tissue (acidosis).

When the fetus experiences hypoxia, it may switch to anaerobic metabolism, which is non-oxygen dependent. The waste product produced during this process is lactic acid. Accumulation of this acid leads to cell death and eventually to acidemia (increase of hydrogen ions in the blood). Should blood flow decrease resulting in significant hypoxia, the peripheral tissues shift into anaerobic metabolism, utilizing glucose as well as any stored glycogen while creating lactic acid. When the amount of lactic acid exceeds fetal buffering capacity, metabolic acidosis is the result. Should the hypoxia become severe enough (or prolonged enough), metabolic acidosis may occur not only in the peripheral tissues, but also in the vital organs (brain, heart, adrenals) where blood flow was initially redistributed as a protective mechanism. Once metabolic acidosis reaches these vital organs, the fetus is at risk for organ damage. Because clinicians cannot directly measure metabolic *acidosis* (tissues), cord gases are evaluated for *acidemia* (blood) as the blood levels represent what is happening in the tissues. Most clinicians use the terms *acidosis* and *acidemia* interchangeably in clinical practice, but it is important to note that when reviewing the fetal response to ongoing hypoxemia, the progression is always hypoxemia → hypoxia → metabolic acidosis → metabolic acidemia.

Shortly after birth, blood is sometimes drawn from the umbilical vein and one of the umbilical arteries. The umbilical vein represents oxygen supply available to the fetus, and the arterial blood best represents fetal usage of oxygen because it is the end point of fetal metabolism as blood returns to the placenta.

Respiratory acidosis occurs when an elevated P_{CO_2} level is present. An elevated P_{CO_2} indicates that the fetus is still processing oxygen via aerobic metabolism. It can develop rapidly in the fetus during acute hypoxia but can also be corrected rapidly when carbon dioxide is allowed to diffuse. Base excess with acidemia, during anaerobic metabolism, can become elevated. With a normal P_{CO_2}, it may reflect a prolonged hypoxic insult (Tucker et al., 2009).

Table 9–2 contains normal values for umbilical cord blood. Note that greater absolute values for base deficit or excess (bicarbonate concentration, which increases to compensate for greater hydrogen ion concentration) are associated with acidemia. Also, acidemia is determined by the pH level. Our goal for a vigorous infant at birth is a pH of 7.1 or higher and a base excess of more than −12 (base deficit of 12 or less) (Lyndon et al., 2015).

NICHD Criteria for Interpretation of FHR Patterns

A variety of systems and terminology have been used in the interpretation of FHR patterns. The FHR should be interpreted within the context of the overall clinical circumstances. Clinical conditions that impact FHR patterns include gestational age, prior results of fetal assessment, medications, maternal medical conditions, and fetal conditions. FHR patterns are dynamic and transient and require frequent assessment. A careful review of current evidence has resulted in a new recommendation for FHR interpretation in the intrapartum period from NICHD based on a three-tier category system (see Critical Component: Three-Tier FHR Interpretation System) for use in the interpretation of EFM during the intrapartal period.

● Category I FHR tracings are normal. They are strongly predictive of a well-oxygenated, nonacidotic fetus with a normal fetal acid-base balance. They may be followed in a routine manner and no action is required.

● Category II FHR tracings are indeterminate. They are not predictive of abnormal fetal acid-base status, yet there is not adequate evidence to classify them as Category I or III. They require evaluation and continued surveillance and reevaluation in the context of the clinical circumstances.

● Category III FHR tracings are abnormal. They are predictive of abnormal fetal acid-base status and require prompt evaluation. Depending on the clinical situation, efforts to resolve the underlying cause of the abnormal FHR pattern should be made expeditiously and should include intrauterine resuscitation or potentially expediting birth.

A more complex five-tier system has also been proposed to standardize management of FHR (Parer & Ikeda, 2007).

CRITICAL COMPONENT

Three-Tier FHR Interpretation System
Category I Normal
FHR tracings include *all* of the following:

- Baseline rate 110 to 160 bpm
- Baseline variability moderate
- Late or variable deceleration absent
- Early decelerations absent or present
- Accelerations absent or present

Category II Indeterminate
FHR tracings include all FHR tracings not categorized as Category I or III. They include *any* of the following:

- Bradycardia not accompanied by absent variability
- Tachycardia
- Minimal baseline variability
- Absent baseline variability not accompanied by recurrent decelerations
- Marked baseline variability
- Absence of induced accelerations after fetal stimulation
- Recurrent variable decelerations with minimal or moderate baseline variability
- Prolonged decelerations greater than 2 minutes but less than 10 minutes
- Recurrent late decelerations with moderate baseline variability
- Variable decelerations with other characteristics, such as slow return to baseline "overshoots" or "shoulders"

Category III Abnormal
FHR tracings that are *either*:

- Absent variability with any of the following:
  - Recurrent late decelerations
  - Recurrent variable decelerations
  - Bradycardia
- Sinusoidal pattern

Macones et al., 2008.

TABLE 9–2	Normal Umbilical Cord Blood Gas Values		
ARTERIAL CORD BLOOD MEASURES	**NORMAL VALUES**	**TARGET VALUES**	
pH	7.20–7.29	≥7.10	
P_{CO_2} (mm Hg)	49.2–56.3	<60	
HCO_3 (mEq/L) bicarbonate	22–24	>22	
Base excess (mEq/L)	2.7–8.3	>−12	
P_{O_2} (mm Hg)	15–24	>20	

Cypher, 2015.

CRITICAL COMPONENT

Five-Tier FHR Interpretation System

The HR five-tier system is based on the five-color system developed by Drs. Parer and Ikeda. The intent of their system is to standardize management of different FHR tracings. The system divides all FHR tracings into one of five categories: green (no acidemia, no intervention required), blue, yellow, orange, or red (evidence of actual or impending fetal asphyxia, rapid delivery recommended). Each color has assigned to it (1) risk of acidemia, (2) risk of evolution to a more serious pattern, or (3) recommended action.

The NICHD's three-tier system of classifying FHR tracings has been criticized for having too wide a range of tracings in Category II. Some researchers and clinicians believe that the five-tier color-coded system classifies EFM tracings more effectively, and it is being adopted by an increasing number of hospitals in the United States.

Category		Risk of Acidemia	Risk of Evolution	Action	Risk of Acidemia Related to Variability, Baseline Heart Rate, and Recurrent Decelerations											
					Decelerations		Recurrent variables			Recurrent late			Prolonged		
I	Green	0	Very low	none											
IIA	Blue	0	Low	Inform M.D. Conservative measures			Mild	Moderate	Severe	Mild	Moderate	Severe	Mild	Moderate	Severe
IIB	Yellow	0	Moderate	Increased surveillance Conservative measures	None	Early	All else	Last 30-60 sec and touch 70 BPM OR last > 60 sec and touch 80 BPM	Last 1-2 min and touch 70 BPM OR last > 2 min and touch 80 BPM	< 15 BPM below baseline	15-44 BPM below baseline	> 45 BPM below baseline	> 80 BPM	80 to 70 BPM	≤ 70 BPM
IIC	Orange	Acceptably low	High	Prepare for possible urgent delivery											
III	Red	Unacceptably high	Not a consideration	Deliver											

Moderate variability (normal)														
FHR	Tachycardia													
	Normal	(110-160 BPM)												
	Mild bradycardia	(> 80 BPM)												
	Moderate bradycardia	(80 to 70 BPM)												
	Severe bradycardia	(≤ 70 BPM)												

Minimal variability														
FHR	Tachycardia													
	Normal	(110-160 BPM)												
	Mild bradycardia	(> 80 BPM)												
	Moderate bradycardia	(80 to 70 BPM)												
	Severe bradycardia	(≤ 70 BPM)												

Absent variability														
FHR	Tachycardia													
	Normal	(110-160 BPM)												
	Mild bradycardia	(> 80 BPM)												
	Moderate bradycardia	(80 to 70 BPM)												
	Severe bradycardia	(≤ 70 BPM)												
	Sinusoidal													
	Marked variability													

REFERENCE: Parer JT, Ikeda T.A. Framework for standardized management of intrapartum fetal heart rate patterns. *Am J Obstet Gynecol*. 2007 Jul;197(1):26 e1-6 PMD: 17618744
Parer JT, Hamilton EF. Comparison of 5 experts and computer analysis in rule-based fetal heart rate interpretation. *Am J Obstet Gynecol*. 2010 Nov; 203(5):451.e1-7. Epub 2010 July 15.PMD: 20633869
Coletta, J, Murphy, E, Rubeo, Z, et al. (2012). The 5-tier system of assessing fetal heart rate tracings is superior to the 3-tier system in identifying fetal academia. *Am J Obstet Gynecol*; 206:226.e1-5.

FHR AND CONTRACTION PATTERN INTERPRETATION

Three major areas are assessed when interpreting FHR pattern: FHR baseline, periodic and episodic changes, and uterine activity.

- Interpretation of FHR baseline includes:
  - Baseline rate.
  - Baseline variability.
- Interpretation of periodic and episodic changes includes:
  - Accelerations.
  - Decelerations (early, variable, late, and prolonged).
- Interpretation of uterine activity includes:
  - Frequency.
  - Duration.
  - Intensity.
  - Resting tone.
  - Relaxation time between UCs.

Baseline Fetal Heart Rate

Baseline FHR is the mean FHR rounded to increments of 5 bpm during a 10-minute window, excluding accelerations, decelerations, or marked variability (Table 9–3; Fig. 9–5). There must be at least 2 minutes of identifiable baseline segments (not necessarily contiguous) in a 10-minute period or the baseline for that period is indeterminate.

Characteristics

- The normal range is 110 to 160 bpm.
- FHR baseline above 160 bpm for at least 10 minutes is tachycardia.
- FHR baseline below 110 bpm for at least 10 minutes is bradycardia.

Medical Management

- Assess the baseline over a 10-minute period.

Nursing Actions

- Assess the baseline over a 10-minute period.

Fetal Tachycardia

Tachycardia is a FHR above 160 bpm that lasts for at least 10 minutes (Fig. 9–6A).

- Tachycardia may be a sign of early fetal hypoxemia, especially with decreased variability and decelerations. Deceleration area is the most predictive electronic fetal monitoring pattern for acidemia, and combined with tachycardia for significant risk of morbidity (Cahill AG, Tuuli MG, Stout MJ, et al., 2018)
- If tachycardia persists above 200–220 bpm, fetal demise may occur.
- Fetal tachycardia >200 bpm may be an arrhythmia

TABLE 9–3 Intrauterine Resuscitation

GOAL	TECHNIQUES/METHODS
Promote fetal oxygenation	• Lateral positioning (left or right side) • IV fluid bolus of ≥500 cc lactated Ringer's solution • Discontinue oxytocin, remove dinoprostone insert, or withhold next dose of misoprostol • Alter pushing to every other contraction or every third contraction, or temporarily stop pushing (during second stage of labor) • Administer oxygen at 10 L/min via nonrebreather face mask (discontinue as soon as possible based on fetal response)
Reduce uterine activity	• Discontinue oxytocin, remove dinoprostone insert, or withhold next dose of misoprostol • IV fluid bolus of ≥500 cc lactated Ringer's solution • Lateral positioning (left or right side) • If no response, consider administration of 0.25 mg subcutaneous terbutaline
Alleviate umbilical cord compression	• Repositioning • Amnioinfusion (during first-stage labor) • Alter pushing to every other contraction or every third contraction, or temporarily stop pushing (during second stage of labor) • If umbilical cord prolapse is noted, elevate the presenting fetal part while preparations are made for an expedited birth
Correct maternal hypotension	• Lateral positioning (left or right side) • IV fluid bolus of ≥500 cc lactated Ringer's solution • If no response, consider ephedrine 5–10 mg IV push

Lyndon et al., 2015.

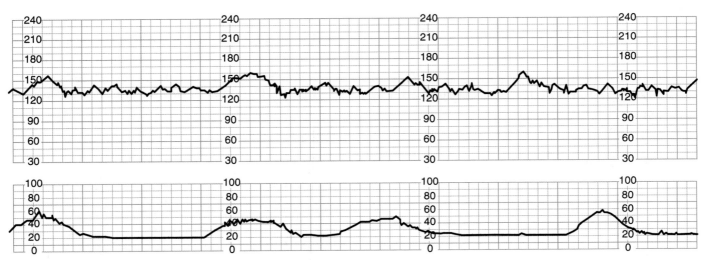

FIGURE 9–5 Normal fetal heart rate with moderate variability. (*Top*) Fetal heart rate. (*Bottom*) Contractions.

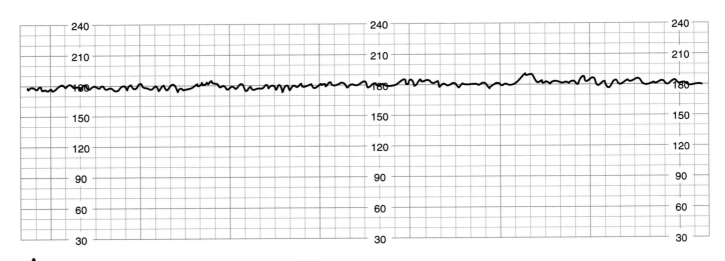

A

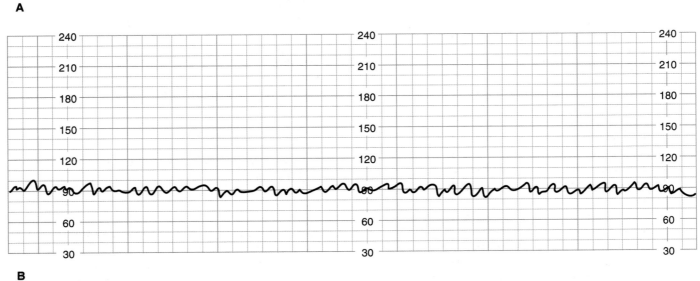

B

FIGURE 9–6 (*A*) Fetal tachycardia. (*B*) Fetal bradycardia.

- Some causes of fetal tachycardia, such as maternal fever or exposure to medications such as terbutaline, do not reflect a risk of abnormal acid-base balance.

Characteristics

- Baseline FHR above 160 bpm that lasts for at least 10 minutes.
- It is often accompanied by a decreased or absent baseline variability due to the relationship to the increased parasympathetic and sympathetic tone.

Causes

Maternal-related causes include:

- Fever.
- Infection.
- Chorioamnionitis.
- Dehydration.
- Anxiety.
- Anemia.
- Medications such as beta-sympathomimetic, sympathomimetic, ketamine, atropine, phenothiazines, epinephrine, terbutaline, and ephedrine.
- Illicit drugs such as cocaine.

Fetal-related causes include:

- Compensatory effort following acute hypoxemia.
- Infection or sepsis.
- Activity/stimulation.
- Chronic hypoxemia.
- Fetal tachyarrhythmia.
- Cardiac abnormalities.
- Anemia.

Medical Management

- Treat the underlying cause of tachycardia, such as antibiotics for infection, antipyretics for fever, or fluids for dehydration.
- Consider delivery.

Nursing Actions

- Assess FHR variability and consider need for position change or oxygen to promote fetal oxygenation.
- Assess maternal vital signs (particularly temperature and pulse), as maternal fever and tachycardia increase FHR.
- Initiate interventions to decrease maternal temperature, if elevated.
  - Give medications as ordered (e.g., antibiotics, antipyretics).
  - Use ice packs to decrease maternal fever.
- Assess hydration by checking skin turgor, mucous membranes, urine specific gravity, and intake and output.
  - Hydrate the woman by oral intake and/or IV fluids.
- Reduce anxiety by explaining, reassuring, and encouraging.
- Decrease or discontinue oxytocin.
- Notify the physician or midwife.

Fetal Bradycardia

Fetal bradycardia is a baseline FHR of less than 110 bpm (Fig. 9–6B).

- A decreased FHR can lead to decreased cardiac output, which causes a decrease in umbilical blood flow that leads to decreased oxygen to the fetus, causing fetal hypoxia.
- Unresolved bradycardia may result in fetal hypoxia and needs immediate intervention.
- Sudden profound bradycardia (less than 80 bpm) is an obstetrical emergency.
- Bradycardia may be tolerated by the fetus if the FHR remains above 80 bpm with variability.
- Bradycardia with normal variability may be benign.
- Bradycardia with loss of variability or late decelerations is associated with current or impending fetal hypoxia (NICHD, 1997a).

Characteristics

- FHR less than 110 bpm for more than 10 minutes

Causes

Maternal-related causes include:

- Supine position.
- Dehydration.
- Hypotension.
- Acute maternal cardiopulmonary compromise (cardiac arrest, seizures).
- Rupture of uterus or vasa previa.
- Placental abruption.
- Medications such as anesthetics and adrenergic receptors.

Fetal-related causes include:

- Fetal response to hypoxia.
- Umbilical cord occlusion.
- Acute hypoxemia.
- Late or profound hypoxemia.
- Hypothermia.
- Hypokalemia.
- Chronic fetal head compression.
- Fetal bradyarrhythmias.

Medical Management

- Intervene related to the cause of bradycardia.
- Consider delivery.

Nursing Actions

- Confirm if EFM is monitoring FHR versus MHR.
- Assess fetal movement.
- Assess the fetal response to fetal scalp stimulation. This is done when FHR is between contractions and when it is determined that baseline has changed.
- Perform a vaginal exam and assess for a prolapsed cord.
- Assess maternal vital signs (especially blood pressure).

- Assess hydration and hydrate as needed to reduce UCs and promote fetal oxygenation.
- Depending on FHR variability and other FHR characteristics, consider:
  - Changing maternal position (left or right lateral) to promote fetal oxygenation.
  - Discontinuing oxytocin to reduce UCs.
  - Giving oxygen 10 L/min via nonbreather face mask to promote fetal oxygenation.
  - Modifying pushing to every other contraction or stop pushing until the FHR recovers to promote fetal oxygenation.
  - Encouraging open glottis pushing efforts.
  - Discouraging prolonged or sustained breath holding with pushing.
  - Supporting the woman and her family.
  - Notifying the physician or midwife.

Baseline Variability

Baseline variability refers to the fluctuations in the baseline FHR that are irregular in amplitude and frequency. Cycles portray the peak to trough (rise and fall) of the heart rate within its baseline range over a minute. It is the most important predictor of adequate fetal oxygenation and fetal reserve during labor (AWHONN, 2015). Baseline variability reflects an intact pathway from the cerebral cortex to the midbrain (medulla oblongata) to the vagus nerve and finally to the heart, and an interaction between the fetal sympathetic and parasympathetic nervous system. Accelerations and decelerations are excluded from the evaluation of baseline variability.

Characteristics

Variability is described as follows:

- Absent: Amplitude range is undetectable (Fig. 9–7A).
- Minimal: Amplitude range is undetectable below 5 bpm range (Fig. 9–7B).
- Moderate: Amplitude from peak to trough, 6 bpm to 25 bpm (Fig. 9–7C). Moderate variability reliably predicts a well-oxygenated fetus with normal acid-base balance at the time.
- Marked: Amplitude range is greater than 25 bpm (Fig. 9–7D).

Minimal or absent variability can occur when the fetus is in a sleep cycle, sedated by certain CNS depressants such as opiates or magnesium sulfate, or has a previous CNS injury. Minimal or absent variability can also be significant for presence of fetal hypoxia or acidosis, especially if persisting 40 minutes despite interventions as listed below (Lyndon et al., 2015).

Causes of Minimal or Absent Variability

- Maternal-related:
  - Supine hypotension
  - Cord compression
  - Uterine tachysystole
  - Drugs (prescription, illicit drugs, alcohol)

- Fetal-related:
  - Fetal sleep
  - Prematurity

Medical Management

- Consider artificial rupture of membranes and more invasive internal monitoring with fetal spiral electrode (FSE).
- Manage cause of decreased variability.
- Consider expedited delivery.

Nursing Actions

- Change the maternal position to promote fetal oxygenation.
- Assess fetal response to fetal scalp stimulation or vibroacoustic stimulation (VAS).
- Assess hydration. Give IV bolus to reduce uterine activity and promote uterine perfusion.
- Discontinue oxytocin to reduce uterine activity.
- Deliver oxygen to the woman at 10 L/min via nonbreather face mask to promote fetal oxygenation.
- Consider invasive monitoring, such as internal FSE.
- Support the woman and her family.
- Notify the physician or midwife and if variability is absent request a bedside evaluation.

Periodic and Episodic Changes

Periodic changes are accelerations or decelerations in the FHR that are related to uterine contractions and persist over time. They include accelerations and four types of decelerations: early, variable, late, and prolonged. Episodic changes are acceleration and deceleration patterns not associated with contractions. Accelerations are the most common episodic change.

Fetal Heart Rate Accelerations

The presence of FHR accelerations is predictive of adequate central fetal oxygenation and reflects the absence of fetal acidemia. They identify a well-oxygenated fetus and require no intervention. The absence of FHR accelerations, especially in the intrapartum period, however, does not reliably predict fetal acidemia.

Characteristics

FHR accelerations are the visually abrupt, transient increases (onset to peak less than 30 seconds) in the FHR above the baseline (Fig. 9–8).

- In a fetus more than 32 weeks' gestation, they are 15 beats above the baseline and last from 15 seconds to less than 2 minutes.
- Before 32 weeks' gestation, accelerations are defined as acceleration of 10 bpm or greater over the baseline FHR for 10 or more seconds.
- Prolonged accelerations are 2 or more minutes but less than 10 minutes.

Causes

- Sympathetic response to fetal movement
- Transient umbilical vein compression

Medical Management

● None

Nursing Actions

● Record accelerations in the woman's labor documentation.

Fetal Heart Rate Decelerations

FHR decelerations are transitory decreases in the FHR baseline. They are classified as early, variable, late, and prolonged decelerations according to their shape, timing, and duration in relationship to the contraction.

● Decelerations are defined as recurrent when they occur with at least 50% of UCs over a 20-minute period.
● Decelerations are defined as intermittent when they occur with fewer than 50% of UCs over a 20-minute period.

Early Decelerations

Early decelerations are visually apparent, usually symmetrical, and have a gradual decrease and return of FHR associated with a

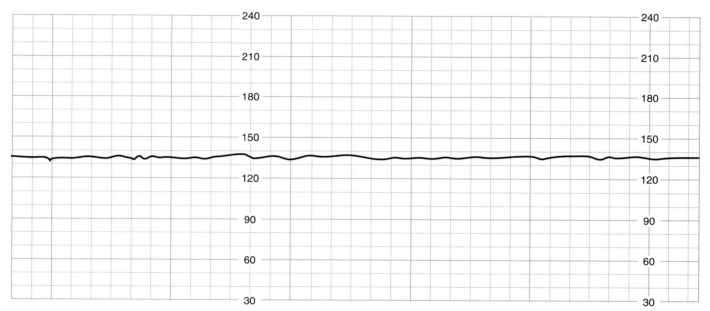

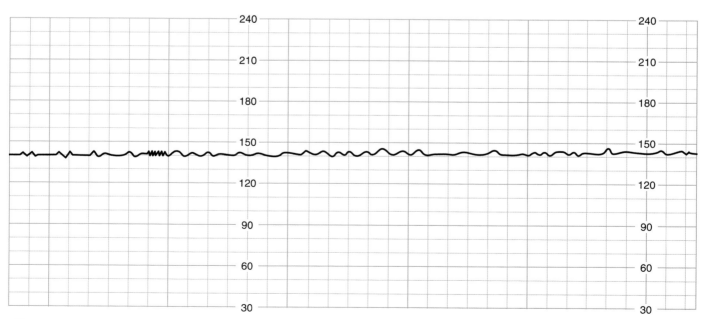

FIGURE 9–7 Types of variability. (**A**) Absent variability (abnormal). (**B**) Minimal variability. (**C**) Moderate variability (normal). (**D**) Marked variability.

Continued

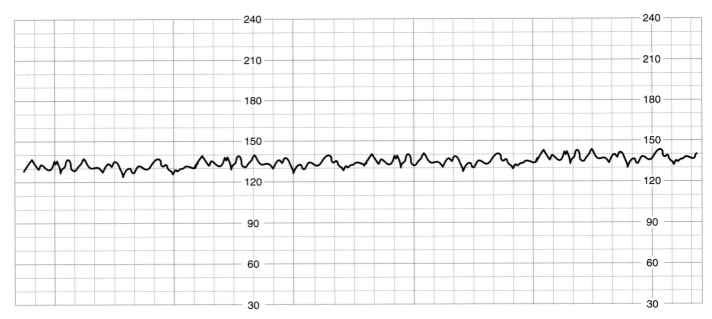

C

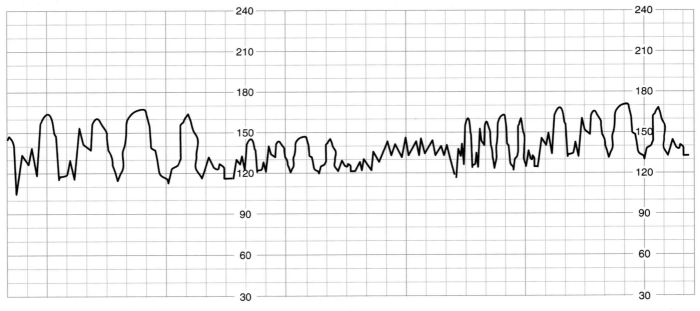

D

FIGURE 9–7 cont'd

UC (Fig. 9–9). They do not occur early or before the contraction starts; thus, this term is something of a misnomer.

Characteristics

● The nadir (the lowest point of the deceleration) occurs at the peak of the contraction.
● Generally, the onset, nadir, and recovery mirror the contraction.

Causes

● When a UC occurs, the fetal head is subjected to pressure that stimulates the vagal nerve.

● Fetal head compression resulting in increased intracranial pressure, decreased transient cerebral blood flow, and corresponding decrease in Po_2 with stimulation of cerebral chemoreceptor (Fig. 9–10).

Medical Management

● None

Nursing Actions

● Early decelerations are benign and no intervention is needed.

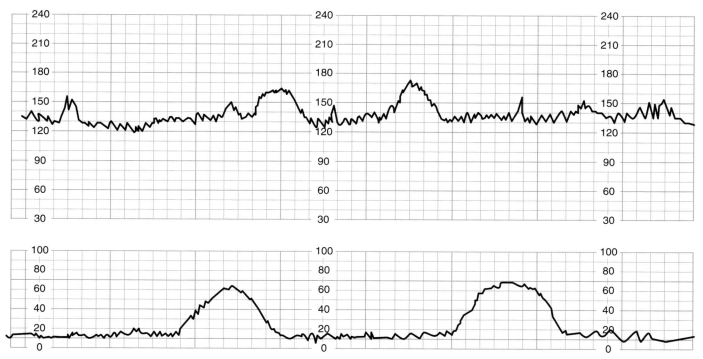

FIGURE 9–8 Fetal heart rate accelerations.

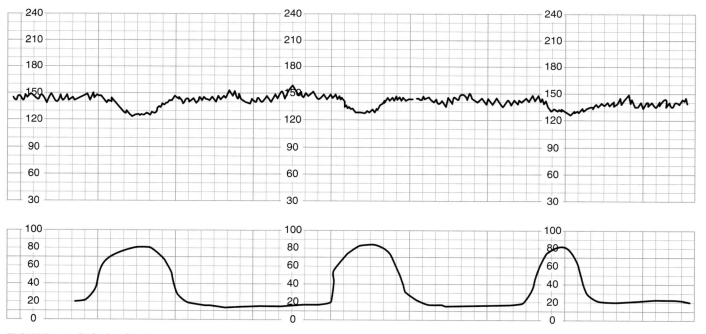

FIGURE 9–9 Early decelerations.

Variable Decelerations

A variable deceleration is a visually apparent abrupt decrease in the FHR of less than 30 seconds from baseline to nadir.

● They are the most common decelerations seen in labor.
● When variable decelerations persist over time, fetal tolerance is confirmed by the presence of variability or accelerations in the FHR (Lyndon et al., 2015).

● Recurrent variable decelerations that become deeper and last longer are more likely to be associated with fetal acidemia (ACOG, 2010).

Characteristics

● They can be periodic or episodic and may vary in duration, depth or nadir, and timing in relation to UCs (Fig. 9–11).

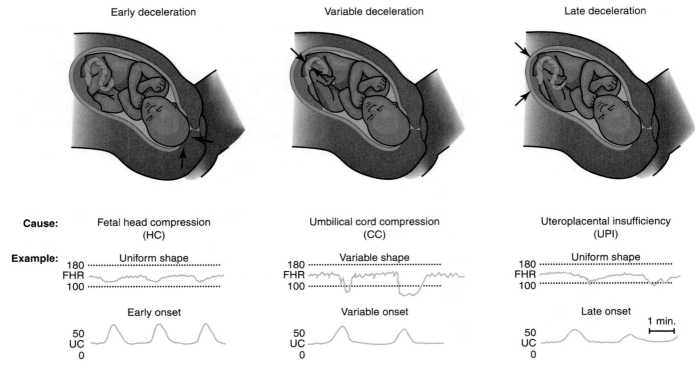

| Early deceleration | Variable deceleration | Late deceleration |

Cause: Fetal head compression (HC) | Umbilical cord compression (CC) | Uteroplacental insufficiency (UPI)

Example: Uniform shape | Variable shape | Uniform shape

FHR 180–100 | FHR 180–100 | FHR 180–100

Early onset | Variable onset | Late onset   1 min.

UC 50–0 | UC 50–0 | UC 50–0

FIGURE 9–10 Causes and examples of periodic decelerations.

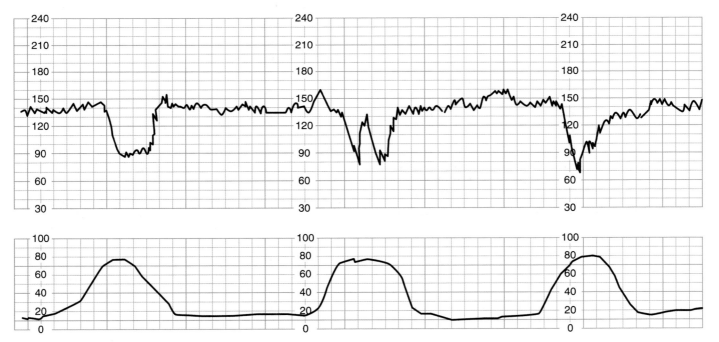

FIGURE 9–11 Variable decelerations.

- The decrease in FHR is at least 15 bpm lasting at least 15 seconds but less than 2 minutes in duration.
- The shape can be a U, W, or V.
- Depth (nadir) of variable deceleration of less than 60 would lead to amnioinfusion intervention in first stage.
- Altering frequency in second stage

- Accelerations at the beginning and end of decelerations ("overshoots") are not associated with acidemia.
- Characteristics of normal variable decelerations include:
  - Duration of less than 60 seconds.
  - Rapid return to baseline.
  - Normal baseline and variability.

- Characteristics of indeterminate or abnormal variable decelerations include:
  - Prolonged return to baseline.
  - Persistence to less than 60 bpm and greater than 60 seconds.
  - Presence of overshoots tachycardia.
  - Repetitive overshoots and absent variability.

Causes

- Umbilical cord occlusion (see Fig. 9–10).
- Umbilical cord compression triggers a vagal response that slows the FHR, usually related to decreased cord perfusion.
- This results in initial compression of the umbilical vein (decreased Po₂ and chemoreceptor stimulation) and then compression of the more muscular umbilical arteries (fetal hypertension with resultant baroreceptors stimulation; remember that hypertension is often accompanied with a corresponding drop in heart rate) (see Fig. 9–11).
- Prolonged cord compression produces a decrease in Po₂ with direct myocardial depression, adrenal activation, and sometimes rebound tachycardia.
- Variable decelerations can also occur with sudden descent of the vertex late in active phase of labor (i.e., head compression).
- These appear different from early decelerations in that they are usually not repetitive or smooth or regular in shape.

Medical Management

- Consider amnioinfusion.
- Consider tocolytics.
- Consider delivery.

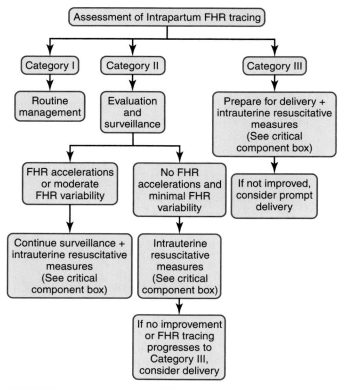

FIGURE 9–12 Management of EFM tracings.

Nursing Actions

- Change the maternal position to promote fetal oxygenation (Fig. 9–12).
- Perform SVE to evaluate cord and labor progress and perform fetal scalp stimulation.
- Perform amnioinfusion if ordered to alleviate umbilical cord compression by increasing volume of fluid in uterus and thereby correcting umbilical cord compression (see Critical Component: Amnioinfusion).
- Administer O₂ at 10 L/min via nonrebreather face mask to improve fetal oxygen status.
- Decrease or discontinue oxytocin.
- Consider need for tocolytic to reduce UCs.
- Consider more invasive monitoring with fetal spiral electrode.
- Modify pushing.
- Support the woman and her family to decrease anxiety or pain.
- Notify the physician or midwife.
- Plan for delivery and care of the neonate.

CRITICAL COMPONENT

Intrauterine Resuscitation Interventions

Interventions for Category II and III indeterminate or abnormal FHR patterns are referred to as intrauterine resuscitation. These interventions maximize uterine blood flow, umbilical circulation, and maternal fetal oxygenation (Lyndon et al., 2015; Simpson, 2004a; Simpson & James, 2005, Simpson, 2015). Interventions to promote fetal oxygenation include:

- Maternal positioning to minimize or correct cord compression, decrease frequency of UCs, and improve uterine blood flow (either left or right).
- Administration of IV bolus of fluid of at least 500 mL of lactated Ringer's to maximize maternal intravascular volume and improve uteroplacental perfusion.
- Correct maternal hypotension with positioning, hydration, and ephedrine as needed.
- Category II and category III tracings require evaluation of the possible etiology.
- Administration of O₂ at 10 L/min via nonrebreather face mask to improve fetal oxygen status. There is some controversy about the values of ogygen administration during labor to inprove fetal heart rate patterns however it remains a common practice (Garite, Nageotte, & Parer, 2015).
- Reduction of uterine activity if UCs are too frequent, as there may be insufficient time for blood to perfuse placenta.
  - Decrease or discontinue oxytocin.
  - Remove cervical ripening agent, if possible.
  - Terbutaline may be used to relax the uterus.
- Amnioinfusion has been used to resolve variable FHR deceleration by alleviating umbilical cord compression as a result of oligohydramnios in the first stage of labor.
  - Amnioinfusion is a procedure in which a saline solution at room temperature is introduced transcervically via an IUPC to correct the FHR decelerations associated with cord compression and/or decreased amniotic fluid.

Continued

- Encourage physiological pushing techniques, alter pushing efforts, or stop pushing, or encourage pushing with every other or every third UC to provide time for fetus to recover when FHR is indeterminate or abnormal during the second stage.
- Support the woman and her family to decrease anxiety or pain, and improve uterine blood flow and maximize oxygenation to fetus.
- Obtain fetal acid-base status if possible with scalp or VAS (the safety and efficacy of VAS in the intrapartal period is debated) or fetal scalp sampling if available. See Chapter 6 for more on VAS.
- Correct maternal hypotension.

Abnormal FHR patterns are associated with fetal acidemia. When this occurs:

- Notify primary provider; the presence of one of the abnormal patterns warrants immediate bedside evaluation by a physician who can initiate a cesarean birth.
- Notify or activate OR, anesthesia, and pediatric teams as indicated.
- Move patient to OR as indicated.

When a Category II or III FHR pattern is identified, initial assessment may also include:

- Assessment of maternal vital signs, especially:
  - Maternal temperature for maternal fever and maternal blood pressure for hypotension.
  - Assessment of uterine activity for uterine tachysystole.
- Cervical exam to assess for:
  - Umbilical cord prolapse
  - Rapid cervical dilation
  - Rapid descent of fetal head

CRITICAL COMPONENT

Amnioinfusion

Amnioinfusion is a therapeutic option when there are recurrent variable decelerations because of decreased amniotic fluid. During amnioinfusion, room temperature normal saline or lactated Ringer's is infused into the uterus transcervically via an intrauterine pressure catheter to increase intraamniotic fluid to cushion the umbilical cord and reduce cord compression. Usually a bolus of 250 to 500 mL is given over a 20- to 30-minute period; sometimes a continuous infusion of 120 to 180 mL/hour may be done for a maximum of 1,000 mL.

Indications: Variable decelerations in first stage of labor

Contraindications: Vaginal bleeding, uterine anomalies, and active infection

Careful monitoring of maternal and fetal response is needed; documentation of fluid infused and fluid returned is also important to avoid iatrogenic polyhydramnios.

Lyndon et al., 2015; Simpson, 2015.

Late Decelerations

Late deceleration is a visually apparent symmetrical gradual decrease of FHR associated with UCs.

- Late decelerations can be a sign of fetal intolerance to labor.
- Fetal tolerance of late decelerations is assessed by evaluating the baseline, the presence of variability, and the presence of accelerations.

Characteristics

- Onset is gradual with onset to nadir at least 30 seconds (Fig. 9–13).
- Nadir (lowest point) of the deceleration occurs after the peak of the contraction.
- In most cases, the onset, nadir, and recovery of the deceleration occurs after the respective onset, peak, and end of the UC.
- Nadir decreases 10 to 20 bpm and rarely 30 to 40 bpm (Freeman et al., 2003).

Causes

- Fetal response to transient or chronic uteroplacental insufficiency (see Fig. 9–10).
- Decreased availability of O_2 because of uteroplacental insufficiency.
- Suppression of the fetal myocardium
- Late decelerations are not completely understood.
  - Usually related to placental insufficiency (in which case they are often accompanied by decreased or absent FHR variability).
  - Late decelerations with moderate variability reflect a compensatory response and are not associated with significant fetal acidemia.
  - Late decelerations with minimal or absent variability reflect hypoxia and represent a risk of significant fetal acidemia.
  - Fetal hypoxia stimulates chemoreceptors when it is acute (i.e., recently occurring) and, if prolonged, results from direct myocardial depression.
  - Maternal-related factors associated with decreased uteroplacental circulation include:
    - Hypotension from regional anesthesia, supine positioning, or maternal hemorrhage
    - Maternal hypertension, gestational or chronic
    - Placental changes affecting gas exchange such as postmaturity or placental abnormalities
    - Decreased maternal hemoglobin or oxygen saturation from severe anemia or cardiopulmonary disease
    - Uterine tachysystole

Medical Management

- Interventions are directed at causes of late decelerations.
- Consider tocolytics.
- Consider delivery.

Nursing Actions

- The degree to which the deceleration is abnormal depends on the status and response of the fetus after the deceleration.

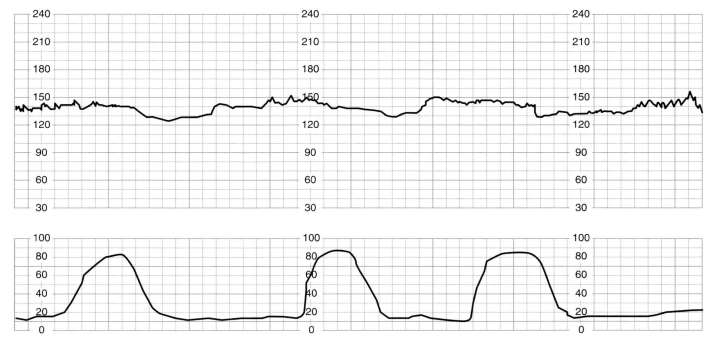

FIGURE 9–13 Late decelerations.

- Change the maternal position to promote fetal oxygenation (see Fig. 9–12).
- Discontinue oxytocin (consider terbutaline) to reduce uterine activity.
- Assess hydration. Give an IV bolus to promote fetal oxygenation.
- Consider fetal scalp stimulation or VAS to assess fetal status (the safety and efficacy of VAS in the intrapartal period is debated; see Chapter 6 for more information on VAS).
- Administer O₂ at 10 L/min via nonrebreather face mask to improve fetal oxygen status.
- Consider more invasive monitoring with fetal spiral electrode.
- Support the woman and her family.
- Notify the physician or midwife.
- Plan for delivery and care of the neonate.

Prolonged Decelerations

Prolonged deceleration is a visually apparent abrupt decrease in FHR below baseline that is greater than 15 bpm, lasting longer than 2 minutes but less than 10 minutes (Fig. 9–14). Prolonged decelerations that are not recurrent and are preceded and followed by normal baseline and moderate variability are not associated with fetal hypoxemia.

Characteristics

- Episodic decelerations that last longer than 2 minutes but less than 10 minutes
- May be abrupt or gradual

Causes

- May be any mechanism that causes a profound change in the fetal O₂
- Interruption of uteroplacental perfusion

- Tachysystole
- Maternal hypotension
- Abruptio placenta
- Interruption of umbilical blood flow
  - Cord compression
  - Cord prolapse
- Vagal stimulation
  - Profound head compression
  - Rapid fetal descent

Medical Management

- Treat the cause of prolonged deceleration.
- Consider amnioinfusion.
- Consider tocolytics.
- Consider delivery.

Nursing Actions

- Assess baseline variability preceding and following deceleration.
- Change the maternal position to improve fetal oxygenation.
- Discontinue oxytocin (consider terbutaline) to decrease the UCs.
- Administer O₂ at 10 L/min via nonrebreather face mask to improve fetal oxygen status.
- Assess hydration. Give an IV bolus to promote fetal oxygenation.
- Perform SVE to assess labor and cord.
- Perform amnioinfusion, if ordered, to alleviate umbilical cord compression.
- Consider more invasive monitoring with fetal spiral electrode.
- Support the woman and her family.
- Notify the physician or midwife.
- Plan for delivery and care of the neonate.

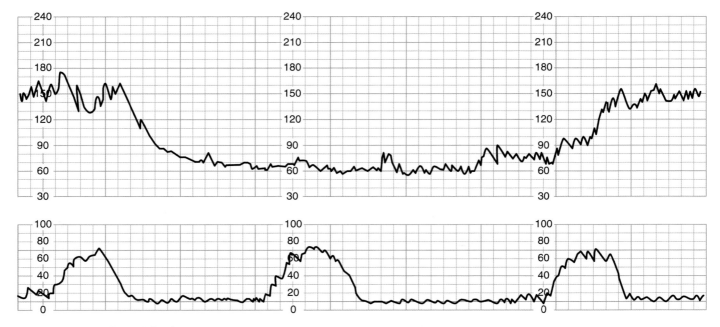

FIGURE 9–14 Prolonged deceleration.

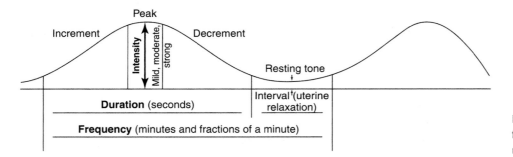

FIGURE 9–15 Example of contraction frequency, duration, intensity, and resting tone.

Uterine Activity and Contraction Patterns

Interpretation of the FHR pattern is done in concurrence with uterine activity. Interpretation of uterine activity includes assessment of the contractions' frequency, duration, and intensity, and the uterine resting tone (Fig. 9–15). Uterine activity can be monitored by palpation or via an IUPC.

- Frequency of contractions is expressed in minutes or seconds and is determined by counting the number of contractions in a 10-minute period, counting from the start of one contraction to the start of the next contraction in minutes. It is recorded in minutes (i.e., frequency of contractions is every 3 minutes). Frequency of contractions can be expressed in a range: for example, UCs every 2 to 3 minutes.
- Duration of contractions is measured in seconds by counting from the beginning to the end of one contraction. Because contractions often vary in their duration, this is typically calculated for several contractions and expressed as a range.
- Intensity is the strength of the contraction and measured by palpation, or internally by an IUPC in mm Hg.

- Resting tone is the pressure in the uterus between contractions. It is measured by an IUPC when internal fetal monitoring is used or by palpation when an external monitor is used. When an IUPC is being used, it is described as the number of mm Hg when the uterus is not contracting and as "soft" if the uterus feels relaxed by palpation.
- Normal: five or fewer contractions in 10 minutes averaged over a 30-minute window (Fig. 9–16A).
- Tachysystole: More than five contractions in 10 minutes over a 30-minute window.

Tachysystole

Tachysystole, formerly called hyperstimulation, is excessive uterine activity. Like duration, frequency of contractions is expressed in minutes and often given in seconds.

- These contraction patterns may contribute to fetal hypoxia.
- Tachysystole should be treated regardless of fetal response.
- Tachysystole can result in decreased uteroplacental blood flow and result in indeterminate or abnormal fetal heart rate patterns.

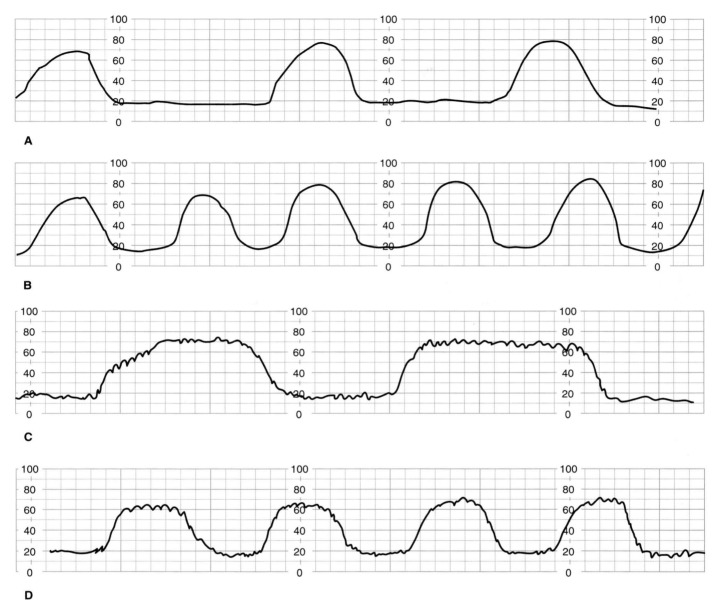

FIGURE 9–16 Examples of UC patterns. (*A*) Normal UCs. (*B*) Tachysystole (<5 UCs 10 minutes). (*C*) Tachysystole (tetanic contraction verified by palpation). (*D*) Tachysystole (inadequate interval of resting tone between UCs).

Characteristics
- More than five contractions in 10 minutes (Fig. 9–16B)
- Contractions lasting 2 minutes or longer (Fig. 9–16C)
- Contractions occurring within 1 minute of each other (Fig. 9–16D)
- Increasing resting tone greater than 20 to 25 mm Hg, peak pressure greater than 80 mm Hg, or Montevideo units greater than 400

Causes
- Tachysystole can be spontaneous or stimulated labor.
- The most common cause is medications used for cervical ripening, induction, and augmentation of labor.
- Abruption may also lead to tachysystole accompanied with increased vaginal bleeding.

- Women with a history of motor vehicle accidents, domestic violence, dehydration, preeclampsia, or methamphetamine use may be at higher risk.

Medical Management
- Manage cause of tachysystole (e.g., discontinuing oxytocin, removing cervical ripening medication). See Chapter 10.

Nursing Actions
- A variety of interventions can effectively reduce uterine activity, such as the following (these practices are known as intrauterine resuscitation):
  - Changing maternal position
  - Providing hydration
  - Using IV fluid bolus
  - Reducing maternal anxiety or pain

- Administering a tocolytic (terbutaline)
- Supporting woman and family

SPECIAL MONITORING CIRCUMSTANCES

In some cases, women require special monitoring to ensure her health and that of the fetus.

Monitoring the Preterm Fetus

As noted in Chapter 7, preterm labor can be defined as the onset of labor at less than 37 weeks' gestation. With the preterm birth rate continuing to rise (Martin, Hamilton, Osterman, Driscoll, & Mathews, 2017), most obstetric units monitor a preterm fetus during the antepartum and intrapartum. Two important points to remember when caring for the mother with a preterm fetus:

- Physiological responses of the preterm fetus depend on the stage of fetal development.
- Physiological responses and tolerance to stress (maternal tachycardia and sepsis) in the preterm fetus can be different (more rapid deterioration) from those in the term fetus.

Some preterm FHR characteristics:

- Baseline is higher but still within normal FHR range.
- Accelerations may be of lower amplitude—accelerations of at least 10 bpm of baseline lasting 10 seconds are considered acceptable for fetus less than 32 weeks' gestation (Macones et al., 2008). However, once the preterm fetus (sometimes as early as 24 to 26 weeks) demonstrates accelerations of 15 bpm above baseline that last for 15 seconds, the fetus is generally held to that criteria in subsequent evaluations.
- Variability may be decreased, although specific parameters have not been quantified (Freeman et al., 2003).
- Variable decelerations may occur more frequently in the preterm fetus even in the absence of contractions (ACOG, 2009). During labor, variable decelerations occur in approximately 70% to 75% of preterm fetuses compared to 30% to 50% in term fetuses (Freeman et al., 2003).
- Late and prolonged decelerations occur at the same frequency in preterm labor as in term labor. Conditions associated with late decelerations, such as IUGR, preeclampsia, and abruption, are more commonly present during preterm labor (Simpson, 2004b).
- Magnesium sulfate (now used for neuroprotection of the preterm fetus rather than tocolytics) decreases FHR variability and acceleration amplitude in preterm infants.
- Beta-sympathomimetics (e.g., terbutaline) are associated with tachycardia in both mother and fetus.
- Indomethacin, other anti-prostaglandin medications, and calcium channel blockers (e.g., Nifedipine) have minimal effect on the preterm fetus.

The preterm fetus is more likely to be subjected to hypoxia, including conditions such as preeclampsia, abruption, and intrauterine infection that frequently are either the indication for or cause of preterm delivery. The loss of variability in a preterm fetus is more predictive of acidosis and depressed Apgar scores at birth than for a term infant (Macones et al., 2008). It is therefore important to continually evaluate trends and continually assess the maternal and fetal condition when making clinical decisions regarding the antepartum and intrapartum management of the preterm fetus.

Monitoring the Woman With Multiple Gestation

Current monitors have the capability of monitoring twins and higher multiples at the same time with two ultrasound transducers on the same monitor. The dual tracings distinguish each fetus by a thicker or darker tracing for one fetus and a thinner or lighter tracing for the other. To more clearly distinguish between the fetuses, their positions on the mother's abdomen can be documented and transducers appropriately labeled. In identifying twins or higher multiples, the more advanced (lower in uterus) fetus is labeled as A, the next one B, and so on. Once the membranes are ruptured, it is recommended that the more advanced fetus is monitored by a scalp electrode to distinguish it from the other fetus. Two monitors are required for higher multiples, with the third fetus on the second monitor, which has an identical clock setting to the first one (Tucker et al., 2009).

At the time of birth, the first twin that is delivered may not necessarily be twin A, especially with cesarean sections. In that case, the medical chart should be written as first twin (B) and second twin (A) or vice versa.

Other Topics

Monitoring of fetal arrhythmias and sinusoidal pattern (a Category III or impending decompensation fetal response) is beyond the scope of this chapter. Resources are cited for more in-depth exploration and advanced concepts in fetal monitoring. Antenatal fetal surveillance and testing are discussed in Chapter 6.

DOCUMENTATION OF ELECTRONIC MONITORING INTERPRETATION— UTERINE ASSESSMENT

Documentation of fetal monitoring consists of the elements described in Table 9–4 and Figure 9–17.

TABLE 9–4   Assessment and Documentation of Electronic Fetal Monitoring

FHR **External/ultrasound**	**UC** **External/tocodynamometry**
• FHR baseline • Baseline variability • Presence of accelerations • Periodic or episodic decelerations	• Frequency • Duration • Palpate strength of UCs and resting tone
Internal/fetal scalp electrode	**Internal/intrauterine pressure catheter**
• FHR baseline • Baseline variability • Presence of accelerations • Periodic or episodic decelerations • FHR dysrhythmias	• Frequency • Duration • Strength of uterine contractions and resting tone (in mm Hg)

Patient Name:		Physician/CNM:			
	DATE:				**KEY**
	TIME:				**Variability** Ab = Absent (undetectable) Min = Minimal (>0 out ≤5 bpm)
Cervix Dilation					Mod = Moderate (6–25 bpm) Mar = Marked (>25 bpm)
Effacement					**Accelerations**
Station					+ = Present and appropriate for gestational age
Fetal Heart Baseline Rate					Ø = Absent
Variability					**Decelerations** E = Early
Accelerations					L = Late V = Variable
Decelerations					P = Prolonged
STIM/pH					**Stim/pH** + = Acceleration in response to stimulation
Monitor Mode					Ø = No response to stimulation
Uterine Activity Frequency					Record number for scalp pH **Monitor mode**
Duration					A = Auscultation/Palpation E = External u/s or toco
Intensity					FSE - Fetal spiral electrode
Resting Tone					IUPC = Intrauterine pressure catheter
Monitor Mode					P = Palpation T = Telemetry
Oxytocin milliunits/min					**Frequency of uterine activity** Ø = None
Pain					Irreg = Irregular
Coping					**Intensity of uterine activity** M = Mild
Maternal Position					Mod = Moderate
O2/LPM/Mask					Str = Strong By IUPC = mm Hg
IV					**Resting tone**
Nurse Initials					R = Relaxed By IUCP = mm Hg
Narrative notes:					**Coping** W = Well S = Support provided For pain use 0–10 scale **Maternal position** A = Ambulatory U = Upright SF = Semi-Fowler's RL = Right lateral LL = Left lateral MS = Modified Sims'

FIGURE 9–17 Example of FHR documentation.

CONCEPT MAP

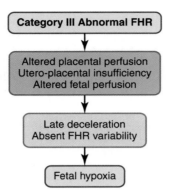

Problem No. 1: Category III FHR
Altered Placental Perfusion-Uteroplacental Insufficiency
Recurrent late decelerations
Absent FHR variability
Category III FHR pattern
Late decelerations and absent FHR variability
Goal: Improve placental perfusion. Fetus will become well perfused and oxygenated; cord gases indicate no respiratory or metabolic acidosis.
Outcome: Fetus will become well perfused and oxygenated; cord gases indicate no respiratory or metabolic acidosis.

Nursing Actions
1. Change maternal position (left, right, lateral, or hands and knees).
2. Administer 500 mL IV bolus of fluid.
3. Perform cervical exam to assess cord prolapse, rapid cervical dilation, or rapid descent of the fetal head.
4. Assess uterine activity for uterine tachysystole.
5. Assess maternal vital signs, especially temperature for maternal fever and blood pressure for hypotension.
6. Administer O_2 at 10 L/min via nonrebreather face mask to improve fetal oxygen status.
7. Consider discontinuing oxytocin if in use.
8. Consider use of terbutaline to stop UCs, unless mother is a drug user, has previous preeclampsia, or has a heart rate greater than 120 bpm.
9. Alter pushing efforts, or stop pushing, or push with every other or every third UC to provide time for fetus to recover when FHR is Category III during second stage.
10. Request an immediate bedside evaluation by a physician or midwife.

Problem No. 2: Maternal anxiety
Woman is crying.
Woman states that she is concerned that baby is going to die.
Patient is G2 P1 at term, 10 cm and pushing.
Goal: Decreased anxiety
Outcome: Patient verbalizes that she feels less anxious.

Nursing Actions
1. Be calm and attentive in interactions with the patient and her family.
2. Explain all procedures and interventions.
3. Explain current fetal status.
4. Assist patient with breathing and relaxation techniques.
5. Encourage the patient and her family to verbalize their feelings regarding concern for the fetus.
6. Remain with the patient and her family.

REFERENCES

Alfirevic, Z., Devane, D., Gyte, G. M. L., & Cuthbert, A. (2017). Continuous cardiotocography (CTG) as a form of electronic fetal monitoring (EFM) for fetal assessment during labour. *Cochrane Database of Systematic Reviews, 2.* doi:10.1002/14651858.CD006066.pub3

American College of Obstetrics and Gynecologists (ACOG). (2009). Intrapartum fetal heart rate monitoring: Nomenclature, interpretation, and general management principles. Practice Bulletin #70. *Obstetrics & Gynecology, 114*(1), 192–202.

American College of Obstetrics and Gynecologists (ACOG). (2010). Management of intrapartum fetal heart rate tracing. Practice Bulletin #116. *Obstetrics & Gynecology, 116*(5), 1232–1240.

American College of Obstetrics and Gynecologists (ACOG). (2017). Approaches to limit intervention during labor and birth. Committee Opinion Number 687. *Obstetrics & Gynecology, 129*(5), 20–28.

Association of Women's Health, Obstetric and Neonatal Nurses (AWHONN). (2015). Fetal heart monitoring position statement. *Journal of Obstetric, Gynecologic, and Neonatal Nursing, 44*(5), 683–686.

Cahill AG, Tuuli MG, Stout MJ, et al. (2018) A prospective cohort study of fetal heart rate monitoring: Deceleration area is predictive of fetal acidemia. *American Journal Obstetrics and Gynecology, 218*:523.e1.

Coletta, J., Murphy, E., Rubeo, Z., & Gyamfi-Bannerman, C. (2012). The 5-tier system of assessing fetal heart rate tracings is superior to the 3-tier system in identifying fetal academia. *American Journal of Obstetrics and Gynecology, 206*(3), 226.e1–5.

Covidien. (2012). Kendal fetal spring electrode, contraindications. Retrieved from www.kendallhg.com/pageBuilder.aspx?contentID150585&webpage-ID=0&topicID=149607&breadcrumbs=0:121623,143502:0

Cunningham, F. G., Leveno, K. J., Bloom, S. L., Spong, C. Y., Dashe, J. S., Hoffman, B. L., . . . Sheffield, J. S. (2014). *Williams obstetrics* (24th ed.). New York, NY: McGraw-Hill.

Cypher, R. (2015). Assessment of fetal oxygenation and acid-base balance. In A. Lyndon & L. Usher Ali (Eds.), *Fetal heart monitoring: Principles and practices* (5th ed.). Dubuque, IA: Kendall Hunt Publishing.

Feinstein, N., Sprague, A., & Trepanier, M. (2008). *Fetal heart rate auscultation* (2nd ed.) Washington, DC: Association of Women's Health, Obstetric and Neonatal Nurses.

Freeman, R. (2002). Problems with intrapartum fetal heart rate monitoring interpretation and patient management. *American College of Obstetricians and Gynecologists, 100*(4), 813–826.

Freeman, R., Garite, T., & Nageotte, M. (2003). *Fetal heart rate monitoring* (3rd ed.). Philadelphia, PA: Lippincott Williams & Wilkins.

Garite TJ, Nageotte MP, Parer JT.(2015) Should we really avoid giving oxygen to mothers with concerning fetal heart rate patterns? *American Journal of Obstretric and Gynecology*; 212(4):459-60, 459.e1. Epub 2015

Joint Commission. (2004). Preventing infant death and injury during delivery. *Sentinel Event Alert, 30*. Retrieved from www.jointcommission.org/assets/1/18/SEA_30.PDF.

Killion, M. M. (2015). Techniques for fetal heart and uterine activity assessment. In A. Lyndon & A. U. Ali (Eds.), *Fetal heart monitoring: Principles and practices* (5th ed.). Dubuque, IA: Kendall Hunt Publishing.

Lyndon, A., & Usher Ali, L, (2015). *Fetal heart monitoring: Principles and practices* (5th ed.). Dubuque, IA: Kendall Hunt Publishing.

Lyndon, A., O'Brien-Abel, N., & Simpson, K. (2014). Fetal assessment during labor. In K. Simpson & P. Creehan (Eds.), *Perinatal nursing* (5th ed.). Philadelphia, PA: Lippincott Williams & Wilkins.

Macones, G., Hankins, G., Spong, C., Hauth, J., & Moore, T. (2008). The 2008 National Institute of Child Health and Human Development Workshop Report on Electronic Fetal Monitoring: Update on definition, interpretation, and research guidelines. *Journal of Obstetric, Gynecologic, & Neonatal Nursing, 37*(5), 510–515.

Martin, J. A., Hamilton, B. E., Osterman, M. J. K., Driscoll, K. A., & Mathews, T. J. (2017). Births: Final data for 2015. *National Vital Statistics Report, 66*(1).

Martis, R., Emilia, O., Nurdiati, D. S., & Brown, J. (2017). Intermittent auscultation (IA) of fetal heart rate in labour for fetal well-bing. *Cochrane Database of Systematic Reviews, 2*. doi: 10.1002/14651858.CD008680.pub2

Menihan, C., & Kopel, E. (2008). *Electronic fetal monitoring: Concepts and applications* (2nd ed.). Philadelphia, PA: Lippincott Williams & Wilkins.

National Institute of Child Health and Human Development (NICHHD). (1997a). Electronic fetal heart rate monitoring: Research guidelines for interpretation. *American Journal of Obstetrics and Gynecology, 177*(6), 1385–1390.

National Institute of Child Health and Human Development (NICHHD). (1997b). Electronic fetal heart rate monitoring: Research guidelines for interpretation. *Journal of Obstetric Gynecology and Neonatal Nursing, 26*(6), 635–640.

Parer, J. T., & Hamilton, E. F. (2010). Comparison of 5 experts and computer analysis in rule-based fetal heart rate interpretation. *American Journal of Obstetrics and Gynecology, 203*(5), 451.e1–7.

Parer, J. T., & Ikeda, T. (2007). A framework for standardized management of intrapartum fetal heart rate patterns. *American Journal of Obstetrics and Gynecology, 197*, 26.e1–26.e6.

Simpson, K. (2004a). Fetal assessment in the adult intensive care unit. *Critical Care Nursing Clinics of North America, 16*, 233–242.

Simpson, K. (2004b). Standardized language for electronic fetal heart rate monitoring. *American Journal of Maternal/Child Nursing, 29*(5), 336.

Simpson, K. (2015). Physiologic interventions for fetal heart rate patterns. In A. Lyndon & L. U. Ali (Eds.), *Fetal heart monitoring: Principles and practices* (5th ed.). Dubuque, IA: Kendall Hunt Publishing.

Simpson, K., & James, D. (2005). Efficacy of intrauterine resuscitation techniques in improving fetal oxygen status during labor. *American College of Obstetricians and Gynecologists, 105*(6), 1362–1368.

True, B. A., & Bailey R. E. (2016). Intrapartum fetal surveillance. Advanced Life Support Obstetrics, Provider Syllabus, American Academy of Family Physicians Pediatrics and American College of Obstetricians and Gynecologists.

Tucker, S., Miller, S., & Miller, D. (2009). *Fetal monitoring, A multidisciplinary approach* (6th ed.). St Louis, MO: Mosby.

High-Risk Labor and Birth

10

Roberta F. Durham RN, PhD
Patrick F. Kilgallen RN, BSN

LEARNING OUTCOMES

Upon completion of this chapter, the student will be able to:

1. Describe the primary causes of dystocia and the related nursing and medical care.
2. Demonstrate understanding of knowledge related to induction of labor and augmentation of labor and vaginal birth after cesarean birth.
3. Identify potential complications of dystocia in labor and related nursing and medical care.
4. Identify and manage high-risk pregnancy, labor, and delivery to promote healthy outcomes for the mother and infant.
5. Describe the key obstetrical emergencies and the related nursing and medical care.

Nursing Diagnoses

- Risk of maternal injury related to interventions implemented for dystocia
- Risk of maternal injury related to obstetrical emergencies
- Risk of fetal injury related to complications of labor and birth
- Anxiety related to labor and birth complications

Nursing Outcomes

- The woman will understand the causes of dystocia and interventions to achieve a safe birth.
- The woman will give birth without maternal or fetal injury.
- The woman will give birth to a healthy infant without complications.
- The woman verbalizes understanding of the situation and plan of care and uses effective coping strategies.

INTRODUCTION

Most pregnant women go into labor spontaneously and have a normal labor and spontaneous vaginal birth. However, interventions to initiate or accelerate labor and birth are increasingly common. This chapter presents problems encountered during labor and birth and interventions related to those complications. Nurses have a key role in identifying complications and implementing nursing actions to achieve a safe birth and improve maternal and neonatal outcomes.

DYSTOCIA

Dystocia is difficult labor that is characterized by abnormally slow labor progress (Cunningham et al., 2014). Abnormal labor results from abnormalities of the power, the passenger, or the passage (American College of Obstetrics and Gynecology [ACOG], 2003). The terms *dystocia* and *failure to progress* are both used to characterize an abnormally long labor. However, this diagnosis is often mistakenly made before the woman has entered the active phase of labor and, therefore, before adequate trial of labor

(Simpson & O'Brien-Abel, 2013). Dystocia is the most common reason for primary cesarean sections (ACOG, 2014c; Queenan, Hobbins, & Spong, 2005). It is associated with the same factors that influence normal labor; these "Ps" are discussed in detail in Chapter 8:

- Powers of labor (uterine contractions and maternal expulsive effort)
- Passenger (fetal presentation, position or development)
- Passage (maternal bony pelvis or soft tissue)

The primary issues impacting nursing care with regard to dystocia are related to uterine factors, which are described in this chapter. Other factors are presented in Chapter 8 and are briefly discussed in the following section. Risk factors for dystocia include:

- Congenital uterine abnormalities such as bicornate uterus.
- Malpresentation of the fetus such as occiput posterior, or face presentation.
- Cephalopelvic disproportion.
- Tachysystole of the uterus with oxytocin.
- Maternal fatigue and dehydration.
- Administration of analgesia or anesthesia early in labor.
- Extreme maternal fear or exhaustion, which can result in catecholamine release interfering with uterine contractility.

Uterine Dystocia

Dystocia, or abnormal labor, includes lack of progressive cervical dilation, lack of descent of the fetal head, or both. Uterine dystocia indicates weak or uncoordinated uterine contractions in labor, characterized as either hypertonic or hypotonic uterine dysfunction.

Hypertonic Uterine Dysfunction

Hypertonic uterine dysfunction is uncoordinated uterine activity. Contractions are frequent and painful but ineffective in promoting dilation and effacement. When this occurs in early labor, it may be referred to as prodromal labor. Women who experience hypertonic uterine dysfunction are at risk for exhaustion related to prolonged labor, and the fetus is at risk for fetal intolerance of labor and asphyxia related to decreased placental profusion.

Risk Factors

- Nulliparous women are more subject to abnormal early labor.

Assessment Findings

- Painful, frequent UCs with inadequate uterine relaxation between UCs with little cervical changes (Fig. 10–1B)
- May be Category II (indeterminate) or Category III (abnormal) fetal heart rate (FHR) related to prolonged labor and inadequate uterine relaxation

Medical Management

- Evaluate labor progress.
- Evaluate cause of labor dysfunction.
- Hydrate to improve uterine perfusion and coordination of UCs.
- Provide pain management to allow the woman to sleep and prevent exhaustion.

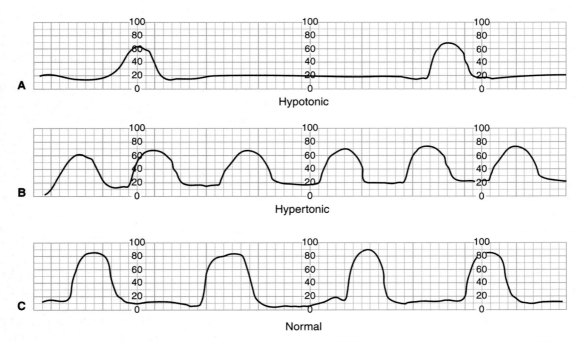

FIGURE 10–1 Hypertonic versus hypotonic versus normal uterine contractions. (**A**) Hypotonic uterine contraction pattern. (**B**) Hypertonic uterine contraction pattern. (**C**) Normal uterine contraction pattern.

Nursing Actions

- Promote rest to try to break the pattern of frequent but ineffective UCs. The pattern typically becomes effective when the woman sleeps for a period of several hours and awakens in a normal labor pattern of active labor. Methods used to promote uterine rest are:
  - Administration of pain medication such as morphine as per order to decrease labor contractions and allow the uterus to rest.
  - Promotion of relaxation.
    - Warm shower or tub bath
    - Quiet environment
    - Minimal interruptions to allow for long period of sleep
- Hydrate the woman with IV or PO fluids if tolerated. Dehydration can result in dysfunctional labor.
- Assess FHR and UCs.
- Evaluate labor progress with a sterile vaginal exam (SVE).
- Inform the woman and family of the progress of labor and explain interventions.
- Inform the care provider of the woman's response and progress in labor.

Hypotonic Uterine Dysfunction

Hypotonic uterine dysfunction occurs when the pressure of the UC is insufficient (intrauterine pressure catheter [IUPC] measurement less than 25 mm Hg) to promote cervical dilation and effacement. Typically, the woman makes normal progress during the latent phase of labor, but during active labor the UCs become weaker and less effective for cervical changes and labor progress (Fig. 10–1A). The woman is at risk for exhaustion and infection related to the prolonged labor, and the fetus is at risk for fetal intolerance of labor and asphyxia. Figure 10–1C shows a normal uterine contraction pattern.

Risk Factors

- Multiparous women often have more problems in the active phase.
- Extreme fear may result in catecholamine release, interfering with uterine contractility.

Assessment Findings

- Decreased frequency, strength, and duration of UCs
- Little or no cervical change
  - Less than 0.5 cm/hr progress in cervical dilation for a primiparous woman in active labor
  - Less than 1 cm/hr progress in cervical dilation for a multiparous woman in active labor
- Increased fear and anxiety levels

Medical Management

- Evaluate labor progression.
- Determine the cause of the dysfunction.
- Consider obstetrical interventions:
  - Augment labor with oxytocin.
  - Perform amniotomy.
  - Perform cesarean birth when other interventions have failed or when there are signs of fetal intolerance of labor.

Nursing Actions

- Assess uterine activity.
- Assess maternal and fetal status.
- Stimulate uterine activity to achieve a normal labor pattern using the following methods:
  - Ambulate and change the position of the woman to promote comfort and labor progress.
  - Hydrate with IV or PO as per orders, as dehydration can result in dysfunctional labor.
  - Administer IV fluids to maximize maternal fluid volume, correct maternal hypotension, and improve placental perfusion.
  - Augment labor with oxytocin as per protocol.
- Evaluate labor progress with SVE.
- Inform the woman and the family of labor progress and explain interventions.
- Provide emotional support. Anxiety levels can increase due to prolonged labor; increased anxiety and fear can interfere with effective UCs.
- Maintain good aseptic technique to minimize the risk of infection if there is rupture of membranes (ROM).
  - Minimize vaginal exams.
  - Maintain perineal cleanliness.
- Inform the care provider of the woman's response and progress in labor.

Active Phase Disorders

In both spontaneous and induced labor, the diagnosis of an arrest disorder should not be made before the patient has entered the active phase. The definitions of arrest disorders vary somewhat from published criteria, as more recent findings regarding labor progress challenge our long-held practices based on the Friedman curve. For example, the active phase of labor is now classified at 6 cm dilation (rather than the previously recognized 4 cm), and multiparous women appear to have a steeper acceleration phase than previously thought (Spong, Berghella, Wenstrom, Mercer, & Saade, 2012).

The current working definition of arrest of labor in the first stage in spontaneous labor (ACOG, 2014c) uses a dilation of more than or equal to 6 cm dilation with membrane rupture and one of the following:

- 4 hours or more of adequate contractions (e.g., more than 200 Montevideo units)
- 6 hours or more of inadequate contractions and no cervical change

As long as fetal and maternal status are reassuring, cervical dilation of 6 cm should be considered the threshold for the active phase of most women in labor. Before 6 cm of dilation is achieved, standards of active phase progress should not be applied. Further, cesarean delivery for active phase arrest in the first stage of labor should be reserved for women at or beyond 6 cm of dilation with ruptured membranes who fail to progress despite 4 hours of adequate uterine activity, or at least 6 hours of oxytocin administration with inadequate uterine activity and no cervical change (ACOG, 2014c). Before diagnosing arrest of labor in the second stage, if the maternal and fetal conditions permit, allow for the following:

● At least 2 hours of pushing in multiparous women
● At least 3 hours of pushing in nulliparous women

Longer durations may be appropriate in certain situations (e.g., with the use of epidural analgesia or with fetal malposition) if progress is being documented (ACOG, 2014c) (Box 10–1).

Second Stage Disorders

The second stage of labor begins when the cervix becomes fully dilated and ends with delivery of the neonate. Parity, delayed pushing, use of epidural analgesia, maternal body mass index (BMI), birth weight, occiput posterior position, and fetal station at complete dilation all have been shown to affect the length of the second stage of labor (ACOG, 2014c). Additionally, the duration of the second stage was approximately 1 hour longer in women who received epidural analgesia than in those who did not.

The literature supports that for women, longer time in the second stage of labor is associated with increased risks of morbidity and a decreasing probability of spontaneous vaginal delivery. However, this may be due to provider actions and interventions. Given the available literature, before diagnosing arrest of labor in the second stage and if the maternal and fetal conditions permit, at least 2 hours of pushing in multiparous women and at least 3 hours of pushing in nulliparous women should be allowed according to current ACOG guidelines. Inadequate expulsive forces occur in the second stage of labor when the woman is not able to push or bear down. It was previously thought that limiting the second stage to 2 hours was essential to decrease fetal

morbidity and mortality. It is now known that waiting beyond 2 hours is safe for the fetus and the 2-hour time frame is no longer clinically valid (see Box 10–1).

● The fetus is at higher risk for asphyxia related to prolonged second stage of labor.
● The woman with a prolonged second stage, beyond 4 hours, is at risk for operative vaginal birth and perineal trauma.

Risk Factors

● Maternal exhaustion
● Epidural anesthesia because woman may not feel the urge to push

Assessment Findings

● Inadequate or ineffective pushing with little or no descent of the fetal head with expulsive pushing efforts
● Potential for Category II (indeterminate) or Category III (abnormal) FHR

Medical Management

● Evaluate the woman's progress, maternal-fetal status, and likelihood of vaginal birth.
● Augment with oxytocin.
● Assist birth with vacuum or forceps.
● Perform cesarean birth when other interventions are ineffective or signs of fetal intolerance to labor.

Nursing Actions

● Assess fetal descent.
● Evaluate fetal response to expulsive pushing.
● Facilitate the second stage of labor by doing the following:
   ● Coaching the woman in bearing-down efforts
   ● Minimizing the Valsalva maneuver by using open glottis push strategies detailed in Chapter 8
   ● Maintaining adequate pain relief for the woman with labor epidurals
   ● Changing the maternal position to a more upright position to facilitate fetal descent
   ● Supporting the woman's involuntary pushing efforts

Precipitous Labor and Birth

Precipitous labor is a labor lasting fewer than 3 hours from onset of labor to birth. The current rate of precipitous labor for women is 2.4% (Cunningham et al., 2014; Martin et al., 2011). Women who experience a precipitous labor often have higher anxiety and pain levels related to the rapid and intense labor experience. Precipitous labor and/or birth places the woman at risk for postpartum hemorrhage related to uterine atony or lacerations. It places the fetus/neonate at risk for hypoxia and at risk for central nervous system (CNS) depression related to hypoxia from rapid birth.

Risk Factors

● Grand multiparity
● History of precipitous labor

BOX 10–1 | Definitions of Arrest Disorders

First-Stage Arrest

Spontaneous labor: greater than 6 cm dilation with membrane rupture and more than 4 hours of adequate contractions (e.g., more than 200 Montevideo units) or more than 6 hours if contractions are inadequate with no cervical change

Induced labor: greater than 6 cm dilation with membrane rupture or greater than 5 cm without membrane rupture and more than 4 hours of adequate contractions (e.g., more than 200 Montevideo units), or more than 6 hours if contractions are inadequate with no cervical change

Second-Stage Arrest

No progress (descent or rotation) for 4 hours or more in nulliparous women with an epidural, 3 hours or more in nulliparous women without an epidural, 3 hours or more in multiparous women with an epidural, 2 hours or more in multiparous women without an epidural

Spong, Berghella, Wenstrom, Mercer, & Saade, 2012.

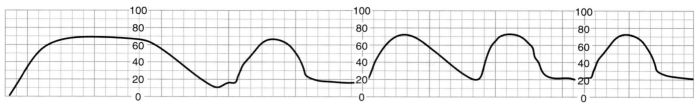

Tachysystole (tetanic contractions)

FIGURE 10–2 Tetanic uterine contractions.

Assessment Findings

● Hypertonic UCs (tetanic UCs) occurring every 2 minutes or more frequently, lasting greater than 60 seconds and strong (Fig. 10–2).
● Potential for Category II (indeterminate) or Category III (abnormal) FHR and nursing actions are based on FHR pattern (see Chapter 9).
● Rapid cervical dilation such that labor is less than 3 hours.

Medical Management

● Prepare for and stand by for precipitous birth.

Nursing Actions

● Remain in the room with the woman since birth is often very rapid with precipitous labor.
● Monitor FHR and UCs every 15 minutes.
● Assess labor progress and cervical change closely with SVEs.
    ● Assess the cervix if the woman states she feels pressure or feels like the baby is coming. This may be a sign of impending birth.
● Support the woman and the family. This type of labor can be frightening, overwhelming, and painful.
● Anticipate potential maternal postpartum complications such as hemorrhage and lacerations.
● Anticipate potential neonatal complications such as hypoxia and CNS depression related to rapid birth.
● Prepare for delivery.

Fetal Dystocia

Fetal dystocia may be caused by excessive fetal size, malpresentation, multifetal pregnancy, or fetal anomalies. The fetus can move through the birth canal most effectively when the head is flexed and is presenting anterior to the woman's pelvis (occiput anterior position). This allows the smallest diameter of the fetal head to enter the maternal pelvis and the most flexible part of the fetal body, the back of the neck, to adapt to the curve of the birth canal. When the fetal position is other than flexed and vertex of the fetus is large in comparison to the maternal pelvis, labor may be difficult and vaginal birth a challenge. Complications of fetal dystocia are:

● Neonatal asphyxia related to prolonged labor.
● Fetal injuries, such as bruising.
● Maternal lacerations.
● Cephalopelvic disproportion (CPD).

CRITICAL COMPONENT

Fetopelvic/Cephalopelvic Disproportion

Fetopelvic disproportion arises from diminished pelvic capacity, excessive fetal size, or both (Cunningham et al., 2014). Cephalopelvic disproportion is a condition in which the size, shape, or position of the fetal head prevents it from passing through the lateral aspect of the maternal pelvis *or* when the maternal pelvis is of a size or shape that prevents the descent of the fetus through the pelvis. A diagnosis of CPD often necessitates a cesarean birth. CPD can rarely be diagnosed until labor has progressed for some time.

The success of any labor depends on the complex interrelationship of several factors:

· Fetal size, presentation, and position
· Size and shape of the maternal pelvis
· Quality of the UCs

Risk Factors

● Contraction or narrowing of the pelvic inlet, the midpelvis, or the pelvic outlet
● Abnormal fetal presentation or position such as asynclitism, face, brow presentation, or breech or transverse lie (Table 10–1)
● Fetal anomalies, such as hydrocephalus, and/or any other fetal anomaly that interferes with fetal descent through the birth canal
● Fetal macrosomia; birth weight greater than 4,500 g

Assessment Findings

● FHR may be heard above the umbilicus versus in the lower uterine segment; this is a sign that the fetus may be in position other than vertex.
● The SVE reveals buttocks or face when malpresentation is the cause of dystocia.
● The presenting part is not engaged in the maternal pelvis.
● There is no fetal descent through the pelvis.

Medical Management

● Confirm the fetal position with SVE and ultrasound.
● Determine the type of obstetrical interventions, such as use of vacuum extractor, forceps, or need for cesarean birth.

TABLE 10–1   Malpresentation of the Fetus

MALPRESENTATION	DESCRIPTION	IMPLICATIONS
Occiput posterior	The occiput of the fetus is in the posterior portion of the pelvis rather than the anterior. As the fetus moves through the birth canal, the occiput bone presses on the woman's sacrum. Rotation of fetal head may occur during fetal descent.	Prolonged labor and prolonged second stage Severe back pain
Face presentation	Fetal head is in extension rather than flexion as it enters the pelvis.	Labor and pushing may be prolonged. Cesarean delivery may be indicated. The neonate's face may have extensive bruising.
Brow presentation	Fetal head presents in a position midway between full flexion and extreme extension. This causes the largest diameter of the head to engage in the pelvis.	Prolonged second stage of labor
Shoulder presentation/compound presentation	Shoulder presentation: The fetal spine is vertical to the maternal pelvis. Compound presentation: One or more fetal extremities accompany the presenting part.	Higher risk of prolapsed cord. Cesarean delivery is typically indicated.

TABLE 10–1   Malpresentation of the Fetus—cont'd

MALPRESENTATION	DESCRIPTION	IMPLICATIONS
Breech presentations: Frank breech 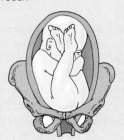 Complete breech 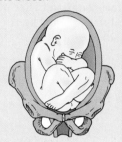 Footling breech (single) 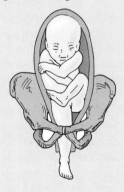 Footling breech (double) 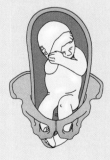	Frank breech: Thighs flexed alongside body, feet are close to the head. Complete breech: One or both knees are flexed. Footling breech: Either one (single footling) or both (double footling) feet present before the buttocks.	Dysfunctional labor Fetal injury Increased risk of prolapsed cord. Typically, cesarean birth is indicated.

Nursing Actions

● Perform Leopold's maneuver as described in Chapter 8 to determine the fetal position.
● Assess the location of the FHR.
● Assess the fetal position with SVE.
● Alert the care provider if there is any question regarding fetal presentation, position, or absence of fetal descent.

Pelvic Dystocia

Pelvic dystocia is related to the contraction of one or more of the three planes of the pelvis. During the prenatal period, the care provider determines the general pelvic size and configuration by vaginal examination. Pelvic measurements are not typically done. Descent and engagement of fetal head in labor indicate adequate pelvic inlet. The outcome of labor is dependent on the interrelationship of the size and shape of the pelvis, fetal size, presentation and position, and quality of the UCs.

The three contractions of the pelvic planes are:

● Inlet contraction, which occurs when the widest part of the pelvis is small.
● Midpelvis contraction, which is related to prominent ischial spines, convergent pelvic side walls, and a narrow sacrosciatic notch; this may arrest the descent of the vertex.
● Outlet contraction, which can be estimated by measuring the transverse diameter of the pelvis. Normally, the antero-posterior diameter is 14 cm.

Risk Factors

● Small pelvis
● Abnormal pelvic shape

Assessment Findings

● Delayed descent of fetal head

Medical Management

● Evaluate the pelvis for contraction of one or more of the planes of the pelvis.
● Evaluate the descent and engagement of the fetal head.

Nursing Actions

● Perform SVE to evaluate the progress of labor and fetal descent into pelvis (i.e., check station).

LABOR INTERVENTIONS

Most pregnant women go into labor spontaneously at term (37 to 42 weeks' gestation) and progress through the labor and birth experience without complications. Increasingly, the approach to labor has shifted from a natural process to one that should be "managed" by the woman, nurse, and care provider. Management of labor has resulted in an increase in labor interventions, including induction of labor (which may also include cervical ripening) and augmentation to speed up labor. This section reviews interventions to induce (initiate) and augment (strengthen) labor.

Labor interventions are medically indicated when either the condition or safety of the woman or fetus would be improved with birth. Because spontaneous labor is associated with fewer complications than induced labor, induction of labor without a medical indication is discouraged.

Despite risks to the woman and fetus (such as increased rates of cesarean birth), labor interventions such as elective induction are at an all-time high. Because of the potential risks associated with induction of labor, elective induction should be undertaken only after fully informing the woman of risks and benefits and establishing a gestational age of 39 weeks or greater. The nurse providing care for the woman during cervical ripening, induction, or augmentation of labor should be aware of the indications, actions, expected results, and potential risks of each agent. Before any agent is used, maternal status and fetal well-being should be established and cervical status should be assessed and documented (Simpson & Knox, 2009).

SAFE AND EFFECTIVE NURSING CARE: Patient Education

Go the Full 40

One source of information women can use when considering childbearing options is the Association for Women's Health Obstetric and Neonatal Nurses' (AWHONN's) "Don't Rush Me . . . Go the Full 40" consumer-awareness campaign, launched in 2012. It seeks to empower women to make labor and delivery decisions that are in their best interests and is designed to help women understand 40 key reasons for carrying her baby to term, challenging the common myth that it's okay for babies to be born just a little early. In fact, babies need the benefit of a full-term pregnancy. Inducing labor before 40 weeks is associated with prematurity, cesarean surgery, hemorrhage, and infection. Babies born before 37 completed weeks of gestation are at risk for breathing problems, feeding issues, jaundice, low blood sugar, and problems stabilizing their own body temperature. (www.health4mom.org; http://www.health4mom.org/category/healthy-pregnancy/go-the-full-40-zone/ http://www.health4mom.org/a/40_reasons121611)

Healthy Mom&Baby, the consumer magazine from AWHONN, can also be helpful for women considering induction.

Labor Induction

Induction of labor is the deliberate stimulation of UCs before the onset of spontaneous labor to facilitate a vaginal delivery. Induction of labor refers to techniques for stimulating uterine contractions to accomplish delivery prior to the onset of spontaneous labor. After nearly 20 years of consecutive increases, induction of labor for singleton births reached a high of 23.8% in 2010, then declined in 2011 (23.7%) and 2012 (23.3%). Since 2006, births delivered at less than 39 weeks have declined (down 12%), and births at 39 weeks or more have increased (up 9%) (Osterman & Martin, 2014). Data show that outcomes for newborns are greatly improved when gestation is longer than 39 weeks. Yet studies indicate that almost a third of babies delivered in the United States are electively delivered—most for convenience. This impacts short-term neonatal morbidity. New guidelines are being set by the Joint Commission to decrease elective inductions of labor prior to 39 weeks' gestation. Labor induction should be performed only for medical indication; if done for nonmedical indications, the gestational age should be 39 weeks or more, and the cervix should be favorable (Bishop score of 8 or higher), especially in the nulliparous patient (Spong et al., 2012) (Box 10–2).

The nurse may face a dilemma when women are admitted for induction or cervical ripening without documented indications for it. It is the nurse's responsibility to ensure that the woman is fully informed by her provider before beginning a procedure (Simpson, 2013). If it is apparent during admission that the woman is not fully informed about the intended method of labor induction, the

CRITICAL COMPONENT

Elective Induction of Labor

It is estimated that 25% to 50% of inductions are elective or nonmedical. Prior to elective induction, fetal maturity must be confirmed to be 39 weeks or greater by the following:

1. Ultrasound before 20 weeks' gestation confirms gestational age of 39 weeks or greater.
2. Fetal heart tones have been documented as present by Doppler for 30 weeks.
3. It has been 36 weeks since a positive serum or urine pregnancy test was confirmed.

According to the American College of Obstetricians and Gynecologists (ACOG), for certain medical conditions, available data and expert opinion support optimal timing of delivery in the late-preterm or early-term period for improved neonatal and infant outcomes. However, for nonmedically indicated early-term deliveries, such an improvement has not been demonstrated. Morbidity and mortality rates are greater among neonates and infants delivered during the early-term period compared with those delivered between 39 and 40 weeks' gestation. Nevertheless, the rate of nonmedically indicated early-term deliveries continues to increase in the United States. They recommend implementing a policy to decrease the rate of nonmedically indicated deliveries before 39 weeks' gestation. In addition, AWHONN states that until we better understand the complex physiology of the hormones involved in labor and birth and the implications of interrupting this powerful hormonal process, it is advisable to limit induction and augmentation of labor to situations for which there are medical indications.

ACOG, 2011; AWHONN, 2014.

BOX 10–2 | Criteria, Indications, and Contraindications for Labor Induction and Cervical Ripening

Criteria

- Gestational age, cervical status, pelvic adequacy, fetal size, and fetal presentation should be assessed.
- Any potential risks to the mother and fetus should be considered.
- The medical record should document that a discussion was held between the pregnant woman and her health care provider about the indications; the agents and methods of labor induction, including the risks, benefits, and alternative approaches; and the possible need for a repeat induction or cesarean birth.
- A nulliparous woman undergoing elective induction of labor with an unfavorable cervix should be counseled about a twofold increased risk of cesarean birth.
- Cervical ripening and induction agents should be administered by trained personnel familiar with their effects on mother and fetus.
- Prostaglandin preparations should be administered where uterine activity and FHR can be monitored continuously for an initial observation period. FHR monitoring should be continued if regular uterine contractions persist.
- FHR and uterine contractions should be monitored closely during induction and augmentation as for any high-risk patient in active labor.
- A physician capable of performing a cesarean birth should be readily available.
- For women undergoing trial of labor after Cesarean (TOLAC), induction of labor for maternal or fetal indications remains an option.
- Misoprostol should not be used for third trimester cervical ripening, or for labor induction in women who have had a cesarean birth or major uterine surgery.

Indications

Indications for induction of labor are not absolute but should take into account maternal and fetal conditions; gestational age; and assessment of the cervix, pelvis, and fetal size and presentation. Following are examples of maternal or fetal conditions that may be indications for induction of labor:

- Abruptio placentae
- Chorioamnionitis (intraamniotic infection)
- Fetal demise
- Gestational hypertension
- Preeclampsia, eclampsia
- Premature rupture of membranes
- Post-term pregnancy

Continued

BOX 10–2—cont'd

- Maternal medical conditions (e.g., diabetes mellitus, renal disease, chronic pulmonary disease, chronic hypertension, or antiphospholipid syndrome)
- Fetal compromise (e.g., severe fetal growth restriction, iso-immunization, oligohydramnios)

Labor may also be induced for logistical reasons (e.g., risk of rapid labor, distance from the hospital, or psychosocial indications). In such circumstances, at least one of the following criteria should be met, or fetal lung maturity should be established:

- Ultrasound measurement at less than 20 weeks' gestation supports gestational age of 39 weeks or greater.
- Fetal heart tones have been documented as present for 30 weeks by Doppler ultrasonography.
- It has been 36 weeks since a positive serum or urine human chorionic gonadotropin pregnancy test result.
- Testing for fetal lung maturity should not be performed and is contraindicated when delivery is mandated for fetal or maternal indications. Conversely, a mature fetal lung maturity test result before 39 weeks' gestation, in the absence of appropriate clinical circumstances, is not an indication for elective labor induction.

Contraindications

Generally, the contraindications for labor induction are the same as those for spontaneous labor and vaginal birth. They include, but are not limited to, the following:

- Vasa previa or complete placenta previa
- Transverse fetal lie
- Umbilical cord prolapse
- Previous classical cesarean birth
- Active genital herpes infection
- Previous myomectomy entering the endometrial cavity

Simpson, 2013.

health care provider who ordered the induction or their physician designee should be notified and should speak to the woman either on the telephone or in person about the potential risks and benefits of the process and ensure that her questions and concerns have been addressed before proceeding (Simpson, 2013).

Women considering labor induction should be told that it is not an isolated intervention. The decision for labor induction often results in a cascade of other interventions and activities that have the potential to negatively affect the childbirth process. Labor induction in the United States leads to an intravenous (IV) line, bed rest, and continuous electronic fetal monitoring (EFM), and frequently amniotomy, significant discomfort, epidural analgesia/anesthesia, and a prolonged stay on the labor unit. The use of oxytocin and prostaglandin agents increases the risk of fetal compromise during labor and birth, mainly as a result of uterine

tachysystole and prolonged stay in the labor unit (Simpson, 2013; Simpson & Atterbury, 2003; Simpson & O'Brien-Abel, 2013).

Numerous methods of labor induction have been proposed as being effective in initiating labor. When the decision has been made to induce labor, the next important question raised is how to induce labor. When deciding on the method of induction, certain clinical factors are considered, including parity, status of membranes (ruptured or intact), status of the cervix (favorable or unfavorable), and history of previous cesarean births.

All these factors or clinical situations are considered important to the provider's decision about which method of labor induction should be used. Labor induction is thought to be less successful when the cervix is unfavorable (not ripe). It is more successful in parous women than in nulliparous women. Little attention has been given to the combination of these factors, which may be important to women and clinicians when attempting to make informed decisions about induction of labor (Kelly et al., 2009).

The nurse providing care for the woman during cervical ripening and induction and augmentation of labor must be aware of appropriate indications for the use of each mechanical method and pharmacological agent, as well as their actions, expected results, and potential risks. Additionally, before any cervical ripening or labor induction agent is used, maternal status and fetal well-being should be established and findings from an assessment of the cervix, pelvis, fetal size, and presentation documented in the medical record by the provider and an estimation of fetal weight/size and assessment of the maternal pelvis should be determined and documented by the provider (AAP & ACOG, 2012).

CRITICAL COMPONENT

Problems With Mistimed Induction of Labor

Accurate dating of pregnancy using early prenatal care and ultrasonography is advised before cervical ripening and induction of labor. Mistimed cervical ripening and induction can result in unplanned iatrogenic preterm birth, and recent evidence documents increased neonatal morbidity in babies born prior to 39 weeks' gestation but after 37 weeks' gestation. Current ACOG guidelines recommend against elective induction of labor before 39 completed weeks of pregnancy, unless medical indications for earlier delivery are noted. Elective inductions account for about half of all inductions and 10% of deliveries.

ACOG recommends that dating be confirmed with at least one of the following:

- Ultrasonography dating at less than 20 weeks' gestation is consistent with gestational age of 39 weeks or more.
- Fetal heart tones have been documented in the patient's medical records for at least 30 weeks by Doppler ultrasonography.
- 36 weeks have passed since a positive urine or serum pregnancy test for human chorionic gonadotropin.

In the United States, the national cost for preterm labor, undelivered, exceeds $360 million in total expenditures per year.

Preterm labor hospitalization costs are in excess of $820 million. However, the direct economic cost is only a fraction of the ultimate cost of delivery of children who are preterm. The cost of immediate newborn care for preterm infants has been estimated at $5 billion annually, and long-term health costs are also very high (Goldberg, 2015). Avoiding unintentional preterm birth is an essential element of safe induction of labor.

Oxytocin Induction

A pharmacological method for labor induction is administration of oxytocin, which is the most common induction agent used worldwide. It has been used alone, in combination with amniotomy, or after cervical ripening with other pharmacological or nonpharmacological methods. Before the introduction of prostaglandin agents, oxytocin was used as a cervical ripening agent as well.

- Endogenous oxytocin is a peptide synthesized by the hypothalamus that is transported to the posterior lobe of the pituitary gland, where it is released in the maternal circulation in response to vaginal and cervical stretching. The release of oxytocin stimulates UCs.
- Synthetic oxytocin is identical to endogenous oxytocin.
- Uterine response to oxytocin usually occurs within 3 to 5 minutes after IV administration begins, with a half-life of 10 minutes (Simpson, 2013).
- Considerable controversy exists related to dose and rate increase intervals when oxytocin is used for induction of labor.

There was a trend to use higher doses of oxytocin, termed "active management of labor" (see Box 10–1). This dosing regimen is based on research conducted in the 1970s in Dublin, Ireland. However, current evidence supports lower-dose infusions (Simpson, 2013), with research reporting more successful vaginal births, fewer operative vaginal deliveries, and less tachysystole and lower cesarean birth rates. Continued increases in oxytocin rates over a long period during induction can result in oxytocin receptor desensitization or downregulation, making oxytocin less effective in producing normal UCs (Simpson, 2013). See Box 10–2 for more on indications and contraindications.

Indications

- Post-term pregnancy
- Pregnancy-induced hypertension
- Preeclampsia/eclampsia
- Maternal medical conditions (e.g., diabetes mellitus, renal disease, chronic pulmonary disease, cardiac disease, chronic hypertension)
- Premature rupture of membranes (PROM)
- Chorioamnionitis
- Fetal stress or compromise, such as severe intrauterine growth restriction (IUGR), oligohydramnios, or isoimmunization

- Fetal demise
- History of rapid labors/distance from the hospital
- Psychosocial considerations

Contraindications

- Any contraindications for vaginal birth
- Previous vertical (classical) uterine scar or prior transfundal uterine scar
- Placental abnormalities such as complete placenta previa or vasa previa
- Abnormal fetal position
- Umbilical cord prolapse
- Active genital herpes
- Pelvic abnormalities

Risks Associated With Inductions

- Tachysystole leading to Category II (indeterminate) or Category III (abnormal) FHR pattern is the primary complication of oxytocin in labor.
- Failed induction of labor: Failure to generate regular (e.g., every 3 minutes) contractions and cervical change after at least 24 hours of oxytocin administration, with artificial membrane rupture if feasible.
- Side effects of oxytocin use are primarily dose related; tachysystole and subsequent FHR decelerations are common side effects (ACOG, 2011).
- Water intoxication can occur with high concentrations of oxytocin with large quantities of hypotonic solutions, but usually only with prolonged administration with at least 40 mU/min.

Assessment Findings

- The woman understands the indication for induction.
- Assessment findings and prenatal records reflect an indication for induction.
- If elective induction, confirmed gestational age of at least 39 weeks.

Medical Management

- Advise of indication for induction of labor and order induction of labor as per institutional protocol.
- Be available to respond to complications.

CRITICAL COMPONENT

Administering Oxytocin in Labor

Nursing responsibility during oxytocin infusion involves careful titration of the drug to the maternal-fetal response. The titration process includes decreasing the dosage rate or discontinuing the medication when contractions are too frequent, discontinuing the medication when fetal status is indeterminate or abnormal, and increasing the dosage rate when uterine activity and labor progress are inadequate. Often during oxytocin infusion, physicians and nurses are focused on the rate-increase section

Continued

of the protocol while ignoring the clinical criteria for dosage increases. For example, if cervical effacement is occurring or if the woman is progressing in labor as expected, based on parity and other individual clinical factors, there is no need to increase the oxytocin rate, even if contractions appear to be mild and infrequent. Labor progress and maternal-fetal response to the medication should be the primary considerations (Simpson, 2013). The goal of oxytocin use in labor is to establish uterine contraction patterns that promote cervical dilation of about 1 cm/hr once in active labor.

Generally, the UC pattern consists of:

- 3 UCs in 10 minutes, lasting 40 to 60 seconds, intensity of 25 to 75 mm Hg with IUCP with resting tone less than 20 mm Hg with 1 minute between each UC.
- Oxytocin is administered intravenously and is piggybacked to a mainline IV solution at the port most proximal to the venous site.
- Oxytocin is *always* infused via a pump.
- There is variation in the concentrations of oxytocin, and it should be prepared by the pharmacy, as it is a high-alert medication.
- Typical concentrations are:
  - 10 units of oxytocin in 1,000 mL of lactated Ringer's result in an infusion rate of 1 mU/min = 6 mL/hr.
  - 20 units of oxytocin in 1,000 mL of lactated Ringer's result in an infusion rate of 1 mU/min = 3 mL/hr.
- Current dose recommendations are for low-dose oxytocin starting at 0.5 mU/min and increasing the dose by 1 to 2 mU/min every 30 to 60 minutes until adequate labor progress is achieved (i.e., cervical effacement or cervical dilation of 0.5 to 1 cm/hr) and regular UCs every 2 to 3 minutes lasting 45 to 60 seconds.
  - Generally, starting doses of 1 to 2 mU/min with increases in 1 to 2 mU/min increments every 30 to 60 minutes are most appropriate and commonly used.
  - Nursing responsibilities during oxytocin infusion involve careful titration of the drug to the maternal and fetal response.
  - The titration process includes decreasing dosage rates or discontinuing infusion when UCs are too frequent.
  - Discontinuing oxytocin when FHR is abnormal (Simpson, 2013; Simpson & O'Brien-Abel, 2013).
  - Increasing doses when UCs are inadequate; however, the lowest possible dose should be used to achieve labor progress (Simpson & Atterbury, 2003).
- Once active labor is established, oxytocin should be discontinued to avoid downregulation. Contemporary labor patterns suggest that the active phase of first-stage spontaneous labor likely does not start until 6 cm for nulliparous women and 5 cm for multiparous women (Simpson, 2013).

- Maternal-fetal response to oxytocin is the primary consideration. If the frequency, intensity, duration, or resting tone of the contraction is increased by oxytocin, this can impede uterine blood flow and can cause fetal compromise, resulting in a Category II or Category III FHR pattern. Thus, oxytocin must be administered with careful monitoring and prompt recognition and interventions for tachysystole to prevent fetal acidosis.
  - Avoid tachysystole because it frequently results in Category II (indeterminate) or Category III (abnormal) FHR pattern.
  - Continuous EFM is typically used with oxytocin administration.
  - In the absence of risk factors, intermittent auscultation is permitted with evaluation of FHR and UCs at least every 30 minutes in active labor and every 15 minutes in the second stage.
- For Category II (indeterminate) or Category III (abnormal) FHR pattern, interventions include the following actions:
  - Discontinue oxytocin.
  - Change maternal position to left lateral position.
  - Initiate IV hydration of at least 500 mL lactated Ringer's.
  - Administer O_2 by nonrebreather mask at 10 L/min.
  - Consider terbutaline if no response.
  - Notify provider, observe, and reevaluate.
  - Notify the provider and request bedside evaluations for Category III abnormal FHR.
  - Assess emotional response of patient and support person to induction of labor. Provide information and reassurance as needed to alleviate feelings of failure.
  - Assess patient's level of fear and provide information and reassurance.
- If oxytocin has been discontinued for 20 to 30 minutes, the FHR is reassuring, and no uterine tachysystole is present, oxytocin may be restarted at half the rate that caused tachysystole and gradually increased every 30 minutes based on maternal-fetal response. If oxytocin has been discontinued for more than 30 to 40 minutes, exogenous oxytocin is metabolized; therefore, oxytocin must be restarted at the initial dose (2 mU per minute) (ACOG, 2011).
- Terminate the oxytocin infusion if there is tachysystole of the uterus, as defined above; precipitous labor; nonreassuring fetal heart rate pattern; if the provider is unexpectedly unavailable; inability to monitor patient's FHR or uterine contraction at recommended intervals; desired labor pattern. If unable to continuously monitor FHR during an epidural administration, stop oxytocin infusion and restart infusion at half strength and increase per protocol once FHR continuous monitoring can be reestablished (ACOG, 2011).

Nursing Actions

- Ensure informed consent has been obtained by providing information about induction and discussing the agents, methods, options, and risks (Gilbert, 2011). Nurses can play an important role in advocating for women who want to wait for labor to progress naturally but face pressure from their families or obstetric providers to undergo nonmedically indicated induction. Nurses can also play an important role in ensuring women have the information needed to make informed decisions regarding labor augmentation (AWHONN, 2014).
- Review prenatal record with woman for indication for labor induction.
- If intermittent auscultation can be done appropriately, it is an acceptable method for labor management if the heart rate remains within normal limits (Category I of the FHR categories).
- In the presence of risk factors, continuous EFM is recommended and FHR should be evaluated and documented every 15 minutes in active labor and every 5 minutes in the second stage.
- Monitor strength, frequency, and duration of UCs as an indicator of oxytocin efficacy Q 30 min.
- Evaluate uterine resting tone by palpation or IUPC pressure below 20 mm Hg to ensure uterine relaxation between contractions.
- Decrease or discontinue oxytocin in the event of uterine tachysystole or indeterminate or abnormal fetal status. The current recommendation when decreasing oxytocin is to lower the dose by half.
- Assess FHR in response to UCs (see Chapter 9).
- Monitor labor progress with SVE for cervical dilation and fetal descent. Cervical change of 1 cm/hr indicates sufficient progress.
- Assess the character and amount of amniotic fluid.
- Assess the character and amount of bloody show.
- Assess the maternal response, including level of discomfort and pain and effectiveness of pain management and labor support Q 30 min.
- Assess vital signs (VS) per policy, generally Q 2 hr.
- Assess input and output (I&O) for fluid overload; output should mirror intake. Signs and symptoms of fluid overload include decreased urine output, edema, increased blood pressure (BP), and pulmonary edema.
- Ensure adequate hydration, assess I&O Q 8 hr.
- Greater than 50% of all legal settlements involved perinatal cases, with 40% to 50% of these cases related to management of oxytocin (Jonsson, Norden-Lindeberg, & Hanson, 2007). Nurses must minimize the risk of patient harm by being well-educated regarding oxytocin risks as well as being proactive with interventions when there is evidence of tachysystole or abnormal FHR patterns.
- Follow the constitutions of chain of command if nursing disagrees with the plan of care (Gilbert, 2011).
- During the infusion of the oxytocin, the attending or another licensed provider who has assumed responsibility for the patient's care shall be available within 30 minutes to manage any complications that may arise. A physician with privileges to perform a cesarean section should be readily available (ACOG, 2011).

SAFE AND EFFECTIVE NURSING CARE: Understanding Medication

Oxytocin: High-Alert Medication

In 2007, IV oxytocin was designated as a high-alert medication. Drugs in this category carry a heightened risk of causing significant patient harm when they are used in error. Errors with high-alert medications may or may not be more common than with other drugs; however, patient injury and consequences of associated errors may be more devastating.

Patient injury from drug therapy is the single most common type of adverse event that occurs in the inpatient setting (Agency for Healthcare Research & Quality, 2001; Institute for Healthcare Improvement, 2007). When medication errors result in patient injury, there are significant costs to the patient, the health care providers, and the institution. Special considerations and precautions are required before and during administration of high-alert medications (Institute for Safe Medication Practices, 2007). This is significant for perinatal care providers because oxytocin is a drug that they use quite frequently. Errors that involve IV oxytocin administration for labor induction or augmentation are most commonly dose-related and often involve lack of timely recognition and appropriate treatment of excessive uterine activity (i.e., tachysystole) (Clark, Simpson, Knox, & Garite, 2009). Other types of oxytocin errors involve mistaken administration of IV fluids with oxytocin for IV fluid resuscitation during Category II or III FHR patterns and/or maternal hypotension and inappropriate elective administration of oxytocin to women who are less than 39 completed weeks' gestation. Oxytocin medication errors and subsequent patient harm is generally preventable (Simpson & Knox, 2009). The perinatal team can develop strategies to minimize risk of maternal-fetal injuries related to oxytocin administration consistent with safe care practices used with other high-alert medications. As with other high-alert medications, the lowest possible dose to achieve the desired therapeutic effect should be used (Simpson, 2013).

1. Requirement that women having elective labor induction be at least 39 completed weeks' gestation
2. Standard order sets and protocols that reflect a standardized clinical approach to labor induction and augmentation based on current pharmacological and physiological evidence
3. Standard concentration of oxytocin prepared by the pharmacy
4. Standard definition of uterine tachysystole that does not include a Category III or II (abnormal or indeterminate) FHR pattern (a contraction frequency of more than five in 10 minutes, a series of single contractions lasting 2 minutes or more, contractions of normal duration occurring within 1 minute of each other)
5. Standard treatment of oxytocin-induced uterine tachysystole guided by fetal status

Agency for Healthcare Research and Quality, 2001; Clark et al., 2009; Institute for Healthcare Improvement, 2007; Institute for Safe Medication Practices, 2007; Simpson & Knox, 2009.

CRITICAL COMPONENT

Tachysystole

Tachysystole is excessive uterine activity and can be either spontaneous or induced. It is defined as more than five contractions in 10 minutes, averaged over 30 minutes (ACOG, 2009a, 2011; Macones, Hankins, Spong, Hauth, & Moore, 2008). Additional features of excessive uterine activity include contractions lasting 2 minutes or longer, contractions of normal duration occurring within 1 minute of each other, or insufficient return of uterine resting tone between contractions via palpation or intraamniotic pressure above 25 mm Hg between contractions via IUPC (ACOG, 2009a).

The placenta serves as the fetal lungs in utero. Uteroplacental circulation allows oxygen to be exchanged for the carbon dioxide and waste products from the fetus. During a contraction, the myometrial pressure exceeds the arterial pressure and the uterine blood flow is interrupted, causing a cessation in oxygen delivery to the placenta and the fetus. The fetus can withstand the stresses of labor during recurring periods of transient hypoxemia through a physiological compensatory mechanism known as the fetal oxygen reserve. However, if contractions are either too long or too strong, hypoxemia may result. Complications of uterine tachysystole for the fetus include hypoxia that can lead to acidemia, worsening to acidosis, ultimately leading to brain damage and even fetal death (Kunz, Loftus, & Nichols, 2013).

Tachysystole, previously referred to as hyperstimulation, is excessive uterine activity and is the most concerning side effect of oxytocin because it can result in a progressive adverse effect on fetal status (Simpson & O'Brien-Abel, 2013) (Fig. 10–3). UCs cause an intermittent decrease in blood flow in the intervillous space where oxygen exchange occurs. The decreased intervillous blood flow associated with tachysystole leads to decreased oxygen to the fetus. Tachysystole can result in progressive deterioration in fetal status and hypoxemia that result in an abnormal fetal heart rate. Tachysystole may result in abruptio placenta or uterine rupture, which are rare complications (ACOG, 2009a).

Tachysystole is defined as:

- Five or more UCs in 10 minutes over a 30-minute window.
- A series of single UCs lasting 2 minutes or longer.
- UCs occurring within 1 minute of each other.

- Insufficient return of uterine resting tone between contractions via palpation or intraamniotic pressure above 25 mm Hg between contractions via IUPC.

Nursing actions for tachysystole with Category I (normal) FHR pattern:

- Maternal repositioning (left or right lateral)
- IV fluid bolus of at least 500 mL lactated Ringer's (unless contraindicated)
- Oxygen 10 L/min via nonrebreather mask
- If uterine activity has not returned to normal after 10 to 15 minutes, decrease oxytocin rate by at least half; if uterine activity has not returned to normal after 10 to 15 more minutes, discontinue oxytocin until uterine activity is normal.

Resume oxytocin after resolution of tachysystole. If oxytocin has been discontinued for less than 20 to 30 minutes, the FHR is normal, and the contraction frequency, intensity, and duration are normal, resume oxytocin at no more than half the rate that caused the tachysystole, and gradually increase the rate as appropriate based on unit protocol and maternal-fetal status. If the oxytocin is discontinued for more than 30 to 40 minutes, resume oxytocin at the initial dose ordered.

Nursing actions for tachysystole with a Category II (indeterminate) or Category III (abnormal) FHR pattern would also include(Lyndon & Ali, 2008):

- Discontinuing oxytocin and notifying the provider.
- Maternal repositioning (left or right lateral).
- Administering IV fluid bolus of at least 500 mL lactated Ringer's (unless contraindicated).
- Giving O_2 at 10 L/min by nonrebreather mask.
- Notifying provider of actions taken and maternal-fetal response.
- With category III FHR pattern request an immediate bedside evaluation.
- Considering terbutaline if no response to above measures.

Resume oxytocin after resolution of tachysystole. If oxytocin has been discontinued for less than 20 to 30 minutes, the FHR is normal, and the contraction frequency, intensity, and duration are normal, resume oxytocin at no more than half the rate that caused the tachysystole, and gradually increase the rate as appropriate based on unit protocol and maternal-fetal status. If the oxytocin is discontinued for more than 30 to 40 minutes, resume oxytocin at the initial dose ordered (Simpson, 2013).

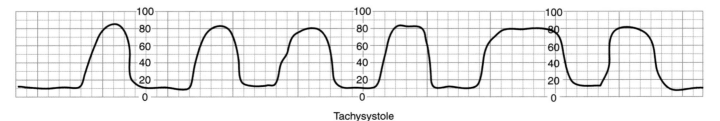

Tachysystole

FIGURE 10–3 Uterine tachysystole (hyperstimulation).

Cervical Ripening

Cervical ripening is the process of physical softening, thinning, and dilating of the cervix in preparation for labor and birth (Simpson, 2013). The cervix, composed of connective tissue, is typically closed until labor begins. At the onset of labor, it undergoes rapid changes, including ripening, effacement, and dilation (Fig. 10–4A and B).

Cervical ripening typically begins prior to the onset of labor contractions and is necessary for cervical dilation and the passage of the fetus. A series of complex biochemical processes, ending with rearrangement and realignment of the collagen molecules, allow the cervix to ripen. The cervix thins, softens, relaxes, and dilates in response to uterine contractions, allowing the cervix to easily pass over the presenting fetal part during labor.

Because cervical status is the most important predictor of successful labor induction, it is crucial for cervical status to be assessed before beginning this process. Typically, cervical status is assessed via the Bishop score (Table 10–2). A Bishop's score greater than 8 generally confers the same likelihood of vaginal delivery with induction of labor as that following spontaneous labor, and thus has been considered to indicate a favorable cervix

TABLE 10–2   Bishop Score to Assess Cervical Ripeness

	0	1	2	3
Dilation cm	0	1–2	3–4	5–6
Effacement %	0%–30%	40%–50%	60%–70%	80%
Station	–3	–2	–1/0	+1/+2
Consistency of cervix	Firm	Medium	Soft	
Cervical position	Posterior	Medium	Anterior	

Bishop, 1964.

(see Fig. 10–4A). Conversely, a Bishop's score of 6 or less has been used to denote an unfavorable cervix in many studies and has been associated with a higher risk of cesarean delivery when labor is induced compared with spontaneous labor (Fig. 10–4B). A score of 6 or more is considered favorable for successful induction of labor. However, when the score is unfavorable (a Bishop score of less than 6), cervical ripening is usually considered. A mechanical or pharmacological cervical ripening agent may be used. These agents can also sometimes stimulate labor.

Mechanical Cervical Ripening

Mechanical cervical ripening methods are devices that are inserted through the vagina and into the cervix to promote cervical dilation. They are among the oldest methods to initiate labor. More recently, pharmacological prostaglandins have partially replaced mechanical methods (Jozwiak et al., 2012). These methods have a lower risk of tachysystole compared to pharmacological methods. Examples of mechanical cervical ripening methods are:

- Hygroscopic dilators (Laminaria, Lamicel, or Dilapan): Several products are available that can be placed in the cervix and promote dilation by water absorption. Laminaria is made from dried seaweed. Commercial products, such as Dilapan and Lamicel, are produced from synthetic hygroscopic material. Several dilators are inserted into the cervix— as many as will fit—and they expand over 12 to 24 hours as they absorb water. Absorption of water from the cervical tissue leads to expansion of the dilators and opening of the cervix, which releases local prostaglandin. They function similarly as the balloon catheter. Women do not need prophylactic antibiotics for the balloon catheter or hygroscopic dilators, unless specific indications exist such as need for subacute bacterial endocarditis prophylaxis. Today, they are used primarily during pregnancy termination rather than for cervical ripening in term pregnancies (Simpson, 2013).
- Balloon catheters: A 30-mL to 50-mL Foley catheter filled with saline is effective in inducing cervical ripening and dilation. The catheter is placed in the uterus and the balloon is filled.

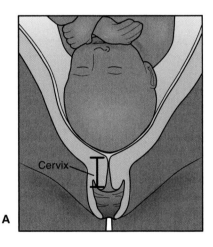

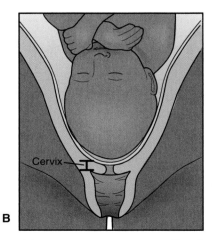

FIGURE 10–4 (*A*) Unripe cervix, cervix is not effaced or dilated. (*B*) Ripe cervix, cervix is 100% effaced and 1 cm dilated.

Direct pressure is then applied to the lower segment of the uterus and the cervix. Balloon catheters appear to be effective for pre-induction cervical ripening by causing direct pressure and overstretching of the lower uterine segment and cervix, as well as stimulating local prostaglandin release (Simpson, 2013).

Indications

- When the woman has little or no cervical effacement
- When pharmacological methods are contraindicated, such as women with prior uterine incision

Contraindications

- Active herpes
- Fetal malpresentation
- Nonreassuring fetal surveillance
- History of prior traumatic delivery
- Regular contractions
- Unexplained vaginal bleeding
- Placenta previa
- Vasa previa
- Prior uterine myomectomy involving the endometrial cavity or classical cesarean delivery
- A history of a prior low transverse cesarean delivery was considered a contraindication to induction of labor. According to the ACOG Practice Bulletin on vaginal birth after previous cesarean delivery, induction of labor is not contraindicated in women with a prior low transverse cesarean delivery; however, use of prostaglandins should be avoided in these patients due to a significantly increased risk of uterine rupture. A relative contraindication to cervical ripening is ruptured membranes. No current evidence shows that cervical ripening followed by delayed induction of labor reduces the rate of cesarean delivery.

Risks Associated With Mechanical Cervical Ripening

- Higher infection rate
- Premature rupture of membranes (PROM)

Assessment Findings

- The cervix is unripe based on SVE and Bishop score.
- Prenatal record reflects indications for induction.

Medical Management

- The physician or midwife places the mechanical dilators, which usually stay in place for 6 to 12 hours before being removed by the care provider.

Nursing Actions

- Obtain informed consent following an informative discussion as to the procedure, and so on.
- Prepare the patient and assist with the insertion procedure.
- Instruct the patient that she might experience discomfort or cramping during insertion.
- Provide ongoing emotional and informational support and encourage relaxation.
- Record the type of dilator and number of dilators or the size of the balloon placed.
- Assess onset of UCs.
- Assess FHR.

- Assess maternal temperature, as the woman is at higher risk for infection.
- Assess for ROM and vaginal bleeding.
- Assess maternal and fetal status as per institutional policy.

Pharmacological Methods of Cervical Ripening

Pharmacological methods of cervical ripening in preparation for labor induction include a variety of hormonal preparations (Table 10–3). These preparations, which are placed in or near the cervix, produce cervical ripening by causing softening and thinning of the cervix. Occasionally these agents can stimulate labor contractions. A review of research on the use of prostaglandins concluded there is an improvement in labor stimulation in vaginal birth rates in 24 hours, no increase in operative birth rates, and significant improvements in cervical favorability within 24 to 48 hours when using prostaglandins (Kelly, Kavanagh, & Thomas, 2003).

Indications

- See indications for induction.

Risks Associated With Pharmacological Methods of Cervical Ripening

- Tachysystole of the uterus

Assessment Findings

- Unripe cervix based on SVE and Bishop score of 6 or less
- Prenatal record reflecting indication for induction

Medical Management

- Determine the need for cervical ripening.
- The ACOG Committee on Obstetrics Practice recommends that misoprostol not be used to induce labor after previous cesarean section or major uterine surgery, due to a significant risk of uterine rupture.
- Insert the pharmacological agent.
  - Administration of the agent should be done at or near the labor and birthing unit.

Nursing Actions

- Obtain informed consent.
- Evaluate the prenatal record for indications and contraindications for induction (see Box 10–2).
- The major risk of the above prostaglandin preparations is uterine hyperstimulation. The woman and fetus must be monitored for contractions, fetal well-being, and changes in the cervical Bishop score.
- Document baseline cervical exam and Bishop score with SVE.
- Obtain baseline FHR.
- Monitor FHR and uterine activity as indicated based on medication and institutional policies.

Sweeping or Stripping the Membranes

Sweeping or stripping the membranes involves digital separation of the chorionic membrane from the wall of the cervix and lower

TABLE 10–3   Pharmacological Cervical Ripening Agents

MEDICATION	CERVIDIL (DINOPROSTONE INSERT)	MISOPROSTOL PGE₁ (CYTOTEC)
Dose	10 mg controlled released vaginal insert with string for removal after 12 hours	25 mcg inserted in the posterior vaginal fornix Q3–6 hrs. Not to exceed 50 mcg. A recent review reports the possibility of rare but serious adverse events, particularly uterine rupture, with misoprostol use. Oral administration is not as effective.
Nursing actions	Can be placed by perinatal nurse. Woman should remain supine or lateral position for 2 hours after insert. Continuous FHR and UC monitoring while medication is in place and for 15 minutes after removal. Oxytocin should be delayed for 30–60 minutes after removal.	Continuous FHR and UC monitoring. Oxytocin should be delayed until at least 4 hours after last dose.
Contraindications	Not recommended for women with previous cesarean section or uterine scar.	Not recommended for women with previous cesarean section or uterine scar.
Actions	UCs after 5–7 hours, tachysystole can occur within 1 hour in up to 5% of patients. Remove if tachysystole or Category II or III FHR.	Wide variations in onset of UCs. Peak action 1–2 hours. Tachysystole more common with misoprostol than with prostaglandins or oxytocin.

Simpson, 2013; Simpson & O'Brien-Abel, 2013.

uterine segment during a vaginal exam done by a primary care provider to stimulate labor. The exact mechanism of action is unclear, but it is commonly believed it releases prostaglandins and may cause maternal oxytocin release. It is most effective in first-time pregnancies with an unripe cervix.

Manual separation of the amniotic membranes from the cervix is thought to induce cervical ripening and the onset of labor. The mechanism is unknown, but mechanical disruption of this tissue has been postulated to increase local prostaglandins by the induction of phospholipase A2 in the cervical and membrane tissues. Such a postulation is certainly consistent with the known stimulation of cervical ripening by prostaglandins.

Membrane sweeping, which involves the digital separation of the membranes from the lower uterine segment during pelvic examination with a dilated cervix, is associated with a decreased risk of late-term and post-term pregnancies. Although some studies of membrane sweeping have yielded conflicting results, the most recent Cochrane Review demonstrated that membrane sweeping was associated with a significant reduction in the number of pregnancies that progressed beyond 41 weeks of gestation and that membrane sweeping may promote the onset of labor. When performed in unselected women, sweeping the membranes reduces the risk of post-term pregnancy and the use of other methods of induction of labor (Boulvain, Stan, & Irion, 2009). Women with late-term or post-term pregnancies who are considering membrane sweeping should be counseled that the procedure can be associated with vaginal bleeding and maternal discomfort. Contraindications to membrane sweeping include placenta previa and other contraindications to labor and vaginal delivery. There is insufficient data on the risks of membrane sweeping in women who are colonized with group B streptococci (GBS). Therefore, the decision to perform membrane sweeping in these women should be based on clinical judgment (ACOG, 2014b).

- The procedure is usually done in the care provider's office.
- The care provider is responsible for explaining the procedure and its risks.
- The FHR should be assessed before and after the procedure.
- The woman might experience some spotting after the procedure.
- The woman might experience mild cramping immediately after the procedure.

Indications

- See indications for oxytocin induction.

Risks Associated With Membrane Sweeping

- Infection
- Bleeding from undiagnosed placental problem
- Unplanned ROM

Assessment Findings

- Intact membranes
- Presenting part engaged
- Term gestation

Amniotomy

Amniotomy is the artificial rupture of membranes (AROM) to induce or augment labor with an amnihook during a SVE (Fig. 10–5A and B). Amniotic fluid release increases the conversion of prostaglandins following the amniotomy.

Amniotomy is most typically used to augment or shorten labor but may also be used to induce labor. There is insufficient evidence to support the value of this as a sole intervention for induction (Bricker & Luckas, 2000). This procedure is done by the primary care provider and only if an emergency delivery can be performed nearby (Gilbert, 2011). It is most effective in multiparous women who are dilated to 2 cm or more. Amniotomy in early labor increases the risk of cesarean birth for abnormal FHR.

Indications

- To stimulate labor

Contraindications

- Fetal head not engaged in the maternal pelvis
- Maternal infection such as HIV, viral hepatitis, or active genital herpes

Risks Associated With Amniotomy

- Severe variable decelerations
- Bleeding from undiagnosed vasa previa or other placental abnormality
- Umbilical cord prolapse when presenting part is not engaged

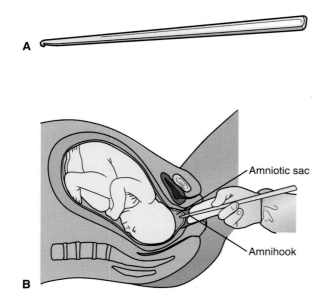

FIGURE 10–5 Amnihook and AROM procedure.

- Intraamniotic infection increases with duration of the rupture.
- A Cochrane Review of trials noted early intervention with amniotomy and oxytocin appears to be associated with a modest reduction in cesarean births (Wei et al., 2013).

Assessment Findings

- The woman leaks amniotic fluid vaginally.

Medical Management

- The procedure is done by the primary care provider with a SVE when head is engaged in the pelvis.

Nursing Actions

- Assess the FHR before, during, and immediately following ROM because of the risk of umbilical cord prolapse.
- Offer comfort and support to the woman, as the procedure may be uncomfortable.
- Assess the color, amount, and odor of amniotic fluid.
- Monitor FHR and UC pattern.
- Document the time of the AROM as well as the indication for amniotomy; amount, color, and odor of amniotic fluid; FHR characteristics before amniotomy; fetal response after the procedure; cervical status; and fetal station.
- Assess maternal temperature every 4 hours or more frequently if signs and symptoms of infection occur.
- Administer pericare, as the woman continues to leak fluid after AROM.
- Typically, nurses do not perform an amniotomy. There may be individual institutional policies allowing nurses to perform AROM under specific criteria.

External Cephalic Version

External cephalic version (ECV) refers to a procedure in which the fetus is rotated from the breech to the cephalic presentation by manipulation through the mother's abdomen (Fig. 10–6). It is typically performed as an elective procedure in nonlaboring women at or near term to improve their chances of having a vaginal cephalic birth. Women most likely to opt for ECV are those who are well informed, encouraged to undergo the procedure, believe in its safety, and desire a vaginal birth. Women may choose not to undergo ECV because of fear of the procedure, incomplete information, and preference for scheduled cesarean delivery (ACOG, 2016).

The effectiveness of ECV is based on its ability to increase the proportion of fetuses in cephalic presentation at birth and decrease the frequency of cesarean delivery. The effectiveness of ECV at term was illustrated by a 2015 systematic review of eight randomized trials (Hofmeyr, Kulier, & West, 2015). The procedure is done by the primary care provider and only if an emergency delivery can be performed nearby (Gilbert, 2011).

Indications

- To position a fetus to vertex

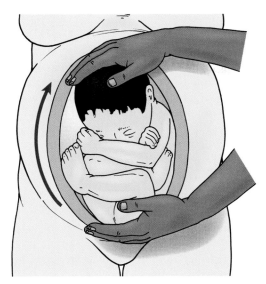

FIGURE 10–6 External cephalic version.

Contraindications

● Placental abnormalities

Risks Associated With ECV

● Severe variable decelerations
● Umbilical cord compression

Assessment Findings

● Leopold's maneuver indicates nonvertex presentation and FHR may be located in upper maternal abdomen.

Medical Management

● The procedure is done by the primary care provider with a SVE when head is engaged in the pelvis. The current recommendation for ECVs at term could reduce the need for cesarean delivery and prevent unnecessary prematurity at the expense of a potentially small increase in cesarean delivery risk.

Nursing Actions

● Fetal well-being and contraction pattern should be assessed by a nonstress test or biophysical profile before and after the procedure (ACOG, 2016). Testing should continue for at least 30 minutes after the procedure. Anti-D immune globulin should be given to Rh-negative mothers who have no plans for delivery within 72 hours after ECV.
● Offer comfort and support to the woman, as the procedure may be uncomfortable.
● Parenteral tocolysis (beta agonist) should be used if there are no contraindications.
● ECV should be attempted only in settings in which cesarean delivery services are readily available.

Labor Augmentation

Augmentation of labor is the stimulation of uterine contractions when spontaneous contractions have failed to result in progressive cervical dilation or descent of the fetus (Simpson, 2013). Wide variations in labor progress and duration occur among women in labor, and there is no consensus among experts as to the appropriate length of labor. The terms *dystocia* and *failure to progress* are sometimes used to characterize an abnormally long labor. Many providers believe there is benefit to decreasing the length of labor through augmentation with oxytocin (Simpson, 2013). Data on augmentation are usually similar to the induction rate (Menacker & Martin, 2008); thus, based on reported data, about half the women laboring in the United States have artificial labor stimulation (AWHONN, 2014). Generally, maternal-fetal status and individual clinical situations are the basis for labor management decisions. According to ACOG, contraindications to augmentation are similar to those for labor induction and may include placenta or vasa previa, umbilical cord presentation, prior classical uterine incision, active genital herpes infection, pelvic structural deformities, or invasive cervical cancer.

Labor augmentation is the stimulation of ineffective UCs after the onset of spontaneous labor to manage labor dystocia. All the principles of oxytocin induction apply to the use of oxytocin for augmentation of labor.

Lower doses of oxytocin are required for augmentation of labor because cervical resistance is lower in women in labor who have some cervical effacement and dilation. This may not be indicated in induction protocols, as some protocols have been influenced by research on active management of labor (Box 10–3).

Indications

● To strengthen and regulate UCs
● To shorten the length of labor

Contraindications

● Any contraindications for vaginal birth
● Previous vertical (classical) uterine scar or prior transfundal uterine scar
● Placental abnormalities such as complete placenta previa or vasa previa
● Abnormal fetal position
● Umbilical cord prolapse
● Active genital herpes
● Pelvic abnormalities

Risks Associated With Augmentation

● Tachysystole leading to a Category II or Category III FHR pattern is a primary complication of oxytocin in labor.

Assessment Findings

● Prolonged labor
● Inadequate UCs and inadequate labor progress

BOX 10–3 | Indications and Contraindications for Labor Augmentation

Indications

Augmentation refers to stimulation of uterine contractions when spontaneous contractions have not resulted in progressive cervical dilation, or descent of the fetus. Expectations for labor progress should be based on the most recent data regarding what constitutes normal progress of labor, based on parity and other maternal factors.

- Before augmentation, assessment of maternal pelvis and cervix and fetal position, station, and well-being should be performed.
- Augmentation should be considered if the frequency of the contractions is less than 3 contractions per 10 minutes, or if the intensity of contractions is less than 25 mm Hg above baseline, or both.

Contraindications

Contraindications to augmentation of labor are similar to those for induction of labor and may include, but are not limited to, the following:

- Placenta or vasa previa
- Umbilical cord presentation
- Prior classical uterine incision
- Active genital herpes infection
- Pelvic structural deformities
- Invasive cervical cancer

Simpson, 2013.

Medical Management

- Determine the need for labor augmentation.
- Be available to respond to complications of using oxytocin to augment labor.

Nursing Actions

- Administer low-dose oxytocin starting at 0.5 mU/min and increasing the dose by 1 to 2 mU/min every 30 to 60 minutes as recommended.
- Monitor FHR and UCs. FHR and UCs are typically continuously monitored, but intermittent monitoring is within the standard of care (see Chapter 9).
- Follow the same principles of nursing care for induction of labor.
- Decrease or discontinue oxytocin in the event of uterine tachysystole or Category II (indeterminate) or Category III (abnormal) FHR.

Complementary Therapies to Stimulate Labor

Over decades, many strategies have been proposed to initiate and/or augment labor. For example, acupuncture may stimulate the uterus. Other practices include bowel stimulation with castor oil or an enema to increase prostaglandin production. Cochrane Reviews of complementary therapies indicate further research is needed to determine the effectiveness of most therapies to stimulate or induce labor (Kelly, Kavanagh, & Thomas, 2001). Complementary therapies may include:

- Herbal preparations:
  - Black cohosh
  - Blue cohosh
  - Evening primrose oil
  - Raspberry leaves may be taken orally to promote prostaglandin or oxytocin production.
- Sexual intercourse:
  - Semen contains prostaglandin to open the cervix, and orgasm may be associated with prostaglandin and oxytocin release.

OPERATIVE VAGINAL DELIVERY

Operative vaginal delivery is a vaginal birth that is assisted by vacuum extraction or forceps. In the United States, 3.1% of all deliveries in 2015 were accomplished via an operative vaginal approach (Martin, Hamilton, Osterman, Driscoll, & Mathews, 2017). Forceps deliveries accounted for 0.56% of vaginal births, and vacuum deliveries accounted for 2.58% of vaginal births. However, there is a wide range in the prevalence of operative vaginal delivery both across and within geographic regions in the United States (1% to 23%), which suggests that evidence-based guidelines for operative vaginal delivery are either inadequate or randomly applied, or familiarity and expertise with the technique is declining (Wegner & Bernstein, 2017).

Use of forceps and vacuum extraction continued to decline in 2015. Use of either method of instrumental delivery decreased from 3.21% in 2014 to 3.14% in 2015 (down from 9.01% in 1990). Use of forceps remains the rarer method, essentially remaining steady in 2015 at 0.56% (from 0.57% in 2014), compared with vacuum extraction, which declined from 2.64% to 2.58%. (Martin, Hamilton, Osterman, Driscoll, & Mathews, 2017). Since 1996, the rate of cesarean birth has increased and the percentage of operative vaginal deliveries with either forceps or vacuum extraction has decreased 45% over 10 years, from 9.4% to 4.5% (Martin et al., 2011).

Indications for operative vaginal delivery are to improve maternal or fetal status by shortening the second stage of labor. Facilitating birth and shortening the second stage of labor can be performed only by care providers with hospital privileges for these procedures. Although sometimes indicated, operative vaginal birth is not without risk of complications to the woman and the fetus. Specific guidelines for the use of forceps and vacuum extraction

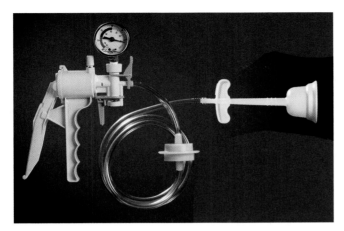

FIGURE 10–7 Vacuum device. *Source: © CooperSurgical.*

are provided, and use of only *one* method, either forceps or vacuum, for an individual patient is recommended. If attempts are unsuccessful, the physician proceeds with a cesarean birth. While operative vaginal delivery is acceptable in appropriate circumstances, it requires an operator who understands the indications and prerequisites and is skilled in the technique. For this reason, the diminishing training and experience in operative vaginal delivery nationally is of concern (ACOG, 2014c; Spong et al., 2012).

Vacuum-Assisted Delivery

Vacuum-assisted delivery or vacuum extraction is a birth involving the use of a vacuum cup on the fetal head to assist with delivery of the head (Fig. 10–7). The cup is placed on the fetal head and suction is increased gradually until a seal is formed. Gentle traction is then applied to deliver the fetal head (Fig. 10–8).

The rate of vacuum-assisted delivery, which had increased by 77% between 1989 (3.5%) and 1997 (6.2%), has since decreased to below 3% (Martin et al., 2017). Some advantages to the use of vacuum over forceps include:

- Easier application.
- Less anesthesia required.
- Less maternal soft tissue damage.
- Fewer fetal injuries.

Current guidelines for vacuum application are as follows:

- The fetal head needs to be engaged and the cervix completely dilated.
- There should be a maximum of three attempts for a period of 15 minutes: the "three-pull rule."
- Cup detachment from the fetal head (pops off the vacuum) is a warning sign that too much pressure or ineffective force is being exerted on the fetal head.
- The physician should proceed with a cesarean birth when vacuum attempts are not successful.

Indications

- Suspicion of immediate or potential fetal compromise
- Need to shorten the second stage for maternal benefit

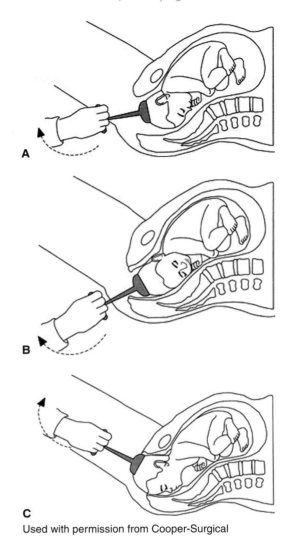

A

B

C

Used with permission from Cooper-Surgical

FIGURE 10–8 Vacuum delivery. *Source: © CooperSurgical.*

- Prolonged second stage
  - Nulliparous woman with lack of continuing progress for 3 hours with regional anesthesia, or for 2 hours without anesthesia
  - Multiparous woman with lack of continuous progress for 2 hours with regional anesthesia, or for 1 hour without regional anesthesia (ACOG, 2015)

Risks for the Woman

- Vaginal and cervical lacerations
- Extension of episiotomy
- Hemorrhage related to uterine atony, uterine rupture
- Bladder trauma
- Perineal wound infection

Risks for the Newborn

- Cephalohematoma (15%) and therefore increased risk of jaundice (Fig. 10–9)

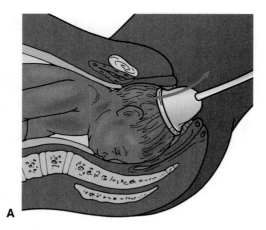

A

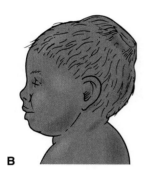

B

FIGURE 10–9 Cephalohematoma.

- Intracranial hemorrhage and retinal hemorrhage
- Scalp lacerations or bruising (10%)

Assessment Findings

- Fetus at 36 weeks' gestation and the fetal head is engaged, at least 0 station in the maternal pelvis (Cunningham et al., 2014)

Medical Management

- Explain the procedure and obtain the woman's consent.
- Place the vacuum appropriately.
- Routine use of episiotomy is no longer recommended because of prolonged healing, increased pain, and potential for third- and fourth-degree tears (ACOG, 2015).
- After three unsuccessful attempts, proceed with a cesarean birth.
- The recommendations of the manufacturer of the vacuum device should be followed.

Nursing Actions

- Assess the woman's comfort level.
- Urinary bladder may be emptied by provider or nurse to decrease risk of trauma.
- Educate and reassure the woman and her family.
- Anticipate potential complications for the woman and the newborn.

- Pump up the vacuum manually to the pressure indicated on the pump, not to exceed 500 to 600 mm Hg.
  - Cup detachment (pop off) is a warning sign that too much ineffective force is being exerted on the fetal head.
- Pressure should be released between contractions.
- The vacuum procedure should be timed from insertion of the cup into the vagina until the birth, and the cup should not be on the fetal head for longer than 15 to 20 minutes.
  - Adherence to the guidelines for the vacuum device related to pressure and maximum time will minimize the nurse's liability in vacuum-assisted vaginal births.

Forceps-Assisted Delivery

Forceps-assisted birth is one in which an instrument is used to assist with delivery of the fetal head, typically done to improve the health of the woman or the fetus. The rate of forceps delivery has decreased over the last 20 years from 5.55% to only 1% (Martin et al., 2011). Outlet forceps are used when the head is visible on the perineum and the skull has reached the pelvic floor, and rotation is less than 45 degrees (Fig. 10–10). Low forceps are used when the skull is at +2 station or lower in the maternal pelvis and not on the pelvic floor and rotation is greater than 45 degrees (Fig. 10–11). Only outlet and low forceps are currently recommended for use in assisting delivery.

Indications

- The fetal head engaged and the cervix is completely dilated.
- There is suspicion of immediate or potential fetal compromise.
- To shorten the second stage for maternal benefit (e.g., maternal exhaustion and/or fetal compromise)
- Prolonged second stage
  - Nulliparous woman with lack of continuing progress for 3 hours with regional anesthesia, or for 2 hours without anesthesia
  - Multiparous woman with lack of continuous progress for 2 hours with regional anesthesia, or for 1 hour without regional anesthesia
- High level of regional anesthesia that inhibits pushing

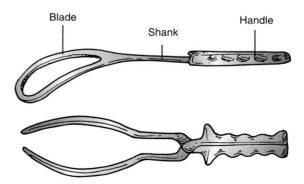

Blade   Shank   Handle

FIGURE 10–10 Outlet forceps.

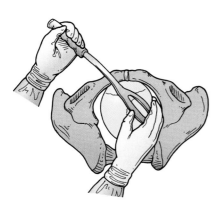
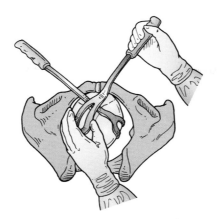
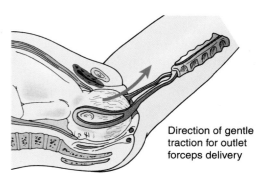

Direction of gentle traction for outlet forceps delivery

FIGURE 10–11 Forceps delivery.

● Maternal cardiac or pulmonary disease that contraindicates pushing efforts

Risks for the Woman

● Vaginal and cervical lacerations
● Extension of episiotomy
● Hemorrhage related to uterine atony, uterine rupture
● Perineal hematoma
● Bladder trauma
● Perineal wound infection

Risks for the Newborn

● Cephalohematoma
● Nerve injuries, including craniofacial and brachial plexus injuries
● Skin lacerations or bruising
● Skull fractures
● Intracranial hemorrhage

Assessment Findings

● The cervix is completely dilated and the membranes are ruptured.
● The fetal head is engaged.
● The woman has adequate anesthesia.

Medical Management

● Use only on a fetus that is at least 34 weeks' gestation (ACOG, 2015).
● Explain the procedure and obtain the woman's consent.
● Routine use of episiotomy is no longer recommended because of prolonged healing, increased pain, and potential for third- and fourth-degree tears (ACOG, 2015).
● Place forceps appropriately.

Nursing Actions

● Assess the woman's anesthesia level and comfort level.
● Insert a straight catheter to empty the bladder to decrease the risk of bladder trauma and increase room for the fetal head and forceps.

● Provide emotional support for the woman and her partner, since use of forceps can increase anxiety level.
● Document the type of forceps, number of applications, and time of application.
● Anticipate potential complications for the woman and the neonate.

OPERATIVE BIRTH

Cesarean birth is a common operation performed on women, with reported rates varying across the world (Fig. 10–12). In developed countries, cesarean birth accounts for 21.3% of births in the United Kingdom; 23% in Northern Ireland; 23.3% in Australia; 32.9% in the United States; and more than 50% in some private hospitals in Chile, Argentina, Brazil, and Paraguay (Viswanathan et al., 2006). The cesarean section rate in the United States is 60% higher than the 1996 rate of 20.7%. Based on current data, 49.5% of women age 40 or

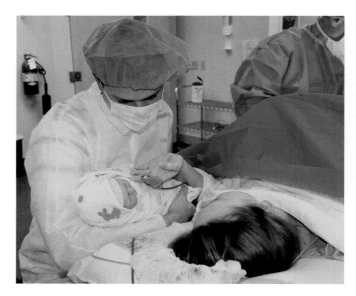

FIGURE 10–12 Family in cesarean birth.

older deliver by cesarean section (Martin et al., 2011). The benefits and harms of elective cesarean birth, repeat cesarean birth, and vaginal birth after cesarean (VBAC) are under vigorous debate. Because cesarean birth accounts for one-third of births in the United States, Chapter 12 is devoted to care of cesarean woman and their families. Despite recommendations from ACOG on the safety of this, there has been a decrease in the rate of VBAC, which fell from 4% to 1% of all deliveries in 2008. At the same time, the rate of repeat C-section nearly doubled. As a result, nearly all childbirths after a previous C-section (91%) were a repeat C-section (Podulka, Stranges, & Steiner, 2011).

Vaginal Birth After a Cesarean

VBAC is used to describe labor and vaginal birth in a woman who has had a prior cesarean birth. A trial of labor after cesarean (TOLAC) offers women the opportunity to achieve a VBAC. Evidence suggests that benefits of VBAC outweigh risks in women with lower uterine transverse cesarean birth who have no contraindications for a vaginal birth. Benefits of VBAC include shorter recovery time and overall lower morbidity and mortality, including less blood loss, fewer infections, and fewer thromboembolic problems (ACOG, 2010). Additionally, ACOG notes for those considering larger families, VBAC may avoid potential future maternal consequences of multiple cesarean deliveries such as hysterectomy, bowel or bladder injury, transfusion, infection, and abnormal placentation such as placenta previa and placenta accreta.

According to ACOG, most women with one previous cesarean birth with a low transverse incision are candidates for vaginal birth after cesarean birth and should be counseled about VBAC and offered a trial of labor (ACOG, 2010). This is reported to be related to more conservative ACOG practice guidelines, legal pressure, and the continuing debate over the harms and benefits of vaginal birth compared with cesarean birth and an increase in repeat cesarean births. VBAC is associated with a small but important risk of uterine rupture, and that risk increases with the number of previous cesarean births. The following are important definitions regarding VBAC delivery:

- A TOLAC is a planned attempt to labor by a woman who has previously undergone a cesarean delivery and desires a subsequent vaginal delivery.
- A VBAC is a "successful" trial of labor resulting in a vaginal birth.
- A TOLAC may result in either a "successful" VBAC or a "failed" trial of labor resulting in a repeat cesarean delivery.
- A repeat cesarean delivery (RCD) may be planned and scheduled beforehand and thus is an elective repeat cesarean delivery (ERCD). If the woman who plans an ERCD enters spontaneous labor before the scheduled date, this is still considered an ERCD even if delivery is unscheduled. The woman with a failed TOLAC undergoes a RCD that is unplanned and unscheduled.

Benefits of VBAC

The benefits of a TOLAC resulting in a VBAC include the following:

- Shorter length of hospital stay and postpartum recovery (in most cases)
- Fewer complications, such as postpartum fever, wound or uterine infection, thromboembolism (blood clots in the leg or lung), need for blood transfusion
- Fewer neonatal breathing problems

Risks of VBAC

The risks of an attempted VBAC or TOLAC include the following:

- Risk of failed TOLAC without a VBAC resulting in RCD in about 20% to 40% of women who attempt VBAC.
- Risk of rupture of uterus resulting in an emergency cesarean delivery. The risk of uterine rupture may be related in part to the type of uterine incision made during the first cesarean delivery. A previous transverse uterine incision has the lowest risk of rupture (0.2% to 1.5% risk). Vertical or T-shaped uterine incisions have a higher risk of uterine rupture (4% to 9% risk). It is important to remember that the direction of the skin incision does not indicate the type or direction of the uterine incision; a woman with a transversal (bikini) skin incision may have a vertical uterine incision.
- While women who attempt TOLAC and VBAC have a low risk of uterine rupture, the risk of uterine rupture is higher with VBAC than with RCD.
- The risk of fetal death is very low with both VBAC and ERCD, but the likelihood of fetal death is higher with VBAC than with ERCD. Maternal death is very rare with either type of delivery.

Candidates for TOLAC/VBAC

- Both ACOG and the National Institutes of Health (NIH) suggest that a TOLAC to attempt a VBAC is an acceptable option for a woman who has undergone one prior cesarean delivery with a low transverse uterine incision, assuming there are no other conditions that would normally require a cesarean delivery such as placenta previa.
- ACOG further suggests that a woman with two prior low transverse uterine incisions, or a woman with a twin pregnancy, or a woman who requires induction of labor may also be considered candidates for VBAC with appropriate counseling.
- TOLAC with anticipated VBAC should be attempted only in those facilities capable of performing emergency cesarean deliveries and those with an appropriate nursing staff, anesthesia team, operating room, and obstetrician or other surgeon immediately available in case an emergency cesarean delivery becomes necessary.
- A woman considering VBAC should discuss with her health care provider the risks and benefits of VBAC versus ERCD, and the discussion should include plans for intervention in

case of uterine rupture or another indication for an emergency cesarean delivery.

● Unlike most medical decisions in which patients are comparing risks and benefits for themselves, the pregnant patient must compare risks and benefits for both herself and her fetus, and the risks and benefits for these two individuals sometimes do not align. A decision that increases maternal risk may be associated with fetal benefit.

● Good, consistent evidence exists indicating that a woman who has had only one previous cesarean delivery using a transverse lower segment hysterotomy incision has the lowest risk of uterine scar separation during a subsequent trial of labor; thus, TOLAC is a reasonably safe option for delivery for these women. In this setting, the body of evidence suggests a TOLAC success rate of 60% to 80%, with an estimated uterine rupture rate of 0.4% to 0.7%. Success rates are higher in patients with additional characteristics, such as a prior vaginal delivery (Cunningham & Wells, 2017).

Management During Labor

In many ways, a woman who attempts VBAC is managed similarly to other women anticipating a vaginal delivery. A fetal monitor may be used to observe the baby's heart rate and monitor for early signs of fetal distress. Medications to induce labor or improve contractions (e.g., oxytocin) are used cautiously since they can increase the risk of uterine rupture. If problems occur during labor, a cesarean delivery will likely be recommended. Waiting for spontaneous labor, thus avoiding cervical ripening agents and oxytocin, appears to significantly decrease the risk of uterine rupture for women attempting VBAC. ACOG supports the use of oxytocin for induction and augmentation of labor in women with a previous cesarean delivery. Misoprostol (prostaglandin E1) should not be used for cervical ripening or labor induction in the third trimester in women with prior uterine incisions and use of other prostaglandins is also strongly discouraged.

VBAC Success Rates

In general, 60% to 80% of women considered candidates for a TOLAC to attempt a VBAC will have a successful vaginal birth (Cunningham & Wells, 2017). Factors that increase the chances for a successful VBAC include:

● A previous vaginal delivery, especially a previous VBAC.
● Spontaneous onset of labor (labor is not induced).
● Normal progress of labor, including dilation and effacement (thinning) of the cervix.
● Prior cesarean delivery performed because the baby's position was abnormal (e.g., breech).
● Only one prior cesarean delivery.
● The prior cesarean delivery was performed early in labor, and not after full cervical dilatation.

A woman with a singleton gestation who has undergone only one previous cesarean delivery performed using a transverse lower segment hysterotomy incision has the lowest risk of uterine scar separation during a subsequent trial of labor; thus, TOLAC is a reasonably safe option for delivery for these women. In this setting, TOLAC success rates are 60% to 80%, with an estimated uterine rupture rate of 0.4% to 0.7%. Success rates are higher in patients with additional characteristics, such as a previous successful TOLAC, previous vaginal delivery, previous cesarean delivery for nonvertex presentation, and in women with spontaneous onset of labor (Cunningham & Wells, 2017).

Indications

● One or two prior low transverse cesarean births with no other uterine scars
● Experts suggest a TOLAC to attempt a VBAC is an acceptable option for a woman who has undergone one prior cesarean delivery with a low transverse uterine incision.
● Guidelines also suggest that a woman with two prior low transverse uterine incisions, a woman with a twin pregnancy, or a woman who requires induction of labor may also be considered candidates for VBAC with appropriate counseling.
● One or two TOLAC with anticipated VBAC should be attempted only in those facilities capable of performing emergency cesarean.
● Clinically adequate pelvis
● Physician and OR team immediately available to perform emergent cesarean birth.

Contraindications

● Prior vertical (classical) or T-shaped uterine incision or other uterine surgery (Fig. 10–13)
● Previous uterine rupture
● Pelvic abnormalities
● Medical or obstetric complications that preclude a vaginal birth
● Inability to perform an emergent cesarean birth if necessary because of insufficient personnel such as surgeons, anesthesia, or facility

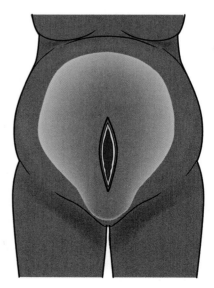

FIGURE 10–13 Vertical uterine incision.

Risks Associated With VBAC

- Uterine rupture and complications associated with uterine rupture (1%)
  - Waiting for spontaneous labor and avoiding use of prostaglandins and oxytocin reduces the risk of uterine rupture.
- A failed TOLAC is associated with more complications than elective repeat cesarean delivery.
- Uterine rupture or dehiscence is the outcome associated with TOLAC that most significantly increases the chance of additional maternal and neonatal morbidity.
- Neonatal morbidity is higher in the setting of a failed TOLAC than in a VBAC.

Assessment Findings

- Records confirm prior transverse uterine scar.

Medical Management

- Explain the risks and benefits of VBAC.
- Induction of labor for maternal or fetal indications remains an option in women undergoing TOLAC.
- Use of misoprostol for cervical ripening is contraindicated.
- The physician and surgical team must be available to perform a cesarean birth if necessary.

Nursing Actions

- Review the prenatal record for documentation of prior uterine scar because VBAC is contraindicated in vertical uterine incisions.
- Closely and continuously monitor uterine activity and FHR.
- Assess the progress of labor.
- Provide information, reassurance, and support to the woman.
- Report any complaints of severe pain and be alert to signs of uterine rupture such as vaginal bleeding and ascending station of fetal presenting part.

OBSTETRIC COMPLICATIONS

Complications during birth can emerge abruptly without warning or risk factors. More often, they are a result of pregnancy-associated or preexisting risks. Regardless, women experiencing complications in labor and birth need special attention and support provided by nurses in the perinatal setting.

Pregnancy-Related Complications in Labor

Most pregnancy-related complications have the potential to impact labor. For example, diabetic women in labor need continuous glucose monitoring because hyperglycemia impacts placental perfusion. Another example is preeclampsia, where vasospasm related to the pathophysiology of preeclampsia also diminishes perfusion and impacts both maternal and fetal outcomes. Refer to Chapter 7 for management and care of patients with these disorders. Several pregnancy-related complications are presented here as examples.

CRITICAL COMPONENT

Nursing Care and Support for Birth Complications

Perinatal nurses can have a profound influence on the labor and birth care provided in the hospital setting, thereby influencing birth outcomes (Adams, Stark, & Low, 2016). Ideally, a hospital perinatal nurse is present with a family for the entire labor and birth process. In a high-risk pregnancy, the woman and her family may be known to the nurses and the same nurse may care for the woman over several days. In this situation, the nurse has an opportunity to form a stronger bond with the patient and enhance trust and therapeutic communication through continuity of care.

Nurses are responsible for assessing maternal and fetal well-being; administering procedures and monitoring their effectiveness; providing nursing interventions to assist with a laboring woman's physical, emotional, and spiritual needs; rendering care related to the birth process, whether vaginal or cesarean; initiating newborn care; and providing care during the early postpartum period. Perinatal nurses also provide advocacy and teaching for women during the birth process, communication with health care providers, and documentation (Adams et al., 2016).

When a woman is experiencing complications in labor or during birth, they experience increased fear and anxiety for themselves and their baby. Effective therapeutic communication with the woman and her family is essential and may help the woman to remain an active decision maker. Women experiencing complications or emergencies need ongoing information they can understand, reassurance, and physical, emotional, and spiritual support to help them to navigate the sometimes treacherous path of labor and birth.

The complexity of communication between mothers and health care team members during labor and birth increases the potential for error and safety issues. The combination of physiological, emotional, relational, and contextual factors that influence labor contribute to the challenge of communication, and nuanced and quickly evolving situations make it more difficult to maintain the shared understanding necessary for successful teamwork. Unrecognized differences in clinical goals and divergent understandings of risks and benefits may increase safety threats (Jacobson, Zlatnik, Kennedy, & Lyndon, 2013).

Post-Term Pregnancy and Birth

Post-term pregnancy refers to a pregnancy that has reached or extended beyond 42 weeks' gestation, dated from the last menstrual period; a late-term pregnancy is defined as one that has reached between 41 0/7 weeks and 41 6/7 weeks of gestation. In 2011, the overall incidence of post-term pregnancy in the

United States was 5.5% (Hamilton, Martin, & Ventura, 2012). About 5% to 10% of pregnancies continue beyond 294 days (42 completed weeks) and are described as being "post-term" or "postdate" (Cunningham et al., 2014). The incidence of post-term pregnancies may vary by population, in part as a result of differences in regional management practices for pregnancies that go beyond the estimated date of delivery. Accurate determination of gestational age is essential for accurate diagnosis and appropriate management of late-term and post-term pregnancies. Antepartum fetal surveillance and induction of labor have been evaluated as strategies to decrease the risks of perinatal morbidity and mortality associated with late-term and post-term pregnancies (ACOG, 2014b). The etiology of most pregnancies that are late-term or post-term is unknown. However, several risk factors for post-term pregnancy have been identified, including nulliparity, prior post-term pregnancy, carrying a male fetus, and maternal obesity (ACOG, 2014b).

Postmaturity refers to the abnormal condition of the newborn resulting from prolonged pregnancy. Both the woman and infant are at increased risk of adverse events when the pregnancy continues beyond term. After 41 weeks, neonatal and postneonatal death risk increase significantly (Gülmezoglu, Crowther, & Middleton, 2006). ACOG (2014b) concludes that induction of labor between 41 0/7 and 42 0/7 weeks can be considered and induction of labor after 42 0/7 weeks and by 42 6/7 weeks of gestation is recommended based on evidence of an increase in perinatal morbidity and mortality

The risk of stillbirth increases beyond 41 weeks. Additional fetal risks of post-term pregnancies include macrosomia, which increases the likelihood of operative vaginal deliveries, cesarean deliveries, and shoulder dystocia, as well as neonatal seizures, meconium aspiration syndrome, and low 5-minute Apgar scores. Oligohydramnios is more common in post-term pregnancies and has been associated with cord compression, FHR abnormalities, meconium-stained amniotic fluid, and fetal acidosis. Maternal risks are generally those associated with macrosomia and related dysfunctional labors, including severe perineal lacerations, infection, and postpartum hemorrhage:

- Induction of labor with an unfavorable cervix
- Cesarean birth
- Prolonged labor
- Postpartum hemorrhage
- Traumatic birth

It is likely that some of these unwanted outcomes result from intervening when the uterus and cervix are not ready for labor. First-trimester pregnancy ultrasound is associated with a reduced incidence of post-term pregnancy, possibly by avoiding incorrect dating and misclassification of postdates. Induction of labor is widely practiced to try to prevent the problems mentioned above and to improve the health outcome for women and their infants.

- Labor induction may itself cause problems, especially when the cervix is not ripe.
- The ideal timing for induction of labor is not clear. In the past, there was a tendency to await spontaneous labor until 42 completed weeks.

- Current practice is to offer induction of labor between 41 and 42 weeks. Data indicating an increased risk of stillbirth at or beyond 41 weeks' gestation and initiation of antepartum fetal surveillance at or beyond 41 weeks' gestation is common (ACOG, 2014b).

The gestational age and the cervix being unfavorable (unripe) may affect the success of the induction of labor and result in an increase in cesarean birth rates.

- When the cervix is favorable (usually a Bishop score of 6 or more), induction is often carried out via oxytocin and AROM.
- If the cervix is not favorable, usually a prostaglandin gel or tablet is placed in the vagina or cervix to ripen the cervix and to initiate the UCs and labor. Many protocols are used with varying repeat intervals and transition to oxytocin and amniotomy depending on the onset of UCs and progress of cervical dilation.

Risks to the Mother

Risks to the mother are related to the larger size of post-term fetuses and include difficulties during labor, an increase in injury to the perineum (including the vagina, labia, and rectum), and an increased rate of cesarean birth with its associated risks of bleeding, infection, and injury to surrounding organs (Norwitz, 2017). Obstetric complications are more likely with increased gestational age, and risks of severe perineal laceration, infection, postpartum hemorrhage, and cesarean delivery increase in women with late-term and post-term pregnancies. In addition, some studies suggest that maternal anxiety is increased as pregnancies approach the post-term period (ACOG, 2014b).

Risks to the Fetus

- Stillbirth or neonatal death: The incidence of stillbirth or infant death is increased in pregnancies that continue beyond 42 weeks. However, the risk is relatively small, with only 4 to 7 deaths per 1,000 deliveries. By comparison, the risk of stillbirth or infant death in pregnancies between 37 and 42 weeks is 2 to 3 per 1,000 deliveries.
- Macrosomia: Post-term fetuses have a greater chance of developing complications related to larger body size (macrosomia), which is defined as weighing more than 4,500 grams, or about 10 pounds. There is a twofold increase in macrosomia believed to contribute to the increased risks of operative vaginal delivery, cesarean delivery, and shoulder dystocia observed in post-term pregnancies.
- Fetal dysmaturity: Also called *post-maturity syndrome,* this refers to a fetus whose growth in the uterus after the due date has been restricted, usually due to a problem with delivery of placental blood flow to the fetus. Postmaturity syndrome complicates 10% to 20% of post-term pregnancies. Post-mature fetuses have decreased subcutaneous fat and lack vernix and lanugo. Meconium staining of the amniotic fluid, skin, membranes, and umbilical cord often is seen in association with a post-mature newborn.

● Oligohydramnios: This occurs more frequently in post-term pregnancies than in pregnancies at less than 42 weeks' gestation. Pregnancies complicated by oligohydramnios have an increased risk of FHR abnormalities, umbilical cord compression, meconium-stained fluid, umbilical cord artery blood pH of less than 7, and lower Apgar scores (ACOG, 2014b). Oligohydramnios has been commonly defined as a single deep vertical pocket of amniotic fluid of 2 cm or less (not containing umbilical cord or fetal extremities) or an amniotic fluid index of 5 cm or less.

● Meconium aspiration: Beyond term, the fetus is more likely to have a bowel movement, called meconium, into the amniotic fluid. If the fetus is stressed, there is a chance it will inhale some of this meconium-stained amniotic fluid; this can cause breathing problems when the baby is born.

● Prolonged pregnancy: This results in a decrease in amniotic fluid volume and may impact fetal status because amniotic fluid cushions the fetus and cord from pressure and injury and amniotic fluid volume is an indicator of placental function.

● Decreased placental reserve: This occurs as the placenta begins to age, as there are increased areas of infarction and deposition of calcium and fibrin within its tissue (Fig. 10–14).

● Meconium-stained fluid: This occurs in 25% to 30% of post-term pregnancies. This creates an increased risk for meconium aspiration of the neonate at birth (Cunningham et al., 2014).

● Fetal macrosomia: There is an increased risk for this as the fetus increases in size, approximately 1 ounce per day after term.

Assessment Findings

● Category II or III FHR related to decreased amniotic fluid and uteroplacental insufficiency with aging placenta
● Meconium-stained fluid
● Women report increased anxiety and frustration with prolonged pregnancy
● Fetal macrosomia

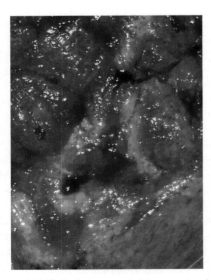

FIGURE 10–14 Calcified placenta are white areas in placenta.

Medical Management

● Antenatal surveillance
● Induction of labor offered at 41 weeks' gestation

Nursing Actions

● Review the plan of care with the woman.
● Confirm prolonged pregnancy on the prenatal record.
● Anticipate management with induction of labor and possible cervical ripening agents.
● Monitor FHR because of increased incidence of uteroplacental insufficiency.
● Assess amniotic fluid for amount and meconium staining with ROM (see Concept Map for post-term pregnancy and labor induction).

CRITICAL COMPONENT

Post-Dates and Post-Term Induction of Labor

Because late-term and post-term pregnancies are associated with an increased risk of perinatal morbidity and mortality, induction of labor between 41 and 42 weeks' gestation can be considered. Induction of labor after 42 0/7 weeks and by 42 6/7 weeks of gestation is recommended given evidence of an increase in perinatal morbidity and mortality (ACOG, 2014a). Membrane sweeping is associated with a decreased risk of late-term and post-term pregnancies. Initiation of antepartum fetal surveillance at or beyond 41 weeks' gestation may be indicated, and a trial of labor after cesarean delivery is an option for uncomplicated post-term pregnancies (ACOG, 2014a).

ACOG, 2014a.

Meconium-Stained Fluid and Birth

In 10% to 20% of deliveries, there is meconium in the amniotic fluid. In utero, meconium passage results from neural stimulation of a maturing gastrointestinal (GI) tract, usually due to fetal hypoxic stress. As the fetus approaches term, the GI tract matures, and vagal stimulation from head or spinal cord compression may cause peristalsis and relaxation of the rectal sphincter, leading to meconium passage. Meconium-stained amniotic fluid may be aspirated by the fetus before or during labor and delivery. Aspiration of meconium results in respiratory distress that in severe cases can be life-threatening. There is strong suggestive evidence that prevention of meconium aspiration, by its removal from the respiratory tract, can ameliorate or prevent the majority of cases of severe meconium aspiration syndrome (MAS). This aspiration induces hypoxia via four major pulmonary effects: airway obstruction, surfactant dysfunction, chemical pneumonitis, and pulmonary hypertension (Geis, 2017).

Risks Associated With Meconium-Stained Fluid

● MAS in the neonate

Assessment Findings

● Meconium-stained amniotic fluid

Medical Management

● All infants with meconium in the amniotic fluid should have their nose, mouth, and pharynx suctioned as soon as the head is delivered (intrapartum suctioning) regardless of whether the meconium is thin or thick.

Nursing Actions

● Alert the neonatal team, as meconium-stained amniotic fluid is a condition that requires notification and availability of an appropriately credentialed team with full resuscitation skills, including endotracheal intubation.
● Infants with meconium-stained amniotic fluid, regardless of whether they are vigorous or not, should no longer routinely receive intubation. However, meconium-stained amniotic fluid is a condition that requires the notification and availability of an appropriately credentialed team with full resuscitation skills, including endotracheal intubation. Resuscitation should follow the same principles for infants with meconium-stained fluid as for those with clear fluid (ACOG 2017a).

Multiple Gestation Birth

The patient with a multiple gestation pregnancy is at higher risk for many complications during the intrapartum period, including preterm birth, preeclampsia, and hemorrhage. With a mean gestational delivery age of 35 weeks for twins, 32 weeks for triplets, and 29.5 weeks for quadruplets, preparing for delivery of multiples is both high-risk and complex (Malone & D'Alton, 2014). Decisions on method of delivery are dependent on numerous factors, including number of fetuses; position of presentation of fetuses, particularly the presenting fetus (twin A); and fetal weight. If the first twin is in a vertex presentation, vaginal delivery may be attempted. It is common for women to be delivered by cesarean birth with twins, though in some cases both twins can be born vaginally or twin A vaginally and twin B by cesarean. There are three routes for twin births: both vaginal, both by cesarean, or twin A vaginally and twin B by cesarean. Common practice in high-order multiple gestations is cesarean delivery at a rate of nearly 95% (Parfitt, 2016). See Chapter 7 for more on multiple gestation pregnancy and Chapter 9 for fetal monitoring with multiples.

Risks Associated With Multiple-Gestation Labor and Delivery

● Preterm labor
● Labor dystocia
● Antepartum hemorrhage (i.e., abruptio placentae) (Parfitt, 2016)
● Stillbirth

Assessment Findings

● Multiple fetuses may be assessed by Leopold's maneuver, but ultrasound is the most definitive assessment of more than one fetus, as well as fetal position (Parfitt, 2016).

● Auscultation may show more than one fetal heartbeat (Bowers, 2014).

Medical Management

● Method of delivery is determined based on fetal presentation, subsequent fetal position, and other medical considerations (AAP & ACOG, 2012; Malone & D'Alton, 2014). Ultrasound is done upon admission to confirm fetal presentations and placental locations.
● Hospital birth with a Level II or Level III nursery
● Two experienced obstetricians or one OB and one certified nurse-midwife
● Delivery is done in a surgical suite.

Nursing Actions

● Provide anticipatory guidance related to procedures and the birth. Discuss the number of persons and personnel present at the birth of multiples (Bowers, 2014). Explore the parents' birth plans and desires.
● Ensure placement of large-bore IV for fluid replacement in case of hemorrhage or need for emergency fluid replacement and anesthesia administration (Parfitt, 2016).
● Continuous FHR monitoring for each fetus and once membranes are ruptured, internal monitoring for twin A.
● Have a hemorrhage cart and/or medications available.
● Anesthesia provider, circulating nurse, and scrub nurse should be present.
● Ensure ultrasound access to confirm position of twin B after birth of twin A.
● Neonatal team should be present for each twin.
● Have type and cross-match blood available.

Stillbirth/Intrauterine Fetal Demise

Stillbirth, or intrauterine fetal demise (IUFD), is defined as a fetal death after 20 weeks' gestation (Parfitt, 2016). According to the Centers for Disease Control and Prevention (CDC) and the National Center for Health Statistics, approximately 26,000 fetal deaths past 20 weeks' gestation occur in the United States annually (MacDorman, Kirmeyer, and Wilson, 2012).

Further discussion of the care of families experiencing an IUFD can be found related to postpartum nursing care in Chapter 17.

Risk Factors

● Although maternal and gestational factors play a role in determining risk factors for stillbirth/IUFD, nearly half of cases have an unknown etiology.
● Risk for fetal mortality is greater among adolescents younger than age 15 and women older than 45 (MacDorman et al., 2012).
● Disparities in fetal mortality among women of different races demonstrate an association between IUFD and both low-income and minimal access to quality health care; however, the disparity remains unexplained. Health care access and socioeconomic and education levels also play a vital role.

- Severe medical maternal complications with diabetes, renal disease, cardiovascular disease, thyroid disease, connective tissue disease and autoimmune disease, malnutrition, maternal trauma, placental abruption, obesity.
- Drug and alcohol use (Troiano, Chez, & Harvey, 2013).
- Post-term pregnancy (more than 2 weeks beyond the estimated date of delivery).
- Extreme prematurity, congenital or genetic abnormalities, making the fetus incompatible with life, or cord accidents.
- Infections such as human parvovirus B19, syphilis, streptococcal, and listeria (Troiano et al., 2013).

Risks Associated With Intrauterine Fetal Demise

- Prolonged retention of the dead fetus may lead to the development of disseminated intravascular coagulation (DIC) in the mother and puts the mother at higher risk for infection, which can result in sepsis or endometritis.

Assessment Findings

- Decreased or absent fetal movement for several hours or more
- Symptoms related to underlying cause of stillbirth
- IUFD is confirmed by visualization of the fetal heart with absence of heart activity on ultrasound (ACOG, 2009b).

Medical Management

- Induction of labor within 24 to 48 hours of confirmed diagnosis
- Stillborn delivery
- Vaginal misoprostol if less than 28 weeks
- Cervical ripening and induction of labor (Troiano et al., 2013)

Nursing Actions

- The emotional worry from the time of suspecting a problem to an actual diagnosis can be devastating for a woman, her family, and the health care team. Women bond with their fetus and feel deep sadness from this loss.
- Provide anticipatory guidance in slow, small increments. When communicating with family and staff, the term *stillbirth* is preferred over *fetal demise* or *death* (Parfitt, 2016). Talk to the patient and family directly and give simple explanations.
- Allow the patient to make decisions related to the plan of care.
- During the admission process, it is crucial that a woman have the support of people who will be there both mentally and physically.
- To maintain a woman's comfort and sense of control, nurses can find out how she would like to birth and what pain management options, either epidural or intravenous narcotic, she would like to consider prior to starting any medications (Sousou & Smart, 2015). Provide comforting touch to the patient.
- Continuity of care; prevent unnecessary moves from labor room to delivery room to recovery room.

- To maintain privacy and comfort, a place card of an appropriate image should be hung on the door to notify all staff and personnel of the woman's status and minimize unnecessary interruptions.
- Offer the opportunity for mother and family to hold and touch the infant and allow unlimited time with infant after delivery (Parfitt, 2016).
- Provide the patient and family with mementos such as baby clothing, photos of baby with family and patient, measuring tape, baby comb, blanket, footprints, and handprints.
- In caring for a family with IUFD, nurses are part of an interdisciplinary team that also includes physicians, midwives, social workers, chaplains, geneticist, genetic counselors, lactation specialists, funeral directors, volunteers, and psychologists (Sousou & Smart, 2015).
- The interdisciplinary team must be mindful of the approach taken when caring for grieving families and should be available both physically and emotionally while anticipating and meeting the needs of the family.
- Nurses can build trust with the women and families they care for while keeping in mind that decisions made are based on each woman's or family's unique cultural and individual identity.
- Suggestions for helping grieving families include listening more than talking, allowing for silence, being genuine and caring, allowing them to express their feelings, and listening to their story without passing judgment (Sousou & Smart, 2015).
- It is important for health care professionals to not use any clichés that belittle the situation; they should not avoid discussing the experience or the baby, nor provide advice or make commentary about the situation.
- Rituals related to the perinatal bereavement process may include naming the infant, having a spiritual blessing or baptism, and arranging a memorial or burial service.
- Mementos are an important part of grieving and memory boxes can be created on behalf of the family by nursing staff. Items often included are photographs of the infant, locks of hair, name bracelets, footprints, measuring tape, name certificates, quilts, clothing, poems, or sympathy cards.

Intraamniotic Infection/ Chorioamnionitis/Triple 1

Intraamniotic infection (IAI), also referred to as chorioamnionitis, is an infection with resultant inflammation of any combination of the amniotic fluid, placenta, fetus, fetal membranes, or decidua (ACOG, 2017b). Chorioamnionitis refers to a heterogeneous group of conditions that includes inflammation as well as infections of varying degrees of severity and duration. Inflammation includes a reaction that results in tissue edema, swelling, and irritation. Infection includes inflammation with concurrent invasion of bacteria, virus, fungus, or another infectious agent. Often a diagnosis of chorioamnionitis is made when any combination (or even one) of the following elements is noted: maternal fever, maternal or fetal tachycardia or both, elevated maternal white blood cell (WBC) count, uterine tenderness, and purulent fluid or purulent discharge from the cervical os. However, the presence of one (or even more than one) of these signs and symptoms does not necessarily indicate intrauterine infection or chorioamnionitis is present (Higgins et al., 2016).

The term intraamniotic infection is commonly used since infection often involves the amniotic fluid, fetus, umbilical cord or placenta, and the fetal membranes. To clarify this issue, an expert panel recommended new terminology that differentiates the mere presence of fever from infection, inflammation, or both, and clarifies that inflammation can occur without infection. Therefore, given the historical inconsistency in use, experts proposed to discontinue the intrapartum use of the term chorioamnionitis and instead use *intrauterine inflammation or infection or both* or *Triple I.*

Isolated maternal fever is defined as maternal oral temperature 102.2°F (39°C) or greater on any one occasion, and it is a documented fever that should be reported to the health care team. If the oral temperature is between 100.4°F (38°C) and 102.2°F (39°C), repeat the measurement in 30 minutes; if the repeat value remains at least 100.4°F (38°C), it is a documented fever and should be reported (Higgins et al., 2016).

Suspected Triple I is fever without a clear source plus any of the following:

- Baseline fetal tachycardia (greater than 160 beats per minute [bpm] for 10 min or longer, excluding accelerations, decelerations, and periods of marked variability)
- Maternal white blood cell count greater than 15,000 per mm^3 in the absence of corticosteroids
- Definite purulent fluid from the cervical os

Confirmed Triple I is all of the above as well as at least one of the following:

- Amniocentesis-proven infection through a positive Gram stain
- Low glucose or positive amniotic fluid culture
- Placental pathology revealing diagnostic features of infection

Fever in the absence of any of these criteria should be categorized as "isolated maternal fever." Isolated maternal fever can include but is not limited to fever secondary to epidural anesthesia, prostaglandin use, dehydration, hyperthyroidism, and excess ambient heat. In the clinical situation of labor with fever and unknown GBS status at 37 weeks' gestation or greater, intrapartum prophylaxis should be initiated as per CDC guidelines. Clinical use of the term chorioamnionitis is outdated and overused and implies the presence of infection. Use of the phrase maternal chorioamnionitis has significant implications for both mother and neonate. The expert panel recommended the use of new terminology, specifically Triple I, with the term chorioamnionitis restricted to pathological diagnosis.

Risk Factors

- Migration of cervicovaginal flora through the cervical canal is the most common pathway for this infection. Intraamniotic infection often is polymicrobial in origin, commonly involves aerobic and anaerobic bacteria, and frequently originates from the vaginal flora (ACOG, 2017b).
- Prolonged rupture of membranes.
- Obstetric risk factors for intraamniotic infection at term have been delineated, including low parity, multiple digital examinations, use of internal uterine and fetal monitors, meconium-stained amniotic fluid, and the presence of certain genital tract pathogens (e.g., group B streptococcal infection and sexually transmitted infections) (ACOG, 2017b).

Risks Associated With Triple I

- For the mother, intrauterine infection may lead to serious complications such as sepsis, prolonged labor, wound infection, need for hysterectomy, postpartum endometritis, postpartum hemorrhage, adult respiratory distress syndrome, intensive care unit admission, and, in rare instances, maternal mortality (ACOG, 2017b; Higgins et al., 2016).
- Intraamniotic infection can be associated with acute neonatal morbidity, including neonatal pneumonia, meningitis, sepsis, and death, as well as long-term infant complications such as bronchopulmonary dysplasia and cerebral palsy. Risk of neonatal infection increases as the duration of ruptured membranes lengthens.

Assessment Findings

- Fetal tachycardia (greater than 160 bpm for 10 minutes or longer)
- Maternal WBC count greater than 15,000 in the absence of corticosteroids
- Purulent fluid from the cervical os (cloudy or yellowish thick discharge confirmed visually on speculum examination to be coming from the cervical canal)
- Biochemical or microbiologic amniotic fluid results consistent with microbial invasion of the amniotic cavity
- Be alert for and report characteristic clinical signs and symptoms of chorioamnionitis, including:
  - Maternal fever (intrapartum temperature higher than 100.4°F [37.8°C]).
  - Significant maternal tachycardia (greater than 120 bpm).
  - Fetal tachycardia (greater than 160 to 180 bpm).
  - Purulent or foul-smelling amniotic fluid or vaginal discharge.
  - Uterine tenderness.
  - Maternal leukocytosis (total blood leukocyte count greater than 15,000 to 18,000 cells/μL).
  - Hypotension.
  - Diaphoresis.
  - Cool or clammy skin.

Medical Management

- Administration of intrapartum antibiotics is recommended whenever an intraamniotic infection is suspected or confirmed. Antibiotics should be considered in the setting of isolated maternal fever unless a source other than intraamniotic infection is identified and documented (ACOG, 2017b).
- The choice of antimicrobial agents in the case of suspected Triple I should be guided by the prevalent microorganisms

causing intrauterine infection. In general, a combination of ampicillin and gentamicin should cover most relevant pathogens. The use of intrapartum antibiotic treatment given either in response to maternal group B streptococcal colonization or in response to evolving signs of intraamniotic infection during labor has been associated with a nearly 10-fold decrease in GBS-specific neonatal sepsis (ACOG, 2017b).

● Controlling the maternal temperature with antipyretics and judicious hydration may be required.

Nursing Actions

● Communicate findings of maternal tachycardia, fetal tachycardia, maternal white blood cell count greater than 15,000, maternal GBS status, duration of rupture of membranes, duration of labor, purulent fluid, amniotic fluid evaluation, highest maternal temperature, epidural anesthesia use, prostaglandin use, antimicrobial agent(s) used, antipyretic used, spontaneous preterm birth, and/or prior spontaneous preterm birth to all members of the obstetrical and neonatal teams.

● Administer antipyretics and antibiotics as ordered.

Pregestational Complications Impacting Intrapartal Period

Maternal morbidity includes physical and psychological conditions that result from or are aggravated by pregnancy and have an adverse effect on a woman's health (Behling & Renaud, 2015). The most severe complications of pregnancy, generally referred to as severe maternal morbidity (SMM), affect more than 50,000 women in the United States every year. Based on recent trends, this burden has been steadily increasing (Callaghan, Creanga, & Kuklina, 2012). The consequences of the increasing SMM prevalence are wide-ranging and include higher health service use, higher direct medical costs, extended hospitalization stays, and long-term rehabilitation. For example, labor complicated by cardiovascular disease is potentially dangerous to maternal and fetal outcomes. Marked hemodynamic changes in labor have a profound effect on the women in labor, placental perfusion, and fetal status.

Extensive discussion of specific pregestational complications and their management in labor is beyond the scope of this text, but the impact of obesity in labor is presented as an exemplar in the following section. Refer to Chapter 7 for additional information on management of pregestational complications.

Maternal Obesity

The World Health Organization and the National Institute of Health define obesity as a BMI of 30 or greater. Maternal obesity was first recognized as a risk factor in pregnancy more than 50 years ago. A global epidemic of obesity is unfolding, including an even greater prevalence in African American and Mexican American women, resulting in new challenges for the management of obesity in up to 34% of pregnant women aged 20 to 39 years old (ACOG, 2015). The obstetric complications of maternal obesity are generally related to issues of maternal pre-pregnancy obesity rather than excessive weight gain during pregnancy. Maternal obesity is

a well-established risk factor for the development of preeclampsia, gestational diabetes, and thrombosis. However, the impact on pregnancy also translates to complications in labor, including spontaneous abortion, labor induction, cesarean births, endometritis, and failed vaginal birth after cesarean. Obesity in labor also puts the laboring woman at increased risk of emergent complications of wound rupture or dehiscence, with a twofold increase in maternal morbidity and fivefold increase in neonatal injury associated in TOLAC (ACOG, 2015). Obesity in the female population is such a prevalent problem that the implications relative to pregnancy often are unrecognized or overlooked. Therefore, an understanding of the management of obesity during labor is essential to maternal and neonatal health, and it is currently recommended that every perinatal department have policies and practices specific to this patient population (ACOG, 2015; Maher, 2014).

Risks at Delivery

● Abnormal progress of labor
● Fetal macrosomia
● Shoulder dystocia
● Higher rates of operative vaginal birth and cesarean birth
● Performing epidural or spinal anesthesia on morbidly obese patients may be extremely problematic.
● Not only do obese women experience higher rates of failed vaginal birth after cesarean (VBAC), but obese women who have a VBAC experience higher rates of infection.
● Increased risk of hemorrhage.
● Intraoperative challenges and complications can include difficulty with IV access, difficulty monitoring blood pressures, prolonged cesarean surgical and recovery time, poor operative exposure, difficulty with transfers, increased aspiration, and thromboembolitic risk.
● Increased postoperative complications, including wound infection, delayed wound healing, excessive blood loss, deep vein thrombosis, and endometritis (ACOG, 2015).

Assessment Findings

● Delayed descent of fetal head, abnormal labor progress, or labor dystocia (Parfitt, 2016)

Nursing Actions

● Anticipate impact of pregnancy complications listed above on labor and birth.
● Challenges caring for obese women in labor can include difficulty gaining IV access, difficulty with monitoring blood pressures, fetal heart tones (FHTs), and UCs, and transferring or moving patients.
● Anticipate the need for additional staff for position changes, monitoring and assistance at birth, and transfer and transport (Maher, 2014; Parfitt, 2016).
● Assess progress of labor; internal monitoring may be necessary.
● Ensure that all equipment is available for labor, delivery, possible cesarean, and recovery, and check that equipment weight limits are adequate to support patient's weight.

- Facilitate patient positioning for administering epidural analgesia to obese women.
- A sensitive and empathic approach to the woman and her family is essential to meet the specialized needs of an obese woman in labor, birth, and recovery.

OBSTETRICAL EMERGENCIES

Obstetrical emergencies are urgent clinical situations that place either the maternal or fetal status at risk for increased morbidity and mortality. Intrapartum emergencies may be related to one or more maternal, fetal, uterine, cord, and/or placental factors. The physiological effects of intrapartum emergencies on the woman and fetus may create rapid deterioration in oxygenation and perfusion. Intrapartum emergencies may place the woman and fetus at risk of exceeding their oxygen and perfusion reserves. Interventions are directed at stabilizing maternal status, which in turn stabilizes fetal status.

Perinatal nurses practice in an environment where emergencies will occur. Preparation for these situations requires allocation of resources and supplies, planning, and collaboration. Inpatient emergencies can be mitigated by a rapid response team that has designated roles, streamlined communication, prompt access to emergency supplies, and ongoing education and training. Specific criteria or triggers used to activate a rapid response team should be defined to reflect the populations cared for by the institution and disseminated among interprofessional staff. Protocols with standardized interventions and on-site drills will improve the care given in an emergency. Prompt recognition of and response to critical clinical scenarios, teamwork, and training enhance patient safety and mitigate the severity of adverse outcomes (ACOG, 2014a). We can improve management of hospitalized patients with the use of a rapid response team that has designated roles, streamlined communication, prompt access to emergency supplies, and ongoing education and training (ACOG, 2014a). Tools include:

- Availability of appropriate emergency supplies in a resuscitation cart (crash cart) or kit
- Development and implementation of a rapid response team
- Development and implementation of protocols that include clinical triggers
- Use of standardized communication tools for huddles and briefs such as SBAR (situation, background, assessment, recommendation)
- Implementation of emergency drills and simulations

Severe maternal morbidity (SMM) includes unexpected outcomes of labor and delivery that result in significant short- or long-term consequences to a woman's health. It is not entirely clear why SMM is increasing, but changes in the overall health of the women giving birth may be contributing to increases in complications. For example, increases in maternal age, prepregnancy obesity, four preexisting chronic medical conditions,

CRITICAL COMPONENT

Examples of Trigger Threshold Parameters

Some events, referred to as "triggers," mandate further actions by the health care team according to protocol, such as bringing the attending physician to the patient's bedside immediately. Some emergencies are preceded by a period of instability during which timely intervention may help avoid disaster. OB emergency teams, sometimes referred to as OB stat team for obstetrical emergencies, are rapid response teams in labor and delivery. Nurses need to recognize that certain changes in a patient's condition can indicate an emergency that requires immediate intervention. A "red" trigger typically mandates an immediate bedside evaluation and a "yellow" trigger indicates further clinical evaluation (ACOG, 2014a).

	Red trigger	Yellow trigger
Temperature; °C	<35 or >38	35–36
Systolic BP; mm Hg	<90 or >160	150–160 or 90–100
Diastolic BP; mm Hg	>100	90–100
Heart rate; beats.min^{-1}	<40 or >120	100–120 or 40–50
Respiratory rate; breaths.min^{-1}	<10 or >30	21–30
Oxygen saturation; %	<95	

and cesarean delivery have been documented (CDC, 2017b). In the United States, the pregnancy-related mortality ratio rose from 10 deaths per 100,000 live births in 1990 to 17.8 deaths per 100,000 live births in 2011 to 15.9 deaths per 100,000 live births in 2012 (CDC, 2017a), which is more than double the 1978 rate of 7.2 deaths per 100,000 live births. Significant racial disparity exists in the pregnancy-related mortality ratio; for example, black women have a pregnancy-related mortality risk three times greater than that of white women (CDC, 2017a). Additionally, complications associated with delivery and specifically for postpartum hemorrhage have increased 75% (Callaghan et al., 2012). Identifying potential problems early, developing written protocols that outline a clear plan of response for common emergencies, and using mock drills to train staff in protocol responses can help ensure that no tasks are redundant or omitted and ultimately create a more controlled environment that promotes positive health outcomes (Roth, Parfitt, Hering, & Dent, 2014). Communication and teamwork are essential parts of safety and improving patient outcomes. Effective, patient-centered communication facilitates interception and correction of potentially harmful conditions and errors. All team members, including women, their families, physicians, midwives, and nurses, have roles in identifying the potential for harm during labor and birth (Lyndon et al., 2015).

CRITICAL COMPONENT

Intrapartum Care Communication

Intrapartum care is inherently dynamic and nuanced, and crucial communication gaps can occur. Road signs may be unclear or change quickly, leading care providers to have completely different interpretations of clinical situations and divergent ideas of the right thing to do. Conflicting approaches are easily exacerbated by the dynamic nature of labor; differences of opinion and prioritization occur with some regularity (Lyndon et al., 2014). Key steps toward improving communication include assuming the best motives of others, recognizing that we all make assumptions that reflect our own worldviews, seeking first to understand others' views and then to be understood, and avoiding stereotyping. Differences of opinion and judgment occur naturally in complex situations such as labor and birth. Ensuring that patients' interests are the focus of action at all times serves as a powerful resource for proactive problem solving (Lyndon et al., 2015). Communication issues, most notably between providers, were identified in 41% of cases and included the lack of timely acknowledgment and effective communication. Other factors were the lack of appreciation for clinical significance or decline, variation in willingness to escalate concerns about care, and poor communication due to lack of team structure and function that often led to delays in care management and effective response.

Shoulder Dystocia

Shoulder dystocia is an unpredictable and unpreventable obstetric emergency that places the laboring mother and neonate at risk of injury and complications (ACOG & SFMFM, 2017c). Shoulder dystocia refers to difficulty encountered during delivery of the shoulders after the birth of the head. Shoulder dystocia often occurs when the passage of the anterior shoulder is obstructed by the symphysis pubis. It also results from an impaction of the posterior shoulder on the maternal sacral promontory (ACOG & SFMFM, 2017c). The anterior shoulder or, more rarely, both shoulders become impacted above the pelvic rim. The first sign is a retraction of the fetal head against the maternal perineum after delivery of the head, sometimes referred to as turtle sign. This impaction of the fetal shoulders may lead to a prolonged delivery time of more than 60 seconds. Because shoulder dystocia is an unpredictable obstetrical emergency that can result in serious fetal morbidity and even mortality, it must be readily recognized and successfully managed. Several techniques that have been proven to assist delivery exist, and there is evidence that a systematic approach can improve outcomes (ACOG, 2017c).

Neonatal morbidity includes brachial plexus injuries, clavicle fracture, neurological injury related to asphyxia, and even death. Reduction in the interval of time from delivery of the head to the body is crucial to fetal outcome. Most experts note that more than a 5-minute delay in head to body interval may result in fetal hypoxemia and acidosis. It is estimated that a newborn can survive for approximately 6 minutes before irreversible brain and organ damage occurs. The incidence of shoulder dystocia ranges from reports of 0.2% to 3% (ACOG & SFMFM, 2017c). Studies have found that prepregnancy, antepartum, and intrapartum risk factors fail to accurately predict the possibility of shoulder dystocia. Additionally, there is no clear evidence to support the use of prophylactic maneuvers to prevent shoulder dystocia (Athukorala, Middleton, & Crowther, 2006).

Risk Factors Associated With Shoulder Dystocia

- Fetal macrosomia (weight greater than 4,500 grams)
- Maternal diabetes
- History of shoulder dystocia
- Prolonged second stage
- Excessive weight gain

Risks Associated With Shoulder Dystocia for the Mother

- Maternal complications include severe perineal lacerations, including fourth-degree lacerations, maternal symphyseal separation and peripheral neuropathy, sphincter injuries, infection, bladder injury, or postpartum hemorrhage (ACOG, 2017c).

Risks Associated With Shoulder Dystocia for the Neonate

- Delay in delivery of the shoulders results in compression of the fetal neck by the maternal pelvis. This impairs fetal circulation and results in possible increased intracranial pressure, anoxia, asphyxia, and neurological injury. Although infrequent, some cases of shoulder dystocia may result in neonatal encephalopathy and even death. The duration of the shoulder dystocia alone has not been shown to be an accurate predictor of neonatal asphyxia or death (ACOG, 2017c).
- Most shoulder dystocia cases are alleviated without injury to the fetus. Brachial plexus injuries and fractures of the clavicle and humerus can occur and usually resolve without long-term complications. However, the presence of a brachial plexus injury is not evidence that shoulder dystocia has occurred (ACOG, 2017c).

Assessment Findings

- The first sign is a retraction of the fetal head against the maternal perineum after delivery of the head, sometimes referred to as turtle sign.
- Delay in delivery of shoulders after delivery of head.

Medical Management

When shoulder dystocia is suspected, the first intervention that should be attempted is the McRoberts maneuver because it is a simple, logical, and effective technique. This is performed by two assistants each grasping a maternal leg and then sharply flexing the thigh back against the maternal abdomen, which causes cephalad rotation of the symphysis pubis and flattening of the lumbar lordosis that can free the impacted shoulder. Pressure is applied above the pubic bone with the palm or fist; then the pressure is directed on the anterior shoulder both downward (to below the pubic bone) and laterally (toward the fetus's face or sternum) to abduct and rotate the anterior shoulder. Fundal pressure should be avoided, as it may further complicate impaction of the shoulder and also may cause uterine rupture.

If both the McRoberts maneuver and suprapubic pressure are unsuccessful, delivery of the posterior arm may be considered as the next maneuver to manage shoulder dystocia (ACOG, 2017c). The Woods corkscrew maneuver progressively rotates the posterior shoulder 180 degrees to disimpact the anterior shoulder.

Nursing Actions

- Explain the situation to the woman and the family and explain the interventions to resolve dystocia and the importance of the woman's assistance with maneuvers. Request the mother not to push.
- Request assistance, as additional nurses may be needed to implement maneuvers to resolve dystocia.
- Insert a straight catheter into the woman to empty the bladder if it is distended to make more room for the fetus.
- A variety of techniques may be used to free the impacted shoulder from beneath the symphysis pubis (ACOG, 2017c); pressure can be applied above the pubic bone or laterally to the pubic bone to dislodge the anterior shoulder and push it beneath the symphysis (Fig. 10–15).
- The mother should not push except when instructed to and only when it is believed the shoulder has been released.
- The McRoberts maneuver consists of sharply flexing the thigh onto the maternal abdomen to straighten the sacrum (Fig. 10–15).
- Fundal pressure is controversial and not indicated in shoulder dystocia.
- Notify the neonatal team.
- Prepare for neonatal resuscitation.
- Document the series of interventions and clinical events with time intervals (Simpson & O'Brien-Abel, 2013).

Prolapse of the Umbilical Cord

Prolapse of the umbilical cord occurs when the cord lies below the presenting part of the fetus (Fig. 10–16A–C). The cord may prolapse in front of the presenting part, into the vagina, or through the introitus. Occult prolapse is when the cord is palpated through the membranes but does not drop into the vagina. When cord prolapse occurs, it is typically with AROM or spontaneous rupture of membranes (SROM), when the presenting part is not engaged in the pelvis. The cord becomes entrapped against the presenting part and circulation is occluded, resulting in FHR bradycardia. A loop of cord may be palpated or visualized in the vagina. An emergency cesarean birth is typically done to improve neonatal outcomes with a prolapsed cord. The overall incidence of umbilical cord prolapse ranges from 0.1% to 0.6% (ACOG, 2014a). Although an uncommon obstetric emergency, with umbilical cord prolapse, the initial response can greatly impact the quality of maternal and infant outcomes (Phelan & Holbrook, 2013).

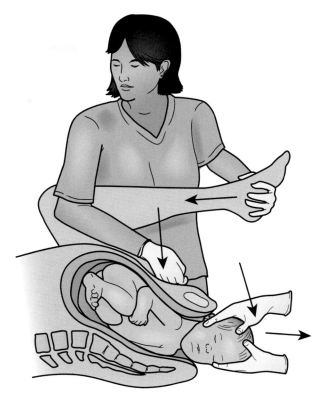

FIGURE 10–15 McRoberts maneuver and suprapubic pressure. When fetal shoulders become impacted under the maternal symphysis pubis, the nurse should initiate the McRoberts maneuver by hyperextending the birthing woman's legs onto her abdomen and simultaneously providing suprapubic pressure to assist the fetus in adducting the arms closer to the body in an attempt to release the impacted shoulders.

Risk Factors for Prolapse of the Umbilical Cord Related to the Fetus

- Malpresentation of the fetus (such as breech), fetal anomalies, intrauterine growth restriction and small for gestational age (IUGR/SGA), unengaged presenting part

Risk Factors Related to Pregnancy

- The primary iatrogenic cause is artificial rupture of membranes (AROM).
- Polyhydramnios, multiple gestation, spontaneous ROM, preterm ROM, and grand multiparity

Risks Associated With Prolapse of the Umbilical Cord

- Total or partial occlusion of the cord, resulting in rapid deterioration in fetal perfusion and oxygenation, causes fetal hypoxia, and if not treated swiftly, can lead to long-term sequela, disability, or death (Phelan & Holbrook, 2013).

Assessment Findings

Umbilical cord prolapse can be occult or overt. Occult prolapse is neither visible nor palpable, and occurs when the cord passes

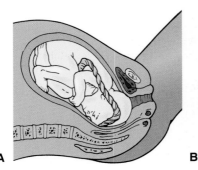
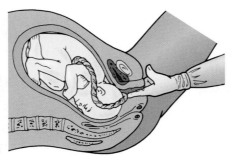
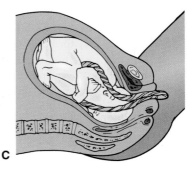

FIGURE 10–16 Prolapsed cord. (**A**) Occult. The cord cannot be seen or felt during a vaginal examination. (**B**) Complete. During a vaginal examination, the cord is felt as a pulsating mass. (**C**) Frank. The cord precedes the fetal head or feet and can be seen protruding from the vagina.

through the cervix alongside the presenting part of the fetus (Fig. 10–16A). In a case of overt prolapse, the cord presents before the fetus and is visible or palpable within the vagina or even past the labia (Phelan & Holbrook, 2013) (Fig. 10–16B&C). Prolapse of the umbilical cord frequently leads to compression, which causes FHR decelerations, including severe sudden deceleration, often with prolonged bradycardia or recurrent moderate-to-severe variable decelerations (Phelan & Holbrook, 2013).

Medical Management

- Vaginal birth or operative vaginal delivery may be attempted if birth is imminent.
- Perform emergency cesarean section.

Nursing Actions

- Elevation of the presenting part. Occlusion of the cord may be partially relieved by lifting the presenting part off the cord with a vaginal exam. The examiner's hand remains in the vagina, lifting the presenting part off the cord until delivery by cesarean (Fig. 10–17).
- Request assistance, notify the health care provider, and request an immediate bedside evaluation.
- Explain to the woman and family that interventions are necessary to expedite delivery. Ensure the woman understands the importance of her assistance.
- Recommend position changes such as knee-chest position or Trendelenburg to try to relieve pressure on the occluded cord

(Fig. 10–18), administer O₂ at 10 L/min by mask, and give IV fluid hydration bolus.
- Discontinue oxytocin and consider administration of a tocolytic agent to decrease uterine activity.
- Move toward emergency delivery. If birth is imminent, the provider may proceed with vaginal delivery. If birth is not imminent, anticipate and prepare for emergency cesarean section.

Vasa Previa/Ruptured Vasa Previa

Vasa previa occurs when fetal vessels unsupported by placenta or umbilical cord traverses the membranes over the cervix. Vasa previa is defined as abnormal fetal blood vessels that run through the fetal membranes, over or near the endocervical os, and are unprotected by the placenta or umbilical cord (Silver, 2015). It is uncommon and occurs in 1 in 2,500 to 5,000 pregnancies.

The condition usually results from velamentous insertion of the cord into the membranes rather than the placenta or from vessels running between lobes of the placenta with one or more accessory lobes (Fig. 10–19A, B). If undiagnosed, it is associated with perinatal mortality of 60% (Oyelese, 2007). Pressure on unprotected vessels by the presenting part can lead to fetal asphyxia and death.

Ruptured vasa previa refers to the rupture of the unprotected fetal vessels running through the membranes and over the cervix (Oyelese, 2007). ROM frequently leads to rapid fetal exsanguination (Cunningham et al., 2014). This is the result of fetal-neonatal hemorrhage if fetal vessels tear in the process of spontaneous or artificial rupture of membranes and labor itself. Because the entire fetal blood volume is usually less than 100 mL/kg, emergent bleeding is often rapid. Also, there is a theoretical risk of compromised blood flow to the fetus from

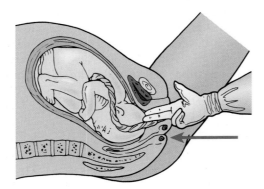

FIGURE 10–17 Vaginal examination with prolapsed cord, lifting presenting part off the cord.

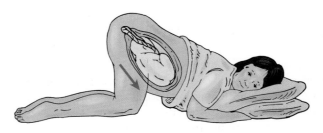

FIGURE 10–18 Knee-chest position with prolapsed cord.

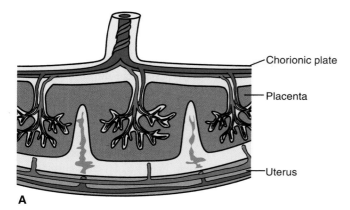

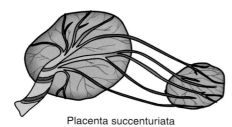

Placenta succenturiata

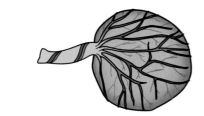

Marginal insertion of the cord

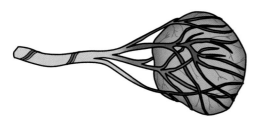

B

Velamentous insertion of the cord

FIGURE 10–19 (*A*) Normal insertion of umbilical cord into chorionic plate. Normally the umbilical cord inserts near the center of the chorionic plate, which stabilizes the fetal vessels as they leave the umbilical cord. Like the roots of a tree, the fetal vessels branch over the surface of the chorionic plate and then dive into the placental parenchyma. (*B*) Illustration depicting abnormalities of umbilical cord insertion into the placenta. With a velamentous insertion of the umbilical cord into the membranes or with a succenturiate lobe, fetal vessels, within the chorionic membranes and unprotected by the placenta, may course across the cervix and result in a vasa previa.

the compression and subsequent occlusion of these compromised vessels by the presenting part of the fetus (Silver, 2015). A recent report with a very few documented cases of vasa previa (*N* = 19) demonstrated some improved neonatal outcomes and survival (Dunn, Nassr, Moaddab, Eppes, & Shamshirsaz, 2017).

Risk Factors for Vasa Previa

- Low-lying placenta or a placenta previa
- Pregnancies in which the placenta has accessory lobes
- Multiple gestation
- Pregnancies resulting from in vitro fertilization

Risks Associated With Vasa Previa

- Fetal asphyxia from cord compression
- Fetal death from exsanguination

Assessment Findings

- Vasa previa is most commonly diagnosed when ROM is accompanied by vaginal bleeding or fetal distress or death, but increasingly it is diagnosed by antenatal ultrasonography.

Medical Management

- If diagnosed prenatally with ultrasound, cesarean birth prior to labor and ruptured membranes improves neonatal outcomes. Recommendations include planned cesarean birth at 35 weeks, which improves neonatal survival to 95% (Nahum, 2016; Oyelese, 2007). It is generally accepted that delivery be performed by cesarean before the onset of labor or ROM (Silver, 2015).
- If diagnosed in labor, urgent cesarean delivery should be undertaken in cases of vaginal bleeding with suspected vasa previa.

Nursing Actions

- If a woman is diagnosed by ultrasound during pregnancy, she may be admitted to the hospital for surveillance, given corticosteroids to promote fetal lung maturity, and scheduled for planned cesarean birth at 35 weeks. Nursing care related to antenatal hospitalization for high-risk pregnancy is detailed in Chapter 7.
- If bleeding occurs with SVE by the nurse, an immediate bedside evaluation by the provider is indicated because urgent cesarean delivery should be accomplished in cases of vaginal bleeding with suspected vasa previa.

Rupture of the Uterus

Rupture of the uterus is a partial or complete tear in the uterine muscle. In complete uterine rupture, all the layers of the uterine wall are separated. In incomplete uterine rupture (uterine dehiscence), the uterine muscle is separated but the visceral peritoneum is intact. Uterine rupture is a rare obstetric emergency most commonly associated with VBAC. From 1976 to 2012, 25 peer-reviewed publications described the incidence of uterine rupture, and these reported 2,084 cases among 2,951,297 pregnant women, yielding an overall uterine rupture rate of 1 in 1,146 pregnancies (0.07%) (Nahum, 2016). Studies show a 0.7% incidence of uterine rupture in women attempting TOLAC (Parfitt, 2016). The uterus with no surgical history that is spontaneously contracting is not likely to rupture. Therefore, avoiding induction of labor may substantially decrease risk of uterine rupture in mothers attempting a TOLAC/VBAC (Parfitt,

2016). Other risk factors are previous vertical uterine scar, previous abortions, abdominal trauma, multifetal gestation, and uterine tachysystole.

Signs and symptoms of uterine rupture are related to internal hemorrhage and reflected in both the maternal and fetal status, in relationship to the extent of the rupture. The condition usually becomes evident because of signs of fetal compromise and maternal hypovolemia related to hemorrhage. If the fetal presenting part is in the pelvis, loss of station may occur, which is detected with a vaginal exam. Maternal and fetal outcomes and survival depend on prompt identification and surgical intervention. Fetal mortality with uterine rupture is reported at 5% to 7% and maternal mortality is as low as 1% in developed countries (Nahum, 2016).

Risks Associated With Rupture of the Uterus

- Potential effects on the woman and fetus include hypovolemic shock, infection, hypoxemia, acidosis, neurological damage, and possible death.
- Maternal complications are primarily due to hypovolemia as a result of hemorrhage.
- Complications to the fetus may be due to uteroplacental insufficiency, placental abruption, cord compression, asphyxia, and/or hypovolemia.

Assessment Findings

- Severe tearing sensation, burning or stabbing pain, and contractions
- Uterine tachysystole and/or hypertonus and vaginal bleeding
- Maternal assessment findings may include signs and symptoms of hypovolemic shock, such as hypotension, tachypnea, tachycardia, and pallor.
- Fetal response is related to hemorrhage and placental separation and may include sudden fetal bradycardia or prolonged late or variable decelerations present even prior to the onset of abdominal pain or vaginal bleeding (Parfitt, 2016).
- Ascending station of the fetal presenting part

Medical Management

- Perform emergency cesarean birth and control maternal hemorrhage. Hysterectomy may be necessary. Transfusions may be needed.

Nursing Actions

- Explain to the woman and her family the interventions that will expedite delivery and the importance of their assistance for the best possible outcome.
- Request assistance and notify the medical provider and request immediate bedside evaluation.
- Gain/maintain large-bore IV access. Stabilize the woman with O_2, IV fluids, and blood products.
- Maintain the woman in the lateral position to maximize urine blood flow (Parfitt, 2016).
- Prepare for emergency cesarean birth.
  - Insert Foley catheter, as bladder rupture is associated with uterine rupture (Parfitt, 2016).

Anaphylactic Syndrome/ Amniotic Fluid Embolism

Anaphylactic syndrome, also known as amniotic fluid embolism, is an often fatal complication that can occur during pregnancy, labor, birth, or the first 24 hours postbirth. Though rare, anaphylactoid syndrome is among the leading five causes of pregnancy-related deaths in the United States (Farsight, Jaimez-Carranza, & Coleman, 2017), with a maternal mortality rate ranging between 61% and 86% (Jones & Clark, 2013). Further, among patients who survive, the majority (85%) have permanent neurological injury (Jones & Clark, 2013). This obstetric emergency is both unpreventable and unpredictable (Stanley Sundin & Bradham Mazac, 2017). It is hypothesized that an embolism forms when the amniotic fluid that contains fetal cells, lanugo, and vernix enters the maternal vascular system. In some patients, this can trigger an anaphylactic reaction that results in cardiorespiratory collapse. Signs and symptoms of anaphylactoid syndrome are related to anaphylactic shock and cardiopulmonary collapse. This syndrome is discussed more completely in Chapter 14.

- The diagnosis is considered unmistakable with the signs and symptoms of sudden dyspnea, hypotension, and DIC that presents during labor or immediately after birth (Clark, 2014).
- Maternal mortality is a potential complication and if concomitant with cardiac arrest, chances of survival are less than 10% (Clark, 2014).

Risk Factors Associated With Anaphylactoid Syndrome

- Advanced maternal age 35 years or older
- Use of oxytocin for medical induction of labor
- Cesarean delivery
- Placental abnormalities (e.g., previa, abruption)
- Uterine rupture
- Assisted operative vaginal delivery (vacuum, forceps)
- Eclampsia
- Polyhydramnios
- Cervical laceration

Risks Associated With Anaphylactoid Syndrome

- Adult respiratory distress syndrome
- Heart failure
- DIC
- Multisystem organ failure

Assessment Findings

- Rapid onset of respiratory distress that occurs during labor, delivery, or 30 minutes postdelivery (Parfitt, 2016) with severe hypoxia, hypotension, cyanosis, loss of consciousness, foaming at the mouth, pulmonary edema, uncontrolled bleeding from uterus, IV sites, or any other incisions due to coagulopathy, seizures, cardiac arrest, and prolonged late decelerations or bradycardia resulting from fetal hypoxia.

Medical Management

- Manage cardiopulmonary arrest, hypotension, and coagulopathy.

- Management goals:
  - Improve oxygenation
  - Optimize cardiac output
  - Correct coagulopathy
  - Deliver fetus

Nursing Actions

- Careful assessment, maternal pulse oximetry, maintain patent IV access, left uterine displacement, notification of OB team, implement advanced cardiac life support (ACLS) protocols, documentation
- Recognize life-threatening diagnosis, and ask for help and an immediate bedside evaluation. Activate L&D code team.
- Prepare for emergent interventions such as rapid sequence intubation. Stabilize woman with O_2 and IV fluids and blood products (Parfitt, 2016).
- Maintain continuous FHR monitoring.
- Prepare for emergency delivery.

Disseminated Intravascular Coagulation

Disseminated intravascular coagulation is a syndrome that occurs when the body is breaking down blood clots faster than it can form a clot. This quickly depletes the body of clotting factors, leading to hemorrhage, and can rapidly lead to maternal death. DIC is always a result of another pathological process or injury and is the final common pathway of coagulation dysregulation (DeLoughery, 2015). DIC can be triggered by a myriad of adverse obstetric events that include placental abruption, amniotic fluid embolism, sepsis syndrome, acute fatty liver of pregnancy, severe preeclampsia, hemolysis, elevated liver enzymes, low platelet count syndrome, and massive obstetric hemorrhage (Cunningham & Nelson, 2015).

During pregnancy, maternal leukocytes are in a higher state of activation than in nonpregnant women and have characteristics akin to sepsis. However, they are well controlled during pregnancy, and it has been proposed that the trophoblast plays a role in the maintenance of the balanced systemic maternal inflammation during pregnancy. Nevertheless, in cases of sepsis caused by an infectious agent or septic abortion and at least in some of the cases of amniotic fluid embolism, this equilibrium is disturbed and the mother develops DIC (Erez, Mastrolia, & Thachil, 2015).

DIC is a dire obstetrical emergency that is a significant cause of maternal morbidity and mortality and is associated with up to 25% of maternal deaths (Cunningham & Nelson, 2015). Prompt recognition and understanding of the underlying mechanisms of disease leading to this complication is essential for successful management and positive outcome (Erez et al., 2015). Women who experience DIC are transferred to the critical care unit and a perinatologist manages the care. This is discussed more completely in Chapter 14.

CRITICAL CARE IN PERINATAL NURSING

Critical care intrapartum nursing may be required when a woman has a preexisting condition or a maternal or fetal complication develops during pregnancy. The ability of a hospital to deliver this high level of care may vary; because high-risk and critically ill women may be encountered in any setting, all intrapartum nurses should be prepared to identify and participate in stabilizing critically ill women for transport to a tertiary care center or intensive care unit (AWHONN, 2008). Intrapartum nurses who care for critically ill women receive additional education and undergo didactic and verification of learning and clinical skills beyond the scope of this chapter. Most critically ill pregnant women are cared for in adult intensive care units or in specialized obstetric critical care units. No matter where the care is delivered, a comprehensive plan of care should address the unique physiological needs of the pregnant woman. Therefore, it is essential that when indicated, critical care and perinatal nurses collaborate to coordinate care for this unique population. Women who have any of the disorders or diseases presented in the high-risk didactic content have the potential to become critically ill if their condition deteriorates.

Nurses are often the first members of the health care team to detect subtle signs and symptoms of developing complications; thus, their contribution to the rescue process is crucial. A nurse's role in alerting the team and mobilizing its response has a direct impact on the ultimate outcome.

Women considered low risk can become acutely ill with little warning, requiring rapid assessment, emergent mobilization of the team, and intervention to support the optimal outcomes (Behling & Renaud, 2015). Women may have obstetric or non-obstetric conditions, which can be complicated by the presence of a fetus and a myriad of potential comorbidities.

The maternal code protocol was developed in accordance with the American Heart Association's (AHA) ACLS algorithms (Vanden Hoek et al., 2010). There are OB-specific additions to the ACLS algorithms from the AHA that are pertinent to the maternal code protocol. For example, displacement of the uterus during cardiopulmonary resuscitation facilitates blood return to the heart and is critical to return of spontaneous circulation. Fetal monitor components should be removed prior to defibrillation or cardioversion to decrease potential risks of arcing and damage to monitor components. Hand placement for chest compressions should be slightly higher on the maternal chest due to cardiac displacement during pregnancy. Early advanced airway should be considered and performed by an experienced professional, as intubation of pregnant patients can be difficult. Mock code drills utilizing the maternal code protocol have assisted in keeping nurses' skills current in performing ACLS steps that are rarely implemented.

When unexpected crises occur on the OB unit, nurses and other clinicians must act quickly and take appropriate steps to ensure best health outcomes. Use of protocols during mock emergency drills can assist in educating staff on critical steps that must be taken while maintaining a calm, collected setting, thus creating a positive learning environment. In the event these drills become reality, preparation that has occurred through use of these protocols can promote a controlled atmosphere with optimal results for both the women experiencing a health crisis and the health care staff caring for them (Roth et al., 2014).

Concept Map

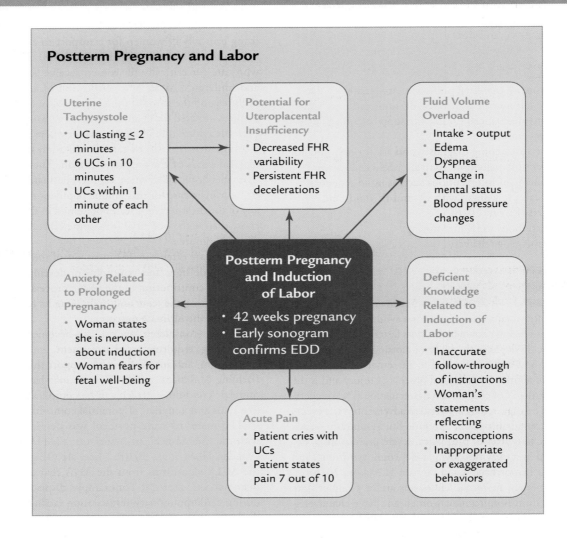

Postterm Pregnancy and Labor

Uterine Tachysystole
- UC lasting ≤ 2 minutes
- 6 UCs in 10 minutes
- UCs within 1 minute of each other

Potential for Uteroplacental Insufficiency
- Decreased FHR variability
- Persistent FHR decelerations

Fluid Volume Overload
- Intake > output
- Edema
- Dyspnea
- Change in mental status
- Blood pressure changes

Anxiety Related to Prolonged Pregnancy
- Woman states she is nervous about induction
- Woman fears for fetal well-being

Postterm Pregnancy and Induction of Labor
- 42 weeks pregnancy
- Early sonogram confirms EDD

Deficient Knowledge Related to Induction of Labor
- Inaccurate follow-through of instructions
- Woman's statements reflecting misconceptions
- Inappropriate or exaggerated behaviors

Acute Pain
- Patient cries with UCs
- Patient states pain 7 out of 10

Problem No. 1: Uterine tachysystole

Goal: Decreased uterine activity

Outcome: Patient will have decreased contractions.

Nursing Actions
1. Evaluation of uterine contraction strength, frequency, and resting tone duration by palpation or IUPC
2. Evaluation of uterine resting tone by palpation or IUPC pressure above 25 mm Hg
3. Assessment of FHR in response to uterine contractions
4. Turn oxytocin down or off in the event of uterine tachysystole or indeterminate or abnormal fetal heart rate
5. Maternal position change
6. IV bolus of at least 500 mL of lactated Ringer's
7. O₂ administration by mask at 10 L/min
8. If no response, consider terbutaline
9. Notify provider

Problem No. 2: Knowledge deficit related to induction of labor

Goal: Patient understands indication and process of labor induction.

Outcome: Patient states she understands indication and process of induction of labor.

Nursing Actions
1. Explain all procedures.
2. Encourage verbalization of questions.
3. Practice active listening.
4. Provide emotional support.
5. Make needed referrals to social services and mental health specialists if needed.

Problem No. 3: Anxiety related to prolonged pregnancy

Goal: Decreased anxiety

Outcome: Patient verbalizes that she feels less anxious.

Nursing Actions

1. Explain all information and procedures in lay language and repeat information prn.
2. Provide autonomy and choices.
3. Encourage patient and family to verbalize their feelings regarding prolonged pregnancy by asking open-ended questions.
4. Be calm and reassuring in interactions with the patient and her family.
5. Explore past coping strategies.

Problem No. 4: Fluid volume overload related to prolonged oxytocin

Goal: Fluid balance

Outcome: Patient maintains fluid balance.

Nursing Actions

1. Auscultate the lung sounds.
2. Assess I&O.
3. Maintain IV fluids as ordered.
4. Calculate intake of all fluids.
5. Measure output including emesis and urine.
6. Assess edema.

Problem No. 5: Acute pain related to UCs

Goal: Decreased pain

Outcome: Patient will state that pain is improved.

Nursing Actions

1. Assess level, location, and type of pain.
2. Sustain physical presence, eye contact.
3. Provide verbal encouragement, reassurance, and praise.
4. Provide comfort measures such as ice chips, fluids, food, and pain medications.
5. Provide hygiene, including mouth care, pericare, and changing underpads.
6. Assist with position changes.
7. Provide reassuring touch, massage.
8. Apply heat and cold.
9. Encourage hydrotherapy via shower or tub if no ROM.
10. Provide an environment that is conducive to relaxation, such as low lights, decreased noise.
11. Teach patient relaxation and breathing techniques.

Problem No. 6: Potential for uteroplacental insufficiency Category II or III FHR

Goal: Maintain normal FHR

Outcome: FHR pattern is Category 1, baseline is normal with moderate variability and accelerations.

Nursing Actions

1. Assess FHR baseline variability and for decelerations.
2. Change the mother's position.
3. IV bolus of at least 500 mL of lactated Ringer's
4. O_2 at 10 L/min by mask
5. Turn oxytocin down or off.
6. Notify the provider.
7. Request bedside evaluation if the FHR is Category III.

Case Study

As a labor and delivery nurse, this is your second shift caring for Mallory Polk. She is a 42-year-old, single, African American attorney whom you admitted yesterday at 32 weeks' gestation with the diagnosis of preterm labor. She was treated with magnesium sulfate and betamethasone. Tonight, when you come on your shift at 7:00 p.m., she remains on magnesium sulfate but is contracting regularly and at 3:20 a.m. has SROM for clear fluid. At 4:00 a.m. her cervix is 5 cm/90%/+1. At this time, the magnesium sulfate is discontinued and normal spontaneous vaginal birth anticipated because of advanced preterm labor. Over the next hour Mallory is contracting every 2 to 3 minutes and coping well with uterine contractions. Her sister, Allison, is at the bedside providing labor support. The FHR baseline is 140s, with average variability, occasional accelerations, and no decelerations. At 5:15 a.m., Mallory feels the urge to have a bowel movement and you do an SVE. Her vaginal exam reveals that she is 10 cm/100%/+1.

Who needs to be notified of your significant assessment findings?
What would you report?

Within 15 minutes of your report, her physician arrives, confirms your assessment that Mallory is completely dilated, and wants her to start pushing. You coach Mallory to begin pushing with her next contraction.

What are your priorities in nursing care for Mallory?
Discuss the rationale for the priorities.
State nursing diagnosis, expected outcome, and interventions related to this problem.
What would you anticipate as Mallory's teaching needs?

Over the next hour, Mallory's contractions slow to every 7 minutes and she is open-glottis pushing and feels the urge to bear down with the peak of contractions. An SVE reveals descent of the fetal head is +2 station. You request the physician to come to the bedside to evaluate fetal descent. After her physician evaluates Mallory, she requests oxytocin augmentation to increase the frequency of her contractions. You initiate oxytocin augmentation at 1 mU/min per physician orders.

Discuss the risk associated with oxytocin augmentation.
Outline nursing actions when caring for a patient with oxytocin augmentation.
What teaching would you include related to oxytocin augmentation?

Within 30 minutes of starting the oxytocin, Mallory is having UCs every 1 to 2 minutes lasting 45 to 55 seconds, moderate to palpation

Continued

with a relaxed uterus between contractions. The FHR baseline is 140s with variable decelerations to 90s for 40 seconds with UCs, and FHR variability is moderate.

What are your priorities in nursing care?
Discuss the rationale for the priorities and nursing actions.
What are your nursing actions based on your assessment?
State nursing diagnosis, expected outcomes.

Over the next hour, Mallory's contractions are every 3 to 4 minutes and she is pushing with contractions and has a strong urge to bear down with contractions. The FHR is 140s with moderate variability and variable decelerations to 100 bpm for 30 seconds with contractions and open-glottis pushing. Her SVE reveals fetal descent to +3 station.

What are your immediate priorities in nursing care for Mallory?
Discuss the rationale for the priorities.

REFERENCES

Adams, E. D., Stark, M. A., & Low, L. K. (2016). A nurse's guide to supporting physiologic birth. *Nursing and Womens Health, 20*(1), 76–85. Retrieved from nwhjournal.org.

Agency for Healthcare Research and Quality. (2001). Reducing and preventing adverse drug events to decrease hospital costs. Publication No. 01-0200. Washington, DC: Author.

American Academy of Pediatrics & American College of Obstetricians and Gynecologists. (2012). *Guidelines for perinatal care* (7th ed.). Elk Grove, IL: Authors.

American College of Obstetricians and Gynecologists (ACOG). (2003). Dystocia and augmentation of labor. Practice Bulletin No. 49. *Obstetrics & Gynecology, 102*(6), 1445–1454.

American College of Obstetricians and Gynecologists (ACOG). (2009a). ACOG Committee on Practice Bulletins—Obstetrics. Practice Bulletin No. 107: Induction of labor. *Obstetrics & Gynecology, 114*(2 Pt 1), 386–397. doi:10.1097/AOG.0b013e3181b48ef5.

American College of Obstetricians and Gynecologists (ACOG). (2009b). Management of stillbirth. Practice Bulletin No. 102. *Obstetrics & Gynecology, 113*(3), 748–761.

American College of Obstetricians and Gynecologists (ACOG). (2010). Vaginal birth after previous cesarean delivery. Practice Bulletin No. 115. *Obstetrics & Gynecology, 116*(2 Pt 1), 450–463.

American College of Obstetricians and Gynecologists (ACOG). (2011). Optimizing protocols for obstetrics: Oxytocin for induction. Washington, DC: Author.

American College of Obstetricians and Gynecologists (ACOG). (2014a). Committee Opinion No. 590: Preparing for clinical emergencies in obstetrics and gynecology. *Obstetrics & Gynecology, 123*, 722–725.

American College of Obstetricians and Gynecologists (ACOG). (2014b). Management of late-term and post-term pregnancies. Practice Bulletin No. 146. *Obstetrics & Gynecology, 124*, 390–396.

American College of Obstetricians and Gynecologists (ACOG). (2014c). Safe prevention of the primary cesarean delivery. *Obstetrics & Gynecology, 123*, 693–711.

American College of Obstetricians and Gynecologists (ACOG). (2015). Operative vaginal delivery. Practice Bulletin No. 154. *Obstetrics & Gynecology, 126*, 1118.

American College of Obstetricians and Gynecologists (ACOG). (2016). External cephalic version. Practice Bulletin No. 161. *Obstetrics & Gynecology, 127*, e54–61.

American College of Obstetricians and Gynecologists (ACOG). (2017a). Committee Opinion No. 689: Delivery of a newborn with meconium-stained amniotic fluid. *Obstetrics & Gynecology, 129*, e33–4.

American College of Obstetricians and Gynecologists (ACOG). (2017b). Committee Opinion No. 712: Intrapartum management of intraamniotic infection. *Obstetrics & Gynecology, 130*, e95–101.

American College of Obstetricians and Gynecologists, & Society for Maternal-Fetal Medicine. (2017c). Shoulder dystocia. Practice Bulletin No. 178. *Obstetrics & Gynecology, 129*(5), e123–132.

Association for Women's Health, Obstetric and Neonatal Nurses (AWHONN). (2008). *Basic high risk and critical care intrapartum nursing clinical competencies and education guide* (4th ed.). Washington, DC: AWHONN.

Association for Women's Obstetric and Neonatal Nurses (AWHONN). (2014). Position statement: Nonmedically indicated induction and augmentation of labor. Washington, DC: AWHONN.

Athukorala, C., Middleton, P., & Crowther, C. A. (2006). Intrapartum interventions for preventing shoulder dystocia. *Cochrane Database of Systematic Reviews, 4.* doi:10.1002/14651858.CD005543.pub2.

Behling, D. J., & Renaud, M. (2015). Development of an obstetric vital sign alert to improve outcomes in acute care obstetrics. *Nursing for Women's Health, 19*(2), 128–141.

Bishop, E. H. (1964). Pelvic scoring for elective induction. *Obstetrics & Gynecology, 24,* 266–268.

Boulvain, M., Stan, C. M., & Irion, O. (2009). Membrane sweeping for induction of labour. *Cochrane Database of Systematic Reviews, 1.* doi:10.1002/14651858.CD000451.pub2

Bowers, N. A. (2014). Multiple gestation. In K. R. Simpson & P. A. Creehan (Eds.), *Perinatal nursing* (4th ed., pp 272–314). Philadelphia, PA: Wolters Kluwer/Lippincott Williams & Wilkins.

Bricker, L., & Luckas, M. (2000). Amniotomy alone for induction of labour. *Cochrane Database of Systematic Reviews, 4.* doi:10.1002/14651858.CD002862.

Callaghan, W. M., Creanga, A. A., & Kuklina, E. V. (2012). Severe maternal morbidity among delivery and postpartum hospitalizations in the United States. *Obstetrics & Gynecology, 120*(5), 1029–1036. doi:10.1097/AOG.0b013e31826d60c5

Centers for Disease Control and Prevention. (2017a). Pregnancy mortality surveillance system. Retrieved from www.cdc.gov/reproductivehealth/maternalinfanthealth/pmss.html.

Centers for Disease Control and Prevention. (2017b). Severe maternal morbidity in the United States. Division of Reproductive Health, National Center for Chronic Disease Prevention and Health Promotion. Retrieved from www.cdc.gov/reproductivehealth/MaternalInfantHealth/SevereMaternalMorbidity.html.

Clark, S. L. (2014). Amniotic fluid embolism. *Obstetrics & Gynecology, 123*(2 pt 1), 337–348.

Clark, S., Simpson, K., Knox, G., & Garite, T. (2009). Oxytocin: New perspectives on an old drug. *American Journal of Obstetrics & Gynecology, 200*(1), 35.e1–35.e6.

Cunningham, E., Leveno, K., Bloom, S., Spong, C., Dashe, J., Hoffman, B., . . . Sheffield, J. (2014). *Williams obstetrics* (24th ed.). New York, NY: McGraw-Hill.

Cunningham, F. G., & Nelson, D. B. (2015). Disseminated intravascular coagulation syndromes in obstetrics. *Obstetrics & Gynecology, 126*(5), 999–1011.

Cunningham, F. G., & Wells, C. E. (2017). Patient education: Vaginal birth after cesarean delivery (VBAC) (beyond the basics). Retrieved ttps://www.uptodate.com/contents/vaginal-birth-after-cesarean-delivery-vbac-beyond-the-basics

DeLoughery, T. G. (2015). Disseminated intravascular coagulation. In *Hemostasis and Thrombosis* (3rd ed., pp. 39–42). Springer International Publishing. DOI: 10.1007/978-3-319-09312-3_8

Dunn, T., Nassr, A., Moaddab, A., Eppes, C., & Shamshirsaz, A. (2017). Vasa previa: Maternal and early neonatal outcomes in the new era of obstetrical care [13K]. *Obstetrics & Gynecology May,* doi:0.1097/01.AOG.0000514606.70935.d2

Erez, O., Mastrolia, S. A., & Thachil, J. (2015). Disseminated intravascular coagulation in pregnancy: Insights in pathophysiology, diagnosis and management. *American Journal of Obstetrics & Gynecology, 213*(4), 452–463.

Farsight, A. Y., Jaimez-Carranza, N. M., & Coleman, C. R. (2017). Multidisciplinary response to amniotic fluid embolism. *Journal of Obstetric, Gynecologic & Neonatal Nursing, 46*(3), S56–S57.

Geis, G. M. (2017). Meconium aspiration syndrome. Medscape. Retrieved https://emedicine.medscape.com/article/974110-overview

Gilbert, E. (2011). Labor and delivery at risk. In S. Mattson & J. Smith (Eds.), *Core curriculum for maternal-newborn nursing* (4th ed.). Thousand Oaks, CA: Sage.

Goldberg, A. E. (2015). Cervical ripening. Medscape. Retrieved https://emedicine.medscape.com/article/263311-overview

Gülmezoglu, A. M., Crowther, C. A., & Middleton, P. (2006). Induction of labour for improving birth outcomes for women at or beyond term. *Cochrane Database of Systematic Reviews, 4.* doi:10.1002/14651858.CD004945.pub2.

Hamilton, B. E., Martin, J. A., & Ventura, S. J. (2012). Births: Preliminary data for 2011. *National Vital Statistics Reports, 61*(5).

Higgins, R. D., Saade, G., Polin, R. A., Grobman, W. A., Buhimschi, I. A., Watterberg, K.... Tse, N. K. for the Chorioamnionitis Workshop Participants. (2016). Evaluation and management of women and newborns with a maternal diagnosis of chorioamnionitis: Summary of a workshop. *Obstetrics & Gynecology, 127*(3), 426–436.

Hofmeyr, G. J., Kulier, R., & West, H. M. (2015). External cephalic version for breech presentation at term. *Cochrane Database of Systematic Reviews.* CD000083.

Institute for Healthcare Improvement. (2007). *Prevent harm from high alert medications: How to guide.* Cambridge, MA: Author.

Institute for Safe Medication Practices. (2007). *High-alert medications.* Huntingdon Valley, PA: Author.

Jacobson, C. H., Zlatnik, M. G., Kennedy, H. P., & Lyndon, A. (2013). Nurses' perspectives on the intersection of safety and informed decision making in maternity care. *Journal of Obstetric, Gynecologic & Neonatal Nursing, 42*(5), 577–587.

Jones, R., & Clark, S. L. (2013). Amniotic fluid embolism (anaphylactoid syndrome of pregnancy). In N. Troiano, C. Harvey, & B. Chez (Eds.), *High risk and critical care obstetrics* (3rd ed., pp. 316–325). Washington: DC: Association of Women's Health, Obstetric and Neonatal Nursing.

Jonsson, M., Norden-Lindeberg, S., & Hanson, U. (2007). Analysis of malpractice claims with a focus on oxytocin use in labour. *Acta Obstetricia et Gynecologica, 86,* 315–319.

Jozwiak, M., Bloemenkamp, K., Kelly, A., Mol, B., Irion, O., & Boulvain, M. (2012). Mechanical methods for induction of labour. *Cochrane Database of Systematic Reviews, 3.* doi:10.1002/14651858.CD001233.pub2.

Kelly, A. J., Alfirevic, Z., Hofmeyr, G. J., Kavanagh, J., Neilson, J. P., & Thomas, J. (2009). Induction of labour in specific clinical situations: Generic protocol. *Cochrane Database of Systematic Reviews, 2.* doi:10.1002/14651858.CD003398.pub2.

Kelly, A. J., Kavanagh, J., & Thomas, J. (2001). Castor oil, bath and/or enema for cervical priming and induction of labour. *Cochrane Database of Systematic Reviews, 2.* doi:10.1002/14651858.CD003099.

Kelly, A. J., Kavanagh, J., & Thomas, J. (2003). Vaginal prostaglandin (PGE2 and PGF2a) for induction of labour at term. *Cochrane Database of Systematic Reviews, 4.* doi:10.1002/14651858.CD003101.

Kunz, M. K., Loftus, R. L., & Nichols, A. M. (2013). Incidence of uterine tachysystole in women induced with oxytocin. *Journal of Obstetric, Gynecologic & Neonatal Nursing, 42,* 12–18. doi:10.1111/j.1552-6909.2012.01428.x

Lyndon, A., & Ali, L. U. (Eds.). (2008). *Fetal heart rate monitoring: Principles and practice* (4th ed.). Dubuque, IA: Kendal/Hunt.

Lyndon, A., Johnson, M. C., Bingham, D., Napolitano, P. G., Joseph, G., Maxfield, D. G., & O'Keeffe, D. F. (2015). Transforming communication and safety culture in intrapartum care. A multi-organization blueprint. *Journal of Obstetric, Gynecologic, & Neonatal Nursing, 44,* 341–349. doi: http://dx.doi.org/10.1111/1552-6909.12575

Lyndon, A., Zlatnik, M. G., Maxfield, D. G., Lewis, A., McMillan, C., & Kennedy, H. P. (2014). Contributions of clinical disconnections and unresolved conflict to failures in intrapartum safety. *Journal of Obstetric, Gynecologic & Neonatal Nursing, 43*(1), 2–12. doi:10.1111/1552-6909.12266.

MacDorman, M. F., Kirmeyer, S. E., & Wilson, E. C. (2012). Fetal and perinatal mortality, United States, 2006. *National Vital Statistics Report, 60*(8).

Macones, G. A., Hankins, G. D. V., Spong, C. Y., Hauth, J., & Moore, T. (2008). The 2008 National Institute of Child Health and Human Development workshop report on electronic fetal monitoring: Update on definitions, interpretation, and research guidelines. *Journal of Obstetric, Gynecologic and Neonatal Nursing, 37,* 510–515. doi: 10.1111/j.1552-6909.2008.00284.x

Maher, M. A. (2014). Obesity in pregnancy. In K. Simpson & P. Creehan (Eds.), *Perinatal nursing* (4th ed.). Philadelphia, PA: Lippincott, Williams & Wilkins.

Malone, F. D., & D'Alton, M. E. (2014). Multiple gestation: Clinical characteristics and management. In R. K. Creasy, R. Resnik, J. D. Iams, C. J. Lockwood, T. R. Moore, & M. F. Green (Eds.), *Creasy & Resnik's maternal-fetal medicine: Principles and practice* (7th ed., pp. 756–784). Philadelphia, PA: Elsevier/Saunders.

Martin, J. A., Hamilton, B. E., Osterman, M. J., Driscoll, A. K., & Mathews, T. J. (2017). Births: Final data for 2015. *National Vital Statistics Reports, 66*(1), 1.

Martin, J., Hamilton, B., Ventura, S., Osterman, M., Kirmeyer, S., Mathews, T., & Wilson, E. (2011). Birth: Final data for 2009. *National Vital Statistic Reports, 57,* 1.

Menacker, F., & Martin, J. A. (2008). Expanded health data from the new birth certificate, 2005. *National Vital Statistics Reports, 56*(13).

Nahum, G. G. (2016). *Uterine rupture in pregnancy.* Medscape. Retrieved https://reference.medscape.com/article/275854-overview

Norwitz, E. R. (2017). Patient education: Post-term pregnancy (Beyond the Basics). Up To Date https://www.uptodate.com/contents/postterm-pregnancy-beyond-the-basics Retrieved

Osterman, M. J., & Martin, J. A. (2014). Recent declines in induction of labor by gestational age. *NCHS Data Brief, 1.*

Oyelese, Y. (2007). Placenta previa, placenta accreta and vasa previa. In J. Queenan (Ed.), *High risk pregnancy.* Washington, DC: ACOG.

Parfitt, S. (2016). Labor and delivery at risk. In Mattson & Smith (Eds.), *AWHONN, core curriculum for maternal newborn nursing* (6th ed.). St. Louis, MO: Elsevier.

Phelan, S. T., & Holbrook, B. D. (2013). *Umbilical cord prolapse.* Royal College of Obstetricians and Gynaecologists. Author.

Podulka, J., Stranges, E., & Steiner, C. (2011). Hospitalizations related to childbirth, 2008. HCUP Statistical Brief #110. Retrieved from http://hcup-us.ahrq.gov/reports/statbriefs/sb110.pdf.

Queenan, J., Hobbins, J., & Spong, C. (2005). *Protocols in high risk pregnancies.* Malden, MA: Blackwell.

Roth, C. K., Parfitt, S. E., Hering, S. L., & Dent, S. A. (2014). Developing protocols for obstetric emergencies. *Nursing for Women's Health, 18*(5), 378–390.

Silver, R. M. (2015). Abnormal placentation: Placenta previa, vasa previa, and placenta accreta. *Obstetrics & Gynecology, 126*(3), 654–668.

Simpson, K. (2013). *Cervical ripening labor induction and labor augmentation of labor* (4th ed.). Washington, DC: AWHONN.

Simpson, K., & Atterbury, J. (2003). Trends and issues in labor induction in the United States: Implications for clinical practice. *Journal of Obstetric, Gynecologic & Neonatal Nursing, 32,* 767–779.

Simpson, K., & Knox, G. (2009). High-alert medication: Implications for perinatal patient safety. *Maternal Child Nursing, 34*(1).

Simpson, K. R., & O'Brien-Abel, N. (2013). Labor and birth. In K. R. Simpson & P. A. Creehan (Eds.). *AWHONN's perinatal nursing* (4th ed., pp. 343–444). Philadelphia, PA: Lippincott Williams & Wilkins.

Sousou, J., & Smart, C. (2015). Care of the childbearing family with intrauterine fetal demise. *Nursing for Women's Health, 19*(3), 236–247.

Spong, C. Y., Berghella, V., Wenstrom, K. D., Mercer, B. M., & Saade, G. R. (2012). Preventing the first cesarean delivery: Summary of a joint Eunice Kennedy Shriver National Institute of Child Health and Human Development, Society for Maternal-Fetal Medicine, and American College of Obstetricians and Gynecologists workshop. *Obstetrics & Gynecology, 120*(5), 1181–1193. doi: 10.1097/AOG.0b013e3182704880

Stanley Sundin, C., & Bradham Mazac, L. (2017). Amniotic fluid embolism. *American Journal of Maternal Child Nursing, 42*(1), 29–35. doi:10.1097/NMC.0000000000000292

Troiano, N. H., Chez, B. F., & Harvey, C. D. (2013). *AWHONN's high risk and critical care obstetrics.* Philadelphia, PA: Lippincott Williams & Wilkins.

Vanden Hoek, T. L., Morrison, L. J., Shuster, M., Donnino, M., Sinz, E., Lavonas, E. J. . . . Gabrielli, A. (2010). Part 12: Cardiac arrest in special situations: 2010 American Heart Association Guidelines for Cardiopulmonary Resuscitation and Emergency Cardiovascular Care. *Circulation, 122*(18 Suppl 3), S829–861. doi:10.1161/CIRCULATIONAHA.110.971069.

Viswanathan, M., Visco, A., Hatmann, K., Wechter, M., Gartlehner, G., Wu, J. . . . Lohr, K. N. (2006). Cesarean delivery on maternal request. *Evidence Report/Technology Assessment,* Full Rep (133), 1–138.

Wegner, E., & Bernstein, I. (2017). Operative vaginal birth. Retrieved

Wei, S., Wo, B. L., Qi, H. P., Xu, H., Luo, Z.C. Roy, C., & Fraser, W. D. (2013). Early amniotomy and early oxytocin for prevention of, or therapy for, delay in first stage spontaneous labour compared with routine care. *Cochrane Database of Systematic Reviews, 8.* doi:10.1002/14651858.CD006794.pub4.

Intrapartum and Postpartum Care of Cesarean Birth Families

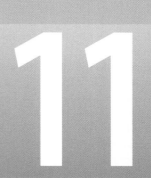

Nancy Irland, DNP, MSN, CNM
Kara Johnson, DNP, RNC-OB, CNS

LEARNING OUTCOMES

Upon completion of this chapter, the student will be able to:

1. Identify factors that place a woman at risk for cesarean birth.
2. Discuss the preoperative nursing care and medical and anesthesia management for cesarean births.
3. Describe the intraoperative nursing care and medical and anesthesia management for cesarean births.
4. Discuss the postoperative nursing care of cesarean birth with women and their families.
5. Identify potential intraoperative and postoperative complications related to cesarean birth and nursing actions to reduce risk.

Nursing Diagnoses

- At risk for low self-esteem related to perceived failure of life event
- At risk for injury related to surgical procedure and effects of anesthesia
- At risk for fluid volume deficit related to blood loss and oral fluid restriction
- At risk for acute pain related to surgical incision
- At risk for infection related to surgical incision, tissue trauma, or prolonged rupture of membranes
- At risk for altered parent-infant attachment related to surgical intervention

Nursing Outcomes

- Parents will verbalize understanding of factors that contributed to the need for cesarean birth.
- The woman will experience an uncomplicated intraoperative period and postoperative recovery.
- The woman will have adequate urinary output and normal amounts of lochia.
- The woman will verbalize a pain level she finds acceptable on a pain scale of 0 to 10.
- The woman will be afebrile and the abdominal incision site will be free of infection.
- The parents will hold the infant close to the body and demonstrate appropriate attachment behavior and care for infant needs.

INTRODUCTION

Cesarean birth, also referred to as cesarean section, C-section (C/S), or surgical birth, is an operative procedure in which the fetus is delivered through an incision in the abdominal wall and the uterus. Approximately one-third of pregnant couples experience a cesarean birth. The percentage of cesarean births has increased from 20.7% in 1996 to 31.9% in 2016 and reflects a 54% increase over a 19-year period (Hamilton, Martin, & Ventura, 2011; Hamilton, Martin, Osterman, Driscoll, & Rossen, 2017). The rate of cesarean birth peaked in 2009 and stabilized between 2009 and 2014. The prevalence of cesarean birth has slowly declined since 2014, but rates have continued to increase for older women. High rates of cesarean births are partially attributed to:

- Decrease in vaginal birth after cesarean section (VBAC) rates.
- Decrease of vacuum and forceps-assisted deliveries.

- Increase in number of fetuses in breech position delivered by cesarean.
- Increase in the number of cesarean deliveries on maternal request (CDMR). CDMR is a cesarean section performed at the request of the woman before the start of labor and in the absence of maternal or fetal medical conditions that present a risk for labor (American College of Obstetricians and Gynecologists [ACOG], 2013).
- Increase in the labor inductions, especially for nulliparous women or women with an unfavorable cervix.
- Increase in the average maternal age at delivery. Women aged 35 and older are often referred to as having a "geriatric pregnancy" or a pregnancy with advanced maternal age. This pregnant population, especially those with their first pregnancy at this age, is at risk for cesarean birth. Nearly half of cesarean births occur in women aged 40 and older.
- Increase in malpractice litigation is perceived as contributing to the cesarean rate.

The needs and experiences of cesarean birth couples are distinctly different from those of couples who experience a vaginal birth. These differences include increased length of hospitalization, longer period of physical recovery, increased pain, and increased negative emotional responses to the childbirth experience. Couples who experience a planned cesarean birth versus an unplanned cesarean birth often face additional challenges. Women who experience an unplanned cesarean birth may have feelings of guilt and failure for not achieving a vaginal birth. Reports of these feelings have decreased as cesarean births have become more common.

CRITICAL COMPONENT

Cesarean Delivery on Maternal Request (CDMR)

- There is insufficient evidence to fully evaluate the benefits and risks of CDMR as compared to planned vaginal delivery; more research is needed.
- CDMR is not recommended for women desiring several children, as the risks of placenta previa, placenta accreta, and gravid hysterectomy rise with each cesarean delivery.
- CDMR should not be performed prior to 39 weeks' gestation because of the significant danger of neonatal complications that include respiratory distress, hypothermia, hypoglycemia, and NICU admission.
- CDMR should not be motivated by the unavailability of effective labor pain management.

ACOG, 2013.

INDICATIONS FOR CESAREAN BIRTH

Cesarean births are performed for maternal and/or fetal reasons. As shown in Box 11–1, labor arrest and nonreassuring fetal tracing are the leading reasons for primary cesarean births in the

BOX 11–1 | Indications for Cesarean Birth

1. Labor arrest: 34%
2. Nonreassuring fetal tracing: 23%
3. Malpresentation: 17%
4. Multiple gestation: 7%
5. Maternal-fetal: 5%
6. Macrosomia: 4%
7. Other obstetric indications: 4%
8. Preeclampsia: 3%
9. Maternal request: 3%

Barber et al., 2011.

United States. The major maternal medical indications for a cesarean birth are:

- Previous cesarean birth.
- Placental abnormalities.
- Mechanical impediment of the progress of labor or arrest of active labor.
- Cephalopelvic disproportion, which occurs when ineffective uterine contractions lead to prolonged first stage of labor *or* when the size, shape, or position of the fetal head prevents it from passing through the maternal pelvis *or* when the maternal bony pelvis is not large enough or appropriately shaped to allow for fetal descent.
- Previous uterine surgery (i.e., surgeries that involve an incision through the myometrium of the uterus).
- Preexisting or pregnancy-related maternal health factors such as:
  - Cardiac diseases.
  - Severe hypertension, preeclampsia.
  - Severe diabetes mellitus.
  - Obesity.

The major fetal medical indications for a cesarean birth are:

- Malpresentation or malposition of fetus such as:
  - Breech presentation.
  - Transverse lie.
  - Persistent occiput posterior position.
  - Fetal hand preceding the fetal head.
  - Asynclitism—oblique malpresentation of the fetal head.
- Category II or III fetal heart rate (FHR) pattern
- Multiple gestation

CRITICAL COMPONENT

Obesity and Cesarean Births

"Obese pregnant women are at increased risk for cesarean delivery, failed trial labor, endometritis, wound rupture or dehiscence, and venous thrombosis" (ACOG, 2015).

Obesity also increases a woman's risk of complications related to anesthesia. These include:

- Difficulty in placement of spinal or epidural anesthesia related to loss of landmarks due to increased body size.
- Impaired respirations for 2 hours following placement of spinal anesthesia.
- Difficulty in placement of endotracheal tube due to increased tissue and edema.

Recommendations include:

- Administration of broad-spectrum antimicrobial prophylaxis to decrease risk of infection.
- Use of pneumatic compression devices and low-molecular-weight heparin to decrease risk of venous thrombosis.

ACOG, 2015.

Preventing the First Cesarean Birth

One in three infants born in the United States is delivered by cesarean birth. The leading driver of both the rise and variation is first-birth cesarean deliveries performed during labor. With the large increase in primary cesarean deliveries, repeat cesarean delivery has emerged as the largest single indication. The economic costs, health risks, and negligible benefits for most mothers and newborns of these higher rates highlight the need for a quality improvement, multistrategy approach, including clinical improvement strategies with careful examination of labor management practices; payment reform to eliminate negative or perverse incentives; education to recognize the value of vaginal birth; and full transparency through public reporting and continued public engagement (Main et al., 2012).

Reserving labor induction primarily for medical indication is key to reduce cesarean delivery rates. If an induction is done for nonmedical indications, the gestational age should be at least 39 weeks or more and the cervix should be favorable, especially in the nulliparous woman. Review of the current literature demonstrates the importance of adhering to appropriate definitions for failed induction and arrest of labor progress. The diagnosis of failed induction should only be made after an adequate attempt. Adequate time for normal latent and active phases of the first stage and for the second stage should be allowed as long as the maternal and fetal conditions permit. The adequate time for each of these stages appears to be longer than traditionally estimated by the well-known Friedman curve. Operative vaginal delivery with forceps or vacuum extractor are acceptable when indicated and can safely prevent cesarean delivery in appropriate situations (Caughey, Cahill, Guise, & Rouse, 2014).

Main and colleagues (2012) concluded that national attention to the problem of unnecessary cesarean deliveries is a public health concern in the search for value and quality in U.S. health care. There is currently no evidence to demonstrate that a 31.9%

cesarean delivery rate is beneficial to women or their infants. Rather, this rate exposes women and infants to unnecessary risks in the perinatal period and long term and results in considerable unnecessary health care costs.

CRITICAL COMPONENT

Interventions and Strategies for Preventing Primary Cesarean Births

1. Implement the American College of Obstetricians and Gynecologists (ACOG) and the Society for Maternal-Fetal Medicine's definition and management of labor dystocia.
2. Develop standardized fetal heart rate interpretation and management.
3. Use cervical ripening agents when labor is induced in women with an unfavorable cervix.
4. When inducing labor, allow longer duration of latent phase (up to 24 hours) and administer oxytocin for at least 12 to 18 hours after membrane rupture before performing cesarean section for failed induction.
5. Use nonmedical interventions such as continuous labor support by nurse or doula.
6. External cephalic version for breech presentation.
7. No elective inductions until 39 weeks.
8. Trial labor for women with twin gestations when first twin is in a vertex presentation.

Coughey et al., 2014.

CLASSIFICATION OF CESAREAN BIRTHS

Cesarean births are classified as either scheduled (planned) or unscheduled (unplanned). Unscheduled cesarean births include emergent, urgent, and nonurgent cesarean births.

- Scheduled cesarean births occur before the onset of labor. Common reasons for a scheduled cesarean birth are:
  - Previous cesarean birth.
  - Maternal or fetal health conditions that place the woman or fetus at risk during labor and/or vaginal birth.
  - Malpresentation, such as breech presentation, diagnosed before labor.
  - CDMR.
- Emergent cesarean birth indicates an immediate need to deliver the fetus (e.g., prolapse of umbilical cord or rupture of uterus).
- Urgent cesarean birth indicates a need for rapid delivery of the fetus, such as with malpresentation diagnosed after onset of labor or placenta previa with mild bleeding and fetal heart rate with Category I FHR.
- Nonurgent cesarean birth indicates a need for cesarean birth related to complications such as failure to progress (cervix does not fully dilate) and failure to descend (fetus does not descend through the pelvis) with Category I FHR.

RISKS RELATED TO CESAREAN BIRTH

Maternal deaths related to cesarean birth have decreased in the United States due to improved surgical techniques, anesthetic care, and the availability of blood transfusions and antibiotic therapy, but this procedure still poses a risk to both the woman and her fetus. Women who experience cesarean births are at higher risk for postpartum infection, hemorrhage, thromboembolic disease, and maternal death. Maternal death is most often related to intrapartum or postpartum hemorrhage. Neonates are at higher risk for fetal injury during surgery, low Apgar scores, and respiratory distress.

Risks Related to Repeat Cesarean Birth

The most significant long-term complication of repeat surgical birth is placenta accreta. The spectrum of placenta accreta includes:

- Accreta: The placenta does not penetrate the entire thickness of the uterine muscle.
- Increta: The placenta extends farther into the myometrium.
- Percreta: The placenta extends fully through the uterine wall and may attach to other internal organs, such as the intestine or bladder.

In all forms of placenta accreta, the placenta does not separate from the uterine wall after delivery, potentially leading to excessive hemorrhage, disseminated intravascular coagulopathy, organ failure, and, in severe cases, death. Typically, a hysterectomy is needed to control a massive hemorrhage.

CRITICAL COMPONENT

Trial of Labor After Cesarean Section

Women who had a previous cesarean section and want more than two children are encouraged to attempt a vaginal birth after cesarean section (VBAC). Although this comes with risks of its own, it avoids the risks of abdominal surgery, future abnormal placental implantation, and infection. The labor process in this situation is called a trial of labor after cesarean section.
ACOG, 2010.

PERIOPERATIVE CARE

Perioperative perinatal nursing incorporates the skills of the specialties of obstetrics, surgery, and postanesthesia care to provide safe and comprehensive care to women who have had cesarean births. In most hospitals, cesarean births are performed in an operating room in the obstetrics department and labor and delivery nurses care for the family throughout the perioperative experience. Preoperative care may vary based on the urgency of the cesarean birth.

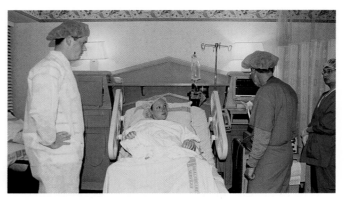

FIGURE 11-1 Couple awaiting scheduled cesarean section.

Scheduled Cesarean Birth

Couples are admitted to the labor and birthing unit the day of surgery (Fig. 11–1). Diagnostic laboratory work, such as complete blood count (CBC), platelet count, urinalysis, blood type, and cross match, may be completed a few days before admission.

CRITICAL COMPONENT

Evidence-Based Practice Guidelines

Nursing specialty organizations such as the Association of Women's Health, Obstetric and Neonatal Nurses (AWHONN) facilitate the use of research findings in clinical practice through the development of evidence-based practice guidelines. One such guideline is AWHONN's perioperative care of the pregnant woman. This guideline describes evidence-based practice to ensure the following:

1. Patient safety measures for perioperative care of the pregnant woman
2. Family-centered education and care practices
3. Assessment and interventions appropriate during preoperative, intraoperative, and postoperative periods for women undergoing cesarean birth

Medical Management

- Preoperatively, the surgeon will explain the reason for the cesarean birth and what it involves prior to hospital admission and obtain surgical consent.
- The surgery is scheduled.
- Presurgical diagnostic laboratory tests, such as CBC, blood type, and Rh, are ordered.
- If the woman's medical record is not available to the hospital electronically, a paper copy of her prenatal record and provider orders are faxed to the birthing unit to be placed in her hospital chart.
- Education is provided about which current medications the woman should take or eliminate on the day of surgery.
- To prevent postoperative infection, many providers recommend that the woman take at least one preoperative shower

at home, using an antiseptic agent on the night prior to the scheduled procedure.

Anesthesia Management

- The anesthesia provider (anesthesiologist or certified registered nurse anesthetist) meets with the couple during the admission process and before the woman is transferred to the operating room.
- The anesthesia provider reviews the prenatal record.
- The anesthesia provider completes an anesthesia history and physical, discusses anesthesia options with the couple, and answers their questions regarding anesthesia and the procedure.

Nursing Actions

- Complete the appropriate admission assessments (including baseline vital signs) and required preoperative forms.
- Obtain laboratory testing per orders, such as CBC, platelets, and type and screen. A delay in lab results can result in a delay in surgery.
- Obtain a baseline fetal heart rate monitor strip of at least 20 minutes before and after administration of regional anesthesia, if possible.
- Review the prenatal chart for factors that place the woman at risk during or after cesarean birth and ensure that physician and anesthesia provider are aware of risk factors such as low platelet count.
- Verify that the woman has been NPO for 6 to 8 hours before surgery, or per hospital protocol.
- Ensure that all required documents, such as prenatal record, current laboratory reports, and consent forms, are in the woman's chart.
- Assess the woman's knowledge and educational needs and provide preoperative teaching that includes what she and her partner can expect before, during, and after the cesarean birth.
- Identify and respect the cultural values, choices, and preferences of the woman and her family and individualize care to meet the needs of the woman and her family.
- Start an IV line and administer an IV fluid preload as per orders.
- Insert a Foley catheter as per order. Insertion is preferably done in the operating room after placement of the spinal or epidural and before the prep.
- Trim the lower abdominal and upper pubic regions with clippers prior to entering operating room (OR).
- Administer preoperative medications per orders. This might include sodium citrate to neutralize stomach acids. Famotidine or metoclopramide may be used to reduce the incidence of nausea or vomiting.
- Prepare the partner or the support person who plans to be present for the birth for the experience by providing appropriate surgical attire to wear in the operating room.
- Instruct the partner or the support person as to where he or she will sit and what he or she can anticipate regarding sights, sounds, and smells typical of an operating room.

- Provide emotional support for the couple as they wait to be transferred to the operating room.
- Complete the surgery checklist, which includes removal of jewelry, eyeglasses/contact lenses, and dentures. Eyeglasses can be given to the support person to bring into the operating room so the woman can use them to see her newborn baby.

CRITICAL COMPONENT

Antibiotic and Venous Thromboembolic Prophylaxis

- Administration of narrow-spectrum prophylactic antibiotics should occur within 60 minutes prior to the skin incision (AWHONN, 2011). Antibiotics of choice include cefazolin, or for women with penicillin and cephalosporin allergy, clindamycin with gentamicin may be given.
- Perform an assessment for risk of venous thromboembolism (VTE) and classify the woman based on VTE classification guidelines. Preoperative anticoagulant therapy may be necessary for women classified as moderate or high-risk or with a history of recurrent thrombosis.
- Apply sequential compression devices prior to surgery.

CRITICAL COMPONENT

IV Fluid Preload Before Anesthesia

An IV fluid preload of 500 to 1,000 mL is given before administration of spinal or epidural anesthesia to increase fluid volume and decrease risk of hypotension related to effects of anesthetic agent (AWHONN, 2011; Cunningham et al., 2014).

The use of prewarmed IV fluids in women having a cesarean birth results in an increased maternal core temperature, improved neonatal umbilical arterial pH, and improved Apgar scores (Munday, Hines, Wallace, Chang, & Yates, 2014).

Unscheduled Cesarean Birth

Unscheduled cesarean births usually have an urgent or emergent cause, such as fetal intolerance of labor or placental problems. The woman and her family are usually highly anxious and have fears that either the woman and/or infant's health is in danger. Due to the urgency of the cesarean birth, there may not be time to fully explain the reasons for the procedure. Therefore, the woman and her partner or support person need an opportunity during the immediate postpartum period to review the events leading up to the cesarean birth.

Medical Management

- Determine the need for a cesarean birth.
- Explain the reason for the cesarean birth.
- Explain the surgical procedure and obtain consent.

Anesthesia Management

- The anesthesia provider completes an anesthesia history and physical and discusses anesthesia options with the woman.

This may not occur until the woman is transferred to the operating room based on the amount of time between the decision for need of cesarean birth and transfer to the operating room.

- The anesthesia provider determines the need for a platelet count.
- The anesthesia provider explains the procedure and addresses the woman's and support person's questions and concerns.

Nursing Actions

- Notify the anesthesia, labor and delivery team, and neonatal personnel of the impending cesarean birth.
- Initiate continuous electronic FHR monitoring.
  - Expected findings: Category II or Category III FHR pattern when the cesarean section is related to fetal intolerance of labor.
- Administer oxygen when indicated (i.e., signs of fetal intolerance of labor).
- Assess the woman's vital signs.
  - Expected findings:
    - The woman's blood pressure is slightly elevated related to anxiety level.
    - There is a potential increase in temperature and pulse rate due to infection and/or dehydration related to prolonged labor and rupture of membranes.
- Start an IV and administer IV fluid preload as per orders.
- Ensure labs are completed as ordered; CBC, platelets, and type and screen or type and cross match.
- Complete and witness surgical and anesthesia consent forms.
- Insert a Foley catheter as ordered. Insertion may be done in the operating room after placement of the spinal or epidural anesthesia and before prep, unless the FHR indicates immediate delivery. In that situation, the catheter may be inserted in the woman's room before transfer to the operating room.
- If hair needs to be removed because it interferes with surgical site, hair clippers are used on the pubic region so that no hair is visible when the woman's legs are together. This should be done in the labor room and not in the operating room.
- Ensure that all required documents are in the woman's chart.
- Complete the surgical checklist.
- Facilitate the transition to unscheduled surgical birth in a timely manner. Guidelines in all hospitals that provide OB care should have the capability of responding to obstetrical emergencies within 30 minutes. Hence the 30-minute "decision to incision rule."
- Assess the couple's emotional response to the need for a cesarean birth.
  - Expected findings
    - Couples and family may experience high levels of anxiety based on fear of injury to the woman and/or unborn child.
    - Couples are not emotionally or mentally prepared for cesarean birth.
    - Couples and family have a knowledge deficit regarding cesarean birth and anesthesia options.
  - Couples and family ask questions regarding cesarean birth and anesthesia options.
- Help ensure the woman and her support person(s) receive information appropriate to the circumstances. Reinforce reason for cesarean section and address questions.
- Provide emotional support during transitional process from labor to preparation for surgery.
- Facilitate couple's communication with entire health care team to decrease fear, anxiety, and distress.
- Facilitate presence of woman's support person during preoperative preparation and surgical procedure because emotional support decreases anxiety.
- Review with the couple what to expect during and after the cesarean birth. Explain that the woman may feel pressure or pulling as her baby is being born.
- Prepare the partner or support person who plans to attend the birth as to what to anticipate in the operating room and provide him or her with proper surgical garb to wear in the operating room.

INTRAOPERATIVE CARE

The complete intraoperative team includes a surgeon, an anesthesia provider, a surgical first assist, a circulating nurse, and neonatal staff. The circulating nurse is responsible for patient safety. This generally includes responsibility for positioning the woman safely, assuring all time-outs and consents are completed appropriately, confirming the presence of newborn care providers at the birth, maintaining a correct count of surgical sponges, and labeling surgical specimens correctly and confirming their disposition to pathology or medical waste. The woman and her family will be anxious about the cesarean birth, whether it is a scheduled or unscheduled procedure. It is often the woman's first surgical experience, which can increase the anxiety level for both the woman and her partner. To help decrease anxiety, it is best if the nurse who admitted the woman for a scheduled cesarean section or the nurse who cared for the couple during labor continues to care for them during the surgery as the circulating nurse.

Complications

Intraoperative complications are rare because of advances in obstetrical anesthesia and surgical techniques. Women who are healthy during pregnancy are at low risk for complications. Intraoperative complications may include:

- Hemorrhage: Increased morbidity and mortality rates are associated with intraoperative and postpartum hemorrhage, which can result in hypovolemic shock, disseminated intravascular coagulation, renal and/or hepatic failure, and possibly the need for emergency hysterectomy.
- Bladder, ureter, and bowel trauma.
- Maternal respiratory depression related to anesthesia.
- Maternal hypotension related to anesthesia, which increases the risk for fetal acidemia.
- Inadvertent injection of the anesthetic agent into the maternal bloodstream; the woman may experience ringing in her

ears, metallic taste in her mouth, and hypotension that can lead to unconsciousness and cardiac arrest.

Anesthesia Management

- Determine the method of anesthesia based on the following factors:
  - Which one is the safest and most comfortable for the woman
  - Which has the least effect on the fetus/neonate
  - Which provides the optimal conditions for the surgery
- Methods of anesthesia
  - Spinal anesthesia is the preferred method for scheduled cesarean sections or for laboring women who do not have an epidural in place (Fig. 11–2). Spinal anesthesia, which is faster than an epidural to place, provides a full sensory and motor block.
  - Epidural anesthesia is used for laboring women who have an epidural in place for labor pain management and who then require a cesarean birth (see Fig. 11–2). Women with epidurals may feel tugging and pulling during the procedure because epidurals are not as dense and do not provide full sensory and motor block.
  - General anesthesia, which is rarely used and carries increased risks, is indicated in the following situations:
    - Rapid delivery is imperative
    - Severe hemorrhage
    - Seizures
    - Failed spinal
- Contraindications for epidural or spinal anesthesia
  - Low platelet count is the most common contraindication, especially with women who have preeclampsia and/or HELLP (hemolysis, elevated liver enzymes, and low platelets) syndrome.
  - Infection or dermatological issues of concern at the proposed site of needle insertion
  - Uncorrected maternal hypovolemia
  - The woman's refusal or inability to cooperate with the procedure
  - Spine abnormalities, injuries, and/or surgeries
  - Sepsis
- Administration of anesthesia
  - Bupivacaine is the preferred anesthetic agent for spinal and epidural blocks.
  - Preservative-free morphine or fentanyl is administered intrathecally to provide postoperative analgesia.
  - Epidural or spinal anesthesia may be administered with the woman sitting on the operating room table or lying on her side. When the woman is lying down, position her with a hip tilt to maintain uterine displacement before, during, and after administration of anesthesia. This will decrease the risk of aortocaval compression related to compression on the aorta and inferior vena cava by the gravid uterus.
- Monitor vital signs and oxygen saturation.
  - Expected findings:
    - Vital signs and oxygen saturation within normal limits with potential mild increase in blood pressure due to anxiety

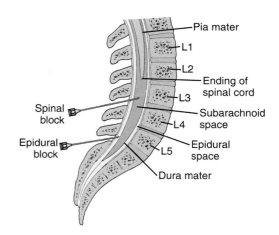

FIGURE 11–2 Spinal and epidural placements.

- Hypotension following administration of the anesthetic agent
- Monitor level of anesthesia, effectiveness of anesthesia, and complications.
  - Gastric aspiration: Aspiration of gastric contents can lead to pneumonitis. This is a potential complication of general anesthesia. Additional conditions that may increase the risk of aspiration include:
    - Morbid obesity.
    - Diabetes.
    - Difficult airway (Apfelbaum et al., 2013).
- Monitor blood loss, accomplished when the circulating nurse weighs lap sponges for a quantified blood loss (QBL) and reports findings to the surgical team. A QBL of up to 1,000 mL is expected in a cesarean birth.
- Administer antibiotics when indicated, generally within 1 hour of the incision time.
- Administer oxytocin after the delivery of the placenta to minimize bleeding.

Medical Management

- Two primary operative techniques are used for cesarean births. Most often, a Pfannenstiel incision, or "bikini cut," is the skin incision. This is a transverse skin incision made at the level of the pubic hairline (Fig. 11–3A). Typically, a lower uterine segment incision is performed on the uterus (Fig. 11–3C). The second operative technique, the classical cesarean delivery, is a vertical abdominal wall skin incision and vertical incision in the body of the uterus (Fig. 11–3 B and D). This technique is rare and is used in emergent cesarean births when immediate delivery is critical.
- The neonate is delivered through the uterine and abdominal incisions (Fig. 11–4). Following the delivery of the neonate, the placenta is manually removed. The uterus may be lifted out of the abdominal cavity or left in place while the uterine incision is repaired. The abdominal tissues and incision are repaired.

Nursing Actions

- Conduct a pre-procedure informational process according to facility policy. Include assessments, comments, and lab work.

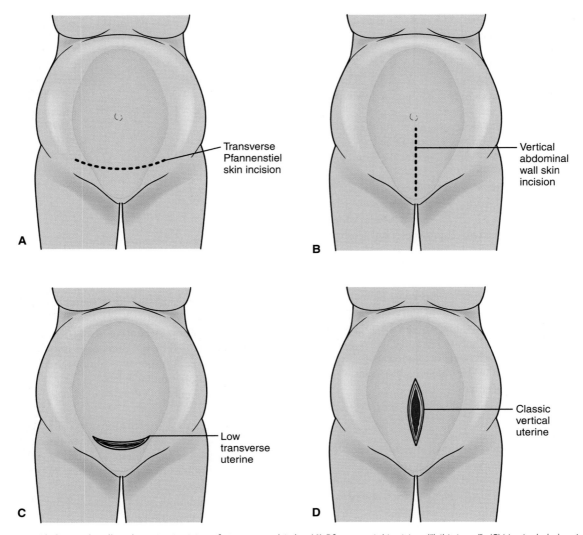

FIGURE 11–3 Abdominal wall and uterine incisions for cesarean births. (*A*) Pfannenstiel incision ("bikini cut"). (*B*) Vertical abdominal wall skin incision. (*C*) Low transverse uterine incision. (*D*) Classic vertical uterine incision.

- Position woman with a hip tilt to maintain uterine displacement before, during, and after administration of anesthesia to decrease the risk of aortocaval compression related to compression on the aorta and inferior vena cava due to weight of the gravid uterus.
- Continue external FHR monitoring until abdominal preparation is initiated. Remove the fetal scalp electrode (FSE) after abdominal surgical preparation is done and before delivery. FSE should not be removed until MD orders it.
- Conduct a time-out before administering anesthesia and before initial incision for validating correct patient, site, and procedure.
- Assist the woman into the proper position for epidural or spinal anesthesia.
- Reposition the woman after epidural or spinal anesthesia into a supine position with a left lateral tilt to decrease the pressure from the uterus on the inferior vena cava and maintain placental perfusion.

- Assess FHR after anesthesia placement.
- Apply the grounding device to the woman's thigh.
- Insert Foley.
- Perform abdominal skin prep using sterile technique.
- Secure the woman to the operating room table with a strap over her upper legs.
- Perform the duties of the circulating nurse, including instrument count, needle count, and sponge count.
- Check equipment used for the newborn to ensure it is in working order and all supplies are readily available for care of the neonate.
- Assess the couple's response to the cesarean birth.
  - Expected findings:
    - Anxiety levels increase related to operating room environment and impending surgery.
    - Couples may have concerns related to potential injury to the woman from anesthesia and/or surgery.
    - The woman may feel abdominal pressure as the neonate is being delivered.

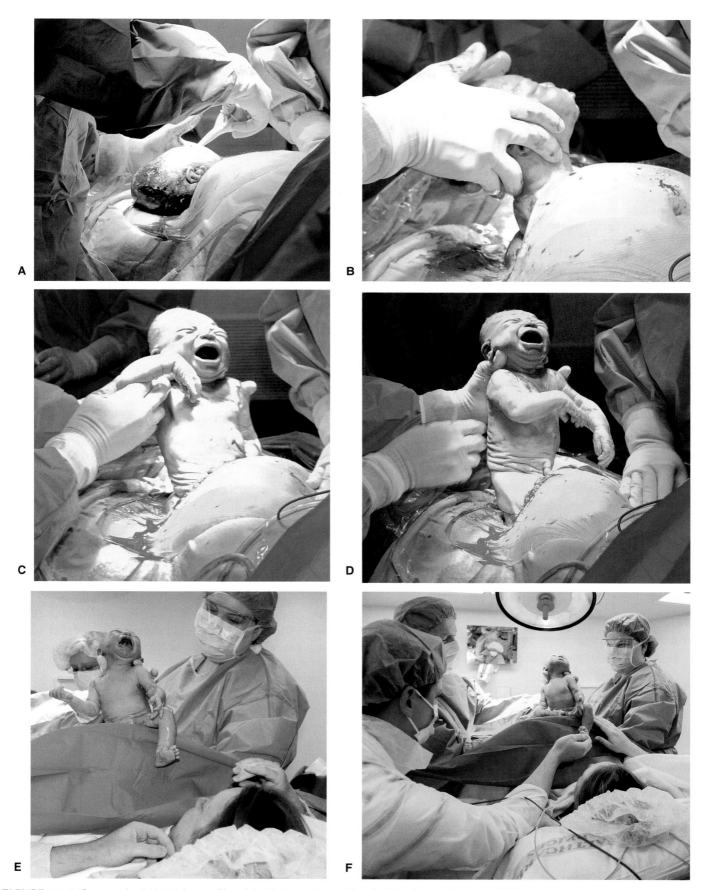

FIGURE 11–4 Cesarean birth. (*A*) Delivery of head. (*B*) Delivery of shoulders. (*C, D*) Delivery of body. (*E, F*) Mom and Dad meeting their daughter.

- Position the partner or support person on a stool next to the woman's head. Instruct the partner or support person to remain seated on the stool. This may prevent falling if the person feels faint.
- Instruct the partner or support person as to what he or she can and cannot touch.
- Provide emotional support to the woman and her partner or support person.
- Facilitate care for the neonate. Neonatal care is usually performed by the neonatal personnel (neonatal nurse, nurse practitioner, and/or neonatologist) who are present for the birth.
  - At least one person skilled in neonatal resuscitation should be available whose only responsibility is to receive and care for the baby.
  - Expected finding: The neonate's 1- and 5-minute Apgar scores are 7 or above unless there is fetal intolerance of labor before the birth.
- Record the time of delivery of the neonate and delivery of the placenta.
- Whenever possible, the newborn should remain in the operative suite with the mother.
- Complete identification bands and place on the neonate and parents before the neonate leaves the operating room.
- Ensure that new parents have an opportunity to see and hold their newborn. In many birthing units, the neonate, if stable, remains in the operating room and skin-to-skin contact is initiated. The neonate is then transferred to the labor and delivery recovery room with the woman and her partner or support person.
- Transfer unstable neonate to the nursery and encourage the partner or support person to accompany the newborn to the nursery. Neonatal personnel are responsible for transferring unstable neonates.
- Address parents' questions regarding the health of their newborn.
- Complete intraoperative documentation.

Evidence-Based Practice: Skin-to-Skin Contact During Cesarean Birth

Schneuder, L., Crenshaw, J., & Gilder, R. (2017). Influence of immediate skin-to-skin contact during cesarean surgery on rate of transfer of newborn to NICU for observation. *Nursing for Women's Health, 21*, 28–33.

A retrospective analysis was conducted to determine if immediate skin-to-skin contact during cesarean birth influenced the proportion of newborns transferred to the NICU for observation. Data was collected for the 2 years prior to implementing skin-to-skin contact immediately during cesarean birth (in the operating room) and for the first 3 years following implementation.

Inclusion criteria: Scheduled and nonemergent cesarean births between 37 and 42 weeks' gestation that occurred within 2 years preceding implementation and the first 3 years following implementation.

Sample: The sample included 2,841 newborns; 1,070 were born before implementation and 1,771 were born after implementation. The mean gestational age was 39 weeks and the mean birth weight was 3,401 g.

Results: The proportion of newborns transferred to NICU for observation was significantly lower after implementing skin-to-skin contact immediately following the birth. Prior to implementation, 5.6% of newborns were transferred to NICU for observation; after implementation, 1.75% were transferred.

Nursing implication: Early and continuous contact with the newborn facilitates parent-infant bonding and attachment. Skin-to-skin contact in the operating room significantly decreases the percentage of newborns who are separated from their parents due to transfers to the NICU for observation.

CRITICAL COMPONENT

Universal Protocol for Preventing Wrong Patient, Wrong Site, Wrong Person Surgery

Joint Commission Standard PC 13.20 EP 9 states that "the site, procedure, and patient are accurately identified and clearly communicated using active communication techniques, during a final verification process such as time-out before the start of any surgical or invasive procedure" (Joint Commission, 2003).

The operating room circulating nurse assists in actively verifying that this is the correct patient and procedure when time-out is called immediately before the epidural or spinal procedure begins and immediately before the surgical incision is made to verify that it is the correct site, procedure, and patient.

POSTOPERATIVE CARE

The recovery time following a cesarean birth is longer compared to vaginal delivery due to the tissue trauma related to surgical intervention. The usual hospital stay is 3 days, with full recovery from surgery taking 6 weeks or longer. The maternal morbidity rate is increased twofold with cesarean delivery compared with vaginal delivery (Cunningham et al., 2014). Principal sources of complications are infection, hemorrhage, and thromboembolism. There is a twofold increase in rehospitalization. Rates of complications vary based on status of cesarean and emergency versus planned. Rates of infection with emergency cesarean are reported at 12%, wound complications at 1.2%, and operative injury at 0.5% (Cunningham et al., 2014).

Complications

Women who enter pregnancy in a healthy state and have experienced a healthy pregnancy are at low risk for complications. In contrast, women who experience a prolonged labor, multiple interventions such as internal monitoring, or prolonged rupture of membranes are at higher risk for postoperative complications. These include the following:

- Hemorrhage: Postpartum hemorrhage is most often identified in the intraoperative period or within the first few hours post-op.
- Anemia related to blood loss
- Deep vein thrombosis
- Pulmonary embolism
- Paralytic ileus
- Hematuria related to bladder trauma
- Infections of the bladder, endometrium, and incision
- Severe headache related to method of anesthesia

CRITICAL COMPONENT

Postoperative Complications

A multidisciplinary team approach is needed to provide care to women experiencing postoperative complications. Nurses have a key role in recognizing deteriorating conditions in the postoperative period. The most common preventable errors related to cesarean births are failure to recognize and act upon changes in vital signs and failure to act on postpartum hemorrhage.

- Pulmonary embolism presents as an acute event. Signs and symptoms are dyspnea, tachypnea, chest tightness, shortness of breath, hypotension, and decreasing oxygen saturation levels.
- Increased morbidity and mortality rates are associated with postpartum hemorrhage due to hypovolemic shock, disseminated intravascular coagulation, renal and/or hepatic failure, and the possible need for emergency hysterectomy.
- Surgical site infection rate is estimated to be 3% to 15%. Signs include serous or purulent drainage, erythema, fever, pain, and wound dehiscence.
- Endometritis is usually diagnosed within the first few days after delivery. Fever is the most common sign. Other signs include chills, uterine tenderness, and foul-smelling lochia.

AWHONN, 2011.

Immediate Postoperative Care

The woman and her newborn are transferred from the operating room to the labor and delivery postanesthesia care unit (PACU) or to her labor room following the cesarean birth. Immediate assessment and monitoring of maternal and newborn status is influenced by the type of anesthesia and preoperative or intraoperative complications. It focuses on maternal and fetal oxygenation, ventilation, circulation level of consciousness, and body temperature. The purpose of PACU care is to stabilize vital signs, bleeding, pain, itching, and nausea and to monitor anesthesia level. One RN should be assigned solely to the care of the mother and one nurse assigned to her newborn until the critical elements are completed, such as report, assessments, and stable vital signs.

Equipment comparable to that in the main PACU should be available for the care of post-op OB patients.

- Blood loss and uterine tone are monitored closely in the PACU. Hospital policy may be to weigh on a scale pads and chux for more accurate measurement of QBL (1gram = 1 mL).
- Input and output (I&O) is monitored.
- Active warming measures are used to prevent hypothermia.
- Facility-based scoring system is used to determine the appropriate timing for discharge from the recovery room.

First 24 Hours After Birth

Medical management, anesthesia management, and nursing actions in the first 24 hours after birth are as follows.

Medical Management

- Assess for involutional changes and signs of potential complications.
- Assess pulmonary function: assess for atelectasis and pneumonia.
- Assess for ileus, cholecystitis, persistent nausea and vomiting, and intestinal obstruction.
- Medical orders are usually standardized. These orders include:
  - IV therapy.
  - Medications such as analgesics and stool softeners.
  - Antibiotic therapy for the woman at risk for infection related to prolonged rupture of membranes, prolonged labor, or elevated temperature during labor.
  - Progression of diet.
  - Removal of the Foley catheter, generally at 12 hours postsurgery.
  - Activity level.
- Immediate care of the newborn is the same for vaginal delivery and is detailed in Chapters 8 and 15.

Anesthesia Management

- When intrathecal morphine is used for postoperative pain management, the anesthesia provider manages the woman's pain for the first 24 hours and administers medications to counteract side effects of intrathecal opioids.

SAFE AND EFFECTIVE NURSING CARE: Understanding Medication

Preservative-Free Morphine
- Indication: Severe pain
- Action: Alters perception of and response to painful stimuli and produces generalized CNS depression
- Common side effects: Respiratory depression, itching, hypotension, nausea and vomiting, and urinary retention
- Route and dose: Administered intrathecally by anesthesiologist or CRNA; 5–10 mg

Vallerand & Sanoski, 2017.

CRITICAL COMPONENT

Maternal Respiratory Depression Related to Intrathecal Morphine

Severe respiratory depression (3% occurrence) is a life-threatening adverse reaction to intrathecal morphine.

- Naloxone and resuscitative equipment must be available whenever intrathecal morphine is administered and during the 24 hours postoperative after injection.
- Respiratory rate and level of sedation are monitored for the first 24 hours postoperative after administration. Normal respiratory rate is 12 to 18 breaths per minute.
- An initial dose of 0.4 to 2 mg of naloxone is administered intravenously for severe respiratory depression. Dose can be repeated every 2 to 3 minutes for a total of 10 mg.
- Respiratory resuscitation is initiated immediately and continued until normal respiratory function returns.

Nursing Actions

After a cesarean birth, most women recover in the labor and birthing recovery unit instead of the postanesthesia unit of the main OR. Nursing actions are similar to those when caring for a woman who had a vaginal birth, with emphasis on the following:

- Review prenatal, labor, and intrapartal records for risk factors.
- Monitor vital signs as per protocol.
  - Monitor respiratory rate, heart rate, blood pressure, pain, pulse oximetry, and level of sedation every hour for the first 24 hours after administration of intrathecal morphine.
  - Monitor for hemorrhage (increased bleeding, increased pulse, decreased blood pressure).
- Assess the fundus and lochia per protocol.
- Assess abdominal dressing for signs of bleeding.
- Assess woman's level of pain and use pharmacological and nonpharmacological interventions for pain management. Evaluate effectiveness of pain management interventions.
- Monitor for side effects of intrathecal morphine and provide appropriate interventions. The primary side effects and interventions are:
  - Pruritus: Administer medication as ordered, such as naloxone or diphenhydramine.
  - Nausea/vomiting: Administer medication as ordered, such as naloxone or metoclopramide.
  - Urinary retention: Occurs after removal of catheter: Administer naloxone or catheterize as ordered.
  - Respiratory depression: Administer oxygen as needed and/or naloxone as ordered.
- Monitor the level of sensation.
- Monitor for seizures, spinal headache, and neurological deficits (e.g., prolonged decreased sensation in legs).

- Auscultate lungs, encourage coughing and deep breathing, and assist woman in using incentive spirometry.
- Monitor intake and urinary output (per Foley catheter and for the first 24 hours following catheter removal).
- Advance diet as tolerated.
- Regulate IV fluids as ordered.
  - Oxytocin is added to IV fluids initially, to reduce the risk of postpartum hemorrhage related to uterine atony.
- Facilitate skin-to-skin contact with parents and infant.
- Assist the woman into a comfortable position for infant feeding.
- Assist with infant care and provide teaching as indicated.
- Provide emotional support by actively listening to the couple recall their birth experience and addressing their questions and concerns.

CRITICAL COMPONENT

Sudden Unexpected Newborn Collapse (SUNC)

SUNC is a rare event when a healthy-appearing, full-term infant suddenly experiences respiratory and cardiac arrest. Infants are at greatest risk during the first few hours of life. To decrease risk of SUNC during skin-to-skin contact, the nurse should place the infant on the mother's chest; confirm that the mother is in a semi-Fowler's position or higher and that the baby is not prone. The newborn's face should be turned to the side. Newborn prone position on the mother's chest, especially if the mother is on her back, can contribute to SUNC (Ferrarello & Carmichael, 2016).

Expected Assessment Findings

- Vital signs are within normal limits.
- Lochia is moderate to scant.
- The fundus is firm and midline and generally 1 to 2 cm above the umbilicus initially, moving down throughout the woman's hospital stay.
- The abdominal dressing is dry.
- The catheter is draining clear/yellow urine. A small amount of blood in the urine may be present when there has been trauma to the bladder during the procedure.
- The IV site is free of signs of infiltration or inflammation.
- The pain level is below 3 on a pain scale of 0 to 10, or within the woman's chosen number.
- The woman gradually regains full motor and sensory function as the effects of the anesthetic agent decrease.
- The woman sits at the bedside for short periods of time.
- The woman may experience itching, nausea, or decreased respirations related to side effects of morphine. Itching and nausea are the most common side effect of morphine. Itching varies from a facial rash to a full-body rash. Antihistamines are given to promote comfort.
- The woman feeds her newborn with or without assistance.
- The partner and family assist in care of the newborn.

- The couple may be tired and need time to rest.
- Women with unplanned cesarean births may experience guilt or a sense of failure or disappointment.
- Couples with unplanned cesarean births may ask questions about the cesarean birth and the events leading up to it.
- The couple will want time alone with their newborn.
- The couple will call family and friends, informing them of the birth.

24 Hours Postoperative to Discharge

The following medical management and nursing actions take place before the mother and baby are discharged.

Medical Management

- Assess the woman for involutional changes and signs of potential postoperative complications.
- Administer antibiotic therapy for women who experienced a prolonged labor or prolonged rupture of membranes or who are febrile.
- Remove abdominal dressing and assess for signs of dehiscence and infection (redness, tenderness, swelling). The dressing is usually removed on the first postoperative day.
- Provide discharge instructions.

Nursing Actions

Nursing actions are similar to those when caring for a woman who had a vaginal birth with addition to and/or emphasis on the following:

- Monitor vital signs as per protocol, generally every 4 hours.
- Assess breath sounds.
- Instruct the woman to deep breaths and cough every 2 hours.
- Instruct the woman on the use of an incentive spirometer if ordered.
- Assess postoperative pain and medicate as indicated.
- Use nonpharmacological pain management strategies.
- Assess the fundus and lochia per protocol. Use gentle pressure when assessing the fundus, as the woman's abdomen will be tender.
- Monitor for signs of hemorrhage and infection.
- Assess the abdominal dressing or surgical wound for drainage and signs of infection.
- Administer antibiotics as ordered.
- Remove the Foley catheter as ordered when the woman can ambulate to the bathroom. This generally occurs 8 to 12 hours postsurgery. Ensure woman voids at least 200 to 300 mL after urinary catheter removal and inform the provider if she cannot. Avoid overdistention of the bladder to reduce risk of subinvolution and hemorrhage.
- Assist the woman with ambulation.
- Encourage oral fluid intake to assist in hydration.

- Discontinue IV fluids as ordered, generally when the woman can take adequate fluids by mouth without nausea.
- Assess bowel sounds and allow the woman to eat regular desired foods unless ordered otherwise. Patients who eat solid foods early rather than waiting for the presence of bowel sounds have shown earlier return of bowel function (Saad et al., 2016).
- Provide information on nutrition to promote tissue healing.
- Assist the woman into a comfortable position for infant feeding. Breastfeeding mothers may be more comfortable in a side-lying position or football hold, which prevents pressure on the abdomen.
- Assist the woman with infant care.
- Facilitate mother-infant attachment by bringing the infant to the woman and ensuring the woman's comfort.
- Instruct the family that they need to assist the woman with infant care and housework, as she needs 6 weeks to recover from surgery.
- Provide opportunities for the family to ask questions about their cesarean birth experience.
- Provide teaching on infant care, postoperative care, and postpartum care.
- Remove staples before discharge per protocol. Instruct woman to make an appointment at her provider's clinic/office for staple removal, if staples not removed in the hospital.

Expected Assessment Findings

- Vital signs and glucose levels are within normal limits. Temperature elevations may be a sign of infection.
- Lung sounds are clear bilaterally.
- The woman deep breathes and coughs every 2 hours while awake.
- Pain level is 3 or below, or reflects the woman's chosen number on a pain scale of 0 to 10 with the use of nonpharmacological and pharmacological interventions.
- The fundus is firm and midline at one finger breadth below the umbilicus.
- Lochia is moderate to scant.
- The abdominal incision is clean, intact, approximated, and free of redness, edema, ecchymosis, and drainage.
- The woman spontaneously voids at least 200 mL within 2 to 3 hours of Foley removal.
- The woman ambulates to the bathroom and in the hallways.
- Bowel sounds are present and the woman reports passing gas.
- The woman is able to tolerate oral fluids and food.
- The woman is able to feed her newborn with or without assistance.
- The couple cares for the needs of their newborn.
- The woman may remain in the taking-in phase longer, as her focus is on pain control and integration of the birthing experience.
- Couples talk about their cesarean birth experience with staff, family, and friends.

Clinical Pathway for Scheduled Cesarean Birth

Focus of Care	Preoperative and After Initial Transfer to the OR	Intraoperative	Immediate Postoperative First 2 hours	First 24 Postoperative Hours	Postoperative 24 Hours to Discharge
Assessments	Review prenatal record for risk factors. Complete admission assessments per protocol. Assess the couple's emotional responses.	Vital signs are monitored by the anesthesia provider. Apgar score on neonate by neonatal personnel. Assess the neonate per protocol.	Assess per protocol level of consciousness (orientation to time, place, person). Assessments to be done every 15 minutes for the first hour, or as ordered: VS, color, O$_2$ sat, sensory motor function, presence or absence of oozing on dressing, fundal height, tone, location, and lochia. Assessments every hour for the first 4 hours or per protocol: urinary output, and bladder distention, I&O. Newborn assessments per protocol usually every 30 minutes for the first 2 hours.	Monitor VS as ordered, usually every hour × 4, then every 4 hours until stable, and then every 8 hours until discharge. Monitor respirations and sedation level as per postintrathecal morphine administration protocol—usually every hour for the first 24 hours. Assess the level and location of pain. Assess abdominal dressing for bleeding and/or drainage. Monitor I&O. Monitor ability to void. Monitor for signs of potential postpartum hemorrhage. Review laboratory test reports such as H&H, CBC. Monitor for signs of potential infections. Complete post-anesthesia assessments. Assess for adverse reaction related to intrathecal morphine, such as decreased respirations, itching, and vomiting, and intervene as per protocol.	Assess as per protocol, usually every 4 hours. Assess incisional site for drainage and signs of infection.
Activity Level	Ambulatory until Foley inserted and sequential compression devices are placed on her legs.	Bed rest	Bed rest	Bed rest until complete return of motor and sensory sensation/ function (generally 6–12 hours). Following return of motor and sensory sensation, the woman is assisted on short walks and may sit in a chair for short periods. Assistance may be required for pericare and ADLs.	Up independently Encourage the woman to ambulate to encourage bowel activity and reduce risk of blood clots. May require minimal assistance with pericare and ADLs.

Clinical Pathway for Scheduled Cesarean Birth—cont'd

Focus of Care	Preoperative and After Initial Transfer to the OR	Intraoperative	Immediate Postoperative First 2 hours	First 24 Postoperative Hours	Postoperative 24 Hours to Discharge
Education	Provide information on surgical procedure, anesthesia, and what to expect during cesarean birth and postoperatively. Keep the couple and their family informed on surgical time.	Provide information to the woman and her support person on woman's and neonate's condition.	Provide information to the woman and her support person on woman's and neonate's condition.	Begin teaching on care of the neonate and of the woman's needs during the postpartum period.	Continue teaching and preparing the couple for discharge. Provide postoperative discharge teaching.
Elimination	After the spinal anesthesia is completed, insert the Foley catheter and connect to continuous drainage.	Foley catheter connected to continuous drainage.	Monitor I&O	Foley catheter to continuous drainage for the first 8–12 hours. Remove the Foley catheter as ordered, generally 12 hours after surgery. Assist the woman to the bathroom and measure voiding.	Assist the woman to the bathroom and measure voiding at least 2 times after catheter removed, if sufficient quantity.
Emotional Needs	The couple may be anxious and excited. Provide emotional support and address questions and concerns.	The couple may be anxious and excited. Address the couple's concerns and questions. Provide an opportunity for the woman to hold the neonate skin-to-skin immediately after the birth, for as long as possible. If the neonate is transferred to the nursery before surgery is over, encourage the partner or support person to accompany the neonate to the nursery.	The couple may be anxious and excited. Address the couple's concerns and questions. Provide an opportunity for the family to be with their neonate.	Couples may be excited and tired. Address the couple's concerns regarding cesarean birth and the woman's and neonate's condition. Provide opportunities for the couple to share their experience and emotional responses to the birth.	Provide opportunities for couple to share their thoughts and feelings regarding taking on care of the neonate and/or breastfeeding.

Continued

Clinical Pathway for Scheduled Cesarean Birth—cont'd

Focus of Care	Preoperative and After Initial Transfer to the OR	Intraoperative	Immediate Postoperative First 2 hours	First 24 Postoperative Hours	Postoperative 24 Hours to Discharge
Medications	Administer preoperative medications per protocol. This may include IV or oral antacids and/or antibiotics.	The anesthesia provider administers oxytocin and other medications as needed throughout surgery.	Administer medications as ordered by anesthesia provider, including medications for treatment of intrathecal morphine side effects such as pruritus and nausea/vomitive.	Administer medications as ordered (i.e., stool softeners, Rhogam for Rh-negative women if indicated, Rubella for non-immune women, etc.).	Administer medications as ordered (i.e., stool softeners, etc.).
Nutrition	NPO Insert IV. Administer IV fluid preload.	NPO IV fluids	Ice chips, clear fluids, IV fluids Assist mother to breastfeed the neonate.	Advance to regular diet as ordered, or as woman tolerates. Assist with breastfeeding if indicated.	Diet as tolerated. Provide information on the role of nutrition in postpartum recovery and breastfeeding. Assist with breastfeeding if indicated.
Pain Management	Anesthesia provider meets with the couple to discuss anesthesia options.	Anesthesia provider inserts the epidural or spinal catheter and administers anesthetic agents. Anesthesia provider, or nurse removes the epidural catheter.	Anesthesia provider is responsible for prescribing medication for pain management in PACU.	Administer oral pain medications as ordered by surgeon. Intrathecal morphine administered via epidural catheter by pump after the birth of the neonate. Anesthesia provider is responsible for prescribing medication for pain management and treatment of intrathecal morphine side effects for the first 24 hours postop.	Per MD orders

Case Study

You are assigned to care for a couple who is scheduled to have a repeat cesarean birth. Lisa is a gravida 2 para 1, 25-year-old woman. Her husband, Joe, is 27 years old and plans to accompany Lisa into the operating room. Their first cesarean birth was due to cephalopelvic disproportion. Lisa and Joe have a healthy 3-year-old daughter, Sara, who is excited about having a baby brother.

Describe the nursing action for the preoperative period.

You transfer the couple to the operating room on the labor and birthing unit. You will be the circulating nurse. Spinal anesthesia is used for the cesarean birth.

Describe the major nursing action during the intraoperative period.
Describe the anesthesia management during this period of time.

Lisa experiences an uncomplicated cesarean birth and delivers a 3,800-gram baby boy with Apgar scores of 9 and 9. Lisa and her

son are transferred to the OB recovery room where you continue to care for the family. Lisa plans to breastfeed her son.

Describe the major nursing actions during the immediate postoperative recovery period.

The following day you are assigned to Lisa and her family in the postpartum unit. The shift report indicates that Lisa's lungs are clear; bowel sounds are present, fundus firm at 1 above U. Lisa's Foley catheter was removed at 10:00 the night before. During the night, she ambulated to the bathroom twice and voided 450 mL each time. She is tolerating fluids and would like scrambled eggs for breakfast. Her H&H are 30 and 10.2. She is having difficulty with breastfeeding. She complained of pain of 6 on a 10-point pain scale.

List the expected assessment findings for this period of time.
Discuss the nursing actions based on the shift report.
Discuss the major nursing action for couples and their newborn in preparation for discharge.

REFERENCES

American College of Obstetricians and Gynecologists (ACOG). (2010). Committee Opinion No. 115: Vaginal birth after previous cesarean delivery. *Obstetrics & Gynecology, 116*(2 Pt 1), 450–463.

American College of Obstetricians and Gynecologists (ACOG). (2013). Committee Opinion No. 559: Cesarean delivery on maternal request. *Obstetrics & Gynecology, 121*(4), 904–907.

American College of Obstetricians and Gynecologists (ACOG). (2015). Obesity in pregnancy. Practice Bulletin No. 156. *Obstetrics & Gynecology, 126*, e112–e126.

Apfelbaum, J., Hagberg, C., Caplan, R., Blitt, C., Connis, R., Nickinovich, D., & Ovassapian, A. (2013). Practice guidelines for management of the difficult airway: An updated report by the American Society of Anesthesiologists Task Force on Management of the Difficult Airway. *Anesthesiology, 118*(2), 251–270. doi:10.1097/ALN.0b013e31827773b2.

Association of Women's Health, Obstetric and Neonatal Nurses (AWHONN). (2011). *Evidence-based clinical practice guideline: Perioperative care of the pregnant woman.* Washington, DC: Author.

Barber, E., Lundsberg, L., Belanger, K., Pettker, C., Funai, E., & Illuzzi, J. (2011). Indications contributing to the increasing cesarean delivery rates. *Obstetrics & Gynecology, 118*, 29–38.

Caughey, A., Cahill, A., Guise, J., & Rouse, D. (2014). ACOG/SMFM obstetric care consensus safe prevention of the primary cesarean delivery. *American Journal of Obstetrics & Gynecology, 210*, 179–193.

Cunningham, F., Leveno, K., Bloom, S., Spong, C., Dashe, J., Hoffman, B., . . . Sheffield, J. (2014). *Williams obstetrics* (24th ed., pp. 587–608). New York, NY: McGraw-Hill.

Ferrarello, D., & Carmichael, T. (2016). Sudden unexpected postnatal collapse of the newborn. *Nursing for Women's Health, 20*(3), 268–275. doi:10.1016/j.nwh.2016.03.005.

Hamilton, B., Martin, J., Osterman, M., Driscoll, A., & Rossen, L. (2017). *Births: provisional data for 2016.* Retrieved from www.cdc.gov/nchs/data/vsrr/report002.pdf.

Hamilton, B., Martin, J., & Ventura, S. (2011). Births: Preliminary data for 2010. *National Vital Statistics Reports, 60*(2).

Joint Commission. (2003). Universal protocol for preventing wrong site, wrong procedure, wrong person surgery. Retrieved from www.jointcommission.org/patientsafety/universalprotocol/

Main, E. K., Morton, C. H., Melsop, K., Hopkins, D., Giuliani, G., & Gould, J. B. (2012). Creating a public agenda for maternity safety and quality in Cesarean delivery. *Obstetrics & Gynecology, 120*, 1194–1198.

Munday, J., Hines, S., Wallace, K., Chang, A., & Yates, P. (2104). A systematic review of the effectiveness of warming interventions for women undergoing cesarean sections. *Worldviews of Evidence-Based Nursing, 11*, 383–393.

Saad, A. F., Saoud, F., Diken, Z. M., Hegde, S., Kuhlmann, M. J., Wen, T. S., . . . Costantine, M. M. (2016). Early versus late feeding after cesarean delivery: A randomized controlled trial. *American Journal of Perinatology, 33*(4), 415–419. doi:10.1055/s-0035-1565918.

Schneuder, L., Crenshaw, J., & Gilder, R. (2017). Influence of immediate skin-to-skin contact during cesarean surgery on rate of transfer of newborn to NICU for observation. *Nursing for Women's Health, 21*, 28–33.

Vallerand, A., & Sanoski, C. (2017). *Davis's drug guide for nurses* (15th ed.). Philadelphia, PA: F.A. Davis.

The Postpartal Period

Postpartum Physiological Assessments and Nursing Care

12

Melissa Goldsmith, PhD, RNC-MNN
Roberta F. Durham, RN, PhD

LEARNING OUTCOMES

Upon completion of this chapter, the student will be able to:

1. Describe the physiological changes that occur during the postpartum period.
2. Identify the critical elements of assessment and nursing care during the postpartum period.
3. Describe safe and effective nursing care during the postpartum period.
4. Describe the critical elements of discharge teaching.

Nursing Diagnosis

- Pain related to tissue trauma secondary to vaginal delivery
- Pain related to uterine involution secondary to vaginal delivery
- Pain related to congestion, increased vascularity, and milk accumulation secondary to breast engorgement
- At risk for infection related to perineal tissue trauma
- At risk for infection (mastitis) related to altered skin integrity and milk stasis
- At risk for fluid volume deficit related to hemorrhage from uterine atony
- At risk for impaired urinary elimination related to decreased sensation, tissue trauma
- At risk for constipation related to hormonal effects on smooth muscles
- At risk for knowledge deficit regarding health promotion postbirth related to lack of information

Nursing Outcomes

- The woman will report adequate pain control.
- The woman will remain free from symptoms of infection.
- The woman's fundus will remain firm with scant to moderate lochia.
- The woman will spontaneously void within 2 to 4 hours postbirth.
- The woman will eat a nutritious diet high in fiber and roughage and will drink a minimum of 10 glasses of fluid per day (80 ounces).
- The woman will verbalize an understanding of major components of health promotion.
- The woman will identify signs of complications that must be reported to the health care provider.
- The woman will have a plan for postpartum follow-up care.

INTRODUCTION

The postpartum period is the 6-week period after childbirth; a time of rapid physiological changes within the woman's body as it returns to a prepregnant state. Women who are healthy at conception and experience a low-risk pregnancy, labor, and birth are at low risk for complications during the postpartum period. After birth, a woman and her family must adapt to many physical, social, and psychological changes, influenced by childbirth, changing hormones, and caring for the baby. The postpartum period is a time of joy and excitement, but this "fourth trimester" also presents considerable challenges for women due to lack of sleep, fatigue, pain, breastfeeding difficulties, stress, depression, and adapting to the new role of motherhood. The focus of this chapter is the physiological aspects of postpartum nursing care (Box 12–1), including assessment of postpartum physiological changes:

- Providing comfort and restoring physiological functions affected by childbirth
- Assessing for early signs of potential complications
- Promoting health and education

Psychological adaptations in the postpartum period are presented in detail in Chapter 13. Perinatal mood and anxiety disorders in their most severe forms can be tragic and preventable causes of maternal and infant mortality. Perinatal mood and anxiety disorders and their sequelae can be addressed by actively screening women, having a plan in place for treatment or referral for those who screen positive, and actively engaging women, their families, and supporters in recognizing symptoms and seeking help in a timely manner (Kendig et al., 2017). Although there is no specific recommendation, some units have begun screening in the immediate postpartum period with standardized tools such as the Edinburg postpartum depression scale. However, screening alone does not improve perinatal outcomes. Systems must be in place to ensure consistent screening with appropriate assessment tools, interventions, and monitoring for women with identified perinatal mood and anxiety disorders.

Maternal Mortality

Maternal mortality is the death of a woman from complications of pregnancy and childbirth occurring up to 1 year postpartum. In a report using data from 2010, the United States ranked 49th out of 184 countries for maternal mortality (Central Intelligence Agency, 2016) and is one of eight countries in which maternal mortality rates have been on the rise in recent years. Although the most current U.S. pregnancy-related mortality rate shows a slight decrease in maternal deaths, from 17.8 deaths per 100,000 live births in 2011 to 15.9 deaths per 100,000 live births in 2012 (Centers for Disease Control and Prevention [CDC], 2016b), this rate is more than double the 1987 rate of 7.2 deaths per 100,000 births. Increased rates may be related to improvements in reporting, but the number is still high for a country with readily available medical care. The CDC and the Department of Health and Human Services Office of Disease Prevention and

Health Promotion have set national health goals published in *Healthy People 2020*, several of which relate to the postpartum period (Table 12–1).

THE REPRODUCTIVE SYSTEM

The reproductive system, which includes the uterus, cervix, vagina, and perineum, undergoes dramatic changes after childbirth. Women are at risk for hemorrhage and infection. Nursing assessments and interventions are aimed at reducing these risks; see "Clinical Pathway for Uncomplicated Vaginal Delivery" for more details.

Uterus

After delivery of the placenta, the uterus begins the process of involution by which it returns to its nearly prepregnant size, shape, and location and the placental site heals. This occurs through uterine contractions, atrophy of the uterine muscle, and a decrease in the size of uterine cells. Involution of the uterus takes between 6 and 8 weeks postdelivery (Cunningham et al., 2014; Smith, 2018). Primiparous women usually do not experience discomfort related to uterine contractions during the postpartum period because the uterus remains contracted (Cunningham et al., 2014). Multiparous women or women who are breastfeeding may experience "afterpains" caused by strong intermittent uterine contractions during the first few postpartum days. Afterpains are moderate to severe cramp-like pains related to the uterus working to remain contracted and/or the increase of oxytocin released in response to infant suckling. The intensity of afterpains will typically decrease after the third postpartum day (Cunningham et al., 2014). The uterus must be contracted during the postpartum

---

BOX 12–1 | Overview of the Postpartum Assessment

The following should be assessed per the health care provider's order or unit protocol.

- Vital signs, pain, breath and heart sounds
- Laboratory findings, such as CBC, rubella status, and Rh status
- Breasts
- Uterus
- Bladder
- Bowel
- Lochia
- Episiotomy, lacerations, perineum, hemorrhoids
- Lower extremities
- Emotions, bonding with infant, fatigue, psychosocial factors

TABLE 12–1 *Healthy People 2020* Objectives Related to the Postpartum Period

OBJECTIVE	BASELINE	TARGET
Reduce the rate of maternal mortality	12.7 maternal deaths per 100,00 live births	11.4 maternal deaths per 100,000
Reduce maternal illness and complications due to pregnancy (complications during hospital labor and delivery)	31.1% of pregnant females experienced complications during hospitalized labor and delivery.	28%
Increase the proportion of infants that are breastfed:		
Ever	74%	81.9%
At 6 months	43.5%	60.6%
At 1 year	22.7%	34.1%
Reduce postpartum smoking relapse among women who quit smoking during pregnancy.	No baseline data provided	No target provided
Increase the number of women giving birth who attend a postpartum care visit with a health care worker.	No baseline data provided	No target provided
Increase the proportion of pregnancies that are intended.	51.0%	56%
Reduce the proportion of females experiencing pregnancy despite use of reversible contraceptive method.	12.4%	9.9%
Reduce the proportion of pregnancies conceived within 18 months of a previous birth.	35.3%	31.7%
Reduce pregnancy rates among adolescent females.	40.2%	36.2%

U.S. Department of Health and Human Services Office of Disease Prevention and Health Promotion, 2012.

period to decrease the risk of postpartum hemorrhage. The contracted uterine muscle compresses the open vessels at the placental site and decreases the amount of blood loss.

Nursing Actions

- Assess the uterus for location, position, and tone of the fundus.
  - After the third stage of labor, assess the uterus:
    - Every 15 minutes for the first hour.
    - Every 30 minutes for the second hour.
    - Every 4 hours for the next 22 hours.
    - Every shift after the first 24 hours or as stated in hospital/unit protocols.
    - More frequently if the assessment findings are not within normal limits.
  - Frequent assessment of uterine tone and placement allows for the identification of potential complications such as uterine atony (decreased uterine muscle tone) that may lead to postpartum hemorrhage (Cunningham et al., 2014).
    - The risk for postpartum hemorrhage is the greatest within the first hour following delivery (Cunningham et al., 2014).
    - Primary (early) postpartum hemorrhage occurs during the first 24 hours after birth.
    - Secondary (late) postpartum hemorrhage may occur from 24 hours to 12 weeks postdelivery but is most prevalent during the first 7 to 14 days following birth (Cunningham et al., 2014).
    - See Chapter 14 for more information about the care of the woman with postpartum hemorrhage.
- Before assessment, inform the woman that you will be palpating her uterus to evaluate for normal involution and bleeding.
- Explain the procedure.
- Instruct the woman to void.
  - Rationale: An over-distended bladder can result in uterine displacement and atony (James, 2014). Encouraging the woman to void prior to uterine assessment will allow for an accurate assessment of uterine placement and tone.
- Provide privacy.
- Lower the head and foot of the bed so that the woman is in a supine position and flat.
- Remove her peripads to evaluate lochia at the same time the fundus is palpated.
- Support the lower uterine segment by placing one hand just above the symphysis pubis (Fig. 12–1).
  - Rationale: Pregnancy stretches the ligaments that hold the uterus in place. Fundal pressure could result in uterine

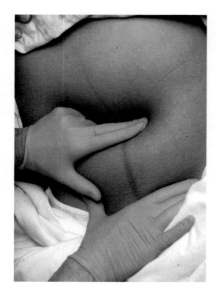

FIGURE 12–1 Nurse supporting lower uterine segment while assessing the postpartum uterus.

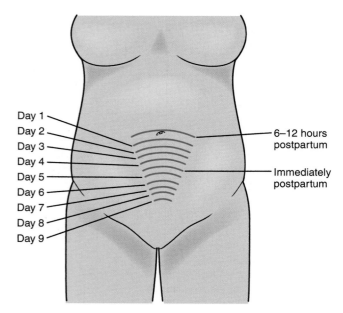

FIGURE 12–2 Location of fundus at 6 to 12 hours postpartum and 1 to 9 days postpartum.

inversion (James, 2014). Supporting the lower uterine segment may prevent uterine inversion during fundal assessment or massage.

● Locate the fundus with the other hand using gentle downward pressure and assess the position, tone, and location of the fundus.

● The fundus may be firm (contracted) or soft (boggy) in tone.

  ● A boggy uterus indicates that the uterus is not contracting and places the woman at risk for excessive blood loss. If the uterus is boggy, the nurse should:

    ● Massage the fundus with the palm of the hand, as fundal massage stimulates contraction of the uterus (Smith, 2018).

      ● Rationale: Fundal massage stimulates contraction of the uterus (Smith, 2018).

    ● Give oxytocin as per the physician's or midwife's postpartum orders.

      ● Rationale: Oxytocin promotes contraction of the uterus by stimulating its smooth muscle, which prevents and controls postpartum hemorrhage (Wilson et al., 2014).

    ● Notify the physician or midwife if the uterus does not respond to massage and postpartum orders have been implemented.

    ● Lack of response to fundal massage and oxytocin administration may indicate complications such as retained placental tissue or birth trauma (Hobel & Lamb, 2016). Continued uterine atony can lead to postpartum hemorrhage and requires assessment and potentially further treatment by the woman's health care provider.

  ● Measure the distance between the fundus and umbilicus with your fingers. Each finger breadth equals 1 cm.

  ● Determine the position of the uterus.

    ● Rationale: A uterus that is shifted to the side may indicate a distended bladder. This interferes with uterine contractibility, which places the woman at risk for uterine atony and increases her risk of hemorrhage (James, 2014).

  ● If the uterus is deviated, soft, or elevated above the umbilicus, the immediate action is to explain to the patient the need for her to void and to assist her to the bathroom. Reassess the uterine position after the woman has voided and returned to her bed. If the patient is unable to void, urinary catheterization may be necessary.

Expected assessment findings include the following (Fig. 12–2):

● Immediately after birth, the uterine fundus is palpated midway between the umbilicus and symphysis pubis and is firm and midline. In the next few hours it is palpated at the umbilicus.

● Within 12 hours after birth of the placenta, the fundus is located at the level of the umbilicus or 1 cm above the umbilicus and is firm and midline.

● 24 hours after birth of placenta, the fundus is located at 1 cm below the umbilicus and is firm and midline.

● The uterus descends 1 cm per day; by day 14 the fundus has descended into the pelvis and is not palpable.

● Subinvolution is the failure of the uterus to involute/descend as expected. Causes include retained placental fragments, infection, and over-distended uterus (e.g., from a large baby). Subinvolution may lead to prolonged or excessive bleeding during the postpartum period (Cunningham et al., 2014).

The nurse should also provide information regarding afterpains, uterine cramps caused by the contraction, and relaxation of the uterus as it decreases in size.

CRITICAL COMPONENT

Uterine Atony (Boggy Uterus)

Uterine atony is the most common cause of postpartum hemorrhage. Because hemostasis associated with placental separation depends on myometrial contraction, atony is treated initially by uterine massage, followed by drugs that promote uterine contraction.

- A boggy uterus is a sign that the uterus is not contracted.
- Risk of excessive blood loss and/or hemorrhage is increased.
- The immediate action is to massage the fundus with the palm of your hand in a circular motion until firm and reevaluate within 5 to 10 minutes.
- If the uterus does not respond to massage, follow the standing order for oxytocin and notify the physician or midwife.

SAFE AND EFFECTIVE NURSING CARE: Understanding Medication

Oxytocin (Pitocin)

Oxytocin stimulates the upper segment of the myometrium to contract rhythmically, which constricts spiral arteries and decreases blood flow through the uterus. Oxytocin is an effective first-line treatment for postpartum hemorrhage. As a high-alert medication, IV oxytocin premixed bags should be prominently and clearly labeled and stored separately to prevent a 1,000 mL bag of oxytocin being mistaken for a plain 1,000 mL bag of resuscitation bolus (Association of Women's Health, Obstetric and Neonatal Nurses [AWHONN], 2015a).

Universal Active Management of Third Stage of Labor

- Increase IV oxytocin rate, 500 mL/hour of 10 to 40 units/500–1,000 mL solution.
- Titrate infusion rate to uterine tone, up to 500 mL as needed.
- Indication: Postpartum control of bleeding.
- Action: Stimulates uterine smooth muscle to produce uterine contraction.
- Adverse reactions with IV use: coma, seizures, hypertension, hypotension, water intoxication.
- Administer via IV infusion using an IV infusion pump, or via the intramuscular (IM) route if the patient does not have IV access.
- Premixed bags of IV fluid containing oxytocin should be clearly marked with bright labels and stored in a different area than plain IV fluid bags.
- Suggested administration: 20 units of oxytocin in 1 L of normal saline or lactated Ringer's.

- Bolus at a rate of 1,000 mL/hr for 30 minutes (10 units of oxytocin), immediately after birth followed by a maintenance dose of 125 mL/hr for 3.5 hours.
- Women who delivered by cesarean section or who are at high risk for postpartum hemorrhage may require continuation of oxytocin administration for greater than 4 hours. Duration and dosage is based on assessment of fundal tone and amount of vaginal bleeding (AWHONN, 2015a).
- For postpartum bleeding, a total of 10 to 40 units may be infused intravenously at a rate of 20 to 40 mU/min, depending on the patient's condition (Wilson et al., 2014).
- For patients without IV access, administer 10 units of oxytocin IM.
- Nursing actions/implications: Monitor vital signs frequently; assess fundal position, tone, and location; assess lochia color amount and odor; assess for signs of water intoxication (drowsiness, headache, anuria); and teach patient that oxytocin will cause uterine cramping.
- Have other uterotonics on hand such as methylergonovine (Methergine), misoprostol (Cytotec), and carboprost (Hemabate).

AWHONN, 2015a; Vallerand & Sanoski, 2013; Wilson et al., 2014.

- Afterpains occur within the first few days and typically decrease 3 days after delivery.
- They occur more commonly with multiparous women and increase with each additional pregnancy/birth.
- The condition may increase when breastfeeding during the first few postpartum days.
- Comfort measures include the following:
  - Encourage patient to empty bladder, as a distended bladder can increase afterpains.
  - Apply warm blanket to abdomen.
  - Relaxation techniques and warm compresses can interfere with the transmission and sensation of pain.
  - Analgesics such as ibuprofen are effective in relieving uterine cramping (Isley & Katz, 2016).

The Endometrium

The endometrium, the mucous membrane that lines the uterus, undergoes exfoliation and regeneration after the birth of the placenta through necrosis of the superficial layer of the decidua and regeneration of the decidua basalis into endometrial tissue. Lochia is a bloody discharge from the uterus that contains red blood cells, sloughed off decidual tissue, epithelial cells, and bacteria (Cunningham et al., 2014). The placental site heals by exfoliation, which involves the sloughing of necrotic endometrial tissue and the regeneration of the endometrium at the placental site (Cunningham et al., 2014; Smith, 2018). This process prevents scarring of the endometrial tissue (James, 2014). Lochia undergoes changes that reflect the healing stages of the uterine placental site (Table 12–2). Uterine contractions constrict the vessels around the placental site and help decrease blood loss.

TABLE 12–2   Stages and Characteristics of Lochia

STAGE	TIME FRAME	EXPECTED FINDINGS	DEVIATIONS FROM NORMAL
Lochia rubra	Days 1–3	Bloody with small clots	Large clots
		Moderate to scant amount	Heavy amount; saturates pad within 1 hour (sign of possible hemorrhage), excessively heavy, saturates a pad in 15 minutes
		Increased flow on standing or breastfeeding	Foul odor (sign of infection)
		Fleshy odor	Placental fragments
Lochia serosa	Days 4–10	Pink or brown color	Continuation of rubra stage after day 4
		Scant amount	Heavy amount; saturates pad within 1 hour (sign of possible hemorrhage), excessively heavy; saturates pad within 15 minutes
		Increased flow during physical activity	Foul odor (sign of infection)
		Fleshy odor	
Lochia alba	Day 10	Yellow to white in color	Bright red bleeding, saturates pad within 1 hour (sign of possible late postpartum hemorrhage)
		Scant amount	Foul odor (sign of infection)
		Fleshy odor	

A primary complication is metritis, which is an infection of the endometrial tissue (see Chapter 14).

Nursing Actions

- Assess lochia for color, amount, and odor at the same time the uterus is assessed.
  - Rationale: Frequent assessment of lochia in the early postpartum period allows the nurse to monitor blood loss and identify if bleeding is excessive, determine if clots are present, and assess for signs of infection.
    - Lochia is described as scant, light, moderate, or heavy (Fig. 12–3).
      - Scant is less than 1 inch on the pad.
      - Light is less than 4 inches on the pad.
      - Moderate is less than 6 inches on the pad.
      - Heavy is when the pad is saturated within 1 hour; excessively heavy is when a pad is soaked within 15 minutes.
- Assess for clots, which occur when the lochia has been pooling in the lower uterine segment.
  - Small clots should be noted in the patient chart.
  - A clot the size of an egg or larger should be weighed and findings reported to the physician or midwife (Suplee et al., 2016), as large clots can interfere with uterine involution.
    - 1 g in weight equals 1 mL of blood loss.
  - Clots should be examined for the presence of tissue.
    - Retained placental tissue can interfere with uterine involution and lead to excessive bleeding (Hobel & Lamb, 2016).

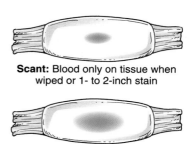

Scant: Blood only on tissue when wiped or 1- to 2-inch stain

Light: 4-inch or less stain

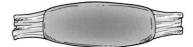

Moderate: Less than 6-inch stain

Heavy: Saturated pad

FIGURE 12–3 Comparison of heavy, moderate, light, and scant lochia on pads.

- Assess for color of lochia. Initial lochia for the first 3 days is rubra, which is red and bloody. The next stage of lochia is serosa, which is pink or brown. The final stage is alba, which is clear or whitish.
- Assess for odor. Lochia has a fleshy odor and smells similar to menstrual blood.

Expected assessment findings are further described in Table 12–2.

Patient Education

- Teach the woman how to assess the fundus and explain the normal process of involution.
- Teach the woman how to massage her uterus if boggy and instruct her to notify the nurse while in the hospital and health care provider after discharge.
  - Rationale: Secondary hemorrhage often occurs after the patient has been discharged. To prevent serious complications, women should understand the normal progression of lochia and uterine involution, and report abnormal amounts of bleeding.
- Provide information on the normal stages of lochia.
- Explain that the flow of lochia can increase when getting up in the morning or after sitting for prolonged periods of time due to vaginal pooling of lochia or from excessive physical activity.
  - Instruct the woman to notify the nurse, physician, or midwife if she experiences an increase in the amount of lochia, if the color of lochia changes back to bright red after the rubra stage is over, or if the lochia has a foul odor.
  - Rationale: Lochia should decrease in amount every day. Foul-smelling lochia could indicate the development of an infection. An increase in lochia or the return of bright red bleeding may be signs of secondary hemorrhage (Cunningham et al., 2014).
- Provide information for reducing the risk of infection such as instructing the patient to change the peripad frequently from the front to back, wash hands before and after changing pads, and use a peri-bottle to keep the area clean.
  - Rationale: Lochia is a medium for bacterial growth. Frequent pad changes and hand washing are actions aimed at preventing infection.
- Document the stage amount and odor of lochia and interventions.

CRITICAL COMPONENT

Excessive Bleeding and Early Warning Signs

Each year in the United States, almost 3% of all births result in postpartum hemorrhage, often signified by heavy lochia. Immediate nursing actions include the following:

- Assess the position, tone, and location of the fundus.
- If the uterus is boggy, massage it.
- If the uterus is boggy and displaced to the side, instruct the patient to void and reevaluate.
  - Ambulate the patient to the bathroom and measure the void. A good void is at least 300 cc.
- Quantify blood loss (QBL) by weighing all blood-soaked peripads and materials.
  - 1 g equals 1 mL of fluid.
  - QBL provides an accurate estimation of blood loss.
  - A scale with an attached laminated card with the dry weights of peripads/chux should be available on units

providing care to postpartum patients (AWHONN, 2015b)

- Notify the midwife or physician of excessive bleeding and QBL.

Continued heavy bleeding with firm fundal tone may indicate the presence of a genitourinary tract laceration or hematoma of the vulva or vagina (Hobel & Lamb, 2016). Be alert to early warning signs. It is important to verify isolated abnormal measurements, particularly for blood pressure, heart rate, respiratory rate, and oxygen saturation. Urgent bedside evaluation is usually indicated if any of these values persist for more than one measurement, present with additional abnormal parameters, or recur more than once (Box 12–2).

While awaiting the arrival of the evaluating clinician, the bedside nurse should follow basic resuscitation principles:

- Achieve free-flowing appropriate venous access
- Increase frequency of vital signs
- Left uterine displacement if woman is still pregnant
- Supplemental oxygen therapy

Appropriate standing orders are needed to allow the bedside nurse to administer these resuscitative measures

Mhyre et al., 2014; AWHONN 2015b.

BOX 12–2 | The Maternal Early Warning Criteria

MEASURE	VALUE
Systolic blood pressure (mm Hg)	<90 or >160
Diastolic blood pressure (mm Hg)	>100
Heart rate (bpm)	<50 or >120
Respiratory rate (breaths per min)	<10 or >30
Oxygen saturation on room air, at sea level %	<95
Oliguria, mL/hr for ≥ 2 hrs	<35
Maternal agitation, confusion, or unresponsiveness	
Woman with preeclampsia reporting a nonremitting headache or shortness of breath	

Vagina and Perineum

- The vagina and perineum experience changes related to the birthing process that may include edema, mild stretching, minor lacerations, major tears, and/or episiotomies.
- A first-degree laceration involves the vaginal mucous membranes and the perineal skin.
- A second-degree laceration involves the vaginal mucous membranes, perineal skin, and the fascia of the perineal body.
- A third-degree laceration involves the perineal skin, vaginal mucous membranes, fascia of the perineal body, and the rectal sphincter.

- A fourth-degree laceration involves the perineal skin and fascia, vaginal mucous membranes, rectal sphincter, and the rectal mucosa and lumen.
- A midline episiotomy is an incision that is midline on the perineum. This type of incision tends to heal more quickly and cause less pain then a mediolateral episiotomy.
- A mediolateral episiotomy is an incision that is made at a 45-degree angle to the perineum.

See Chapter 8 for further discussion of lacerations and episiotomy.

The woman may experience mild to severe pain, depending on the degree and type of vaginal and/or perineal trauma. Women who have a third- or fourth-degree laceration, an episiotomy, or hemorrhoids may require a stool softener or laxative to facilitate bowel movements (Isley & Katz, 2016). The primary complication is infection at the laceration or episiotomy site. Lacerations can tear posteriorly toward the rectum, causing difficulty with bowel movements. Lacerations can also tear anteriorly toward the urethra, causing swelling and possibly difficulty with urination. The vagina and perineum undergo healing and restoration during the postpartum period. Immediately after delivery, the vaginal walls are smooth, but rugae are reestablished within 3 weeks of delivery (James, 2014).

Nursing Actions

- The perineum is assessed when the fundus and lochia are checked in the postdelivery period (James, 2014). After that, the perineum is assessed every shift using the acronym REEDA (redness, edema, ecchymosis, discharge, approximation of edges of episiotomy or laceration).
  - Rationale: Frequent assessment of the perineum using the REEDA scale will allow identification of potential complications, such as excessive swelling, infection, hematoma, and excess bleeding (James, 2014). See Chapter 14 for more information about lacerations and hematoma.
- Explain the procedure.
- Provide privacy.
- Lower the head and foot of the bed so that the woman is in a supine position and flat.
- Remove her peripads to evaluate labia and perineum anteriorly.
- Assist the woman to her side and separate the buttocks to expose the perineum and rectum for assessment.
  - Rationale: Assess the perineum anteriorly, then place the woman in the side-lying position to inspect the perineal area and assess the amount of lochia present on the entire peripad. While the woman is in the side-lying position, assess the rectal area for hemorrhoids.
- Expected assessment findings:
  - Mild edema
  - Minor ecchymosis
  - Approximation of the edges of the episiotomy or laceration if visible; most lacerations are internal and not visible.
  - Mild to moderate pain

- Assess for discomfort and provide comfort measures.
  - Apply ice to the perineum, or encourage the use of cold sitz baths for the first 24 to 48 hours to manage swelling (East et al., 2012).
    - Rationale: Ice causes local vasoconstriction, which decreases edema and provides an anesthetic effect (Cunningham et al., 2014; Isley & Katz, 2016).
  - Encourage the woman to lie on her side.
    - Rationale: The side-lying position decreases pressure on the perineum.
  - Instruct the woman to tighten her gluteal muscles as she sits down and to relax muscles after she is seated.
    - Rationale: This helps cushion the perineum and increases comfort when assuming a sitting position.
  - Instruct the woman to wear peripads snugly to prevent rubbing.
  - Instruct the woman to take warm sitz baths, starting 24 hours after delivery twice a day for 20 minutes.
    - Rationale: Warm sitz baths promote circulation, healing, and comfort (Cunningham et al., 2014).
  - Administer a topical anesthetic per the physician's or midwife's order.
    - Rationale: Topical anesthetics may relieve localized discomfort (Cunningham et al., 2014).
  - Administer analgesia per the physician's or midwife's order and assess adequacy of pain relief within 30 minutes. Note the patient's acceptable pain level, as sometimes we cannot achieve 0 pain. Analgesics such as ibuprofen are effective in treating perineal pain (Isley & Katz, 2016).
- Reduce the risk for infection.
  - Instruct the woman to use a peri-bottle with warm water and rinse the perineum after elimination.
  - Instruct the woman to change the peripad frequently.
  - Instruct the woman to properly dispose of soiled pads and to wash her hands.
    - Rationale: Lochia is a medium for bacterial growth. Frequent pad changes and hand washing will reduce the risk for infection.

CRITICAL COMPONENT

Assessment and Management of Pain in the Postpartum Period

Pain in the postpartum period may result from uterine contractions/afterpains, perineal trauma, lacerations, episiotomy, nipple pain caused by improper infant latch, breast engorgement, hemorrhoids, and general soreness related to the work of labor and birth (Isley & Katz, 2016; James, 2014).

Pain is considered the fifth vital sign and should be assessed routinely when vital signs are done, when the patient complains of pain, before and after a painful procedure, and before and after implementation of a pain management intervention (Wilkinson & Treas, 2011). Assess pain using an appropriate pain scale per agency protocol. Many scales measure pain intensity, duration, quality, location, factors that make pain better or worse, and acceptable level of pain. The culture of the woman influences her response to pain, and pain behaviors are culturally bound. Sometimes pain measurement tools that rely on numbers or any kind of linear format, such as a row of faces, may not work well across cultures. Through careful listening and probing, nurses can uncover what is really happening with each patient's pain.

Examples of nonpharmacological interventions include:

- Ice packs
- Warm compresses
- Sitz baths
- Repositioning
- Showering
- Topical treatments, such as witch hazel pads and anesthetic sprays applied to localized perineal discomfort.
  Pharmacological interventions may include:
- NSAIDs such as ibuprofen (for mild to moderate pain):
  - Ibuprofen (Motrin) may be administered with food or milk to decrease GI upset. Give with a full glass of water.
  - Patients with asthma, nasal polyps, or who are allergic to aspirin are at risk for hypersensitivity to ibuprofen.
  - Route and dose for ibuprofen: PO; 400 to 800 mg every 4 to 6 hours PRN, maximum 24-hour dose 3,200 mg/day. Assess pain before and 30 minutes after administration.
- Opioid analgesics may be used for moderate to severe pain. These medications are often used in combination with a nonopioid medication for added analgesic effect.

Breasts

During pregnancy, the breasts undergo changes in preparation for lactation. After delivery, there is a decrease in estrogen and progesterone and an increase in prolactin (Cunningham et al., 2014). Prolactin stimulates breast milk production. When the infant suckles, the posterior pituitary releases oxytocin, resulting in the milk ejection reflex, also called the let-down reflex (Cunningham et al., 2014).

Immediately after delivery, breast fullness is normal. While breast tissue may be swollen, it is soft and nontender (James, 2014). Around the third postpartum day, both breastfeeding and nonbreastfeeding women experience some degree of primary breast engorgement, an increase in the vascular and lymphatic system of the breasts that precedes the initiation of milk production. The woman's breasts become larger, firm, warm, and tender, and the woman may feel a throbbing pain in the breasts. Primary engorgement subsides within 24 to 48 hours (Box 12–3).

Women who breastfeed experience subsequent breast engorgement related to distention of milk glands that is relieved by having the baby suckle or by expressing milk. Colostrum, a clear, yellowish fluid, precedes milk production and is secreted after delivery. It is higher in protein and lower in carbohydrates than breast milk and contains immunoglobulins G and A, which provide protection for the newborn during the early weeks of life. The secretion of colostrum continues for 5 days to 2 weeks postdelivery, during which time there is a transition to mature milk (Cunningham

et al., 2014). Mature milk contains proteins, carbohydrates, fat, minerals, vitamins, hormones, and immunological substances such as secretory IgA, lymphocytes, and growth factor (Cunningham et al., 2014). The composition of breast milk changes during the feeding and throughout the course of feedings during the day. For example, the fat content of mature milk increases two to three times throughout a breastfeeding session (Newton, 2016).

A primary complication associated with breastfeeding is mastitis, which is an infection of the breast (for more, see Chapter 14). Breastfeeding and lactation are discussed in more detail in Chapter 16.

Nursing Actions for the Breastfeeding Woman

- Inspect and palpate the breasts for signs of engorgement: tenderness, firmness, warmth, and/or enlargement.
  - Expected assessment findings:
    - During the first 24 hours postpartum, the breasts are soft and nontender.
    - On postpartum day 2, the breasts are slightly firm and nontender.
    - On postpartum day 3, the breasts are firm, tender, and warm to touch.
- Assess the nipples for signs of irritation and nipple tissue breakdown.
  - Rationale: Signs of irritation and tissue breakdown are cracked, blistered, or reddened areas. Skin breakdown of the nipples is often associated with an improper infant latch. Nipple soreness is a primary reason that women stop breastfeeding, so this complaint should be addressed (Janke, 2014). Additionally, skin breakdown can be an entry point for bacteria (Cunningham et al., 2014). See Chapter 16 for interventions to prevent/treat nipple irritation and breakdown.
- Assess for plugged milk ducts (see Box 12–3).

Nursing Actions for the Nonbreastfeeding Woman

- Assess the breasts for primary engorgement.
  - Inspect and palpate the breasts for signs of engorgement: tenderness, firmness, warmth, and/or enlargement.
    - Rationale: In women who choose not to breastfeed, milk leakage, breast pain, and engorgement may be experienced between 1 and 4 days postdelivery (James, 2014).
  - Expected assessment findings:
    - During the first 24 hours postpartum, the breasts are soft and nontender.
    - On postpartum day 2, the breasts are slightly firm and nontender.
    - On postpartum day 3, the breasts are firm and tender.

Patient Education

- Instruct the woman to wear a supportive bra or sports bra 24 hours a day until her breasts become soft. Teach

BOX 12-3 | Breast Care and Assessment

Common findings include:

- Breast engorgement: caused by an increase in the vascular and the lymphatic systems within the breast and milk accumulation.
- Physiological engorgement:
  - Breasts are swollen.
- Pathological engorgement:
  - Breasts are hard, swollen, red, and tender/painful.
  - Breasts feel warm to the touch.
  - Woman may feel a throbbing sensation in the breasts.
  - Woman may have an elevated temperature.
  - Infant may have difficulty latching on due to the severe engorgement (Newton, 2016).
- Treatment for breastfeeding women:
  - Frequent feedings to empty the breasts and to prevent milk stasis
  - Warm compresses to the breast and breast massage to facilitate the flow of milk prior to feeding sessions
  - Express milk by breast pump or manually if the infant is unable to nurse (i.e., preterm infant)
  - Ice packs after feedings to reduce inflammation and discomfort
  - Analgesics for pain management
  - Wear a supportive bra
- Prevention and treatment for nonbreastfeeding women
  - Wear a supportive bra
  - Avoid stimulating the breast
  - Ice packs to breast
  - Analgesics for pain management
  - Subsides within 48 to 72 hours (Janke, 2014)
- Plugged milk ducts are associated with inadequate emptying of the breasts and stasis of the milk (Janke, 2014).
- Symptoms: palpation of tender breast lumps the size of peas (Janke, 2014)
- Treatments:
  - Frequent feedings
  - Changing infant feeding positions (Janke, 2014)
  - Application of warm compresses to breast or taking a warm shower prior to feeding session
  - Massaging the breasts prior to feeding session
- Continued milk stasis or unresolved plugged milk ducts can lead to mastitis and potential breast abscess (Janke, 2014).
- Patient education
  - Encourage the woman to wear a supportive but nonconstrictive bra.
  - Instruct the woman to examine her nipples before feedings for signs of irritation.
  - After feeding, the woman should expose her nipples to air.
  - Improper latch should be adjusted to decrease nipple tissue breakdown (James, 2014).
  - Instruct the woman to feed her infant frequently on demand or express milk if she is experiencing breast engorgement.
  - Encourage the woman to wash her hands frequently and to keep her breasts clean to prevent infection.
- Provide information on mastitis.
  - Mastitis typically occurs at 3 to 4 weeks postbirth.
  - The infection may be caused by bacterial entry through cracks in the nipples and is associated with milk stasis, engorgement, long intervals between feedings, stress, and fatigue (Janke, 2014).
  - Symptoms include fever, chills, malaise, flulike symptoms, unilateral breast pain, and redness and tenderness in the infected area.
  - The woman needs to report symptoms to her health care provider.
  - A culture of the breast milk may be ordered prior to starting the woman on antibiotics.
  - Treatment: Empty the affected breast, antibiotic therapy, analgesia, rest, adequate nutrition, and hydration.
  - The woman should continue to breastfeed or pump her breasts as per the physician's or midwife's recommendation.
  - The woman should apply moist heat to the affected breast before breastfeeding.
  - Document findings, interventions, and evaluation.

the woman to avoid expressing milk or stimulating the breasts.
- Rationale: Atrophy in milk-secreting cells of the breasts can be caused by back pressure in the milk ducts that occurs when the breasts are not emptied (Janke, 2014).
- Instruct the woman who is experiencing engorgement to:
  - Apply ice to the breasts.
  - Not express milk because this stimulates milk production.
  - Avoid heat to the breast because this can stimulate milk production.
  - Take an analgesic for pain.
- Document findings and interventions.

THE CARDIOVASCULAR SYSTEM

Women experience an average blood loss of 200 to 500 mL through vaginal birth. This has a minimal effect on a woman's system due to pregnancy-induced hypervolemia. Stroke volume and cardiac output increase during the first few postpartum hours as blood that was shunted through the uteroplacental unit returns to the maternal system. Cardiac output is elevated for 24 to 48 hours after delivery and returns to prepregnant levels within 10 days (Cunningham et al., 2014).

After delivery, plasma volume initially decreases due to blood loss, then increases due to shifts from the extracellular to vascular space (Isley & Katz, 2016). Along with a decrease in the total blood volume, this often results in a transient anemia that typically resolves by 8 weeks after delivery (Isley & Katz, 2016). White blood cell (WBC) levels may increase to 30,000/mm within a few hours of birth as the result of the stress of labor and birth, and return to normal levels within 7 days (Cunningham et al., 2014).

Women are at risk for thromboembolism related to the increase of circulating clotting factors during pregnancy (Isley & Katz, 2016). Clotting factors slowly decrease after delivery of the placenta and return to normal ranges within the first 2 postpartum weeks. A potentially life-threatening complication of thrombus formation is pulmonary emboli (James, 2014).

Risk of orthostatic hypotension, a sudden drop in the blood pressure when the woman stands up, increases during the first postpartum week due to decreased vascular resistance in the pelvis.

- Explain cause and incidence of orthostatic hypotension.
- Instruct the woman to rise slowly to a standing position.
- Assist the woman when ambulating during the first few hours postbirth.
- Assist the woman to a sitting position if she becomes dizzy or faint.
- Ammonia ampule may still be used in some facilities if the woman faints but is often not available.
- Assess for excessive blood loss.

Most women will experience an episode of feeling cold and shaking during the first few hours following birth. This phenomenon, called postpartum chills, is related to vascular instability.

Nursing Actions

- Assess pulse and blood pressure:
  - Every 15 minutes for the first hour after delivery.
  - Every 30 minutes for the second hour.
  - Every 4 hours for the next 22 hours.
  - Every shift after the first 24 hours or as stated in hospital/unit protocols.
    - Rationale: Hemodynamic changes occur during labor and delivery and in the postpartum period, including rapid changes in blood volume and cardiac output. Assessment of pulse and blood pressure is important to identify potential complications such as excessive blood loss, orthostatic hypotension, infection, and gestational hypertension/preeclampsia. An elevated pulse may indicate excessive blood loss, fever, or infection (James, 2014).
- Assess for excessive blood loss. Expected findings include:
  - Pulse and blood pressure within normal ranges. However, after delivery there may be a transient 5% elevation in the woman's systolic and diastolic blood pressure (Isley & Katz, 2016).
  - Bradycardia may occur postdelivery and in the early postpartum period, and is considered normal (James, 2014).

- Assess for orthostatic hypotension. Women are at risk for orthostatic hypotension during the first postpartum week when standing from a seated or prone position.
  - Explain cause and incidence of orthostatic hypotension.
  - Instruct the woman to rise slowly to a standing position.
  - Assist the woman when ambulating during the first 24 hours postbirth.
  - Assist the woman to a sitting position if she becomes dizzy or faint.
  - Use an ammonia ampule if the woman faints.
  - Check lab values such as a complete blood count (CBC), if ordered.
    - Rationale: Components of the CBC, such as the hematocrit and hemoglobin, are assessed in cases where excessive blood loss has occurred. The hematocrit measures the concentration of red blood cells in the blood (Kee, 2009). Hemoglobin decreases by 1 to 1.5 g/dL and hematocrit decreases 3% to 4% per 500 mL of blood loss (James, 2014).
  - Expected assessment findings:
    - Blood loss within normal ranges
    - Hemoglobin and hematocrit within normal ranges
    - Anemia is not unusual during the postpartum period and is diagnosed if the hemoglobin is less than 11 g/dL and the hematocrit is less than 32%. Women may receive an oral iron supplement (ferrous sulfate) to treat postpartum anemia (Samuels, 2016).
    - Pulse rate should be within normal limits; however, in some women bradycardia may occur. Blood pressure should be within normal limits. An increase in pulse rate may be an indicator of excessive blood loss or infection (James, 2014). Elevated blood pressure of 140/90 or greater may indicate preeclampsia (James, 2014).
- Assess lower extremities for venous thrombosis.
  - Rationale: Increased coagulability associated with pregnancy continues into the postdelivery period. Additionally, venous stasis may occur when there is limited mobility in the immediate postpartum period. These factors lead to an increased risk of venous thrombosis (Isley & Katz, 2016).
  - Assess the calves and the groin area for tenderness, edema, and sensation of warmth each shift. Compare pulses in both extremities. Measure the calf width if thromboembolism is suspected (James, 2014).
    - Rationale: Symptoms of deep vein thrombosis include muscle pain; tenderness; palpation of a hard, cordlike vessel; swelling of veins; edema; and decreased blood circulation to the affected area.
  - Expected assessment findings:
    - No tenderness or sensation of warmth.
- Assess for postpartum chills.
  - Assess temperature.
  - Women who are experiencing chills with temperature within normal ranges may be offered a warm blanket and reassurance that it is normal.
  - Women who are experiencing chills with elevated temperature should be evaluated further for possible infection, and the physician or midwife needs to be notified.

Patient Education

- Instruct the woman on ways to reduce risk of orthostatic hypotension. Women should be accompanied by the nurse during ambulation in the early postpartum period.
  - Rationale: Orthostatic hypotension places the patient at risk for fainting and falls.
- Encourage frequent ambulation.
  - Rationale: Early and frequent ambulation prevents deep vein thrombosis by preventing stasis of blood in the lower extremities (Cunningham et al., 2014).
- Instruct the woman not to cross her legs (James, 2014).
- Apply compression stockings per provider orders for women with a history of blood clots (James, 2014).

THE RESPIRATORY SYSTEM

Chest wall compliance returns after the birth of the infant as diaphragm pressure is reduced. The respiratory system returns to a prepregnant state by the end of the postpartum period.

Nursing Actions

- Assess the respiratory rate:
  - Every 15 minutes for the first hour.
  - Every 30 minutes for the second hour.
  - Every 4 hours for the next 22 hours.
  - Every shift after the first 24 hours or as stated in hospital/unit protocols.
- Assess breath sounds.
  - Rationale: Women who received oxytocin, large amounts of intravenous fluids, or tocolytics such as magnesium sulfate or terbutaline; had multiple birth, infection, or preeclampsia; or who were on bed rest are at risk for pulmonary edema (James, 2014).
- Expected assessment findings:
  - Within normal limits. The respiratory rate in the postpartum period is typically in the range of 12 to 20 breaths per minute (bpm). The Pao$_2$ should be 95% or higher (James, 2014).
  - Breath sounds clear.
- Document findings and intervention.

THE IMMUNE SYSTEM

The immune system, which is suppressed during pregnancy, returns to normal in the postpartum period (Isley & Katz, 2016). It is common for the postpartum woman to experience mild temperature elevations during the first 24 hours postbirth related to muscular exertion, exhaustion, dehydration, or hormonal changes. A temperature greater than 100.4°F (38°C) after the first 24 hours on two occasions may be indicative of postpartum infection and requires further evaluation.

Women who are rubella nonimmune should be immunized for rubella before discharge (Cunningham et al., 2014). Women may be required to sign a consent form prior to administration of the vaccine. Women may also receive vaccinations such as Tdap (tetanus, diphtheria, and pertussis), hepatitis B, varicella, and influenza if needed in the postpartum period (American College of Obstetricians and Gynecologists [ACOG], 2013, 2018; CDC, 2016a).

Rh isoimmunization occurs when an Rh-negative woman develops antibodies to Rh-positive blood related to exposure to Rh-positive blood either by blood transfusion or during pregnancy with a Rh-positive fetus. Women who are sensitized produce IgG anti-D (antibody), which crosses the placenta and attacks the fetal red blood cells, causing hemolysis. Rh isoimmunization is preventable.

SAFE AND EFFECTIVE NURSING CARE: Understanding Medication

Rubella Immunization

- Women who contract rubella during the first trimester have a 90% chance of transmitting the virus to their fetuses.
- Fetuses exposed to rubella during the first trimester are at risk for birth defects that include deafness, blindness, heart defects, and mental retardation.
- Postpartum women who are rubella-nonimmune should be immunized for rubella before discharge. The measles, mumps, and rubella vaccine is often given.
- Women who are immunized should avoid pregnancy for 4 weeks, although the risk of the fetus developing birth defects from the vaccine is extremely low.

  CDC, 2016a.

SAFE AND EFFECTIVE NURSING CARE: Understanding Medication

Prevention of Rh Isoimmunization

Rho immune globulin is given to Rh-negative women at 28 weeks' gestation. Rh-negative women who gave birth to an Rh-positive neonate are screened for anti-Rh antibodies (Coombs' test). A second injection of Rho immune globulin is given to the woman in the postpartum period if her baby is Rh positive and she is Coombs' negative.

Medication
Rh (D) Immune Globulin (RhoGAM, Rhophylac)

- Indication: Administered to Rh-negative women who have given birth to an Rh-positive neonate
- Action: Prevents production of anti-Rh (D) antibodies
- Adverse reactions: Pain at the injection site, anemia, allergic reaction
- Route and dose: 300 mcg Rhogam IM only, or Rhophylac, 300 mcg IV or IM within 72 hours postbirth

• Nursing actions: Confirm that the mother is Rh negative and the infant is Rh positive prior to administration. Observe patient for 20 minutes after administration for signs of an allergic reaction. Rh immune globulin may interfere with the immune response to live vaccinations (e.g., measles, mumps, rubella [MMR]). The administration of live vaccines should be delayed for 3 months following administration.

Vallerand & Sanoski, 2013; Wilson et al., 2014.

Nursing Actions

● Assess temperature:
  ● Every 15 minutes for the first hour.
  ● Every 30 minutes for the second hour.
  ● Every 4 hours for the next 22 hours.
  ● Every shift after the first 24 hours or as stated in hospital/unit protocols.
    ● Rationale: Assessing the postpartum patient's temperature allows health care providers to monitor for complications such as infection.
● For temperature elevations of less than 100.4°F (38°C) during the first 24 hours postbirth:
  ● Encourage the woman to drink 8 to 10 glasses of fluid, or at least 64 ounces a day (James, 2014).
  ● Promote relaxation and rest
  ● Reassess 1 hour after intervention
    ● Rationale: Slight temperature elevations during the first 24 hours postpartum are likely associated with dehydration (Whitmer, 2011).
● For temperature elevations 100.4°F (38°C) or higher after 24 hours postbirth:
  ● Encourage the woman to drink a minimum of 10 glasses of fluids a day (James, 2014).
  ● Notify the physician or midwife of the elevated temperature and anticipate further evaluation. Notify the nursery of the maternal temperature elevation (James, 2014).
    ● Rationale: A temperature of 100.4°F (38°C) on two different occasions after the first 24 hours postdelivery is a sign of infection (James, 2014).
● Administer rubella vaccine as indicated.
● Administer other needed vaccines as ordered.
● Administer Rho(D) immune globulin (Rhophylac or RhoGAM) as indicated.
● Document findings and interventions.

THE URINARY SYSTEM

Women are at risk for urinary complications after birth. Transient stress incontinence associated with impaired pelvic muscle function involving the urethra may occur in the first 6 weeks postpartum (Isley & Katz, 2014; James, 2014). Many factors are associated with stress urinary incontinence, including pregnancy, multiparity, perineal trauma, infant size, length of second stage labor, and pushing techniques that increase pressure on the pelvic floor (James, 2014). Primary complications are bladder distention and cystitis.

Bladder Distention

Bladder distention, rapid bladder filling, incomplete emptying, and inability to void are common during the first few days postbirth (Cunningham et al., 2014). These are related to administration of intravenous fluids in the postdelivery period, decreased sensation of the urge to void due to anesthesia or analgesia, edema around the urethra, perineal lacerations or episiotomy, operative vaginal delivery, or bladder trauma (Cunningham et al., 2014; Mulder, Oude Rengerink, Van der Post, Hakvoort, & Roovers, 2016). Diuresis caused by decreased estrogen levels occurs within 12 hours after birth and aids in the elimination of excess tissue fluids. During this time urine output may be 3,000 cc or more per day (James, 2014).

Nursing Actions

● Assist the woman to the bathroom and encourage her to void within 2 to 4 hours postbirth.
  ● Rationale: Early voiding decreases the risk of cystitis and prevents bladder distention, which could lead to uterine atony and postpartum hemorrhage (James, 2014).
● Assess for urinary disturbances.
● Measure voidings postbirth. The woman should be able to void at least 300 cc within 2 to 4 hours of delivery.
  ● Rationale: Various birth-related factors, such as the stretching of the urethra, displacement of the bladder, birth trauma–associated neural dysfunction, and anesthesia, may interfere with the return of urinary function. Rapid filling of the bladder associated with the administration of IV fluids during labor and delivery and postpartum diuresis can lead to overdistention of the bladder (James, 2014). Measuring voidings allows the nurse to identify inadequate output and problems with urinary elimination.
  ● If voiding is less than 150 mL, the nurse must palpate for bladder distention, as this is indicative of urinary retention. Signs of bladder distention include uterine atony, displacement of the uterus above the umbilicus to the right, increased lochia, and fullness in the suprapubic area (James, 2014). Incomplete emptying of the bladder can lead to uterine atony and postpartum hemorrhage. Urinary retention may also lead to cystitis.
  ● A bladder scanner using ultrasound technology may be used to assess for urinary retention or to measure bladder residual volume after a void of less than 150 mL (Buchanan & Beckmann, 2014).
  ● If the woman is unable to spontaneously void and has an over-distended bladder postbirth, she will need to be catheterized (Cunningham et al., 2014; James, 2014; Smith, 2018). An indwelling urinary catheter left in place for 24 hours is recommended when inability to void is related to edema (Cunningham et al., 2014; Smith, 2018).
    ● A straight or "in and out" catheterization may be done if there is little or no edema present and repeated catheterizations are not needed.

- An integrative method when a woman is unable to void is the use of peppermint oil. That entails saturating a cotton ball with peppermint oil and placing it in the "hat" (urine-collection container) with a small amount of water and placing the "hat" on the toilet. Instruct the woman to sit on the toilet. The vapors of the peppermint oil have a relaxing effect on the urinary sphincter.
  - The woman should be able to void within 2 to 4 hours of delivery.
- Rationale: After 24 hours, edema associated with trauma of the bladder and urethra related to birth should decrease (James, 2014).
- Assess for frequency, urgency, and burning on urination.
  - Notify the physician or midwife if the patient reports frequency, urgency, and/or burning on urination.
    - Rationale: These are signs of possible cystitis.
      - Expected assessment findings:
        - The woman spontaneously voids within 2 to 4 hours postbirth.
  - Each voiding is at least 300 mL.
  - The woman does not experience frequency, urgency, and burning on urination.
- Instruct the woman to increase fluid intake to a minimum of 10 glasses per day.
- Document findings and interventions.

Cystitis

Cystitis is a bladder inflammation/infection.
- Symptoms: Frequency, urgency, pain/burning on urination, suprapubic tenderness, hematuria, and malaise
- Treatment: Antibiotic therapy, increased hydration, rest

Evidence-Based Practice: Urinary Incontinence

Woodley, S. J., Boyle, R., Cody, J. D., Mørkved, S., & Hay-Smith, E. J. C. (2017). Pelvic floor muscle training for prevention and treatment of urinary and faecal incontinence in antenatal and postnatal women. *Cochrane Database of Systematic Reviews, 12.* doi:10.1002/14651858.CD007471.pub3

Urinary incontinence is experienced by approximately one-third of women during the postpartum period. Fecal incontinence is less prevalent and may occur after severe perineal trauma during delivery. The purpose of this systematic review was to determine the effectiveness of pelvic floor muscle training (PFMT) in preventing and treating urinary and fecal incontinence in pregnant and postpartum women (Woodley, 2017). This was a review of 38 studies, including randomized controlled trials and quasi-experimental studies that compared voluntary pelvic floor muscle exercises that were taught and supervised by health professionals, compared to usual prenatal or postpartum care, which may have included advice on pelvic floor exercises.

Results:
- Targeting continent antenatal women early in pregnancy and offering a structured PFMT program may prevent the onset of urinary incontinence in late pregnancy and postpartum. However, the cost-effectiveness of this is unknown.

- When PFMT was initiated in early pregnancy by primiparous women, it was effective in reducing the incidence of urinary incontinence in late pregnancy and up to 6 months postpartum.
- When PFMT was started during the antenatal or postpartum period to treat urinary incontinence, it was found to be effective in treating urinary incontinence up to 1 year postdelivery.
- The long-term effects of PFMT are unknown and should be further explored.

THE ENDOCRINE SYSTEM

Abrupt changes occur in the endocrine system after the delivery of the placenta. Estrogen, progesterone, and prolactin levels decrease. Estrogen levels begin to rise after the first week postpartum. For nonlactating women, prolactin levels continue to decline throughout the first 3 postpartum weeks. Menses begins 7 to 9 weeks postbirth. The first menses is usually anovulatory. Ovulation usually occurs by the fourth cycle. The average time for women who are not breastfeeding to return to ovulation is 10 weeks postpartum (James, 2014).

In women who are lactating, prolactin levels increase in response to the infant's suckling. Lactation suppresses menses, likely due to hormonal changes, including elevated prolactin levels (James, 2014). Return of menses depends on the length and amount of breastfeeding. Ovulation is suppressed longer for lactating women than for nonlactating women. The mean time to return to ovulation for women who breastfeed is 17 weeks postdelivery (James, 2014).

Both lactating and nonlactating women should be advised to use contraception when they resume sexual intercourse, as ovulation can precede return of menses. Breastfeeding is not an effective contraceptive method.

Diaphoresis

Diaphoresis occurs during the first few postpartum weeks in response to decreased estrogen levels. This profuse sweating, which often occurs at night, assists the body in excreting the increased fluid accumulated during pregnancy.

Nursing Actions

- Assess for diaphoresis.
  - If present, assess for infection by taking the woman's temperature.
  - Expected assessment findings:
    - Diaphoresis with temperature within normal ranges

Patient Education

- Instruct the woman regarding the cause of diaphoresis.
- Discuss comfort measures such as wearing cotton nightwear.
- Discuss that feelings of warmth, sweating, and chills are signs of fever, a cardinal sign of infection. Women with these symptoms need to differentiate between fever and

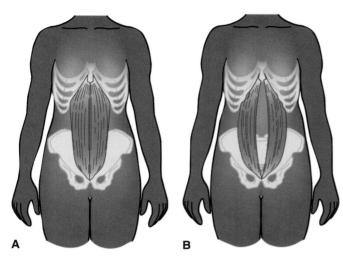

FIGURE 12-4 Diastasis recti abdominis. (**A**) Normal location of rectus muscles of the abdomen. (**B**) Diastasis recti. There is separation of the rectus muscles.

diaphoresis, the latter of which is a normal physiological process.

● Document findings and interventions.

THE MUSCULAR AND NERVOUS SYSTEMS

After birth, the abdominal muscles experience reduced tone and the abdomen appears soft and flabby. Some women experience a separation of the rectus muscle, which is noted as diastasis recti abdominis (Fig.12–4). This separation becomes less apparent as the body returns to a prepregnant state. Women may experience muscular soreness related to the labor and birth experience. Lower body nerve sensation may be diminished for women who have received an epidural during labor. Delay ambulation until full sensation returns.

Nursing Actions

● Assess for diastasis recti abdominis.
  ● The nurse can feel the separation of the rectus muscle when assessing the fundus.
  ● Reassure the woman that this is normal and will diminish over time.
● Assess for muscle tenderness.
  ● Rationale: Muscle soreness may result from positioning during labor and delivery, and generalized muscle use during second stage labor/pushing.
  ● Expected assessment findings:
    ○ Mild to no muscle soreness
  ● Comfort measures for muscle soreness:
    ○ Ice pack to area for 15 minutes
    ○ Heat to area: Applying heat increases circulation, which facilitates healing. Cold packs result in vasoconstriction and decreased swelling. These interventions

may alter the woman's perception of pain according to the gate control theory of pain modulation (Wilkinson & Treas, 2011). Analgesics alter a patient's perception of pain.
    ○ Warm shower
    ○ Analgesia
● Assess for decreased nerve sensation.
  ● Rationale: Epidural or spinal anesthesia causes lack of sensation that may last several hours into the early postpartum period. Regional anesthesia may interfere with urinary elimination and mobility until the effects wear off.
  ● Expected assessment findings:
    ○ Full sensation of lower extremities for women who did not receive an epidural during labor.
    ○ Diminished lower body sensation for women who received an epidural during labor with full sensation returning within a few hours postbirth.
  ● Delay ambulation or assist the woman when ambulating until full sensation has returned.
    ○ Rationale: Women who have received spinal or epidural anesthesia are at risk for falls until full sensation has returned.
● Assess for headache.
  ● If the woman complains of headache, assess the location and quality of the headache (James, 2014).
  ● Notify the woman's health care provider if the headache is associated with signs and symptoms of preeclampsia, or if a postepidural/spinal headache is suspected.
    ○ Rationale: Women who have had spinal or epidural anesthesia may develop headaches related to dural puncture and subsequent leakage of cerebrospinal fluid (CSF) leading to decreased levels of CSF. Headaches related to epidural or spinal anesthesia tend to be worse when the patient is in an upright position and improved when the patient is lying down (Sacks & Smiley, 2014). Headache may also be associated with preeclampsia (James, 2014).
● Assess for fatigue
  ● Rationale: Fatigue is a common complaint among women during the postpartum period. Discomfort and lack of sleep related to infant care activities contribute to feelings of fatigue (James, 2014).
● Promote rest and sleep.
  ● Provide teaching about the importance of sleep and rest.
  ● Encourage the woman to sleep/nap while the baby is sleeping and to prioritize activities with a focus on self- and infant care.
  ● Cluster nursing care such as assessments, interventions, and medication administration.
    ○ Rationale: This minimizes disruptions to the woman's sleep/naps.
  ● Medicate the woman for pain as per orders and/or offer nonpharmacological interventions if appropriate.
    ○ Rationale: Pain interferes with sleep (Wilkinson & Treas, 2011).
● Document findings and interventions.

THE GASTROINTESTINAL SYSTEM

Gastrointestinal muscle tone and motility decrease postbirth with a return to normal bowel function by the end of the second postpartum week.

- Constipation
  - Women are at risk for constipation due to decreased GI motility from the effects of progesterone, decreased physical activity, dehydration and fluid loss from labor, fear of having a bowel movement after perineal lacerations or episiotomy, and perineal pain and trauma.
- Hemorrhoids
  - Women commonly develop hemorrhoids during pregnancy and/or the birthing process. Hemorrhoids often slowly resolve but can be painful. Sometimes hemorrhoids persist postpartum.
- Appetite
  - Women are hungry after the birthing experience and can be given a regular diet, unless they are on a prescribed diet such as for diabetes. Women are exceptionally hungry during the first few postpartum days and may require snacks between meals.
- Weight loss
  - Most women will experience significant weight loss during the first 2 to 3 weeks postpartum. Immediately after birth, women lose approximately 11 to 12 pounds as the result of delivery and blood loss.
  - Diuresis results in the loss of approximately another 5 to 8 pounds postdelivery (Cunningham et al., 2014).
  - The average American woman at the end of 6 months postpartum is approximately 3 pounds above her prepregnancy weight (Cunningham et al., 2014).

Nursing Actions

- Assess bowel sounds at each shift.
  - Notify the physician or midwife if bowel sounds are faint or absent.
    - Rationale: Decreased motility can lead to diminished peristalsis and intestinal obstruction.
- Assess for constipation.
  - Ask the woman if and when she had a bowel movement.
    - Rationale: Constipation is common in the postpartum period. Bowel function usually returns in 2 to 3 days after delivery (James, 2014). Decreased frequency of bowel movements and the passage of hard, dry stools indicate constipation (Turawa, Musekiwa, & Rohwer, 2015).
  - Instruct the woman to increase fluid intake and increase fiber and roughage in diet to decrease risk of constipation. Bring her water and prune juice. Remind her to drink often.
    - Rationale: A diet that includes fiber-rich foods (i.e., fruits, vegetables, whole grains, and legumes) promotes intestinal peristalsis. Adequate fluid intake is necessary when women are encouraged to increase dietary fiber to prevent constipation. Intake of 3,000 mL of fluids a day will soften bowel movements and provide adequate mucus to lubricate the colon (James, 2014).
  - Ask the woman what she did for constipation during pregnancy or in the past and implement these strategies.
  - Encourage ambulation.
    - Rationale: Ambulation promotes intestinal peristalsis and reduces the risk for constipation (Turawa et al., 2015).
  - Administer a stool softener or laxative as per health care provider's orders.
    - Rationale: Stool softeners prevent constipation by increasing water in the stool, promoting stool softening and elimination (Vallerand & Sanoski, 2013). Laxatives are effective in relieving constipation and work by adding bulk to the stools or stimulating the nerves that irritate the intestinal wall (Turawa et al., 2015).
    - Docusate sodium (Colace) is a stool softener that helps incorporate water into the stool and can be administered to prevent constipation.
    - Route and dose: PO; 100 mg twice a day
    - Nursing actions/implications: Administer with a full glass of water or juice; do not administer within 2 hours of other laxatives, such as mineral oil. Effectiveness may take 1 to 3 days after administration.
- Assess for hemorrhoids.
  - Rationale: Hemorrhoids may increase in size during labor and cause discomfort in the postpartum period (James, 2014).
  - Instruct the woman to lie on her side, then separate the buttocks to expose the anus.
  - If hemorrhoids are present:
    - Encourage the woman to avoid sitting for long periods of time by lying on her side.
    - Witch hazel pads or topical anesthetics can be used to reduce discomfort from hemorrhoids (Isley & Katz, 2016; James 2014).
    - Sitz baths are helpful in promoting circulation and reducing pain.
- Assess appetite.
  - Assess the amount of food eaten during meals.
  - Ask the woman if she is hungry.
    - Rationale: In most cases, after a vaginal delivery women can resume eating a regular diet (James, 2014).
- Ask the woman if she is nauseous or has vomited.
  - Rationale: Nausea and vomiting may occur during labor. Additionally, nausea is a common side effect of opioid analgesics commonly used for pain management during labor and delivery (Wilkinson & Treas, 2011).

Patient Education

- Instruct the woman to increase fluid intake and increase fiber and roughage in diet to decrease risk of constipation.
- Provide nutritional education. This is especially important for lactating women and women who had a cesarean birth.

Women who are breastfeeding need to increase caloric intake by 500 to 1,000 calories a day (James, 2014).

● Encourage the woman to ambulate to increase GI motility and decrease risk of gas pains.

● Instruct the woman to increase fluid intake to a minimum of 10 glasses per day.

SAFE AND EFFECTIVE NURSING CARE: Cultural Competence

Food Preferences Across Cultures

Foods and how they are prepared can be significant to women of different cultures. The nurse should:

● Ask women if there are foods that they prefer to eat based on their cultural beliefs; if not available in the hospital, encourage patients to have family members bring home-made dishes.

● In-service training should be provided to staff about cultures that are common to that unit.

FOLLOW-UP CARE

In the weeks after birth, a woman must adapt to multiple physical, social, and psychological changes. She must recover from childbirth, adjust to changing hormones, and learn to feed and care for her newborn. In addition to being a time of joy and excitement, this "fourth trimester" can present considerable challenges for women, including lack of sleep, fatigue, pain, breastfeeding difficulties, stress, depression, lack of sexual desire, and urinary incontinence. Guidelines recommend that all women attend a postpartum follow-up visit 4 to 6 weeks after birth, or sooner if complications are present. However, as many as 40% of women do not attend a postpartum visit. Attendance rates are lower among populations with limited resources.

The comprehensive postpartum visit includes a full assessment of physical, social, and psychological well-being, with screening for postpartum depression using a validated instrument such as the Edinburgh Postnatal Depression Scale. Birth spacing recommendations and reproductive life plans should be reviewed and a commensurate contraceptive method provided. Systems should be in place to ensure that women who desire long-acting reversible contraception or another form of contraception can receive it during the comprehensive postpartum visit if placement wasn't done immediately after birth. Vaccination history should be reviewed and immunizations provided as needed. Women should be asked about common postpartum concerns, including perineal or cesarean wound pain, incontinence, dyspareunia, fatigue, depression, anxiety, and infant feeding problems, and identified concerns addressed. Suggested topics for anticipatory guidance include infant feeding, expressing breast milk if returning to work or school, postpartum weight retention, sexuality, physical activity, and nutrition. Smoking and substance use cessation should be addressed and are discussed in the following section.

DISCHARGE TEACHING

Nurses are the health care providers who perform the most postpartum education in the United States, so it is critical that they work to improve discharge education to provide information that is efficient, timely, and evidence based. When women are discharged after birth, nurses play a vital role in providing them with education on self-care, transitioning home, and caring for a newborn. Many women are unaware of their health needs after giving birth. Women experience many signs and symptoms associated with the normal physiological and psychosocial changes of the postpartum period. Therefore, it is important to help them understand how to differentiate signs and symptoms that are normal from those that are not (Suplee, Kleppel, & Bingham, 2016). Women also need to know why it is necessary and appropriate to proactively seek and obtain care when they are not feeling well and how urgently they should obtain this care based on the types of symptoms they are experiencing. Armed with information about and understanding the postbirth warning signs, women can be empowered to act immediately rather than wait and suffer potentially devastating consequences.

Although the window of opportunity for discharge planning and teaching postpartum women is small and the volume of information to be relayed is substantial, the necessity of providing this critical information cannot be overstated. Nurses can work together within their maternity services to develop best practices to accomplish essential maternal and newborn discharge teaching in the most efficient and effective manner possible. For example, plan discharge teaching over the course of the woman's postpartum stay rather than waiting for day of discharge. Another strategy is to include this information as part of prenatal education. Incorporating a checklist and patient education tool (such as the AWHONN tools) into hospital electronic health record systems and the discharge education process will provide nurses with a resource handout to use when providing evidence-based care education.

The lack of follow-up care for the 40% of women who do not attend these visits represents missed opportunities to improve the health of women who have recently given birth. This poor rate of attendance at postpartum visits further supports the need to take full advantage of the limited postpartum hospital stay by providing consistent discharge education on postbirth warning signs of potentially life-threatening conditions that require immediate medical attention. Discharge teaching for the woman and her family should focus on:

● Signs of complications that need to be reported to the physician or midwife:
  ● Heavy lochia (saturating a pad in 1 hour) indicates possible secondary postpartum hemorrhage (James, 2014).

- The return of bright red, heavy bleeding after lochia has diminished or that becomes serosa or alba, or the passage of clots the size of an egg or larger indicates possible secondary postpartum hemorrhage (Suplee, Klepple, Santa-Donato, & Bingham, 2016).
- Foul-smelling lochia; indicates possible infection.
- Increased temperature (100.4°F [38°C] or higher); indicates possible infection.
- Pelvic or abdominal tenderness/pain; indicates possible infection.
- Frequency, urgency, or burning on urination; indicates possible cystitis.
- Unilateral breast tenderness, warm reddened area; chills and fever; indicates possible mastitis, which often occurs 3 to 4 weeks after delivery (James, 2014).
- Blurry vision, severe headaches, epigastric abdominal pain, fluid retention; may be associated with preeclampsia (Suplee, Kleppel, Santa-Donato, et al., 2016).
- Leg pain, swelling, redness may indicate venous thrombosis. Chest pain and difficulty breathing may be associated with pulmonary embolism (Suplee, Kleppel, Santa-Donato, et al., 2016).
- Thoughts of harming infant or self, difficulty caring for self and/or infant, difficulty sleeping or sleeping too much, and persistent feelings of depression and sadness are associated with postpartum depression (Suplee, Kleppel, Santa-Donato, et al., 2016).
- Expected physical changes
  - Uterine involution, afterpains, progression of lochia
  - Breast changes, engorgement
  - Diaphoresis and diuresis
  - Weight loss
    - Women can expect to lose approximately 12 pounds immediately after delivery, and an additional 5 to 8 pounds due to fluid losses associated with uterine involution and diuresis (Cunningham et al., 2014).
- Self-care
  - Hygiene
  - Perineal care, continue to change pad frequently and use peri-bottle until lochia has stopped
  - Breast care for lactating and nonlactating women
  - Pharmacological and nonpharmacological pain control measures

SAFE AND EFFECTIVE NURSING CARE: Patient Education

AWHONN Postpartum Discharge Teaching Project: Warning Signs

Call 911 for:

Pain in the chest

Obstructed breathing or shortness of breath

Seizures

Thoughts of hurting yourself or baby

Call your provider for:

Bleeding soaking though one pad/hour or passing a clot the size of an egg.

Incision that is not healing

Red or swollen leg that is warm or painful to touch

Temperature of 100.4 or higher

Headache that does not get better even after taking medicine, or bad headache with changes in vision

If you cannot reach your provider, go to an emergency room.

AWHONN, 2016; Suplee, Kleppel, Santa-Donato, & Bingham, 2016.

HEALTH PROMOTION

Health promotion topics for new mothers are as follows. Explain all discharge medications, including dose, frequency, action, and side effects. Stress the importance of following through with postpartum follow-up visits to her physician or midwife as discussed above. Scheduling a postpartum visit before discharge may facilitate the postpartum visit.

Nutrition and Fluids

The nurse must provide instruction about nutritional needs for lactating and nonlactating women.

- Lactating women should increase their caloric intake by 500 to 1,000 calories per day and have a fluid intake of approximately 2 to 3 liters per day.
- Teach lactating women that there is no evidence that an occasional alcoholic drink is harmful (Niebyl, Weber, & Briggs, 2016); however, the long-term effects of daily alcohol use on breastfeeding infants is unknown, so alcoholic beverages should be kept to a minimum. If a woman does drink, she should wait for 2 to 2.5 hours per drink before nursing (TOXNET, 2017).
- Teach the woman how to use MyPlate (www.ChooseMyPlate.gov) and how this can assist in meeting her nutritional needs (Fig. 12–5). Women who are anemic should increase consumption of leafy green vegetables, beans, red meat, poultry, iron-fortified cereal, breads, pasta, and dried fruits such as raisins. To prevent constipation, women who have hemorrhoids, perineal lacerations, or episiotomy should consume foods that add roughage to their diets such as fruits, vegetables, beans, and whole grains. Woman should drink a minimum of 10 glasses of fluids per day, or 80 ounces.

Smoking Cessation and Relapse Prevention

- A goal of *Healthy People 2020* is to reduce postpartum relapse of smoking among women who quit during pregnancy (U.S. Department of Health and Human Services, 2012).

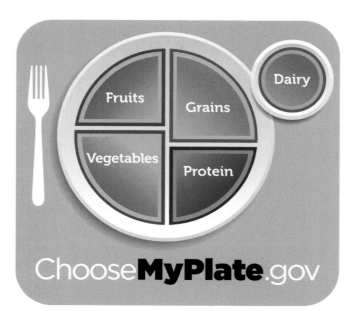

FIGURE 12–5 MyPlate illustrates the five food groups using a familiar mealtime visual, a place setting. Source: United States Department of Agriculture, www.ChooseMyPlate.gov.

● Ask women about tobacco use.
● Teach women about the dangers of smoking (e.g., cancer, lung problems such as chronic obstructive pulmonary disease, osteoporosis).
● Teach women to never allow smoking around their infant/children, as secondhand smoke is associated with problems such as ear infections and respiratory issues.
● Encourage women who quit smoking for pregnancy to remain abstinent. Most women who quit smoking during pregnancy relapse after delivery.
● Advise women who currently smoke to quit. Provide information about resources to assist with cessation, such as counseling services/classes, cessation help lines, and medications.

Activity and Exercise

Physical activity is good for the overall health of postpartum women with no other medical problems. For example, moderate-intensity physical activity, such as brisk walking, keeps their heart and lungs healthy after pregnancy. Physical activity also helps improve mood throughout the postpartum period. Exercise helps maintain a healthy weight, and when combined with eating fewer calories helps with weight loss (CDC, 2015).

Healthy women should get at least 150 minutes (2.5 hours) per week of moderate-intensity aerobic activity such as brisk walking. While 150 minutes each week sounds like a lot of time, women can break it into smaller chunks throughout the week. In fact, it is best to spread activity out during the week, as long as you exercise with moderate or vigorous effort for at least 10 minutes at a time.

● Explain the importance of activity to decrease risk of constipation and to promote circulation and a sense of well-being.
● Instruct the woman about appropriate exercises in the postpartum period, such as walking.

● Encourage the woman to do Kegel exercises to strengthen the pelvic floor.

Rest and Comfort

● Teach the woman the importance of rest in promoting healing and lactation.
● Problem-solve with the woman about ways to increase rest time (e.g., nap when the baby is napping, prioritize activities).
● Encourage the woman to take medications as ordered by the physician or midwife (e.g., vitamins, iron, pain medications).

Evidence-Based Practice: Weight Loss in Women After Childbirth

Amorim Adegboye, A. R., & Linne, Y. M. (2013). Diet or exercise, or both for weight reduction in women after childbirth. *Cochrane Database of Systematic Reviews*, (7). doi: 10.1002/14651858.CD005627.pub3

Gaining weight during pregnancy is a normal occurrence. Postdelivery retention of weight gained during pregnancy is common and has been linked to long-term weight problems and obesity in women. Overweight and obesity may lead to chronic disease and lifelong negative health effects. The purpose of this systematic review was to determine the effectiveness of exercise, diet, or exercise in combination with diet as compared to usual care, in reducing weight postdelivery. The authors reviewed 14 studies; only randomized trials or quasi-randomized trials were included in this review. Additional outcomes that were explored included the effect of interventions on breastfeeding, infant growth, and maternal cardiovascular fitness.
Results:

● Exercise alone improved cardiovascular fitness but did not result in increased weight loss.

● Diet combined with exercise compared to usual care resulted in increased weight loss and improved cardiovascular fitness. Women who participated in this intervention were more likely to return to a healthy weight.

● Diet alone compared to usual care resulted in weight loss.

Diet and/or exercise had no negative effects on breastfeeding or infant growth; however, more research is needed since the sample size included in this review was small.

Contraception

● Assess the couple's desire for future pregnancies.
● Assess satisfaction with previous method of contraception.
● Encourage the patient to discuss contraceptive options with the health care provider. The immediate placement of long-acting reversible contraception (LARC), such as intrauterine devices and contraceptive implants, is an option during the postpartum period (ACOG, 2016). LARC is highly effective in preventing unwanted pregnancy and short intervals between pregnancies (ACOG, 2016).
● Provide information on various methods of contraception (Table 12–3).

TABLE 12–3   Methods of Contraception

METHOD	FAILURE RATE	AVAILABILITY	ADVANTAGES	DISADVANTAGES
Natural Methods				
Abstinence	0%	Readily available	No contraindications Prevents exposure to STIs Readily available	Must be consistently practiced or it is not effective
Natural Family Planning	24%	Handouts and information from care provider Internet access of information Fertility monitoring devices now available	No contraindications or side effects	Must have a regular menstrual cycle and have knowledge/willingness to frequently monitor body functions: temperature, vaginal mucus production and consistency Does not protect against STIs
Withdrawal	22%		No cost or contraindications	Does not protect against STIs Disrupts sexual intercourse
Lactational Amenorrhea Method (LAM)			No cost or contraindications	Requires *exclusive* breastfeeding/infant suckling Using a barrier method with LAM increases effectiveness
Barrier Methods				
Condoms (Male and Female)	18% male condom 21% female condom	Over-the-counter (OTC) purchase	Readily available Protects against STIs No systemic effects	Allergic reactions may occur Barrier methods have higher rate of protection when combined with spermicides Must be applied at time of coitus and may be considered disruptive
Vaginal Sponges	12% if no prior births 24% if previous births	OTC Limited availability No fitting needed Spermicide is added, but must be activated with addition of fluid before insertion	One-time use May be placed before intercourse May leave in for up to 30 hours Protects repeated acts of intercourse	Must be left in place for at least 6 hours postintercourse Irritation, discomfort, and allergic reaction may occur May increase risk for infections, including STIs
Cervical Caps	14% if no prior birth 29% women with prior birth	Provider determines fit based on OB history; no exam needed Limited availability Spermicide must be added before each insertion	No systemic effects Fits snugly over cervix May leave in for up to 48 hours for repeated intercourse No systemic effects	Must be left in place for 6 hours after coitus Does not protect against STIs

TABLE 12–3 Methods of Contraception—cont'd

METHOD	FAILURE RATE	AVAILABILITY	ADVANTAGES	DISADVANTAGES
Diaphragms	12%	Limited availability Must be fitted by provider and must be refitted after birth or a large weight gain	No systemic effects May be placed in anticipation of intercourse Fits over cervix May leave in place for 24 hours for repeated intercourse	Need additional doses of spermicide for repeated intercourse Leave in place for 6 hours after intercourse May increase risk of yeast infection, cystitis, and toxic shock syndrome if use is prolonged
Spermicidal gels, cream suppository, or foam	28%	OTC	No systemic effects Foam may be used for an immediate emergency contraceptive	Allergic reaction Irritation Frequent use contraindicated for individuals at risk for HIV
Hormonal Methods				
Combination Estrogen/Progesterone Oral Contraception	9%	Prescription only Many options available available;12-week pill cycle with menses only 4 times per year	Suppresses ovulation Take one pill a day Many noncontraceptive benefits include reduced risk for: endometrial and ovarian cancer, benign breast disease, anemia, may improve acne	Contraindications to hormonal methods: History of deep vein thrombosis, pulmonary emboli, hypertension, heart disease Women aged 35 or older, who smoke Active cancer Genetic clotting disorders, liver disease May have multiple side effects (nausea, headache, spotting weight gain, breast tenderness, chloasma) Increased risks for blood clots, heart disease, and strokes Do not provide protection against STIs
Emergency Contraceptives (not to be used as regular form of birth control)	9%	Postcoital ingestion of hormones Must take within 72–120 hours of incident OTC for women aged 17 years or older. Prescription only for women younger than 17 years old.	Reduces risk of pregnancy for one-time unprotected intercourse by suppressing ovulation	Side effects include headache, nausea, vomiting, abdominal pain Heavier or lighter menstrual bleeding, fatigue, diarrhea Does not protect against STIs

Continued

TABLE 12–3   Methods of Contraception—cont'd

METHOD	FAILURE RATE	AVAILABILITY	ADVANTAGES	DISADVANTAGES
Progestin only	6%	Prescription only	Take one pill at same time every day Can be used during lactation	Weight gain Irregular bleeding May have minor side effects: nausea, mood changes Does not protect against STIs
Depo-Provera	3%	Injectable every 3 months Prescription only	One injection 4 times a year, Can be used during lactation	Weight gain, decreased bone density Delayed fertility Bleeding abnormalities Headache, mood changes, breast tenderness Does not protect against STIs
Contraceptive patch	9%	Prescription only	Place a new patch weekly for 3 weeks, then remove for 1 week	Risk similar to those for oral contraceptives, including increased risk for thrombotic event Possibly less effective for larger women Possible skin irritation Does not prevent STIs
Vaginal ring	9%	Prescription only	Flexible hormone-filled ring inserted and left in the vagina for 3 weeks, then removed for 1 week Ring can be left in for 28 days, with immediate placement of new ring	Side effects similar to oral contraceptives Vaginal irritation and discharge may occur Does not protect against STIs
Long-Acting Reversible Contraceptives				
Intrauterine Contraceptives (IUCs), Copper Material or Hormone Releasing (Levonorgestrel)	0.8% 0.2%	Prescription Inserted during office visit May also be placed in the hospital during the immediate postpartum period	May be used with lactation Can be used by teens, as well as women with medical problems/contraindications to other hormonal methods Highly effective Long-term contraceptive method; good for 1–10 years Copper-releasing IUC can be used as emergency contraceptive; must be inserted within 7 days of intercourse	Low risk of uterine perforation Contraindicated in women diagnosed and treated for pelvic inflammatory disease (PID) within the prior 3 months Increase of cramping and bleeding in the first few cycles Does not protect against STIs

TABLE 12-3   Methods of Contraception—cont'd

METHOD	FAILURE RATE	AVAILABILITY	ADVANTAGES	DISADVANTAGES
Hormone Implants	.05%	One rod implanted in the arm	Once in place, there is minimal discomfort	Side effects similar to oral contraceptives
		Office procedure	Lasts for several years	Irregular bleeding
		May be placed during the immediate postpartum period in the hospital setting	Can be used during lactation	Skin irritation at site
				Does not protect against STIs
				Must be removed
Sterilization				
Vasectomy	0.15%	Surgical procedure done under local anesthesia in the office or clinic	High rate of effectiveness	Discomfort for 2–3 days
				Difficult to reverse
				Need to use alternative contraceptive method until two postsurgery sperm tests indicate procedure is effective
Tubal ligation	0.5%	Surgical procedure done under general anesthesia	High rate of effectiveness	Bleeding or pain at incision site
				Difficult to reverse
Sterilization implant	0.03%	Office procedure	Implants placed in the fallopian tubes, which causes scar tissue that eventually block the tubes	Another contraceptive method needs to be used until blockage is confirmed, usually 3 months

Shoupe & Mishell, 2016.

CRITICAL COMPONENT

AWHONN Position Statement: Insurance Coverage for Contraceptives

AWHONN supports the inclusion of all contraceptive drugs, devices (including device insertion), and related services that are approved by the U.S. Food and Drug Administration as covered health insurance benefits in public and private plans. AWHONN considers access to widespread, affordable, and acceptable health care, which includes safe and reliable contraceptives, to be a basic human right.

AWHONN, 2016.

Sexual Activity

● Instruct the couple to discuss with the physician or midwife when they can resume sexual intercourse.
  ● General guidelines are to resume sexual intercourse when the lochia has stopped, perineum has healed, and the woman is physically and emotionally ready.
● Explain that an artificial vaginal lubricant might be needed to increase comfort during intercourse due to changes in hormone levels that result in vaginal dryness.
● Explain the importance of using contraception when the couple resumes sexual activity.

Prescribed Medications

Explain all discharge medications, including dose, frequency, action, and side effects.

Clinical Pathway for Uncomplicated Vaginal Delivery

Focus of Care	Postpartum: Admission	Postpartum: First 4 Hours	Postpartum: Greater Than 4 Hours Discharge	Expected Outcomes/ Discharge Criteria
Diagnostic tests	RPR, Hepatitis B surface antigen, rubella, blood type and Rh status documented or drawn if no prenatal record available GBS status documented with appropriate interventions Urine toxicology screenings per policy	Fetal Rh study as indicated (woman Rh-negative and neonate Rh-positive)	CBC as ordered Notify CNM/MD of abnormal results or if the woman is symptomatic	Rubella status known and MMR vaccine given if indicated Rh status known—Rh immune globulin given if indicated CBC within normal ranges Needed vaccinations are given as ordered (flu shots, Tdap, varicella, etc.)
Activity and safety	Moves legs Lifts bottom off bed Needs assistance with initial ambulation Infant security and safety reviewed	Women who received an epidural for labor and/or birth will need assistance with ambulation until return of sensory and motor sensation	Able to stand and walk with minimal assistance	Ambulates without assistance
Treatments and patient care	Assess vital signs Assess level of consciousness Assess fundus, lochia, and perineum Ice to perineum Assess lower extremities for edema, pain, pulses Assess Foley catheter if in place Assess IV site and fluids if in place Assess breast for potential breastfeeding problems	Vital signs as per orders Postpartum physical assessment as per orders/ unit protocol Pericare with each voiding Ice to perineum Input and output while Foley catheter or IV in place Measure first 2 voidings; notify CNM/MD if urine output <30 mL/hr If patient unable to void or voids less than 150 mL, and uterus is above the umbilicus and deviated to the side, consider catheterization	Vital signs as per orders Postpartum physical assessment as per orders Pericare with each voiding Ice to perineum for first 24 hours Assess breast for signs of engorgement and nipple irritation	Vital signs stable and within normal limits Fundus firm, midline, and descending by 1 cm per day Lochia moderate to scant Perineum healing without signs of infection Breasts exhibit physiological changes of lactation Breastfeeding without difficulty Bowel and bladder function within normal limits

Clinical Pathway for Uncomplicated Vaginal Delivery—cont'd

Focus of Care	Postpartum: Admission	Postpartum: First 4 Hours	Postpartum: Greater Than 4 Hours Discharge	Expected Outcomes/ Discharge Criteria
Medications	Maintain IV patency if indicated Oxytocin as indicated to reduce risk of or treat postpartum hemorrhage Analgesics and/or comfort measure as indicated for pain management	IV discontinued if fundus firm and lochia within normal limits Oxytocin discontinued if fundus firm and lochia within normal limits Analgesics and/or comfort measures as indicated for pain management	Analgesics and/ or comfort measure as indicated for pain management Rubella vaccine administered, if indicated, at least 30 minutes before discharge Rh(D) immune globulin administered as indicated Stool softener as ordered	Mild to moderate pain relieved with comfort measures and/or PO analgesia Rubella vaccine administered when indicated Rh(D) immune globulin administered as indicated Discharge medication teaching provided
Nutrition	Regular diet as tolerated PO fluids	Regular diet as tolerated PO fluids	Regular diet as tolerated PO fluids	Maintains adequate diet and fluid intake
Discharge planning/ evaluation of social support	Evaluate need for referrals such as social worker, lactation specialist, and dietitian Explain physical changes Teach self-care and health promotion	Continue to evaluate need for referrals Initiate referrals as indicated Explain physical changes Teach self-care and health promotion	Review discharge preparation with the woman and her family Explain physical and emotional changes Teach self-care and health promotion	The woman and her family have appropriate support on discharge. The woman can provide appropriate self-care. The woman and her family verbalize the importance of follow-up care for both the woman and infant.
Patient/family education	Initiate discharge teaching by assessing immediate learning needs Assist with breastfeeding	Continue discharge teaching based on the woman's/family's learning needs	Complete discharge teaching	The woman and her family verbalize understanding of infant needs and the woman's needs. The woman and her family demonstrate basic well-baby care skills. The woman and her family verbalize understanding of signs and symptoms that warrant contact with the health care provider.

CONCEPT MAP

Knowledge Deficit: Postpartum Self Care

Risk for Disturbed Sleep
* Pain
* Caring for infant
* Feeding infant during the night

Risk for Constipation
* Dehydration
* Decreased intake
* Immobility
* Anesthesia/analgesia
* Hormonal effects of pregnancy

Pain/Impaired Comfort
* Afterbirth pains
* Perineal pain
* Breast engorgement
* Nipple pain
* Muscle soreness

Altered Skin Integrity
* Perineal trauma, lacerations, episiotomy
* Nipple soreness

Knowledge Deficit Postpartum Self Care

Lack of knowledge about physical/physiologic changes of postpartum and related self-care measures

Risk of Bleeding
* Uterine atony
* Retained placenta/tissue
* Perineal trauma: lacerations, hematoma, episiotomy

Risk for Infection
* Altered skin integrity
* Metritis
* Cystitis
* Mastitis

Breastfeeding: Risk for Ineffective
* Improper infant latch
* Anxiety
* Maternal lack of knowledge
* Pain
* Altered skin integrity

Risk for Injury:
* Falls related to orthostatic hypotension
* Falls related to impaired sensation associated with regional anesthesia

Risk for Impaired Urinary Elimination
* Urinary retention
* Lack of bladder tone
* Rapid filling of bladder related to increased IV fluid given during labor and delivery
* Diuresis
* Decreased sensation due to anesthesia
* Trauma to GU tract/edema of urethra etc.

Problem No. 1: Risk for bleeding

Goal: The amount of vaginal bleeding will be within normal limits.

Outcome: The woman's lochia amount will be moderate to small; the woman's fundus is firm and midline. The woman's vital signs will be within normal limits. Urine output will be within normal limits. The woman will verbalize when she will notify the provider if her bleeding is excessive.

Nursing Actions

1. Teach the woman the purpose of fundal checks.
2. Teach the woman to palpate her fundus and massage it if soft.
3. Teach the woman about the normal progression of lochia; what to expect regarding amount, color, and flow.
4. Instruct the woman to notify the nurse or provider if she soaks more than one pad an hour or passes clots.
5. Instruct the woman about the purpose of oxytocin administration; provide information about afterpains.
6. Teach the woman the importance of emptying her bladder every 3 to 4 hours.

Problem No. 2: Risk for impaired urinary elimination

Goal: Spontaneous voids of a sufficient quantity (at least 300 mL per void)

Outcome: The woman will spontaneously void at least 300 mL per void. The woman will state the importance of voiding frequently and adequately. The woman will identify that she will notify the nurse or provider of burning, frequency, or urgency with voiding.

Nursing Actions

1. Explain to the woman that voidings will be measured after delivery.
2. Encourage the woman to void within 2 to 4 hours of delivery and to empty her bladder.
3. Explain to the woman that if she is unable to void, she will need to have a catheter placed to empty her bladder.
4. Instruct the woman to notify the nurse or health care provider if she experiences frequency, burning, or urgency during urination.
5. Encourage the woman to drink 10 glasses of fluids a day (80 ounces) and bring water to the bedside.
6. Teach the woman that diuresis is a normal process and often begins within 12 hours of delivery.

Problem No. 3: Pain/impaired comfort

Goal: Pain or discomfort is adequately controlled.

Outcome: The woman will identify nonpharmacological and pharmacological methods to treat pain and discomfort. The woman's pain/discomfort is adequately controlled.

Nursing Actions

1. Teach the woman to report pain by providing information about the intensity, location, and quality of her discomfort.
2. Provide the patient with nonpharmacological methods of pain control:
   a. Ice packs for 24 to 48 hours
   b. Sitz baths/warm compresses
   c. Peri-bottle
   d. Repositioning
   e. Deep breathing and relaxation
   f. Warm shower
3. Inform the woman about medications ordered and administered for pain (action, dose and frequency, potential side effects).
4. Educate the woman about nonpharmacological methods of pain control.

Problem No. 4: Risk for infection

Goal: Reduce risk of infection.

Outcome: The woman will remain free from signs of infection. The woman will identify ways to prevent infection and when to call the nurse or health care provider for signs of infection.

Nursing Actions

1. Explain the importance of monitoring vital signs and monitor them per protocol.
2. Instruct the woman to call the provider if she has signs of infection such as temperature over 100.4°F (38°C); chills, pain in her abdomen, perineum, or breasts; burning, frequency, or urgency with urination; foul-smelling lochia.
3. Teach the woman the importance of hand washing before and after pericare and after pad changes.
4. If indicated, teach the woman about immunizations that will be given prior to discharge.

Problem No. 5: Risk for injury

Goal: Reduced risk for injury

Outcome: The woman will call for assistance with ambulation until sensation returns to her lower extremities (postepidural) and her blood pressure and pulse are within normal limits. The woman will remain free from injury associated with falls.

Nursing Actions

1. Explain orthostatic hypotension and the importance of requesting assistance in the initial postpartum period.
2. Instruct the woman to rise slowly to a standing position.
3. Advise the woman to ambulate with assistance the first few times up after birth.
4. Instruct the woman to return to bed/sitting position if she becomes dizzy and to call for help.

Problem No. 6: Altered skin integrity

Goal: Regain skin integrity through healing

Outcome: The woman will identify perineal care and comfort measures. The woman will identify signs of perineal infection and will notify her health care provider if she experiences signs of infection.

Nursing Actions

1. Teach the woman that her perineal area will be assessed for redness, bruising, swelling, and drainage. Explain the procedure and position the woman on her side for better visualization of the area.
2. Teach the woman about comfort measures for perineal lacerations/episiotomy such as ice packs during the first 24 to 48 hours and warm sitz baths after the first 24 hours.
3. Instruct the woman on how to use topical treatments that may be ordered by the health care provider.
4. Teach the woman to rinse the perineum with the peri-bottle using warm water after each elimination.
5. Encourage the woman to change peripads frequently, and to wash her hands before and after pad changes to reduce risk of infection.
6. Teach the woman to lie on her side to decrease pressure on her perineum.
7. Instruct the woman to take ordered analgesics as directed to decrease perineal pain.
8. Teach the woman to report signs of perineal infection such as drainage, swelling, pain, and fever to the health care provider.

Problem No. 7: Risk for constipation

Goal: The woman will have regular, soft bowel movements.

Outcome: The woman will state ways to promote regular, soft bowel movements. The woman will not develop constipation.

Nursing Actions

1. Provide fluid and water and prune juice to facilitate hydration.
2. Teach the woman the importance a diet high in fruits, vegetables, and whole grains.
3. Teach the woman the importance of drinking 2,000 to 3,000 mL of fluids daily.

Continued

4. Teach the woman the importance of ambulating several times daily.

5. Instruct the woman to have a bowel movement when she feels the urge.

6. If ordered, teach the woman about stool softeners, laxatives, and so on. Discuss the action, dose and frequency, and potential side effects.

Problem No. 8: Risk for disturbed sleep

Goal: Adequate sleep and rest

Outcome: The woman will be report adequate sleep patterns, and report feeling rested. The woman will identify strategies for getting enough rest and sleep.

Nursing Actions

1. Attempt to cluster care to decrease interruptions.

2. Teach the woman the importance of sleep and rest in healing and recovery from childbirth.

3. Encourage the woman to identify strategies for getting enough sleep, such as sleeping when the baby sleeps and naps, prioritizing activities to focus on self- and infant care, and occasionally delegating infant care and feeding to other family members if possible so that she can rest.

4. Teach the woman ways to treat pain and discomfort to facilitate rest and sleep.

Problem No. 9: Breastfeeding—risk for ineffective feeding

Goal: Effective breastfeeding

Outcome: The woman will identify how to tell if the baby is breastfeeding effectively. The woman will demonstrate proper positioning and technique for breastfeeding her infant. The baby will latch to the mother's nipple properly and demonstrate signs of adequate feedings. The woman will identify community resources to contact for support and assistance with breastfeeding.

Nursing Actions

1. Teach the woman to recognize cues that the baby is hungry.

2. Assist the woman to prepare for a feeding by getting into a comfortable position.

3. Assist the woman in positioning the infant for breastfeeding (cradle hold, cross-cradle hold, football hold, etc.).

4. Teach the woman how to properly get the infant latched to the nipple, and signs of correct latch-on.

5. Teach the woman about the frequency and duration of feedings.

6. Teach the woman how to remove the baby from the breast and how to burp the baby.

7. Teach the woman how to recognize that the baby is receiving adequate feedings.

8. Provide the woman with information about lactation consultant services and community resources available to support breastfeeding after discharge.

Nursing Care Plan

Problem *(Check Appropriate Line)*	Actual or Potential	Action *(Initial Care Provided)*	Expected Outcome/ Discharge Criteria *(Initial Outcomes Obtained)*
Potential or actual postpartum hemorrhage related to: _____ Uterine atony _____ Retained placenta _____ Laceration _____ Hematoma _____ Full bladder _____ Other _____	Initiated by: RN: _____ Date/time _____ ☐ Actual ☐ Potential Change in status: Date/time _____ RN: _____ ☐ Actual ☐ Potential Resolved: Date/time _____ RN: _____	_____ Monitor and assess vital signs, including blood pressure and woman's mental status, lochia flow, and uterine tone per policy. _____ Encourage voiding every 2–3 hours. _____ Massage fundus as needed and instruct the woman on self-assessment. _____ Notify CNM/MD for heavy bleeding/ saturation of one pad in <1 hour. _____ Give medications such as oxytocin, Methergine, or Hemabate per CNM/ MD order. _____ Assist with activity PRN. _____ Notify the provider if the woman has continued excessive bleeding and/or dizziness.	_____ Lochia scant to moderate rubra _____ Fundus firm and at midline _____ No signs or symptoms of postpartum hemorrhage

Nursing Care Plan—cont'd

Problem *(Check Appropriate Line)*	Actual or Potential	Action *(Initial Care Provided)*	Expected Outcome/ Discharge Criteria *(Initial Outcomes Obtained)*
Potential or actual alteration in comfort related to:	Initiated by:	_____ Pain assessment	_____ Pain will be adequately controlled by analgesics and nonpharmacological comfort measures.
_____ Uterine cramping	RN: _____	_____ Provide or assist with nonpharmacological comfort measures for relief	
_____ Incision	Date/time _____		_____ The mother will demonstrate proper positioning of the infant during feedings.
_____ Perineal/rectal pain	☐ Actual	_____ Provide analgesics as ordered	
_____ Breast discomfort	☐ Potential	_____ Assess breastfeeding by observing breastfeeding sessions each shift	
_____ Other _____	Change in status:	_____ Assess latch score	_____ The baby will latch properly during feedings.
Potential or actual alteration in effective breastfeeding	Date/time _____	_____ Assess the breasts/nipples for pain and skin breakdown	
related to:	RN: _____	_____ Assess for psychosocial factors that may interfere with parental bonding with infant	_____ The mother will remain comfortable during breastfeeding.
_____ Poor latch	☐ Actual		
_____ Previous breast surgery	☐ Potential	_____ Assess parental bonding and caretaking behaviors	
_____ Twins or higher-order multiples	Resolved:	_____ Assess the parent's support system	_____ No signs of skin breakdown or trauma on mother's nipples.
_____ Infant with cleft lip/palate	Date/time _____		
_____ Nearly term infant	Initiated by:		_____ Parents will demonstrate signs of bonding with infant:
_____ Infant in NICU	RN: _____		
_____ Patient's health status	Date/time _____		_____ attentive to infant cues and needs
	☐ Actual		
_____ Other _____	☐ Potential		_____ holds infant en face
Potential or actual impaired parent–infant bonding related to:	Change in status:		_____ cuddles infant
	Date/time _____		_____ talks to infant
_____ Adolescent parents	RN: _____		_____ calls baby by name
_____ Substance abuse	☐ Actual		
_____ Domestic violence	☐ Potential		_____ breast feeds/ bottle feeds baby
_____ Social risk factors	Resolved:		
_____ Infant's health status	Date/Time _____		
	RN: _____		
_____ Mother's health status	Initiated by:		
	RN: _____		
_____ Other _____	Date/Time _____		
	☐ Actual		
	☐ Potential		
	Change in status:		
	Date/time _____		
	RN: _____		
	☐ Actual		
	☐ Potential		
	Resolved:		
	Date/time _____		
	RN: _____		

Continued

Nursing Care Plan—cont'd

Problem *(Check Appropriate Line)*	Actual or Potential	Action *(Initial Care Provided)*	Expected Outcome/ Discharge Criteria *(Initial Outcomes Obtained)*
Potential or actual postpartum infection related to: _____ Perineum _____ Uterus _____ Breast _____ GBS _____ Other _____	Initiated by: RN: _____ Date/time _____ ☐ Actual ☐ Potential Change in status: Date/time _____ RN: _____ ☐ Actual ☐ Potential Resolved: Date/time _____ RN: _____	_____ Vital signs monitored per policy _____ CNM/MD notified immediately if any signs or symptoms of infection are present _____ Woman instructed in self-care, including pericare, incisional care, and breast care _____ Woman instructed in signs and symptoms of infection	_____ Woman will exhibit no signs or symptoms of infection (i.e., temperature <100.4°F [38°C], no abnormal discharge, incision clean and dry if present, breasts without redness). _____ Woman will verbalize understanding of signs and symptoms of infection and aware of when to notify CNM/MD.
Potential or actual alteration in elimination related to: _____ Loss of bladder and/or bowel sensation/function following childbirth _____ Other _____	Initiated by: _____ Date/time _____ ☐ Actual ☐ Potential Change in status: Date/time _____ RN: _____ ☐ Actual ☐ Potential Resolved: Date/time _____ RN: _____	_____ Assess and monitor for bladder distention as needed _____ Assess and document initial voidings after delivery to ensure >30 mL/hr without retention in first 6–12 hours _____ If unable to void, catheterize per CNM/MD order _____ Provide instructions on Kegel exercises _____ Encourage early ambulation, adequate fluid intake, diet with roughage to prevent constipation _____ Provide stool softener as ordered	_____ Woman is voiding without difficulty. _____ Fundus is firm and midline. _____ Woman is able to verbalize methods of avoiding constipation and to notify CNM/MD if no stool in 4 days.

Case Study

As the nurse, you admit Margarite Sanchez to the postpartum unit at 10:50 a.m. and receive the transfer report from labor and delivery stating the following:

- Patient is a 28-year-old G3 P2 Hispanic woman who gave birth at 8:39 a.m., vaginal delivery with a second-degree laceration.
- She received two doses of Nubain in labor at 2:15 a.m. and at 4:40 a.m. for pain relief in active labor.
- Both mother and baby are stable.
- The mother's bleeding in labor and delivery was moderate.
- VS are 120/68-72-20-98.2
- Ms. Sanchez did not void in labor and delivery.
- Ms. Sanchez nursed her baby for 15 minutes on each breast after the birth.

José, her husband, has accompanied her to the unit.

Detail the aspects of your initial assessment.

As part of the physical assessment, you discover her fundus is 2 cm above the umbilicus and deviated to the left; her lochia is moderate, saturating one-third of the pad during transfer; and her perineum is swollen.

What are your immediate priorities in nursing care for Margarite Sanchez?

Discuss the rationale for the priorities.

Initial teaching would include the following:

At 5 hours postpartum, Margarite rates her perineal pain at 6 on a scale of 0 to 10.

State the nursing diagnosis, expected outcome, and interventions related to this problem.

The next day you are assigned to care for the Sanchez family. Your report from the previous shift indicated that:

- Her vital signs were within normal limits.
- She had voided once during the night.

- Her fundus was 1 cm below the umbilicus.
- Lochia was scant to moderate.
- She breastfed her infant twice.

Margarite informs you that she experienced night sweats.

Discuss your nursing actions, including rationales.

You are anticipating that she will be discharged in the afternoon.

Discuss your plan for discharge teaching, indicating the priority needs with rationales.

REFERENCES

American College of Obstetricians and Gynecologists (ACOG). (2013). ACOG Committee Opinion No. 566: Update on immunization and pregnancy: Tetanus, diphtheria, and pertussis vaccination. *Obstetrics & Gynecology, 121*(6), 1411–1414.

American College of Obstetricians and Gynecologists. (2018). *Influenza vaccination during pregnancy* (ACOG Publication No. 732). e109–14. Retrieved from: https//www.acog.org

American College of Obstetricians and Gynecologists (ACOG). (2016). Committee Opinion No. 670: Immediate postpartum long-acting reversible contraception. *Obstetrics & Gynecology, 128*(2), e32–37.

Amorim Adegboye, A., & Linne, Y. (2013). Diet or exercise, or both for weight reduction in women after childbirth. *Cochrane Database of Systematic Reviews,* (7). doi:10.1002/14651858.CD005627.pub3

Association of Women's Health, Obstetric and Neonatal Nurses (AWHONN). (2015a). Guidelines for oxytocin administration after birth: AWHONN practice brief number 2. *Nursing for Women's Health, 19*(1), 99–101.

Association of Women's Health, Obstetric and Neonatal Nurses (AWHONN). (2015b). Quantification of blood loss: AWHONN Practice Brief number 1. *Nursing for Women's Health, 19*(1), 96–98.

Association of Women's Health, Obstetric and Neonatal Nurses (AWHONN). (2016). Insurance coverage for contraception. Retrieved from www.awhonn.org

Buchanan, J., & Beckmann, M. (2014). Postpartum voiding dysfunction: Identifying the risk factors. *Australian and New Zealand Journal of Obstetrics and Gynecology, 54,* 41–45. doi:10.1111/ajo.12130

Centers for Disease Control (CDC). (2013). Updated recommendations for use of tetanus toxoid, reduced diphtheria toxoid, and acellular pertussis vaccine (Tdap) in pregnant women-advisory committee on immunization practices (ACIP) 2012. *Morbidity and Mortality Weekly, 62,* 131–134.

Center for Disease Control (2015). Healthy Pregnant or Postpartum Women. Retrieve from: www.cdc.gov/physicalactivity/basics/pregnancy/index.html

Centers for Disease Control (CDC). (2016a). *Maternal vaccines: Part of a healthy pregnancy.* Retrieved from www.cdc.gov/vaccines/pregnancy/pregnant-women/index.html.

Centers for Disease Control (CDC). (2016b). *Pregnancy surveillance system.* Retrieved from www.cdc.gov/reproductivehealth/maternalinfanthealth/pmss.html.

Central Intelligence Agency. (2016). *The world factbook.* Retrieved from www.cia.gov/library/publications/resources/the-world-factbook/rankorder/2223rank.html.

Cunningham, F., Leveno, K., Bloom, S., Song, C., Dashe, J., Hoffman, M., . . . Sheffield, J. (2014). *William's obstetrics* (24th ed.). New York, NY: McGraw-Hill.

East, C., Begg, L., Henshall, N., Marchant, P., & Wallace, K. (2012). Local cooling for relieving pain from perineal trauma sustained during childbirth. *Cochrane Collaboration, 9.*

Hobel, C., & Lamb, A. (2016). Obstetric hemorrhage: Antepartum, intrapartum, and postpartum. In N. F. Hacker, J. C. Gambone, & C. Hobel (Eds.), *Hacker and Moore's essentials of obstetrics and gynecology* (6th ed., pp. 136–144). New York, NY: Elsevier.

Isley, M., & Katz, V. (2016). Postpartum care and long term health considerations. In S. G. Gabbe, J.R. Niebyl, L. J. Simpson, M. B. Landon, H. L. Galan, E.

R. M Juaniax, . . . W. A. Grobman (Eds.), *Obstetrics: Normal and problem pregnancies* (7th ed., pp. 499–516). New York, NY: Elsevier.

James, D. (2014). Postpartum care. In K. Simpson & P. Creehan (Eds.), *AWHONN: Perinatal nursing* (4th ed., pp. 530–577). Philadelphia, PA: Lippincott, Williams & Wilkins.

Janke, J. (2014). Infant nutrition. In K. Simpson & P. Creehan (Eds.), *AWHONN: Perinatal nursing* (4th ed., pp. 626–655). Philadelphia, PA: Lippincott, Williams & Wilkins.

Kee, J. (2009). *Laboratory and diagnostic tests with nursing implications* (6th ed.). Upper Saddle River, NJ: Pearson.

Kendig, S., Keat, J., Hoffman, C., Kay, L., Miller, E., Moore-Simas, T., . . . Lemieux, L. (2017). Consensus bundle on maternal mental health: perinatal depression and anxiety. *Journal of Obstetric, Gynecologic & Neonatal Nursing, 46*(2), 272–281.

Mhyre, J., D'Oria, R., Hameed, A., Lappen, J., Holley, S., Hunter, S., . . . D'Alton, M. (2014). The maternal early warning criteria: A proposal from the National Partnership for Maternal Safety. *Journal of Obstetric, Gynecologic, and Neonatal Nurses, 43,* 771–779 and *Obstetrics & Gynecology 124,* 782–787.

Mulder, F., Oude Rengerink, K., Van der Post, J., Hakvoort, R., & Roovers, R. (2016). Delivery related risk factors for covert postpartum urinary retention after vaginal delivery. *International Urogynecology Journal, 27,* 55–60. doi:10.1007/s0092-015-2768-8

Niebyl, J., Weber, R., & Briggs, G. (2016). Drugs and environmental agents in pregnancy and lactation: Teratology, epidemiology. In S. G. Gabbe, J. R. Niebyl, L. J. Simpson, M. B. Landon, H. L. Galan, E. R. M. Juaniax, . . . W. A. Grobman (Eds.), *Obstetrics: Normal and problem pregnancies* (7th ed., pp. 499–516). New York, NY: Elsevier.

Newton, E. (2016). Lactation and breastfeeding. In S. G. Gabbe, J. R. Niebyl, L. J. Simpson, M. B. Landon, H. L. Galan, E. R. M. Juaniax, . . . W. A. Grobman (Eds.), *Obstetrics: Normal and problem pregnancies* (7th ed., pp. 499–516). New York, NY: Elsevier.

Sacks, A., & Smiley, R. (2014). Post-dural puncture headache: The worst common complication in obstetric anesthesia. *Seminars in Perinatology, 38,* 386–394.

Samuels, P. (2016). Hematologic complications of pregnancy. In S. G. Gabbe, J. R. Niebyl, L. J. Shoupe, & D. Mishell (Eds.), *The handbook of contraception: A guide for practical management.* New York, NY: Humana Press.

Shoupe, D., & Mishell, D. (2016). *The handbook of contraception: A guide for practical management.* Switzerland: Springer International Publishing Humana Press.

Smith, R. (2018). Normal postpartum changes. In R. P. Smith, & F. H. Netter's (Eds.), *Netter's obstetrics and gynecology* (3rd ed., pp. 440–442). New York, NY: Elsevier.

Suplee, P., Kleppel, L., & Bingham, D. (2016). Discharge education on maternal morbidity and mortality provided by nurses to women in the postpartum period. *Journal of Obstetric, Gynecologic & Neonatal Nursing, 45*(6), 894–904.

Suplee, P., Kleppel, L., Santa-Donato, A., & Bingham, D. (2016). Improving postpartum education about warning signs of maternal morbidity and mortality. *Nursing for Women's Health, 20,* 554–567.

TOXNET. (2017). *Lactmed: Alcohol.* Retrieved from: https://toxnet.nlm.nih.gov/cgi-bin/sis/search2/f?./temp/~33QCpE:1.

Turawa, E., Musekiwa, A., & Rohwer, A. (2015). Interventions for preventing postpartum constipation. *Cochrane Databases of Systematic Reviews, 9.* doi:10.1002/14651858.CDO11625.pub2

U.S. Department of Health and Human Services Office of Disease Prevention and Health Promotion. (2012). *Healthy People 2020 topics and objectives.* Retrieved from: https://www.healthypeople.gov/

Vallerand, A., & Sanoski, C. (2013). *Davis's drug guide for nurses* (13th ed.). Philadelphia, PA: F.A. Davis.

Whitmer, T. (2011). Physical and psychological changes. In S. Mattson & J. Smith (Eds.), *Core curriculum for maternal-newborn nursing* (4th ed.). St. Louis, MO: Elsevier.

Wilkinson, J., & Treas, L. (2011). *Fundamentals in nursing* (2nd ed.). Philadelphia, PA: F.A. Davis.

Wilson, B., Shannon, M., & Shields, K. (2014). *Pearson nurse's drug guide.* Boston, MA: Pearson.

Woodley, S. J., Boyle, R., Cody, J. D., Morkved, S., & Hay-Smith, E. J. C. (2017). Pelvic floor muscle training for prevention and treatment of urinary and faecal incontinence in antenatal and postnatal women. *Cochrane Database of Systematic Reviews, 12.* doi:10.1002/14651858.CD007471.pub3

Transition to Parenthood

Linda Chapman, RN, PhD

LEARNING OUTCOMES

Upon completion of this chapter, the student will be able to:

1. Describe the process of "becoming a mother."
2. Identify factors that influence women and men in their role transitions to mother and father.
3. Discuss bonding and attachment.
4. Identify factors that affect the family dynamics.
5. Describe nursing actions that support couples during their transition to parenthood.

Nursing Diagnosis

- Knowledge deficit related to role of parent due to being a first-time parent
- At risk for situational self-esteem disturbance due to new parenting role
- At risk for altered family processes related to incorporation of a new family member
- At risk for altered parent–infant attachment related to anxiety of being a new parent

Nursing Outcomes

- Parents will verbalize an understanding of parental role expectations and responsibilities.
- Parents will verbalize stressors of new role.
- Parents will demonstrate positive comments and actions when interacting with family members.
- Parents will hold the infant close to the body, attend to the infant's needs, and interact with the infant.

INTRODUCTION

The postpartum period is a time of both physiological and psychological adjustments. As the woman is adjusting to the numerous physiological changes within her body, she and her partner are adjusting to their new roles as parents and the effect these new roles have on their relationship and the family unit (Fig. 13–1). This chapter focuses on the psychological, emotional, and developmental changes that take place during the transition to parenthood.

TRANSITION TO PARENTHOOD

The transition to parenthood is a dynamic developmental process that begins with the knowledge of pregnancy and continues throughout the postpartum period as the couple takes on their new or expanded roles of mother and father. Whether this is the first child or tenth child, this transition is a major life event that is both exciting and stressful, producing developmental challenges

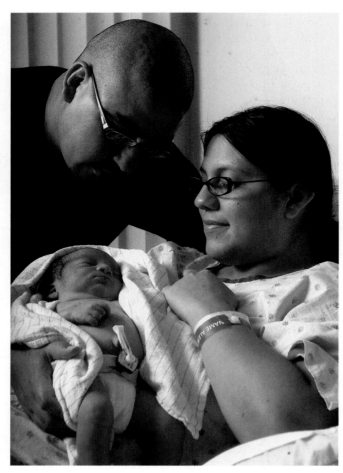

FIGURE 13–1 Mother and father getting acquainted with their new son.

for the individual, the couple's relationship, and family members. It is common for new parents to experience:

● Increased stress related to learning the role of mother or father, childcare tasks, financial concerns, work-family conflict, and chronic fatigue.
● Decreased satisfaction within their couple relationship.
● Decrease in sexual and intimate activities.

Each individual deals with the growth, realization, and preparation of becoming a parent in different ways. Personal values, societal expectations, and cultural beliefs influence how an individual takes on the role of parent. Transition to parenthood is fostered or hampered by many factors, some of which include:

● Previous life experiences: Previous experiences caring for infants and children can foster a smoother transition to parenthood.
● How they were parented: A positive feeling of how they were parented can enhance the transition to parenthood.
● Length and strength of the relationship between partners: A strong relationship between the couple can foster a smoother transition to parenthood.
● Financial considerations: Financial concerns can cause stress and hamper the transition to parenting.

● Educational levels: Decreased ability to read and comprehend information regarding child care may hamper the couple's ability to gain knowledge in the care of the infant.
● Support systems: A lack of positive support in the care of the woman and infant can increase stress and hamper the transition to parenting.
● Desire to be a parent: A lack of desire to be a parent can hamper the transition to parenting.
● Age of parents: Adolescent parents may have a more difficult transition to parenthood.

The transition to parenthood involves taking on the role of mother or father, viewing the child as an individual with his or her own personality, and incorporating the new child into the family system.

Evidence-Based Practice: Maternal and Paternal Fatigue

Loutzenhiser, L., McAuslan, P., & Sharpe, D. (2015). The trajectory of maternal and paternal fatigue and factors associated with fatigue across the transition to parenthood. *The Australian Psychological Society, 19,* 15–27.

This longitudinal study assessed parental fatigue and factors associated with fatigue that included parental stress, parental sleep quality, infant negativity, and infant sleep duration. Additionally, parental general health and depressive symptoms were measured. The sample consisted of 108 cohabitating mother–father couples expecting their first child. Data were collected during the third trimester and at 1, 3, and 6 months postbirth.

Results:

● High levels of prenatal fatigue were associated with higher levels of postpartum fatigue for both the mother and father.
● Maternal and paternal fatigue increased following the birth and remained consistent over 6 months.
● Mothers were more fatigued than fathers.
● Poor sleep quality was associated with fatigue for both mothers and fathers.
● Poor sleep quality in mothers was associated with higher levels of stress and depressive symptoms.
● Poor quality of sleep for fathers was associated with shorter duration of infant sleep.
● Age was not associated with postpartum fatigue for either mother or father.
● Younger mothers reported high levels of stress and depressive symptoms than older mothers.
● Neither family income nor length of couple relationship was associated with fatigue.

Nursing actions:

● Assess levels of fatigue for both the mother and father during the postpartum period.
● Promote rest by providing uninterrupted time during the postpartum hospitalization.
● Promote resting during postpartum hospitalization by clustering nursing care to allow for periods of uninterrupted times for resting.
● Provide information on strategies to decrease fatigue during the prenatal period and postnatal periods.
● Assist mothers in managing stress and depressive symptoms. This is more beneficial to improving their sleep quality than focusing on infant sleep patterns.

Parental Roles

Individuals have many roles throughout their lifetimes. Children take on the roles of son or daughter, sister or brother, grandchild, and student. Additional roles are acquired with age, and roles change over time as the individual matures and new roles are added. The role of mother or father evolves and changes over time as the child grows and additional children are added to the family. Each new role has expectations and responsibilities that the individual must learn in order to be successful in the role.

Couples are given the title of mother and father with the birth of their child but must learn the expectations and responsibilities of these roles.

- Examples of parental role expectations are that others will acknowledge the person as being a parent or that the child will obey the parents.
- Examples of responsibilities are that the parents will love and protect their child.

Knowledge of these expectations and responsibilities is acquired through intentional learning (formal instructions) and incidental learning (observing others in the role). Most individuals have little intentional/instructional learning regarding the role of mother or father and must rely on incidental learning of these expectations and responsibilities. Examples of incidental learning of the parental role are:

- Observing other individuals who are mothers and fathers.
- Recalling how they were parented.
- Watching movies or television programs that have mothers and/or fathers as characters.

The process of learning and developing parental roles should start during the pregnancy. Partners who learn together during the pregnancy have better outcomes when they take on the role of parents. Providing couples with written information regarding different styles of parenting roles allows the expectant couple to learn about parenting behaviors. The expectant couple can then discuss parenting issues and mutually agree on expectations and responsibilities for their new roles.

Expected Findings

- Parents identify changing roles and are willing to make lifestyle changes to accommodate the changes.
- Parents identify with the parental roles.
- Parents discuss what the roles mean to them.
- Couples incorporate a third person, the infant, into their relationship.
- Couples support each other in mutual caregiving tasks.

Nursing Actions

Nursing actions are directed at supporting the couple as they take on their role of mother or father. Nursing actions include:

- Providing an environment that is conducive to rest, such as uninterrupted periods of time so that parents can sleep.
  - Adequate rest can increase the couple's ability to take in new information and develop new skills.
- Providing culturally sensitive care.
  - Mother and father role expectations and responsibilities vary based on cultural backgrounds.
- Active listening; encourage the parents to talk about their expectations of each other in their respective role of mother or father.
  - Having realistic and mutually agreed upon expectations decreases the level of stress within the relationship.
- Providing parental education on infant care with a variety of educational strategies such as handouts, videos, and demonstrations of procedures (burping, swaddling, entertaining, and stimulating the infant).
  - Information needs to be appropriate and relevant for the couple.
- Providing positive feedback for parents' infant care behaviors.
  - New parents are insecure regarding infant care and need to know they are correctly interacting with and caring for their infant.
- Providing information on community parenting classes and support groups.
  - This will provide parents opportunities for both intentional and incidental learning.

MOTHERHOOD

Becoming a mother is a term used to describe the process that women undergo in their transition to motherhood and establishment of their maternal identity (Mercer, 2004).

Mercer describes four stages through which women progress in "becoming a mother":

- Commitment, attachment, and preparation for an infant during pregnancy
- Acquaintance with and increasing attachment to the infant, learning how to care for the infant, and physical restoration during the early weeks after birth
- Moving toward a new normal during the first 4 months
- Achievement of a maternal identity around 4 months (Mercer, 2006)

The process of becoming a mother begins during pregnancy but can occur before pregnancy. Some women begin preparing for this role as children when they fantasize about being mothers and role-play motherhood with dolls. Others actively improve their health in preparation for the pregnancy before conceiving (Mercer, 2006).

The process of "becoming a mother" is influenced by:

- How the woman was parented.
- Her life experiences.
- Her unique characteristics.
- Her cultural beliefs.
- The pregnancy experience.
- The birth experience.
- Support from partner, family, and friends.
- The woman's willingness to assume the role of mother.
- The infant's characteristics such as appearance and temperament (Mercer, 1995, 2006).

Nursing Actions

- Review prenatal and labor records for risk factors such as complications during pregnancy and labor and birth.
  - Pregnancy and birth experiences can either enhance or impede the process of becoming a mother.
- Assess the stages of "becoming a mother."
  - Assessment data assists in developing individualized nursing actions.
  - Expected assessment findings:
    - Positive feelings toward being pregnant
    - Positive health behaviors
    - Nurturing behaviors toward the infant
    - Protective feelings toward the infant
    - Increasing confidence in knowing and caring for the infant
    - Establishment of new family routines (Mercer, 2006)
- Provide rooming-in or couplet care to facilitate bonding and attachment.
- Provide private time for the parents to interact with their infant.
- Provide comfort measures for the woman to promote rest and healing.
- Listen to the woman's concerns in order for her to process the incorporation of the infant into her life.
- Provide information on the care of infants.
- Praise the woman for the care she provides her infant.

Evidence-Based Practice: Maternal Adaptation During the Early Postpartum Period

In the 1960s, Reba Rubin conducted qualitative research studies focusing on maternal adaptation during the early postpartum weeks. Her research is the foundation of our understanding of the psychosocial experience of women during the postpartum period. Two concepts identified through her research are "maternal phases" and "maternal touch." Rubin (1984) refined and modified the process as more evidence was linked to maternal adjustments and behaviors and identified areas of development that women progress through to "becoming a mother."

Ramona Mercer, a student and colleague of Rubin, added to and expanded this body of nursing knowledge through numerous research studies that focused on the maternal role. Based on these studies, Mercer (1995) developed the theory of "maternal role attainment," which describes and explains the process women progress through as they become a mother. Based on her previous research and the research of others, Mercer (2004) supports replacing the term *maternal role attainment* with *becoming a mother*. The term *becoming a mother* reflects that the process is not stagnant but continually evolving as the woman and her child are changing and growing.

The theories generated by Rubin's and Mercer's research agendas are the cornerstone of evidence-based knowledge used in establishing nursing guidelines for the care of postpartum women and families.

Maternal Phases

As defined by Rubin (1963b, 1967), a three-phase maternal process occurs during the first few weeks of the postpartum period (Table 13–1). A delay in transitioning through the phases may indicate that the woman is experiencing difficulty in becoming a mother. Factors that can affect the woman's transition through the maternal phases are:

- Medications (e.g., magnesium sulfate or analgesics) that depress the central nervous system (CNS), leading to tiredness and a slow response to stimuli.
- Complications during pregnancy, labor and birth, and/or postpartum (e.g., preterm labor, chronic illness, difficult birth, or cesarean birth) can cause the woman's focus to shift to her health and well-being, and/or to resolving feelings of disappointment.
- Cesarean births can cause increased discomfort that interferes with the woman's ability to care for her infant.
- Pain causes a shift of maternal attention from focusing on caring for baby to seeking pain relief for self.
- Preterm infants or infants who experience complications can cause additional stress on the woman and delay her transition through the phases.
- Mood disorders such as depression cause the woman's focus to be more on self and less on the infant.
- Lack of support from the partner and/or support system may lead to maternal exhaustion.
- Adolescent mothers, who are more focused inwardly and on peer relationships than on care of the infant.
- Lack of financial resources, which forces the woman to focus on obtaining basic needs rather than on her infant.
- Cultural beliefs, which can influence the woman's behavior and the amount of time she spends in each phase. In some cultures, for example, women are expected to rest rather than be actively involved in care or decision making during the first few months of the infant's life.

Nursing Actions

- Review prenatal and labor records for factors that might delay progression through the maternal phases.
- Assess for maternal phases.
  - Assessment data assists in developing individualized nursing actions.
  - Expected assessment findings:
    - Taking-in behaviors during the first 24 to 48 hours
    - Taking-hold behaviors from 24 to 48 hours through the first few weeks after birth
  - Nursing care during the taking-in phase is directed by the nurse because the woman is more dependent during this phase and has difficulty making decisions.
  - Nursing care during the taking-hold phase is directed more by the woman, as she is becoming more independent and has an increased ability to make decisions.
- Provide comfort measures such as backrubs, uninterrupted periods of rest, and analgesics.
- Adapt teaching to reflect the maternal phase.
  - During the taking-in phase, teaching is directed to immediate learning needs and is provided in short sessions, as the woman's focus is on self versus learning about the care of the infant.
  - During the taking-hold phase, praise the woman for her learning, as she is eager to learn but can become frustrated with not being able to master a new task quickly.

TABLE 13–1   Maternal Phases

TAKING-IN PHASE	TAKING-HOLD PHASE	LETTING-GO PHASE
The taking-in phase, a period of dependent behaviors, occurs during the first 24 to 48 hours after birth and includes the following maternal behaviors:	The taking-hold phase, the movement between dependent and independent behaviors, follows the taking-in phase. It can last weeks and includes the following maternal behaviors:	In the letting-go phase, the movement from independence to the new role of mother is fluid and interchangeable with the taking-hold phase. Maternal characteristics during this phase are:
• The woman is focused on her personal comfort and physical changes.	• The focus moves from self to the infant.	• Grieving and letting go of old relationship behaviors in favor of new ones.
• The woman relives and speaks of the birth experience.	• The woman begins to be independent.	• Incorporating the infant into her life whereby the baby becomes a separate entity from her.
• The woman adjusts to psychological changes.	• The woman has an increased ability to make decisions.	• Accepting the infant as he or she really is.
• The woman is dependent on others for her and her infant's immediate needs.	• The woman is interested in the infant's cues and needs.	• Giving up the fantasy of what it would/could have been.
• The woman has a decreased ability to make decisions.	• The woman gives up the pregnancy role and initiates taking on the maternal role.	• Independence returns; may go back to work or school.
• The woman concentrates on personal physical healing (Rubin, 1963b, 1967).	• The woman is eager to learn; it is an excellent time to initiate postpartum teaching.	• May have feelings of grief, guilt, or anxiety.
	• The woman begins to like the role of "mother."	• Reconnection/growth in relationship with partner (Rubin, 1963b, 1967).
	• The woman may have feelings of inadequacy and being overwhelmed.	
	• The woman needs verbal reassurance that she is meeting her infant's needs.	
	• The woman may show signs and symptoms of baby blues and fatigue.	
	• The woman begins to let more of the outside world in (Rubin, 1963b, 1967).	

FATHERHOOD

Men's preparation for the role of father is vastly different from women's preparation for motherhood. In general, men do not fantasize about being a father, nor do they role-play being a father during childhood. During pregnancy, men mentally evaluate how they were fathered and how they want to father, but the reality of becoming a father may not occur until the child is born (May, 1982). Additionally, expectant fathers often picture themselves parenting older children rather than infants (Dayton et al., 2016).

Evidence-Based Practice: Expectant Fathers' Beliefs and Expectations

Dayton, C., Buczkoski, R., Murik, M., Goletz, J., Hicks, L., Walsh, T., & Bocknek, E. (2016). Expectant fathers' beliefs and expectations about fathering as they prepare to parent a new infant. *Social Work Research, 40,* 225–237.

The purpose of this qualitative study was to gain a deeper understanding of expectant fathers' experiences as they prepared to parent a new infant. Forty-four expectant fathers were interviewed during their partner's third trimester. Five major themes emerged from the data:

1. Being there: Men talked about the importance of being present in their child's life.

2. Fathering older children: Men talked more frequently about parenting older children versus infants. They focused on father roles with children beyond infant and toddler periods.

3. Preparation for life in society: Men talked about the importance of fathers preparing their children to be successful in their community and society. They identified their father roles as educator and life coach, providing emotional support to their children in dealing with life's challenges, serving as a positive role model, and facilitating their children's engagement within the community.

4. Heaviness of the fathering role: Men described fathering as an extremely difficult task that included being responsible for another life and the importance of providing financial and concrete support to their children,

5. Parenting support: Men indicated that they relied on women versus men for support in their role as father. The women were usually their partner, their mother, or other female relatives.

Implications:

1. Providing opportunities for expectant fathers to talk about their preparation and feelings regarding their new and emerging role of father.

2. Father involvement that begins in pregnancy is associated with positive maternal and infant outcomes. The provision of prenatal and postpartum education interventions can assist men in understanding the importance of early father involvement in the care of their infant and its effect on the infant's development. Early parenting behaviors include rocking, soothing and carrying their infant.

The meaning of "father" varies based on the man's interpretation of the role and its expectations and responsibilities. This is influenced by:

● How he was fathered.
● How his culture defines the role.
  ● In some cultures, men are not expected to be involved in the birthing process and/or care of the infant.
● By friends and family, and by his partner.

The man's partner has a major influence on the degree of the man's involvement in infant and child care. For the man to be an involved father, his partner needs to share this desire and to be supportive.

Becoming a father evolves over time as the man has increasing contact with his infant, increasing knowledge of infant and infant care, and increasing experiences in infant care. Factors that influence the man's transition to fatherhood are:

● Developmental and emotional age.
● Cultural expectations.
● Relationship with his partner.
● Knowledge and understanding of fatherhood.
● Previous experiences as a father.
● The way he was fathered.
● Financial concerns.
● Support from partner, friends, and family.

Nursing Actions

● Provide information on infant care and infant behavior.
● Demonstrate infant care such as diapering, feeding, and holding.
  ● Providing information and demonstrating infant care skills enhances the father's comfort in caring for his infant.
● Praise the father for his interactions with his infant.
  ● Praising can encourage continued interactions with his infant.
● Provide opportunities for the father to talk about the meaning of fathering.
  ● Talking about the meaning of fathering assists in identifying his beliefs regarding the role.
● Facilitate a discussion with the father and his partner to identify mutual expectations of the fathering role.
  ● Mutually agreed-upon expectations can decrease the level of stress within the relationship.

ADOLESCENT PARENTS

Adolescence is the transition between childhood and adulthood. This is a very challenging time, as the individual experiences many physiological, psychological, and social changes. Adolescent parenting is a stressful life experience in that the adolescent is taking on the role responsibilities of being a mother or father while at the same time working through the developmental tasks of being a teenager. Additionally, adolescent parents have few life experiences that prepare them for the role conflicts and strain experienced by first-time parents.

Adolescent mothers often live with their parents or other relatives following the birth of their child, while adolescent fathers tend to not live with the adolescent mother and their child. Adolescent parents, due to having fewer life experiences and coping skills, are more likely to use harsher parenting practices such as yelling and screaming (Urban Child Institute, 2014). The children of adolescent parents have more difficulty in acquiring cognitive and language skills and social and emotional skills (Urban Child Institute, 2014).

Nursing Actions

Nursing actions are directed at supporting the adolescent parents in developing childcare behaviors and learning to cope with the stress of parenting, as well as increasing the adolescent father's involvement in the support, care, and nurturing of his child. These nursing actions include the following:

● Assess level of knowledge.
  ● Information needs to be appropriate and relevant for the individual and/or couple for learning to occur.
● Present information at an age-appropriate level.
  ● Learning styles and teaching strategies are different for young teens and older teens. Information needs to be provided in a manner that will engage the adolescent parent in the learning process.
● Include the adolescent father in infant care teaching sessions.
  ● Adolescent fathers need information and encouragement in developing care behaviors.
● Involve the maternal grandparent in teaching sessions focused on infant care.
  ● Grandparents need a review of infant care since most teen mothers live with their parents during the first year.
● Discuss with the adolescent parents their expectations of each other regarding child care and support.
  ● Realistic and mutually agreed-upon expectations decrease the level of stress within the relationship.
● Involve adolescent fathers in prenatal care based on adolescent mother's comfort level.
  ● Adolescent fathers who are involved during the prenatal period have greater involvement with infants following the birth.

Evidence-Based Practice: Adolescent Parents

Jacobs, F., Easterbrooks, A., Goldberg, J., Mistry, J., Bumgarner, E., Raskin, M., Fosse, N., & Fauth, R. (2016). Improving adolescent parenting: results from a randomized controlled trial of a home visiting program for young families. *American Journal of Public Health, 106,* 342–349.

This randomized controlled research study aimed to estimate the effects of a home-visiting program serving first-time adolescent parents on parenting, child development, educational attainment of parents, family planning, and maternal health and well-being. The sample included 704 first-time adolescent mothers who were randomly assigned to the intervention group and the control group.

The intervention group participated in the Healthy Families Massachusetts (HFM) home visiting services. Weekly home visits were made for the first 6 months following the birth. The home visits included goal setting, curriculum-based activities, support tailored to individual families, routine development and health screenings, and linkages to medical and other services needed. The control group did not receive HFM home visiting services but were provided information about child development and referrals to other services. Data was collected at three points: T1, enrollment; T2, 12 months after enrollment; and T3, 24 months after enrollment.

Results:

- Positive parenting: No difference between the two groups with respect to likelihood of child maltreatment.

- Optimal child health and development: No difference between the two groups.

- Educational attainment and employment: HFM mothers were twice as likely to finish at least 1 year of college. There was no difference between the groups in terms of employment.

- Prevention of repeat pregnancies: HFM mothers were more likely to report use of condoms than the control group. There was no difference between the groups' use of hormonal birth control or likelihood of second birth.

- Parental health and well-being: HFM mothers were significantly less likely to participate in risky behaviors, such as substance abuse, fighting, and unprotected sex. They were also less likely to use marijuana.

Implications for nursing care: Public health programs that include home visits can lower risky behaviors in adolescent mothers and increase their likelihood of attending and completing college.

SAME-SEX PARENTS

In the United States, 4.4% of female adults and 3.7% of male adults identify as lesbian, gay, bisexual, or transgender (LBGT) (Gallup, 2017). The number of millennials, the present childbearing generation, who identify themselves as LGBT has increased from 5.8% in 2012 to 7.3% in 2016 (Gallup, 2017). The percentage of Americans' satisfaction with acceptance of gays and lesbians in the United States has risen from 38% in 2002 to 56% in 2015, and the percentage of dissatisfied Americans has decreased from 55% in 2002 to 42% in 2012 (Gallup, 2012). These statistics indicate an increasing acceptance of the homosexual lifestyle. These trends also indicate that there are an increasing number of lesbian women of childbearing age.

Prior to conception, lesbian couples have discussions similar to those of heterosexual couples regarding parenting philosophies, child care, and work arrangements, but unlike heterosexual couples, lesbian couples must decide which woman will become the child's biological mother. This decision is based on which woman desires to be pregnant and may be influenced by age and health of each partner, career goals, and which woman's insurance covers the cost of reproductive technology and the pregnancy/childbirth medical care (Amato & Jacob, 2010; Wojnar & Katzenmeyer, 2014). In some cases, both women want to conceive a child and decide that one will conceive the first child and the other will conceive the second child.

Once the couple has decided who will conceive, they must decide how they will conceive. Most lesbian couples use artificial insemination (AI) and thus must decide whether they want a known or unknown sperm donor. They will gather information about

sperm banks and obtaining sperm. Lesbian couples share similar feelings as heterosexual couples who are using AI. They often find the process to be stressful due to the monitoring of ovulation and the timing of insemination, and the process becomes more stressful when pregnancy does not occur within the first few months of AI (Amato & Jacob, 2010; Wojnar & Katzenmeyer, 2014).

During the postpartum hospitalization, the couple needs information regarding care of their infant and of the postpartum woman. The postpartum couple views themselves as coparents and plans to equally share in the care of their child. It is important to include both women in teaching sessions regarding infant care. Most lesbian mothers breastfeed their infants and it is not uncommon for both mothers to breastfeed their infant (see Critical Component below). It is important for nurses to ask the mothers if they both plan to breastfeed and if so, assist both in breastfeeding and provide information on induction of lactation and use of lactation supplementation.

CRITICAL COMPONENT

Induction of Lactation

Several methods can be used to induce lactation for nonbirthing mothers. These include hormonal therapy, manual and/or electric pumping of the breast, use of an at-breast supplementation device, or a combination of these methods. The nonbirthing mother should begin preparing her breasts for lactation several months before the birth of the baby. The following website by Breastfeeding USA provides additional information for nonbirthing women who desire to breastfeed: https://breastfeedingusa.org/content/article/breastfeeding-your-adopted-baby-0.

Lesbian couples take on the role of birth mother and comother during their transition to parenting. They will experience similar stress-producing issues as heterosexual couples as they take on their new roles, but research findings indicate that lesbian parents report less parental stress than heterosexual couples (Borneskog, Lampic, Sydsjo, Bladh, & Svanberg, 2014). Lesbian couples report lower parental stress related to feelings of incompetence as a parent and social isolation compared to heterosexual couples (Borneskog et al., 2014). Most lesbian couples are egalitarian in their roles and equally share in the care of their infant (Borneskog et al., 2014). These relationship traits might influence the lower levels of parental stress.

The non-childbearing mother, who is not visibly pregnant, might experience stress related to "invisibility and lack of support from their work or social community" (McManus, Hunter, Renn, 2006). This is enhanced if the non-childbearing mother has not "come out" at work or in her social community. The non-childbearing mother experiences another stressor related to parental rights, as rights for the nonbirth mother vary from state to state. Even when the couple is legally married, the non-childbearing mother may not automatically have parental rights. It is recommended that the non-childbearing mother legally adopt the couple's child.

Children raised by lesbian parents are well adjusted and have similar emotional, social, and cognitive development as children of heterosexual parents. A longitudinal study by Farr compared adoptive children of same-sex couples and heterosexual couples, collecting data when the children were preschool age and then 5 years later. The results from this study indicated no difference between the children of same-sex parents and heterosexual parents. Same-sex-parented children were well adjusted at each data collection point. The same-sex parents were capable in their parenting role and satisfied with their couple relationship (Farr, 2017).

Nursing Actions

- Self-assessment of the nurse's attitudes, beliefs, and knowledge of homosexuality
  - Personal beliefs, attitudes, and knowledge can have a positive or negative influence on patient–nurse interactions and nursing care.
  - Nurses need to be respectful of people with diverse lifestyles.
- Assess the couple's knowledge of infant care and parenting roles.
  - Important to evaluate couple's knowledge level and then reinforce and add to the knowledge base
- Include both mothers in teaching sessions that focus on infant care.
  - Lesbian couples tend to be egalitarian in their roles and equally share the care of their infant (Lindsey, 2015).
- Clarify if both mothers are planning to breastfeed their infant; if so, provide breastfeeding teaching and support to each mother.
  - Often both mothers will breastfeed their infant and both need assistance.
- Encourage both mothers to hold infant and engage in infant care.
  - Bonding and attachment is important for each parent's mother–child relationship.

BONDING AND ATTACHMENT

Bonding and attachment between parents and children are critical factors in the transition to parenting and parental role attainment. Bonding is defined as the emotions that begin during pregnancy or shortly after birth between the parent and the infant (Klaus & Kennell, 1982). Bonding is unidirectional from parent to infant. Attachment is an emotional connection that forms between the infant and his or her parents (Bowlby, 1969). It is bidirectional from parent to infant and from infant to parent. Attachment has a lifelong impact on the developing individual. The quality of this attachment influences the person's physical and emotional development and is the foundation for the formation of future relationships. With each interaction, the parent and infant become more acquainted with each other, recognizing and becoming sensitive to each other's behaviors. This leads to reciprocal behaviors and emotional bonds between parent and infant over time (Table 13–2).

Bonding and Attachment Behaviors

Bonding and attachment are affected by time, proximity of parent and infant, whether the pregnancy is planned/wanted, and the ability of the parents to process through the necessary development tasks of parenting. Other factors that influence bonding and attachment behaviors are:

- The knowledge base of the couple.
- Past experience with children.
- Maturity and educational levels of the couple.
- Type of extended support system.
- Maternal/paternal expectations of the pregnancy.
- Maternal/paternal expectations of the infant.
- Cultural expectations.

Risk Factors for Delayed Bonding and/or Attachment

- Maternal illness during pregnancy and/or the postpartum period that interferes with the woman's ability to interact with her infant
- Neonatal illness such as prematurity that necessitates separation of the infant from the parents
- Prolonged or complicated labor and birth that leads to exhaustion for both the woman and her partner
- Fatigue during the postpartum period related to lack of rest and sleep

TABLE 13–2   Bonding and Attachment Behaviors

BONDING BEHAVIORS UNIDIRECTIONAL: PARENT → INFANT	ATTACHMENT BEHAVIORS BIDIRECTIONAL: PARENT ↔ INFANT
En face	Parents respond to the infant's cry.
Calls baby by name	The infant responds to the parents' comforting measures.
Cuddles baby close to chest	Parents stimulate and entertain the infant while awake.
Talks/sings to baby	Parents become "cue sensitive" to the infant's behavior.
Kisses the baby	
Breastfeeds the baby or holds the baby close when bottle-feeding	

- Physical discomfort experienced by women postbirth
- Age and developmental age of the woman, such as adolescent or developmentally challenged
- Outside stressors not related to pregnancy or childbirth (e.g., concerns with finances, poor social support system, or need to return to work soon after the birth)

Nursing Actions

- Review the prenatal and labor record for risk factors that place woman/couple at risk for delayed bonding/attachment.
- Assess for risk factors that could delay bonding and attachment.
    - Early identification of couples at risk can lead to early interventions to enhance bonding/attachment.
- Assess cultural beliefs.
    - Type of interactions between parents and infants can vary based on cultural beliefs.
- Assess for bonding and attachment by observation of parent–infant interaction.
    - Assessment data provides information for individualizing nursing actions.
    - Expected assessment findings:
        - Parents hold the infant close.
        - Parents refer to the infant by name or proper sex.
        - Parents respond to the infant's needs.
        - Parents speak positively about the infant.
        - Parents appear interested in learning about the infant.
        - Parents ask appropriate questions about infant care.
        - Parents appear comfortable holding and caring for the infant.
    - Maladaptive assessment findings:
        - Parents call the infant "it."
        - Parents avoid eye contact with the infant (this can be viewed as adaptive based on culture).
        - Parents do not respond to the infant's cries.
        - Parents are emotionally unavailable to the infant.
        - Parents allow others to care for the infant, showing no interest (this can be viewed as adaptive based on culture).
        - Parents demonstrate poor feeding techniques such as propping bottles, not burping the infant, or seeming to be uncomfortable and/or irritated when nursing.
- Teach parents about bonding and attachment and the importance of these to the child's development of future relationships.
    - Understanding why it is important enhances likelihood of increased bonding and attachment behaviors by parents.
- Instruct parents regarding the importance of parents responding to the infant's cues such as crying, cooing, and movement.
    - Attachment is bidirectional.
- Promote bonding and attachment by:
    - Initiating early and prolonged contact between the parent and infant (Fig. 13–2).
    - Initiating rooming-in or couplet care.
    - Providing positive comments to parents regarding their interactions with the infant.
    - Encouraging mothers to breastfeed.

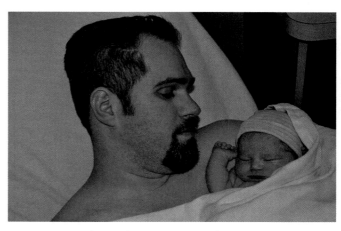

FIGURE 13–2 Skin-to-skin contact can enhance bonding and attachment.

- Encouraging the woman and her partner to talk about their birth experience and feelings regarding becoming parents.
- Promote attachment between mothers and infants separated due to either maternal illness or neonatal complications by:
    - Recommending that family members take pictures of the infant and bring them to the mother to keep in her room.
    - Assisting parents to the NICU or nursery so that they can see and touch their infant.
    - Providing opportunities for parents to care for the infant in the NICU or nursery.
    - Instructing the woman on breast milk pumping and encouraging her to bring breast milk to the NICU for use with her infant.
    - Informing parents that they can call the NICU or nursery any time of the day or night and talk with the nurse caring for their infant.

PARENT–INFANT CONTACT

Early contact between the parents and their infant fosters the development of attachment and integration of the infant into the maternal and paternal relationship. Continued contact and interaction provide the avenue for the parents and infant to learn more about each other. As they interact and perform their roles, they find themselves becoming more aware of the cues that make them respond to each other. This interaction cycle of behavior is called reciprocity, a biorhythmic or inherent rhythm that exists between the parents and infant and becomes stronger with each interaction and the passing of time. This sequence of events strengthens the bonding and attachment processes that are the foundation for all the child's future relationships as he or she grows.

Maternal Touch

New mothers begin to progress through the transition of maternal touch with the first physical contact with their infants (Rubin, 1963a). Most mothers do not instantly feel close to their infants and progress through three stages before feeling

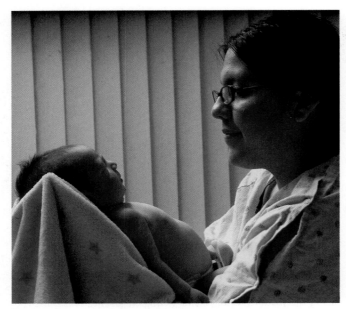

FIGURE 13–3 Mother and son in en face position.

comfortable holding her infant close to her body. In the earlier stages, the breastfeeding woman can feel awkward in holding her infant close to feed. Progression through the stages usually occurs over a few hours when a mother has early and continuous contact with her infant. It can take several days if the mother has limited contact with her infant, which can occur if the infant is ill and admitted to an intensive care nursery. These stages, as described by Rubin, are:

● Initial stage: The woman touches her infant tentatively with her fingertips.
● Second stage: The woman, as she becomes more comfortable with herself as a mother, uses her hand to stroke her infant's head or body.
● Final stage: The mother holds her infant in her arms and brings her infant close to her body.

Rubin's maternal touch is a component of the acquaintance process through which mothers and infants transition. Mothers go through multiple stages of awareness during early contact with their infants. The first time the new mother touches and meets her infant, she is excited about her infant's features and verbally responds to sounds and expressions the baby makes. Later, after the new mother enters the final stage of maternal touch, she will hold her infant en face, a position in which the mother and infant are face-to-face with eye contact (Fig. 13–3). The en face position provides a positive connection that facilitates the bonding process. Some cultures believe that you should not gaze into the infant's eyes.

CRITICAL COMPONENT

Paternal–Infant Contact

The new father, when holding his child for the first time, may feel awkward and uncomfortable and have a fear of injuring the baby. These feelings will decrease over time with continued contact with the infant.

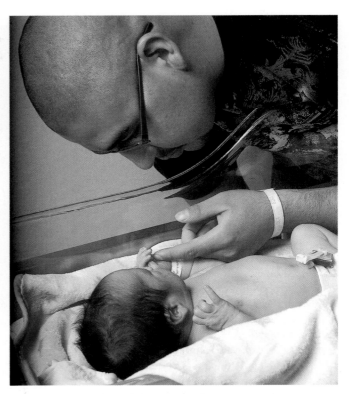

FIGURE 13–4 Father exhibiting sign of engrossment by gazing at his son.

Paternal–Infant Contact

In the 1980s, studies provided data that promoted and supported fathers' involvement in the birth of their infants. When expectant fathers participated in the labor and birth of their children in roles that were comfortable for them, they had a greater sense of belonging, which led to deeper engagement in the father role. Reinforcement of this type of involvement has had positive benefits to the family unit and strengthened early and positive parental involvement in the bonding and attachment process. Early physical contact with the infant provides an opportunity for the new father to become comfortable touching and holding, which fosters a more active role in caring for his infant.

New fathers experience an intense preoccupation about and interest in their infants. Greenberg and Morris (1974) identified these behaviors as engrossment (Fig. 13–4). These behaviors can vary based on the cultural beliefs of the couple.

Evidence-Based Practice: The Infant's Impact on the Father

Greenberg, M., & Morris, N. (1974). Engrossment: The infant's impact upon the father. *American Journal of Orthopsychiatry, 44,* 520–531.

In their research of new fathers, Greenberg and Morris identified the concept of engrossment that new fathers experience during the postpartum period in relationship to their infants. They defined engrossment as an absorption, preoccupation, and interest with their infants. New fathers can be observed gazing at their infants for prolonged periods of time as if they are in a hypnotic trance. Greenberg and Morris described seven characteristics of engrossment:

- A visual awareness of the infant: Seeing their infant as attractive
- A tactile awareness of the infant: Having a desire to touch the infant
- An awareness of and positive comments about their infant's distinct features
- A perception that their infant is perfect
- A strong attraction to their infant
- A feeling of strong elation
- An increase of self-esteem

Nursing Actions for Parent–Infant Contact

- Assess for stages of maternal touch.
  - Assessment data assists in developing individualized nursing care.
  - Expected findings:
    - Tentatively touching her infant's extremities with her fingertips
    - Progressing to fuller touch and examination of the infant
    - Verbalizing positive comments about the infant
    - Snuggling and providing comfort to the infant
    - En face positioning to interact with the infant (varies based on cultural beliefs)
- Assess paternal–infant interactions.
  - Expected findings (varies based on cultural beliefs)
    - Spends prolonged periods of time gazing at the infant
    - Assists with infant care
    - Holds the infant close to the body
    - Expresses delight in his infant's features
    - Verbally and physically expresses love and joy for both his infant and his partner
  - Maladaptive findings (may be viewed as adaptive based on cultural beliefs)
    - Displays little or no interest in the infant
    - Makes negative comments about or to the infant
    - Ignores the infant's needs and cues
    - Displays sadness or anger to the partner or infant
    - Does not spend time with the infant or is emotionally absent
    - Experiences mood swings
    - Has conflict between family members over the infant
- Provide early, continuous, and uninterrupted periods of time for parents to see, hold, and interact with their infant.
  - Bonding and attachment occur over time and with continued contact.
- Facilitate rooming-in, which provides the opportunity for the infant and father to stay in the mother's room throughout the hospital stay.
- Promote parental interaction with the infant by delaying unnecessary procedures.
- Provide adequate rest periods for the parents. This ensures they have the stamina and rest to take care of and provide emotional support to each other.
- Provide comfort measures to assist the parents in feeling rested and relaxed.

- Explain to new parents that they may not feel comfortable holding the infant close and that these feelings will decrease with increasing contact with their infant.
- Role model en face positioning.
- Role model appropriate behaviors by calling the infant by name and identifying normal infant behaviors.
- Use therapeutic listening and provide positive feedback to parents when they are verbalizing their feelings about their infant.
- Educate parents about the infant's unique behaviors and temperament.
- Educate and give information to both parents using multiple models of learning.
  - Teaching strategies need to fit the learning style of the parents.
- Provide culturally sensitive care to the family unit.
  - The way parents interact with their infant can vary based on cultural beliefs.

SAFE AND EFFECTIVE NURSING CARE: Cultural Competence

Cultural beliefs influence the ways parents relate to and care for their infants, including the role of fathers during the postpartum period and care of infants. An awareness of variations across cultural practices is an important component in providing appropriate care. Cultural beliefs can influence:

- The degree of the father's involvement in infant care.
- The role extended family members have in the care of the infant and new mother.
- The method of infant feeding.
- Foods that are eaten and foods that are avoided during the postpartum period.
- When a woman can bathe and wash her hair.
- When the baby is named and who names the baby.

COMMUNICATION BETWEEN PARENT AND CHILD

Communication is a bidirectional process that involves a sender and a receiver. People communicate through verbal and written words and through their eyes, ears, faces, and body gestures. Infants can see, hear, and smell; respond to their environments; and display displeasure. They engage in behaviors designed to evoke a response from individuals in their environments. They rely on vocal noises such as crying and cooing, as well as facial expressions and body movements to participate actively in relationship-building with other humans. The challenge to parents is learning the cues infants use to communicate their needs and pleasures.

Nurses are in the unique position to provide information about the infant's ability to communicate. They can help parents identify infant behaviors and offer appropriate interventions to promote positive interactions. The following are examples of infant communication styles and cues:

- Crying
- Cooing
- Facial expressions
- Eye movements
- Smelling
- Cuddling
- Arm and leg movements
- Entrainment, a phenomenon in which the infant moves his or her arms and legs in rhythm with speech patterns of an adult.

Responding to and encouraging infant communication assists the infant in developing communication and language skills. The parents' ability to recognize their infant's positive response cues fosters their confidence in their parenting skills. Teaching parents how to identify their infant's unique cues and behaviors promotes a positive relationship that empowers the dyad to continue to grow and learn as the infant matures and adds new skills and insights into the relationship.

Parents who are aware of and start to understand infant behaviors by becoming cue-sensitive will be able to identify:

- The best times to communicate with their infant.
- Ways to comfort.
- Methods to help infant self-comfort.
- When the infant is overstimulated and how to provide quiet times during these periods of fussiness.

Infants have very acute senses when interacting with their parents. Infants who are placed on their mothers' abdomens will crawl to the breast. Infants also interact with their parents by responding to voices and touch. They look en face and root when stimulated. These initial interactions and ongoing interactions lead to synchrony events, which are reciprocal actions between parents and infants that show mutual expressions of contentment. These interactions are very pleasurable for parents and infants. Examples of synchrony events are:

- The mother holding the infant in an en face position. The response to this action is that they gaze into each other's eyes and talk, coo, or smile at each other.
- The father placing his finger in the infant's hand. The infant grabs the father's finger and they gaze at each other.

CRITICAL COMPONENT

Positive Interactions Between Parents and Infants

Infants have the ability to communicate, to interact, and to be stimulated by early interactions. Depending on the state of awareness, infants can respond positively by becoming more alert or can respond negatively by crying. Nurses who understand infant behaviors, infant states of awareness, and communication cues can identify and promote positive interactions between parents/caregivers and their infants through role modeling and parent education (Table 13–3).

TABLE 13–3   Infant States

STATES	BEHAVIORS	ACTIONS
Deep sleep	Minimal body twitches and eye movement; cycles between deep and light sleep	Do not try to wake up or feed infant.
Light sleep	More active body movement; may smile	More easily aroused and stimulated
Drowsy	Awakens easily; can be rocked back to sleep or made more awake	May enjoy being held and cuddled
		Responds to gentle stimuli
		May self-comfort by sucking
Quiet alert	Eyes open; quiet and attentive	Best time for interacting
Active alert	More sensitive to stimuli, active body movement; may be tired or hungry or need changing	Decrease stimuli.
		Provide a quiet environment.
		Provide comfort measures.
		The infant may attempt to self-comfort.
Crying	Grimaces, cries, or whimpers	The infant may self-comfort.
		Meet infant needs.

Nursing Actions

- Review prenatal, labor and birth, and postpartum records for factors that might delay or hinder parent–infant communication and provide early interventions.
- Assess parent–infant interactions.
  - Expected findings:
    - Parents gently touch their infant and hold the infant close to the body.
    - Parents talk to or sing to their infant.
    - Parents, when culturally acceptable, hold their infant en face.
    - Parents respond to their infant's cues for interaction and care.
    - The infant responds to his or her parents' touch and voice.
  - Role model communication with infant.
    - Parents learn through incidental and intentional learning.
  - Praise parents for their interactions with their infant.
  - Provide teaching on infant communication:
    - The infant's ability and need to communicate
    - Eye contact, when culturally appropriate
    - Synchronized interactions
    - Recognizing and interpreting the infant's cues
    - Entrainment
    - Infant alertness states

FAMILY DYNAMICS

Family dynamics are the unique ways in which family members interact and participate within the family. Adaptation to these dynamics determines the cohesiveness, or lack thereof, in the family unit.

There are several types of relationships and family compositions. The family structure can be as small as the mother and infant, or as large as two or more generations plus extended family members. Each has its own unique dynamics and structure that present challenges and offers rewarding experiences to nurses who come into contact with these various family compositions. Examples of family compositions include:

- Married or nonmarried male–female couples.
- Married and nonmarried same-sex couples.
- Adoptive couples.
- Adolescent women with partner, mother, and/or grandmother as support system.
- Adolescent women without support system.
- Single adult women with no partner.
- Blended families.

The time immediately after childbirth is filled with emotional changes for the partners and family members. Family members are redefining who they are as individuals and their roles within the family. Adjustments within the couple's relationship and family unit occur as the couple and family members

incorporate and make room for the newest family member. Couples make adjustments within their relationship and learn how to support each other in their roles as parents. They reprioritize their other responsibilities and roles to fit their new roles and responsibilities. Siblings take on the role of older brother or sister and adjust to the decreased amount of time the parents have to interact with and care for them.

The family unit is affected and influenced by changes both within and outside the family. Outside influences, such as friends and relatives, may have positive or negative effects on the family. The couple needs to determine which resources are helpful and which are stressful, and from whom they can seek positive assistance. Nursing care is directed at assisting families in identifying their needs and adjustment during this period of transition.

Coparenting

Coparenting is "a conceptual term that refers to the ways that parents and/or parental figures relate to each other in the role of parents" (Feinberg, 2003, p. 96). Coparenting:

- Occurs when the parents have shared responsibilities in child rearing.
- Consists of support for each other and coordination they exhibit in child rearing.
- Does not imply that parenting roles are or should be equal in responsibilities or authority (Feinberg, 2003).
- Develops during the transition to parenthood and is influenced by:
  - The parent's beliefs, values, desires, and expectations.
  - The individual's cultural background and the dominant culture of the society (Feinberg, 2003).
  - The infant's temperament (Davis, Schoppe-Sullivan, Mangelsdorf, & Brown, 2009).

Evidence-Based Practice: Effect of Infant Temperament on Coparenting

Davis, E., Schoppe-Sullivan, S., Mangelsdorf, S., & Brown, G. (2009). The role of infant temperament in stability and change in the coparenting across the first year of life. *Parenting: Science and Practice, 9*, 143–159.

In this longitudinal study of 56 two-parent families, the researchers collected data at infants' age of 3.5 months and 13 months. Data included (1) observational assessments of coparenting and (2) mothers' and fathers' perceptions of their infant's temperament difficulties.

Results:

- Infant difficulty reported by fathers at 3.5 months was associated with a decrease in supportive coparenting behavior.
- Supportive coparenting behaviors observed in fathers at 3.5 months was associated with a decrease in reported infant difficulties.

Recommendations:

- Early interventions to enhance coparenting are essential for families with temperamentally difficult infants.

Multiparas

The maternal role changes and becomes more complex with each additional child. Multiparas may have more knowledge and practice regarding the care of infants, but they usually experience more exhaustion and have less help than with their first child. In a classic 1979 article, Ramona Mercer described the unique concerns of multiparas:

- Concerns for her other children
  - Will her other children feel abandoned?
- Concerns about being able to love the new child
  - Does she have the capacity to love this new child as she does her other child?
- Concerns for her ability to care for more than one child
  - Does she have the time and energy to care for an additional child?
- Concerns about her ability to get rest and sleep
  - Will she be able to find time for sleep and rest?
- Concerns about having help at home to care for her and her expanding family
  - Will family members and friends be willing to help her with a second child?

It is important that nurses who care for multiparous women provide them with opportunities to express their concerns, fears, and doubts in caring for and loving another child. Nurses can facilitate this transition by providing reassurance and suggesting strategies in caring for an additional child. Strategies for caring include:

- Spending quality time with the older child when the infant is sleeping.
- Carrying the infant in a sling to free hands for doing things with the older child.
- Having prepared meals ready to use during the day.
- Encouraging the partner to take on more responsibility for cleaning, cooking, and caring for the older child.

Sibling Rivalry

The addition of a new family member can be a stressful life event for siblings within the family unit. They will need to adjust in their young lives in response to the incorporation of the infant within the family. Depending on the age of the siblings and birth order, children experience varying degrees of feeling displaced. Younger children experience a sense of loss over no longer being the "baby" of the family. Older children may have a sense of increased responsibility due to their parents' expectation that they assist in caring for younger children.

Preparing for the new family addition should begin during pregnancy as the parents talk about the expected new baby (see Chapter 5). Providing opportunities for children to feel the fetus move and hear the fetal heartbeat are concrete ways to assist children in understanding the upcoming event. Discussion on what it will mean to have a new baby in the family can also help in adjustment.

Siblings should be introduced to their new brother or sister as soon as possible and spend time with mother and baby during the postpartum hospitalization. They should be allowed to hold and touch the new baby with supervision (Fig. 13–5).

Nursing Actions for Family Dynamics

Introducing a new member into the family can be stressful for each member of the family. The majority of nursing actions are aimed at reducing stress within the family and on family members. Nursing actions include the following:

- Review the records for relationship issues, pregnancy history, and delivery summary.
  - Complications encountered during pregnancy and/or labor and birth can have a negative effect on family dynamics.
- Assess for prior experiences with infants.

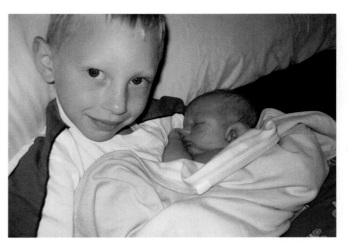

FIGURE 13–5 Big brother meets the new family member.

- Assess for maladaptive behaviors and make referrals to social services or the community health nurse as indicated.
- Respect cultural beliefs and incorporate them in the nursing care.
  - How an individual interacts within the family unit is influenced by his or her cultural beliefs.
- Provide information of the potential adjustments parents, couples, and siblings will encounter as they incorporate the infant into the family.
- Assist parents in identifying ways to assist their other children in their adjustments to the new family member.
- Provide positive verbal reinforcement for their family interactions.
- Provide opportunities for family members to talk about the adjustments within the family.
  - Increased communication can decrease misunderstanding.
- Provide opportunities for couples to talk about the adjustments within their couple relationship and ways to enhance their relationship.

PARENTS WITH SENSORY OR PHYSICAL IMPAIRMENTS

Parents with sensory impairments such as visual loss or diminished hearing, or those with physical impairments such as decreased mobility, present challenges to nurses and other health care professionals. These challenges can turn into opportunities to creatively adapt nursing care to meet the needs of these parents. It is important that health care professionals be aware of the rights of individuals with disabilities, provide information in ways they can understand, and provide care that is sensitive to their needs.

Visual impairment, auditory impairment, and physical impairment vary in degree. Visual impairment ranges from visual loss, where the person can read large print, to complete blindness, where the person has no usable vision. Auditory impairment ranges from mild to profound hearing loss. Those with mild hearing loss have enough hearing to carry on a conversation under ideal conditions. People with profound hearing loss usually rely on sign language to communicate and will not be able to converse orally with hearing people. Physical impairment can range from dependency on a cane to loss of motor control in the arms and legs.

CRITICAL COMPONENT

Working With Parents With a Sensory or Physical Impairment

It is important to treat parents with sensory or physical impairments as people and not as disabilities. They have the same capacity to love and nurture their infant. They have the same need for information and assistance in learning to care for their infant. They are aware of their limitation due to their impairment and, in most cases, have already developed strategies for caring for the infant. Nurses need to assess parents for their knowledge level and their plans for caring for their infants and then modify nursing care to meet the needs of the new parents.

Nursing Actions

For visually impaired parents, nursing actions are as follows:

- When reporting, use the person's name. Do not refer to her as the "blind woman in room 211."
- When entering a room, address the person by name and introduce yourself and anyone else who is in the room.
- When leaving a room, announce your departure and indicate if others are staying or leaving.
- Speak directly to the person in a clear manner. Do not exaggerate word pronunciation or speak in a loud voice.
- Keep doors, cabinets, and closets closed to prevent injury.
- Use sighted-guide when assisting with ambulation (the visually impaired person holds the elbow of the sighted person when walking). Avoid shoving, pushing, or grabbing unless in an emergency.
- Do not pull on the person's cane to direct her.
- Do not play with a seeing-eye dog while it is in harness. Ask permission to touch the dog.
- Orient the person to the area of the room or new location after you have guided her to this new area.
  - At a given point (the door or bed), orient the room by describing its contents in logical sequence of progressive order (e.g., "To the right as you lie in the bed is the nightstand with the phone and call button; beside that is the bed curtain and then a chair. Next to the chair is the door to the bathroom").
- Describe the location of food on a plate according to the clock face (e.g., "Potatoes are at 2:00, meat is at 5:00"). Ask the woman if she needs assistance.
- Offer to read printed material or ask for the preferred manner for receiving information that is in printed form.
- Provide space for Braillers and other special equipment used by the woman.
- Provide teaching in a manner the parents can understand. Example of teaching instructions:
  - Instruct the parents in diapering by having them diaper their child while you explain the steps.
- Provide discharge teaching and instructions in Braille or on audiotape.

For Hearing-Impaired Parents:

- Face the parents when speaking to them.
- Be articulate but do not exaggerate pronunciation.
- Speak in a normal voice volume.
- Be within 6 to 8 feet of the parents when speaking to them. Make sure that light from windows is behind the parents.

- Avoid putting your hand over your mouth or turning your back to the parents when you are speaking.
- When communicating information with the use of illustrations, provide time for parents to study the illustrations.
- If there is more than one speaker, take turns speaking with clear indications as to who is speaking.
- Minimize background noises (e.g., turn off volume of TV, close the door to the room).
- If there is misunderstanding, do not repeat words louder; instead use synonyms or other words that mean the same thing.
- Provide discharge teaching and information in written form that parents can easily understand.
- Use graphics and visuals when available.
- Ensure a registered interpreter for the deaf person is present when discussing medical information and teaching. When using an interpreter:
  - Allow sufficient time for the interpreter to complete a thought.
  - Speak directly to the patient and not to the interpreter.
  - Avoid saying, "Tell him/her . . ."
  - Check the parent for understanding or if he or she is getting too much information.
  - Allow time for questions and concerns.
- A head nod by the parent may have different meanings, such as "yes" or "continue"; it may not mean that the parent understands.
- Flick lights on and off to get the attention of the parent. Do not shout, wave, or touch to get his or her attention.
- Be aware that hearing aids amplify sound 6 to 10 times, so shouting and loud noises can be uncomfortable.
- Provide closed-captioned TV, TDD/TTY (telephone device for deaf), writing pad, and implements.
- Discuss with the parents how they have adapted their home for the infant.
  - Some parents will use a device that causes a light to flash in response to the infant's cry, thus alerting parents to check on their infant.
  - Some parents might use closed-circuit TV to monitor the infant while in another room.

For Parents With Physical Impairments:

- Provide standard ADA-required facilities, such as raised toilets, wheelchair-accessible rooms and hallways, and easy-to-use call buttons.
- Keep the environment free of clutter.
- Assess the type of assistance needed by asking the parents.
- Discuss the type of assistance parents will need in caring for their infant at home.
- Assist parents in infant care.
- Assist parents in developing strategies to adapt infant care to their limitations.

- Make referrals to social services when indicated for additional assistance.

CRITICAL COMPONENT

Assisting Parents With an Impairment

Nurses can best assist parents who have sensory or physical impairments by exploring, identifying, and implementing techniques, tools, and alternative ways to:
- Facilitate bonding and attachment.
- Teach parents about infant care.
- Promote a safe environment for the infant.
- Enhance the family dynamics.

POSTPARTUM BLUES

Postpartum blues, also known as baby blues, occur during the first few postpartum weeks, last for a few days, and affect the majority of women. During this period, the woman feels sad and cries easily but is still able to take care of herself and her infant. (Postpartum psychological complications are discussed in Chapter 14.)

Possible causes of postpartum blues include:

- Changes in hormonal levels.
- Fatigue.
- Stress from taking on the new role of mother.

Signs and symptoms of postpartum blues are:

- Anger.
- Anxiety.
- Mood swings.
- Sadness.
- Weeping.
- Difficulty sleeping.
- Difficulty eating.

Nursing Actions

- Provide information to the couple regarding postpartum blues. The nurse should:
  - Explain that this occurs in the majority of postpartum women.
  - Explain the importance of rest in reducing stress.
  - Explain to the woman's partner the importance of emotional and physical support during this period of time.
  - Explain that the woman or family should seek assistance from the health care provider if the symptoms persist beyond 4 weeks or if symptoms concern the woman or her family, as she may be experiencing postpartum depression.

Clinical Pathway for Transition to Parenthood

Focus of Care	Postpartum Admission	Postpartum 4 to 24 Hours	Postpartum 24 to 48 Hours	Discharge Criteria
Emotional status	Taking-in phase	Progressing toward the taking-hold phase	Taking-hold phase. The woman shows more independence in managing her own and the infant's care.	The woman is able to provide self-care. The woman demonstrates increased confidence in infant care.
Nursing action	Provide care and comfort to the woman. Provide positive reinforcement of appropriate behaviors. Discuss the infant's unique capabilities. Provide early and consistent contact with the infant to facilitate bonding.	Encourage the woman and her family to participate in self- and infant care. Encourage extended infant contact. Observe for bonding and attachment behaviors. Begin discharge education.	Observe for bonding and attachment behaviors, noting any signs of maladaptive behaviors. Provide written/visual information on infant behaviors and characteristics. Teach methods for comforting the infant.	Positive bonding and attachment behaviors noted. Parents express understanding of infant behaviors and cues. Parents express positive understanding of how to care for the infant. Provide resources for parents to call as needed.
Family dynamics	Parents demonstrate beginning bonding behaviors. Parents begin introducing the infant to the extended family.	Parents demonstrate positive bonding and attachment behaviors. Extended family demonstrate positive/supportive behaviors toward the infant.	Parents continue to demonstrate bonding and attachment behaviors. Extended family demonstrates positive behaviors toward infant and parents.	Parents demonstrate positive adaptive behaviors.

CONCEPT MAP

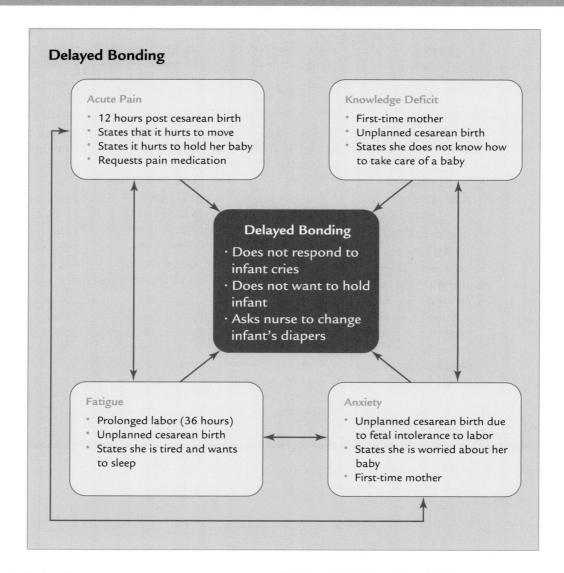

Delayed Bonding

Acute Pain
- 12 hours post cesarean birth
- States that it hurts to move
- States it hurts to hold her baby
- Requests pain medication

Knowledge Deficit
- First-time mother
- Unplanned cesarean birth
- States she does not know how to take care of a baby

Delayed Bonding
- Does not respond to infant cries
- Does not want to hold infant
- Asks nurse to change infant's diapers

Fatigue
- Prolonged labor (36 hours)
- Unplanned cesarean birth
- States she is tired and wants to sleep

Anxiety
- Unplanned cesarean birth due to fetal intolerance to labor
- States she is worried about her baby
- First-time mother

Problem No. 1: Acute pain

Goal: Minimal pain

Outcome: Woman reports that her pain is controlled at a level at or below 2 on a 10-point scale.

Nursing Actions
1. Assess level, location, and type of pain.
2. Assist woman into a comfortable position.
3. Administer pain medications based on assessment data as per orders.
4. Provide an environment that is conducive to relaxation (i.e., low lights, decreased noise, and uninterrupted rest periods).
5. Teach woman relaxation techniques.
6. Demonstrate position when holding infant that promotes maternal comfort (i.e., woman lying on her side with infant next to her, avoiding external pressure on woman's abdomen).

Problem No. 2: Knowledge deficit

Goal: Improved knowledge of infant care

Outcome: By time of discharge, mother will state she feels comfortable caring for her infant.

Nursing Actions
1. Assess women's level of knowledge regarding infant care and cesarean births to identify learning needs and level of understanding.
2. Provide information at woman's level of understanding.
3. Create an environment that is conducive of learning (i.e., turn off TV, close door to room, help mother into a comfortable position).
4. Medicate for pain, if needed, prior to teaching sessions to promote comfort.

5. Provide information on infant care, bonding and attachment, and post-cesarean birth recovery during several short teaching sessions.
6. Assist woman with infant care (i.e., bring infant to her so she can change diaper).
7. Praise mother for infant care behaviors.

Problem No. 3: Fatigue
Goal: Increased level of energy
Outcome: Woman states that she feels rested.

Nursing Actions

1. Assess level of fatigue.
2. Create an environment that is conducive to rest and sleep by:
   a. Clustering nursing activities to increase the amount of uninterrupted time.
   b. Providing pain management techniques (e.g., pain medications, back rubs).
   c. Closing door to room and dimming lights.
   d. Assisting woman into comfortable position.
3. Explain importance of rest in the healing process.
4. Provide information on high-energy foods.

Problem No. 4: Anxiety
Goal: Decreased level of anxiety
Outcome: Woman states that she feels comfortable holding and caring for infant.

Nursing Actions

1. Assess the woman's beliefs, attitudes, concerns, and questions regarding infant care and mothering.
2. Discuss with the woman her labor and birth experience and clarify reasons for cesarean birth and any misconceptions.
3. Discuss with the woman the health of her infant and address her concerns.
4. Encourage the woman to hold infant by:
   a. Explaining the importance of mother–infant contact.
   b. Helping her into a comfortable position.
   c. Bringing infant to her.
5. Praise the woman for her infant care behaviors.

Case Study

As the nurse in the postpartum unit, you are caring for the Sanchez family. Margarite gave birth to a healthy boy 5 hours ago. Both she and her son are stable. She breastfed her son for 15 minutes after the birth.

You notice that she is lightly touching the top of her infant's head with her fingertips. She comments that she does not feel comfortable holding her baby close to her body for breastfeeding.

Discuss your nursing actions that are based on your knowledge of maternal touch.
List the maternal phase and expected maternal behaviors for this period of time.
List five expected bonding behaviors for this period of time.

The next day you are again assigned to care for the Sanchez family. Mom and baby are stable. José, Margarite's husband, is present during the shift. Margarite and José voice concern about integrating their infant into the family.

Discuss your nursing actions that reflect an understanding of the couple's transition to parenthood.
Discuss specific strategies to decrease sibling rivalry.

Margarite tells you that she thinks she experienced postpartum depression with her first baby. She tells you that she cried a lot during the first week at home but was able to care for herself and her infant.

Discuss the appropriate nursing actions in response to her concerns.

REFERENCES

Amato, P., & Jacob, M. (2010). Can two eggs make a baby? Fertility options for lesbians. In S. Dibble & P. Robertson (Eds.), *Lesbian health 101.* San Francisco, CA: UCSF Nursing Press.

Borneskog, C., Lampic, C., Sydsjo, G., Bladh, M., & Svanberg, A. (2014). How lesbian couples compare with heterosexual in vitro fertilization and spontaneous pregnant couples when it comes to parenting stress? *ACTA Paediatrica, 103,* 537–545.

Bowlby, J. (1969). *Attachment and loss. Vol. 1. Attachment.* New York, NY: Basic Books.

Davis, E., Schoppe-Sullivan, S., Mangelsdorf, S., & Brown, G. (2009). The role of infant temperament in stability and change in coparenting across the first year of life. *Parenting: Science and Practice, 9,* 143–159.

Dayton, C., Buczkoski, R., Murik, M., Goletz, J., Hicks, L., Walsh, T., & Bocknek, E. (2016). Expectant fathers' beliefs and expectations about fathering as they prepare to parent a new infant. *Social Work Research, 40,* 225–237.

Farr, R. (2017). Does parental sexual orientation matter: A longitudinal follow-up of adoptive families with school-aged children. *Developmental Psychology, 53,* 252–264.

Feinberg, M. (2003). The internal structure and ecological context of coparenting: A framework for research and intervention. *Parenting: Science and practice, 3,* 95–131.

Gallup. (2012). U.S. acceptance of gay/lesbian relations is the new normal. Retrieved from www.gallup.com/poll/154634/Acceptance-Gay-lesbian--relations-new-nrmal.aspx?version=print.

Gallup. (2017). In U.S., more adults identifying as LGBT. Retrieved from www.gallup.com/poll/201731/lbgt-identification-rises.aspx?version=print.

Greenberg, M., & Morris, N. (1974). Engrossment: The newborn's impact upon the father. *American Journal of Orthopsychiatry, 44,* 520–531.

Jacobs, F., Easterbrooks, A., Goldberg, J., Mistry, J., Bumgamer, E., Raskin, M., . . . Fauth, R. (2016). Improving adolescent parenting: Results from a randomized controlled trial of a home visiting program for young families. *American Journal of Public Health, 106,* 342–349.

Klaus, M., & Kennell, J. (1982). *Parent–infant bonding.* St. Louis, MO: C. V. Mosby.

Lindsey, L. (2015). *Gender roles: A sociological perspective* (6th ed.). New York, NY: Routledge.

Loutzenhiser, L., McAuslan, P., & Sharpe, D. (2015). The trajectory of maternal and paternal fatigue and factors associated with fatigue across the transition to parenthood. *Australian Psychological Society, 19,* 15–27.

May, K. (1982). Three phases of father involvement in pregnancy. *Nursing Research, 31,* 337–342.

McManus, A., Hunter, L., & Renn, H. (2006). Lesbian experiences and needs during childbirth: Guidance for health care providers. *Journal of Obstetric, Gynecologic, & Neonatal Nursing, 1,* 13–23.

Mercer, R. (1979). Having another child: "She's a multip—she knows the ropes." *Journal of Maternal Child Nursing, 4,* 301–304.

Mercer, R. (1995). *Becoming a mother: Research from Rubin to the present.* New York, NY: Springer.

Mercer, R. (2004). Becoming a mother versus maternal role attainment. *Journal of Nursing Scholarship, 36,* 226–232.

Mercer, R. (2006). Nursing support of the process of becoming a mother. *Journal of Obstetric, Gynecologic & Neonatal Nursing, 35,* 649–651.

Rubin, R. (1963a). Maternal touch. *Nursing Outlook, 11,* 828–831.

Rubin, R. (1963b). Puerperal change. *Nursing Outlook, 9,* 753–755.

Rubin, R. (1967). Attainment of the maternal role. Part 1. Processes. *Nursing Research, 16,* 237–346.

Rubin, R. (1984). *Maternal identity and the maternal experience.* New York, NY: Springer.

Urban Child Institute. (2014). How adolescent parenting affects children, families, and communities. Retrieved from www.urbanchildinstitute.org/articles/editorials/how-adolescent-parenting-affects-children-families-and-communities

Wojnar, D., & Katzenmeyer, A. (2014). Experiences of preconception, pregnancy, and new motherhood for lesbian nonbiological mothers. *Journal of Obstetric, Gynecologic, & Neonatal Nursing, 45,* 50–60.

High-Risk Postpartum Nursing Care

14

Kara Johnson, DNP, RNC-OB, CNS
Nancy Irland, DNP, RN, CNM
Roberta F. Durham, RN, PhD

LEARNING OUTCOMES

Upon completion of this chapter, the student will be able to:

1. Describe the primary causes of postpartum hemorrhage and the related nursing actions and medical care.
2. Describe the primary postpartum infections and the related nursing actions and medical care.
3. Describe the primary postpartum psychological complications and the related nursing actions and medical care.

Nursing Diagnoses

- At risk for hemorrhage related to uterine atony, lacerations, retained placental tissue, or hematoma
- At risk for infection related to tissue trauma or prolonged rupture of membranes
- At risk for mood disorders related to stress, hormonal changes, lack of rest, or lack of social support

Nursing Outcomes

- The woman's fundus will remain firm, and lochia will be within normal range.
- The woman will remain asymptomatic of infection.
- The woman will indicate that she feels supported by her family.

INTRODUCTION

The postpartum period is a critical time to ensure women and their newborns are healthy. It is important to closely monitor a woman's health during this recovery time—especially if she experienced complications during pregnancy or childbirth—as over half of maternal deaths occur during the first days, weeks, and months after childbirth. Even healthy women who give birth are at risk for these complications. The most common yet preventable causes of severe maternal morbidity and maternal mortality include obstetric hemorrhage, infection, severe hypertension, and venous thromboembolism. Each of these will be addressed in this chapter.

Most women do not experience complications during the postpartum period, but when they do, it can be life-threatening and disruptive to the family unit. Most complications occur after discharge and may require readmission to the hospital. Many hospitals do not allow the infant to be readmitted with the mother, so readmission to the hospital for treatment of complications can interfere with the attachment process and increase stress within the family.

A focus of postpartum nursing care is to reduce women's risks for complications related to childbirth and identify complications early for prompt interventions. Women need to be evaluated by their health care provider when a complication is suspected.

CRITICAL COMPONENT

Risk Reduction for Postpartum Complications

Reducing a woman's risk for postpartum complications is a major component of postpartum nursing care. Nursing actions to reduce risk are:

- Reviewing the prenatal and intrapartum records for risk factors such as anemia, long labor, and operative vaginal delivery and addressing these risk factors in planning care.
- Assessing for signs of a postpartum complication and intervening appropriately.
  - *Early identification and treatment decreases the impact of the complication.*
- Assisting the woman with ambulation.
  - *Ambulation decreases risk of venous thromboembolism.*
- Preventing overdistended bladder.
  - *Overdistended bladder can place the woman at risk for uterine atony, neurogenic bladder, and/or cystitis.*
- Using good hand washing techniques by health care workers, patients, and visitors.
- Promoting health with appropriate diet, fluids, activity, and rest.

Severe maternal morbidity (SMM) includes unexpected perinatal outcomes that result in significant short- or long-term consequences to a woman's health. It is not entirely clear why SMM is increasing, but changes in the overall health of the population of women giving birth may be a contributing factor. This includes documented increases in maternal age, pre-pregnancy obesity, preexisting chronic medical conditions, and cesarean deliveries. Over the past decade, severe maternal morbidity in the United States has increased by 75% for complications associated with delivery, specifically for postpartum hemorrhage (Callaghan, Creanga, and Kuklina, 2012). As noted in Chapter 10, identifying potential problems early, developing written protocols that outline a clear plan of response for common emergencies, and using mock drills to train staff in protocol responses can help ensure that no tasks are redundant or omitted and ultimately create a more controlled environment that promotes positive health outcomes. Communication and teamwork are an essential part of safety and improving patient outcomes. Effective, patient-centered communication facilitates interception and correction of potentially harmful conditions and errors. All team members, including women, their families, physicians, midwives, and nurses, have roles in identifying the potential for harm during labor and birth (Lyndon, Lagrew, Shields, Main, & Cape, 2015).

A current national initiative to improve outcomes is the Safe Motherhood Initiative (see Box 14–1), which is focused on the following measures:

- Early opportunities exist to assess risk for, anticipate chances of, and plan for an obstetric hemorrhage.
- Multidisciplinary coordination and preparation, particularly with the blood bank, is critical to provide safe obstetrical care.

BOX 14–1 | Maternal Safety Bundle: Obstetric Hemorrhage

Maternal Safety Bundle Obstetric Hemorrhage

A leading cause of maternal morbidity and mortality is failure to recognize excessive blood loss during childbirth (Joint Commission, 2010). Women die from obstetric hemorrhage because effective interventions are not initiated early enough. Hemorrhage is the most frequent cause of severe maternal morbidity and preventable maternal mortality and therefore is an ideal topic for the initial national maternity patient safety bundle. These safety bundles outline critical clinical practices that should be implemented in every maternity unit (ACOG, 2015a; Main et al., 2015).

Obstetric Hemorrhage: Key Elements 4 Rs

Obstetric Hemorrhage Safety Bundle From the National Partnership for Maternal Safety, Council on Patient Safety in Women's Health Care

Readiness (Every Unit)

- Hemorrhage cart with supplies, checklist, and instruction cards for intrauterine balloons and compressions stitches
- Immediate access to hemorrhage medications (kit or equivalent)
- Establish a response team—who to call when help is needed (blood bank, advanced gynecologic surgery, other support and tertiary services)
- Establish massive and emergency release transfusion protocols (type-O negative/uncross-matched)
- Unit education on protocols, unit-based drills (with post-drill debriefs)

Recognition and Prevention (Every Patient)

- Assessment of hemorrhage risk (prenatal, on admission, and at other appropriate times)
- Measurement of cumulative blood loss (formal, as quantitative as possible)
- Active management of the third stage of labor (department-wide protocol)

Response (Every Hemorrhage)

- Unit-standard, stage-based, obstetric hemorrhage emergency management plan with checklists
- Support program for patients, families, and staff for all significant hemorrhages

Reporting and Systems Learning (Every Unit)

- Establish a culture of huddles for high-risk patients and post-event debriefs to identify successes and opportunities
- Multidisciplinary review of serious hemorrhages for systems issues
- Monitor outcomes and process metrics in perinatal quality improvement (QI) committee

ACOG, 2015a. Retrieved from https://safehealthcareforeverywoman.org/patient-safety-bundles/obstetric-hemorrhage

- A standardized approach to obstetric hemorrhage includes a clearly defined, staged checklist of appropriate actions to be taken in an emergency that can help to improve patient outcomes.

HEMORRHAGE

Postpartum hemorrhage (PPH) is a blood loss greater than 500 mL for vaginal deliveries and greater than 1,000 mL for cesarean deliveries with a 10% drop in hemoglobin and/or hematocrit (Harvey & Dildy, 2012). Patients with PPH are treated using a two-pronged approach: (1) resuscitation and management of obstetric hemorrhage and potential hypovolemic shock and (2) identification and management of the underlying cause(s) of the hemorrhage.

CRITICAL COMPONENT

Quantification of Blood Loss After Birth

Normal blood loss for a vaginal birth is approximately 500 mL within 24 hours. Visual estimation of blood loss (EBL) is common practice in obstetrics; however, the inaccuracy of EBL has been well established and blood loss can be underestimated by up to 50% (AWHONN, 2014b). AWHONN recommends that cumulative blood loss be formally measured or quantified after every birth. Inaccurate measurement of postpartum blood loss has the following implications:

Underestimation can lead to delay in delivering lifesaving hemorrhage interventions.

Overestimation can lead to costly, invasive, and unnecessary treatments such as blood transfusions that expose women to unnecessary risks.

Direct measurement of blood loss can be accomplished by two complementary approaches. The easiest is to collect blood in calibrated, under-buttocks drapes for vaginal birth. The second approach is to weigh blood-soaked items and clots. These items can be collected in a single bag and weighed using a gravimetric method. By using this method, the weight of dry pads is subtracted from the total weight to obtain an estimate of blood loss. Weigh all blood-soaked materials and clots to determine cumulative volume.

AWHONN, 2014b; Main et al., 2015.

The primary source of blood loss is from the placental site. The increase of blood volume and red blood cells (RBC) during pregnancy normally compensates for the blood loss that occurs following the detachment of the placenta. Additionally, physiological changes during pregnancy and immediately after the expulsion of the placenta decrease the amount of blood loss from the placental site. These physiological changes include the following:

- Hypercoagulability
  - Factor VIII complex increases during pregnancy.
  - Factor V increases following placental separation.

- Platelet activity increases during pregnancy.
- Fibrin formation increases during pregnancy.
- Contractions of the uterine myometrium
  - Blood vessels that supply the placental site pass through the myometrium, an interlacing network of smooth muscle fibers.
  - Contractions of the myometrium compress the blood vessels at the placental site, thus decreasing the amount of blood loss.

An estimated 5% of postpartum women will experience a PPH (Harvey & Dildy, 2012). Major complications of PPH include hemorrhagic shock related to hypovolemia, disseminated intravascular coagulation (DIC), organ failure, and death. The primary causes of PPH in descending order of frequency are the "4 Ts":

- Tone: uterine atony
- Tissue: retained placental fragments
- Trauma: lower genital track lacerations
- Thrombin disorders: disseminated intravascular coagulation (Table 14–1).

PPH is classified as primary (early) and secondary (late) hemorrhage. Primary PPH occurs within the first 24 hours after childbirth and is caused by uterine atony, lacerations, or hematomas. Secondary PPH occurs 24 hours to 6 weeks postdelivery and is caused by hematomas, subinvolution, or retained placental tissue.

Risk Factors

- Neonatal macrosomia: birth weight greater than 4,000 g
- Placenta previa or placenta accreta
- Multiple gestation
- Previous cesarean or uterine surgery
- Polyhydramnios
- High parity
- Prior PPH
- Operative vaginal delivery: use of forceps or vacuum extractor
- Augmented or induced labor
- Ineffective uterine contractions during labor: prolonged first and second stage of labor
- Precipitous labor and/or birth
- Chorioamnionitis
- Maternal obesity
- Congenital or acquired coagulation defects

CRITICAL COMPONENT

Examples of Threshold Parameters

Clinical situations such as postpartum hemorrhage or infection mandate further actions by the health care team according to protocol, such as bringing the attending physician to the patient's bedside immediately. Some clinical emergencies are preceded by a period of instability during which timely intervention may help avoid disaster. OB emergency teams, sometimes referred to as OB stat team for obstetrical emergencies, are

Continued

rapid response teams in the perinatal department. Perinatal nurses need to recognize that certain changes in a patient's condition can indicate an emergency that requires immediate intervention. A "red" trigger typically mandates an immediate bedside evaluation and a "yellow" trigger indicates further clinical evaluation (American College of Obstetricians and Gynecologists [ACOG], 2014).

Careful assessment and interpretation of maternal vital signs are critical in patient care during active bleeding. Obstetric patients, however, may not show signs and symptoms usually observed in nonpregnant patients with hemorrhage until approximately one-third of the woman's entire blood volume is lost (Harvey & Dildy, 2012).

	Red Trigger	Yellow Trigger
Temperature; °C	<35 or >38	35–36
Systolic blood pressure (BP); mm Hg	<90 or >160	150–160 or 90–100
Diastolic BP; mm Hg	>100	90–100
Heart rate; beats.min^{-1}	<40 or >120	100–120 or 40–50
Respiratory rate; breaths.min^{-1}	<10 or >30	21–30
Oxygen saturation; %	<95	

TABLE 14–1 Precipitating Factors for Hemorrhage—the 4 Ts

	MEDICAL FACTORS	SIGNS AND SYMPTOMS	NURSING ACTIONS
Tone (uterine atony)	• Large baby • High parity • Rapid labor • Fever • Fibroids	• Bleeding may be slow and steady, or profuse • Large, boggy uterus • Clots	• Assist the uterus to contract via massage and/or medications • Monitor bleeding—weigh pads and chux (1 gm = 1 mL) • Maintain fluid balance (may need second IV, Foley catheter) • Monitor vital signs and labs; blood type and screen if ordered • Administer oxygen 10–12 L via face mask • Keep patient warm
Tissue	• Retained or abnormal placenta	• In addition to the above, uterus may not respond to interventions • Uterus may remain larger than normal • Strings of tissue may be seen in the blood	• Call provider to assess; D&C may be needed • Monitor for signs of shock • Administer oxygen if indicated
Trauma	• Lacerations	• Firm uterus with continued bleeding • Steady trickle of unclotted, bright red blood	• Call provider to evaluate, locate, and repair laceration • Monitor vital signs and lochia • Weigh pads and chux to monitor blood loss
	• Hematoma (may be vulvar, vaginal, cervical, or retroperitoneal)	• Firm uterus • Sudden onset of painful perineal pressure • Bulging area just under the skin • Difficulty voiding or sitting	• Assess for visible hematoma • Call provider to assess • Anticipate possible excision and ligation if >3 cm • Consider indwelling catheter • Continue to assess vital signs, blood loss, and fluid maintenance • Pain management, including ice to the area
Thrombin disorders	• Preeclampsia • Stillbirth	• Disseminated (systemic) intravascular coagulopathy (DIC) • Oozing from IV sites • Nosebleeds • Petechiae • Bleeding gums • Hypotension and other signs of shock • Abnormal clotting lab values	• Early recognition is key factor in survival • Confirm accurate blood loss estimates • Monitor lab values, vital signs, intake and output • Manage systemic manifestations such as volume replacement, platelets IV, oxygen by mask at 10 L/min

CRITICAL COMPONENT

Indications of Primary PPH

- A 10% decrease in the hemoglobin and/or hematocrit postbirth
- Saturation of the peripad within 15 minutes
- A fundus that remains boggy after fundal massage
- Tachycardia (late sign)
- Decrease in blood pressure (late sign)

Because failure to recognize and intervene related to obstetric hemorrhage can result in severe maternal morbidity and even mortality, protocols are used to stage obstetric hemorrhage and outline a protocol and standard line of care. Box 14–2 presents the elements of common obstetric hemorrhage protocols.

Blood transfusion or cross-matching is warranted for certain obstetric events (Box 14–3). In cases of severe obstetric

---

BOX 14–2 | Staging Obstetric Hemorrhage: Elements of Common Protocols

Stage 1

Hemorrhage: Blood loss >500 mL vaginal OR blood loss >1,000 mL cesarean with normal vital signs and lab values

Initial Steps

Ensure 16G or 18G IV access

Increase IV fluid (crystalloid without oxytocin)

Insert indwelling urinary catheter

Fundal massage

Medications

Increase oxytocin, additional uterotonics

Oxytocin (Pitocin), 10–40 units per 500–1,000 mL solution

Methylergonovine (Methergine), 0.2 mg IM (may repeat)

15-methyl PGF2α (Hemabate, Carboprost), 250 mcg IM (may repeat in q15 minutes, maximum 8 doses)

Misoprostol (Cytotec), 800–1,000 mcg PR 600 mcg PO or 800 mcg PL

Blood Bank

Type & cross-match 2 units RBCs

Action

Determine etiology and treat. Consider 4 Ts—tone (i.e., atony), trauma (i.e., laceration), tissue (i.e., retained products), and thrombin (i.e., coagulation dysfunction)

Prepare operating room, if clinically indicated (optimize visualization/examination)

Stage 2

Hemorrhage: Continued bleeding EBL up to 1,500 mL OR >2 uterotonics with normal vital signs and lab values

Initial Steps

Mobilize additional help

Place second IV (16–18G)

Draw STAT labs (CBC, coagulation studies, fibrinogen)

Prepare OR

Medications

Continue Stage 1 medications

Blood Bank

Obtain 2 units RBCs (DO NOT wait for labs. Transfuse per clinical signs/symptoms). Thaw 2 units fresh frozen plasma

ACTION

Escalate therapy with goal of hemostasis

Huddle and move to Stage 3 if continued blood loss and/or abnormal vital signs

Stage 3

Hemorrhage: Continued bleeding with EBL >1,500 mL OR >2 units RBCs given OR patient at risk for occult bleeding/coagulopathy OR any patient with abnormal vital signs/labs/oliguria

Initial Steps

Mobilize additional help

Move to operating room

Announce clinical status (vital signs, cumulative blood loss, etiology)

Outline and communicate plan

Medications

Continue Stage 1 medications

Blood Bank

Initiate massive transfusion protocol (if clinical coagulopathy, add cryoprecipitate, consult for additional agents)

Action

Achieve hemostasis, interventions based on etiology

Stage 4

Hemorrhage: Cardiovascular collapse (massive hemorrhage, profound hypovolemic shock, or amniotic fluid embolism)

Initial Steps

Mobilize additional resources

Medications

ACLS

Blood Bank

Simultaneous aggressive massive transfusion

Action

Immediate surgical intervention to ensure hemostasis (hysterectomy)

ACOG, 2013b, 2015a; AWHONN, 2013; Main et al., 2015.

BOX 14–3 | Massive Transfusion Protocol

Blood Bank: Massive Transfusion Protocol

To provide safe obstetric care institutions must:

- Have a functioning massive transfusion protocol (MTP).
- Have a functioning emergency release protocol (a minimum of 4 units of O-negative/uncross-matched RBCs).
- Have the ability to obtain 6 units PRBCs and 4 units FFP (compatible or type specific) for a bleeding patient.
- Have a mechanism in place to obtain platelets and additional products in a timely fashion.

Example of a Blood Bank: Massive Transfusion Protocol

I. Patient Currently Bleeding and at Risk for Uncontrollable Bleeding

1. Activate MTP—call (add number) and say, "Activate massive transfusion protocol"

2. Nursing/anesthesia draw stat labs

   a. Type and crossmatch

   b. Hemoglobin and platelet count, PT(INR)/PTT, fibrinogen, and ABG (as needed)

II. Immediate Need for Transfusion (type and cross-match not yet available)

Give 2 to 4 units O-negative PRBCs ("OB emergency release")

III. Anticipate Ongoing Massive Blood Needs and Obtain Massive Transfusion Pack

Administer as needed in the following ratio 6:4:

6 units PRBCs

4 units FFP

1 apheresis pack of platelets

IV. Initial Lab Results

If normal → anticipate ongoing bleeding → repeat massive transfusion pack → bleeding controlled → deactivate MTP

If abnormal → repeat massive transfusion pack → repeat labs → consider cryoprecipitate and consultation for alternative coagulation agents (prothrombin complex concentrate, recombinant Factor VIIa, tranexamic acid)

ACOG, 2015a.

hemorrhage, at least 4 units of blood products may be necessary to save the life of a maternity patient. Hospitals are encouraged to coordinate efforts with their laboratories, blood banks, and quality improvement departments to determine the appropriateness of transfusion and quantity of blood products necessary for these patients.

Uterine Atony

Uterine atony, decreased tone in the uterine muscle, is the major cause of primary PPH. Uterine contractions constrict the open vessels at the placental site and assist in decreasing blood loss. When the uterus is relaxed, the vessels are less constricted and the woman experiences increased blood loss from the placental site. Uterine atony often occurs in women:

- Whose uterus was overdistended by a multiple pregnancy or large fetus.
- Who have given birth more than five times.
- Who had prolonged or dysfunctional labor with or without oxytocin augmentation.

Assessment Findings

- Soft (boggy) fundus versus firm fundus
- Saturation of the peripad within 15 minutes
- Slow and steady or sudden and massive bleeding
- Presence of blood clots
- Pale color and clammy skin
- Anxiety and confusion
- Tachycardia
- Hypotension

Medical Management

- Medications used for active bleeding: oxytocin, methylergonovine, misoprostol, and carboprost to stimulate uterine contractions
  - After expulsion of the placenta, oxytocin may be given intramuscularly or in an intravenous solution titrated as indicated.
- Bimanual compression of the uterus per provider (Fig. 14–1)
- IV therapy initially to reduce risk of hypovolemia
  - Isotonic, non-dextrose crystalloid solutions (normal saline or lactated Ringer's solution)
  - A ratio of 3 to 1—3 liters of IV solution for each liter of estimated blood loss
  - Blood replacement to reduce risk for hemorrhagic shock

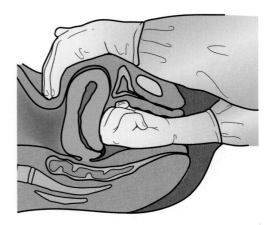

FIGURE 14–1 Bimanual compression of the uterus.

- Platelets, fresh frozen plasma, and cryoprecipitate replacement in management of massive obstetric hemorrhagic shock
- Nonsurgical interventions such as uterine packing with gauze or uterine tamponade
  - Uterine tamponade: A catheter device with a 300 mL balloon is inserted into the uterus via the vagina. The catheter balloon is filled with approximately 300 mL saline, enough to exert pressure on vessels at placental site and stop the bleeding.
- Surgical interventions such as dilation and curettage (D&C) and/or hysterectomy may be indicated when all other treatments have failed to contract the uterus.

Nursing Actions

- Review prenatal and intrapartum records for PPH risk factors and closely monitor women who are at risk for uterine atony.
- Assess for a displaced uterus. This will generally be to the patient's left. An overdistended bladder can displace the uterus and cause it to relax. When the uterus is displaced to the side during fundal exam:
  - Assist the woman to the bathroom to void, then reassess the location and firmness of the fundus and the amount and characteristics of the lochia.
  - Catheterize the woman if she is unable to void or is experiencing small, frequent voidings.
  - Use bladder scanner to assess urine volume.
- Assess the fundus for degree of firmness. If boggy:
  - Massage uterus and reassess every 5 to 15 minutes (Fig. 14–2).
  - Put baby to breast to initiate release of oxytocin.
- Assess lochia for amount and clots.
  - Express clots, which can interfere with uterine contraction.
  - Weigh bloodied pads and linens to obtain an accurate amount of blood loss: 1 g = 1 mL of blood.
- Review laboratory tests such as hemoglobin and hematocrit (H&H).

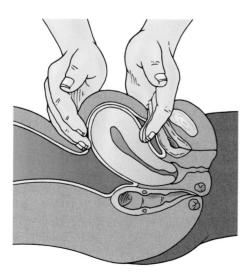

FIGURE 14–2 Fundal massage.

- Notify physician or midwife of abnormal assessment findings and/or test results.
  - Establish IV site with large-bore intravenous catheter.
  - Administer oxytocin, methylergonovine, misoprostol, and/or carboprost to stimulate uterine contractions as ordered.
  - Start and monitor blood transfusions as ordered and per protocol.
- Provide emotional support and teaching to both the woman and her support system, since PPH can increase the anxiety and stress levels of the woman and her family.

SAFE AND EFFECTIVE NURSING CARE: Understanding Medication

Uterotonics

The use of uterotonics for the prevention of PPH during the third stage of labor is recommended for all births (World Health Organization, 2012). Oxytocin is the recommended uterotonic drug for the prevention of PPH. Oxytocin should be used for management of third stage of labor for all births (AWHONN, 2014a).

Oxytocin (Pitocin)

- Classification: hormone/oxytocic
- Route: Oxytocin should be administered only by the intramuscular (IM) or intravenous (IV) route, not by IV push. As a high-alert medication, IV oxytocin premixed bags should be infused via an IV infusion pump to control administration.
- Prominently and clearly label with bright-colored labeling.
- Store separately to prevent a 1,000-mL IV bag with oxytocin being mistaken for a plain 1,000-mL bag used for IV fluid resuscitation bolus.
- Administer IV oxytocin by providing a bolus dose followed by a total minimum infusion time of 4 hours after birth. For women who are at high risk for a postpartum hemorrhage, continuation beyond 4 hours is recommended. Rate and duration should be titrated according to uterine tone and bleeding.
- Common dosing is 20 units oxytocin in 1 L normal saline or lactated Ringer's solution with an initial bolus rate of 1,000 mL/hour bolus for 30 minutes (equals 10 units) followed by a maintenance rate of 125 mL/hour over 3.5 hours (equals remaining 10 units).
- Give oxytocin 10 units IM in women without IV access.
- Actions: Stimulates uterine smooth muscle that produces intermittent contractions. Has vasopressor and antidiuretic properties.
- Indications: Control of PP (postpartum) bleeding after placental expulsion.

Methylergonovine (Methergine)

- Classification: oxytocic/ergot alkaloids
- Route/dosage: IM 200 mcg (0.2 mg) every 2 to 4 hours up to 5 doses.

- Actions: Directly stimulates smooth and vascular smooth muscles causing sustaining uterine contractions.
- Indications: Prevent or treat PP hemorrhage/uterine atony/ subinvolution. Contraindicated in hypertensive patients.

Carboprost—Tromethamine (Hemabate)
- Classification: Prostaglandin
- Route/dosage: IM 250 mcg injected into a large muscle or the uterus.
- Actions: Contraction of uterine muscle
- Indications: Uterine atony

Misoprostol (Cytotec)
- Classification: antiulcer/prostaglandins
- Route/dosage: PO/rectally 200 to 1,000 mcg
- Actions: Acts as a prostaglandin analogue; causes uterine contractions.
- Indications: To control PP hemorrhage. This medication is used off label and is not yet approved by the FDA for this use.

  AWHONN, 2014a; McGovern, Bingham, & Didley, 2019; Vallerand, Sanoski, & Deglin, 2017.

Lacerations

Lacerations of the cervix, vagina, labia, and perineum can occur during childbirth and are the second most common cause of primary PPH. Lacerations often occur in women who:

- Give birth to large babies (fetal macrosomia).
- Experience an operative vaginal delivery, such as use of forceps or vacuum extraction.
- Experience a precipitous labor and birth.

Assessment Findings

- A firm uterus that is midline with heavier than normal bleeding
- Bleeding that is usually a steady stream without clots
- Tachycardia
- Hypotension

Medical Management

- Visual inspection of cervix, vagina, perineum, and labia
- Surgical repair of laceration

Nursing Actions

- Review labor and birth records for possible risk factors and frequently monitor women who are at higher risk for lacerations.
- Monitor vital signs.
- Monitor blood loss.
  - Weigh bloodied pads and linens to obtain accurate amount of blood loss: 1 g = 1 mL of blood.
- Notify the physician or midwife of increased bleeding with a firm fundus.

- Administer medications for pain management as ordered.
- Prepare the woman for a pelvic examination.
- Provide emotional support to the woman and her family.

Hematomas

Hematomas occur when blood collects within the connective tissues of the vagina or perineal areas related to a vessel that ruptures and continues to bleed (Fig. 14–3). It is difficult to determine the degree of blood loss since the blood is retained within the tissue; thus, PPH may not be diagnosed until the woman is in hypovolemic shock. Trauma caused by episiotomies, use of forceps, and prolonged second stage of labor is the most common cause of hematomas.

Assessment Findings

- Women express severe pain in the vaginal/perineal area, and the intensity of pain cannot be controlled by standard postpartum pain management.
- Presence of tachycardia and hypotension.

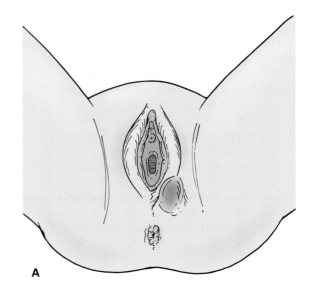

A

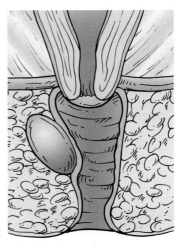

B

FIGURE 14–3 (*A*) Vulvar hematoma. (*B*) Vaginal wall hematoma.

- Hematomas in the vagina cannot be visualized by the nurse. When located in the vaginal area, women will express severe pain, a heaviness or fullness in the vagina, and/or rectal pressure.
- Hematomas in the perineal area present with swelling, discoloration, and tenderness.
- Hematomas can become large enough to displace the uterus and cause uterine atony, which can increase the degree of blood loss even though the blood is not visible externally.

Medical Management

- Small hematomas are evaluated and monitored without surgical intervention.
- Large hematomas are surgically excised and the blood evacuated. The open vessel is identified and ligated.
  - Women experience immediate relief from pain once the blood has been evacuated.

Nursing Actions

- Review the chart for risk factors and closely monitor women at risk for a hematoma.
- Apply ice to the perineum for the first 24 hours to decrease the risk of hematoma.
- Assess the degree of pain by using a pain scale.
  - Severe vaginal/perineal pain is a primary symptom of hematoma.
  - Ask women who verbally or nonverbally indicate increased pain if they are experiencing any heaviness or fullness in their vaginal or rectal areas.
- Monitor for decrease in blood pressure and an increase in pulse rate, symptoms that indicate shock.
- Administer prescribed analgesia for pain management.
- Review laboratory reports such as H&H, as a decrease in H&H may be an indication of blood loss.
- Notify the physician or midwife of nursing assessment findings for further evaluation.
- Provide emotional support and teaching to both the woman and her family, as increasing pain can increase anxiety and stress levels.

Subinvolution of the Uterus

Subinvolution of the uterus means the uterus does not decrease in size and does not descend into the pelvis (arrest or delay of involution). This usually occurs later in the postpartum period. Subinvolution of the uterus can occur in women who have fibroids or endometritis or who have retained placental tissue.

Assessment Findings

- The uterus is soft and larger than normal for the days postpartum.
- Lochia returns to the rubra stage and can be heavy.
- Back pain is present.

Medical Management

- Ultrasound evaluation to identify intrauterine tissue or subinvolution of the placental site (ACOG, 2017b).

- Medical intervention depends on the cause of the subinvolution.
  - A D&C is performed for retained placental tissue.
  - Methergine PO is prescribed for fibroids.
  - Antibiotic therapy is initiated for endometritis.

Nursing Actions

- Review prenatal and labor records for risk factors.
- Monitor women who are at risk for subinvolution of the uterus more frequently.
- Patient education is the primary action, as PPH from subinvolution usually occurs after discharge.
  - Provide education on involution and signs to report, such as increased bleeding, clots, or a change in the lochia to bright red bleeding.
  - Provide education on ways to reduce risk for infection, such as changing peripads frequently, hand washing, nutrition, adequate fluid intake, and adequate rest.
  - Explain to women who have fibroids that they are at risk for subinvolution. Provide instruction on the proper use of discharge medication, since these women are usually discharged with an order for Methergine PO.

Retained Placental Tissue

Retained placental tissue is the primary cause of secondary postpartum hemorrhage. It occurs when small portions of the placenta called cotyledons remain attached to the uterus during the third stage of labor. Manual removal of the placenta increases the risk of retained placental tissue. The retained placental tissue can interfere with involution of the uterus, potentially leading to endometritis and subinvolution of the uterus.

Assessment Findings

- Profuse bleeding that suddenly occurs after the first postpartum week
- Subinvolution of the uterus
- Elevated temperature and uterine tenderness if endometritis is present
- Pale skin color
- Tachycardia
- Hypotension

Medical Management

- D&C is performed to remove retained placental tissue.
- IV antibiotic therapy may be prescribed because of the increased risk for endometritis.

Nursing Actions

- Patient education is a primary intervention, as PPH from retained placental fragments usually occurs after discharge.
  - Instruct women to report to their health care provider any sudden increase in lochia, bright red bleeding, elevated temperature, or uterine tenderness.

Nursing Actions Following a PPH

- Because failure to recognize and intervene related to obstetric hemorrhage can result in severe maternal morbidity and even mortality, protocols are used to stage obstetric hemorrhage and outline a protocol and standard line of care. See Box 14–2 for the elements of common obstetric hemorrhage protocols.
- Assess the fundus and lochia every hour and PRN for the first 4 hours and then PRN.
- Instruct the woman on how to assess the fundus, how to do fundal massage, and the signs of PPH that should be reported to the health care provider.
- Increase oral and IV fluid intake to decrease risk of hypovolemia.
- Explain the importance of preventing bladder distention to reduce the risk for further PPH.
- Assist with ambulation since there is an increase of orthostatic hypotension related to blood loss.
- Anticipate the risk of fatigue related to blood loss.
- Provide uninterrupted rest periods while in the hospital.
- Provide an opportunity for the woman and her support system to talk about their experiences with PPH, as they may have related feelings of fear, anxiety, and stress.
- Provide information on foods high in iron and the importance of eating a high-iron diet to decrease the risk of anemia.
- Review the H&H laboratory report. Notify the physician or certified nurse-midwife (CNM) of abnormal results.

COAGULATION DISORDERS

A variety of complications can occur during the postpartum period related to alterations in the clotting mechanisms, including disseminated intravascular coagulation, anaphylactoid syndrome of pregnancy (sometimes referred to as amniotic fluid embolism), and thrombosis.

Disseminated Intravascular Coagulation

Disseminated intravascular coagulation (DIC) is a syndrome in which the coagulation pathways are hyperstimulated. When this occurs, the woman's body breaks down blood clots faster than it can form them, quickly depleting the body of clotting factors and leading to hemorrhage and death.

- DIC is a complication of an underlying pathological process called anaphylactoid syndrome of pregnancy.
- Women who experience DIC are transferred to critical care units, and a perinatologist, when available, manages their care.

Risk Factors

- Abruptio placenta, the primary cause of DIC
- HELLP (hemolysis, elevated liver enzymes, and low platelets) syndrome
- Anaphylactoid syndrome of pregnancy
- Hemorrhage

Assessment Findings

- Prolonged, uncontrolled uterine bleeding
- Bleeding from the IV site, incision site, gums, and bladder
- Purpuric areas at pressure sites, such as blood pressure cuff site
- Abnormal clotting study results, such as low platelets and activated partial thromboplastin time
- Increased anxiety
- Signs and symptoms of shock related to blood loss:
  - Pale and clammy skin
  - Tachycardia
  - Tachypnea
  - Hypotension

Medical Management

Medical management focuses on optimizing hemodynamic function and improving overall tissue oxygenation while identifying and eliminating the underlying pathology (Sisson & Mann, 2013).

- Laboratory tests (e.g., fibrinogen levels, prothrombin time [PT], partial thromboplastin time [PTT], and platelet count) to assess for abnormal clotting
- Identification of the primary cause of bleeding and intervention based on this knowledge
- IV therapy
- Blood replacement
- Platelet transfusion
- Fresh frozen plasma
- Cryoprecipitate
- Oxygen therapy

Nursing Actions

- Reduce risk of DIC.
  - Review prenatal and labor records for risk factors.
  - Monitor women more frequently who are at risk for DIC.
  - Assess for PPH and intervene appropriately. Early intervention can decrease the risk of DIC.
  - Monitor vital signs and immediately report to the MD or CNM abnormal findings, such as an increase in heart rate, a decrease in blood pressure, and a change in quality of respirations.
- Obtain IV site with large-bore intracatheter as per orders.
  - Administer IV fluids as ordered.
- Administer oxygen as ordered.
- Obtain laboratory specimens as ordered.
- Review laboratory results and notify the physician of results.
- Start blood transfusion as ordered.
- Provide emotional support and information to the woman and her family to decrease level of anxiety.
- Facilitate transfer to ICU.

Anaphylactoid Syndrome of Pregnancy

Anaphylactoid syndrome of pregnancy, also referred to as amniotic fluid embolism (AFE), is a rare but often fatal complication that can occur during pregnancy, labor and birth, or the first 24 hours postbirth. It is a two-stage process that occurs when amniotic fluid containing fetal cells, lanugo, and vernix enters the maternal vascular system. Amniotic fluid within the vascular system initiates a cascading process that leads to cardiorespiratory collapse and DIC. Women usually die within a few hours of symptom onset.

The process that causes the fluid to enter the maternal vascular system is not clearly understood. Areas of potential entry points of amniotic fluid are:

- The cervix, following rupture of amniotic membranes.
- Site of placental separation.
- Site of uterine trauma—lacerations that occur during the labor and delivery process (Jones & Clark, 2013).

Numerous risk factors, such as induction of labor, abruptio placenta, and placenta previa, have been postulated, but there are no reliable risk factors that predict AFE (Jones & Clark, 2013).

Assessment Findings

- Dyspnea
- Seizures
- Hypotension
- Cyanosis
- Cardiopulmonary arrest
- Uterine atony that causes massive hemorrhage and leads to DIC
- Cardiac and respiratory arrest

Medical Management

- No scientific data exists to support any intervention that improves maternal prognosis with anaphylactoid syndrome of pregnancy.
- The focus is on maintaining cardiac and respiratory function, stopping the hemorrhage, and correcting blood loss.
- Complete blood count (CBC), platelet count, arterial blood gases, fibrinogen, and prothrombin time are a few of the laboratory tests that might be ordered.
- Blood type and screen for possible transfusion
- Chest x-ray exam
- Blood replacement, packed red blood cells, and platelets
- Transfer to the critical care unit.
- A heart-lung bypass machine, when available, may be used to help stabilize the woman.

Nursing Actions

- Monitor for signs of anaphylactoid syndrome of pregnancy.
- Notify the physician immediately of assessment data so that early interventions can be initiated.
- Administer oxygen.
- Establish two IV sites with large-bore intracatheters: one for IV fluid replacement and one for blood replacement.
- Obtain laboratory specimens as ordered.
- Administer blood replacement as ordered.

- Provide emotional support to the woman and her support system.
- Call code and initiate CPR when indicated.
- Facilitate transfer to ICU.

Venous Thromboembolic Disease

Venous thromboembolism (VTE) is a blood clot that starts in a vein. It is the third leading vascular diagnosis after heart attack and stroke, affecting about 300,000 to 600,000 Americans each year. There are two types of VTE: deep vein thrombosis (DVT), which is a clot in a deep vein, usually in the leg but sometimes in the arm or other veins, and pulmonary embolism (PE), which occurs when a DVT clot breaks free from a vein wall, travels to the lungs, and blocks blood supply. Blood clots in the thigh are more likely to break off and travel to the lungs than blood clots in the lower leg or other parts of the body; thus, they are a larger concern.

Thromboembolism is a blood clot that can potentially block blood flow and damage the organs, a leading cause of maternal morbidity and mortality in the United States. The risk of venous thrombosis and pulmonary embolism in otherwise healthy women is considered highest during pregnancy and postpartum (Cunningham et al., 2014). Pregnancy is a hypercoagulable state with increased fibrin generation, increased coagulation factors, and decreased fibrinolytic activity. Venous stasis in the lower extremities, increased blood volume, and compression of the inferior vena cava and pelvic veins with advancing gestation all combine to increase risk five times over nonpregnant women. About 80% of thromboembolic events during pregnancy are venous, with pulmonary embolism and other VTE responsible for 1.1 deaths per 100,000 deliveries, or 9% of all maternal deaths in the United States (ACOG, 2011).

Physiological and anatomical changes during pregnancy increase the risk for thromboembolism postpartum. Hypercoagulability, increased venous stasis, decreased venous outflow, uterine compression of the inferior vena cava and pelvic veins, reduced mobility, and changes in levels of coagulation factors normally regulating hemostasis all result in an increased thrombogenic state. Risk factors for VTE unrelated to pregnancy include a personal history of VTE, thrombophilia, obesity, hypertension, and smoking (ACOG, 2011). Medical conditions such as diabetes, heart disease, hypertension, renal disease, sickle-cell disease, smoking, or serious infections can also increase the risk for VTE (AAP & ACOG, 2012). Classic signs of DVT are dependent edema, abrupt unilateral leg pain, erythema, low-grade fever, and positive Homan's sign (i.e., pain with dorsiflexion of foot). A PE may present with shortness of breath, tachypnea, tachycardia, dyspnea, pleural chest pain, fever, and anxiety.

Objective tests for DVT include Doppler ultrasound, magnetic resonance venography, and pulsed Doppler study. Chest x-ray, CT, and electrocardiography are used to diagnose PE. ACOG recommends preventive treatment with anticoagulant medication for women who have had an acute VTE during pregnancy, a history of thrombosis, or those at significant risk for VTE during pregnancy and postpartum, such as women with high-risk acquired or inherited thrombophilias. Women with a history of thrombosis should be evaluated for underlying causes to determine whether anticoagulation medication is appropriate during pregnancy. Most women who take anticoagulation medications before pregnancy will need to continue during pregnancy and postpartum. Treatment goals include prevention of further clot propagation, prevention of PE, and prevention of further venous thromboembolism.

- Anticoagulation therapy is required for women experiencing a DVT during pregnancy with heparin compounds titrated to achieve a PTT of 1.5 to 2.5 times control values. IV anticoagulation should be maintained for at least 5 to 7 days, after which treatment is converted to subcutaneous heparin (Cunningham et al., 2014).
- Early reviews concluded that low-molecular-weight heparins (LMWH) are safe and effective for use throughout pregnancy. ACOG concluded that risks associated with LMWH use were rare and that no cause-and-effect relationship has been established between LMWH and congenital anomalies or maternal hemorrhage (Cunningham et al., 2014).
- Treatment of PE is to stabilize a woman with a life-threatening PE and transfer to ICU. Thromboembolitic therapy and catheter or surgical embolectomy may be done.

Nursing Actions

- Begin ambulation after symptoms dissipate (Cunningham et al., 2014).
- Administer elastic stockings.
- Manage pain, administering pain medication as needed.
- Teach woman how to administer heparin subcutaneously to her abdomen.
- Instruct woman to report side effects such as bleeding gums, nosebleeds, easy bruising, or excessive trauma at injection site.
- Venous thromboembolism bundle is discussed in detail in Chapter 7.

INFECTIONS

Postpartum infections comprise a wide range of entities that can occur after vaginal and cesarean births or during breastfeeding. In addition to trauma sustained during the birth process or cesarean procedure, physiological changes during pregnancy contribute to the development of postpartum infections (Wong, 2017). An estimated 6% of postpartum women will experience a postpartum infection (Wong, 2017), causing an estimated 12.7% of maternal deaths (Centers for Disease Control [CDC], 2017). Common sites for infections during the postpartum period are the uterus, bladder, breast, and incision site. Most of these infections can be easily treated when identified at an early stage. Infections that are not identified and treated at an early stage can lead to serious complications such as abscess formation, cellulitis, thrombophlebitis, and septic shock.

The following are risk factors for postpartum infections:

- History of cesarean delivery
- Premature rupture of membranes
- Frequent cervical examination
  - Sterile gloves should be used in examinations. Other than a history of cesarean delivery, this risk factor is most important in postpartum infection.
- Internal fetal monitoring
- Preexisting pelvic infection, including bacterial vaginosis
- Diabetes
- Nutritional status
- Obesity

Complications of postpartum infection may include:

- Scarring
- Infertility
- Sepsis
- Septic shock
- Death

Endometritis

Endometritis, also referred to as metritis, is an infection of the endometrium, myometrium, and/or parametrial tissue that usually starts at the placental site and spreads to encompass the entire endometrium. Approximately 2% of women who experience a vaginal birth and 15% of women who experience a cesarean birth develop endometritis. The uterine cavity is usually sterile until the rupture of the amniotic sac. As a consequence of labor, delivery, and associated manipulations, anaerobic and aerobic bacteria can contaminate the uterus. Endometritis is an infection of the uterus characterized by postpartum fever, midline lower abdominal pain, and uterine tenderness. Also, purulent lochia, chills, headache, malaise, and/or anorexia may be present.

Risk Factors

- Cesarean birth is a primary risk factor
- Prolonged rupture of membranes
- Prolonged labor
- Internal fetal and uterine monitoring
- Meconium-stained fluid
- Multiple cervical exams during labor
- Obesity

Assessment Findings

- Elevated temperature greater than 100.4°F (38°C) with or without chills
- Midline lower abdominal pain or discomfort
- Uterine tenderness
- Tachycardia
- Subinvolution
- Malaise
- Headache
- Chills
- Lochia heavy and foul-smelling when anaerobic organisms are present
  - Foul-smelling lochia is a later sign that occurs when the entire endometrium is involved.
  - Lochia is scant and odorless when beta-hemolytic streptococcus is present.

Medical Management

Endometritis is usually treated with broad-spectrum IV antibiotics and rest. Blood cultures to identify the causative organism of endometritis are done if the patient does not respond to empiric therapy. White blood cell (WBC) counts are monitored.

- CBC to assess for leukocytosis (WBC count greater than 20,000/mm^3)
- Endometrial cultures
- Blood cultures
- Urinalysis to rule out urinary tract infection, which can present with similar symptoms
- Antibiotic therapy
  - Mild cases: Oral antibiotic therapy
  - Moderate to severe cases: IV antibiotic therapy, which is discontinued after the woman is afebrile for 24 hours.
  - Improvement should be noted within 72 hours of initiation of antibiotic therapy.

Nursing Actions

- Reduce risk of endometritis.
  - Educate the woman regarding proper hand-washing techniques to reduce spread of bacteria.
  - Instruct the woman in proper pericare and to wipe perinium front to back.
  - Instruct the woman to change her peripad every 3 to 4 hours or sooner because lochia is a medium for bacterial growth.
  - Encourage early ambulation by explaining how ambulation reduces the risk of infection by promoting uterine drainage.
  - Encourage intake of fluids to rehydrate by explaining to the woman that maintaining adequate hydration can reduce her risk for infections. Woman should have a minimum fluid intake of 3,000 mL/day (James, 2014).
  - Educate the woman on a diet high in protein and vitamin C, which aids in tissue healing.
- Monitor WBC count. However, it is important to remember that this is normally elevated after delivery for a short period; continued monitoring of the WBC count is required in identifying endometritis and is likely to show a left shift and increasing number of neutrophils.
- Monitor for signs and symptoms of endometritis.
  - Report assessment data of possible endometritis and abnormal laboratory reports to physician and/or midwife for further evaluation.
- Administer antibiotics as ordered.
- Provide pain management measures.
- Provide emotional support to the woman and her family.
- Discharge teaching
  - Provide information on discharge medications.
  - Provide information on signs and symptoms to report to health care provider.

Urinary Tract Infection

Urinary tract infections (UTIs) are common during the postpartum period. A woman's urethra and bladder are often traumatized during labor and birth due to intermittent or continuous catheterizations and the pressure of the infant as it passes through the birth canal. Additionally, the bladder and urethra lose tone after delivery, making the retention of urine and urinary stasis common. The risk of developing a UTI is high. Women may also develop a UTI due to epidural anesthesia or vaginal procedures. Bacteria most frequently found in UTIs are normal bowel flora, including *Escherichia coli, Klebsiella, Proteus,* and *Enterobacter* species. Any form of invasive manipulation of the urethra (e.g., Foley catheterization) increases the likelihood of a UTI. Cystitis is a lower urinary tract infection. It is easily treated, but if left untreated or if treatment is delayed, the woman is at risk for pyelonephritis. Patients with UTIs often complain of frequent, urgent, and/or painful urination with suprapubic pain. A low-grade fever and hematuria may also be present. UTIs are treated with antibiotics, but it is important that these patients drink adequate fluids to flush bacteria out of the system.

Risk Factors

- Epidural anesthesia, which decreases the woman's ability to feel the urge to void, leading to an increased risk for an overdistended bladder
- Overdistended bladder or incomplete emptying of the bladder, which can cause an increase of bacterial growth in the bladder
- Urinary catheter inserted during the labor process
- Neonatal macrosomia, which can cause edema around the urethra
- Operative vaginal deliveries, forceps, or vacuum extractor, which can cause edema around the urethra
- Intrapartal vaginal exams and the birth process, which can contaminate the urethra with bacteria

Assessment Findings

- Low-grade fever (101.3°F [38.5°C])
- Burning on urination
- Suprapubic pain
- Urgency to void
- Small, frequent voidings—less than 150 mL per voiding

Medical Management

- Urinalysis, CBC, and urine culture and sensitivity
- Antibiotics (usually PO) started before culture results

Nursing Actions

- Risk reduction for UTI
  - Assist the woman to the bathroom to void within a few hours after birth. This will flush bacteria out of the urethra.
  - Catheterize the woman if she is unable to void within 2 to 3 hours postbirth.
  - Remind the woman to void every 3 to 4 hours; she may not feel the urge to void during the first 24 to 48 hours following birth.

- Measure voidings for the first 24 hours, assessing for complete emptying of the bladder. Each voiding should be equal to or greater than 150 mL.
- Change peripads at least every 3 to 4 hours. Soiled peripads can encourage growth of bacteria that can enter the urethra.
- Remind postpartum women to drink a minimum of 3,000 mL/day (AWHONN, 2006).
- Encourage foods that increase acidity in urine, such as cranberry juice, apricots, and plums.
- Monitor for signs and symptoms of UTI.
  - Report findings of possible UTI to the physician or CNM for further evaluation.
- Obtain laboratory specimens as ordered.
- Administer antibiotics as ordered.
- Push oral hydration.
- Discharge teaching
  - Provide information on proper use of discharge medications.
  - Provide information on signs and symptoms of cystitis and report these changes to the health care provider.

Mastitis

Mastitis is an inflammation/infection of the breast tissue that is common among lactating women. It usually occurs in just one breast, most often in the upper outer breast quadrant. Although it usually occurs in the first 3 to 6 months of breastfeeding, it can happen at any time. The most common organism reported in mastitis is *Staphylococcus aureus*. The organism usually comes from the breastfeeding infant's mouth or throat. Patients with mastitis have very tender, engorged, erythematous breasts, and infection is frequently unilateral. Mastitis is generally self-limiting, and continued breastfeeding can help clear up the infection and condition. It does not harm the baby. If antibiotic therapy is indicated, the infection generally resolves within 24 to 48 hours of antibiotic therapy. Abscess formation can occur in 10% of women who develop mastitis.

Risk Factors

- History of mastitis with a previous infant
- Cracked and/or sore nipples
- Using only one position for breastfeeding, which may reduce emptying of the breast
- Wearing a tight-fitting bra
- Poor nutrition
- Ample milk supply and reduction in the number of feedings

Assessment Findings

- Breast tenderness or warmth to the touch
- Generally feeling ill (malaise)
- Breast swelling and hardness
- Pain or a burning sensation continuously or while breastfeeding
- Skin redness, often in a wedge-shaped pattern
- Fever of 101°F (38.3°C) or greater

Medical Management

- Oral antibiotics therapy for 10 to 14 days
- Culture of expressed milk from affected breast if infection does not resolve

Nursing Actions

- Risk reduction:
  - Mastitis is less likely to occur with complete emptying of the breasts and good breastfeeding technique. Thus, postpartum nurses must teach breastfeeding patients proper latch-on technique and stress regular breastfeeding and allowing complete emptying of both breasts. Breastfeeding patients are also encouraged to avoid missing feedings and allowing the breasts to become engorged.
  - Treatment for mastitis typically involves antibiotic therapy and regular breastfeeding or pumping the breast. Nurses can encourage these patients to apply cold or warm compresses to ease discomfort and to take analgesics as needed. Mastitis usually resolves quickly if patients continue to breastfeed or pump regularly.
  - Explain to the woman the importance of washing her hands before feeding to decrease spread of bacteria.
  - Proper hand-washing technique by hospital personnel
  - Teach the woman methods to decrease nipple irritation and tissue breakdown, such as correct infant latch-on and removal from the breast, more than one breastfeeding position, and air-drying nipples after feedings (refer to Chapter 16 for additional information).
  - Teach the woman the importance of a healthy diet and adequate fluids to decrease risk for any infection.
  - Recommend that the patient consider a larger bra size as breast size changes.
  - Recommend massaging the breast during breastfeeding, especially over tender areas and under the armpit, a common location of engorgement.
  - Empty both breasts fully during breastfeeding.
- Palpate and inspect the breasts for signs of mastitis.
  - Report assessment data of possible mastitis to physician or CNM.
- Administer antibiotics as ordered.
- Administer analgesia as ordered.
- Apply warm compresses to the affected area for comfort and promotion of circulation.
- Instruct the woman to continue to breastfeed or to massage and express milk from the affected breast to promote continuation of milk flow.
- Explain to the woman that it is very common for lactating women to experience mastitis and that it is easily treated when identified early.

Wound Infections

Wound infections can occur at the laceration site, episiotomy site, and cesarean incision site. Aseptic technique throughout childbirth and postpartum is critical in decreasing the woman's risk for wound infections. Most often, the etiologic organisms associated with perineal cellulitis and episiotomy site infections are *Staphylococcus* or *Streptococcus* species and gram-negative organisms, as in endometritis. Postpartum patients with wound infections typically have wounds that exhibit redness, warmth, poor wound approximation, tenderness, and pain. If untreated, these patients may develop a fever and other symptoms of an infection, such as malaise. Blood cultures may be obtained to isolate the causative organism. Antibiotics will typically be administered, and drainage of the wound may be necessary.

Patients must be taught about proper hand washing and encouraged to maintain adequate fluid intake and increased protein intake to assist in wound healing. Wound infections can be intensely painful, especially in the perineum. Therefore, the nurse assists these patients in managing pain with analgesics and positioning.

Risk Factors

- Obesity
- Diabetes
- Malnutrition
- Long labor
- Prolonged operative time during cesarean section
- Premature rupture of membranes
- Preexisting infection, including chorioamnionitis
- Immunodeficiency disorders
- Corticosteroid therapy
- Poor suturing technique

Assessment Findings

- Erythema
- Heat
- Swelling
- Tenderness
- Purulent drainage
- Low-grade fever
- Increased pain at incision or laceration site

Medical Management

- Obtain a culture specimen from the wound or laceration if indicated.
- For mild to moderate wound infections that do not have purulent drainage:
  - Administer oral antibiotic therapy.
  - Apply warm compresses to area.
- Wound infections with purulent drainage:
  - Open and drain the wound.
  - IV antibiotic therapy.

Nursing Actions

- Assess perineum or surgical incision for REEDA (redness, edema, ecchymosis, discharge, approximation of edges of episiotomy or laceration). Inform physician or midwife of abnormal assessment data.
- Assess vital signs.
- Obtain laboratory specimens such as cultures as ordered.

- Review laboratory reports and notify the physician or midwife of abnormal results.
- Administer antibiotics as ordered.
- Pain management
  - Administer analgesia for fever and discomfort as ordered.
  - Apply hot packs for abdominal wounds or sitz bath for perineal wounds to promote comfort and circulation.
- Use proper hand-washing technique before and after contact with the wound.
- Provide education on proper diet, fluids, and rest that can decrease the risk for infection and assist in the healing process.
- Provide information on proper use of discharge medications.

CRITICAL COMPONENT

AWHONN Health Information Technology for the Perinatal Setting

The Association of Women's Health, Obstetric and Neonatal Nurses (AWHONN) recognizes the vital role of health information technology in the health care delivery system in the United States. Interoperability is particularly important in the obstetric environment because the patient changes venues for care as she progresses through pregnancy, intrapartum, and postpartum. Many hospital information systems—such as admission, discharge, transfer; laboratory; pharmacy; critical care; and the emergency room—must efficiently interface. The ability to provide quality care safely and efficiently becomes compromised as the perinatal nurse navigates through multiple discordant systems. Additionally, important information from the patient's prenatal record may not populate her intrapartum and postpartum records or the newborn's record, further adding to inefficiency, fragmentation, and potential for error (AWHONN, 2011).

MANAGEMENT OF PREGNANCY COMPLICATIONS IN THE POSTPARTUM PERIOD

The postpartum period is a critical time to ensure women and their newborns are recovering from birth and are adapting and healthy. It is important to closely monitor a woman's health during this recovery time, particularly if she experienced complications during pregnancy.

Acute Onset of Severe Hypertension Postpartum

Women in the postpartum period with acute-onset, severe systolic (greater than or equal to 160 mm Hg) hypertension, severe diastolic (greater than or equal to 110 mm Hg) hypertension, or both require urgent antihypertensive therapy. The goal is not to normalize BP but to achieve a range of 140–150/90–100 mm Hg to prevent repeated, prolonged exposure to severe systolic hypertension. In the event of a hypertensive crisis with prolonged uncontrolled hypertension, maternal stabilization should occur before delivery even in urgent circumstances. Treatment with first-line agents should be expeditious and occur as soon as possible within 30 to 60 minutes of confirmed severe hypertension to reduce the risk of maternal stroke.

IV labetalol and hydralazine have long been considered first-line medications for the management of acute-onset, severe hypertension in pregnant women and women in the postpartum period. Immediate-release oral nifedipine also may be considered as a first-line therapy, particularly when IV access is not available.

It is important to note differences in recommended dosage intervals between these options, which reflect differences in their pharmacokinetics. Protocols should be followed for maternal monitoring of blood pressure every 5 to 15 minutes. None of the recommended drugs require cardiac monitoring.

Although all three medications are appropriately used for the treatment of hypertensive emergencies in pregnancy, each agent can be associated with adverse effects. Parenteral hydralazine may increase the risk of maternal hypotension (systolic BP 90 mm Hg or less). Parenteral labetalol may cause neonatal bradycardia and should be avoided in women with asthma, heart disease, or congestive heart failure. Nifedipine has been associated with an increase in maternal heart rate, and with overshoot hypotension (ACOG, 2017a). Extensive discussion of preeclampsia is in Chapter 7.

Management of Diabetes Postpartum

Diabetes is a complex disorder caused by various pathological mechanisms in the secretion of and/or response to insulin. The result is hyperglycemia, which in turn damages organ systems. Hyperglycemia during pregnancy affects 7% to 18% of all pregnant women (ACOG, 2013a). Diabetes can incur significant morbidity and mortality for the mother, fetus, and the newborn into adulthood. Diabetes in all forms is the most common metabolic disease complicating pregnancy and postpartum.

Diabetes, more than almost any other disease or condition, requires patient collaboration and partnership to ensure successful management and follow-up (AWHONN, 2016). Women with diabetes can provide the information about their food choices, activity, compliance with blood glucose (BG) monitoring, and medication administration that health care professionals need to make collaborative decisions about course and treatment. However, not all women are aware of the importance of this information. Further, many women with diabetes may lack understanding of their role and influence on BG management. Therefore, education and empowerment is critical from the outset, and appropriate postpartum follow-up is essential (AWHONN, 2016). Women with chronic medical conditions such as diabetes should be counseled regarding the importance of follow-up with their primary care provider in a timely fashion for ongoing coordination of care. It is important that women with diabetes be counseled that these disorders are associated with a higher lifetime risk of maternal cardiometabolic disease.

Pregestational Diabetes

Insulin requirements for the pregestational diabetic woman decrease in the immediate postpartum period. With oral intake, subcutaneous insulin doses can resume, typically at prepregnancy normal glucose tolerance postpartum doses (Daley, 2014). Women with diabetes are at higher risk for complications such as infection and should be closely monitored for mastitis, endometritis, and wound infections. Breastfeeding is highly encouraged. Benefits include a reduction in the risk of developing type 2 diabetes mellitus (T2DM) for women with gestational diabetes mellitus (GDM), especially with exclusive breastfeeding (avoid formula supplementation) and longer duration of lactation. Utilization of 500 kcal per day for lactation may lead to improved pregnancy weight loss.

Gestational Diabetes

Most women with gestational diabetes return to normal glucose tolerance postpartum (Daley, 2014). Although the carbohydrate intolerance of GDM frequently resolves after delivery, up to one-third of affected women will have diabetes or impaired glucose metabolism at postpartum screening, and it has been estimated that 15% to 50% will develop type 2 diabetes later in life (ACOG, 2013). Postpartum screening at 6 to 12 weeks is recommended for all women who had GDM to identify women with diabetes mellitus (DM), impaired fasting glucose levels, or impaired glucose tolerance. Follow-up is essential to ensure normal fasting glucose values.

Nursing Actions

The nurse must counsel women with a history of GDM that they have a sevenfold increased risk of developing type 2 diabetes compared with women with no GDM history (ACOG, 2013a). Counseling can be provided to women with a history of GDM to modify risk factors such as obesity with weight reduction and exercise. Women should also be informed they are at high risk for developing GDM with subsequent pregnancies. For women who may have subsequent pregnancies, more frequent screening can detect abnormal glucose metabolism before pregnancy and provides an opportunity to ensure preconception glucose control (ACOG, 2013a). Women should be encouraged to discuss their GDM history and need for screening with their health care providers.

Exercise or increased activity is recommended for women with a high risk of diabetes, such as those with a history of GDM. Exercise independent of weight loss has a role in preventing or delaying the development of overt diabetes, due to the resulting decrease in insulin resistance. Additionally, inactivity is a risk factor for the development of T2DM (AWHONN, 2016).

Explore challenges related to the prevention of overt diabetes. Strategies include:

- Assessing knowledge, risk perception, self-efficacy, current prevention behaviors, and intention to change behavior.
- Identifying barriers to health promoting behaviors and solutions to promote behavior change.
- Identifying social support (including family/support system) in education, counseling, and problem solving.

- Designing interventions that are individualized and easily accessible, such as phone counseling and computer-based education.
- Providing information about resources such as exercise classes and diet advice.
- Providing links as needed to dietitians, primary care providers, and mental health professionals to ensure ongoing support.
- Breastfeeding, which is strongly recommended after delivery for all women with pregestational diabetes mellitus or gestational diabetes mellitus.
- Schedule a follow-up appointment 2 to 6 weeks postdischarge with the provider who managed diabetes during pregnancy.

Maternal Obesity Postpartum

Mothers who are obese are at risk for complications postpartum regardless of method of birth, including increased incidence of infection and wound complications. Maternal obesity, defined by a body mass index (BMI) of 30 or higher, has long been recognized as a risk factor in pregnancy. Being overweight or obese during pregnancy is associated with many adverse outcomes, including miscarriage, impaired glucose tolerance, and sleep apnea (Opray, Grivell, Deussen, & Dodd, 2015). Obesity during pregnancy increases the risk of morbidity and mortality for both the mother and baby and is a well-established risk factor for the development of comorbid conditions such as preeclampsia, gestational and type 2 diabetes, and thrombosis (ACOG, 2015b). Obesity-related complications during pregnancy are associated with future metabolic dysfunction in these women. Forty-six percent of obese pregnant women have gestational weight gain that exceeds the Institute of Medicine pregnancy weight gain guidelines. Excess gestational weight gain is a significant risk factor for postpartum weight retention. This further increases the risk of metabolic dysfunction and pregravid obesity in future pregnancies. Pregravid obesity is associated with early termination of breastfeeding, postpartum anemia, and depression (ACOG, 2015b). Obesity is a risk factor for venous thromboembolism in the general medical population.

For prevention of venous thromboembolism in very-high-risk groups, pharmacological thromboprophylaxis should be considered in addition to pneumatic compression devices.

Nursing Actions

- Precisely assess the uterus. Tone and lochia may be difficult due to maternal size (Maher, 2014).
- Measure and record height and weight of woman and calculate BMI.
- Reinforce information on maternal complications postpartum and postop associated with obesity.
- Because postpartum presents an ideal time during which to initiate simple healthy behaviors, such as walking and proper diet that can be maintained after birth, offer suggestions and encouragement for lifestyle changes.
- Provide referrals to dietitian for nutritional counseling and reinforce guidelines for diet and weight loss (Cunningham et al., 2014). Interpregnancy weight loss in women who are obese may decrease the risk of a large-for-gestational-age neonate in a subsequent pregnancy. Behavioral interventions employing diet and exercise can improve postpartum weight reduction in contrast to exercise alone.
- Women who are obese may need additional support breastfeeding.
- Encouraging the woman to sleep in a sitting position may help, as effects of obesity on the respiratory system are decreased in this position.
- Making appropriate environmental changes to accommodate the larger patient, such as assuring that patient beds, and chairs can support at least 400 pounds.

POSTPARTUM FOLLOW-UP

At discharge from maternity care, the woman should receive contact information for her postpartum care team and written instructions regarding the timing of follow-up postpartum care. Women are recommended to have a comprehensive postpartum visit within the first 6 weeks after birth. This visit will include a full assessment of physical, social, and psychological well-being and a discussion of the desired form of contraception. At the conclusion of the postpartum visit, the woman and her provider determine who will assume primary responsibility for her ongoing care. If responsibility is transferred to another primary care provider, the obstetric care provider is responsible for ensuring that there is communication with the primary care provider so that he or she can understand the implications of any pregnancy complications for the woman's future health and maintain continuity of care. Postpartum patients and their families are instructed to call the health care provider if the woman experiences any of the following:

- Fever
- Foul-smelling lochia
- Large blood clots (golf ball–sized or bigger) or bleeding that saturates a pad in 1 hour
- Discharge, erythema, or severe pain from incisions or stitched areas
- Hot, red, painful areas on the breasts or legs
- Bleeding and/or severe pain in the nipples or breasts
- Severe headaches and/or blurred vision
- Chest pain and/or dyspnea without exertion
- Frequent, painful urination
- Signs of depression

A postpartum care plan should be reviewed, updated, and discussed with women after the birth. Women are often uncertain about whom to contact for postpartum concerns. Up to one in four postpartum women did not have a phone number for a health care provider to contact for concerns about themselves or their infants (ACOG, 2016a). The care plan includes contact information and written instructions on the timing of follow-up postpartum care. Just as a health care professional or health care practice leads the woman's care during pregnancy, a primary maternal care provider should assume responsibility for her postpartum care.

The comprehensive postpartum visit is typically scheduled between 4 and 6 weeks after delivery. However, there is considerable variation in recommendations for timing of postpartum visits. Early follow-up is recommended for women with hypertensive disorders of pregnancy, with blood pressure evaluation no later than 7 to 10 days postpartum; other experts have recommended follow-up at 3 to 5 days. Early follow-up also may be beneficial for women at high risk of complications, such as postpartum depression, cesarean or perineal wound infection, lactation difficulties, or chronic conditions (ACOG, 2016a). These visits, which in some cases may be conducted through home nursing evaluations, are essential for follow-up.

The postpartum visit provides an opportunity for women to ask questions about their labor, childbirth, and complications. Complications should be discussed with respect to risks for future pregnancies, and recommendations should be made to optimize maternal health during the interconception period. It is important that women with gestational diabetes, hypertensive disorders of pregnancy, or preterm birth be counseled that these disorders are associated with a higher lifetime risk of maternal cardiometabolic disease (ACOG, 2016a).

POSTPARTUM PSYCHOLOGICAL COMPLICATIONS

A women's psychological state is affected during the postpartum period by hormonal changes, lack of sleep, and the stress of integrating a new person into the woman's life and the family unit. Most women experience postpartum blues, which are short-term and require no medical intervention (see Chapter 13). Approximately 15% of women will experience major mood disorders that have a profound effect on their ability to care for themselves and/or their infants. Mood disorders during the first year after childbirth have a negative effect on the mother–infant relationship (Milgrom & Holt, 2014). Two major mood disorders are postpartum depression and postpartum psychosis. These disorders require management by mental health professionals.

Perinatal mood and anxiety disorders are among the most common mental health conditions encountered by women of reproductive age. When left untreated, perinatal mood and anxiety disorders can have profound adverse effects on women and their children, ranging from increased risk of poor adherence to medical care, exacerbation of medical conditions, loss of interpersonal and financial resources, smoking and substance use, suicide, and infanticide. Perinatal mood and anxiety disorders are associated with increased risks of maternal and infant mortality and morbidity and are recognized as a significant patient safety issue. In 2015, the Council on Patient Safety in Women's Health Care convened an interdisciplinary workgroup to develop an evidence-based patient safety bundle to address maternal mental health. The focus of this bundle is perinatal mood and anxiety disorders (Box 14–4). The bundle is modeled after other bundles released by the Council on Patient Safety in Women's Health Care and provides broad direction for incorporating perinatal mood and anxiety disorder screening, intervention, referral, and

follow-up into maternity care practice across health care settings (Kendig et al., 2017).

The primary role of the perinatal nurse is assessing for early signs of potential mood disorders and reporting these findings to the woman's health care provider for further evaluation and treatment. Assessing for postpartum mood disorders and anxiety disorders should be included in the nurse's postpartum assessments.

BOX 14–4 | Maternal Safety Bundle: Depression and Anxiety

Maternal Mental Health: Perinatal Depression and Anxiety Patient Safety Bundle, Council on Patient Safety in Women's Health Care

Perinatal mood and anxiety disorders in their most severe forms can be tragic and preventable causes of maternal and infant mortality. Perinatal mood and anxiety disorders and their sequelae can be addressed by actively screening women, having a plan in place for treatment or referral for those who screen positive, and actively engaging women, their families, and supporters in recognizing symptoms and seeking help in a timely manner. Everyone must work together to remove the stigma that still surrounds mental health disorders. The elements of the bundle are general so that they can be adapted for a variety of settings. The purpose is to provide a consistent approach to recognition and treatment of perinatal mood and anxiety disorders.

Readiness (Every Clinical Care Setting)

- Identify mental health screening tools to be made available in every clinical setting (outpatient obstetric clinics and inpatient facilities).

- Establish a response protocol and identify screening tools for use based on local resources.

- Educate clinicians and office staff on use of the identified screening tools and response protocol.

- Identify an individual who is responsible for driving adoption of the identified screening tools and response protocol.

Recognition and Prevention (Every Woman)

- Obtain individual and family mental health history (including past and current medications) at intake, with review and updates as needed.

- Conduct validated mental health screening during appropriately timed patient encounters, to include both during pregnancy and in the postpartum period.

- Provide appropriately timed perinatal depression and anxiety awareness education to women and family members or other support persons.

Response (Every Case)

- Initiate a stage-based response protocol for a positive mental health screening result.

- Activate an emergency referral protocol for women with suicidal or homicidal ideation or psychosis.

- Provide appropriate and timely support for women as well as family members and staff as needed.
- Obtain follow-up from mental health care providers on women referred for treatment (this should include release of information forms).

Reporting and Systems Learning (Every Clinical Care Setting).
- Establish a nonjudgmental culture of safety through multidisciplinary mental health rounds.
- Perform a multidisciplinary review of adverse mental health outcomes.
- Establish local standards for recognition and response to measure compliance, understand individual performance, and track outcomes.

ACOG, 2016b.

Evidence-Based Practice: Postpartum Depression

Dennis, C., & Dowswell, T. (2013). Psychosocial and psychological interventions for preventing postpartum depression. *Cochrane Database of Systematic Reviews, 2*. Art. No.: CD001134. doi:10.1002/14651858.CD00134.pub3.

This systemic review aimed to assess the effect of diverse psychosocial and psychological interventions compared with usual antepartum, intrapartum, or postpartum care. Twenty-eight randomized controlled research studies involving a total of 17,000 women were included in the review.

Results:
Women who received a psychosocial or psychological intervention were significantly less likely to develop postpartum depression compared to women who received standard care. Beneficial interventions were:

- Professionally based postpartum home visits.
- Lay- or peer-based postpartum telephone support.
- Interpersonal psychotherapy.
- Those provided by various health professionals and lay individuals and were similarly beneficial.
- Those specifically targeted at "at-risk" mothers.

Authors' conclusions:
Psychosocial and psychological interventions significantly reduce the number of women who develop postpartum depression. Beneficial interventions include professionally based postpartum home visits, telephone-based peer support, and interpersonal psychotherapy.

Postpartum Depression

Depression, the most common mood disorder in the general population, is approximately twice as common in women as in men, with its initial onset peaking during the reproductive years (ACOG, 2015c). Perinatal depression, which includes major and minor depressive episodes that occur during pregnancy or in the first 12 months after delivery, is one of the most common medical complications during pregnancy and the postpartum period,

affecting one in seven women (ACOG, 2015c). Perinatal depression and other mood disorders, such as bipolar disorder and anxiety disorders, can have devastating effects on women, infants, and families. In fact, maternal suicide exceeds hemorrhage and hypertensive disorders as a cause of maternal mortality. Perinatal depression often goes unrecognized because changes in sleep, appetite, and libido may be attributed to normal pregnancy and postpartum changes. In addition to clinicians not recognizing such symptoms, women may be reluctant to report changes in their mood (ACOG, 2015b). Data indicates that fewer than 20% of women in whom postpartum depression was diagnosed had reported their symptoms to a health care provider. Therefore, it is important for clinicians to ask the pregnant or postpartum patient about her mood.

Postpartum depression (PPD) is a mood disorder characterized by severe depression that occurs within the first 6 to 12 months postpartum and affects an estimated 11.5% of postpartum women (Ko, Rockhill, Tong, Morrow, & Farr, 2017). PPD affects the woman, her partner, and other children within the family unit. Women who receive proper treatment will recover from PPD, but they grieve over the lost time with their infants (AWHONN, 2006). A major difference between postpartum blues and PPD is that PPD is disabling; the woman is unable to safely care for herself and/or her baby (Table 14–2).

PPD is classified as a major depressive disorder when the woman has a depressed mood or a loss of interest or pleasure in daily activities for at least 2 weeks in addition to four of the following symptoms:

- Significant weight loss or gain: a change of more than 5% of body weight in a month
- Insomnia or hypersomnia
- Changes in psychomotor activity: agitation or retardation
- Decreased energy or fatigue
- Feelings of worthlessness or guilt
- Decreased ability to concentrate; inability to make decisions

Risk Factors

- History of depression before pregnancy
- Depression or anxiety during pregnancy
- Inadequate social support
- Poor quality relationship with partner
- Life and child care stresses
- Complications of pregnancy and/or childbirth
- Single
- Low socioeconomic status

Assessment Findings

- Sleep and appetite disturbance
- Fatigue greater than expected when caring for a newborn
- Despondency
- Uncontrolled crying
- Anxiety, fear, and/or panic
- Inability to concentrate
- Feelings of guilt, inadequacy, and/or worthlessness
- Inability to care for self and/or baby
- Decreased affectionate contact with the infant

TABLE 14–2   Major Differences Between Postpartum Blues and Postpartum Depression

POSTPARTUM BLUES	POSTPARTUM DEPRESSION
Symptoms disappear without medical intervention.	Requires psychiatric interventions.
Occurs within the first 2 weeks postpartum.	Occurs within the first 12 months postpartum.
Able to safely care for self and baby.	Unable to safely care for self and/or baby.

- Decreased responsiveness to the infant
- Thoughts of harming baby
- Thoughts of suicide

Medical/Psychiatric Management

- Mild PPD
  - Interpersonal psychotherapy (Yonkers, Vigod, & Ross, 2011)
- Moderate PPD
  - Interpersonal psychotherapy
  - Antidepressants (Yonkers, Vigod, & Ross, 2011).
- Severe PPD or suicidal ideation
  - Intense psychiatric care
  - Crisis interventions
  - Interpersonal psychotherapy
  - Antidepressants
  - Electroconvulsive therapy (Yonkers, Vigod, & Ross, 2011)

Nursing Actions

- Review prenatal record for risk factors.
- Monitor mother–infant interactions more closely for women at risk for PPD.
- Anticipatory guidance: Teach the woman and her partner signs of PPD that should be reported to her health care provider.
- Be supportive and encouraging in interactions.
- Provide the woman with information regarding postpartum support groups and other community resources to assist her with parenting issues and to provide support.
- Postpartum support by health care professionals can mitigate the onset of postpartum mood disorders (Yonkers, Vigod, & Ross, 2011).

Postpartum Psychosis

Postpartum psychosis (PPP), a variant of bipolar disorder, is the most serious type of postpartum mood disorder. Postpartum psychosis is relatively rare, with prevalence in the general population of 0.1% to 2.6% per 1,000 births (Jones, Chandra, Dazzan, & Howard, 2014; VanderKruik et al., 2017). The onset of symptoms is rapid and can occur as early as 2 to 3 days after childbirth. The patient develops frank psychosis, cognitive impairment, and grossly disorganized behavior that represents a complete change from previous functioning. Hormonal shifts, obstetrical complications, sleep deprivation, and increased environmental stress can all contribute to the onset of

symptoms (Sit, Rotherschild, & Wisner, 2006). Women with PPP require immediate hospitalization and evaluation, as they are at risk for injuring themselves or their infants. The rapid and accurate diagnosis of postpartum psychosis is essential to expedite appropriate treatment and to allow for quick, full recovery, prevention of future episodes, and reduction of risk to the mother and her children and family (Sit, Rotherschild & Wisner, 2006).

Risk Factors

- Women with known bipolar disorder
- Personal or family history of bipolar disorder or affective disorder (Jones et al., 2014).

Assessment Findings

- Paranoia, grandiose or bizarre delusions, usually associated with the baby
- Mood swings
- Extreme agitation
- Depressed or elated moods
- Distraught feelings about ability to enjoy infant
- Confused thinking
- Strange beliefs, such as that she or her infant must die
- Disorganized behavior (Engqvist, Ferszt, Ahlin, & Nilsson, 2009; Sit et al., 2006)

Medical/Psychiatric Management

- Hospitalization to the psychiatric unit
- Psychiatric evaluation
- Antidepressant and antipsychotic drug treatment
- Psychotherapy
- Electroconvulsive therapy

Nursing Actions

AWHONN recommends that health care facilities caring for childbearing women provide education to professional nurses on the symptoms of postpartum depressive disorders. Patients should be screened for this potentially disabling condition. In addition, nurses should be aware of the treatment options for women suffering from postpartum depressive disorders so these patients can obtain treatment as early as possible when the condition occurs (AWHONN, 2008).

- Review the prenatal record for risk factors or psych history, including affective disorders or bipolar disorder.

- Educate women who are at risk and their support system of early signs of PPP, such as mood swings, hallucinations, and strange beliefs, and instruct them to contact the health care provider if symptoms are present.
- Early detection and treatment can prevent a major episode (Wesseloo et al., 2016).

Paternal Postnatal Depression

Most new fathers experience feelings of happiness and excitement, but some experience depression. Paternal postnatal depression (PPND) is estimated to occur in 1% to 8% of new fathers during the first 6 months following childbirth. During the first few months postpartum, the man's testosterone levels decrease and estrogen levels increase. Lower levels of testosterone are linked with depression in men. PPND can have a negative effect on the couple's relationship and on the father–child relationship, and it can have a long-term negative effect on the mental well-being of the child (Melrose, 2010). Signs and symptoms of PPND are not as apparent as they are with maternal PPD.

CRITICAL COMPONENT

Paternal Postnatal Depression

PPND often goes undiagnosed and untreated for the following reasons:

- The man or health care provider fails to recognize signs and symptoms of PPND
- Lack of guidelines for assessing and treating PPND
- The man downplaying the degree to which the symptoms affect his life and relationships
- The man's reluctance to discuss his depression symptoms with friends, family, or health care professionals
- The man resisting mental health treatment; worried about stigma of depression
- Few existing programs that address PPND

Signs and Symptoms

- The man may withdraw from social interactions.
- The man may be cynical in his interactions and experience irritable moods.
- The man may demonstrate avoidance behaviors such as spending more time away from the family.
- The man's affect may appear to be anxious or mad versus sad.

Risk Factors

- Maternal PPD is the primary risk factor.
- Depressive symptoms during partner's pregnancy

- Unplanned and/or unexpected pregnancy
- Baby with health or feeding problems
- Lack of social support
- Excessive stress about becoming a father
- Preexisting mental health disorder
- Stressful life event (e.g., death of his parent)

Assessment Findings

- Irritable
- Overwhelmed
- Frustrated
- Indecisive
- Avoidance of social situations
- Cynical
- Increased alcohol consumption
- Drug use
- Domestic violence

Medical Management

- Interpersonal psychotherapy
- Antidepressant medications

Nursing Actions

- Provide information on PPND to the man and his partner.
- Stress the importance of seeking professional help if he is experiencing symptoms of PPND.
  - Explain that PPND can have negative long-term effects on his child.

Evidence-Based Practice: Parental Psychological Health

Barlow, J., Smailagic, N., Huband, N., Roloff, V. & Bennett, C. (2014). Group-based parent training programs for improving parental psychosocial health. *Cochrane Database of Systematic Review, 5.* Art. No.: CD002020. doi: 10.1002/14651858.CD002020.pun4.

The aim of this systematic review was to address whether group-based programs are effective in improving parental psychosocial well-being. The review included 48 studies that involved 4,937 participants.

Results:

- Group-based programs led to statistically significant short-term improvements in depression, anxiety, stress, anger, guilt, confidence, and satisfaction with relationship partner.
- At 6 months, only stress and confidence continued to be significant.
- At 1 year, none of the measures were significant.

Authors' conclusions:
The findings of the review support the use of parenting program to improve the short-term psychosocial well-being of parents.

CONCEPT MAP |

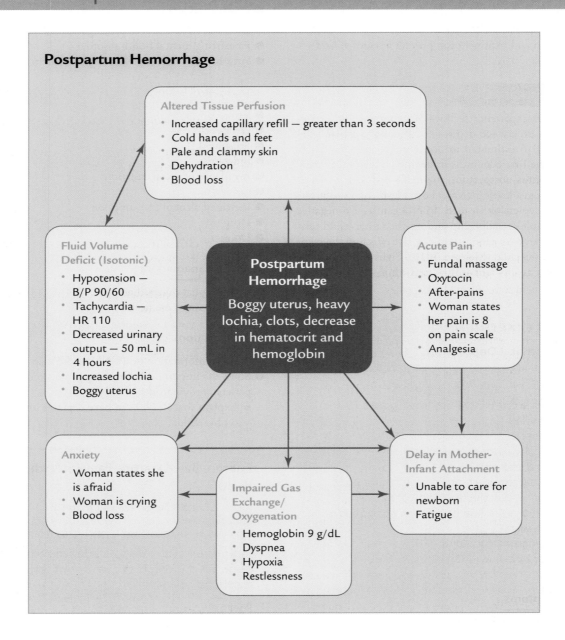

Postpartum Hemorrhage

Altered Tissue Perfusion
- Increased capillary refill — greater than 3 seconds
- Cold hands and feet
- Pale and clammy skin
- Dehydration
- Blood loss

Fluid Volume Deficit (Isotonic)
- Hypotension — B/P 90/60
- Tachycardia — HR 110
- Decreased urinary output — 50 mL in 4 hours
- Increased lochia
- Boggy uterus

Postpartum Hemorrhage
Boggy uterus, heavy lochia, clots, decrease in hematocrit and hemoglobin

Acute Pain
- Fundal massage
- Oxytocin
- After-pains
- Woman states her pain is 8 on pain scale
- Analgesia

Anxiety
- Woman states she is afraid
- Woman is crying
- Blood loss

Impaired Gas Exchange/ Oxygenation
- Hemoglobin 9 g/dL
- Dyspnea
- Hypoxia
- Restlessness

Delay in Mother-Infant Attachment
- Unable to care for newborn
- Fatigue

Problem No. 1: Fluid volume deficit (isotonic)

Goal: Increase fluid volume

Outcome: The woman's blood pressure and heart rate will be within normal ranges, and intake and output will be within 200 mL of each other by the end of the shift.

Nursing Actions

1. Assess fundus for firmness: massage if boggy.
2. Assess lochia for amount, color, and clots.
3. Instruct and remind the woman to drink lots of fluids.
4. Initiate IV therapy as ordered.
5. Initiate oxytocin therapy as ordered.
6. Assess intake and output.

7. Assist the woman to the bathroom every 3 to 4 hours.
8. Monitor blood pressure and pulse every 2 hours.
9. Assess skin turgor and mucous membranes every 4 hours.

Problem No. 2: Altered tissue perfusion

Goal: Normal tissue perfusion

Outcome: Blood pressure and pulse within normal limits; capillary fill less than 3 seconds.

Nursing Actions

1. Every 2 hours, monitor vital signs, capillary refill, and motor and sensory status.

2. Compare post-hemorrhage Hgb/Hct with results on admission to labor.
3. Administer oxygen as per orders and monitor oxygen saturation levels.

Problem No. 3: Anxiety
Goal: Decreased anxiety
Outcome: The woman verbalizes that she feels less anxious.

Nursing Actions
1. Be calm and reassuring in interactions with the woman and her family.
2. Explain all procedures.
3. Teach the woman relaxation breathing techniques.
4. Encourage the woman and family to verbalize their feelings regarding recent hemorrhage by asking open-ended questions.

Problem No. 4: Delay in mother–infant attachment
Goal: Positive mother–infant attachment
Outcome: The woman will hold the infant close, respond to the infant's needs, and state she enjoys her baby.

Nursing Actions
1. Encourage rooming in.
2. Assist the woman with infant care as needed.
3. Encourage holding of infant by assisting the woman into a comfortable position and placing the infant in her arms.
4. Praise the woman for positive mother–infant interactions.
5. Provide information on infant care.

Problem No. 5: Acute pain
Goal: Decreased pain
Outcome: The woman will state that pain is within her chosen numerical level on pain scale.

Nursing Actions
1. Assess level, location, and type of pain.
2. Prevent overdistention of the bladder by reminding the woman to void every 3 to 4 hours.
3. Administer pain medications based on assessment data as ordered.
4. Provide an environment that is conducive to relaxation, such as low lights, decreased noise, and uninterrupted rest periods.
5. Teach the woman relaxation techniques.

Problem No. 6: Impaired gas exchange/oxygenation
Goal: Maintain oxygenation
Outcome: Oxygen saturation is 98% and respiratory rate and pattern are within normal limits.

Nursing Actions
1. Monitor respirations, breath sounds, and oxygen saturation.
2. Provide oxygen by mask as ordered.
3. Instruct and assist the woman with deep breathing and coughing to decrease the risk of pneumonia.
4. Initiate iron replacement therapy as ordered.
5. Provide nutritional information on foods high in iron such as green leafy vegetables.

Case Study

You are a nurse working in the postpartum unit. You are assigned Mallory Polk, a 42-year-old African American woman. (Refer to the Case Study in Chapters 7 and 10 for antepartum and intrapartum data.)

Summary of Labor and Delivery Record
Mallory was admitted 2 days ago at 31 weeks' gestation for preterm labor. She was given magnesium sulfate to delay delivery and provide fetal neuroprotection, and received two doses of betamethasone for lung maturity. She spontaneously delivered a 1,559-gram boy with Apgar scores of 5/7 at 1 and 5 minutes, respectively. Her baby is experiencing mild signs of respiratory distress and is in the NICU.

Postpartum Report
Mallory is 4 hours postbirth and has an IV of 500 mL lactated Ringer's solution with 30 units of oxytocin running at 100 mL/min in her left arm. She voided in the recovery unit 2 hours after birth.

Assessment Findings
Vital signs: Temperature 98.6°F (37°C); pulse 106 bpm; respirations 14 breaths/min; BP 110/70 mm Hg
Fundus is at the umbilicus and boggy.
Lochia is heavy.

Based on your assessment findings and Mallory's history, what are your immediate nursing actions?

Discuss the rationale for your nursing actions.

You reevaluate Mallory 10 minutes after your initial nursing actions. Her fundus is firm, midline, and 1 finger breadth below the umbilicus with scant lochia. You continue to monitor Mallory and 15 minutes later her fundus is boggy with heavy lochia. The fundus becomes firm after massage. You increase the rate of oxytocin to 150 mL/min. Her pulse is 118 bpm and blood pressure is 100/60 mm Hg. You notify her CNM and report your findings.

Detail the aspects of your assessment findings that you will report to the CNM.

The CNM orders an injection of methergine 0.2 mg IM now.

Discuss your nursing actions and rationale for actions.

Discuss the assessment data needed to determine effectiveness of medical and nursing actions.

You note that in her prenatal chart she has a diagnosis of fibroids.

Discuss the implications of the diagnosis as it relates to your nursing care and discharge teaching plan.

REFERENCES

American Academy of Pediatrics and the American College of Obstetricians and Gynecologists. (2012). *Guidelines for Perinatal Care* (7th ed.). Elk Grove Village, IL: Author.

American College of Obstetricians and Gynecologists (ACOG). (2011). Thromboembolism in Pregnancy. Practice Bulletin No. 123. *Obstetrics & Gynecology, 118*(3), 718–729. doi:10.1097/AOG.0b013e3182310c4c

American College of Obstetricians and Gynecologists (ACOG). (2013a). Gestational diabetes mellitus. Practice Bulletin No. 137. *Obstetrics & Gynecology, 122,* 406–416.

American College of Obstetricians and Gynecologists (ACOG). (2013b). Postpartum hemorrhage from vaginal delivery. Patient Safety Checklist Number 10. Retrieved from https://www.acog.org/Clinical-Guidance-and-Publications/Patient-Safety-Checklists-List

American College of Obstetricians and Gynecologists (ACOG). (2014). Safe prevention of the primary cesarean delivery. Obstetric Care Consensus No. 1. *Obstetrics & Gynecology, 123,* 693–711.

American Congress of Obstetricians and Gynecologists (ACOG). (2015a). Maternal Safety Bundle Obstetric Hemorrhage. Safe Motherhood Initiative. Author. Washington, D.C.

American College of Obstetricians and Gynecologists (ACOG). (2015b). Obesity in pregnancy. Practice Bulletin No. 156 *Obstetrics & Gynecology, 126,* 112–126.

American College of Obstetricians and Gynecologists (ACOG). (2015c). Screening for perinatal depression. Committee Opinion No. 630. *Obstetrics & Gynecology, 125,* 1268–1271.

American College of Obstetricians and Gynecologists (ACOG). (2016a). Optimizing postpartum care. Committee Opinion No. 666. *Obstetrics & Gynecology, 127,* 187–192.

American College of Obstetricians and Gynecologists (ACOG). (2016b). Patient safety bundle: Maternal mental health: Perinatal depression and anxiety. Retrieved from http://safehealthcareforeverywoman.org/patient-safety-bundles/maternal-mental-health-depression-and-anxiety/.

American College of Obstetricians and Gynecologists (ACOG). (2017a). Emergent therapy for acute-onset, severe hypertension during pregnancy and the postpartum period. Committee Opinion No. 692. *Obstetrics & Gynecology, 129,* e90–95.

American College of Obstetricians and Gynecologists (ACOG). (2017b). Postpartum hemorrhage. Practice Bulletin. *Obstetrics & Gynecology, 108,* 1039–1046.

Association of Women's Health, Obstetric and Neonatal Nursing (AWHONN). (2008). The role of the nurse in postpartum mood and anxiety disorders. Washington, DC: Author.

Association of Women's Health, Obstetric and Neonatal Nurses (AWHONN). (2011). AWHONN position statement: Health information technology for the perinatal setting. *JOGNN, 40,* 383–385.

Association of Women's Health, Obstetric and Neonatal Nurses (AWHONN). (2013). Postpartum Hemorrhage Project: A multi-hospital quality improvement program. https://cdn.ymaws.com/www.awhonn.org/resource/resmgr/PDFs/PPH/PPHPoster.pdf

Association of Women's Health, Obstetric and Neonatal Nurses (AWHONN). (2014a). Guidelines for oxytocin administration after birth: Practice Brief No. 2. *Journal of Obstetric, Gynecologic, & Neonatal Nursing, 44,* 161–164. doi:10.1111/1552-6909.12528

Association of Women's Health, Obstetric and Neonatal Nurses (AWHONN). (2014b). Quantification of Blood Loss: AWHONN Practice Brief No. 1. *Journal of Obstetric, Gynecologic, & Neonatal Nursing, 44,* 158–160. doi:10.1111/1552-6909.12519.

Association of Women's Health, Obstetric and Neonatal Nurses (AWHONN). (2016). The nursing care of the woman with diabetes in pregnancy evidence-based clinical practice guideline. Evidence-Based Clinical Practice Guideline Development Team.

Barlow, J., Smailagic, N., Huband, N., Roloff, V. & Bennett, C. (2014). Group-based parent training programs for improving parental psychosocial health. *Cochrane Database of Systematic Review, 5.* Art. No.: CD002020. doi: 10.1002/14651858.CD002020.pun4.

Callaghan, W. M., Creanga, A. A., & Kuklina, E. V. (2012). Severe maternal morbidity among delivery and postpartum hospitalizations in the United States. *Obstetrics & Gynecology, 120*(5), 1029–1036. doi:10.1097/AOG.0b013e31826d60c5

Centers for Disease Control (CDC). (2017). Maternal mortality surveillance system. Retrieved from www.cdc.gov/reproductivehealth/maternalinfanthealth/pmss.html.

Cunningham, E., Leveno, K., Bloom, S., Spong, C., Dashe, J., Hoffman, B., . . . Sheffield, J. (2014). *Williams obstetrics* (24th ed.). New York, NY: McGraw-Hill.

Daley, J. (2014). Diabetes in pregnancy. In K. Simpson & P. Creehan (Eds.), *Perinatal nursing* (4th ed.). Philadelphia, PA: Lippincott, Williams & Wilkins.

Dennis, C., & Dowswell, T. (2013). Psychosocial and psychological interventions for preventing postpartum depression. *Cochrane Database of Systematic Reviews, 2.* Art. No.: CD001134. doi:10.1002/14651858.CD00134.pub3.

Engqvist, I., Ferszt, G., Ahlin, A., & Nilsson, K. (2009). Psychiatric nurses' descriptions of women with postpartum psychosis and nurses' response—an exploratory study in Sweden. *Issues in Mental Health Nursing, 30,* 23–30.

Harvey, C., & Dildy, G. (2012). Obstetric hemorrhage. AWHONN Monograph. Association of Women's Health Obstetrics and Neonatal Nursing, Washington, D.C.

James, D. (2014). Postpartum care. In K. Simpson & P. Creehan (Eds.), *Perinatal nursing* (4th ed., pp. 473–520). Philadelphia, PA: Wolters Kluwer/Lippincott, Williams & Wilkins.

Jones, I., Chandra, P. S., Dazzan, P., & Howard, L. M. (2014). Bipolar disorder, affective psychosis, and schizophrenia in pregnancy and the post-partum period. *Lancet, 384*(9956), 1789–1799. doi:10.1016/S0140-6736(14)61278-2

Jones, R., & Clark, S. (2013). Amniotic fluid embolus. In N. Troiano, C. Harvey, & B. Chez. *High risk and critical care obstetrics* (3rd ed., pp. 316–325). Philadelphia, PA: Wolters Kluwer/Lippincott, Williams & Wilkins.

Kendig, S., et al. (2017). Consensus bundle on maternal mental health: Perinatal depression and anxiety. *Journal of Obstetric, Gynecologic & Neonatal Nursing, 46*(2), 272–281.

Ko, J. Y., Rockhill, K. M., Tong, V. T., Morrow, B., & Farr, S. L. (2017). Trends in postpartum depressive symptoms—27 states, 2004, 2008, and 2012. *MMWR Morbidity and Mortality Weekly Report, 66,*153–158. http://dx.doi.org/10.15585/mmwr.mm6606a1

Lyndon, A., Lagrew, D., Shields, L., Main, E., & Cape, V. (2015). Improving health care response to obstetric hemorrhage. California Maternal Quality Care Collaborative Toolkit to Transform Maternity Care. Published by the California Maternal Quality Care Collaborative.

Lyndon, A., Zlatnik, M. G., Maxfield, D. G., Lewis, A., McMillan, C., & Kennedy, H. P. (2014). Contributions of clinical disconnections and unresolved conflict to failures in intrapartum safety. *Journal of Obstetric, Gynecologic & Neonatal Nursing, 43*(1), 2–12. doi:10.1111/1552-6909.12266.

Maher, M. A. (2014). Obesity in pregnancy. In K. Simpson & P. Creehan (Eds.), *Perinatal nursing* (4th ed.). Philadelphia, PA: Lippincott, Williams & Wilkins.

Main, E. K., Goffman, D., Scavone, B. M., Low, L. K., Bingham, D. Fontaine, P. L., . . . Levy, B. S. (2015). National partnership for maternal safety: Consensus bundle on obstetric hemorrhage. *Journal of Obstetric, Gynecologic & Neonatal Nursing, 44,* 462–470. doi:10.1111/1552-6909.127

McGovern, B., Bingham, D., & Dildy, G. A., 3rd. (2019). Obstetric hemorrhage. In N. H. Troiano, P. M. Witcher, & S. McMurtry Baird (Eds.), *High-risk & critical care obstetrics* (4th ed., pp. 258–285). Philadelphia, PA: Wolters Kluwer.

Melrose, S. (2010). Parental postpartum depression: How can nurses help? *Contemporary Nurse, 34,* 199–210.

Milgrom, J., & Holt, C. (2014). Early intervention to protect the mother-infant relationship following postnatal depression: Study protocol for a randomised controlled trial. *Trials, 15,* 385. doi:10.1186/1745-6215-15-385

Opray, N., Grivell, R. M., Deussen, A. R., & Dodd, J. M. (2015). Directed preconception health programs and interventions for improving pregnancy outcomes for women who are overweight or obese. *Cochrane Database of Systematic Reviews, 7.* Art. No.: CD010932. doi:10.1002/14651858.CD010932.pub2.

Sisson, M., & Mann, M. (2013). Disseminated intravascular coagulation in pregnancy. In N. Troiano, C. Harvey, & B. Chez (Eds.). *High risk and critical care obstetrics* (3rd ed.). Philadelphia, PA: Wolters Kluwer/Lippincott, Williams & Wilkins.

Sit, K., Rotherschild, A., & Wisner, K. (2006). A review of postpartum psychosis. *Journal of Women's Health, 15,* 352–368.

Vallerand, A., Sanoski, C., & Deglin, J. (2017). *Davis's drug guide for nurses* (15th ed.). Philadelphia, PA: F.A. Davis.

VanderKruik, R., Barreix, M., Chou, D., Allen, T., Say, L., Cohen, L., and on behalf of the Maternal Morbidity Working Group (2017). *BMC Psychiatry* 17:272. doi:10.1186/s12888-017-1427-7

Wambach, K., & Riordan, J. (2016). Breast related problems. In *Breastfeeding and human lactation* (5th ed., pp. 319–356). Burlington, MA: Jones & Bartlett Publishers.

Wesseloo, R., Kamperman, A. M., Munk-Olsen, T., Pop, V. J. M., Kushner, S. A., & Bergink, V. (2016). Risk of postpartum relapse in bipolar disorder and postpartum psychosis: A systematic review and meta-analysis. *American Journal of Psychiatry, 173*(2), 117–127. doi.org/10.1176/appi.ajp.2015.15010124

Wong, A. (2017). Pregnancy, postpartum infections. *eMedicine.* Retrieved from: http://emedicine.medscape.com/article/796892-overview.

World Health Organization. (2012). WHO recommendations for the prevention and treatment of postpartum haemorrhage. Retrieved from www.who.int/reproductivehealth/publications/maternal_perinatal_health/9789241548502/en/index.html.

Yonkers, K., Vigod, S., & Ross, L. (2011). Diagnosis, pathophysiology, and management of mood disorders in pregnancy and postpartum women. *Obstetrics & Gynecology, 117,* 961–977.

The Neonatal Period

Physiological and Behavioral Responses of the Neonate

15

Linda Chapman, RN, PhD

LEARNING OUTCOMES

Upon completion of this chapter, the student will be able to:

1. Identify the changes that occur during the transition from intrauterine to extrauterine life and the related nursing actions.
2. List the critical elements of neonatal assessment.
3. List the critical elements of neonatal gestational age assessments.
4. Discuss methods used in neonatal pain management.
5. Describe the nursing care for neonates during the first week of life.
6. Describe the common laboratory and diagnostic tests for neonates.
7. Discuss the nursing actions that support parents in the care of their newborn.
8. Describe the most common therapeutic and surgical procedures used for neonates and the related nursing care.
9. Discuss the importance of incorporating knowledge of cultural beliefs, customs, and newborn variations in the care of the parents and newborn.

Nursing Diagnoses

- At risk for altered body temperature related to decreased amounts of subcutaneous fat and/or large body surface
- At risk for infections related to tissue trauma and/or poor hand-washing techniques by health care providers and parents
- At risk for impaired gas exchange related to transitioning from fetal to neonatal circulation, cold stress, and/or excessive mucus production
- At risk for fluid volume deficit related to limited oral intake
- At risk for knowledge deficit related to first-time parenting and/or limited learning resources

Nursing Outcomes

- The neonate's temperature will be within normal limits, and the skin will be pink and feel warm to the touch.
- The neonate will not exhibit signs or symptoms of an infection.
- The neonate's respiratory rate and heart rate will be within normal ranges and the airway will remain clear.
- The neonate will void six times daily.
- Parents will respond to their newborn's needs.

INTRODUCTION

The neonatal period is from birth through the first 28 days of life. During these few weeks, the neonate transitions from intrauterine to extrauterine life and adapts to a new environment. Most neonates who are term and whose mothers experienced a healthy pregnancy and low-risk labor and birth accomplish this transition with relative ease (Fig. 15–1).

The focus of nursing care during this time is to protect and support neonates as they undergo numerous physiological changes and adapt to extrauterine life. This is accomplished by:

- Maintaining body heat.
- Maintaining respiratory function.
- Decreasing risk for infection.
- Assisting parents in providing appropriate nutrition and hydration.
- Assisting parents in learning to care for their newborn.

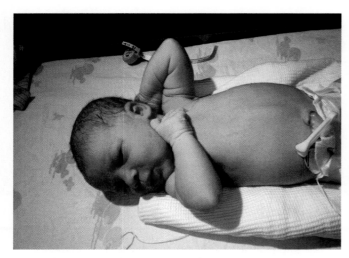

FIGURE 15–1 Neonate 15 minutes after birth transitioning to extrauterine life.

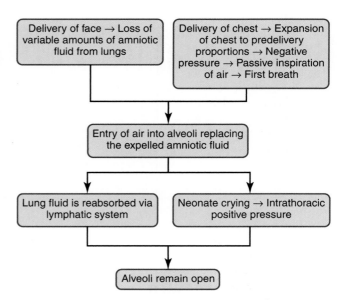

FIGURE 15–2 Transition to extrauterine pulmonary function: Mechanical stimuli.

TRANSITION TO EXTRAUTERINE LIFE

The transition to extrauterine life begins at birth when the umbilical cord is clamped and the neonate takes the first breath. This initiates various changes within the neonate's physiological systems, each of which must adapt to the changes that occur during this transition. The most critical and dynamic changes occur in the respiratory and cardiovascular systems. Other systems that undergo significant changes are thermoregulatory, metabolic, hepatic, gastrointestinal, renal, and immune systems.

The Respiratory System

The establishment of extrauterine respirations is the most critical and immediate physiological change that occurs in the transition from fetus to neonate. This change is initiated by compression of the thorax, which forces amniotic fluid from the lungs; lung expansion; increase in alveolar oxygen concentration; and vasodilatation of the pulmonary vessels. The primary factors that initiate extrauterine respirations are mechanical stimuli (Fig. 15–2) and chemical stimuli (Fig. 15–3). Sensory stimuli such as exposure to temperature changes, sounds, lights, and touch also influence respirations by stimulating the respiratory center of the medulla. The presence of surfactant, a phospholipid, within the alveoli assists in the establishment of functional residual capacity. This residual capacity helps keep the alveolar sacs partially open at the end of exhalation, which decreases the amount of pressure and energy required on inspiration (see Chapter 17). The initiation of respiration affects pulmonary circulation and gas exchange as follows:

● First breath → ↑ alveolar oxygen tension (Pao_2) and ↓ arterial pH → dilation of pulmonary arteries → ↓

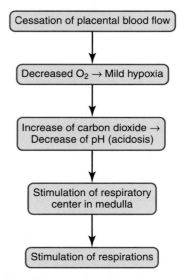

FIGURE 15–3 Transition to extrauterine pulmonary function: Chemical stimuli.

pulmonary vascular resistance → ↑ blood flow through pulmonary vessels → ↑ oxygen and carbon dioxide exchange within the lungs

Two factors that negatively affect the transition to extrauterine respirations are:

● Decreased surfactant levels related to immature lungs.
● Persistent hypoxemia and acidosis that leads to constriction of the pulmonary arteries.

Approximately 10% of neonates require some degree of assistance with respirations at the time of delivery, and 1% require extensive resuscitation.

CRITICAL COMPONENT

Signs of Fetal Respiratory Distress

- Cyanosis
- Abnormal respiratory pattern such as apnea and tachypnea
- Retractions of the chest wall
- Grunting
- Flaring of nostrils
- Hypotonia

The Circulatory System

The transition from fetal circulation to neonatal circulation begins rapidly within seconds of the clamping of the umbilical cord and the initiation of the first breath. Fetal circulation is discussed in Chapter 3. The transition to neonatal circulation is strongly influenced by the changes within the respiratory system. The decrease in pulmonary vascular resistance causes an increase in pulmonary blood flow, and the increase in systemic vascular resistance influences the cardiovascular changes (Fig. 15–4).

The three major fetal circulatory structures that undergo changes are the ductus venosus, foramen ovale, and the ductus arteriosus.

- The ductus venosus, which connects the umbilical vein to the inferior vena cava, closes by day 3 of life and becomes a ligament. Blood flow through the umbilical vein stops once the cord is clamped.
- The foramen ovale, which is an opening between the right atrium and the left atrium, closes when the left atrial pressure is higher than the right atrial pressure. Significant neonatal hypoxia can cause a reopening of the foramen ovale. This closure occurs when:
  - Increased Pao_2 → decreased pulmonary pressure → increased pulmonary blood flow → increased pressure in left atrium → closure of foramen ovale.
- The ductus arteriosus, which connects the pulmonary artery with the descending aorta, usually closes within 15 hours postbirth. It will remain open when the lungs fail to expand or when Pao_2 levels drop. Closure occurs when:
  - The pulmonary vascular resistance becomes less than system vascular resistance → left to right shunt → closure of ductus arteriosus.

The Thermoregulatory System

The fetus is surrounded in amniotic fluid that maintains a fairly constant environmental temperature based on the maternal body temperature. Once the neonate enters the extrauterine world, he must adapt to changes in the environmental temperatures. The neonate's responses to extrauterine temperature changes during the first few weeks are delayed and place the neonate at risk for cold stress. A neutral thermal environment (NTE) is needed to support the infant during this transition. NTE is

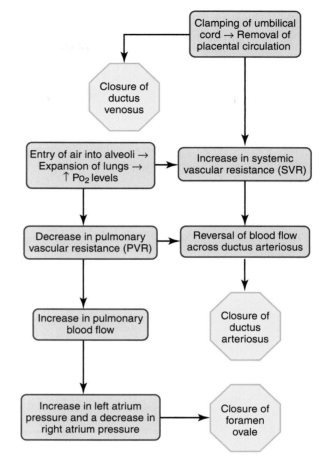

FIGURE 15–4 Transition to neonatal circulation.

an environment that maintains body temperature with minimal metabolic changes and/or oxygen consumption. NTE decreases possible complications related to the delayed response to environmental temperature changes.

The neonate responds to cold by:

- An increase in metabolic rate.
- An increase of muscle activity.
- Peripheral vascular constriction.
- Metabolism of brown fat.

Brown adipose tissue (BAT), also referred to as brown fat or nonshivering thermogenesis, is a highly dense and vascular adipose tissue. Full-term neonates possess large amounts of BAT, while preterm neonates, children, and adults have smaller amounts (Blackburn, 2012). BAT is located in the neck, thorax, axillary area, intrascapular areas, and around the adrenal glands and kidneys. BAT reserves are rapidly depleted during periods of cold stress.

BAT promotes:

- An increase in metabolism.
- Heat production through intense lipid metabolic metabolism of BAT.
- Heat transfer to the peripheral system (Blackburn, 2012).

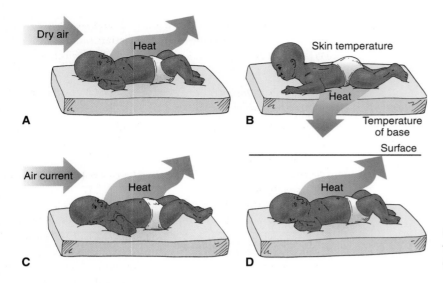

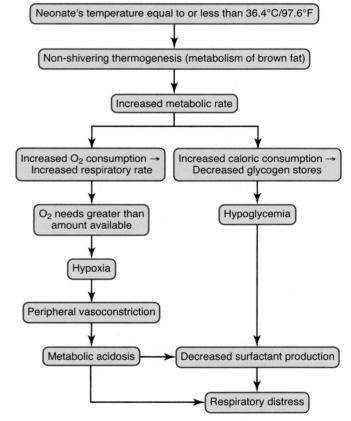

FIGURE 15–5 The four mechanisms of heat loss in the newborn. (*A*) Evaporation. (*B*) Conduction. (*C*) Convection. (*D*) Radiation.

Neonates are at higher risk for thermoregulatory problems related to:

- Higher body-surface-area-to-body-mass ratio.
- Higher metabolic rate.
- Limited and immature thermoregulatory abilities.

Factors that negatively affect thermoregulation are:

- Decreased subcutaneous fat.
- Decreased BAT in preterm neonates.
- Large body surface.
- Loss of body heat from evaporation, conduction, convection, and/or radiation (Fig. 15–5):
  - Evaporation: Loss of heat that occurs when water on the neonate's skin is converted to vapors, such as during bathing or directly after birth
  - Conduction: Transfer of heat to cooler surface by direct skin contact, such as cold hands of caregivers or cold equipment
  - Convection: Loss of heat from the neonate's warm body surface to cooler air currents, such as air conditioners or oxygen masks
  - Radiation: Transfer of heat from the neonate to cooler objects that are not in direct contact with the neonate, such as cold walls of the isolette or cold equipment near the neonate

Cold Stress

Cold stress is a term that describes excessive heat loss that leads to hypothermia and results in the utilization of compensatory mechanisms to maintain the neonate's body temperature (Fig. 15–6). Cold stress occurs when there is a decrease in environmental temperature that causes a decrease in the neonate's body temperature which can lead to respiratory distress.

Possible consequences of cold stress are:

- Hypoglycemia.
- Metabolic acidosis.
- Decreased surfactant production.
- Respiratory distress that can lead to neonatal death.

FIGURE 15–6 Cold stress.

- Hypoxemia.
- Increased indirect bilirubin.
- Delayed transition from fetal to neonatal circulation.
- Weight loss.

Risk Factors

- Prematurity
- Small for gestational age

- Hypoglycemia
- Prolonged resuscitation efforts
- Sepsis
- Neurological, endocrine, or cardiorespiratory problems

Signs and Symptoms

- Axillary temperature at or below 36.5°C (97.7°F)
- Cool skin
- Lethargy
- Pallor
- Tachypnea
- Grunting
- Hypoglycemia
- Hypotonia
- Jitteriness
- Weak suck

Nursing Actions

Preventive actions should include the following:

- Dry the neonate thoroughly immediately after birth to decrease heat loss due to evaporation.
- Remove wet blankets from the neonate's direct environment to decrease heat loss due to radiation, evaporation, and conduction.
- Place a stocking cap on the neonate's head to decrease heat loss due to radiation and convection (Fig. 15–7).
- Skin-to-skin contact with the mother with a warm blanket over the mother and neonate decreases heat loss due to radiation and conduction.
- Use prewarmed blankets and clothing to decrease heat loss due to conduction.
- Swaddle in warm blankets to decrease heat loss due to convection and radiation.
- Prewarm radiant warmers and heat shields to decrease heat loss due to conduction.
- Delay initial bath until the neonate's temperature is stable to decrease heat loss due to evaporation.
- Place the neonate away from air vents to decrease heat loss due to convection.

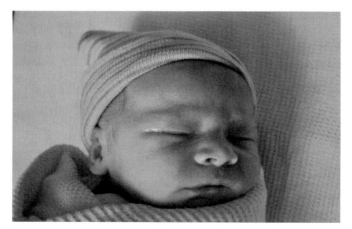

FIGURE 15–7 Stocking cap is placed on the neonate's head to reduce heat loss due to radiation and convection.

- Place the neonate away from outside walls and windows to decrease heat loss due to convection radiation.
- Maintain an NTE to decrease heat loss due to convection and radiation.

Actions when the neonate displays signs/symptoms of cold stress include the following:

- Place a stocking cap on the neonate's head.
- Skin-to-skin contact with the mother with a warm blanket over both the mother and neonate when there is a mild decrease in temperature; reassess temperature as per institutional protocol.
- Swaddle in warm blankets; reassess temperature as per institutional protocol, which is generally every 30 minutes until stable.
- Place the naked neonate under a preheated radiant warmer.
  - Attach the servo-controlled probe on the neonate's abdomen or other body surface that is closest to the radiant source. It is recommended not to place probe over BAT areas, but there are too few research studies to view this as evidenced-based practice (Blackburn, 2012).
  - Increase the temperature by 1°C (1.8°F) until 36.5°C (97.8°F).
  - Monitor the neonate's temperature, respiratory rate, and heart rate every 5 minutes when rewarming.
  - Assess and adjust the neonate's fluid requirement; fluids may need to be increased to compensate for insatiable water loss.
- Monitor temperature as per institutional protocol.
- Obtain a heel stick to assess for hypoglycemia (glucose below 40 mg/dL) and treat for hypoglycemia based on glucose level.

The Metabolic System

Large quantities of glycogen are stored by the fetus during pregnancy in preparation for meeting energy requirements when transitioning from intrauterine to extrauterine life. Immediately after birth, the neonate becomes independent of the mother's metabolism and must balance the amount of insulin production with glucose availability. Glucose values normally decrease about 1 hour postbirth, and then values rise and stabilize by 2 to 3 hours postbirth (Blackburn, 2012). Optimal range for plasma glucose is 70 to 100 mg/dL.

Hypoglycemia (blood glucose level below 40 mg/dL in the neonate) is common during the transitional time, especially in neonates of diabetic mothers. During intrauterine life, neonates of diabetic mothers produce high levels of insulin in response to the high levels of circulating maternal glucose. The neonate's insulin level remains higher than normal, leading to hypoglycemia.

CRITICAL COMPONENT

Hypoglycemia

Hypoglycemia is defined as a blood glucose level below 40 mg/dL in the neonate.

Risks for Hypoglycemia

- Neonates of diabetic mothers
- Neonates weighing more than 4,000 g or large for gestational age

- Post-term neonates
- Preterm neonates
- Small-for-gestational-age neonates
- Hypothermia
- Neonatal infection
- Respiratory distress
- Neonatal resuscitation
- Birth trauma

Signs and Symptoms

- Jitteriness
- Hypotonia
- Irritability
- Apnea
- Lethargy
- Temperature instability

Nursing Actions

- Monitor for signs and symptoms of hypoglycemia.
- Assess blood glucose level with use of glucose monitor.
- Assist the woman to either breastfeed or formula feed her infant. IV infusion of a dextrose solution or buccal 40% dextrose gel is used when hypoglycemia persists.
- Maintain NTE to decrease risk of cold stress.

The Hepatic System

The liver is an extraordinary organ with multiple functions, producing enzymes that act as a catalysis for chemical reactions (Scanlon & Sanders, 2015). Functions of the liver include:

- Carbohydrate metabolism:
    - The liver regulates the blood glucose levels by converting excessive glucose to glycogen (insulin and cortisol facilitate this process) and converting glycogen to glucose when glucose levels are low.
- Amino acid metabolism.
- Lipid metabolism.
- Synthesis of plasma proteins.
- Blood coagulation:
    - Coagulation factors II, VII, IX, and X are synthesized in the liver. Vitamin K influences the activation of these factors. During intrauterine life, the fetus receives vitamin K from its mother. After birth, the neonate experiences a decrease in vitamin K and is at risk for delayed clotting and for hemorrhage. Vitamin K is synthesized in the intestinal flora, which is absent in the newborn. The intestinal flora develops after the introduction of microorganisms, which usually occurs with the first feedings.
    - A vitamin K injection is given as a prophylaxis to decrease the risk of bleeding related to vitamin K deficiency. The decline of maternally acquired vitamin K levels is greater in breastfed neonates, neonates with a history of perinatal asphyxia, and neonates of mothers who are on warfarin (Blackburn, 2012).

- Conjugation of bilirubin
    - There is an increase in the neonate's red blood cell (RBC) turnover (shorter RBC life span) and an increased RBC count at birth. These factors contribute to a proportionally greater amount of bilirubin production. There are two forms of bilirubin: indirect and direct.
        - Indirect bilirubin (unconjugated bilirubin), a fat-soluble substance, is produced from the breakdown of red blood cells (RBCs). It is converted to direct bilirubin (conjugated bilirubin), a water-soluble substance, by liver enzymes. Direct bilirubin is in a form that can be excreted in the urine and stool.
        - Hyperbilirubinemia is a condition in which there is a high level of unconjugated bilirubin in the neonate's blood related to the immature liver function, high RBC count that is common in neonates, and an increased hemolysis caused by the shorter life span of fetal RBCs. Hyperbilirubinemia is categorized into physiological jaundice and pathological jaundice (see Chapter 17).
- Phagocytosis by Kupffer cells (macrophages)
    - The Kupffer cells destroy old RBC, pathogens, and other foreign material that enter the liver via the circulatory system. Many of the bacteria that reside in the normal flora of the colon are harmful outside of the colon. The Kupffer cells will destroy these bacteria when they enter the liver via the bloodstream (Scanlon & Sanders, 2015).
- Storage of fat-soluble vitamins A, D, E, and K and iron
    - The formation of new RBCs is suppressed during the first few weeks postbirth. During this time, the liver stores iron from destroyed RBCs. This iron is used when RBC formation is resumed (Blackburn, 2012).
- Detoxification
    - The smooth endoplasmic reticulum (SER) of the liver produces enzymes that detoxify harmful substances such as medications (Blackburn, 2012). The neonate has a reduced number of SER → decreased ability to detoxify medication → increased risk of toxic effects from medications.

SAFE AND EFFECTIVE NURSING CARE: Understanding Medication

Phytonadione (Vitamin K, AquaMEPHYTON)

- Indication: Prevention of hemorrhagic disease in neonate
- Action: Vitamin K is required for the hepatic synthesis of blood coagulation factors II, VII, IX, and X.
- Common side effects: erythema, pain, and swelling at injection site
- Route and dose: IM; 0.5 to 1 mg within 1 hour of birth

Vallerand & Sanoski, 2017.

The Gastrointestinal System

The neonate's gastrointestinal system is functionally immature but rapidly adapts to demands for growth and development through ingestion, digestion, and absorption of nutrients, as well as eliminations of waste. Gastric capacity for the first few days is approximately 5 to 10 mL and increases to 60 mL by day 7. Stomach-emptying time is 2 to 4 hours, requiring the neonate to feed at that interval. Neonates may appear uninterested in feeding during the first few days.

The characteristics of stools and stool patterns vary depending on the type, frequency, and amount of feeding and the age of the neonate (Table 15–1). Breastfed neonates tend to have more stools per day than formula-fed neonates. It is not uncommon for the neonate to pass 4 to 8 stools per day. Constipation usually does not occur in breastfed neonates and can occur in bottle-fed infants when formula is not properly diluted. The types of stools are:

● Meconium stool: begins to form during the fourth gestational month and is the first stool eliminated by the neonate. It is sticky, thick, black, and odorless. It is first passed within 24 to 48 hours.
● Transitional stool: begins around the third day and can continue for 3 or 4 days. The stool transitions from black to greenish black, to greenish brown, to greenish yellow. This phase of stool characteristics occurs in both breastfed and formula-fed neonates.
● Breastfed stool: yellow and semiformed. Later it becomes a golden yellow with a pasty consistency and has a sour odor.
● Formula-fed stool: drier and more formed than breastfed stools. It is a paler yellow or brownish yellow and has an unpleasant odor.
● Diarrheal stool: loose and green.

The Renal System

Two major functions of the kidneys are control of fluid and electrolyte balance and excretion of metabolic waste. During fetal life, these functions are assumed by the placenta. Once the cord is clamped, the neonate's kidneys must take on these functions. Initially the neonate's kidneys are immature and place the neonate, especially preterm neonates, at risk for:

● Overhydration: The glomerular filtration rate (GFR) is initially low in the neonate but doubles by 2 weeks of age (Blackburn, 2012).
   ● Decreased GFR → ↓ ability to excrete water → ↑ risk of overhydration and water intoxication
● Dehydration: This can occur due to the neonate's kidneys' limited ability to concentrate urine.
● Electrolyte disorders: Examples include hyponatremia and hypernatremia in the preterm neonate. Increased sodium loss can occur in increased water loss, which increases risk of hyponatremia. Dehydration related to excessive sodium intake increases risk for hypernatremia (Blackburn, 2012).
● Drug toxicity: The limited abilities of the kidneys can affect the excretion of drugs from the neonate's systems and increase the risk of side effects and toxicity (Blackburn, 2012).

Full-term neonates excrete 15 to 60 mL/kg of urine per day for the first few days of life. Urinary output increases to 250 to 400 mL by the end of the first month of life (Blackburn, 2012). Neonates usually lose 5% to 10% of birth weight during the first week of life due to diuresis. A delay or decrease in urinary output can occur in neonates whose mothers received magnesium sulfate during labor. Magnesium sulfate blocks neuromuscular transmissions and can cause urinary retention (Blackburn, 2012).

The Immune System

The immune system protects the body from invasion by foreign materials such as bacteria and viruses (Scanlon & Sanders, 2015). Before rupture of membranes, fetuses live in the sterile environment of the maternal uterus and rely on the maternal immune system to protect them from pathogenic organisms. During the transition from extrauterine life, neonates begin the process of developing normal microbial flora and must respond

TABLE 15–1 Minimum Number of Wet Diapers and Stools During First Month

NEONATE'S AGE	NUMBER OF WET DIAPERS	NUMBER OF STOOLS	TYPE OF STOOL
Day 1	1	1	Meconium—sticky, thick, and black
Day 2	2	3	Meconium—sticky, thick, and black
Day 3	5–6	3	Transitional—looser greenish black/greenish brown
Day 4	6	3	Yellow, soft, and watery
Day 5 → 1 month	6	3	Breastfed stool or formula-fed stool

DHHS, 2009.

to colonization by potential pathogenic bacteria (Blackburn, 2012). Neonates are first exposed to organisms from the maternal genital tract during the birthing process. The maternal genital track may contain group B streptococcus and *Escherichia coli*, which can result in neonatal sepsis (see Chapter 17). Neonates are at risk for infections related to:

- Immature defense mechanism.
- Lack of experience with and exposure to organisms, which leads to a delayed response to antigens.
- Breakdown of skin and mucous membranes, which provides a portal of entry for bacteria (Blackburn, 2012).

Major components of the immune system are as follows:

- Active humoral immunity is the process in which B cells detect antigens and produce antibodies against them. Active humoral immunity is further classified as:
  - Acquired immunity that develops from vaccination.
  - Natural immunity that develops from exposure to antigens, after which the individual produces antibodies.
- Passive immunity, which is not permanent, is acquired either naturally or artificially.
  - An example of natural passive immunity is the placental transmission of antibodies from the mother to the fetus. This provides protection for the neonate during the first few months of life from the pathogens to which the mother has been exposed.
  - An example of artificial passive immunity is gamma globulin, which provides immediate protection for a short time.
- Lymphocytes are white blood cells that are primarily composed of T cells and B cells.
  - The number of T cells within the neonate's system is comparable to that in adults, but their functional abilities are decreased, which delays the response to microorganisms (Blackburn, 2012).
  - The functional abilities of B cells are also hyporesponsive (Blackburn, 2012).

- Immunoglobulins are classified as IgG, IgA, IgM, IgD, and IgE (Table 15–2).
  - Maternal IgGs are the primary antibodies that cross the placenta and enter the fetal system and provide passive immunity for the neonate (Blackburn, 2012).
  - The maternal transfer of IgG antibodies protects the neonate from bacterial and viral infections for which the mother has developed antibodies, such as rubella, tetanus, and diphtheria (Blackburn, 2012).

NEONATAL ASSESSMENT

A neonatal assessment should be done within 2 hours after birth. This initial assessment provides the baseline data for the neonate, evaluates the neonate's transition to extrauterine life, and assists in determining the course of nursing and medical care. The initial assessment includes a general survey, physical assessment, gestational assessment, and pain assessment.

CRITICAL COMPONENT

Methods of Reducing Heat Loss During Assessments

The thermoregulatory systems of neonates respond more slowly to external temperature changes than those of adults. Prevention of heat loss is critical when doing assessments. Methods to reduce heat loss during assessments include:

- Ensuring that the room is warm and free of air drafts.
- Placing the neonate under a warming unit to help maintain an NTE or assessing the neonate in the mother's arms. Skin-to-skin contact between the mother and neonate can decrease the amount of heat loss.
- Keeping the neonate wrapped and exposing only the body area that is being checked when doing assessments in an open crib or in a parent's arms.

TABLE 15–2 Classes of Immunoglobulins

NAME	LOCATION	FUNCTION
IgG	Blood	Crosses the placenta to provide passive immunity for newborns
	Extracellular fluid	Provides long-term immunity after recovery or a vaccine
IgA	External secretions (tears, salvia, etc.)	Present in breast milk to provide passive immunity for breastfed infants
		Found in secretions of all mucous membranes
IgM	Blood	Produced first by the maturing immune system of infants
		Produced first during an infection (IgG production follows)
		Part of the ABO blood group
IgD	B lymphocytes	Receptors on B lymphocytes
IgE	Mast cells or basophils	Important in allergic reaction (mast cells release histamine)

Scanlon & Sanders, 2015.

Preparation for Assessment

- Review the prenatal record and birth record for factors that could place the neonate at risk for complications. Examples of risk factors are:
  - Maternal malnutrition prior to and/or during pregnancy.
  - Maternal age younger than 16 or older than 35 years.
  - Chronic maternal illnesses such as diabetes and hypertension.
  - Hypertensive disorders of pregnancy.
  - Labor and birth before 38 weeks' gestation.
  - Labor longer than 24 hours.
  - Operative delivery: Use of forceps or vacuum extractor.
  - Medications during labor that affect the central nervous system (CNS), such as magnesium sulfate and analgesia/anesthesia.
  - Prolonged rupture of membranes (longer than 24 hours).
  - Meconium-stained amniotic fluid.
  - Placental abnormalities.
  - Apgar score 7 or below at 5 minutes.
- Gather the equipment needed for the assessment: latex gloves, measuring tape, infant stethoscope, thermometer, scale for weighing, and documentation records.
- Ensure that assessment is done in an NTE (i.e., close doors to prevent drafts and regulate room temperature).
- Inform the parents of the assessment and invite them to watch. This is especially helpful for the woman's partner.

General Survey

- A general survey of the neonate is completed before the physical assessment. This survey is best completed while the neonate is quiet.
- Observe the respiratory pattern and assess respirations and breath sounds. It can be difficult to assess respiratory rate once the neonate responds to being handled (cries) during the physical assessment.
- Observe posture.
- Assess the skin for color, birth trauma, and birthmarks.
- Observe the level of alertness/activity.
- Assess muscle tone and posture.

Physical Assessment

Typically, the physical assessment starts with the head and ends with the legs and feet and includes assessing reflexes that are unique to neonates (Tables 15–3, 15–4, and 15–5).

Gestational Age Assessment

Gestational age assessment of the neonate is based on the mother's menstrual history, prenatal ultrasonography, and/or neonatal maturational examination. The calculation of gestational age by instruments such as Dubowitz neurological exam or Ballard scale of physical and neuromuscular maturity assists in predicting potential problems and establishing plan of care based on gestational age. Most hospital nurseries have written policies on which neonates should routinely be assessed

for gestational age. Gestational age assessment is commonly completed on:

- Neonates who are preterm, born before 37 weeks based on the maternal menstrual history, or post-term, born after 42 weeks by dates.
- Neonates who weigh less than 2,500 g or more than 4,000 g.
- Neonates of diabetic mothers.
- Neonates whose condition requires admission to a neonatal intensive care unit (NICU).

The Dubowitz neurological exam is a standardized tool that assesses 33 responses in four areas:

- Habituation (the response to repetitive light and sound stimuli)
- Movement and muscle tone
- Reflexes
- Neurobehavioral items

The Ballard Maturational Score (BMS) is calculated by assessing the physical and neuromuscular maturity of the neonate. It can be completed in less time than the Dubowitz neurological exam and consists of six evaluation areas for neuromuscular maturity and six items of observed physical maturity (Table 15–6). The examination determines weeks of gestation and classifies the neonate as preterm (less than 37 weeks), term (37 to 42 weeks), or post-term (older than 42 weeks).

The scores from these exams provide a gestational age that is graphed based on weight, length, and head circumference to determine if the neonate is average for gestational age, small for gestational age (SGA), or large for gestational age (LGA) (Fig. 15–8).

- SGA is a term used for neonates whose weight is below the 10th percentile for gestational age.
- LGA is a term used for neonates whose weight is above the 90th percentile for gestational age.

Pain Assessment

Neonates are subjected to a variety of painful stimuli during their transition to extrauterine life (e.g., injections, heel sticks for blood samples, and circumcision). In the past, health care providers believed that neonates did not experience the sensation of pain, so little attention was given to assessing and reducing pain in the neonate. In the 1990s, researchers began to address this lack of knowledge by gaining a better understanding of neonatal pain, developing tools that assess for neonatal pain, and determining appropriate and safe pain management for neonates.

The 1995 National Association of Neonatal Nurses (NANN) position statement on pain management in infants says that "all health care professionals who care for neonates/infants need ongoing education in the assessment and management of neonatal pain and that neonates/infants be protected from the adverse effects of pain" (NANN, 1995).

Pain assessment is part of the nursing care of neonates (Box 15–1). Several pain scales, such as Premature Infant Pain Profile (PIPP) and Neonatal Infant Pain Scale (NIPS), have been developed to assess for neonatal pain. Pain assessment tools commonly look at state of arousal, cry, motor activity, respiratory

(text continues on p. 27)

TABLE 15–3   Neonatal Assessment by Area/System

AREA OR SYSTEM	TECHNIQUE AND ASSESSMENT	EXPECTED FINDINGS FOR TERM NEONATE	DEVIATIONS FROM NORMAL
Posture	Unwrap the newborn and observe posture when the neonate is quiet.	Extremities are flexed.	Extension of extremities often related to prematurity; effects of medications given to mother during labor such as magnesium sulfate and analgesics/anesthesia; birth injuries; hypothermia; or hypoglycemia
Head circumference	Measure by placing tape around the head just above the ears and eyebrows. Measurement is usually recorded in centimeters.	33–35.5 cm (13–14 in.)	Microcephaly: Head circumference is below the 10th percentile of normal for newborns gestational age. This is often related to congenital malformation, maternal drug or alcohol ingestion, or maternal infection during pregnancy. Macrocephaly: Head circumference is >90th percentile. This can be related to hydrocephalus.
Chest circumference	Measure by placing tape around the chest over the nipple line.	30.5–33 cm (12–13 in.) or 2–3 cm less than head circumference	
Length	Measure the length of body by securing tape on a flat surface. Place the top of neonate's head at the top of the tape. Extend the body and one leg. Measurement is taken from the top of the head to the bottom of the heel.	45.7–53 cm (18–21 in.)	Molding may interfere with accurate assessment of length. Neonates whose length is <45 cm should be further assessed for causes such as intrauterine growth restriction or prematurity.
Weight	Clean scale before use. Place clean paper on the scale. Set the scale at zero. Place the naked neonate on the scale. Record the neonate's weight. Do not leave the neonate unattended while weighing.	2,500–4,000 g (5 lb 8 oz–8 lb 13 oz) Weight loss of 5%–10% of birth weight during the first week is normal. This is due to water loss through urine, stools, and lungs and an increase in metabolic rate. It is also related to limited fluid intake. The neonate will regain birth weight within 10 days.	Weight above the 90th percentile is common in neonates of diabetic mothers. Weight below the 10th percentile is due to prematurity, intrauterine growth restriction, malnutrition during the pregnancy.

TABLE 15–3   Neonatal Assessment by Area/System—cont'd

AREA OR SYSTEM	TECHNIQUE AND ASSESSMENT	EXPECTED FINDINGS FOR TERM NEONATE	DEVIATIONS FROM NORMAL
Temperature	Place a clean temperature probe in the axillary area. Axillary temperatures are preferred because of the risks of tissue trauma, perforation, and cross-contamination associated with the rectal temperature method (Blackburn, 2012).	36.5°C–37.2°C (97.7°F–99°F) Axillary	Hypothermia or hyperthermia is related to infection, environmental extremes, and/or neurological disorders.
Respirations	Assess respiratory rate by observing the rise and fall of the chest and abdomen for 1 full minute.	30–60 breaths per minute Slightly irregular Diaphragmatic and abdominal breathing Rate increases when crying and decreases when sleeping.	Periods of apnea >15 seconds Tachypnea that may be related to sepsis, hypothermia, hypoglycemia, or respiratory distress syndrome. Respirations <30; may be related to maternal analgesia and/or anesthesia during labor.
Pulse	Assess apical pulse rate by auscultating for 1 full minute. Assess rate and rhythm. Use of a stethoscope designed for neonates is recommended.	110–160 bpm Rate increases (to 180 bpm) with crying and decreases (to 90 bpm) when asleep. Murmurs may be heard; most are not pathological and disappear by 6 months.	Tachycardia (>160 bpm) indicates possible sepsis, respiratory distress, congenital heart abnormality. Bradycardia (<100 bpm) indicates possible sepsis, increased intracranial pressure, or hypoxemia.
Blood pressure	Blood pressure is not a routine part of neonatal assessment. Requires the use of specially designed equipment for neonates. The blood pressure is obtained from either the arm or the leg of the neonate.	50–75/30–45 mm Hg	
Integumentary/skin	Inspect the skin for color, intactness, bruising, birth marks, dryness, rashes, warmth, texture, and turgor. Inspect nails. Stork bite	Skin is warm with acrocyanosis (cyanosis of hands and feet). Milia are present on the bridge of the nose and chin (see Table 15–4). Lanugo is present on the back, shoulders, and forehead, which decreases with advancing gestation (see Table 15–4). Peeling or cracking is often noted on infants >40 weeks' gestation. Mongolian spots, also referred to as congenital dermal melanocytosis (see Table 15–4)	Jaundice within the first 24 hours is pathological (see Chapter 17). Pallor occurs with anemia, hypothermia, shock, or sepsis. Greenish/yellowish vernix indicates passage of meconium during pregnancy and/or labor. Persistent ecchymosis or petechiae occurs with thrombocytopenia, sepsis, or congenital infection. Abundant lanugo is often seen in preterm neonates.

Continued

TABLE 15–3   Neonatal Assessment by Area/System—cont'd

AREA OR SYSTEM	TECHNIQUE AND ASSESSMENT	EXPECTED FINDINGS FOR TERM NEONATE	DEVIATIONS FROM NORMAL
Integumentary/skin (continued)		Hemangiomas such as salmon-colored patch (stork bites), nevus flammeus (port-wine stain), and strawberry hemangiomas are developmental vascular abnormalities. Stork bites are found at the nape of the neck, on the eyelid, between the eyes, or on the upper lip. They deepen in color when the neonate cries. They disappear within the first year of life. Nevus flammeus are purple- to red-colored flat areas that can be located on various portions of the body. These do not disappear. Strawberry hemangiomas are raised bright red lesions that develop during the neonatal period. They spontaneously resolve during early childhood. Erythema toxicum, newborn rash (see Table 15–4).	Thin and translucent skin, and increased amounts of vernix caseosa are common in preterm neonates. Nails are longer in neonates >40 weeks' gestation. Pilonidal dimple: A small pit or sinus in the sacral area at top of crease between the buttocks; the sinus can become infected later in life.
Head	Note the shape of the head. Inspect and palpate fontanels and suture lines. Inspect and palpate the head for caput succedaneum and/or cephalohematoma (see Table 15–4). 	Molding present (see Table 15–4). Fontanels are open, soft, intact, and slightly depressed. They may bulge with crying. The anterior fontanel is diamond shaped, approximately 2.5–4 cm (closes by 18 months of age). The posterior fontanel is a triangle shape that is approximately 0.5–1 cm (closes between 2 and 4 months). May be difficult to palpate due to excessive molding. There are overriding sutures when there is increased molding.	Fontanels that are firm and bulging and not related to crying are a possible indication of increased intracranial pressure. Depressed fontanels are a possible indication of dehydration. Bruising and laceration at the site of the fetal scalp electrode or vacuum extractor. Presence of caput succedaneum and/or cephalohematoma (see Table 15–4).
Neck	Lift the chin to assess the neck area. 	The neck is short with skin folds. Positive tonic neck reflex (see Table 15–5).	Webbing is a possible indication of genetic disorders. Absent tonic neck reflex is an indication of nerve injury.

TABLE 15–3   Neonatal Assessment by Area/System—cont'd

AREA OR SYSTEM	TECHNIQUE AND ASSESSMENT	EXPECTED FINDINGS FOR TERM NEONATE	DEVIATIONS FROM NORMAL
Eyes	Assess the position of the eyes. Open the eyelids and assess color of sclera and pupil size. Assess for blink reflex, red light reflex, and pupil reaction to light.	Eyes are equal and symmetrical in size and placement. The neonate is able to follow objects within 12 inches of the visual field. Edema may be present due to pressure during labor and birth and/or reaction to eye prophylaxes. The iris is blue-gray or brown. The sclera is white or bluish white. Subconjunctival hemorrhages related to birth trauma. Pupils are equally reactive to light. Positive red light reflex and blink reflex. No tear production (tear production begins at 2 months). Strabismus and nystagmus related to immature muscular control.	Absent red light reflex indicates cataracts. Unequal pupil reactions indicate neurological trauma. Blue sclera is a possible indication of osteogenesis imperfecta.
Ears	Inspect the ears for position, shape, and drainage. Hearing test is done before discharge.	Top of the pinna is aligned with external canthus of the eye. Pinna without deformities, well formed and flexible. The neonate responds to noises with positive startle signs. Hearing becomes more acute as Eustachian tubes clear. Neonates respond more readily to high-pitched vocal sounds.	Low-set ears are associated with genetic disorders such as Down syndrome. Absent startle reflex is associated with possible hearing loss.
Nose	Observe the shape of the nose. Inspect the opening of the nares.	The nose may be flattened or bruised related to the birth process. Nares should be patent. Small amount of mucus. Neonates primarily breathe through their noses.	Large amounts of mucus drainage can lead to respiratory distress. A flat nasal bridge is seen with Down syndrome. Nasal flaring is a sign of respiratory distress.

Continued

TABLE 15–3   Neonatal Assessment by Area/System—cont'd

AREA OR SYSTEM	TECHNIQUE AND ASSESSMENT	EXPECTED FINDINGS FOR TERM NEONATE	DEVIATIONS FROM NORMAL
Mouth 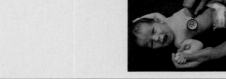 Thrush	Inspect lips, gums, tongue, palate, and mucous membranes. Open the mouth by placing gentle pressure on the lower lip. Test for rooting, sucking, swallowing, and gag reflexes (see Table 15–5).	Lips, gums, tongue, palate, and mucous membranes are intact, pink, and moist. Reflexes are positive. Epstein's pearls are present (see Table 15–4).	Natal teeth, which can be benign or related to congenital abnormality (see Table 15–4). Thrush, a fungal infection, can be contracted during vaginal birth. It appears as white patches on the mucous membranes of the mouth. Thin philtrum may be indicative of fetal alcohol syndrome. Cleft lip and/or palate, which is a congenital abnormality in which the lip and/or palate does not completely fuse (see Chapter 17).
Chest/lungs	Inspect shape, symmetry, and chest excursion. Inspect the breast for size and drainage. Auscultate breath sounds. 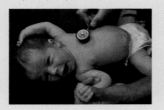	The chest is barrel-shaped and symmetrical. Breast engorgement is present in both male and female neonates related to the influence of maternal hormones and resolves within a few weeks. Clear or milky fluid from nipples related to maternal hormones. Lung sounds are clear and equal. Scattered crackles may be detected during the first few hours after birth. This is due to retained amniotic fluid, which will be absorbed through the lymphatics.	Pectus excavatum (funnel chest) is a congenital abnormality. Pectus carinatum (pigeon chest) can obstruct respirations. Chest retractions are a sign of respiratory distress. Persistent crackles, wheezes, stridor, grunting, paradoxical breathing, decreased breath sounds, and/or prolonged periods of apnea (>15–20 seconds) are signs of respiratory distress. Decreased or absent breath sounds are often related to meconium aspiration or pneumothorax.
Cardiac	Auscultate heart sounds; listen for at least 1 full minute. Palpate peripheral pulses.	Point of maximal impulse (PMI) at the 3rd or 4th intercostal space. S_1 and S_2 are present. Normal rhythm with variation related to respiratory changes. Murmurs in 30% of neonates, which disappear within 2 days of birth. Peripheral pulses are present and equal. The femoral pulse may be difficult to palpate.	Dextrocardia: Heart on the right side of the chest. Displaced PMI occurs with cardiomegaly. Persistent murmurs indicate persistent fetal circulation or congenital heart defects.

TABLE 15–3   Neonatal Assessment by Area/System—cont'd

AREA OR SYSTEM	TECHNIQUE AND ASSESSMENT	EXPECTED FINDINGS FOR TERM NEONATE	DEVIATIONS FROM NORMAL
Abdomen	Inspect size and shape of the abdomen. Palpate the abdomen, assessing for tone, hernias, and diastasis recti. Auscultate for bowel sounds. Inspect the umbilical cord. 	The abdomen is soft, round, protuberant, and symmetrical. Bowel sounds are present but may be hypoactive for the first few days. Passage of meconium stool within 24-48 hours postbirth. The cord is opaque or whitish blue with two arteries and one vein, and covered with Wharton's jelly. The cord becomes dry and darker in color within 24 hours postbirth and detaches from the body within 2 weeks.	Asymmetrical abdomen indicates a possible abdominal mass. Hernias or diastasis recti are more common in African American neonates and usually resolve on their own within the first year. One umbilical artery and vein is associated with heart or kidney malformation. Failure to pass meconium stool is often associated with imperforated anus or meconium ileus.
Rectum	Inspect the anus.	The anus is patent. Passage of stool within 24-48 hours.	Imperforated anus requires immediate surgery. Anal fissures or fistulas.
Genitourinary: female	Place thumbs on either side of the labia and gently separate tissue to visually inspect the genitalia. Assess for the presence and position of clitoris, vagina, and urinary meatus. 	Labia majora covers labia minora and clitoris. Labia majora and minora may be edematous. Blood-tinged vaginal discharge related to the abrupt decrease of maternal hormones (pseudomenstruation). Whitish vaginal discharge in response to maternal hormones. The neonate urinates within 24 hours. The urinary meatus is midline and an uninterrupted stream is noted on voiding.	Prominent clitoris and small labia minora are often present in preterm neonates. Ambiguous genitalia; may require genetic testing to determine sex. No urination in 24 hours may indicate a possible urinary tract obstruction, polycystic disease, or renal failure.

Continued

TABLE 15–3   Neonatal Assessment by Area/System—cont'd

AREA OR SYSTEM	TECHNIQUE AND ASSESSMENT	EXPECTED FINDINGS FOR TERM NEONATE	DEVIATIONS FROM NORMAL
Genitourinary: male	Inspect the penis, noting the position of the urinary meatus. Inspect and palpate the scrotum to assess for testicles. With the thumb and forefinger of one hand, palpate each testis while the other thumb and forefinger are placed over the inguinal canal to prevent the ascent of testes during assessment. Start at the upper aspect of the scrotum and move away from the body.	The urinary meatus is at the tip of the penis. The scrotum is large, pendulous, and edematous with rugae (ridges/creases) present. Both testes are palpated in the scrotum. The neonate urinates within 24 hours with an uninterrupted stream. 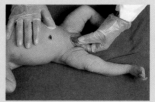	Hypospadias: The urethral opening is on the ventral surface of penis. Epispadias: The urethral opening is on the dorsal side of penis. Undescended testes: testes not palpated in the scrotum. Hydrocele is enlarged scrotum due to excess fluid. No urination in 24 hours may indicate possible urinary tract obstruction, polycystic disease, or renal failure. Ambiguous genitalia may require genetic testing to determine sex. Inguinal hernia.
Musculoskeletal 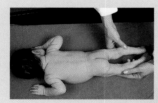	Inspect extremities, spine, and gluteal folds. Palpate the clavicles. Perform the Barlow and Ortolani maneuvers. 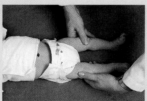 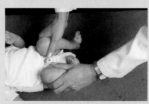 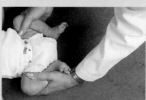 Assessing range of motion for arm is especially important if there was shoulder dystocia during the birthing process.	Arms are symmetrical in length and equal in strength. Legs are symmetrical in length and equal in strength. 10 fingers and 10 toes. Full range of motion of all extremities. No clicks at joints. Equal gluteal folds. C curve of spine with no dimpling.	Polydactyly: Extra digits may indicate a genetic disorder. Syndactyly: Webbed digits may indicate a genetic disorder. Unequal gluteal folds and/or positive Barlow and Ortolani maneuvers are associated with congenital hip dislocation. Decreased range of motion and/or muscle tone indicates possible birth injury, neurological disorder, or prematurity. Swelling, crepitus and/or neck tenderness indicates possible broken clavicle, which can occur during the birthing process in neonates with large shoulders. Simian creases, short fingers, wide space between big toe and second toe are common with Down syndrome.

TABLE 15–3   Neonatal Assessment by Area/System—cont'd

AREA OR SYSTEM	TECHNIQUE AND ASSESSMENT	EXPECTED FINDINGS FOR TERM NEONATE	DEVIATIONS FROM NORMAL
Neurological	Assess posture. Assess tone. Test newborn reflexes (see Table 15–5).	Flexed position Rapid recoil of extremities to the flexed position Positive newborn reflexes	Hypotonia: Floppy, limp extremities indicate possible nerve injury related to birth, depression of CNS related to maternal medication received during labor or to fetal hypoxia during labor, prematurity, or spinal cord injury. Hypertonia: Tightly flexed arms and stiffly extended legs with quivering indicate possible drug withdrawal. Paralysis indicates possible birth trauma or spinal injury. Tremors are possibly due to hypoglycemia, drug withdrawal, cold stress.

Dillon, 2007; Mattson & Smith, 2016.

TABLE 15–4   Common Newborn Characteristics

CHARACTERISTIC	APPEARANCE	SIGNIFICANCE
Acrocyanosis	Hands and/or feet are blue.	Response to cold environment. Immature peripheral circulation
Circumoral cyanosis	A benign localized transient cyanosis around the mouth.	Observed during the transitional period; if it persists, it may be related to a cardiac anomaly.
Mottling	A benign transient pattern of pink and white blotches on the skin.	Response to cold environment.
Harlequin sign	One side of body is pink and the other side is white.	Related to vasomotor instability.

Continued

TABLE 15–4   Common Newborn Characteristics—cont'd

CHARACTERISTIC	APPEARANCE	SIGNIFICANCE
Mongolian spots	Flat, bluish discolored area on the lower back and/or buttock. Seen more often in African American, Asian, Hispanic, and Native American infants.	Might be mistaken for bruising. Need to document size and location. Resolves on own by school age.
Erythema toxicum	A rash with red macules and papules (white to yellowish-white papule in center surrounded by reddened skin) that appear in different areas of the body, usually the trunk area. Can appear within 24 hours of birth and up to 2 weeks.	Benign Disappears without treatment.
Milia	White papules on the face; more frequently seen on the bridge of the nose and chin.	Exposed sebaceous glands that resolve without treatment. Parents might mistake these for whiteheads. Inform parents to leave them alone and let them resolve on own.
Lanugo	Fine, downy hair that develops after 16 weeks' gestation. The amount of lanugo decreases as the fetus ages. Often seen on the neonate's back, shoulders, and forehead.	Gradually falls out. The presence and amount of lanugo assist in estimating gestational age. Abundant lanugo may be a sign of prematurity or genetic disorder.

TABLE 15–4   Common Newborn Characteristics—cont'd

CHARACTERISTIC	APPEARANCE	SIGNIFICANCE
Vernix caseosa 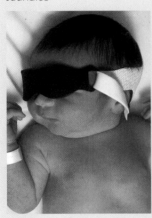	A protective substance secreted from sebaceous glands that covered the fetus during pregnancy. It looks like a whitish, cheesy substance. May be noted in auxiliary areas and genital areas of full-term neonates.	The presence and amount of vernix assists in estimating gestational age. Full-term neonates usually have none or small amounts of vernix.
Jaundice 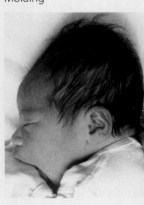	Yellow coloring of skin. First appears on the face and extends to the trunk and eventually the entire body. Best assessed in natural lighting. When jaundice is suspected, the nurse can apply gentle pressure to the skin over a firm surface such as nose, forehead, or sternum. The skin blanches to a yellowish hue.	Jaundice within the first 24 hours is pathological; usually related to problem of the liver (see Chapter 17). Jaundice occurring after 24 hours is referred to as physiological jaundice and is related to increased amount of unconjugated bilirubin in the system (see Chapter 17).
Molding	Elongation of the fetal head as it adapts to the birth canal	Resolves within 1 week.

Continued

TABLE 15–4   Common Newborn Characteristics—cont'd

CHARACTERISTIC	APPEARANCE	SIGNIFICANCE
Caput succedaneum 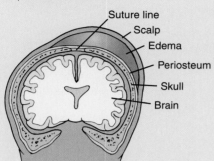	A localized soft tissue edema of the scalp It feels "spongy" and can cross suture lines.	Results from prolonged pressure of the head against the maternal cervix during labor. Resolves within the first week of life.
Cephalhematoma 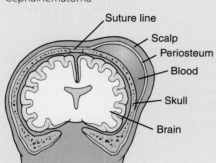	Hematoma formation between the periosteum and skull with unilateral swelling. It appears within a few hours of birth and can increase in size over the next few days. It has a well-defined outline. It does not cross suture lines.	Related trauma to the head due to prolonged labor, forceps delivery, or use of vacuum extractor. Can contribute to jaundice due to the large amounts of red blood cells being hemolyzed. Resolves within 3 months.
Epstein's pearls 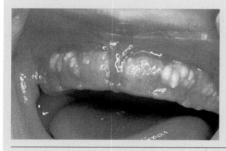	White, pearl-like epithelial cysts on gum margins and palate	Benign and usually disappears within a few weeks.
Natal teeth 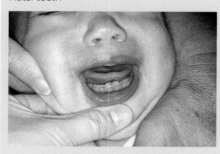	Immature caps of enamel and dentin with poorly developed roots Usually only one or two teeth are present.	They are usually benign, but can be associated with congenital defects. Natal teeth are often loose and need to be removed to decrease the risk of aspiration.

Dillon, 2007.

TABLE 15–5   Newborn Reflexes

REFLEX	HOW ELICITED	EXPECTED RESPONSE	ABNORMAL RESPONSE
Moro Present at birth; disappears by 6 months	Jar the crib or hold the baby in a semi-sitting position and let the head slightly drop back. 	Symmetrical abduction and extension of arms and legs, and legs flex up against trunk. The neonate makes a "C" shape with thumb and index finger.	A slow response might occur with preterm infants or sleepy neonates. An asymmetrical response may be related to temporary or permanent birth injury to clavicle, humerus, or brachial plexus.
Startle Present at birth; disappears by 4 months	Make a loud sound near the neonate. 	Same as Moro response	Slow response when sleeping Possible deafness Possible neurological deficit
Tonic neck Present between birth and 6 weeks; disappears by 4 to 6 months	With the neonate in a supine position, turn the head to the side so that the chin is over the shoulder. 	The neonate assumes a "fencing" position with arms and legs extended in the direction in which the head was turned.	Response after 6 months may indicate cerebral palsy.
Rooting Present at birth; disappears between 3 and 6 months	Brush the side of a cheek near the corner of the mouth. 	The neonate turns the head toward the direction of the stimulus and opens the mouth. Instruct mothers who are lactating to touch the corner of the neonate's mouth with a nipple and the infant will turn toward the nipple for feeding.	May not respond if recently fed. Prematurity or neurological defects may cause weak or absent response.
Sucking Present at birth; disappears at 10–12 months	Place a gloved finger or nipple of a bottle in the neonate's mouth. 	Sucking motion occurs.	May not respond if recently fed. Prematurity or neurological defects may cause weak or absent response.

Continued

TABLE 15–5   Newborn Reflexes—cont'd

REFLEX	HOW ELICITED	EXPECTED RESPONSE	ABNORMAL RESPONSE
Palmer grasp Present at birth; disappears at 3–4 months	The examiner places a finger in the palm of the neonate's hand. 	The neonate grasps fingers tightly. If the neonate grasps the examiner's fingers with both hands, he or she can be pulled to a sitting position.	Absent or weak response indicates a possible CNS defect; or nerve or muscle injury.
Plantar grasp Present at birth; disappears at 3–4 months	Place a thumb firmly against the ball of the infant's foot. 	Toes flex tightly down in a grasping motion	Weak or absent may indicate possible spinal cord injury.
Babinski Present at birth; disappears at 1 year	Stroke the lateral surface of the sole in an upward motion. 	Hyperextension and fanning of toes	Absent or weak may indicate a possible neurological defect.
Stepping or dancing Present at birth; disappears at 3–4 weeks	Hold the neonate upright with feet touching a flat surface. 	The neonate steps up and down in place.	Diminished response may indicate hypotonia.

Dillon, 2007.

TABLE 15–6   Ballard Maturational Assessment

NEUROMUSCULAR MATURITY	PHYSICAL MATURITY
Posture	**Skin**
Assess the position the neonate assumes while lying quietly on the back.	The examiner inspects the neonate's chest and abdominal skin areas for texture, transparency, thickness, and peeling/cracking.
The more mature, the greater degree of flexion in legs and arms.	A preterm neonate's skin is smooth, thin, and translucent (numerous veins visible).
	A full-term neonate's skin is thicker and more opaque with some degree of peeling.
Square Window	**Lanugo**
Assess the degree of the angle created when the examiner flexes the neonate's hand toward the forearm.	The examiner assesses the amount of lanugo on the neonate's back.
The more mature, the greater the flexion.	Lanugo begins to form around the 24 weeks' gestation. It is abundant in preterm neonates and decreases in amount as the neonate matures.
Arm Recoil	**Plantar Creases**
With the neonate in a supine position, the examiner fully flexes the forearm against the neonate's chest for 5 seconds. The examiner extends the arms and releases them.	The examiner inspects the bottom of the feet for location of creases.
The more mature, the faster the arms return to the flexed position (recoil).	The more creases over the greater proportion of the foot, the more mature the neonate.
Popliteal Angle	**Breast Tissue**
With the neonate in a supine position and pelvis flat, the examiner flexes the neonate's thigh to the abdomen. The leg is then extended. The angle at the knee is estimated.	The examiner assesses the degree of nipple formation. The size of the breast bud is measured by gently grasping the tissue with thumb and forefinger and measuring the distance between thumb and forefinger.
The lesser the angle, the greater the maturity.	The greater the degree of nipple formation and size of the breast bud, the greater the maturity.
Scarf Sign	**Ear Formation**
With the neonate in a supine position, the examiner takes the neonate's hand and moves the arm across the chest toward the opposite shoulder. The examiner notes where the elbow is in relationship to the midline of the chest.	The examiner assesses the ear for form and firmness.
	The more defined the ear is and the firmer it is, the more mature the neonate.
The more preterm, the more the elbow crosses the midline.	
Heel to Ear	**Genitalia**
	Male:
With the neonate in a supine position, the examiner takes the neonate's foot and moves it toward the ear.	The examiner palpates the scrotum for the presence of testes and inspects the scrotum for appearance.
The lesser the flexion (the farther the heel is from the ear), the greater the maturity.	The greater the descent of the testes and the greater degree of rugae (creases), the greater the maturity.
	Female:
	The examiner moves the neonate's hip one half abduction and visually inspects the genitalia.
	The more the labia majora covers the labia minora and clitoris, the greater the maturity.

Neuromuscular Maturity

	-1	0	1	2	3	4	5
Posture							
Square Window (Wrist)	-90°	90°	60°	45°	30°	0°	
Arm Recoil		180°	140°-180°	110°-140°	90°-110°	<90°	
Popliteal Angle	180°	160°	140°	120°	100°	90°	<90°
Scarf Sign							
Heel To Ear							

Physical Maturity

Skin	sticky friable transparent	gelantinous red translucent	smooth pink visible veins	superficial peeling or rash, few veins	cracking pale areas rare veins	parchment deep cracking no vessels	leathery cracked wrinkled
Lanugo	none	sparse	abundant	thinning	bald areas	mostly bald	
Plantar Surface	heel-toe 40–50 mm:-1 <40 mm:-2	>50 mm no crease	faint red marks	anterior transverse crease only	creases ant. 2/3	creases over entire sole	
Breast	imperceptible	barely perceptible	flat areola no bud	stippled areola 1–2 mm bud	raised areola 3–4 mm bud	full areola 5–10 mm bud	
Eye/ear	lids fused loosely:-1 tightly:-2	lids open pinna flat stays folded	sl. curved pinna; soft; slow recoil	well-curved pinna; soft but ready recoil	formed and firm instant recoil	thick cartilage ear stiff	
Genitals (Male)	scrotum flat, smooth	scrotum empty faint rugae	testes in upper canal rare rugae	testes descending few rugae	testes down good rugae	testes pendulous deep rugae	
Genitals (Female)	clitoris prominent labia flat	prominent clitoris small labia minora	prominent clitoris enlarging minora	majora and minora equally prominent	majora large minora small	majora cover clitoris and minora	

Maturity Rating

Score	Weeks
-10	20
-5	22
0	24
5	26
10	28
15	30
20	32
25	34
30	36
35	38
40	40
45	42
50	44

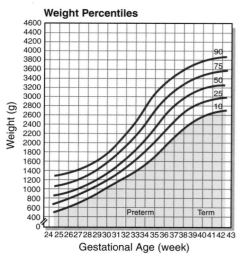

Weight Percentiles

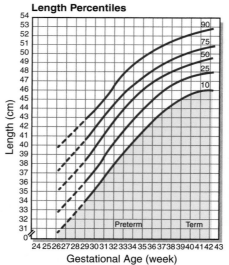

Length Percentiles

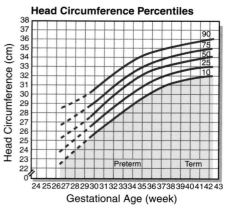

Head Circumference Percentiles

Classification of Infant*	Weight	Length	Head Circ.
Large for gestational age (LGA) (>90th percentile)			
Appropriate for gestational age (AGA) (10th to 90th percentile)			
Small for gestational age (SGA) (<10th percentile)			

*Place an "X" in the appropriate box (LGA, AGA, or SGA) for weight, for length, and for head circumference.

FIGURE 15–8 Ballard Gestational Age Assessment Tool.

BOX 15-1 | ASPMN Position Statement: Pain Assessment in the Patient Unable to Self-Report

"The American Society for Pain Management Nursing (ASPMN) positions that all persons with pain deserve prompt recognition and treatment. Pain should be routinely assessed, reassessed, and documented to facilitate treatment and communication among health care clinicians. In patients who are unable to self-report pain, other strategies must be used to infer pain and evaluate interventions."

Herr, Coyne, McCaffery, Manworren, & Merkel, 2011.

pattern, and facial expressions. Some tools may also include blood pressure and oxygen saturation level. The tool used for assessment varies based on hospital policies and procedures.

BEHAVIORAL CHARACTERISTICS

The neonate is a biosocial being with unique behavioral characteristics that affect parent–infant attachment (see Chapter 13). Infant temperament has a major influence on the parent–infant relationship. Temperament can vary from an infant being an "easy" baby to a "fussy" baby. Most infants vacillate between the two extremes of temperament. Some infants are more sensitive to stimulus and are difficult to comfort, but most infants respond to parents' efforts to comfort. Infant temperaments that match the expectations of the parents foster parent–infant attachment, whereas those who do not match parents' expectations can hamper the parent–infant attachment (see Chapter 13 for additional information).

Periods of Reactivity

Neonates experience predictable behavior during the first 6 to 8 hours of extrauterine life, referred to as periods of reactivity. Neonates will transition between periods of activity and inactivity. Each of the periods is characterized by predictable behaviors.

Initial Period of Reactivity

This period of reactivity occurs in the first 15 to 30 minutes postbirth. The neonate is alert and active and vigorously responds to external stimuli.

- Respirations are irregular and rapid and can be as high as 90 breaths per minute; the heart rate is rapid and can be as high as 180 beats per minute (bpm).
- The neonate may exhibit momentary grunting, flaring, and retractions.
- The neonate may experience brief periods of apnea and brief periods of cyanosis.
- The amount of oral mucus increases.

Period of Relative Inactivity

This period of relative inactivity begins approximately 30 minutes after birth and lasts 2 hours when the infant enters a sleep state and becomes unresponsive to external stimuli. Respiratory rate and heart rate decrease and can fall slightly below normal range, and oral mucus production decreases.

Second Period of Reactivity

The second period of reactivity follows the period of relative inactivity and lasts 2 to 8 hours. Neonates vacillate between active alert and quiet alert states. The neonate is more responsive to external stimuli. There are periods of rapid respirations and increased heart rate in response to stimuli and activity. There is an increase in bowel activity and the neonate may pass meconium stool.

The initial period of activity provides an opportunity for the parents and neonate to respond to each other. It is an ideal time to initiate breastfeeding. The neonate is not responsive during the period of inactivity and will not be interested in feeding/sucking. During the second period of reactivity, the neonate is interested in feeding/sucking, and this is another ideal time for breastfeeding.

Brazelton Neonatal Behavioral Assessment Scale

The Brazelton Neonatal Behavioral Assessment Scale (BNBAS) is used to assess the neonate's neurobehavioral system. The BNBAS was originally developed as a research tool and has been adapted for use in the clinical setting. The BNBAS is not routinely performed on healthy neonates. It is composed of 28 behavior items and 18 reflex items divided into six categories:

- Habituation: The development of decreased sensitivity to a repeated stimulus such as light, sound, or heel stick. It is a protective mechanism against overstimulation. Habituation may not be fully developed in premature neonates or in neonates with CNS abnormalities or injuries.
- Orientation: The ability of the neonate to focus on visual and/or auditory stimuli. The neonate will turn his or her head in the direction of sound or will follow a visual stimulus. This response is diminished in premature neonates.
- Motor maturity: The ability of the neonate to control and coordinate motor activity. Normal findings are smooth, free movement with occasional tremors. Movement is jerky in premature neonates and/or in neonates with CNS abnormalities or injuries.
- Self-quieting ability: The ability of the neonate to quiet and comfort self. It is accomplished by sucking on the fist/hand or attending to external stimuli. The ability is diminished in neonates with neurological injuries or in those exposed to drugs in utero.
- Social behaviors: The ability of the neonate to respond to cuddling and holding. These behaviors are diminished or absent in neonates with neurological injuries or in neonates exposed to drugs in utero.

- Sleep/awake states: These are also referred to as infant states or behavior states. There are two sleep states and four awake states.
  - Deep sleep: During this state, there is no body movement except for an occasional startle reflex. This reflex is delayed in response to external stimuli. External stimuli are less likely to cause a change in state. The eyes are closed and there are no eye movements. Breathing is smooth and even.
  - Light sleep: During this state, there is random body movement. Rapid eye movement (REM) is present. The neonate responds to external stimuli with a startle reflex and with a possible change of state. Breathing is irregular.
  - Drowsy: During this state, there is intermittent body movement. Eyes open and close and have a dull and heavy-lidded appearance. Breathing is irregular. Response to sensory stimuli is delayed. External stimuli will most likely cause a change in state. Breathing is irregular.
  - Alert: During this state, the neonate's eyes are wide open with a bright look and focus on the sources of stimuli. There is a delay in response to stimuli and minimal body movement. Respirations are regular.
  - Eyes open: During this state, there is a considerable body movement with periods of fussiness. The eyes are open. The neonate responds to external stimuli with increased startle reflexes and motor activity. Breathing is irregular.
  - Crying: During this state, there is high motor activity and intense crying. It is difficult to calm the neonate. The eyes are opened or tightly closed. Breathing is irregular (Brazelton & Nugent, 1995).

NURSING CARE OF THE NEONATE

Nursing care of the neonate during hospitalization is divided into two time frames. The first is the fourth stage of labor, from birth through the first 4 hours of extrauterine life. The second is from 4 hours of age to discharge.

Nursing Actions During the Fourth Stage of Labor

The changes that occur in the neonate's body during the transition to extrauterine life require frequent assessments and monitoring to identify early signs of physiological compromise. Early identification of complications or difficulty with transition allows for earlier initiation of nursing and medical actions to support the neonate in a healthy transition. The following nursing actions occur in the labor/delivery/recovery room and/or nursery, depending on hospital policies and health state of the neonate.

- Review prenatal and intrapartal records for factors that place the neonate at risk, such as prolonged rupture of membranes (risk of infection), meconium-stained fluid (risk of respiratory distress), and gestational diabetes (risk of hypoglycemia).

- Decrease risk of cold stress by:
  - Drying the neonate immediately after birth to prevent excessive heat loss through evaporation.
  - Discarding wet blankets and placing the neonate on dry, warm blankets or sheets.
  - Placing a stocking cap on the neonate's head to decrease the risk of heat loss through convection.
  - Placing the neonate in the mother's arms with skin-to-skin contact and a warm blanket over mother and baby or placing the neonate under a preheated radiant warmer.
- Support respirations by clearing the mouth and nose of excessive mucus with a bulb syringe when indicated (see Chapter 16).
- Use universal precautions. Wear gloves until after the neonate has been bathed to decrease exposure to blood-borne pathogens from amniotic fluid and maternal blood.
- Obtain the Apgar score at 1 and 5 minutes and initiate appropriate actions based on the score (see Chapter 8).
- Assess vital signs.
  - This is usually done within 30 minutes of birth, 1 hour after birth, and then every hour for the remainder of the recovery period.
  - Vital signs are assessed every 5 to 15 minutes for neonates with signs of distress.
  - The frequency of assessments may vary based on institutional policies and the health of the neonate.
  - Administer O_2 per institutional protocol, if the heart rate is below 100 bpm, cyanosis is present, and/or apnea occurs. Before administration of O_2 the nurse should:
    - Check the airway and apply suction if indicated.
    - Stimulate the neonate by rubbing his or her back.
- Inspect the clamped cord for number of vessels and for bleeding.
- Complete and place identifying bands on the neonate and parents before the neonate is separated from parents (e.g., taken to the nursery or NICU).
- Weigh and measure the neonate.
- Complete a neonatal assessment within 2 hours of birth.
  - Explain to the parents the assessments and procedures performed on their newborn.
- Complete a gestational age assessment as per hospital policies.
- Obtain blood glucose levels by using a glucose monitor.
  - This is done on all neonates who exhibit symptoms of hypoglycemia as well as neonates who are at risk for hypoglycemia.
- Administer erythromycin ophthalmic ointment to each eye.
  - The American Academy of Pediatrics and Centers for Disease Control and Prevention (CDC) recommend that ophthalmic neonatorum prophylaxis be administered to all newborns within 24 hours of birth.
  - Refer to institutional policies for timing of the application of ointment.
- Administer phytonadione IM within 6 hours of birth.
- Support breastfeeding by providing a relaxing environment for the woman and her newborn (Fig. 15–9).
- Bathe the neonate with neutral pH soap. The initial bath is delayed until the neonate's temperature is stable and within

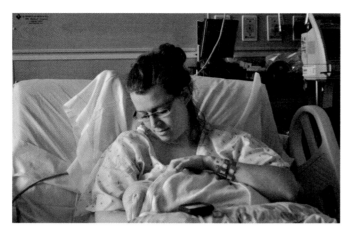

FIGURE 15–9 Newborn breastfeeding during the fourth stage of labor.

normal limits. The timing of the initial bath can vary; refer to hospital policies.

● Promote parent–infant attachment by creating a relaxing environment:
  ● Cluster nursing activities to allow for periods of uninterrupted time for new parents to spend with their newborn.
  ● Dim lights and close room door.
● Notify the neonate's physician or nurse practitioner of the neonate's date and time of birth and assessment findings.

SAFE AND EFFECTIVE NURSING CARE: Understanding Medication

Erythromycin Ophthalmic Ointment (0.5%)
● Indication: Prophylaxis treatment for gonococcal or chlamydial eye infections
● Action: Prevents bacterial growth by inhibiting folic acid synthesis
● Common side effects: Edema and inflammation of eyelids
● Route and dose: Apply a 1/4-inch bead of ointment to lower eyelid of each eye.
● Precaution: Prevent the applicator tip from directly touching the eye by holding the application tube 1/2 inch from the eye.

Vallerand & Sanoski, 2017.

CRITICAL COMPONENT

Promoting Parent–Infant Attachment
The promotion of parent–infant attachment is a critical component of nursing care and needs to occur as soon as possible after birth. Often, nurses allow other nursing actions to take priority over parent–infant attachment or find it is easier to do assessments under the warming unit. Assessments and monitoring of vital signs can be performed in the parent's arms

when the neonate is full-term, the Apgar score is 8 or higher, and there were no signs of fetal distress during labor or at the time of birth. Parent–infant interaction is influenced by the parent's cultural beliefs. It is important for nurses to demonstrate cultural awareness in their nursing care.

Nursing Actions
• Initiate skin-to-skin contact with a warm blanket over the neonate and parent.
• Point out and explain expected neonatal characteristics such as molding, milia, and lanugo.
• Provide alone time for the couple and their neonate by organizing care that allows for uninterrupted time.
• Delay administration of eye ointment until parents have had an opportunity to hold the baby. Once ointment is administered, the neonate is less likely to open his or her eyes and make eye contact with parents.
• Provide nursing care that reflects respect for the parents' cultural beliefs.

CRITICAL COMPONENT

Danger Signs
The following signs may be an indication of an abnormality or complication. Document these signs in the neonatal record and report them to the physician or nurse practitioner:

• Tachypnea (greater than 60 breaths per minute)
• Retractions of chest wall
• Grunting
• Nasal flaring
• Abdominal distention
• Failure to pass meconium stool within 48 hours of birth
• Failure to void within 24 hours of birth
• Convulsions
• Lethargy
• Jaundice within first 24 hours of birth
• Abnormal temperature, either abnormally high or low
• Jitteriness
• Persistent hypoglycemia
• Persistent temperature instability

Nursing Actions From 4 Hours of Age to Discharge

The second stage of neonatal care focuses on monitoring the neonate's adaptation to extrauterine life and helping parents learn about their newborns and how to care for them. The nursing actions listed are for neonates who do not exhibit signs of distress or potential complications.

● Assess vital signs as per hospital policy.
  ● Neonates continue to have difficulty in regulating their body temperature during this period. Vital signs for stable neonates are assessed at least once per shift. The physician or nurse practitioner should be notified when temperature decreases persist.

- Complete neonatal assessment once per shift. The type of assessment varies based on institutional policies.
- Promote parent–infant attachment by providing uninterrupted times with their newborn.
- Promote sibling attachment by providing opportunities for interactions with the newborn, such as having older siblings assist with newborn care or listen to the newborn's heart.
- Prevent infant abduction from the hospital. Prevention begins during the fourth stage of labor and continues throughout the hospitalization. Each hospital has policies and procedures addressing methods to prevent infant abduction. Common steps that are taken are:
  - Taking footprints and photo of infant for identification purposes.
  - Placing armbands on the mother, her partner, and their neonate that contain the same identification number. The bands of neonates should be checked with the bands of the parents at the beginning of each shift and when taking or returning neonates from or to the mother's room.
  - Placing infant security tags and using hospital abduction alarm systems that trigger an alarm, locked doors, and freeze elevators if the infant comes within 4 feet of an exit or elevator.
  - Requiring personnel working in the maternal–newborn units to wear name tags specific to that unit. Name tags should have a photo and name of the person.
  - Instructing parents and family members to not allow anyone to take their newborn if the person does not possess the appropriate identification specific to the maternity unit.
  - Encouraging parents to accompany any person who removes their infant from the mother's room.
  - Placing the neonate's crib on the far side of the room away from the door leading to the hallway.
  - Instructing parents not to leave their newborn in the mother's room unattended. This includes when she is taking a shower.
  - Securing the maternal–newborn units, allowing only visitors with identification to enter.
- Assist parents with infant feeding (see Chapter 16).
- Provide information to parents on newborn care (see Chapter 16).
- Teach parents about normal newborn characteristics (see Table 15–4).
- Instruct parents to place their newborns on their backs to decrease the risk of sudden infant death syndrome (see Chapter 16).

CRITICAL COMPONENT

Hypothermia

Neonates with temperatures below 36.5°C (97.7°F) are at risk for hypothermia.

Nursing actions include the following:

- Parent–infant skin-to-skin contact with a warm blanket over both the neonate and the parent or wrap the neonate in warm blankets.
- If the temperature remains below 36.5°C (97.7°F), place the neonate under a preheated warmer. Unwrap the neonate so that the skin is exposed to the radiant heat. Attach the electronic skin probe. The warmer is set at 1.5°C above the neonate's temperature. Continue to adjust the radiant temperature in relationship to the neonate's temperature.
- Monitor the blood glucose level as per institutional policies, as hypothermia can lead to hypoglycemia.
- Notify the physician or nurse practitioner if the neonate's temperature does not return to normal ranges.
- Document the temperature and actions taken.

SKIN CARE

The skin of a term neonate is smooth, soft, slightly transparent, and has less pigmentation than that of an older child (Blackburn, 2012). The neonate's skin is subjected to a variety of stresses related to the birthing process and transition to extrauterine life. Causes of potential threats to skin integrity are:

- Pressure exerted on the presenting part of the fetus during the labor and birthing process from maternal structures such as the pelvis, causing edema and hematomas.
- Abrasions, bruising, and edema of the skin related to use of vacuum extractors, forceps, and internal fetal monitoring.
- Exposure to bacteria from the maternal genital tract.
- Use of adhesives.
- Drying out and flaking of skin, a natural process that occurs during the first few weeks of life.
- Diaper dermatitis.

Nursing Actions

- Assess skin once per shift and the perineal area at each diaper change. Intact and healthy skin is a first-line defense against infection.
- Decrease risk of diaper dermatitis by changing diapers and cleaning the perineal area with water every 1 to 3 hours. Apply barrier products containing petrolatum and/or zinc oxide at each diaper change for infants at risk for diaper dermatitis (AWHONN, 2013). Apply antifungal creams when fungal infection is present.
- Use adhesives that cause the least amount of trauma. Slowly and gently remove adhesives using moist gauze (AWHONN, 2013).
- Apply emollients to dry and flaking skin every 12 hours as needed (AWHONN, 2013).

SCREENING TESTS

Prior to hospital discharge, screening tests are performed to assist the neonate's health care provider in identifying possible harmful disorders or genetic disorders.

BOX 15–2 | AWHONN Position Statement: Newborn Screening

"The Association of Women's Health, Obstetric and Neonatal Nursing (AWHONN) supports national minimum standards for newborn screening programs. Federal oversight is necessary to guarantee that all newborns have equal access to timely identification and interventions for disorders that have been identified for routine screening. In addition, a combination of federal and state funding should be allocated to initiate and sustain programs that limit the effects of these disorders.

"AWHONN recommends that Newborn Screening programs include the following:

- Health care provider education
- Parent education
- Parental notification and consent, even if tests are mandatory
- Timely screening tests prior to hospital or birthing facility discharge
- Post discharge follow-up for additional screening tests or other services, when appropriate
- Resources for appropriate referrals
- Accurate and consistent systems for data collection
- Access to interventions and treatments indicated by the diagnosis."

AWHONN, 2011.

Newborn Screening

Newborn screenings consist of a blood test and a hearing test. Some states are also including heart defect screening. The blood test screens for infections, genetic diseases, and inherited and metabolic disorders and is performed on all babies born in the United States (Box 15–2). Routine newborn screening (blood test) began in the 1960s when all babies were screened for phenylketonuria (PKU); today, newborns are screened for approximately 30 disorders. Each state has statutes or regulations on newborn screening, and the degree of screening varies from state to state. Specific information on each state's requirements can be accessed at www.babysfirsttest.org/newborn-screening/states.

CRITICAL COMPONENT

Phenylketonuria

PKU is an inborn error of metabolism. Neonates with PKU are unable to metabolize phenylalanine, which is an amino acid commonly found in many foods such as breast milk and formula. This leads to a buildup of phenylpyruvic and phenylacetic acids, which are abnormal metabolites of phenylalanine. The buildup of abnormal metabolites can cause permanent brain damage and death. This can be prevented by early detection and dietary management.

The ideal time of blood collection is at 2 to 5 days of age, which provides time for the neonate to ingest breast milk or formula. Most tests are done within the first 24 to 48 hours of birth due to early hospital discharges. Information pertaining to the test is given to the parents. The blood is obtained from a heel stick and may be collected by nursing or laboratory personnel. To ensure accurate results, a blood test is obtained during the first pediatric clinic appointment.

CRITICAL COMPONENT

Heel Stick

The heel stick is a common procedure performed on neonates. Blood is collected to assess blood glucose, hematocrit, and for newborn screening.

Procedure

1. Provide parents with information on the test or tests that have been ordered for their child.
2. Obtain required consents.
3. Warm the neonate's foot for 10 minutes by wrapping in a warm, moist washcloth. This will help facilitate circulation to the peripheral area.
4. Don gloves.
5. With the nondominant hand, hold the neonate's foot in a dorsiflexed position. The nurse or technician should have a firm grasp of the foot, but the foot should not be squeezed.
6. Clean the heel with alcohol.
7. Puncture the skin in the lateral or medial aspect of the heel to decrease the risk of nerve damage.

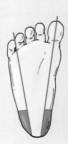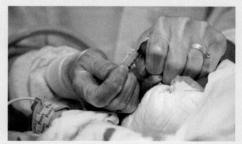

8. Wipe off the first few drops of blood.
9. Allow large drops of blood to form and to fall on the testing material.
10. Clean the puncture area and place a small dressing over it.

Document that blood was collected, the type of test, the site of puncture, and the response of the neonate.

Hearing Screening

Language development begins at birth as neonates are exposed to sounds and voices in their environment. Hearing loss is a common congenital abnormality with a prevalence of 1.6 per 1,000 screened infants. Early detection of hearing loss provides parents the opportunity to seek interventions that foster language development. In 1993, the National Institutes of Health (NIH) recommended that all newborns be screened for hearing loss prior to hospital discharge (NIH, 2017). All states have established Early Hearing Detection and Interventions (EHDI), which mandate that all newborns be screened for hearing loss—96.1% of infants are screened prior to 1 month.

The hearing screening test is usually done in the hospital before discharge by a member of the nursing staff who has completed special training and education in conducting the test.

There are two types of screening tests that may be used either alone or together. The screening tests rely on physiological measures versus behavioral response but do not provide information on the type or degree of hearing impairment. These screening tests are:

- Otoacoustic emissions (OAE) is a painless test that is conducted when the neonate is asleep or lying still. A tiny, flexible ear probe is inserted into the neonate's ear. It records responses of the outer hair cells of the cochlea to clicking sounds coming from the probe's microphone. A referral is made to a hearing specialist when there is no recorded response from the cochlear hair cells.
- Automated auditory brain stem response (AABR) is a painless test conducted when the neonate is asleep or lying still. Disposable electrodes are placed high on the neonate's forehead, on the mastoid, and on the nape of the neck. This screening test assesses electrical activity of the cochlea, auditory nerve, and brain stem in response to sound. A referral to a hearing specialist is recommended for neonates who do not have a positive response to the sound stimuli.

Tests must be conducted in a quiet room. Vernix, blood, and amniotic fluid in the ear can interfere with accurate screening. Neonates who fail the initial screening test are rescreened in 1 month. Diagnostic testing is recommended for neonates who fail the second screening.

THERAPEUTIC AND SURGICAL PROCEDURES

Therapeutic and surgical procedures that healthy newborns may encounter include immunizations and elective circumcisions.

Immunizations

Hepatitis B is spread through contact with blood of an infected person or by sexual contact with an infected person, and it causes inflammation of the liver. The CDC recommends that all neonates be vaccinated for hepatitis B before hospital discharge. The CDC also recommends that neonates who have been or possibly have been exposed to hepatitis B during birth be given both the hepatitis B vaccine and hepatitis B immune globulin (HBIg) within 12 hours of birth. The second dose of hepatitis B vaccine is given at 1 to 2 months of age. The third dose is given at 6 to 18 months of age (see Appendix B).

CRITICAL COMPONENT

Intramuscular Injections
Procedure

1. Review the written orders for the newborn.
2. Inform the parents of the reason for the medication or vaccine.
3. Obtain written consent when required.
4. Follow the five rights of medication administration.
5. Draw up medication or vaccine in a 1-mL syringe with a 25-gauge 5/8 needle.
6. Invite the parents to comfort their infant by stroking the infant's head or hands.
7. Put on gloves.
8. Undo the diaper for full exposure of the leg.
9. Identify the injection site. The preferred site is the vastus lateralis.
10. Clean the area with an alcohol swab and let it dry. It is extremely important to remove all maternal blood and amniotic fluid from the injection site to prevent transmission of blood-borne pathogens.
11. Stabilize the knee with the heel of the hand. Grasp the tissue of the injection site with your thumb and forefinger.
12. Insert the needle at a 90-degree angle.

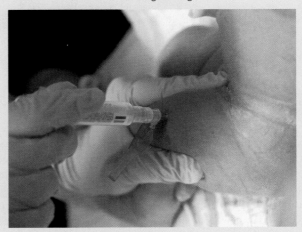

13. Slowly inject medication or a vaccine to decrease the amount of discomfort.
14. Withdraw the needle and rub the site to promote absorption.
15. Place a small dressing over the site.
16. Properly dispose of the needle and syringe.
17. Document date, time, and location of injection.

Circumcision

Male circumcision is an elective surgery to remove the foreskin of the penis. According to a 2015 CDC report, the percentage of newborn circumcisions declined from 1979 to 2010, from 64.5% to 58.3% (CDC, 2015). The decision to circumcise the neonate is made by the parents and is based on their cultural, religious, and personal beliefs. The American Academy of Pediatrics does not recommend routine new-born circumcisions. Circumcisions are done in the hospital before the woman and infant are discharged or later in the pediatric clinic.

Contraindications for circumcision include:

● Preterm neonates.
● Neonates with a genitourinary defect.
● Neonates at risk for bleeding problems.
● Neonates with compromising disorders such as respiratory distress syndrome.

Risks related to circumcision include:

● Hemorrhage.
● Infection.
● Adhesions.
● Pain.

Benefits related to circumcision include decreased incidence of urinary tract infections and sexually transmitted infections.

Three common devices used for circumcisions are Gomco clamp, Mogen clamp, and Plastibell (Fig. 15–10). The Mogen clamp is commonly used by mohels when performing ceremonial circumcisions.

Surgical Procedure

Preoperative care measures are as follows:

● Information regarding benefits and risks of circumcisions, and the procedure is provided by neonate's health care provider.
● Written consent is obtained from the parents.
● Verification that the neonate has voided, as lack of voiding may be related to an anatomical abnormality that contraindicates circumcision.
● The neonate does not eat 2 to 3 hours before the procedure to decrease the risk of vomiting and aspiration during the procedure.
● Acetaminophen is administered 1 hour before procedure per the physician's order for pain management (Box 15–3).

During intraoperative care:

● The neonate is positioned and secured on a specially designed plastic board, often referred to as a circumcision board. The board is padded to promote comfort. The upper part of the neonate is swaddled to promote comfort and reduce heat loss.
● An ear bulb is placed near the neonate to use in case of vomiting or increased mucus.
● The penis is cleansed, and a sterile drape specially designed for circumcision is placed over the trunk.
● A sucrose-dipped pacifier is offered during the nerve block and procedure for pain management.
● The physician administers a penile nerve block.
● The physician applies a Gomco clamp, Mogen clamp, or Plastibell (see Fig. 15–10).

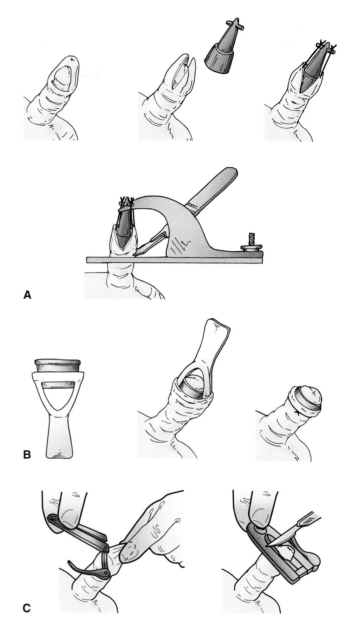

FIGURE 15–10 Removal of the prepuce during circumcision. (*A*) Gomco clamp. (*B*) Plastibell. (*C*) Mogen clamp.

● The physician surgically removes the foreskin with a scalpel.
● Some health care providers, when using a Gomco or Mogen clamp, will apply a petroleum-impregnated gauze around the end of the penis to promote comfort by reducing the amount of irritation caused by friction with the diaper.

Postoperative care includes the following:

● The penis is assessed every 15 minutes for the first hour for signs of bleeding, then every 2 to 3 hours according to hospital policies. The physician is notified when bleeding is present (spots larger than the size of a quarter).
● Acetaminophen PO is administered every 4 to 6 hours.
● Voidings are assessed and documented. The neonate should void within 24 hours after the procedure.

BOX 15–3 | ASPMN Position Statement: Male Infant Circumcision Pain Management

"The American Society for Pain Management Nursing (ASPMN) holds the position that nurses and other healthcare professionals must provide optimal pain management throughout the circumcision process for male infants. Parents must be prepared for the procedure and educated about the infant's pain assessment. They must also be informed of pharmacologic and integrative pain management therapies."

Nursing actions include:

- Administering acetaminophen 1 hour prior to procedure.
- Applying topical anesthetic cream prior to procedure.
- Positioning newborn in a semi-recumbent position on a padded surface with arms swaddled.
- Administering 24% sucrose or breast milk orally 2 minutes before penile manipulation or offering pacifier for non-nutritive sucking if sucrose or breast milk contraindicated.
- Administrating oral acetaminophen for at least 24 hours postprocedure.
- Instructing parents in infant pain assessment and management, and in care of circumcision.

ASPMN, 2011.

Parent Education

- Instruct parents to watch for bleeding and signs of infection and to note when their child voids.
- Inform parents that the gauze will fall off on its own and they should not pull it off. Pulling the gauze off can interfere with the healing process.
- Instruct parents to fasten diapers loosely to promote comfort by decreasing pressure on the surgical site.

- Instruct parents to notify the physician when:
  - Bleeding is present (larger than the size of a quarter).
  - Signs of infection are present.
  - The neonate has not voided within 24 hours.

See Chapter 16 for additional information on neonatal circumcision.

Evidence-Based Practice: Sucrose as Analgesia for Minor Procedural Pain Management in Neonates

Thakkar, P., Arora, K., Das, B., Javadekar, S., & Panigrahi, S. (2016). To evaluate and compare the efficacy of combined sucrose and non-nutritive sucking for analgesia in newborns undergoing minor painful procedure: a randomized controlled trial. *Journal of Perinatology, 36,* 67-70.

The aim of this randomized control study was to evaluate and compare the effectiveness of combined sucrose and non-nutritive sucking (NNS) for pain management for neonates undergoing heel-stick procedures. The sample consisted of 180 full-term neonates with birth weight greater than 2,200 g and older than 24 hours. The neonates were randomized into one of four groups with intervention administered 2 minutes before the procedure.

- Group 1 received 30% sucrose solution PO by sterile syringe.
- Group 2 received NNS, in which sterile gauze was held gently in the neonate's mouth and the palate tickled to stimulate sucking.
- Group 3 received both 30% sucrose and NNS.
- Group 4 received no interventions.

Two minutes before the intervention(s), baseline heart rate and oxygen saturation were recorded. Continuous video recording of the procedure, including heart rate and oxygen saturations, were done throughout the procedure. The Premature Infant Pain Profile (PIPP), which is used on both full-term and preterm infants, was used to evaluate neonates' pain during the procedure.

Results:
The median PIPP score significantly decreased in groups 1, 2, and 3 compared to the non-intervention group (group 4). The combined intervention (group 3) of sucrose and NNS significantly decreased the medium PIPP score compared with groups 1 and 2.

Conclusion:
Use of sucrose and NNS are effective methods of pain management for full-term infants undergoing heel-stick procedures with combined use of sucrose and NNS being more effective.

Clinical Pathway for Full-Term Low-Risk Neonate

DELIVERY DATE AND TIME

Focus of Care	Birth to First Hour	1–4 Hours of Age	4–24 Hours of Age	24 Hours of Age to Discharge
Assessments	Obtain Apgar score at 1 and 5 minutes. Inspect the skin for abrasions or bruises.	Complete neonatal assessment by 2 hours of age. Complete gestational assessment as per hospital policy. Weigh and measure the head, chest, and length.	Assess at the beginning of each shift or per hospital policies. Weigh the newborn each day per hospital policy.	Assess at the beginning of each shift or per hospital policies and before discharge. Weigh the newborn each day per hospital policy.
Thermoregulation	Close the doors to the birthing room. Dry the neonate thoroughly and place in a prewarmed crib or skin-to-skin on the mother's chest with a warm blanket over them. Place a stocking cap over the top of the neonate's head. Assess axillary temperature every 30 minutes or per hospital policy.	Prevent heat loss by maintaining an NTE. Encourage skin-to-skin contact with either parent and with a warm blanket over both the neonate and parent. Wrap the neonate in blankets when in an open crib. Place a stocking cap on the head.	Prevent heat loss by maintaining an NTE. Wrap the neonate in blankets when in an open crib. Place a stocking cap on the neonate's head.	Prevent heat loss by maintaining an NTE. Assist the mother in dressing her infant for discharge in clothing and blankets that help maintain the neonate's normal body temperature.
Respiratory	Clear the nose and mouth of mucus with use of an ear bulb. Assess respirations every 30 minutes. Assess lung sounds. Monitor for signs of respiratory distress: grunting, flaring, retractions.	Keep the nose and mouth free of mucus with use of an ear bulb. Assess respirations every hour. Assess lung sounds. Monitor for signs of respiratory distress: grunting, flaring, retractions.	Assess respirations once per shift. Assess lung sounds once per shift. Monitor for signs of respiratory distress: grunting, flaring, retractions.	Assess respirations once per shift. Assess lung sounds once per shift and before discharge.
Cardiovascular	Assess skin color for cyanosis. Assess heart rate every 30 minutes.	Assess skin color for cyanosis. Assess heart rate every hour.	Assess the heart rate once per shift.	Assess heart rate once per shift and before discharge.
Activity	Assess the level of activity and compare to periods of reactivity. Monitor for signs of hypoglycemia (i.e., jitteriness).	Assess the level of activity and compare to periods of reactivity. Monitor for signs of hypoglycemia (i.e., jitteriness).	Assess the level of activity and compare to periods of reactivity. Monitor for signs of hypoglycemia (i.e., jitteriness).	Assess the level of activity.

Continued

Clinical Pathway for Full-Term Low-Risk Neonate— cont'd

DELIVERY DATE AND TIME

Focus of Care	Birth to First Hour	1–4 Hours of Age	4–24 Hours of Age	24 Hours of Age to Discharge
Nutrition	Ideal time to introduce breastfeeding is when the neonate is in the first period of reactivity.	Breastfeed on demand.	The ideal time for feeding is when the neonate is in the second period of reactivity. Breastfeed or bottle feed on demand; feeding should be every 2–4 hours.	Breastfeed or bottle feed on demand; feeding should be every 2–4 hours.
Elimination	The neonate may or may not void or pass meconium stool.	The neonate may or may not void or pass meconium stool.	The neonate voids within 24 hours. The neonate may or may not pass meconium stool.	The neonate voids a minimum of 2 times on day 2 and 5–6 times on day 3. The neonate passes meconium or transitional stools several times a day.
Medications and immunizations	Inform the parents which medications are being administered and why. Administer vitamin K injection and instill eye ointment as per physician's order.	Inform parents which medications are being administered and why. Administer vitamin K injection and instill eye ointment if not done during first hour as per physician order.	Provide parents with information on hepatitis B vaccine and obtain written consent if required. Administer hepatitis B vaccine as per physician order. Administer hepatitis B immune globulin vaccine when indicated per physician order.	
Special procedures	Heel stick to assess glucose levels as indicated (i.e., jitteriness), LGA, and SGA.	Heel stick to assess glucose levels as indicated (i.e., jitteriness), LGA, and SGA.		Newborn screening tests: Blood sample Newborn hearing Circumcision might be done several hours before discharge.
Family attachment	Delay eye ointment until parents have had the opportunity to hold their newborn. Provide time for parents to see and touch and/or hold the newborn. Explain to partners that they can stay with their newborn while assessments are being completed.	Complete necessary assessments as quickly as possible in order to provide uninterrupted time for parents to hold and be with their newborn. Complete assessments at bedside when possible.	Arrange nursing care to provide uninterrupted time for parents and their newborn. Teach parents about normal newborn characteristics and behavior.	Arrange nursing care to provide uninterrupted time for parents and their newborn.

Clinical Pathway for Full-Term Low-Risk Neonate— cont'd

DELIVERY DATE AND TIME

Focus of Care	Birth to First Hour	1–4 Hours of Age	4–24 Hours of Age	24 Hours of Age to Discharge
Education	Point out normal newborn characteristics such as molding, lanugo, and vernix. Begin education on breastfeeding (e.g., positioning, latching on, releasing suction).	Teaching is kept to a minimum since parents are usually tired during this period of time or want to call family members to announce the birth.	Ideal time for teaching. Provide information on caring for a newborn (see Chapter 16).	Continue teaching parents about the care of their newborn (see Chapter 16). Complete the appropriate hospital discharge teaching forms. Give parents a copy of written discharge instructions. Explain the importance of follow-up well-child checkups and the importance of scheduling their first appointment as recommend by their pediatrician or Pediatric Nurse Practitioner (PNP).
Safety	Place completed ID bands on the neonate, mother, and her partner. Attach infant safety tag. Keep the side of warmer up when not at crib side. Teach parents how to support the head and neck of their neonate. Use the five rights when administering medications. Wear gloves until after the first bath.	Teach parents abduction prevention protocol. Place the neonate on his or her back. Instruct parents not to leave the newborn unattended on a flat surface such as the mother's bed. Teach parents the importance of placing the neonate on his or her back. Wear gloves if there is the possibility of exposure to body fluids.	Provide education on infant safety (see Chapter 16). Follow hospital policies to prevent infant abduction. Wear gloves if there is the possibility of exposure to body fluids.	Review infant safety before discharge. Follow hospital policies to prevent infant abduction. Wear gloves if there is the possibility of exposure to body fluids. Inform parents that a federally approved car seat will be needed to transport the infant home and that it will need to be properly placed in the car.

CONCEPT MAP

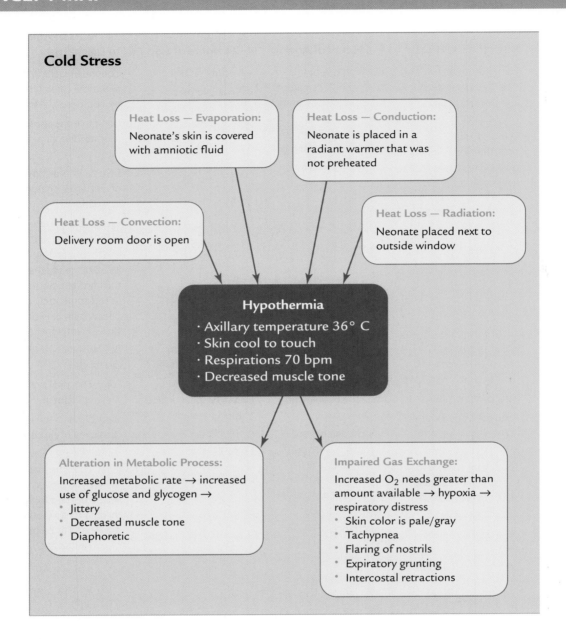

Cold Stress

Heat Loss — Evaporation:
Neonate's skin is covered with amniotic fluid

Heat Loss — Conduction:
Neonate is placed in a radiant warmer that was not preheated

Heat Loss — Convection:
Delivery room door is open

Heat Loss — Radiation:
Neonate placed next to outside window

Hypothermia
· Axillary temperature 36° C
· Skin cool to touch
· Respirations 70 bpm
· Decreased muscle tone

Alteration in Metabolic Process:
Increased metabolic rate → increased use of glucose and glycogen →
* Jittery
* Decreased muscle tone
* Diaphoretic

Impaired Gas Exchange:
Increased O_2 needs greater than amount available → hypoxia → respiratory distress
* Skin color is pale/gray
* Tachypnea
* Flaring of nostrils
* Expiratory grunting
* Intercostal retractions

Problem No. 1: Heat loss due to evaporation
Goal: Maintain a neutral thermal environment (NTE)
Outcome: The neonate's temperature is within normal range.

Nursing Actions
1. Dry neonate's body with warm towel.
2. Remove wet bedding and clothing.
3. Monitor vital signs.

Problem No. 2: Heat loss due to conduction
Goal: Maintain NTE
Outcome: The neonate's temperature is within normal range.

Nursing Actions
1. Skin-to-skin contact with parent with warm blanket over both the neonate and the parent.
2. Preheat warmer prior to use.
3. Use warm blankets.
4. Warm hands prior to touching neonate.
5. Warm equipment prior to contact with neonate.
6. Monitor vital signs.

Problem No. 3: Heat loss due to convection
Goal: Maintain NTE
Outcome: The neonate's temperature is within normal range.

Nursing Actions

1. Close doors to room.
2. Place the neonate away from air vent, windows, and doors.
3. Place a stocking cap on the neonate's head.
4. Warm O_2 when administering oxygen.
5. Monitor vital signs.

Problem No. 4: Heat loss due to radiation

Goal: Maintain NTE

Outcome: The neonate's temperature is within normal range.

Nursing Actions

1. Preheat radiant warmer prior to use.
2. Place the neonate away from cold walls and windows.
3. Keep cold objects away from the neonate.
4. Place stocking cap on the neonate's head.
5. Monitor vital signs.

Problem No. 5: Alteration in metabolic processes—hypoglycemia

Goal: Manage episode of hypoglycemia.

Outcome: The neonate's glucose level is within normal range.

Nursing Actions

1. Monitor for signs and symptoms of hypoglycemia.
2. Monitor glucose levels.
3. Assist the woman with breastfeeding or formula feeding.
   a. Assess glucose levels 30 minutes after feeding.
4. Maintain a NTE.

Problem No. 6: Impaired gas exchange—respiratory distress

Goal: Adequate gas exchange

Outcome: Pao_2 is 60 to 70 mm Hg; $Paco_2$ is 35 to 45 mm Hg; skin color is pink; lung sounds are clear; and no signs of retractions, grunting, or nasal flaring.

Nursing Actions

1. Monitor vital signs, oxygen saturation, and arterial blood gases.
2. Maintain patent airway.
3. Suction airway as indicated.
4. Administer oxygen as per orders.
5. Maintain an NTE.

Case Study

You are assigned to the mother-baby couplet unit, where your patients for the day include the Sanchez family. Margarite is a 28-year-old G3 P2 Hispanic woman who gave birth to a healthy male, Manuel, at 0839. Margarite experienced an uncomplicated labor of 12 hours. Membranes ruptured 7 hours before delivery. She received 2 doses of Nubain during labor. The last dose was given at 0440.

Manuel weighs 3,800 g and is 50 cm in length. His 1- and 5-minute Apgar scores were 8 and 9, respectively. Manuel is 2 hours old. The Ballard score indicates that Manuel is 39 weeks. Margarite breastfed her son for 15 minutes on each breast immediately after the birth.

Your initial shift assessment findings are:

Vital signs: Axillary temperature, 36.2°C (97.2°F); apical pulse, 100 bpm; respirations, 30 breaths per minute.

Skin is warm and pink with acrocyanosis.

Fontanels are soft and flat.

Molding is present.

Lung sounds are clear.

There is mild nasal flaring.

Manuel is in a sleep state and unresponsive to external stimuli.

Based on the above information, discuss the primary nursing diagnoses for baby Manuel.

Discuss the immediate nursing actions for baby Manuel. Provide rationales for your nursing actions.

Thirty minutes later, you note that Manuel is jittery and exhibits signs of hypoglycemia.

List the signs and symptoms of hypoglycemia and related nursing actions.

Several hours later, Manuel's father is present and holding Manuel.

List signs of parent–infant bonding.

Discuss nursing actions that will support parent–infant attachment.

REFERENCES

American Society for Pain Management Nursing (ASPMN). (2011). Position statement: Male infant circumcision pain management. Retrieved from www.aspmn.org/documents/circumcisiom.pdf.

Association of Women's Health, Obstetric and Neonatal Nurses (AWHONN). (2013). *Neonatal skin care* (3rd ed.). Washington, DC: AWHONN.

Blackburn, S. (2012). *Maternal, fetal, and neonatal physiology* (4th ed.). St. Louis, MO: W. B. Saunders.

Brazelton, T., & Nugent, J. (1995). *Neonatal behavioral assessment scale.* London: MacKeith Press.

Centers for Disease Control and Prevention (CDC). (2015). *Trends in circumcision for male newborns in U.S. hospitals: 1979–2010.* Retrieved from www.cdc.gov/nchs/data/hestat/circumcision_2013/circumcision_2013.htm.

Department of Health and Human Services (DHHS). (2009). *How to know if your baby is getting enough milk.* Retrieved from www.womenshealth.gov/publicatins/diaper_checklist.pdf.

Dillon, P. (2007). *Nursing health assessment* (2nd ed.). Philadelphia, PA: F.A. Davis.

Herr, K., Coyne, P., McCaffery, M., Manworren, R., & Merkel, S. (2011). Pain assessment in the patient unable to self-report: Position statement with clinical practice recommendations. *Pain Management Nursing, 12,* 230–250.

Mattson, S., & Smith, J. (2016). *Core curriculum for maternal-newborn nursing* (5th ed.). St. Louis, MO: Elsevier Saunders.

National Association of Neonatal Nursing (NANN). (1995). Position statement on pain management in infants. *Neonatal Network, 14,* 54–55.

National Institutes of Health (NIH). (2017). Your baby's hearing screening. Retrieved from https://www.nidcd.nih.gov/health/your-babys-hearing-screening

Scanlon, V., & Sanders, T. (2015). *Essentials of anatomy and physiology* (7th ed.). Philadelphia, PA: F.A. Davis.

Thakkar, P., Arora, K., Das, B., Javadekar, S., & Panigrahi, S. (2016). To evaluate and compare the efficacy of combined sucrose and non-nutritive sucking for analgesia in newborns undergoing minor painful procedure: A randomized controlled trial. *Journal of Perinatology, 36,* 67–70.

Vallerand, A., & Sanoski, C. (2017). *Davis's drug guide for nurses* (15th ed.). Philadelphia, PA: F.A. Davis.

Discharge Planning and Teaching

16

Sylvia A. Fischer, RN, MSN, CNM, FNP-C
Linda L. Chapman, RN, PhD

LEARNING OUTCOMES

Upon completion of this chapter, the student will be able to:

1. Incorporate principles of teaching and learning when providing newborn care information to parents.
2. Discuss the nutritional needs of newborns and infants.
3. Demonstrate awareness of cultural values in care of newborns.
4. Describe the stages of human milk.
5. Describe the process of human milk production.
6. Develop a teaching plan for breastfeeding.
7. Develop a teaching plan for formula feeding.
8. Provide parents with information regarding newborn care that reflects the assessed learning needs of parents.

Nursing Diagnoses

- Knowledge deficit related to infant feeding due to lack of experience and/or information
- Knowledge deficit related to newborn care due to lack of experience and/or information
- Knowledge deficit related to signs of infant illness related to lack of information

Nursing Outcomes

- The woman will effectively feed her newborn.
- The parents will demonstrate proper care of their newborn.
- The parents will convey they are comfortable with caring for their newborn.
- The parents will list signs of potential infant illness that need to be reported to the health care provider.

INTRODUCTION

Caring for a newborn and raising a child to adulthood are among the most important roles parents will assume in their lifetimes, yet there is little formal education for these responsibilities. Couples' knowledge pertaining to newborn care varies based on their past experiences with children, their cultural beliefs, information gained from friends and relatives, and books they have read or classes they have attended.

Discharge planning and teaching begins during pregnancy, when couples are encouraged to read about infant care and attend infant care classes in preparation for their emerging role as parents. They will also receive educational information from their health care provider. Throughout the postpartum hospital stay, teaching is provided in short sessions to the woman, her partner, and other family caregivers of the newborn. Most hospitals or birthing centers have standard discharge teaching forms that are completed and signed by the woman and the discharge nurse. A written copy of key points of infant care is given to parents on discharge. Prior to discharge, the woman's physicians or midwife will identify care needs for the mother and infant and schedule a follow-up appointment within a few days or up to two weeks based on these assessed needs.

Principles of Teaching and Learning

Teaching plans must be individualized to reflect the needs of the parents. This is accomplished by incorporating teaching-learning principles in the parents' education sessions regarding the care of their newborn. The five rights of teaching should be included in teaching plans for parents (Box 16–1).

NEWBORN NUTRITION AND FEEDING

Breastfeeding and bottle feeding are the two basic methods of infant feeding. Neonates who are unable to suck and/or swallow are gavage-fed (see Chapter 17). The choice between breastfeeding and bottle feeding is influenced by past infant feeding experiences, cultural beliefs, friends and family, health of the woman and baby, support of the partner, perceived health effects, and discussion during pregnancy with a health care provider. Women who desire to breastfeed their infants should begin preparing during the prenatal period by gathering information and support to facilitate a successful experience. Women who choose to bottle feed their infants must gather bottle-feeding equipment prior to the birth of their infants.

Breastfeeding

Human milk is the preferred source of infant nutrition and provides all the nutritional needs an infant requires. It changes as the infant grows to meet individualized growth and development needs (American Academy of Pediatrics [AAP], 2012a). Breastfeeding is the method of infant feeding recommended by the Association of Women's Health, Obstetric and Neonatal Nurses (AWHONN), the American College of Nurse-Midwives (ACNM), American Academy of Pediatrics (AAP), and the American College of Obstetricians and Gynecologists (ACOG) (Box 16–2 and Fig. 16–1). The Baby-Friendly Hospital Initiative was developed to ensure that birthing hospitals are the center of support for breastfeeding. An objective of *Healthy People 2020* is to increase the proportion of infants who are breastfed from 74% to 81.9%. Target goals include increase in the following proportions by 2020:

● Infants breastfed at 6 months from 45.5% to 60.6%.
● Infants breastfed at 1 year from 22.7% to 34.1%.
● Infants who are exclusively breastfed through 3 months from 33.6% to 46.2%.
● Infants who are exclusively breastfed through 6 months from 14.1% to 25.5%.
● Employers that have worksite lactation support programs from 25% to 38% (U.S. Department of Health and Human Services, 2017).

The decision to breastfeed is influenced by the woman's age, educational level, previous infant feeding method, career obligations, support from her partner, and cultural beliefs. The woman's partner plays a significant role in her choice to breastfeed and to continue breastfeeding. Her feelings about and success at

---

BOX 16–1 | The Five Rights of Teaching

When you are making a teaching plan, you can use this as a checklist to ensure that you consider each of the five "rights" of teaching in the plan.

Right Time
● Is the learner ready, free from pain and anxiety, and motivated?
● Do you and the learner have a trusting relationship?
● Have you set aside sufficient time for the teaching session?

Right Context
● Is the environment quiet, free of distractions, and private?
● Is the environment soothing or stimulating, depending on the desired effect?

Right Goal
● Is the learner actively involved in planning the learning objectives?
● Are you and your client both committed to reaching mutually set goals of learning that achieve the desired behavioral changes?
● Are family and friends included in planning so that they can help follow through on behavioral changes?
● Are the learning objectives realistic and valued by the client; do they reflect the client's lifestyle?

Right Content
● Is the content appropriate for the client's needs?
● Is the information new or a reinforcement of information that has already been provided?
● Is the content presented at the learner's level?
● Does the content relate to the learner's life experiences or is it otherwise relevant to the learner?

Right Method
● Do the teaching strategies fit the learning style of the client?
● Do the strategies fit the client's learning ability?
● Are the teaching strategies varied?

Wilkinson & Van Leuven, 2007, p. 530, Box 24–1.

---

breastfeeding are enhanced when her partner supports breastfeeding, assists in the care of the newborn, and does household tasks, thus facilitating the woman's ability to rest and conserve energy.

Benefits of Breastfeeding for the Infant

In the short term, infants who are breastfed have a decreased risk of:

● Gastroenteritis.
● Hospitalization due to respiratory syncytial virus.
● Otitis media.

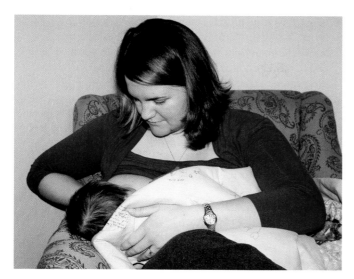

FIGURE 16-1 Breastfeeding enhances mother–infant attachment.

BOX 16-2 | Position Statements on Breastfeeding

"AWHONN supports, protects and promotes breastfeeding as the optimal method of infant nutrition, including the provision of human milk for preterm and other vulnerable infants. Women should be encouraged and supported to exclusively breastfeed for the first six months of an infant's life and continue to breastfeed for the first year and beyond" (AWHONN, 2015a).

"Exclusive breastfeeding—defined as the practice of only giving an infant breast-milk for the first 6 months of life (no food or water)—has the single largest potential impact on child mortality of any preventative intervention" (WHO, 2014).

"Breastfeeding is a natural and beneficial source of nutrition and provides the healthiest start for an infant. In addition to the nutritional benefits, breastfeeding promotes a unique and emotional connection between mother and infant" (AAP, 2012a).

● Necrotizing enterocolitis.
● Sudden infant death syndrome (SIDS).
● Urinary tract infections (AWHONN, 2015b).

Over the long term, breastfed infants are at decreased risk of:

● Asthma.
● Atopic dermatitis.
● Cardiovascular disease.
● Celiac disease.
● Childhood inflammatory bowel disease.
● Obesity.
● Sleep disorders.

Benefits of Breastfeeding for the Woman

Short-term maternal benefits include decreased blood loss and decreased risk of infection. Women who breastfed for longer than 3 months lost more weight than those who did not breastfeed.

Long-term maternal benefits include decreased risk for diabetes, metabolic syndrome, osteoporosis, autoimmune disease, and ovarian and breast cancer. Psychological benefits include enhanced maternal–infant attachment and decreased risk of postpartum depression (AWHONN, 2015b).

CRITICAL COMPONENT

Baby-Friendly Hospital Initiative

The Baby-Friendly Hospital Initiative (BFHI) is a global program that was launched by the World Health Organization (WHO) and the United Nations Children's Fund (UNICEF) in 1991 to encourage and recognize hospitals and birthing centers that offer an optimal level of care for infant feeding and mother/baby bonding (Baby-Friendly USA, 2017).

Hospitals and birthing facilities must adhere to the ten steps to receive and retain designation as being "baby-friendly."

These are the ten steps to successful breastfeeding:

• Have a written breastfeeding policy that is routinely communicated to all health care staff.
• Train all health care staff in the skills necessary to implement this policy.
• Inform all pregnant women about the benefits and management of breastfeeding.
• Help mothers initiate breastfeeding within 1 hour of birth.
• Show mothers how to breastfeed and how to maintain lactation, even if they are separated from their infants.
• Give infants no food or drink other than breast milk unless medically indicated.
• Practice rooming-in: Allow mothers and infants to remain together 24 hours a day.
• Encourage breastfeeding on demand.
• Do not give pacifiers or artificial nipples to breastfeeding infants.
• Foster the establishment of breastfeeding support groups and refer mothers to them on discharge from the hospital or birth center.

Baby-Friendly USA, 2017.

Contraindications for Breastfeeding

● Women with active and untreated tuberculosis
● Women who are receiving diagnostic or therapeutic radioactive isotopes
● Women who are receiving antimetabolites or chemotherapeutic agents
● Women who have herpes simplex lesions on a breast
● Women who are HIV positive
  ● In the developing world, the risks of artificial feedings outweigh the risks of acquiring HIV through breast milk; therefore, women are encouraged to breastfeed.
● Women who use street drugs such as cocaine
● Infants with galactosemia

Composition of Human Milk

Human milk contains all the nutritional needs of the infant. Proteins, carbohydrates, and fats are synthesized in the breasts' alveolar glands.

- Proteins account for approximately 6% of the calories in human milk and are easier to digest than protein in prepared formula.
- Carbohydrates account for approximately 42% of the calories in human milk with lactose as the main carbohydrate.
- Fats account for approximately 52% of the calories in human milk.
- Cholesterol, which is essential for brain development, is higher in human milk.
- Vitamins and minerals are transferred to the human milk from the maternal plasma.

Human milk contains multiple antibodies, enzymes, and immune factors that help protect the infant from common infections. It also stimulates the growth of healthy bacteria in the intestinal system, which inhibits growth of bacteria that can cause diseases.

Stages of Human Milk

There are three stages of human milk as the body establishes the lactation process.

- Stage 1: Colostrum, which is present in the breast starting in the second trimester, is a thick yellowish breast fluid. It has higher levels of protein and lower levels of fats, carbohydrates, and calories than mature human milk. It also contains high levels of immunoglobulins G and A. Since colostrum is thick and is produced in a small amount, newborns will need to nurse more frequently to ensure receipt of the antibodies and antioxidants needed to facilitate immune system development and introduce healthy bacteria into the gastrointestinal system (Simpson & Creehan, 2014). Colostrum acts as a laxative and assists in the passage of meconium.
- Stage 2: Transitional milk consists of colostrum and milk. This stage lasts from 6 to 13 days. During this stage, the milk will gradually change, with decreasing levels of protein and increasing levels of fats, carbohydrates, and calories.

- Stage 3: Mature milk is composed of 20% solids and 80% water. It contains approximately 22 to 23 calories per ounce. Human milk will change to meet the needs of the infant. Milk produced for preterm infants contains twice the amount of protein than milk produced to mothers of full-term infants (Janke, 2014).
  - Foremilk is the milk that is produced and stored between feedings and released at the beginning of the feeding session. It has higher water content.
  - Hind milk is the milk produced during the feeding session and released at the end of the session. It has a higher fat content.

Overview of Milk Production

The woman's body prepares for lactation, or the production of breast milk, as the breasts develop during puberty and undergo further changes during pregnancy. The changes that occur during pregnancy are referred to as mammogenesis. Under the influence of increased estrogen and progesterone during pregnancy, the breasts and areolas enlarge, the mammary glands differentiate, and lobules and alveoli within the breast develop (Janke, 2014). Lactogenesis, a series of changes that transform the mammary epithelial cells from a nonsecretory state to a secretory state, begins during the second trimester.

Milk is produced in the alveolar glands and is transported to the nipple through the lactiferous ducts (Fig. 16–2) and is influenced by hormones and infant suckling.

- Prolactin, the primary hormone responsible for lactation, is produced during pregnancy. High levels of estrogen and progesterone suppress lactation. Once the placenta is expelled, estrogen and progesterone levels decrease and prolactin levels increase, which results in the stimulation of milk production.
- Suckling increases prolactin levels and volume of milk production. Milk production can be viewed as a supply–demand effect. The more milk the infant takes in, the more milk is produced.

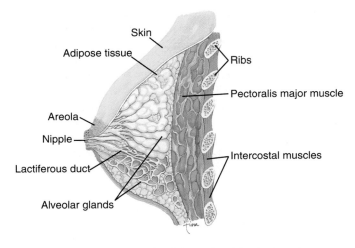

FIGURE 16–2 Mammary gland shown in midsagittal section.

CRITICAL COMPONENT

Lactogenesis

Lactogenesis is the three-phase process a woman's body progresses through in the establishment of milk production.

• Lactogenesis I begins during the second trimester and ends around the second day postpartum. During this phase, the alveolar cells differentiate into lactocytes (milk-producing cells). Under the influence of increasing levels of prolactin, the lactocytes begin to produce colostrum. By postpartum day 1, the breasts are producing 100 mL of colostrum/day.

• Lactogenesis II begins around the third postpartum day. Prolactin levels increase as progesterone levels decrease. These changes and infant suckling stimulate the breast to begin producing large amounts of milk.

• Lactogenesis III: The woman enters this phase when the milk supply is established and the amount of milk is controlled by the suckling and emptying of the breast (supply–demand system). The beginning of this phase varies, typically about 9 to 10 days postpartum (Janke, 2014).

Let-Down Reflex

The let-down reflex or milk-ejection reflex results in milk being ejected into and through the lactiferous duct system. Oxytocin causes the myoepithelial cells of the alveoli to contract, forcing the milk into the duct system. Let-down occurs multiple times during each feeding. The let-down reflex can be inhibited by stress, anxiety, pain, and fatigue and can be stimulated by hearing an infant cry. It can also occur during sexual arousal or activity due to the natural release of oxytocin in response to an orgasm.

Process of Breastfeeding

Breastfeeding is a natural process, with its success dependent on the woman's desire to breastfeed; a supportive environment; and proper positioning, latching on, suckling, and transferring of milk. The breastfeeding experience varies among individuals, viewed by some women as a very positive life experience and by others as a very negative experience. Nurses must understand and respect the woman's feelings about breastfeeding. The nurse can support the woman by providing the information and encouraging her to educate herself on feeding methods that will work for her. Many national and community support programs provide educational materials, classes, and support groups to facilitate a positive outcome. Each breastfeeding session should include the following steps:

1. The mother must determine when to feed the infant. This is facilitated by recognizing hunger cues exhibited by the infant; these typically occur 30 minutes before the infant cries. Offering the breast when early hunger cues are exhibited will reduce the infant's stress and facilitate bonding (Janke, 2014). Hunger clues include:
   - Opening the mouth in response to tactile stimulation.
   - Hand-to-mouth movement.
   - Quiet alert state.
   - Rooting.
   - Sucking sounds or movement.
   - Sucking of fingers or hand.

2. The woman should assume a comfortable position before she starts to feed her infant. Pain and discomfort can prevent or delay the let-down reflex. A sitting position in a chair, which facilitates good body position, is recommended. Other positions are lying on the side or back or sitting in bed.

3. Once comfortable, the woman positions the newborn to facilitate latching on. The newborn is held in a cradle position, a "football" position, or a cross-cradle position. Pillows are used to support the newborn and/or the woman. The front of the newborn completely faces the breast to prevent the newborn's head from being turned. Another way to describe this is that the newborn's ear, shoulder, and hip should be aligned.

4. The woman supports her breast by placing one hand around the breast several inches behind the areola. Supporting the breast takes the weight of the breast away from the newborn's chin and makes latching on easier (AWHONN, 2015b). The woman should avoid pushing down on the breast, which can tip the nipple upward and make the nipples sore.

5. The woman brings the newborn to her breast when the mouth is open wide; the breast should not be brought to the newborn. This assists with latching on. To encourage the newborn to open wide, take advantage of the rooting reflex by touching the newborn's chin to the breast. This signals the newborn to open the mouth. The newborn then reaches up and over the nipple to achieve an asymmetrical latch with more areola visible at the top of the mouth than on the bottom. *Latching on* refers to the newborn's ability to grasp the breast and to effectively suckle. The newborn's mouth is around the areola with the nipple in the back of the newborn's mouth. The lips create a firm seal around the areola (Fig. 16–3).

6. The newborn should feed completely from one side and then be offered the second breast. Many newborns and infants nurse only from one breast at each feeding. It is recommended to start feeding from the breast that the newborn finished on during the previous feeding. This promotes complete emptying of each breast every 6 to 8 hours and facilitates adequate milk supply in each breast.

7. The mother removes the newborn from the breast by gently sliding a clean finger into the corner of the newborn's mouth to break suction (see Fig. 16–3) before removing the newborn from the breast. Proper removal of newborn from the breast is important in decreasing nipple irritation.

8. The newborn should be burped at the end of the feeding session.

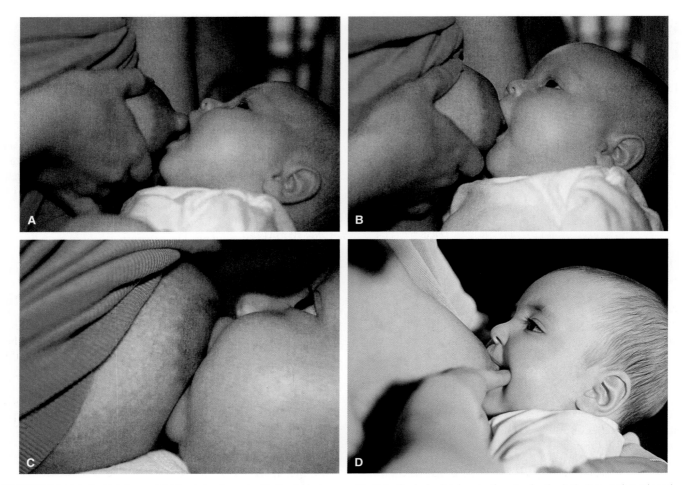

FIGURE 16–3 Infant latch-on. (*A*) Nipple is aligned with the baby's nose. (*B, C*) As the baby latches to the nipple, the baby's mouth is placed 1 to 2 inches beyond the base of the nipple. (*D*) To remove the baby from the breast, the woman inserts her finger into the corner of the baby's mouth to break the seal.

SAFE AND EFFECTIVE NURSING CARE: Patient Education

Signs of Successful Breastfeeding

Nurses should educate patients on the following indicators of successful breastfeeding:

- Latch-on should not be painful after the first few moments of suckling.
- The newborn's tongue is between the lower gum and breast.
- The woman feels a tugging sensation when the newborn begins to suckle.
- Swallowing can be heard.
- Satiation cues include but are not limited to relaxed body, decreased suckling, and sleep.

Patient Education

Lactation consultants are often employed by hospitals to assist women with breastfeeding. While lactation consultants are valuable members of the maternity nursing staff, they do not replace the nurse's responsibility to provide proper breastfeeding teaching and support. The nurse and lactation consultant work together to ensure a positive breastfeeding experience. Before discharge, the woman should be given information on lactation consultants and lactation groups to contact if she has questions or problems.

A primary role of a nurse caring for a woman who is breastfeeding is to facilitate successful breastfeeding by providing information and assisting the woman in her breastfeeding techniques. It is recommended that at least three complete feeding sessions per day during hospitalization be observed by the nurse or lactation consultant to assess the woman's ability to assist her infant with correctly latching on to the breast (AWHONN, 2015b). The Quick Care Guide Breastfeeding Support: Prenatal Care Through the First Year, which is located in Appendix A, is a summary of AWHONN's evidence-based nursing care for breastfeeding women. Refer to this for additional nursing actions.

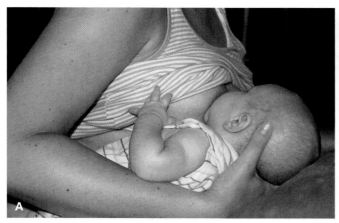 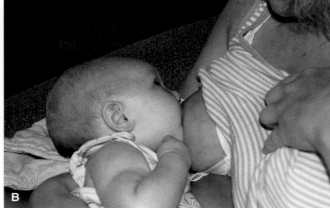

FIGURE 16–4 Positions for breastfeeding. (*A*) Football hold. (*B*) Cradle hold.

CRITICAL COMPONENT

Promoting Optimal Breastfeeding

The nurse and hospital policies can promote optimal breast-feeding by:

- Encouraging early and frequent breastfeeding.
- Providing 24-hour rooming-in for healthy moms and infants.
- Keeping baby warm and close by promoting skin-to-skin contact during feedings.
- Teaching mother about infant hunger cues and to feed on demand versus on schedule or timed feedings.
- Explaining to mother that cluster feeds are normal and they usually occur in the evening, sometimes leading to longer sleep for the infant.
- Keeping the mother comfortable and pain-free.

Janke, 2014.

Maternal and Newborn Positioning

The mother can hold her infant in a variety of positions during feeding sessions, depending on what is most comfortable for both mom and baby. Periodically changing infant's position on the breast can decrease nipple irritation.

- Lying-down position: The woman lies in bed or on the sofa in a comfortable position. Pillows are used to provide proper support of her head and neck. The newborn lies next to the woman on his or her side so that the head is directly facing the nipple. A pillow or rolled blanket can be used to support the newborn in this position.
- Sitting position: The woman sits in a chair or bed with shoulders and back straight to reduce strain on her back and shoulder. The newborn can be held in several different positions. Three common sitting positions are:
  - Cross-cradle position: The newborn's head is supported by the woman's hand, and the newborn's back is against the woman's forearm. The abdomen of the newborn is

facing/touching the woman's abdomen. This is an ideal position to use when the woman is first learning to breast-feed, as it facilitates good head control.
  - Football hold position: The newborn's head is cradled in the woman's hand and the body is supported between the woman's arm and her side. The newborn's head is directly facing the nipple (Fig. 16–4A).
  - Cradle position: The newborn's head is cradled in the crook of the woman's arm. The woman supports the newborn's back with her arm and buttock with her hand. The abdomen of the newborn is facing/touching the woman's abdomen (Fig. 16–4B).

Determining Effective Feeding

Women who are breastfeeding for the first time usually want to know how they can determine if their infant is getting enough milk and if they are breastfeeding properly. Cues that indicate feedings are effective include the following:

- The woman feels physically and emotionally comfortable when feeding her newborn.
- The newborn properly latches on, as indicated by no nipple pain or trauma.
- The newborn suckles and the woman can hear and/or see swallowing, which indicates the transfer of milk.
- The newborn spontaneously releases his or her grip on the breast when satiated.
- The newborn is drowsy and arms and legs are relaxed at the end of the feeding session.
- There are at least eight wet diapers and several stools per day once breast milk has come in and breastfeeding is established.
- The newborn recovers his or her birth weight by 2 weeks of age.

Common tools used to assess and document breastfeeding efforts are LATCH (Table 16–1) and the Bristol Breastfeeding Assessment Tool (BBAT) (Box 16–3).

- The tools assess both the woman and her infant and assist in determining the level of support needed and the type of interventions required for the pair.

TABLE 16–1   Latch Scoring System

	0	1	2
L: Latch	Too sleepy or reluctant No latch achieved	Repeated attempts Hold nipple in mouth Stimulate to suck	Grasps breast Tongue down Lips flanged Rhythmic sucking
A: Audible swallowing	None	A few with stimulation	Spontaneous and intermittent <24 hours old Spontaneous and frequent >24 hours old
T: Type of nipple	Inverted	Flat	Everted (after stimulation)
C: Comfort (breast/nipple)	Engorged Cracked, bleeding, large blisters, or bruises Severe discomfort	Filling Reddened/small blisters or bruises Mild/moderate pain	Soft Tender
H: Hold (positioning)	Full assist (staff holds infant at breast)	Minimal assist (i.e., elevate head of bed; place pillow for support) Teach one side; mother does the other side Staff holds and then mother takes over	No assist from staff Mother able to position/hold infant

Jensen, Wallace, & Kelsay, 1994.

BOX 16–3 | Bristol Breastfeeding Assessment Tool

Bristol Breastfeeding Assessment Tool (BBAT)

The infant and mother are given a score between 0 and 2 on each of the following:

1. Positioning: Infant well supported, tucked into mother on his or her side, nose opposite nipple, and mother is confident in handling infant.

2. Attachment: Infant roots, wide-open mouth, quick latch encompassing a large amount of breast tissue, able to maintain a good latch throughout feeding.

3. Suckling: Establishes effective pattern on both breasts (rapid sucks, then slow with occasional pauses). Infant demonstrates sign of satisfaction and ends feeding.

4. Swallowing: Audible and regular swallowing; no clicks.

Scored separately for pain assessment:

Comfort: Breast and nipples display no visual damage and mom is comfortable.

Ingram, Johnson, Copeland, Churchill, & Taylor, 2015.

- The lower the score, the higher the need for support and education.
- Score can vary from one feeding to the next feeding.

Preventing Nipple Tissue Breakdown

Painful nipples are a primary reason that women stop breastfeeding before the 8th week (Janke, 2014). Nipple irritation can lead to tissue breakdown, which can be a cause of mastitis. Each breastfeeding woman must be taught to inspect her nipples for signs of irritation: redness, bruising, and tissue breakdown. Early interventions can decrease the risk of infection and bleeding. To decrease irritation, the woman should:

- Use proper technique for latching on and releasing suction. Problems with latching on increase the risk for early cessation of breastfeeding (Janke, 2014).
- Apply warm compresses to the breasts/nipples before feeding to enhance the let-down reflex (AWHONN, 2015b).
- Express colostrum or milk and rub it on the nipple and areola at the end of the feeding session.
- Change positions when feeding (e.g., football to cradle hold) to reduce pressure areas on the nipple. The pressure exerted on the nipples by the newborn is not uniform.
- Begin the feeding session on the less sore breast because suckling is more vigorous at the beginning of the feeding session.

● Wash breasts with water only. The woman should avoid use of soaps and alcohol, which cause excessive dryness of the breast/nipple.
● Contact her health care provider if she is experiencing cracked and/or bleeding nipples. The breasts need to be assessed for signs of possible infection.

Comfort and Relaxation

High levels of anxiety and discomfort interfere with successful breastfeeding by preventing or delaying the let-down reflex, which can cause a decrease in milk transfer and a decrease in milk supply. Decreased milk supply is another reason women stop breastfeeding by or before the 8th week (Janke, 2014). Nursing actions that promote comfort and relaxation are:

● Lowering maternal anxiety level by:
  ● Providing the woman/couple with easily understood breastfeeding information over several teaching sessions so she is not overwhelmed by too much information.
  ● Being calm and patient in interactions with the woman/couple during breastfeeding sessions.
  ● Explaining that it can take time for both the woman and newborn to become comfortable with breastfeeding.
  ● Ensuring that the newborn is alert and ready to feed before bringing him or her to the breast. Newborns will not feed well when they are asleep/not ready to feed.
  ● Praising the woman for her decision to breastfeed her infant.
● Providing instructions on methods to reduce pain and to promote comfort:
  ● Explain the relationship of rest, relaxation, and comfort on milk production.
  ● Teach the proper use of analgesics that are recommended by the health care provider and are safe for lactating women.
  ● Demonstrate the use of a "Boppy pillow" or pillows to support both the mother's and newborn's body (Fig. 16–5).
  ● Teach breathing and relaxation techniques.

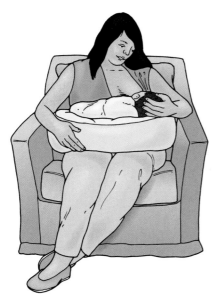

FIGURE 16–5 Boppy pillow.

Nutrition and Fluids

Decreased caloric intake and fluids can decrease milk volume. Lactating women need to consume an additional 500 calories/day over the recommended pre-pregnant requirements due to the increased energy requirement for milk production. They also need to drink a minimum of 2 liters of fluid per day.

● Instruct women to develop a food plan based on My Plate and her food preferences.
● Instruct women to have a glass of fluid next to them and drink it while they are nursing their infant since it is common to become thirsty while nursing.

SAFE AND EFFECTIVE NURSING CARE: Patient Education

My Plate for Breastfeeding Women

Nurses should instruct breastfeeding women to incorporate foods listed below into their diet. These are the best sources for nutrients needed when breastfeeding.

Vegetable Group

Choose fresh, frozen, canned, or dried:

● Carrots
● Sweet potatoes
● Pumpkin
● Spinach
● Cooked greens (such as kale, collards, turnip greens, and beet greens)
● Winter squash
● Red sweet peppers

These vegetables all have both vitamin A and potassium. When choosing canned vegetables, look for "low sodium" or "no salt added" on the label.

Fruit Group

Choose fresh, frozen, canned, or dried:

● Cantaloupe
● Honeydew melon
● Mangoes
● Prunes
● Bananas
● Apricots
● Oranges
● Red or pink grapefruit
● 100% prune juice or orange juice

These fruits all provide potassium, and many also provide vitamin A. When choosing canned fruit, look for those canned in 100% fruit juice or water instead of syrup.

Dairy Group

● Fat-free or low-fat yogurt
● Fat-free milk (skim milk)

Continued

- Low-fat milk (1% milk)
- Calcium-fortified soymilk (soy beverage)

These provide the necessary calcium and potassium and should be fortified with vitamins A and D.

Grains Group
- Fortified ready-to-eat cereals
- Fortified cooked cereals

When buying ready-to-eat and cooked cereals, choose those made from whole grains. Also look for cereals that are fortified with iron and folic acid.

Protein Foods Group
- Beans and peas (e.g., pinto beans, soybeans, white beans, lentils, kidney beans, and chickpeas), pot of beans
- Nuts and seeds (e.g., sunflower seeds, almonds, hazelnuts, pine nuts, peanuts, and peanut butter)
- Lean beef, lamb, and pork
- Oysters, mussels, and crab
- Salmon, trout, herring, sardines, and pollock

NOTE: Do not eat shark, swordfish, king mackerel, or tilefish when you are pregnant or breastfeeding. They contain high levels of mercury.

USDA, 2018

Expressing and Storing Breast Milk

It is important for women to learn how to express milk and how to store milk properly, as most will need to skip a feeding or feedings when they are away from their infant for more than a few hours or when returning to work (Box 16–4). Women can begin expressing and storing milk once they are comfortable with breastfeeding and the milk supply is established. The best time to express milk is at the end of a feeding session. Milk can be expressed by hand or with the use of an electric breast pump.

For manual expression of milk, instruct the woman to:

- Wash her hands before touching her breasts.
- Massage each quadrant of her breast.
- Place her thumb and forefinger so they form the letter *C*, with the thumb at the 12 o'clock position and the forefinger at the 6 o'clock position.
- Push the thumb and finger toward the chest wall.
- Lean over and direct the spray of milk into a clean container.
- Repeat this several times.
- Occasionally massage the distal area of the breast.
- Reposition the thumb and forefinger to the 3 and 9 o'clock positions and repeat the above sequence.

A variety of electric and battery-operated breast pumps are available. Electric pumps can be fitted with bilateral accessory kits so that both breasts can be pumped at the same time. Electric pumps closely simulate the suckling of infants. Instruct women to follow the directions provided with the electric pump of choice. Women's hands and nails should be washed and all equipment properly cleaned before expressing and storing milk.

BOX 16–4 | AWHONN Position Statement: Breastfeeding in the Workplace

"Recognizing the fact that breastfeeding is the optimal form of infant nutrition, AWHONN supports legislation and initiatives that promote and protect lactation in the workplace. AWHONN believes that employers should provide lactating women with break time that permits adequate frequency and duration of milk expression within the workplace."

AWHONN, 2008.

Expressed milk can be stored for use when the woman is not present to breastfeed. Milk must be stored in glass bottles, hard BPA-free plastic containers, or plastic bags designed for storage of breast milk when storing milk for longer than 72 hours. Each container needs to be labeled with the date the milk was expressed. When freezing, it is best to leave an inch of space at the top of the container to allow for the expansion of the milk that occurs during the freezing process. Frozen milk should be stored in the back of the freezer and not on the freezer door.

Breast milk can safely be stored:

- At room temperature (77°F) for up to 6 to 8 hours.
- In the refrigerator for up to 5 days.
- In the freezer that is attached to a refrigerator for 3 to 6 months.
- In a deep freezer for 6 to 12 months (Janke, 2014).

Breast milk should not be heated in the microwave, as it can cause uneven heating or overheating. Overheating by either microwave or stovetop can destroy antibodies within the breast milk. Breast milk is safely thawed by:

- Placing the bottle or bag in the refrigerator overnight.
- Placing it under warm running water.
- Setting it in a container of warm water.

Medications

Instruct the woman to check with her primary care provider and the infant's primary care provider before she takes prescribed and over-the-counter medications, including vitamins and herbal supplements (AWHONN, 2015b). Breastfeeding is not recommended if the woman is taking amphetamines, chemotherapy agents, ergotamines, or statins.

SAFE AND EFFECTIVE NURSING CARE: Understanding Medication

Breastfeeding and Medication

Most medications are safe to take when breastfeeding, but the woman needs to check with her health care provider before taking a new medication. When a medication is prescribed, the provider will choose drugs that have:

- A short half-life.
- High protein binding.
- High molecular weight.
- Low oral bioavailability.

Additional concerns are:

- Is the drug medically necessary?
- Does the drug have proven data of safety for breastfeeding mothers?
- Is the health care provider following proven guidelines?

  Hale & Rowe, 2017.

Bottle Feeding

While breast milk is the recommended form of infant nutrition, some women do not breastfeed for maternal health, newborn health, or personal reasons (Fig. 16–6). Commercially prepared formulas are a nutritious alternative to breast milk. Formulas come in many varieties, including cow's milk or soybean. Vitamin D and other nutrients are added to provide a healthy choice for infants. There are also special formulas for preterm infants and those with different allergies. Formulas come "ready-made" or in powder form and concentrated. They contain 50% more protein than human milk. Vegetable oils are used instead of animal fat to ease digestion. Unfortunately, vegetable oil is void of cholesterol, which is essential for brain development.

Advantages of Formula Feeding

- Provides a pleasurable infant caring experience for the partner, as either parent can feed the infant.
- Provides the opportunity for the woman to leave the infant with other people while she goes out or returns to work without the need to pump breast milk or plan activities around the infant's feeding schedule.
- Decreases the frequency of feedings because digestion of formula is slower than that of human milk.

Disadvantages of Formula Feeding

- Need for increased time to prepare formula
- Increased cost compared to breastfeeding
- Increased risk of infection due to lack of antibodies that are naturally present in human milk
- Increased risk of childhood obesity and insulin-dependent diabetes

Teaching Topics

- Parents should select bottles that are BPA-free and easy to clean.
- Parents can opt for either rubber or silicone nipples.
  - Silicone nipples retain fewer odors and last longer.

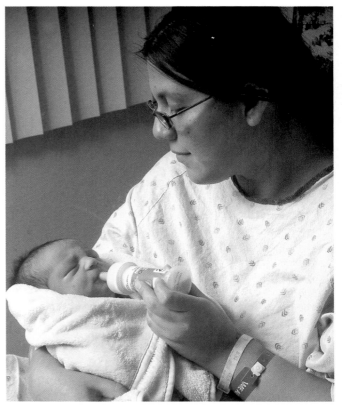

FIGURE 16–6 Bottle feeding is an alternate method of nourishing a newborn.

- Rubber nipples are cheaper but tend to break down faster and retain odors.
- Nipples need to be washed with soapy warm water and rinsed well.
- The rate of flow from the nipples is controlled by either the shape of the hole or the size of the hole. There are three types of flow rates:
  - Slow: designed for newborn infants
  - Medium: designed for infants under 6 months
  - Fast: designed for older infants
- Formulas are available in powder, concentrated, and ready-to-use forms. It is important to instruct the parents to follow the directions provided by the manufacturer when preparing formula.
  - Prolonged overdilution of formulas can cause water intoxication; prolonged underdilution can cause dehydration.
  - Once bottles of formula have been prepared, they need to be kept refrigerated and used within 24 hours to decrease risk of bacterial contamination.
  - Opened cans or bottles of ready-to-use formula need to be kept refrigerated and used within 24 hours to decrease risk of bacterial contamination.
  - Clean bottles, nipples, and can openers in a dishwasher or with hot soapy water.
  - Discard unused formula that remains in the bottle at the end of feeding to decrease risk of bacterial contamination.

CRITICAL COMPONENT

Preparing Infant Formula
- Clean and disinfect the formula preparation area.
- Wash hands.
- Use bottles and nipples that have been washed in hot, soapy water and rinsed well or have been washed in a dishwasher.
- Use boiled non-fluoride water or distilled water to mix with concentrated or powdered formula.
  - The water should be cooled (room temperature) before mixing it with the formula.
  - Well water should be tested for presence of nitrate; if present, bottle water should be used (AAP, 2015c).
- Check the expiration date on the formula packaging.
- Wash, rinse, and dry the top of the formula can.
- Follow directions on the formula packaging for proper dilution of concentrate or amount of powder formula per ounce of water.
- Mix the formula by gently shaking or swirling the bottle.
- Store mixed formula in airtight bottles in the refrigerator for up to 24 hours.
- Warm a refrigerated bottle by placing it in a container filled with warm water.
- Store open containers of ready-to-use, concentrated formula or a prepared bottle in the refrigerator and dispose of after 24 hours.

APP, 2012b.

- Newborns take in 0.5 to 1 ounce (15 to 30 mL) per feeding during the first few days of life. This increases to 2.5 to 3 ounces (75 to 90 mL) per feeding by day 4 and gradually increases to 32 ounces (950 mL) per day.
  - Rule of thumb: 2.5 ounces of formula/1 pound of baby weight/day.
  - Newborns/infants can be fed on demand or at least every 3 to 4 hours.
- Newborns/infants should be held during feedings with the head slightly higher than the trunk of the body. This position can decrease the risk of otitis media. Newborns/infants are usually fed in a cradle holding position.
- Burp the infant halfway through feeding and at end of feeding by tapping/patting the infant on the back for a few minutes. Some infants may not need to burp with each feeding.

CRITICAL COMPONENT

Bottle Feeding
- Mix the formula as directed by the manufacturer.
- Hold the infant close to the body as with breastfeeding.
- Tilt the bottle so that the nipple is full of milk to decrease the amount of air swallowed by the infant.
- Do not prop bottles, as this places infants at higher risk for choking, otitis media, and tooth decay.

- Check the size of the nipple hole.
  - The hole may be too big if the infant has a sudden mouthful of formula and almost chokes, or when you turn the bottle upside down and the milk flows out of the nipple instead of dripping.
  - The hole may be too small if the infant seems to be working hard when sucking or when the bottle is upside down and it takes longer than a second per drip of formula.
- Discard unused formula from the bottle at the end of the feeding.

Nutritional Needs

During the first year of life, the infant experiences rapid growth. The infant will double his or her birth weight by 5 months and triple by age 1. Caloric needs vary based on size of infant, rate of growth, activity, and metabolic rate.

- Infants experience growth spurts at 3 to 5 days, 1 week, 6 weeks, 3 months, and 6 months and require more frequent feedings during these time periods (AWHONN, 2015b).
- Adequate nutritional intake is determined by plotting the weight and length of the infant at each well-child checkup.

Birth to 4 Months

The nutritional requirements for infants are ideally met by breast milk. Iron-fortified infant formula is substituted when the woman is not breastfeeding.

- Breastfeeding is on demand. Newborns usually feed 8 to 12 times per day during the first few weeks, gradually decreasing to 6 to 10 feedings per day. Women produce 500 to 600 mL of breast milk per day during the first few weeks and 700 to 800 mL until semisolid foods are introduced. Milk production decreases once semisolid foods are introduced.
- Formula feeding is either on demand or every 3 to 4 hours. Newborns start with 0.5 to 1 ounce (15 to 30 mL) per feeding and gradually increase to 32 ounces (960 mL) per day.

4 to 6 Months

Feeding breast milk or formula is continued. Introduction of semisolid foods is determined by the physician or nurse practitioner in collaboration with parents. The AAP and WHO guidelines recommend waiting to start solids until 6 months of age to reduce allergy risks. Before 4 to 6 months, the sucking reflex forces semisolid food out of the mouth versus to the back of the mouth. Parents should not introduce semisolid foods until recommended by the health care provider. Infants are ready for semisolid foods when they:

- Can sit independently.
- Can draw in the lower lip as a spoon is removed.
- Indicate hunger by opening the mouth.
- Refuse food by closing the mouth and turning away.

Pureed fruits and vegetables and single-grain cereal such as rice and oats are the first food to be introduced. Cereal should not be given in bottles, as this increases risk of choking and aspiration.

NEWBORN CARE

It is the responsibility of the nursing staff to ensure that couples have adequate knowledge of newborn care to safely care for their child. A teaching plan is developed for all couples based on assessment of their knowledge level and cultural beliefs. Some couples require a minimal amount of teaching while others require intensive education. The following information on infant care is presented in alphabetical order for easier reference.

Bathing

The first few bathing experiences can be stressful for the parents, but over time it typically becomes a very pleasurable experience for both the parents and child (Fig. 16–7). Daily bathing with soap is not necessary and can cause skin irritation. Use of a mild preservative-free soap that has neutral pH is recommended to decrease the risk of skin irritation. The use of soap on the face is not recommended. Genital and rectal areas should be cleaned at each diaper change with water or diaper wipes. The face and neck areas should be cleaned after feedings with plain water.

Bathing is best done before a feeding to decrease the risk of emesis related to jostling during bathing. Gather all items required for bathing (e.g., soap, towels, washcloth, clean clothing, diapers, blankets) before the bath. To maintain the infant's body temperature, bathe the infant in a warm room free of drafts. The bath water temperature should be between 90°F and 100°F. Keep bath time short (5 to 10 minutes) to reduce heat loss (AWHONN, 2013).

Immerse the infant in warm water deep enough to cover the shoulders to ensure even temperature distribution and decreased heat loss due to evaporation. There is controversy regarding when an infant can be immersed in water. Some believe it must be delayed until the cord has fallen off and the cord site is healed,

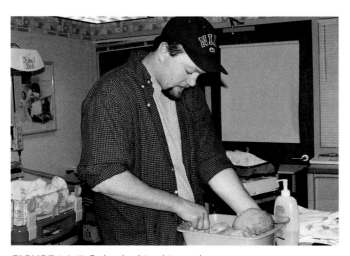

FIGURE 16–7 Father bathing his newborn.

whereas others do not. Follow the institution's policy on newborn bathing. Bathing procedure is as follows:

- Support the infant's head and neck with the parent's forearm.
- Do not leave the infant unattended in bathwater.
- Start from the cleanest area (eyes) and end with the dirtiest area (buttock).
  - An alternative method is trunk-to-head.
- Cleanse eyes from the inner to outer aspects using a clean corner of the washcloth per eye to reduce the risk of transfer of infection from one eye to the other.
- Wash hair and massage the scalp.
- Lift the chin to clean neck folds, where milk often collects.
- Cleanse the upper body.
- Cleanse the lower body.
- Clean female genitals by washing from front to back to decrease the risk of cystitis.
- Elevate the scrotum and cleanse the area.
- Dry the infant and put on a clean diaper and clothes.

Evidence-Based Practice: Trunk-to-Head Bathing

So, H., You, M., Mun, J., Hwang, H., Kim, H., Pyeon, S., Shin, M., & Chang, B. (2014). Effect of trunk-to-head bathing on physiological responses in newborns. *JOGGN, 43*, 742-751.

- The aim of this quasi-experimental design research study was to determine the effects of trunk-to-head bathing versus head-to-trunk bathing on newborns' body temperature, heart rate, and oxygen saturation.

- Study participants included 62 healthy full-term newborns at a university hospital in South Korea. Participants were randomly assigned to experimental (trunk-to-head bathing) and control (head-to-trunk bathing) groups. Measurements of temperature, heart rate, and oxygen saturation were taken before the bath, immediately after the bath, and at 30 minutes and 60 minutes after the bath.

- There was no significant difference in body temperature, heart rate, or oxygen saturation. There was a significant difference in rate that body temperature returned to initial body temperature. Both groups had a 0.2° Celsius temperature drop after bathing. The experimental group returned to initial body temperature more rapidly than control group.

- The researchers concluded that bathing trunk-to-head reduced the time of heat loss from evaporation, as heads were wet for shorter periods of time.

Bulb Syringe

Bulb syringes are used to assist the infant in clearing mucus from the nasopharynx. It is important for parents to learn how to properly use a bulb syringe and should be given opportunities to practice this skill prior to discharge. Newborns should have their own bulb syringe that is cleaned with soapy water and rinsed after each use. The procedure for bulb syringe use is as follows:

- Compress the syringe and insert it into either the nose or the mouth.
  - When using in the mouth, the syringe is placed in each side of the mouth, the roof of the mouth, and the back of the mouth (Fig. 16–8).

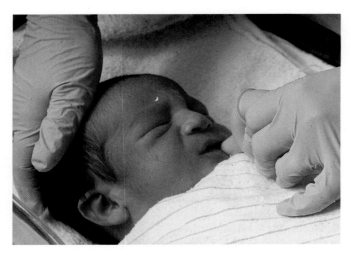

FIGURE 16–8 A bulb syringe in used to remove mucus.

- When using in the nose, the syringe is placed in each nostril.
- Release pressure from the syringe and allow it to slowly expand.
- Remove the syringe from the area.
- Remove the drainage from the syringe by compressing the syringe and forcing the contents into a tissue.
- Repeat until newborn is clear of mucus.

Circumcision Care

The circumcised glans penis (tip of the penis) will appear red and will form yellow crusted areas as it heals; these areas should not be washed off. Parents should check for bleeding every 4 hours for the first 24 hours postprocedure and notify the health care provider of bleeding at the circumcised area. Parents should also notify the health care provider if:

- The newborn has not voided within 24 hours.
- There is bleeding from the circumcised area.
- The entire penis is red, warm, and swollen and/or there is drainage from the surgical site (signs of infection).
- Gomco or Mogen clamp:
  - If the penis adheres to the diaper, soak the area with water until it naturally releases. Do not pull the diaper off the penis. Pulling the gauze off can cause pain and interfere with the healing process.
  - The circumcised area heals within 2 weeks.
- Plastibell method:
  - Do not apply lubricants on the penis when a Plastibell has been used. Lubricants can increase the risk of displacement of the plastic ring.
  - The plastic ring falls off in 7 to 10 days. Parents should not pull it off.

Clothing

The amount of clothing needed varies depending on whether the infant is inside or outside and on the temperature of the environment. The amount and type of clothing can be influenced by cultural beliefs. It is important to explore with parents what they know and believe about infant dressing and educate them on risks related to overheating and overbundling.

Newborns and infants are usually comfortable wearing a diaper, T-shirt, and loose-fitting outfit when inside. The most comfortable clothing for infants is 100% cotton, as synthetic clothing may irritate the skin. Additional layers of clothing or heavier blankets and a hat are used when the infant is outside in cooler weather. The infant's skin must be protected from the sun.

Newborns/infants can become overheated with too many clothes or blankets. Avoid overheating/overbundling infant at sleep time to decrease risk of SIDS. Signs of overheating are:

- Sweating.
- Damp hair.
- Heat rash.
- Rapid breathing.
- Restlessness.

Colic

Colic is uncontrollable crying in healthy infants younger than the age of 5 months and occurs in 20% of infants between 2 and 4 weeks of age (AAP, 2015a). It is common for newborns to have a steady increase in crying until age 6 weeks, when it gradually decreases. This type of pattern is not necessarily colic. Healthy infants who cry for at least 3 hours for 3 or more days a week for at least 3 weeks are considered colicky. The cause of colic is unknown. Symptoms of colic include:

- Infant flexes/curls legs when crying.
- Infant has difficulty/discomfort with bowel movements.
- Infant is more irritable after a feeding.
- Infant is more irritable when placed in crib.
- Infant appears in pain.
- Infant requires frequent cuddling.
- Infant suddenly changes from happy to crying.

Parents should keep a diary of when their infant is awake, asleep, eating, and crying. This will assist the pediatrician or nurse practitioner in determining if crying is related to a medical cause (AAP, 2015a). This will also help the health care provider offer specific methods for soothing the infant. Methods for soothing colicky infants include the following:

- Hold the infant and sway from side to side or walk around with the infant.
- Give the infant a pacifier.
- Swaddle the infant.
- Place the infant (abdomen facing down) over the knees and gently rub or pat the back.
- Place the infant in a baby bouncer.
- Place the infant in a car seat and take him or her for a ride in the car.
- Place the infant in a car seat and put on top of a running clothes dryer. Do not leave the infant unattended on the dryer.
- Place the infant in a stroller and go for a walk.

Caring for an infant with colic can be an emotionally and physically draining experience for the parents. The parents can become increasingly frustrated as their efforts to calm their infant do not seem to work. During these periods of feeling frustrated and overwhelmed, the parents need to take a break from their infant.

CRITICAL COMPONENT

Colic

The AAP has the following advice for parents and caregivers who are feeling frustrated when caring for infants with colic:

- Take a deep breath and count to 10.
- Place your baby in a safe place, such as a crib or playpen without blankets and stuffed animals; leave the room and let your baby cry alone for about 10 to 15 minutes.
- While your baby is in a safe place, consider some actions that may help calm you down:
  - Listen to music for a few minutes.
  - Call a friend or family member for emotional support.
  - Do simple household chores, such as vacuuming or washing the dishes.
- If you have not calmed down after 10 to 15 minutes, check on your baby but do not pick up your baby until you have calmed down.
- When you have calmed down, go back and pick up your baby. If your baby is still crying, retry soothing measures.
- Call your doctor. There may be a medical reason why your baby is crying.
- Try to be patient. Keeping your baby safe is the most important thing you can do. It is normal to feel upset, frustrated, or even angry, but it is important to keep your behavior under control. Remember, it is never safe to shake, throw, hit, slam, or jerk any child—and it never solves the problem.

AAP, 2016d.

Cord Care

The umbilical cord begins to dry once the cord is clamped and cut. The cord clamp is removed 24 hours after birth. Over the next few days, the cord becomes dry, hard, and black. The cord falls off and the site subsequently heals within 2 weeks. Care of the cord includes the following measures:

- The diaper is placed below the cord to facilitate drying of the cord (Fig. 16–9).
- If the cord becomes dirty, clean it with plain water and dry it with a clean, absorbent cloth.
- Parents should contact the health care provider if there is bleeding from the cord site, foul-smelling drainage, redness in the surrounding skin, or fever.

Diapering

Most parents use disposable diapers that come in various sizes based on the weight of the infant; others use cloth diapers, such as all-in-one diapers that contain a cotton diaper, nylon cover, and Velcro

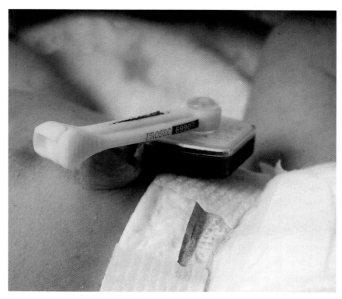

FIGURE 16–9 When diapering, the cord is left exposed.

or snap fasteners. Some parents use a combination of both—cloth at home and disposable when away from home. Diapers need to be changed when they become wet or soiled to prevent skin irritation. Parents should check diapers every few hours to see if they need changing. It is recommended to change the diapers every 1 to 3 hours during the day and at least once at night (AWHONN, 2013). Take the following steps when changing diapers:

- Gather supplies (e.g., clean diaper, clean clothing, and wet washcloth) before placing the infant on a flat surface such as a changing table.
- Unfasten diaper and lower the front of the diaper.
- Lift the infant's bottom using an ankle hold and fold the soiled diaper under the bottom.
- Use water or commercial diaper wipes to clean genital and rectal areas, wiping from front to back for female infants. For male infants, lift the scrotum and wash under it.
- Lift the bottom of the infant with use of an ankle hold, remove the soiled diaper, and then place a clean diaper under the infant.
- Fasten both sides of the diaper so that there is a snug fit.
- Dress the newborn.
- Properly dispose of the diaper.
- Wash hands.

Elimination

The frequency and characteristics of infant stools and urination are important for parents to track during the first few weeks after birth. An infant's stool and urination reflect feeding and hydration. Providing guidelines for what is normal and what to expect can assist parents in early identification of potential feeding and dehydration problems. Teaching plan should include the following:

- Instruct parents on the stages of newborn stools (see Chapter 15).

- Explain that newborns pass several stools per day (see Table 15–1).
- Inform parents that newborns should have at least six wet diapers per day once breastfeeding or bottle feeding has been established (see Table 15–1).
- Inform parents that a newborn's diapers may have a pink stain related to urates, which is a normal occurrence.
  - Urates persisting in more than two diapers may suggest dehydration and weight loss. Parents need to report a continued presence of urates to the physician or nurse practitioner for further evaluation.
- Inform parents that blood may occur on the diaper of female newborns related to a withdrawal of maternal hormones. This is referred to as pseudomenstruation.
- Instruct parents to notify the health care provider if stools are runny and green and/or if infant has fewer than six wet diapers per day.
- Instruct parents to notify the health care provider if the infant becomes constipated. Constipation can be a sign of inadequate intake and needs to be evaluated by the health care provider.

Follow-up Care

Routine follow-up care of the newborn is an essential component of safe infant care and health promotion. Typically, the pediatrician or nurse practitioner will want a newborn follow-up visit within 48 to 72 hours of discharge. The nurse can assist the parents with scheduling the appointment and should reinforce the importance of well-child checkups. The well-child checkups provide an opportunity to:

- Assess the infant's growth.
  - Growth spurts occur at 14 days, 3 weeks, 6 weeks, 3 months, and 6 months. During these growth spurts, infants can be fussy and need to be fed more frequently.
- Assess feeding pattern.
- Assess the developmental level.
- Assess for jaundice.
- Provide the appropriate immunizations (see Appendix B).
- Do follow-up metabolic screening.
- Continue teaching parents about the care of their child and what to expect at each developmental milestone.

The AAP recommends the following:

- First visit within 2 to 4 days after hospital discharge
- Subsequent visits at 1, 2, 4, 6, 9, and 12 months of age.

Kangaroo Care

Kangaroo care, also referred to as skin-to-skin care, is when a parent holds his or her bare-chested infant to their bare chest. Both the parent and the infant are covered with a warm blanket. Benefits for the baby include:

- Stabilization of temperature, heart rate, and breathing.
- Increased weight gain.
- Increased time in deep sleep.

- Decreased crying.
- Longer quiet alert states that facilitate successful breastfeeding sessions.

Benefits for the mother include:

- Decreased stress.
- Increased bonding and emotional attachment to infant.
- Increased milk supply.

Nonnutritive Sucking

Sucking is a pleasurable experience for newborns and infants, whether they are engaged in nutritive sucking (sucking during breastfeeding or bottle feeding) or nonnutritive sucking. Nonnutritive sucking, such as using a pacifier or the infant's fist and fingers, is used to soothe or calm an infant. The parents' choice to use a pacifier is influenced by cultural, societal, and community norms. Pacifiers should not be used to delay feedings or substitute for parental attention. Do not force an infant to take a pacifier.

- Pacifier should not be used with breastfed infants until 1 month of age. This provides the time needed for infants to establish breastfeeding.
  - Pacifiers have been linked to shorter breastfeeding duration.
  - The mouth motions that a newborn uses when breastfeeding, referred to as suckling, are different from the mouth motions (sucking) used with bottle feeding or use of pacifier.
- Pacifier safety measures:
  - Purchase pacifiers that are molded in one piece to prevent it from coming apart.
  - The shield between the nipple and ring should be made of firm plastic with ventilation holes and have a diameter of at least 1.5 inches.
  - Do not tie the pacifier around the infant's neck or to the infant's crib. A cord around the neck places the infant at risk for strangulation.
  - Wash pacifiers with warm soapy water.
  - Replace pacifier when discolored or torn (AAP, 2015d).

Pediatric Abusive Head Trauma

Pediatric abusive head trauma (PAHT) or abusive head trauma (AHT), also referred to as shaken baby syndrome, is an injury to the skull or intracranial contents of an infant or child younger than age 5 caused by inflicted blunt impact and/or violent shaking. There are 1,300 reported cases of PAHT per year; most are in children younger than 6 months and in 25% of the reported cases the child dies. The Centers for Disease Control and Prevention (CDC) examined the trends in the death of children younger than 5 attributed to PAHT. Data was collected from 1999 to 2014. During this time, 2,250 deaths were related to PAHT. The fatal PAHT rate in 2014 was 0.43 per 100,000 children <5 years (Spies & Klevens, 2017). Infant crying is usually the trigger that causes the parent or caretaker to shake or hit the infant's head.

Infants are at higher risk for injury related to violent shaking due to their weak neck muscles and large, heavy heads. When the infant is violently shaken, the brain bounces back and forth against the skull, causing bruising, swelling, and bleeding within the brain tissue. PAHT injuries can cause death or permanent and severe brain damage such as:

● Subdural hematomas
● Hypoxic ischemic encephalopathy (HEI) resulting in:
  ● Cerebral palsy
  ● Seizures
  ● Mental retardation
  ● Learning disabilities (AAP, 2015b)
● Retinal hemorrhage occurs in 85% of cases (AAO, 2015b).

CRITICAL COMPONENT

Outcomes of Pediatric Abusive Head Trauma

Pediatric abusive head trauma (PAHT) or abusive head trauma leads to long-term neurological, cognitive, behavioral, and academic outcomes. According to the CDC, these include:

• Ongoing rehabilitation needs—83%.
• Attention deficits—79%.
• Behavioral disorders—53%.
• Language abnormalities—49%.
• Motor deficits—45%.
• Visual deficits—45%.
• Severe neurological impairment—40%.
• Epilepsy—38%.
• The need for special education—30%.
• Sleep disorders—17%.

Lind et al., 2016.

Symptoms of injury related to PAHT include:

● Extreme irritability.
● Lethargy.
● Poor feeding.
● Breathing problems.
● Convulsions.
● Vomiting.
● Decreased smile or vocalization.
● Increased head circumference.
● Grip-like bruising on arms and chest (Gordy & Kuns, 2013; National Institute of Neurological Disorders and Strokes [NINDS], 2017).

It is important that parents receive PAHT information and strategies to use when their frustration levels are high. The teaching plan should include:

● How shaking causes injury to the infant's brain and eyes.
● The long-term effects of PAHT.
● Information on the stages of infant/childhood development.
● Information on infant crying.
  ● Infants cry for various reasons, such as when they are hungry, uncomfortable, and in pain.

● Infants can cry for no reason that the parents can identify.
● It is normal for infants to cry for 30 to 40 minutes. Sometimes, infant crying may last longer and usual soothing methods will not be effective.
● It is common for infants to cry more in the afternoon and evening.
● Information on soothing crying infants
  ● See the "Soothing Babies" section.
● Information on stress reduction.
  ● Assist parents in identifying ways to cope with their frustrations.
  ● Explain to parent it is normal to feel frustrated when efforts to calm a baby are not effective.
  ● Explain to the parents that it is okay to place their infant in a crib and leave the room for 10 minutes while they regain their composure.
● Information on what to do when feeling overwhelmed.
  ● Ask for help—ask a friend or family member to care for the infant so they can have time to relax and regain composure.
  ● Contact community resources such as Parental Stress Line.

PAHT is preventable. Several prevention programs have been developed by health centers and organizations; these are an important component in decreasing the incidents of PAHT. Each of these programs includes information on causes and effects of AHT, infant crying patterns, and stress-reduction techniques. One of the programs is the Period of PURPLE Crying, available from the National Center on Shaken Baby Syndrome (www.dontshake.org).

SAFE AND EFFECTIVE NURSING CARE: Patient Education

Period of PURPLE Crying Program

The Period of PURPLE Crying is the name given to the National Center on Shaken Baby Syndrome's evidence-based prevention program. The letters PURPLE stand for:

P: Peak of crying—your baby may cry more each week, the most at 2 months, the least in 3 to 5 months.

U: Unexpected—crying can come and go and you do not know why.

R: Resists soothing—your baby may not stop crying no matter what you do.

P: Pain-like face—a crying baby may look to be in pain, even when he or she is not.

L: Long lasting—crying can last as much as 5 hours a day or more.

E: Evening—your baby may cry more in the late afternoon and evening.

National Center on Shaken Baby Syndrome, 2016.

Prevention of Dental Decay

Infants' teeth are susceptible to "baby bottle tooth decay," a condition that occurs when sweetened liquids are given in bottles to infants and allowed to remain in the mouth for a period of time. Within 20 minutes, the sugar from the sweetened liquid responds to mouth bacteria and forms acids that cause dental decay (American Dental Association [ADA], 2017). Infants who fall asleep with a bottle in their mouths or who receive several bottles of sweetened liquids during the day are at higher risk for tooth decay.

CRITICAL COMPONENT

Decreasing the Risk of Baby Bottle Tooth Decay
The ADA (2017) recommends the following to decrease risk of baby bottle tooth decay:

- Do not put infants to bed with a bottle of milk, juice, or sugar water.
- Do not give infants bottles with sugar water or soda.
- Clean the infant's gums with clean gauze after each feeding.
- Brush teeth once the first tooth erupts.
- Consult a dentist regarding fluoride treatments if the water supply does not contain it.
- Begin regular dental appointments by the first birthday.

Safe Sleep

In response to the number of infant deaths attributed to SIDS, in 1992 the AAP recommended that all infants be placed on their backs for naps and night sleeping (Fig. 16–10). Since then, infant deaths attributed to SIDS have decreased by 50%.

In 2011, the AAP expanded its recommendations that focus on all sleep-related infant deaths such as suffocation and strangulation. In 2016, the AAP updated their recommendations for a safe sleeping environment (AAP Task Force, 2016). The National Institute of Child Health and Human Development supports AAP recommendations and instituted the Safe to Sleep campaign, which incorporates the recommendations (see Appendix C).

To reduce the risk of SIDS and other sleep-related infant deaths, the National Institute of Child Health and Human Development (2017) and American Academy of Pediatrics (2016c) recommend the following:

- Always place infants on their backs to sleep, for nap and at night. Once infants can turn on their own from back to front, it is safe to leave them in the position they assume. Infants should not be swaddled once they can move from back to front.
- Use a firm sleep surface covered by a fitted sheet.
- Keep soft objects, toys, and loose bedding out of infant's sleep area.

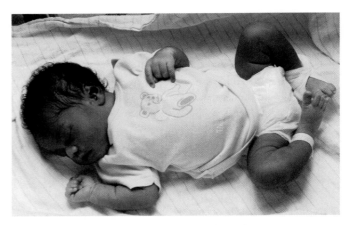

FIGURE 16–10 Place the baby on his back to sleep.

- Cribs, bassinets, and portable cribs need to meet the safety standards of the Consumer Product Safety Commission.
- Infants should sleep in a crib in their parents' room for at least the first 6 months of life. Infants should not sleep in an adult bed, on a couch, or on a chair, whether alone or with anyone else.
- Women should get regular health care during pregnancy and should not smoke, drink alcohol, or use illegal drugs during pregnancy.
- Parents should not smoke or allow smoking around their baby.
- Infants should be breastfed to reduce risk for SIDS.
- Give infants dry pacifiers that are not attached to a string for naps and at night.
- Do not allow infants to overheat during sleep.
- Follow health care provider's guidance on infant vaccines and regular health checkups.
- Avoid products that claim to reduce the risk of SIDS and other sleep-related cause of infant death.
- Give infants plenty of tummy time when they are awake and supervised.

Safety

Parents are responsible for the safety of their children. Newborns and infants are at risk for injury related to falls, ingestion of harmful products, and accidents. An infant safety teaching plan should include education on the following topics.

Infant Car Seats

- Infant car seats need to be used for all infants when traveling in a motor vehicle, including on the day of discharge from the hospital.
- Infants are safest when secured in the backseat. Rear-facing car seats are used with infants until they are 2 years of age or until the child has reached the highest weight or height limit allowed by the manufacturer of the infant seat.
- Parents need to select a car seat that best fits their vehicle and follow the instructions on how to secure the seat to the

vehicle's seat and properly position and secure the infant into it.

- Parents can contact a certified child passenger safety (CPS) technician for assistance in the installation and use of infant car seats before bringing the newborn home. Instruct parents to visit www.seatcheck.org to locate a CPS near their home.
- Each state has laws that govern the use of infant and child car seats. Laws for specific states can be viewed at www.seatcheck.org.
- Instruct parents to never leave their child in a car unattended.

Prevention of Falls

- Instruct parents not to leave their infant on an elevated flat surface without supervision.
- Instruct parents not to leave their infant in an infant car seat on an elevated surface unattended.
- Install gates at stairwells.
- Select a high chair with a wide base to prevent tipping over.

Poisoning Prevention

- Place all cleaning materials in upper cabinets out of the infant's reach.
- Place all medications, including vitamins, in upper cabinets out of the infant's reach.
- Place safety latches on all lower cabinets and keep the cabinet doors closed.
- Remove lead paint from older cribs and infant furniture and walls.
- Never leave infants unattended in rooms or yards.

Accident Prevention

- Keep small objects out of the reach of infants to prevent choking.
- Remove strings and ribbons from bedding, sleepwear, and pacifiers to prevent strangulation.
- Keep plastic bags out of reach.
- Keep all sharp objects in drawers or cabinets and out of the infant's reach.
- Check water temperature used for bathing. Water temperature should be 100°F to 100.4°F (37.8°C to 38°C).
  - Set the water heater thermostat at 120°F or lower.
- Do not leave the infant in the bathtub unsupervised.
- Keep any guns unloaded and locked and out of the infant's reach.
- Install safety devices around swimming pools.
- Do not cook while holding the infant.
- Supervise infants when pets are in the room.
- Ensure infant crib, high chair, and other furniture or play equipment meet current safety standards (i.e., all four sides of cribs are fixed/unmovable).
- Cover electrical outlets.

Sibling Rivalry

There will be some degree of sibling rivalry when a new baby is introduced into the family. Older children will feel the shift of attention from them to the new baby and may react negatively to this change. Toddlers may begin wetting themselves, wanting to use diapers, or crying to get attention. Others may want to drink from a bottle. Some children may hit or pinch their new sibling. Parents can decrease the degree of sibling rivalry using the following methods:

- Start preparing older children during pregnancy for the new family addition by talking to them about becoming an older brother or sister, having them feel the baby kick, and having them around newborn infants (see Chapter 5).
- Have older siblings attend sibling classes offered by some hospitals and agencies.
- Bring older children to the postpartum unit to meet their new sibling.
- Give the older children a gift and tell them it is from their new brother or sister.
- Spend quality time with older children such as reading or playing games.
- Take older children on special outings without the new sibling.
- Teach the older sibling about why babies cry and why mom or dad needs to attend to the baby's cry.

Skin Care

The newborn's skin is delicate and can be irritated easily. The skin should be inspected daily for signs of tissue irritation and breakdown. The following should be included in the teaching plan:

- General skin care
  - Avoid daily bathing with soap.
  - Use cleansers that have neutral pH.
  - Avoid use of adhesives. Removing adhesives can remove the epidermis layer of the skin and lead to a breakdown of the skin barrier.
  - Apply petroleum-based ointments sparingly to dry skin and avoid the head and face.
  - Avoid use of skin ointments with perfume, dyes, and preservatives.
- Diaper dermatitis is common. It can occur when diapers are not changed frequently or when the area is not cleaned thoroughly at each diaper change. It can also occur when there is a change in the infant's diet, when the infant is teething, or when the infant is taking medications that can change the chemistry of the urine and stools.
  - Methods to reduce risk of and treat diaper dermatitis:
    - Change diapers frequently; every 1 to 3 hours during the day and at least once during the night (AWHONN, 2013).
    - Cleanse infant's bottom with water or disposable diaper wipes during each diaper change (AWHONN, 2013).
    - Use petroleum-based or zinc oxide ointments during diaper changes (at the first sign of a rash).
    - Avoid use of powders. Powders increase the risk of bacterial and candidal growth.

- Avoid use of antibiotic ointments, which can increase the risk of allergic skin reactions.
- Expose the infant's bottom to the air while he or she is sleeping.
- Add a half cup of vinegar to the rinse cycle of cloth diapers to help remove soap residues and alkaline irritants.

Soothing Babies

Newborns and infants cry when they are hungry, uncomfortable, bored, exposed to new experiences, or sick. The parents' task is to determine the cause of crying and then respond with appropriate soothing techniques. The parent should check to see if the infant is hungry or needs a diaper change. Parent should check for signs of illness such as rash, elevated temperature, swollen gums; if ill, contact doctor or nurse practitioner. Techniques that can be used to soothe/calm the infant include the following:

- Feed if crying is related to hunger.
- Reposition the infant to a more comfortable position.
- Talk or sing to the infant.
- Swaddle the infant.
- Hold the infant close to the body so he or she can feel the warmth of the parent's body and hear the parent's heartbeat.
- Hold the infant and rock back and forth or walk around the house or dance with the infant.
- Offer the infant a pacifier.
- Place the infant in a stroller and go for a walk.

Several methods for calming infants are available to use when teaching parents ways to calm their infant. One of these methods is the "5 S's."

SAFE AND EFFECTIVE NURSING CARE: Patient Education

Five S's for Soothing Babies

The 5 S's were developed by Dr. Harvey Karp, pediatrician, to help parents in calming their infant:

1. Swaddling
2. Side positioning or stomach position (supervised by adult)
3. Shushing
4. Swinging
5. Sucking

Additional information can be found on Dr. Karp's website, www.happiestbaby.com, or in his book *Happiest Baby Guide to Great Sleep.*

Karp, 2013.

Swaddling

Swaddling means to wrap the infant snugly in a blanket, which provides warmth and a sense of security that can have a calming effect. Parents need to be instructed on the proper method of swaddling. Improper swaddling can increase the infant's risk for SIDS and hip dysplasia. Swaddling should be discontinued around the second month when the infant can roll from front to back (AAP, 2017). Infants who are swaddled and roll from back to front while sleeping are at greater risk for SIDS.

CRITICAL COMPONENT

Hip Dysplasia

When swaddling an infant:

"It's especially important to allow the hips to spread apart and bend up. In the womb, the legs are in a fetal position with the legs bent up across each other. Sudden straightening of the legs to a standing position can loosen the joints and damage the soft cartilage of the socket."

International Hip Dysplasia Institute, 2017.

Swaddling Instructions

- Place the blanket on a flat surface.
- If using a square blanket, fold the top corner over.
- Place the infant on the blanket with the shoulders at the fold line.
- Bring the left arm down and wrap the blanket across the arm and chest. Tuck the blanket under the infant's right side.
- Bring the right arm down and wrap the blanket across the arm and chest. Tuck the blanket under the infant's left side.
- Loosely fold the bottom end of the blanket and tuck behind the infant.
  - The legs should be bent up and out.
  - Leave enough room for the hips to move (International Hip Dysplasia Institute, 2018).
- Check the tightness of swaddle. The parent should be able to get two to three fingers between the infant's chest and the swaddle (AAP, 2017).

Temperature Taking

There are two main methods for assessing an infant's temperature: axillary and rectal. It is important for parents to ask their infant's health care provider their preferred method of assessing the infant's temperature. Digital thermometers are recommended over mercury-filled ones. Parents should take the infant's temperature before calling the health care provider if they feel that their child is sick. The teaching plan should include the following:

- Instruct parents to take an axillary temperature by placing the thermometer in the axillary region and holding the

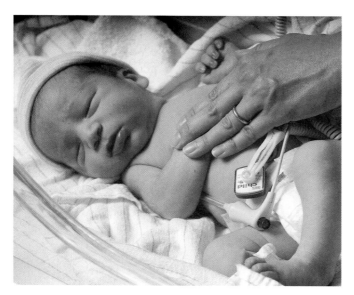

FIGURE 16–11 Placement of thermometer when taking an axillary temperature.

child's arm against his or her side until the thermometer beeps (approximately 1 minute) (Fig. 16–11).
● Teach parents how to take a rectal temperature:
  ● Clean the end of the thermometer with alcohol or soapy water and rinse in cold water.
  ● Lubricate the end of the thermometer with a lubricant such as petroleum jelly.
  ● Place the child on his or her back and hold the legs in a flexed position.
  ● Insert the thermometer no farther than 0.5 inches into the rectum.
  ● Hold the thermometer in place until it beeps.
  ● Remove the thermometer after it has beeped and check the digital reading.
● Teach parents how to read a thermometer.
  ● An elevated temperature might be related to overheating from too many blankets or clothing. Instruct parents to remove some clothing and retake the temperature after 15 to 20 minutes.
  ● Notify the health care provider if the temperature remains elevated (axillary temperature greater than 99°F [37.2°C]).

Uncircumcised Male

Care of the uncircumcised infant includes the following:

● Do not force the foreskin over the penis.
  ● The foreskin fully retracts on its own around 3 years of age.
  ● Forcing the foreskin over the penis or using cotton swabs to clean under the foreskin can damage the inner layer of the foreskin, which can lead to adhesion formation.
● Gently cleanse the penis when bathing the infant and when changing the diaper.
● Once the foreskin naturally retracts (around age 3), gently clean between the foreskin and glans of the penis when bathing the child.

When to Call the Pediatrician or Nurse Practitioner

Parents should notify the infant's health care provider if the infant:

● Has a rectal temperature above 100.4°F (38°C) or axillary temperature above 99°F (37.2°C)
  ● Ask the health care provider which method to use to assess infant's temperature; this will vary based on the health care provider's preferences or hospital and clinics policies.
  ● Use a digital thermometer to take an axillary or rectal temperature.
● Has loss of appetite.
● Is not interested in eating every 3 hours.
● Refuses to eat.
● Is lethargic.
● Is sleepy and not as active as usual.
● Does not wake on own for feedings or is not interested in feeding.
● Does not cry or has weak cry.
● Has watery green stools.
● Is vomiting.
● Has a decrease in the number of wet diapers.
● Has a skin rash.
● Has sunken or bulging fontanels.
● Is bleeding from circumcision site and/or cord site.
● Has a foul odor from the circumcision site and/or cord site.

CONCEPT MAP

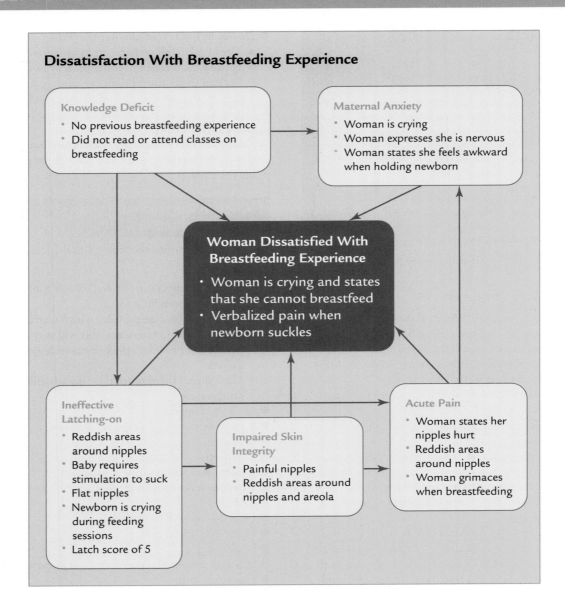

Dissatisfaction With Breastfeeding Experience

Knowledge Deficit
* No previous breastfeeding experience
* Did not read or attend classes on breastfeeding

Maternal Anxiety
* Woman is crying
* Woman expresses she is nervous
* Woman states she feels awkward when holding newborn

Woman Dissatisfied With Breastfeeding Experience
* Woman is crying and states that she cannot breastfeed
* Verbalized pain when newborn suckles

Ineffective Latching-on
* Reddish areas around nipples
* Baby requires stimulation to suck
* Flat nipples
* Newborn is crying during feeding sessions
* Latch score of 5

Impaired Skin Integrity
* Painful nipples
* Reddish areas around nipples and areola

Acute Pain
* Woman states her nipples hurt
* Reddish areas around nipples
* Woman grimaces when breastfeeding

Problem No. 1: Knowledge deficit

Goal: The woman will demonstrate proper breastfeeding techniques before discharge.

Outcome: Establishment of breastfeeding as evidenced by:
* Proper alignment of the baby and woman.
* Proper latch-on.
* LATCH score of 8 or greater.
* Audible swallowing.
* Absence of reddened areas or blisters.
* The woman stating she feels comfortable with breastfeeding.

Nursing Actions
1. Explain that the ideal time to feed is when the baby is in a quiet alert state and demonstrates feeding cues.
2. Provide information on newborn feeding cues, such as sucking movements and sounds, hand-to-mouth movements, and rooting reflects; explain that crying is a late feeding cue (Janke, 2014).
3. Demonstrate different positions for holding the baby when breastfeeding: cross-cradle, cradle, and football positions.
4. Provide information on using pillows in assisting the woman in a comfortable position.
5. Teach the woman how to properly align the baby's body to her body when breastfeeding, by assisting her and the baby in a proper breastfeeding position and explaining how this facilitates effective feeding.
6. Instruct the woman to support her baby's head and neck while the baby nurses.

7. Instruct the woman to bring the baby to her breast and not the breast to the baby.

8. Explain the importance of having the baby's mouth cover most of her areola with her nipple in the back of the baby's mouth.

9. Explain that the woman should feel a tugging sensation as the baby begins to suckle.

10. Explain that she should not experience pain when the baby is suckling. Pain may be an indication that the baby has not properly latched on and needs to be repositioned.

11. Teach the woman that she should hear audible swallowing as a sign that the baby is suckling properly and receiving milk.

12. Instruct the woman to assess her nipples for signs of nipple irritation and provide information on how to decrease the risk of nipple irritation.

13. Demonstrate how to properly remove the baby from her breast by placing a clean finger in the side of the baby's mouth to release the suction.

14. Provide information on lactation consultants and breastfeeding support groups in the community.

Problem No. 2: Maternal anxiety
Goal: Decrease of anxiety level
Outcome: The woman expresses that she feels comfortable with breastfeeding.

Nursing Actions

1. Assess the woman's beliefs, attitudes, concerns, and questions regarding breastfeeding to identify the source of anxiety to assist in identifying areas to address in the action plan.

2. Assess the woman's knowledge of breastfeeding and provide information to increase her knowledge level.

3. Assess the woman's cultural beliefs regarding breastfeeding and incorporate these in the teaching plan.

4. Assess the level of the partner's support for the woman's desire to breastfeed and explain how he or she can assist the woman with breastfeeding.

5. Assess the woman's comfort level and initiate methods to promote comfort such as relaxation techniques, proper positioning for feeding, use of pillows to support the woman and her baby, and ensuring adequate rest and sleep for the woman.

6. Establish an environment that is conducive for the woman to breastfeed, such as a quiet room and privacy.

7. Provide encouragement for the woman by praising her for her decision to breastfeed, for using proper breastfeeding techniques, and for responding to the baby's feeding cues.

8. Reevaluate the woman's level of anxiety by assessing verbal and nonverbal behaviors.

Problem No. 3: Ineffective latching on
Goal: Effective latching on
Outcome: The baby will effectively latch on as evidenced by:
- The baby's mouth covering most of the woman's areola.
- The woman's nipple being in the back of the baby's mouth.

- The baby's lips creating a firm seal around the areola.
- Audible swallowing.
- Absence of reddened areas or blisters.
- LATCH score of 8 or greater.

Nursing Actions

1. Assess the woman's breastfeeding technique.
2. Assess the nipples and areola for signs of irritation.
3. Provide information on latching on.
4. Assist the woman and her baby with proper positioning that facilitates latching on.
5. Instruct the woman to bring the baby to her breast when the baby's mouth is wide open.
6. Instruct the woman to delay use of a pacifier until the baby is able to latch on and breastfeeding is established, which is usually 1 month.

Problem No. 4: Acute pain
Goal: Absence of pain
Outcome: The baby will properly latch on and the woman will state that she is not experiencing pain in the breast area when feeding her baby.

Nursing Actions

1. Assess the level of pain using a pain scale.
2. Assess the breast for signs of irritation, such as reddened areas, blisters, or cracking, and provide information on methods to decrease irritation.
3. Assess the breastfeeding technique by observing the woman during a feeding session.
4. Provide information and assistance to facilitate latching on.
5. Provide information on various positions for holding the baby during feeding sessions.
6. Explain that warm, moist compresses may decrease nipple pain (AWHONN, 2015b).
7. Medicate with analgesia PRN.

Problem No. 5: Impaired skin integrity
Goal: Skin will remain intact.
Outcome: The tissue of the nipples and areola will be intact with no redness or blisters.

Nursing Actions

1. Assess nipples and areolas for signs of irritation.
2. Instruct the woman to inspect her nipples and areolas after each feeding.
3. Assess the woman during feeding sessions for proper breastfeeding techniques.
4. Provide information on proper positioning of the baby for breastfeeding.
5. Provide information on latching on.
6. Instruct the woman to gently rub breast milk around her nipples and areolas after each feeding session.

Case Study

As the nurse, you are caring for Margarite Sanchez, a 28-year-old G3 P2 Hispanic woman who delivered a healthy boy, Manuel. Margarite and her husband have a healthy 2.5-year-old boy. Margarite informs you that she breastfed her older child, José, for 9 months without problems. Her older son was interested in the pregnancy and being a big brother, but he has been crying and is restless and irritable during hospital visits. He also does not want to hold his baby brother and is demanding to be taken to the toy store.

Margarite's husband tells you that he was very involved in the care of his first child.

A circumcision is planned for Manuel the morning of discharge.

Based on your knowledge of the Sanchez family, list the priority learning needs and state the rationale for your selection of learning needs. Describe your teaching plan based on the identified priority learning needs. The plan should include:

- *Preparation of the learning environment.*
- *Methods to assess their learning needs.*
- *Information that will be shared with the couple.*
- *Method for evaluating effectiveness of teaching.*

REFERENCES

American Academy of Ophthalmology (AAO). (2015). *Abusive head trauma/shaken baby syndrome—2015.* Retrieved from www.aao.org/clinical-statement/abusive-head-traumashaken-baby-syndrome.

American Academy of Pediatrics (AAP). (2012a). Breastfeeding and the use of human milk. Policy statement. *Pediatrics, 129,* e827–e835.

American Academy of Pediatrics (AAP). (2015a). *Colic relief tips for parents.* Retrieved from https://www.healthychildren.org/English/ages-stages/baby/crying-colic/Pages/Colic.aspx

American Academy of Pediatrics (AAP). (2015b). *Understanding abusive head trauma in infants and children.* Retrieved from https://www.aap.org/en-us/Documents/cocan_understanding_aht_in_infants_children.pdf

American Academy of Pediatrics (AAP). (2015c). Where we stand: testing of well water. Retrieved from https://www.healthychildren.org/English/safety-prevention/all-around/Pages/Where-We-Stand-Testing-of-Well-Water.aspx

American Academy of Pediatrics (AAP). (2015d). *Pacifier safety.* Retrieved from https://www.healthychildren.org/English/safety-prevention/at-home/Pages/Pacifier-Safety.aspx

American Academy of Pediatrics (AAP). (2016a). *How to calm a fussy baby: Tips for parents and caregivers.* Retrieved from www.healthychildren.org.

American Academy of Pediatrics (AAP). (2016c). SIDS and other sleep-related infant deaths: Evidence based for 2016 update recommendations for safe infant sleeping environment. *Pediatrics, 138,* e20162940

American Academy of Pediatrics (AAP). (2016d). *Why parents and caregivers need breaks from crying babies.* Retrieved from https://www.healthychildren.org/English/ages-stages/baby/crying-colic/Pages/Calming-A-Fussy-Baby.aspx.

American Academy of Pediatrics (AAP). (2017). *Swaddling: Is it safe?* Retrieved from www.healthychildren.org/English/ages-stages/baby/diapers-clothing/Pages/Swaddling-Is-it-Safe.aspx

American Academy of Pediatrics Task Force. (2016). SIDS and other sleep-related infant deaths: Updated 2016 recommendations for a safe infant sleeping environment. *Pediatrics, 138,* e20162938.

American Dental Association (ADA). (2017). *Baby bottle tooth decay.* www.mouthhealthy.org./en/az-topics/b/baby-bottle-tooth-decay

Association of Women's Health, Obstetric and Neonatal Nurses (AWHONN). (2008). *Breastfeeding and lactation in the workplace (position statement).* Washington, DC: Author.

Association of Women's Health, Obstetric and Neonatal Nurses (AWHONN). (2013). *Neonatal skin care* (3rd ed.). Washington, DC: Author.

Association of Women's Health, Obstetric and Neonatal Nurses (AWHONN). (2015a). Breastfeeding (position statement). *Journal of Obstetric, Gynecologic, & Neonatal Nursing, 44,* 145–150.

Association of Women's Health, Obstetric and Neonatal Nurses (AWHONN). (2015b). *Breastfeeding support: Prenatal care through the first year. Evidence-based clinical practice guideline* (3rd ed.). Washington, DC: Author.

Baby-Friendly USA. (2017). Ten steps to successful breastfeeding. Retrieved from www.babyfriendlyusa.org.

Gordy, C., & Kuns, B. (2013). Pediatric abusive head trauma. *Nursing Clinic of North America, 48,* 193–201.

Hale, T., & Rowe, H. (2017). *Medications & mothers' milk.* New York, NY: Springer.

Ingram, J., Johnson, D., Copeland, M., Churchill, C., & Taylor, H. (2015). The development of a new breast feeding assessment tool and the relationship with breast feeding self-efficacy. *Midwifery, 31,* 132–137.

International Hip Dysplasia Institute. (2018). *Hip-healthy swaddling.* Retrieved from https://hipdysplasia.org/developmental-dysplasia-of-the-hip/hip-healthy-swaddling/

Janke, J. (2014). Newborn nutrition. In *Perinatal nursing* (4th ed.). Philadelphia, PA: Wolters Kluwer/Lippincott Williams & Wilkins.

Jensen, D., Wallace, S., & Kelsay, P. (1994). LATCH: A breastfeeding charting system and documentation tool. *Journal of Obstetric, Gynecologic, & Neonatal Nursing, 23,* 27–32.

Karp, H. (2013). *The happiest baby guild to great sleep.* New York, NY: HarperCollins.

Lind, K., Toure, T., Brugel, D., Meyer, P., Laurent-VAnnier, A., & Chevignard, M. (2016). Research article: Extended follow-up of neurological, cognitive, behavioral and academic outcomes after severe abusive head trauma. *Child Abuse and Neglect, 51,* 358–367.

National Center on Shaken Baby Syndrome. (2016). *What is shaken baby syndrome?* Retrieved from https://dontshake.org/purple-crying

National Institute of Child Health and Human Development. (2017). *What is safe sleep environment?* Retrieved from www.nichd.nih.gov/sts/about/environment/room/Pages/text_alternative.aspx

National Institute of Neurological Disorders and Strokes (NINDS). (2017). *NINDS shaken baby syndrome information page.* Retrieved from https://www.ninds.nih.gov/NODE/2816

Simpson, K., & Creehan, P. (2014). *Perinatal nursing* (4th ed.). Philadelphia, PA: Wolters Kluwer/LWW.

So, H., You, M., Mun, J., Hwang, H., Kim, H., Pyeon, S., . . . Chang, B. (2014). Effect of trunk-to-head bathing on physiological responses in newborns. *Journal of Obstetric, Gynecologic, & Neonatal Nursing, 43,* 742–751.

Spies, E., & Klevens, J. (2017). Fatal abusive head trauma among children aged <5 years—United States, 1999–2014. *Morbidity and Mortality Weekly Report, 65,* 20.

United States Department of Agriculture (USDA). (2018). Making healthy choices in each food groups. Retrieved from www.choosemyplate.gov/moms-making-healthy-food-choices.

U.S. Department of Health and Human Services (DHHS). (2017). Healthy People 2020 topics and objectives. Retrieved from https://www.healthypeople.gov/2020/topics-objectives

Wilkinson, J., & Van Leuven, K. (2007). *Fundamentals of nursing.* Philadelphia, PA: F.A. Davis.

World Health Organization (WHO/UNICEF). (2014). Global nutrition targets 2025: Breastfeeding policy brief (WHO/NMH/NHD/14.7). Geneva: World Health Organization.

High-Risk Neonatal Nursing Care

17

Darice Taylor, MSN, RNC ————————————————————

LEARNING OUTCOMES

Upon completion of this chapter, the student will be able to:

1. Describe the physiology and pathophysiology associated with selected complications of the neonatal period.
2. Identify critical elements of assessment and nursing care of the high-risk neonate.
3. Develop a discharge plan for high-risk neonates.
4. Describe the loss and grief process experienced by parents whose infant has died.

Nursing Diagnoses

- Impaired gas exchange related to inadequate surfactant and immature lung tissue
- Risk for ineffective airway clearance related to meconium aspiration
- Ineffective thermoregulation related to prematurity, lack of subcutaneous fat, and environmental temperature
- Imbalanced nutrition related to prematurity; inability to absorb nutrients; decreased perfusion to gastrointestinal tract; postnatal change from high glucose exposure to low glucose exposure and hyperinsulinism; cleft lip/cleft palate
- Risk for infection related to prematurity, exposure to infectious agents, and maternal chorioamnionitis
- Pain related to procedures; birth trauma
- Risk for injury related to lack of oxygen to the brain; prolonged ventilation and oxygen administration; effects of drugs on fetal/neonatal growth and development; birth trauma; hypoglycemia; asphyxia; meconium aspiration; kernicterus
- Risk for ineffective parent/family coping related to infant illness or death
- Grieving related to the infant with a high-risk condition; loss of the dream of the perfect infant; death of the infant
- Risk for impaired parent–infant attachment related to separation

Nursing Outcomes

- The infant exhibits a breathing pattern within normal limits with respiratory rate between 30 and 60 breaths per minute with no signs of respiratory distress.
- The infant maintains temperature within normal limits.
- The infant gains weight, consumes adequate nutritional intake, has adequate output, and is free of signs of hypoglycemia or malnutrition.
- The infant remains free of signs of infection; the white blood cell count is within normal limits and the blood, urine, and cerebrospinal fluid (CSF) cultures are negative.
- The infant exhibits decreased signs of pain after receiving nonpharmacological or pharmacological pain-reduction interventions.
- The infant is free of signs of injury.
- Parents communicate needs, state ability to cope, identify a support system, and ask for help and information when needed.
- Parents identify what to expect during the grieving process.
- Parents visit the infant in the intensive care nursery, demonstrate caregiving behaviors, express interest in the newborn, and respond to the infant's behavioral cues.

INTRODUCTION

Infant mortality rates in the United States have significantly decreased from 47 per 1,000 live births in 1940 to 5.82 per 1,000 in 2014 (Kochanek, Murphy, Xu, & Tejada-Vera, 2016). Although this is a significant decrease, it indicates that 23,215 infants died in 2014, too high an infant mortality rate for a nation with the available wealth and resources possessed by the United States. One of the primary causes of illness and death in the neonate is complications related to prematurity.

This chapter provides an overview of the critical components of care for the high-risk neonate, a subspecialty of maternity nursing. Nurses who elect to work in a neonatal intensive care nursery will need to gain an in-depth knowledge of high-risk neonates through additional readings and classes that focus on the unique needs of high-risk neonates and their parents.

PRETERM NEONATES

Period of gestation and birth weight are the two most important predictors of an infant's health and survival. Prematurity and low birth weight are the second leading causes of infant death in the United States after congenital malformations and chromosomal anomalies (Kochanek et al., 2016). The number of overall preterm births has decreased from 10.44% in 2007 to 9.63% in 2015, but the percentage of late preterm births continues to increase (Martin, Hamilton, Osterman, Driscoll, & Matthews, 2017) (Table 17–1). Preterm is classified as:

● Very preterm: Neonates born at less than 32 weeks' gestation (<32 weeks) (Fig. 17–1).
● Preterm: Neonates born between 32 and 34 weeks' gestation (>32 and <34 weeks).
● Late preterm: Neonates born between 34 and 37 weeks' gestation (>34 and <37 weeks).

The percentage of preterm births based on mother's race are:

● Non-Hispanic black: 13.4%.
● American Indian or Alaska Native: 10.5%.
● Hispanic: 9.1%.
● Non-Hispanic white: 8.9%.
● Asian or Pacific Islander: 8.6% (Martin et al., 2017).

TABLE 17–1   Percentage of Preterm Births

	2007	2015
All Preterm	10.44	9.63
Early Preterm (Less Than 34 weeks)	2.93	2.76
Late Preterm (34 to 36 weeks)	6.82	6.87

Martin et al., 2017.

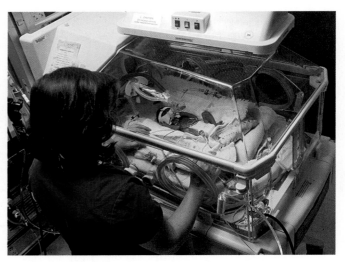

FIGURE 17–1 A very premature neonate born at 27 weeks' gestation.

Prematurity is a primary reason for low birth weight. Classification of birth weight (regardless of gestational age) is as follows:

● Low birth weight: Less than 2,500 g at birth
● Very low birth weight: Less than 1,500 g at birth
● Extremely low birth weight: Less than 1,000 grams at birth

Multiple factors place a woman at risk for preterm labor and birth. Many are modifiable, and many are not (Table 17–2). Common complications related to prematurity are respiratory distress syndrome, retinopathy of prematurity, bronchopulmonary dysplasia, patent ductus arteriosus, periventricular-intraventricular hemorrhage, and necrotizing enterocolitis.

Assessment Findings

● Gestational age by Ballard score is at or below 37 weeks.
● Physical characteristics vary based on gestational age (Fig. 17–2).
   ● Tone and flexion increase with greater gestational age. Early in gestation, resting tone and posture are hypotonic and extended.
   ● The skin is translucent, transparent, and red.
   ● Subcutaneous fat is decreased.
   ● Lanugo is present between 20 and 28 weeks' gestation. At 28 weeks' gestation, lanugo begins to disappear on the face and the front of the trunk.
   ● Creases on the anterior part of the foot are not present until 28 to 30 weeks. As gestation increases, plantar creases increase and spread toward the heel of the foot.
   ● Eyelids are fused in very preterm neonates. Eyelids open between 26 and 30 weeks' gestation.
   ● Overriding sutures are common among premature, low-birth-weight neonates.
   ● The pinna of the ear is thin, soft, flat, and folded.

TABLE 17–2   Risk Factors for Preterm Labor and Birth

NONMODIFIABLE RISK FACTORS	TREATABLE/MODIFIABLE RISK FACTORS
Previous preterm birth	Age at pregnancy <17 or >34 years
Multiple abortions	Unplanned pregnancy
Race/ethnic group	Single
Uterine/cervical anomaly	Low educational level
Multiple gestation	Poverty, unsafe environment
Polyhydramnios	Domestic violence
Oligohydramnios	Life stress
Pregnancy-induced hypertension	Number of implanted embryos in assisted reproduction
Placenta previa (after 22 weeks)	Low pre-pregnancy weight
Diethystilbestrol exposure	Obesity
Short interval between pregnancies	Health problems that can be treated: hypertension, diabetes, clotting problems, anemia
Parity (0 or >4)	Incompetent cervix
Premature rupture of membranes	Genitourinary infection
Bleeding in first trimester	Infection
	Periodontal disease
	Substance/alcohol use
	Cigarette smoking
	Long hours of employment/standing
	Late or no prenatal care
	Air pollution

March of Dimes, 2016.

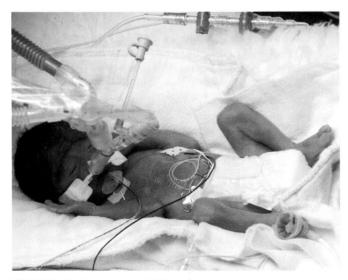

FIGURE 17–2 A neonate at 27 weeks' gestation.

- The testes are not descended and are found in the inguinal canal.
- Tremors and jittery movement may be noted.
- The cry is weak.
- Reflexes may be diminished or absent.
- Immature suck, swallow, and breathing patterns are observed in very premature infants. These neonates may not be able to take adequate oral feedings.
- Apnea (cessation of breathing for 20 seconds or longer) or a shorter pause accompanied by bradycardia (heart rate less than 100 beats per minute [bpm]) are commonly observed (Eichenwald, 2016).
- Hypotension may occur among extremely low-birth-weight infants.
- Heart murmur may be present related to patent ductus arteriosus.
- Anemia is common, especially among very-low-birth-weight babies.

Medical Management

- Lung maturity is determined with lecithin/sphingomyelin (L/S) ratio or phosphatidylglycerol (PG) before elective induction or cesarean birth and for women in preterm labor.
- Corticosteroids, betamethasone or dexamethasone, are administered to the pregnant woman if the woman presents in preterm labor or if preterm birth is anticipated. Evidence suggests that corticosteroid administration results in reduced mortality rates as well as neonatal morbidities such as respiratory distress syndrome (RDS), necrotizing enterocolitis (NEC), and intraventricular hemorrhage (IVH). Corticosteroid administration also reduces the need for respiratory support and the length of stay in the neonatal intensive care unit (NICU) (Wong, Abdel-Latif, & Kent, 2014).
- Cardiorespiratory, oxygen saturation, blood gas, and end CO_2 monitoring
- Respiratory support
  - Nasal continuous positive airway pressure (NCPAP) or intubation
- Laboratory tests
  - Bilirubin level
  - Blood cultures based on risk factors
  - Complete blood count with manual differential
  - Electrolytes
  - Blood glucose
  - Liver function tests
- Medications
  - Sodium bicarbonate to treat metabolic acidosis if present
  - Dopamine or dobutamine for treatment of hypotension
  - Erythropoietin (EPO) administration to stimulate production of red blood cells (RBCs) if indicated
    - The use of EPO reduces the need for RBC transfusions, but there is an increased risk for retinopathy of prematurity (Ohlsson & Aher, 2014).
  - Antibiotic therapy as indicated to decrease risk of infection or treatment of infection
  - Opioids to treat pain associated with procedures that cause moderate to severe pain, such as with surgical procedures
- Blood transfusion if the neonate is anemic or to replace blood loss due to laboratory tests or blood loss during birth (Sherman, 2015a)
- Intravenous fluids as indicated
- Parenteral (intravenous) nutrition if indicated by the neonate's gestational age and/or clinical condition
- Central line if long-term parenteral nutrition is required
- Umbilical artery and umbilical vein catheters
- Information about the neonate's condition, treatment plan, and follow-up care is provided to the parents

Nursing Actions

- Review prenatal, intrapartal, and neonatal histories for any known risk factors that would potentially impact the neonate.
- Participate in resuscitation of the neonate as indicated.
  - The NICU nurse, neonatologist, and/or neonatal nurse practitioner should be present at high-risk births.
- Stabilize and transfer the neonate to the NICU for ongoing specialized care.
- Perform gestational assessment to determine age of neonate if gestational age is unknown or unreliable.
  - Protocols of care differ with gestational age.
- Perform a physical assessment, evaluating for problems associated with prematurity.
  - Nursing care includes the immediate recognition and prioritization of problems to decrease neonatal morbidity and mortality.
- Assess for signs of respiratory distress:
  - Grunting
  - Flaring
  - Retracting
  - Cyanosis
- Provide respiratory support.
  - Maintain a patent airway.
  - Administer oxygen to maintain oxygen saturation within ordered parameters.
    - Oxygen administration may be given using low- or high-flow nasal cannulas, NCPAP, or ventilator.
    - Oxygen is humidified and warmed to prevent drying of mucous membranes and dropping of body temperature. A decrease in body temperature increases body metabolism, which increases the risk for hypoglycemia and respiratory distress.
  - Suction airway as needed to remove secretions, as neonates have a smaller airway diameter, which increases the risk of obstruction.
- Maintain neutral thermal environment by:
  - Drying the infant gently immediately after birth to prevent heat loss from evaporation.
  - Keeping the head covered to prevent heat loss due to radiation and convection.
  - Using plastic barriers made of polyethylene to cover preterm neonates after birth to prevent heat loss and transepidermal water loss
  - Using a chemical warming mattress during resuscitation and transport to the NICU
    - Extremely-low-birth-weight neonates are at high risk for cold stress during the period immediately after birth. Neonates placed in plastic barriers and/or on chemical mattresses immediately after birth have higher admission temperatures upon admission to the NICU (Sharma, 2016).
  - Prewarming radiant warmers, incubators, and linens
  - Controlling environmental temperature with the use of servo control. A temperature-control probe should be placed on the neonate's abdomen to assist in maintaining the neonate's temperature within the normal range (axillary 36.3°C to 36.9°C [97.4°F to 98.4°F]) for premature neonates.
  - Placing the neonate in a double-walled incubator to prevent transepidermal water loss and heat loss

- Encouraging kangaroo care (skin-to-skin care) in stable neonates
- Weaning infants gradually from incubator to an open crib (Brand & Boyd, 2015)
- Assess cardiovascular system.
  - Murmurs
  - Pulses
  - Capillary refill
- Provide cardiovascular support.
  - Monitor blood pressure, oxygen saturation, and blood gases.
  - Obtain and monitor hemoglobin and hematocrit as per order.
  - Administer blood transfusion as per order.
- Assess responses to interventions. These responses may be changes in breathing, oxygen saturation, vital signs, and neonatal behavior.
- Maintain fluid and electrolyte balance.
  - Monitor input and output by:
    - Weighing diapers to determine output.
    - Assessing frequency, color, amount, and specific gravity of urine to determine hydration status.
    - Recording fluid intake and output (I&O) from IV fluids, feedings, chest tubes, urinary catheters, stomas.
  - Restrict fluid intake as per order.
    - Fluid restriction is commonly ordered for neonates with bronchopulmonary dysplasia (BPD) and patent ductus arteriosus (PDA) or other complications that can lead to pulmonary edema.
  - Monitor electrolyte levels as per order.
    - Hyperkalemia (elevated potassium levels), hyponatremia (low sodium level), and hypernatremia (high sodium level) may occur among low-birth-weight infants (Sherman, 2015a).
  - Administer intravenous fluids as per order.
    - Monitor the site of intravenous access for signs of infection, skin breakdown, and infiltration.
  - Add humidity to the neonate's environment to decrease water loss that can occur through the neonate's immature skin, known as transepidermal water loss (TEWL).
    - Humidity added to the environment prevents heat loss, improves skin integrity, decreases TEWL, and promotes electrolyte balance (Sherman, 2015a).
- Meet the neonate's nutrition requirements.
  - Obtain and monitor blood glucose levels as per order.
  - Administer parenteral nutrition (intravenous) if the neonate is unable to receive enteral feedings (via gastrointestinal tract) or is advancing slowly on feeding volumes.
    - Low-birth-weight neonates (less than 2,500 g) and neonates less than 32 weeks' gestation:
      - May lack the ability to digest and absorb feedings.
      - May have an inability to suck, swallow, and breathe.
      - Will most likely require parenteral nutrition (Sherman, 2015a).
  - Administer trophic feedings (small volume enteral feedings) as per order. They are often given while neonates are receiving parenteral feedings to ease the transition to full enteral feedings and enhance gastrointestinal functioning (Sherman, 2015a).
  - Administer enteral feedings orally or by gastric tube (gavage feedings), depending on the infant's gestational age and clinical condition. Most neonates who are older than 34 weeks' gestation usually receive oral feedings soon after birth.
    - Human milk reduces the risk of necrotizing enterocolitis (NEC) and is preferred for enteral feedings (Herrmann & Carroll, 2014).
    - Human milk requires fortification because it does not provide the calories, protein, fat, carbohydrate, potassium, calcium, sodium, and phosphorus that the premature infant needs (Ditzenberger, 2015).
    - Formulas developed specifically for preterm infants are available. These formulas are modified to promote absorption and digestion for babies with immature gastrointestinal functioning and contain the extra calories, protein, minerals, and vitamins required by preterm babies (Ditzenberger, 2015).
- Use proper technique for gavage feedings.
  - When feedings are initiated and before each feeding, assess for signs of feeding tolerance as follows (Ditzenberger, 2015):
    - Check for the presence of bowel sounds.
    - Assess the abdomen for bowel loops and discoloration.
    - Measure abdominal girth.
    - Check for gastric residuals by aspirating stomach contents with the syringe. Note the amount, color, and consistency of the contents.
    - Assess for emesis.
    - Check stools for occult blood as per order.
    - Check stools for reducing substances as per order.
    - Assess stools for consistency, amount, and frequency.
  - Use nonnutritive sucking with a pacifier during gavage feedings. Nonnutritive sucking eases the transition from gavage feeding to bottle feeding and results in decreased length of hospital stay for preterm neonates (Foster, Psaila, & Patterson, 2016).
  - Monitor weight daily. Weight gain of 10 to 20 g per kg/day indicates appropriate growth and caloric intake for a preterm neonate (Ditzenberger, 2015).
  - Monitor length and head circumference weekly.
  - Calculate and monitor intake of fluids, calories, and protein daily (Ditzenberger, 2015). Preterm infants require between 105 and 130 kcal/kg/day.

CRITICAL COMPONENT

Procedure for Gavage Feeding

Gavage feedings are appropriate for neonates who cannot safely receive oral feedings.

1. Use a size 5 to 8 French feeding tube.
2. For orogastric route, measure the tube from the mouth to the ear and from the ear to the lower end of the sternum.

Continued

For nasogastric route, measure from the nose to the ear and from the ear to the lower end of the sternum.

3. Check for proper placement of the tube after each insertion and before each feeding. It is important to check hospital policies since there are various methods used for assessing proper insertions.
4. Use tape to ensure that the tube is secured.
5. Check for residuals before starting the feeding by aspirating stomach contents with the syringe. Note the amount, color, and consistency of the contents.
6. Feedings may be given by gravity or placed on a pump over 30 to 60 minutes.
7. In some cases, continuous tube feedings may be ordered.
8. To remove the feeding tube, pinch it closed and remove it swiftly.
9. Assess the neonate for feeding intolerance throughout feeding.

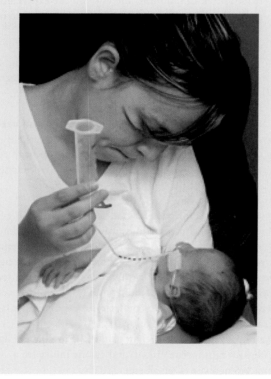

● Transition the neonate from tube feedings to oral feedings.
  ● Transitioning to oral feedings occurs when the neonate:
    ○ Has cardiorespiratory regulation.
    ○ Demonstrates a coordinated suck, swallow, and breathe.
    ○ Demonstrates hunger cues such as bringing hand to the mouth, sucking on fingers.
    ○ Maintains a quiet alert state.
  ● Properly position the neonate for bottle feeding by holding the swaddled baby in a semi-upright or upright position.
  ● Observe the neonate for respiratory status, apnea, bradycardia, oxygenation, and feeding tolerance.

● Pace feeding and allow for breathing breaks since preterm neonates may become fatigued during feedings.
● Support breastfeeding.
  ● Evidence suggests that breast milk decreases the incidence of NEC (Herrmann & Carroll, 2014).
  ● When the neonate is unable to breastfeed, instruct the mother in the use of a breast pump and storage of breast milk.
  ● Encourage the mother to bring breast milk to the NICU so that it can be used for enteral feedings for her infant.
  ● Teach the mother about feeding cues, breastfeeding positions, correct latch, and evaluating the feeding.
    ○ Encourage breastfeeding as frequently as possible to establish successful latching. Infants who successfully breastfeed in the NICU are more likely to continue breastfeeding after discharge (Briere, McGrath, Xiaomei, Brownell, & Cusson, 2016).
  ● Weigh the neonate before and after breastfeeding to monitor intake.
    ○ Many mothers are hesitant to breastfeed their premature or ill neonate because they are afraid the volume will not be adequate. Weighing the neonate before and after breastfeeding can be an accurate way to demonstrate successful breastfeeding and positive mother–infant bonding (Rankin et al., 2016).
  ● See Appendix A for additional nursing actions.
● Administer medications as per order.
● Provide skin care as follows:
  ● Assess for skin breakdown and signs of infection; the thin, fragile skin of the preterm neonate is predisposed to injury (Fig. 17–3).

AWHONN/NANN RBP4 NEONATAL SKIN CONDITION SCORE (NSCS)
Dryness
1 = Normal, no sign of dry skin 2 = Dry skin, visible scaling 3 = Very dry skin, cracking/fissures
Erythema
1 = No evidence of erythema 2 = Visible erythema, <50% body surface 3 = Visible erythema, ≥50% body surface
Breakdown/excoriation
1 = None evident 2 = Small, localized areas 3 = Extensive
Note: Perfect score = 3, worst score = 9
This scoring system, developed for the AWHONN/NANN Neonatal Skin Care Project (RBP4) was adapted from a visual scoring system used in a previous study (Lane and Drost, 1993). It can facilitate assessment of neonatal skin conditions. This tool continues to undergo reliability and validity testing.

FIGURE 17–3 Neonatal Skin Condition Score.

- Use a neutral pH cleanser and sterile water when bathing and only bathe the soiled areas.
- Use adhesives sparingly.
- Change diapers frequently.
- Change positions frequently.
- Apply emollients gently to avoid friction.
- Use water, air, or gel mattresses (Association of Women's Health, Obstetric and Neonatal Nurses [AWHONN], 2013).
- Obtain laboratory test as per orders.
- Assess for signs of jaundice.
- Assess for signs of NEC, such as abnormal vital signs, abdominal distention (increase in abdominal circumference), abdominal discoloration, bowel loops, feeding intolerance, emesis, residuals, bloody stools, and behavioral changes.
- Manage pain to prevent potential long-term sensory disturbances and altered pain responses that may last into adulthood.
  - Frequently assess the neonate for signs of pain, especially during painful procedures. Instruments to measure neonatal pain among preterm neonates are available and should be integrated into routine care.
  - Administer sucrose and promote nonnutritive sucking during painful procedures.
  - Administer opioids as per orders to treat pain associated with procedures that cause moderate to severe pain.
  - Use nonpharmacological interventions such as swaddling, positioning, kangaroo care, and therapeutic touch, and decrease environmental stimulus.
  - Evaluate the effectiveness of nonpharmacological and pharmacological interventions.
- Provide developmentally appropriate care to decrease stress and enhance neurodevelopment.
  - Maintain a quiet setting to decrease negative physiological responses such as apnea and fluctuations in heart rate, blood pressure, and oxygen saturation.
  - Keep lighting dim and change lighting in NICU to simulate night and day.
  - Cluster nursing activities to provide for extended periods of sleep.
  - Avoid clustering painful interventions together.
  - Provide care when the neonate is awake.
  - Provide individualized care based on the neonate's responses and needs.
  - Allow a break in care/stimulation if neonate becomes stressed.
  - Minimize handling for neonates in an unstable condition.
  - Position and swaddle
    - Change the neonate's position slowly and gently.
    - Reposition every 2 to 3 hours. Assess the infant's response to repositioning.
    - Position neonate in the side-lying or prone position (enhances oxygenation and gastric emptying).
    - The head of the bed may be elevated 15 degrees.
    - Swaddle in flexion with arms and hands placed toward the infant's midline.

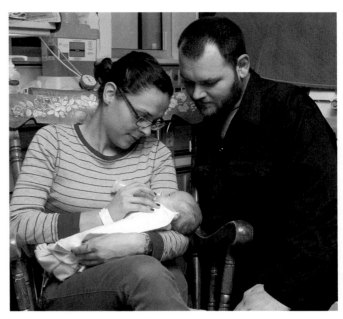

FIGURE 17–4 Parents bottle-feeding their baby.

  - Create a nest with blankets to enhance containment.
  - Avoid swaddling or nesting that is overly restrictive to neonatal movement (Spruill, 2015).
- Encourage kangaroo care (skin-to-skin contact with the parents) for medically stable neonates. Benefits of kangaroo care include the following:
  - Decreases risk of low body temperature.
  - Reduces illness, infection, and pain perception.
  - Improves daily weight gain and mother–infant attachment.
  - Decreases the length of hospital stay (Cho et al., 2016).
- Provide emotional support to parents and family members.
- Involve parents and family in all aspects of the infant's care. This helps to decrease anxiety and fears, thus allowing for an increase in parent–infant bonding.
  - Teach parents what to expect from their preterm infant and how to interpret behavioral cues.
  - Teach parents how to provide care for their infant (Fig. 17–4).
  - Encourage parent–infant bonding by welcoming parents to the NICU and praising them for their involvement with their infant.
  - Teach parents about the infant's condition and involve parents in the plan of care.

RESPIRATORY DISTRESS SYNDROME

Respiratory distress syndrome (RDS) is a life-threatening lung disorder that results from small, underdeveloped alveoli and insufficient levels of pulmonary surfactant. These combined factors can cause an alteration in alveoli surface tension that eventually results in atelectasis. The incidence of RDS decreases with increasing gestational age and affects 90% to 98% of all premature infants born at less than 28 weeks' gestation (Fraser, 2015). The effects of atelectasis are:

- Hypoxemia and hypercarbia.
- Pulmonary artery vasoconstriction.
- Right-to-left shunting through the ductus arteriosus and foramen ovale as the neonate's body attempts to counteract the compromised pulmonary perfusion.
- Metabolic acidosis that occurs from a buildup of lactic acid that results from prolonged periods of hypoxemia.
- Respiratory acidosis that occurs from the collapsed alveoli being unable to rid the body of excess carbon dioxide.

Pulmonary surfactant is a substance composed of 90% phospholipids and 10% proteins. It reduces the surface tension within the lungs and increases the pulmonary compliance that prevents the alveoli from collapsing at the end of expiration. Type II alveolar cells within the lungs begin to produce pulmonary surfactant around 24 to 28 weeks and continue to term. Tests used to evaluate fetal lung maturity are:

- Phosphatidylglycerol (PG):
  - PG is synthesized from mature lung alveolar cells.
  - It is present in the amniotic fluid within 2 to 6 weeks of full-term gestation.
  - The presence of PG indicates lung maturity and a decrease indicates risk of RDS.
- L/S ratio:
  - Lecithin and sphingomyelin are two phospholipids that are detected in the amniotic fluid.
  - The ratio between the two phospholipids provides information on the level of surfactant.
  - An L/S ratio greater than 2:1 in a nondiabetic woman indicates the fetus's lungs are mature.
  - An L/S ratio of 3:1 in a diabetic woman indicates the fetus's lungs are mature.

Complications of RDS

- Patent ductus arteriosus (PDA)
- Pneumothorax
- Bronchopulmonary dysplasia (BPD)
- Pulmonary edema
- Hypotension
- Anemia
- Oliguria
- Hypoglycemia and altered calcium and sodium levels
- Retinopathy of prematurity
- Seizures
- Intraventricular hemorrhage

Assessment Findings

- Respiratory distress varies based on degree of prematurity.
- Respiratory difficulty begins shortly after delivery, and the neonate must work progressively harder at breathing to maintain open terminal airways (Fraser, 2015).
- Tachypnea
  - A respiratory rate greater than 60 breaths per minute

- Intercostal, subcostal, and substernal retractions; seesaw breathing patterns occur.
- Audible expiratory grunting
  - Caused by forcing air past a partially closed glottis
  - Used by the neonate in an attempt to prevent alveolar collapse
  - More pronounced with severe distress
- Nasal flaring
- Increased oxygen levels to maintain a Pao_2 and $Paco_2$ within normal limits.
  - The normal range of Pao_2 is 60 to 70 mm Hg.
  - The normal range of $Paco_2$ is 35 to 45 mm Hg.
- Skin color is gray or dusky.
- Breath sounds on auscultation are decreased. Rales are present as RDS progresses.
- The neonate is lethargic and hypotonic.
- X-ray exam shows a reticulogranular pattern of the peripheral lung fields and air bronchograms.
- Hypoxemia may occur (Pao_2 less than 50 mm Hg).
- Acidosis may result from sustained hypoxemia.
- Tachycardia
  - Heart rate greater than 160 bpm
  - More prevalent if acidosis and hypoxemia are present

Medical Management

- Cardiorespiratory, oxygen saturation, and blood gas monitoring
- Endotracheal tube when clinically indicated
- Exogenous surfactant as indicated for neonates at risk for or with RDS
- Respiratory support as indicated. The mode of ventilation and settings are based on the neonate's condition and arterial blood gas results. Methods of respiratory support include:
  - Continuous positive airway pressure (CPAP) used for neonates who are at risk for RDS or who have RDS. It can be administered by nasal cannula, nasal mask, nasal prongs, endotracheal tube, or nasopharyngeal route.
  - Mechanical ventilation, which is used when CPAP is not effective (use judiciously to avoid damage to lung tissue).
  - High-frequency oscillatory ventilation, which is used when mechanical ventilation has proven unsuccessful.
    - Delivers small volumes of gas at a high rate (greater than 300 breaths/minute)
    - Less traumatic on fragile lung tissue
  - Extracorporeal membrane oxygenation therapy (ECMO), which is a cardiopulmonary bypass machine with a membrane oxygenator that is used when the neonate does not respond to conventional ventilator therapy. Blood shunts from the right atrium and is returned to the aorta, allowing time for the lungs to heal and mature.
- Diagnostic tests
  - Chest x-ray exam to assist in evaluation of RDS
- Laboratory tests
  - Arterial, venous, or capillary blood gases
  - Blood cultures if neonate is at risk for infection
- Medications
  - Antibiotics as indicated

Nursing Actions

Nursing actions for neonates with RDS are similar to actions for preterm neonates, with additional emphasis on the following:

- Provide respiratory support.
  - Maintain a patent airway.
  - Assess for correct placement of endotracheal tube.
    - Listen for equal breath sounds bilaterally, assess for equal chest rise, use commercial end tidal CO_2 detector.
  - Administer oxygen as ordered to maintain oxygen saturation within ordered parameters.
    - Hypoxemia and acidosis may further decrease surfactant production.
  - Minimize oxygen demand by maintaining a neutral thermal environment, clustering care to decrease stress, and treating acidosis as clinically indicated and ordered.
  - Suction airway as needed for removal of secretions, as neonates have a smaller airway diameter, which increases the risk of obstruction.
    - Suctioning may stimulate the vagus nerve, causing bradycardia, hypoxemia, or bronchospasm.

CRITICAL COMPONENT

Surfactant Replacement Therapy Administration

Natural Surfactant
- Composed of calf, pig, or cow lung (minced) combined with lipids
- Examples: Survanta, Curosurf, Infasurf

Synthetic Surfactant
- Example: Exosurf

Action
- Reduces surface tension of the alveoli, thus preventing collapse during expiration
- Enhances lung compliance to allow easier inflation, which decreases the work of breathing

Indications
- Respiratory distress, meconium aspiration syndrome, persistent pulmonary hypertension

Route
- Administered via endotracheal tube

Dosing Regimen (dose and technique vary by product)
- Prophylaxis: Initiated within 15 minutes of birth, based on risk factors of RDS such as gestational age less than 27 to 30 weeks. Multiple doses can be given if indicated.
- Rescue therapy: Treatment of confirmed RDS. Treatment is typically initiated within 8 hours of birth for infants who have increased oxygen demands and need mechanical ventilation.

Adverse Effects
- Bradycardia, decreased oxygen saturation, tachycardia, reflux, gagging, cyanosis, blockage of the endotracheal tube, hypotension

Benefits of Surfactant Therapy
- Prophylactic therapy decreases the occurrence of RDS and mortality in preterm neonates.
- Decreased risk of pneumothorax
- Decreased risk of intraventricular hemorrhage
- Decreased risk of bronchopulmonary dysplasia
- Decreased risk of pulmonary interstitial emphysema

Fraser, 2015.

- Monitor vital signs, oxygen saturation, and blood gas results.
- Maintain neutral thermal environment to decrease the risk of cold stress.
  - Cold stress increases oxygen consumption, may promote acidosis, and may further impair surfactant production.
- Monitor I&O and daily weights.
  - Dehydration impairs ability to clear airways because mucus becomes thickened.
  - Overhydration may contribute to alveolar infiltrates or pulmonary edema.
  - Weight loss and increased urine output may indicate diuretic phase of RDS.
- Promote rest by implementing calming measures or administering ordered sedation.
  - Minimizing stimulation and energy expenditure reduces metabolic rate and oxygen consumption.

BRONCHOPULMONARY DYSPLASIA

Bronchopulmonary dysplasia (BPD) is a chronic lung problem that affects neonates who have been treated with mechanical ventilation and oxygen for problems such as RDS. Neonates who are dependent on oxygen beyond 28 days of life and/or have been on mechanical ventilation are at risk for BPD. This condition leads to decreased lung compliance and pulmonary function secondary to fibrosis, atelectasis, increased pulmonary resistance, and overdistention of the lungs (Bancalari & Walsh, 2015; Fraser, 2015) (Fig. 17–5). Pulmonary edema results from the increased pulmonary vascular resistance. The prognosis for infants with BPD is dependent on the severity of the disease and the infant's overall health status. Long-term outcomes may include prolonged hospitalization, long-term oxygen therapy that may be required after discharge, cerebral palsy, retinopathy of prematurity, and hearing loss.

Risk Factors

- Prematurity
- RDS
- Oxygen toxicity

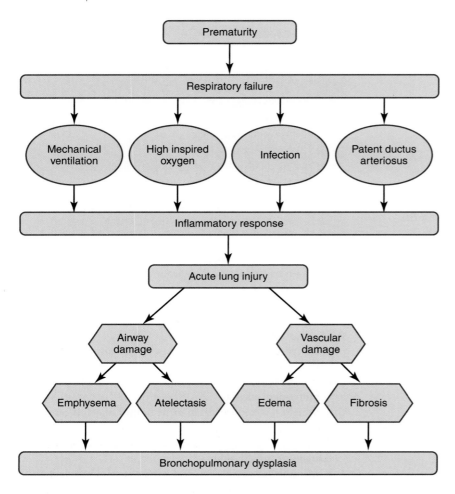

FIGURE 17-5 Bronchopulmonary dysplasia.

- Intubation
- Assisted ventilation with positive pressure
- Lower gestational age and birth weight (less than 32 weeks)
- Infection
- Pulmonary vascular damage secondary to excessive fluid administration, right-to-left shunting associated with patent ductus arteriosus, and increased airway resistance (Bancalari & Walsh, 2015).

Complications

- Pneumonia, upper respiratory infection
- Ear infections
- Congestive heart failure
- Developmental delays
- Cerebral palsy
- Hearing loss
- Retinopathy of prematurity
- Sudden death

Assessment Findings

- Chest retractions
- Audible wheezing, rales, and rhonchi
- Hypoxia
- Respiratory acidosis

- Bronchospasm
- Difficulty weaning from ventilator or increased requirements for ventilator
- Intolerance to fluids: edema, decreased urinary output, and weight gain
- Chest x-ray exam results exhibit cardiomegaly, lung hyperinflation, and infiltrates (Fraser, 2015).

Medical Management

- Diagnostic tests
  - Chest x-ray exam to assess for cardiomegaly, lung hyperinflation, and infiltrates
  - Echocardiogram if cardiac complications are suspected
- Laboratory tests
  - Electrolytes
  - Arterial blood gases
- Medications
  - Bronchodilators: Administered to reduce bronchoconstriction
  - Corticosteroids: Administered to reduce bronchospasm, edema, and inflammation of pulmonary tissue
  - Diuretics: Administered to treat fluid retention and decrease risk for pulmonary edema
- Prophylaxes against respiratory syncytial virus, as infants with BPD are predisposed to this infection

- Chest physiotherapy
- Respiratory assistance and oxygen therapy
- Monitor I&O
- Determine the method of feeding to meet the neonate's nutritional and caloric needs

CRITICAL COMPONENT

Bronchopulmonary Dysplasia

Treatment for BPD is a regimen of support and time: time for the normal repair process within the lungs to improve functioning and time for the infant to grow and thrive.

Nursing Actions

Nursing actions for neonates with BPD are similar to actions for preterm neonates with additional emphasis on the following:

- Provide mechanical ventilation and oxygen administration as per orders.
  - Gradually wean neonate from mechanical ventilation as per orders.
- Provide chest physiotherapy as per orders.
  - This assists to clear secretions from the lungs.
- Provide fluids as ordered.
  - Provide maximum calories with minimal fluid. Fortification of formula or breast milk may be needed to obtain optimal growth.
    - Infants with BPD have a higher metabolic rate at rest (Bancalari & Walsh, 2015).
- Administer medications and monitor for adverse reactions.
- Monitor I&O and daily weights.
  - Infants with BPD are at risk for fluid overload and pulmonary edema.

Patent Ductus Arteriosus

Patent ductus arteriosus (PDA) occurs when the ductus arteriosus remains open after birth (Fig. 17–6). During fetal circulation, the ductus arteriosus connects the pulmonary artery with the descending aorta and shunts blood away from the lungs. Normally, the ductus arteriosus closes within a few hours of birth, but this can take as long as 96 hours. The incidence of PDA among term neonates is 1 in 2,000 live births (Sadowski, 2015). The occurrence of PDA is greater among neonates of lower gestational age and birth weight. It occurs in 45% of neonates who weigh less than 1,750 g and 80% of neonates who weigh less than 1,200 g at birth (Sadowski, 2015). Complications related to PDA are congestive heart failure, chronic lung disease, renal failure, NEC, and intraventricular hemorrhage (Heuchan & Clyman, 2014).

Assessment Findings

- Heart murmur heard at the upper left sternal border (some neonates with PDA may not have an audible murmur)
- Active precordium
- Widened pulse pressure with decreased diastolic blood pressure

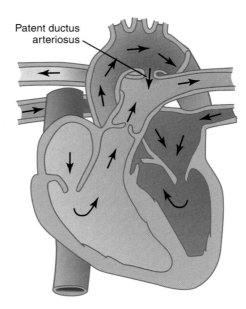

FIGURE 17–6 Patent ductus arteriosus.

- Tachycardia and tachypnea
- Recurrent apnea
- Increased work of breathing
- Bounding pulses
- Difficulty weaning from ventilator support
- Increased demand for oxygen or ventilation
- The presence of a patent ductus arteriosus confirmed by echocardiogram
- Chest x-ray exam may show increased pulmonary vasculature, pulmonary edema, and mild enlargement of the heart (Sadowski, 2015).

Medical Management

The medical treatment of PDA includes managing symptoms with fluid restriction and diuretics.

- Diagnostic tests
  - Echocardiogram to assist in evaluation of PDA
- Medications
  - Diuretics
  - Indomethacin and ibuprofen were frequently used in the past but are rarely used today due to side effects such as gastrointestinal bleeding, decreased glomerular filtration, and decreased urine output.
- Cardiology consultant to determine the method of treatment and need for surgical intervention
- Surgical ligation (suture, clip, or coil) of PDA is indicated for neonates with a hemodynamically significant PDA who do not respond to medical management.

Nursing Actions

Nursing actions for neonates with PDA are similar to actions for preterm neonates with additional emphasis on the following:

- Administer oxygen and mechanical ventilation as per orders.
- Administer medications as per orders.

- Monitor I&O for signs of fluid overload.
  - Fluids may be restricted until PDA is resolved.
  - Infant will be NPO during treatment and surgery.
- Prepare the neonate and family for surgery.

INTRAVENTRICULAR HEMORRHAGE

Intraventricular hemorrhage (IVH) occurs in the germinal matrix tissue surrounding the lateral ventricles of the developing brain. They occur among premature neonates, neonates who experience RDS, and those who experience complications associated with ventilation such as pneumothorax, hypercarbia, and acidosis (deVries, 2015).

IVH occurs in 30% to 40% of infants weighing less than 1,500 g and younger than 32 weeks' gestation. Very few full-term neonates (2% to 3%) experience IVH (Verklan, 2015). Most hemorrhages occur within the first week of life, with 90% occurring within 72 hours after birth (Verklan, 2015).

There are four grades of intraventricular hemorrhage based on the extent of involvement; the higher the grade, the higher the risk for long-term sequelae:

- Grade I: Hemorrhage in germinal matrix
- Grade II: Intraventricular hemorrhage without ventricular dilatation
- Grade III: Intraventricular hemorrhage with ventricular dilatation; clots fill more than 50% of the ventricle
- Grade IV: Extension of blood into cerebral tissue or parenchymal involvement

Risk Factors

- Prematurity, birth at less than 34 weeks' gestation
- Amniotic fluid infection
- Perinatal asphyxia
- RDS, or respiratory failure necessitating ventilatory support
- Increased arterial pressure
- Low 5-minute Apgar score
- Maternal general anesthesia
- Low birth weight
- Alteration of blood pressure, either hypotension or hypertension
- Acidosis, hypercarbia
- Low hematocrit
- Pneumothorax (Verklan, 2015; Shah & Wusthoff, 2016)

The long-term prognosis often depends on the severity of the hemorrhage with death rates of 5% for small hemorrhage, 15% for moderate hemorrhage, and 50% for severe hemorrhage. Neurological problems such as cerebral palsy and delayed mental development occur in 10% of neonates with a small hemorrhage, 40% with a moderate hemorrhage, and 80% with a severe hemorrhage. Approximately 50% of premature infants do not experience neurological problems, and 25% to 30% of very-low-birth-weight neonates who had IVH do not exhibit neurodevelopment problems (Verklan, 2015).

Assessment Findings

- Sudden change in condition
- Bradycardia
- Increased oxygen requirements
- Hypotonia
- Metabolic acidosis
- Shock
- Decreased hematocrit
- Full and/or tense anterior fontanel
- Hyperglycemia
- Signs that bleeding is worsening include:
  - Apnea.
  - Increased need for ventilator support.
  - Drop in blood pressure.
  - Acidosis.
  - Seizures.
  - Full and tense fontanels and rapid increase in head size.
  - Diminished activity or level of consciousness (Verklan, 2015).

Medical Management

- Diagnostic tests
  - Cranial ultrasounds should be performed on all high-risk neonates within the first week of life to assess for IVH.
  - Lumbar puncture to assist in evaluation of IVH. Cerebrospinal fluid is analyzed for RBCs, xanthochromia, decreased glucose, and increased protein (Verklan, 2015).
  - Electroencephalogram (EEG) is done to evaluate seizure activity.
- Laboratory tests
  - Hemoglobin and hematocrit to evaluate extent of bleeding
- Blood transfusions as indicated

Nursing Actions

Nursing actions for neonates with IVH are similar to actions for preterm neonates, with additional emphasis on the following:

- Assess for changes in vital signs, behavior, and neurological status, which may indicate increased intracranial pressure.
- Reduce stress to neonate by maintaining a quiet and dark environment.
- Administer fluid volume replacement slowly to minimize fluctuations in blood pressure.

Evidence-Based Practice: Nursing Strategies to Prevent IVH

Kaspar, A., & Rubarth, L. B. (2016). Neuroprotection of the preterm infant. *Neonatal Network, 35*(6), 391–395. doi:10.1891/0730-0832.35.6.391

Shifts in cerebral perfusion have been linked to the development of IVH, and many studies have evaluated the effects of routine nursing care on fluctuations in cerebral blood flow.

Based on the physiological data and the views of experts in the field, nursing strategies used to decrease cerebral blood flow fluctuations are:

- Supine midline head positioning
- Keep head of bed flat or slightly elevated
- Keep hips below head level with diaper changes
- Maintain temperature within normal range
- Minimize crying
- Minimize stimulation such as light and noise

Conclusion: Implementing nursing strategies to decrease cerebral blood flow fluctuations can decrease the incidence of IVH which promotes better outcomes for the premature infant.

NECROTIZING ENTEROCOLITIS

Necrotizing enterocolitis (NEC) is a gastrointestinal disease that affects neonates. NEC results in inflammation and necrosis of the bowel, usually the proximal colon or terminal ileum, typically occurring after the initiation of enteral feedings (Bradshaw, 2015). Preterm neonates are predisposed to NEC due to:

- Altered blood flow regulation, particularly to the intestines.
- Impaired gastrointestinal host defense when faced with stress/injury to the intestinal tissue.
- Alterations in the inflammatory response (Caplan, 2015).

Ninety percent of NEC cases are among preterm neonates and 5% to 10% of cases occur in neonates who were born at term (Caplan, 2015). In term neonates, NEC is usually associated with problems that result in a decrease in gastrointestinal (GI) blood flow and intestinal ischemia. Examples of these problems are asphyxia, intrauterine growth restriction (IUGR), and polycythemia (Caplan, 2015).

Causes of intestinal ischemia/asphyxia include:

- Hypotension.
- Hypoxia.
- Stress.
- Low body temperature.
- Hypovolemia.
- Polycythemia.
- Patent ductus arteriosus (Bradshaw, 2015).

Risk Factors

- Prematurity
- Bacterial colonization
- Formula feeding (breast milk significantly lowers risk for NEC)
- Intestinal hypoxemia (Caplan, 2015)

Long-Term Outcomes

- NEC is fatal in 10% to 30% of cases.
- 30% will have mild NEC and recover with medical management.
- 25% of neonates with NEC will develop bowel obstruction.
- Short bowel syndrome may occur in neonates who have had surgical treatment.

- Neurodevelopmental problems such as cerebral palsy may develop (Caplan, 2015).

Assessment Findings

Symptoms of NEC typically begin between 3 and 10 days after birth but can occur up to several weeks of age:

- Apnea, bradycardia, and tachycardia
- Respiratory failure
- Hypoxemia
- Unstable temperature
- Hypotension, shock
- Abdominal distention, bloody stools, abdominal tenderness, vomiting, increased gastric residuals, discoloration of abdomen, visible bowel loops
- Lethargy
- Abnormally high or low white blood cell count; thrombocytopenia
- Abnormal electrolyte levels
- Metabolic acidosis
- Abdominal x-ray films of neonates with NEC may show distention of the intestines with gas; gas in one part of the intestine, and lack of gas in other parts; air in the wall of the intestine and/or the portal venous system; dilated loops of bowel; and air in abdomen (Bradshaw, 2015).

Medical Management

- Diagnostic tests
  - Abdominal x-ray exam to assist in evaluation of NEC
  - Serial x-rays to determine worsening or improvement
- Laboratory tests
  - Blood cultures, complete blood count, C-reactive protein, stool cultures, electrolyte panel, arterial blood gases and coagulation studies
- Medications
  - Antibiotics
  - Analgesia
  - Antihypertensives
- Discontinuation of oral feedings, NPO
- Intravenous fluids
- Gastric decompression
  - Replacement of gastric output with normal saline to avoid dehydration

Surgical Management

- Surgical intervention for the removal of necrotic bowel, resection of bowel, or for perforation of bowel related to NEC. A temporary colostomy may be performed.

Nursing Actions

Nursing actions for neonates with NEC are similar to actions for preterm neonates with additional emphasis on the following:

- Assess for abdominal distention, visible bowel loops, emesis, bloody stools, and abnormal vital signs.
  - Early recognition and prompt treatment increases the chances for medical management.

- Withhold feedings as per orders and obtain intravenous access.
- Perform gastric decompression as per orders by placing an orogastric tube and connecting it to low suction.
- Monitor I&O.
  - Maintain circulating blood volume.
  - Maintain adequate hydration.
- Prepare the neonate and family for surgery when indicated.

RETINOPATHY OF PREMATURITY

Retinopathy of prematurity (ROP) is common in premature neonates and those with low birth weight. ROP occurs because the retina is not completely vascularized and is susceptible to stress or injury (Sun, Hellstrom, & Smith, 2015). If injury or exposure to a stressor occurs, the normal vascularization of the retina may be interrupted. Vasoproliferation, an abnormal growth of vasculature, occurs when tissue grows within the retina or extends into the vitreous body. Ultimately, abnormal vascularization and associated bleeding and fluid leakage cause scar tissue that pulls and distorts the retina and displaces the macula (Sun et al., 2015). It also causes retinal folds and can lead to retinal detachment (Sun et al., 2015).

The incidence of ROP increases as gestational age and birth weight decrease. ROP occurs primarily in neonates less than 29 weeks' gestation and in up to 67% of neonates weighing less than 1,251 g (Fraser & Diehl-Jones, 2015). Long-term outcome for this disease depends on the extent of its progression and ranges from full recovery to blindness.

Manifestations of ROP are primarily observed during an eye examination performed by a pediatric ophthalmologist. The International Classification of Retinopathy of Prematurity provides a system of five stages to classify ROP based on the severity of the disease. Stage 4 is partial retinal detachment, and stage 5, the most severe, is complete retinal detachment. The progression of ROP is variable. An aggressive type of ROP called Rush disease can manifest at 3 to 5 weeks postdelivery and progress quickly to complete detachment of the retina. In many cases, ROP evolves slowly and may take a year to become stable (Sun et al., 2015).

Risk Factors

- Prematurity and low birth weight
- Prolonged hyperoxia (exposure to high levels of oxygen) and duration of mechanical ventilation
- Hypoxia, hypercapnia, hypocapnia, and acidosis
- Steroid exposure
- Infection/sepsis
- Patent ductus arteriosus
- Multiple gestation
- Intraventricular hemorrhage
- Blood transfusion
- Maternal diabetes, bleeding, smoking, and hypertension (Fraser & Diehl-Jones, 2015; Sun et al., 2015)

Decreasing risk of ROP includes:

- Continuous monitoring of oxygen to maintain prescribed pulse oximetry parameters.
- Careful use of oxygen during procedures such as suctioning.
- Use of equipment such as oxygen blenders to ensure the exact concentration of oxygen.
- Properly maintaining and calibrating oxygen systems.

Long-term outcomes are as follows:

- 90% of neonates with ROP experience recovery with no or minimal loss of vision.
- Complications such as glaucoma, strabismus, cataracts, amblyopia, retinal detachment, and blindness may occur.
- Corrective glasses may be needed to treat visual acuity deficits (Fraser & Diehl-Jones, 2015; Sun et al., 2015).

Assessment Findings

- Retinal changes noted on ophthalmic examination.

Medical Management

- Eye evaluation for possible ROP completed by the pediatric ophthalmologist for all neonates born before 30 weeks' gestation, or with a birth weight of less than 1,500 g. Neonates who weigh between 1,500 g and 2,000 g at birth with medical complications should also receive an eye exam. The eye examination should occur at 4 to 6 weeks after birth.
- Neonates with immature or abnormal vessel development should have repeated eye exams to monitor progression of the disease (Fraser & Diehl-Jones, 2015).
- The aim of medical treatment is to decrease the risk of blindness. Treatment is determined by the extent of abnormal vessel development and may include:
  - Laser photocoagulation: Laser is used to coagulate the avascular periphery of the retina to prevent vessel proliferation.
  - Cryotherapy: A supercooled probe is used to prevent vessel proliferation by freezing the avascular retina.
  - Vitreoretinal surgery: This is done to reattach the retina (Fraser & Diehl-Jones, 2015).

Nursing Actions

- Reduce the risk for ROP.
  - Administer oxygen to maintain prescribed pulse oximetry parameters.
  - Use oxygen blenders and oxygen-calibrating systems to ensure exact concentration of oxygen.
  - Avoid bright lights by keeping lighting in the nursery at a low level and by covering isolettes and cribs with blankets.

Evidence-Based Practice: Risk Reduction of Retinopathy of Prematurity

Newnam, K. M. (2014). Oxygen saturation limits and evidence supporting the targets. *Advances in Neonatal Care, 14*(6), 403–409. doi:10.1097/ANC.0000000000000150

The aim of this systematic review was to address the question, "What are the recommended oxygen saturation targets for the preterm infant and the preterm infant corrected to term?" Eighteen articles were included in the review.

Results:

- Hypoxia and hyperoxia have both short-term and long-term negative effects of ROP, periventricular leukomalacia, NEC, and BPD.
- Oxygen saturation limits of 87% to 94% were associated with lower incidents of ROP.
- Lower oxygen saturation limits of 85% to 89% were associated with increased risk for neonatal death.
- Higher oxygen saturation rates of 91% to 95% were associated with increased ROP rates.
- Infants are within saturation limits about 31% of the time and require multiple oxygen adjustments hourly.

Conclusions:

Rapid and consistent assessment with appropriate interventions are required to maintain oxygen saturation limits of 87% to 94% to decrease risk of ROP and neonatal death.

POSTMATURE NEONATES

A post-term neonate is one who is delivered after the completion of 41 weeks' gestation. Postmaturity is related to a higher risk of morbidity and mortality (Benjamin & Furdon, 2015). The cause of post-term pregnancies is unknown. Placental insufficiency related to the aging of the placenta may result in postmaturity syndrome, in which the fetus begins to use its subcutaneous fat stores and glycemic stores (Hardy, D'Agata, & McGrath, 2016). Placental function decreases, resulting in altered oxygenation and nutrient transport, which increases the risk for hypoxia and hypoglycemia at the onset of labor. If the placenta continues to function well after term, the result may be a newborn who is large for gestational age (LGA). The risk of macrosomia, or a birth weight above 4,000 to 4,500 g, increases when pregnancy is prolonged.

Risk Factors

- Anencephaly
- History of postterm pregnancies
- First pregnancy
- Grand multiparous women

Complications

- Meconium aspiration: The presence of meconium in the amniotic fluid related to fetal hypoxia places the neonate at risk for meconium aspiration syndrome (discussed later in this chapter).
- Fetal hypoxia: related to placental insufficiency and a decrease in amniotic fluid, which increases the risk of cord compression
- Neurological complications: this includes seizures related to fetal asphyxia during labor and birth due to alteration in oxygenation

- Hypoglycemia: related to alteration in nutrient transport due to decreased placental functioning
- Hypothermia: related to loss of subcutaneous fat related to insufficient nutrient transport through the placenta
  - Polycythemia, a compensatory response, is caused by an alteration in oxygenation associated with placental insufficiency; hematocrit greater than 65% is considered polycythemia in a neonate (Diehl-Jones & Fraser, 2015).
  - Birth trauma related to macrosomia.

Assessment Findings

- Dry, peeling, cracked skin
- Lack of vernix
- Profuse hair
- Long fingernails
- Thin, wasted appearance
- Meconium staining (green or yellow staining on the infant's skin, nail beds, or umbilical cord)
- Hypoglycemia
- Poor feeding behavior

Medical Management

- Oxygen therapy administered for perinatal depression or respiratory distress
- Hematocrit to assess for polycythemia
- Blood glucose monitoring for hypoglycemia

Nursing Actions

- Assess the prenatal record and intrapartum history, including Apgar scores, for risk factors.
- Assess the neonate for:
  - Gestational age with use of gestational age scoring system
  - Birth trauma if neonate is macrosomic
  - Respiratory distress (e.g., grunting, nasal flaring, chest retractions, tachypnea)
  - Cyanosis
  - Oxygen saturation if respiratory distress or cyanosis is present
  - Signs of meconium staining
  - Blood glucose levels
  - Vital signs
  - Weight
  - Gross anomalies
- Monitor for signs of hypoglycemia.
  - Jitteriness, irritability, poor feeding, apnea, grunting, lethargy
- Provide early and frequent feedings if respiratory status is stable.
  - Early and frequent feedings reduce the risk of hypoglycemia.
- Monitor I&O.
  - Post-term infants may be poor feeders and thus are at risk for inadequate fluid intake.

MECONIUM ASPIRATION SYNDROME

Meconium aspiration syndrome is a cause of respiratory failure in term and post-term neonates. Some fetuses pass meconium stool into the amniotic fluid. This occurs when there is a relaxation of the fetus's anal sphincter, usually due to fetal asphyxia in utero. It can also occur with breech presentations and in cephalic presentations without evidence of asphyxia (Blackburn, 2013). Meconium is released into the amniotic fluid in roughly 8% to 29% of deliveries. Of these cases, 5% develop meconium aspiration syndrome (Fraser, 2015).

There is a risk that the fetus can aspirate the meconium-stained fluid at the time of delivery. The presence of meconium fluid in the neonate's lungs can cause a partial obstruction of the lower airways that leads to a trapping of air and a hyperinflation of the airway distal to the obstruction, causing uneven ventilation (Blackburn, 2013). It can also cause a chemical pneumonitis and inhibit surfactant action (Blackburn, 2013). Additionally, the neonate is at risk for pulmonary hypertension due to increased pulmonary vascular resistance. These changes place the neonate at risk for atelectasis.

Assessment Findings

- Meconium-stained amniotic fluid
- Meconium visualized below the vocal cords
- Greenish or yellowish discoloration of the skin, nail beds, and umbilical cord
- Respiratory depression at the time of birth or within a few hours after birth
- Low Apgar scores
- Need for resuscitation after delivery due to perinatal depression
- Signs of respiratory distress such as nasal flaring, grunting, chest retractions
- Chest may appear barrel shaped and overdistended.
- The expiration phase of breathing may be extended.
- Diminished air movement, and the presence of rales and rhonchi assessed on auscultation
- Atelectasis and hyperinflated areas through the lungs noted on chest x-ray
- Arterial blood gas findings may include low PaO_2 despite administration of 100% oxygen, and respiratory and metabolic acidosis in serious cases (Fraser, 2015).

Medical Management

- Suctioning of the oropharynx and the nasopharynx to remove meconium immediately after the delivery of the neonate's head and before the first breath is a common practice. Evidence does not support this practice as effective in preventing meconium aspiration (Blackburn, 2013).
- Arterial blood gases to determine respiratory status and to guide treatment
- Chest x-ray
- Blood glucose monitoring

- Oxygen with or without assisted ventilation depending on the neonate's condition
- Surfactant therapy to decrease risk of need for ECMO (Natarajan, Sankar, Jain, Agarwal, & Paul, 2016)
- Sedatives or paralytic agents to relax neonates who are receiving ventilation
- Antibiotics to treat pneumonia
- Cooling therapy
  - Therapeutic hypothermia reduces cerebral injury and improves neurological outcomes for neonates who experience a hypoxic event and/or asphyxia in utero or during the birthing process (Harris et al., 2014).

Nursing Actions

- Assist with suctioning and resuscitation at the time of delivery.
- Assess neonate for:
  - Respiratory distress such as grunting, flaring, retracting, cyanosis, and tachypnea.
  - Complications of meconium aspiration syndrome, such as acidosis, hypoglycemia, hypocalcemia, pneumonia, pneumothorax, bronchopulmonary dysplasia, and persistent pulmonary hypertension.
  - Neurological problems secondary to asphyxia (Fraser, 2015).
- Administer oxygen and/or assisted ventilation as per order.
- Monitor blood glucose.
  - Complication of respiratory distress is an increased metabolic rate and thus a higher incidence of hypoglycemia.
- Manage ECMO if indicated.
- Manage neonates receiving cooling therapy.

PERSISTENT PULMONARY HYPERTENSION OF THE NEWBORN

Normally after birth, the pulmonary vascular bed relaxes, allowing blood circulation to the lungs. Persistent pulmonary hypertension (PPHN) results when the normal vasodilation and relaxation of the pulmonary vascular bed do not occur. This leads to elevated pulmonary vascular resistance, right ventricular hypertension, and right-to-left shunting of blood through the foramen ovale and ductus arteriosus (Fraser, 2015). PPHN is predominantly a problem among term or near-term neonates who experience hypoxia/asphyxia, RDS, meconium aspiration, sepsis, or congenital lung anomalies such as diaphragmatic hernia (Steinhorn, 2015). Even after the precipitating factor is treated, vasoconstriction and increased vascular resistance may persist, causing decreased pulmonary blood circulation, hypoxemia, lactic acidosis, and acidemia (Fraser, 2015).

Risk Factors

- Hypoxia and asphyxia are the most common risk factors for PPHN
- Low Apgar scores

- RDS, meconium aspiration, pneumonia
- Bacterial sepsis
- Delayed circulatory transition at birth caused by factors such as delayed resuscitation, central nervous system depression, hypothermia
- Hypothermia or hypoglycemia leading to acidosis
  - Polycythemia or hyperviscosity of the blood, which could cause blockages in the pulmonary vascular bed
  - Prenatal pulmonary hypertension associated with premature closure of the ductus arteriosus, or fetal systemic hypertension
  - Underdevelopment of pulmonary vessels associated with congenital anomalies of the lung or heart
  - Abnormal development of pulmonary vessels associated with intrauterine asphyxia or intrauterine meconium aspiration, which leads to increased muscularization of pulmonary vessels that causes increased vascular resistance (Fraser, 2015)

Assessment Findings

- Respiratory issues
  - Slow to breathe, difficult to ventilate
  - Symptoms evident within 12 hours of birth
  - Tachypnea
  - Chest retractions and/or grunting
  - Cyanosis
  - Low Pao_2, even with administration of high levels of oxygen
  - Chest x-ray with infiltrates
- Cardiac issues
  - Hypotension
  - Heart murmur
  - Echocardiogram shows pulmonary hypertension and enlarged right side of the heart
  - Congestive heart failure
- Metabolic issues
  - Hypocalcemia
  - Hypoglycemia
  - Metabolic acidosis (Fraser, 2015)
- Hematological issues
  - Disseminated intravascular coagulation (DIC)
  - Thrombocytopenia
- Possible kidney damage, leading to decreased urine output, proteinuria, and hematuria
- Long-term outcomes after PPHN include:
  - Hearing loss (sensorineural).
  - Neurological deficits.
  - Chronic lung disease.
  - Death (Fraser, 2015).

Medical Management

- Main goal is to correct hypoxia and acidosis.
- Preductal and postductal blood gas or oxygen saturation to distinguish structural heart problems from PPHN.
  - Right to left shunting is suspected when there is a difference of 15 mm Hg or more between the preductal and postductal Pao_2 (Fraser, 2015).

- Echocardiogram to evaluate for cardiac anomalies, right to left shunting of blood, pulmonary resistance, and pulmonary artery pressures.
- Oxygen and conventional mechanical ventilation
  - Hyperoxygenation is often used to keep Pao_2 levels above 90 mm Hg, and hyperventilation is used to keep $Paco_2$ levels in the low normal range, prevent acidosis, and promote decreased pulmonary artery pressure. Hyperventilation causes alkalosis, which has been found to lower pulmonary resistance (Fraser, 2015).
  - If conventional mechanical ventilation is ineffective, high-frequency oscillatory ventilation may be instituted.
  - ECMO if other treatments are not effective
- Intravenous fluids
- Laboratory tests (complete blood count, glucose, electrolytes, calcium, arterial blood gases, blood cultures)
- Umbilical catheter for arterial and venous pressure monitoring, blood gas monitoring, and to administer vasopressors as indicated
- Surfactant therapy
- Nitric oxide therapy
  - Nitric oxide induces vasodilation and reduces pulmonary resistance.
  - Use of nitric oxide has reduced the percentage of neonates with PPHN being placed on ECMO.
- Medications
  - Vasopressors, such as dopamine and nitroprusside, to decrease right to left shunting by maintaining systemic vascular pressure above pulmonary vascular pressure
  - Vasodilators, such as prostaglandins and isoproterenol, to promote pulmonary artery dilation
  - Muscle relaxants to induce paralysis among neonates who resist ventilation
  - Sedatives and analgesics, such as morphine and midazolam (Versed)
  - Antibiotic therapy to decrease risk of and/or treat infection

Nursing Actions

- Review maternal prenatal, intrapartal, and neonatal histories.
- Assess the neonate for respiratory distress, meconium aspiration, and clinical manifestations of PPHN.
- Administer oxygen and mechanical ventilation as ordered.
- Monitor vital signs and pulse oximetry.
- Anticipate the placement of umbilical catheters.
  - Vasoconstriction makes peripheral intravenous access difficult.
  - Arterial blood gases and lab values are easily accessed via an umbilical catheter, thus preventing the infant from receiving painful heel sticks and venipunctures.
  - Multiple intravenous fluids and medications can be administered simultaneously via umbilical catheters.
- Administer IV fluids as per order.
- Administer medications as per order.

- Obtain and monitor results of laboratory tests.
  - Immediate intervention is required for abnormal lab results.
- Keep handling, treatments, suctioning, and stimulation to a minimum, as these can result in decreased PaO_2 levels and vasoconstriction.
- Provide emotional support for parents, incorporate them in care of their infant, and keep them informed of their infant's condition.

SMALL FOR GESTATIONAL AGE AND INTRAUTERINE GROWTH RESTRICTION

A small for gestational age (SGA) infant is one whose weight is less than the 10th percentile for his or her gestational age. Neonates whose growth is not consistent with gestational age may be affected by intrauterine growth restriction (IUGR), caused by a decrease in cell production related to chronic malnutrition. There are two types of IUGR: symmetric and asymmetric.

- Symmetric IUGR, a generalized proportional reduction in the size of all structures and organs except for heart and brain, occurs early in pregnancy and affects general growth. When a complication occurs very early in pregnancy, fewer cells develop, leading to smaller organ size (Benjamin & Furdon, 2015). Symmetric IUGR can be identified by ultrasound in the early part of the second trimester. Conditions that may result in symmetric IUGR include exposure to teratogenic substances, congenital infections, and genetic problems (Benjamin & Furdon, 2015).
- Asymmetric IUGR, a disproportional reduction in the size of structures and organs, results from maternal or placental conditions that occur later in pregnancy and impede placental blood flow. Examples of conditions that may result in asymmetric IUGR include preeclampsia, placental infarcts, or severe maternal malnutrition (Benjamin & Furdon, 2015).

Risk Factors

See Table 17–3 for maternal, fetal, and placental risk factors for IUGR.

Outcomes

Neonates with IUGR are at risk for:

- Labor intolerance related to placental insufficiency and inadequate nutritional and oxygen reserves.
- Meconium aspiration related to asphyxia during labor.
- Hypoglycemia related to inadequate glycogen stores and reduced gluconeogenesis, and an increase in metabolic demands from heat loss, which diminishes glucose stores (Armentrout, 2015).

- Hypocalcemia, defined as serum calcium levels less than 7.5 mg/dL, related to birth asphyxia (Halbardier, 2015).
  - Signs of hypocalcemia are often similar to those of hypoglycemia and include jitteriness, tetany, and seizures.

Assessment Findings

- Physical characteristics of the IUGR neonate include:
  - Large head in relationship to the body.
  - Long nails.
  - Large anterior fontanel.
  - Decreased amounts of Wharton's jelly present in the umbilical cord.
  - Thin extremities and trunk.
  - Loose skin due to a lack of subcutaneous fat.
  - Dry, flaky, and/or meconium-stained skin.
- Weight, head circumference, and length are all below the 10th percentile for gestational age in symmetric IUGR (Benjamin & Furdon, 2015).
- Head circumference and length are appropriate for gestational age; however, the weight is below the 10th percentile for the baby's gestational age in asymmetric IUGR (Benjamin & Furdon, 2015).
- RDS may occur in SGA neonates who are born prematurely or who have aspirated meconium-stained amniotic fluid.
- Hypothermia related to decreased subcutaneous fat and glucose supply, impaired lipid metabolism, and depleted brown fat stores (Benjamin & Furdon, 2015).
- Polycythemia

Medical Management

- Identify IUGR during pregnancy and intervene based on the cause.
- Assess for congenital anomalies.
- Oxygen therapy for perinatal depression and respiratory distress
- Laboratory tests
  - Blood glucose monitoring
  - Hematocrit if polycythemia is suspected
  - Serum calcium levels

Nursing Actions

- Review prenatal and intrapartal records for risk factors.
- Perform a gestational age assessment to determine if neonate is SGA or preterm.
- Assess for respiratory distress.
- Assess the neonate for gross anomalies.
- Assess the skin for color and signs of meconium staining.
  - Infants with meconium staining have an increased risk of respiratory distress.
- Maintain a neutral thermal environment.
  - SGA infants have decreased subcutaneous fat and are more susceptible to hypothermia.
- Decrease risk of hypoglycemia.

TABLE 17–3   Factors Contributing to Intrauterine Growth Restriction

MATERNAL	FETAL	PLACENTAL	ENVIRONMENTAL
Multiple gestation	Female sex	Small placenta	High altitude
Primiparity	Discordant twins	Abnormal cord insertion	Excessive exercise
Grand multiparity	Congenital anomalies	Placenta previa	Exposure to x-ray
Age <15 years	Chromosomal syndromes	Chronic abruptio placenta	Exposure to toxins
Age >45 years	Congenital infections	Placental hemangiomas	
No prenatal care	Rubella		
Low socioeconomic status	Toxoplasmosis		
Nutritional status	Cytomegalovirus		
Low pre-pregnancy weight	Inborn errors of metabolism		
Low weight gain			
Substance abuse			
Smoking			
Vascular disease			
Renal disease			
Cardiac disease			
Preeclampsia			
Chronic hypertension			
Advanced diabetes			
Sickle cell anemia			
Phenylketonuria			
Medications			
Anticonvulsants			
History of stillbirth			
History of preterm birth			
History of IUGR/LBW baby			
Maternal short stature			

Hardy et al., 2016.

- SGA infants are at high risk for hypoglycemia due to their decreased amount of subcutaneous fat and thus are at increased risk of cold stress.
- Assess for signs of hypoglycemia.
- Monitor blood glucose.
- Provide early and frequent feedings.
  - SGA infants may need gavage feedings due to poor suck or inability to finish feedings due to lack of stamina.
- Monitor for hypocalcemia.

- Weigh daily.
  - SGA infants may require higher caloric intake.
- Monitor vital signs.
- Monitor for feeding intolerance.
  - SGA infants are susceptible to NEC due to placental insufficiency.
- Obtain laboratory tests as per orders.
- Teach parents the importance of keeping the baby warm and providing frequent feedings.

LARGE FOR GESTATIONAL AGE

A large for gestational age (LGA) infant has a weight above the 90th percentile for his or her gestational age. Characteristically, LGA infants (Fig. 17–7) are macrosomic and have greater body length and head circumference compared to infants who are appropriate for gestational age.

Risk Factors

- Maternal diabetes
- Multiparity
- Previous macrosomic baby
- Prolonged pregnancy (Hardy et al., 2016)

Outcomes

LGA fetuses and neonates are at risk for:
- Cesarean births.
- Operative vaginal delivery.
- Shoulder dystocia.
- Breech presentation.
- Birth trauma.
- Cephalopelvic disproportion.
- Hypoglycemia.
- Hyperbilirubinemia.

Assessment Findings

- Birth trauma related to shoulder dystocia or breech presentation
  - Fractured clavicle
  - Brachial nerve damage
  - Facial nerve damage
  - Depressed skull fractures
  - Cephalohematoma
  - Intracranial hemorrhage
  - Asphyxia (Hardy et al., 2016)
- Poor feeding behavior

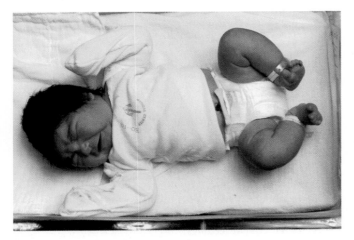

FIGURE 17–7 Large for gestational age neonate.

- Hypoglycemia
- Polycythemia in neonates of diabetic mothers related to a decrease in extracellular fluid and/or fetal hypoxia
- Hyperbilirubinemia that occurs 48 to 72 hours after delivery related to polycythemia, decreased extracellular fluid, or bruising or hemorrhage from birth trauma

Medical Management

- Assessments for birth trauma, hypoglycemia, and respiratory distress
- Laboratory tests:
  - Blood glucose
  - Hematocrit
  - Bilirubin levels when indicated for jaundice

Nursing Actions

- Review prenatal and intrapartal records for risk factors.
- Assess respiratory status.
- Assess neonates for birth traumas such as fractured clavicles, brachial nerve damage, facial nerve damage, and cephalohematoma.
- Obtain and monitor blood glucose per agency protocol.
- Observe for signs of hypoglycemia.
  - LGA infants are at increased risk for hypoglycemia due to depletion of glycogen stores.
- Provide early and frequent feedings to decrease risk for hypoglycemia.
  - LGA infant may feed poorly and require gavage feedings.
- Obtain and monitor hematocrit as per orders.
  - High hematocrit increases the risk for jaundice.
- Assess skin color for signs of polycythemia, which appears as a red, ruddy skin color.
  - Infants of diabetic mothers are at risk for polycythemia.
- Perform a gestational age assessment.
- Observe for jaundice.
  - LGA infants are at higher risk for jaundice due to polycythemia.

HYPERBILIRUBINEMIA

Hyperbilirubinemia, increased levels of bilirubin in the blood, affects more than 60% of term and 80% of preterm neonates (Allen, 2015). Bilirubin exists in two major forms: unconjugated and conjugated. Unbound (unconjugated) bilirubin can deposit into tissue and cross the blood-brain barrier. Conjugated bilirubin is bound to albumin and once bound, is water-soluble. It is nontoxic and can be excreted by the neonate (Allen, 2015). Bilirubin cannot be excreted until it is conjugated.

When serum bilirubin levels are greater than 5 mg/dL, neonates will exhibit visible signs of jaundice. The clinical significance of jaundice is based on the gestational age of the neonate, hours of life, and the total serum bilirubin level (Bradshaw, 2015). Prematurity may result in greater severity of physiological jaundice, and any jaundice among preterm neonates must be evaluated.

A complication of hyperbilirubinemia is kernicterus, an abnormal accumulation of unconjugated bilirubin in the brain cells. Bilirubin accumulates within the brain and becomes toxic to the brain tissue, causing neurological disorders such as deafness, delayed motor skills, hypotonia, and intellectual deficits (Kaplan, Wong, Sibley, & Stevenson, 2015). A goal of medical and nursing actions is to prevent kernicterus through early identification and treatment of hyperbilirubinemia.

Hyperbilirubinemia is categorized into physiological jaundice and pathological jaundice.

Physiological Jaundice

Physiological jaundice results from hyperbilirubinemia that commonly occurs after the first 24 hours of birth and during the first week of life. Common physiological characteristics of the neonate place it at risk for physiological jaundice:

- Increased RBC volume
- RBC life span of 70 to 90 days, compared to 120 days in adults
- High bilirubin production (6 to 8 mg/kg/day)
- Neonates reabsorb increased amounts of unconjugated bilirubin in the intestine due to lack of intestinal bacteria, decreased gastrointestinal motility, and increased beta-glucuronidase (a deconjugating enzyme).
- Decreased hepatic uptake of bilirubin from the plasma due to a deficiency of ligandin, the primary bilirubin binding protein in hepatocytes
- Diminished conjugation of bilirubin in the liver due to decreased glucuronyl transferase activity (Bradshaw, 2015)

Assessment Findings

- Physiological jaundice is typically visible after 24 hours of life.
- Total serum bilirubin levels generally peak on day 3 of life in term neonates and on days 5 or 6 in preterm neonates (Bradshaw, 2015).
- Jaundice is characterized by a yellowish tint to the skin and sclera of the eyes.
  - As total serum bilirubin levels rise, jaundice will progress from the newborn's head down toward the trunk and lower extremities.

Pathological Jaundice

Pathological jaundice results when various disorders exacerbate physiological processes that lead to hyperbilirubinemia of the newborn. Such disorders can result in pathological unconjugated or conjugated hyperbilirubinemia (Table 17–4).

Assessment Findings

- Jaundice that occurs within the first 24 hours of life
- Total serum bilirubin levels that increase by more than 5 mg/dL per day (Kaplan et al., 2015)
- Jaundice lasting more than 1 week in a term newborn or more than 2 weeks in a premature neonate day (Kaplan et al., 2015)
- Risk factors, medical management, and nursing actions are similar for both physiological and pathological jaundice.

Risk Factors for Hyperbilirubinemia

- Maternal factors
  - Asian, Native American, or Greek ethnicity
  - ABO incompatibility (e.g., the woman is blood type O and the neonate is blood type A or B)
  - Rh incompatibility (e.g., the woman is Rh negative and the neonate is Rh positive)
  - Breastfeeding (Table 17–5)
  - Diabetes
  - Use of oxytocin or bupivacaine during labor
- Neonatal factors
  - Delayed cord clamping, which increases RBC volume
  - Hypoxia, acidosis, hypothermia, or hypoglycemia
  - Delayed or infrequent feedings
  - Excessive weight loss after birth
  - Bruising or cephalohematoma
  - Prematurity
  - Bacterial or viral infection (especially toxoplasmosis, syphilis, varicella-zoster, parvovirus B19, rubella, cytomegalovirus, and herpes [TORCH] infections)
  - Previous sibling with hyperbilirubinemia

Medical Management for Hyperbilirubinemia

- Diagnostic tests
  - Total serum bilirubin, with fractionation of serum bilirubin into direct (conjugated bilirubin) and indirect (unconjugated bilirubin) reacting pigments.
  - Antiglobulin (Coombs') test: Used to determine hemolytic disease of the newborn related to Rh or ABO incompatibility
    - Direct antiglobulin (Coombs') test is used to detect abnormal in vivo coating of the neonate's RBCs with antibody globulin (maternal antibodies); when present, the test is considered positive.
  - Transcutaneous bilirubinometry, a noninvasive method to estimate total serum bilirubin levels among term and near-term neonates, is used to identify neonates at risk for developing hyperbilirubinemia (Hardy et al., 2016).
  - Complete blood count assists in management of pathological jaundice.
- Treatment is determined by the level of bilirubin and the age of the neonate in hours (Table 17–6).
- Phototherapy is the most widely used and effective treatment for hyperbilirubinemia.
  - Various types of phototherapy delivery systems are available, including blue lights, white lamps, halogen lamps, fiber-optic blankets, and blue light emitting diodes. The most effective lights are those with high-energy output in the blue-green spectrum (Hardy et al., 2016).
  - Phototherapy results in photoconverting bilirubin molecules to water-soluble isomers that can be excreted in the urine and stool without conjugation in the liver (Maisels, 2015).
  - Total serum bilirubin levels should drop 1 to 2 mg/dL within 4 to 6 hours after the initiation of phototherapy.

TABLE 17–4   Causes of Pathological Hyperbilirubinemia

CAUSES OF PATHOLOGICAL UNCONJUGATED HYPERBILIRUBINEMIA	CAUSES OF CONJUGATED HYPERBILIRUBINEMIA (ALWAYS PATHOLOGIC)
Hemolysis of RBCs	**Hepatitis**
Rh/ABO incompatibilities	Neonatal idiopathic hepatitis
Bacterial and viral infections	Infectious hepatitis
Inherited disorders of RBC/bilirubin metabolism	Toxic hepatitis
Glucose-6-phospate dehydrogenase deficiency	Intestinal obstruction
Sequestered Blood	Ischemic necrosis
Cephalohematoma	Parenteral alimentation
Bruising	Metabolic disorders
Hemangiomas	Hematological disorders
Cerebral, pulmonary, retroperitoneal bleeding	Ductal disturbances in bilirubin excretion:
Decreased hepatic uptake of bilirubin	• Extrahepatic biliary atresia
Decreased hepatic function/perfusion	• Intrahepatic biliary atresia
• Hypoxia	• Bile plug syndrome
• Asphyxia	• Tumors of the liver and biliary tract
• Sepsis	
Increased enterohepatic circulation	
• Delayed feedings	
• Breastfeeding jaundice	
• Breast milk jaundice	
• Intestinal obstructions	
Polycythemia	
Swallowed blood	
Hypothyroidism	
Hypopituitarism	

Kaplan et al., 2015.

CRITICAL COMPONENT

Fiber-Optic Blanket (Bili Blanket)

The bili blanket is a portable phototherapy device that can be used in the hospital or in the home for treatment of hyperbilirubinemia. The blanket, a fiber-optic panel connected to a power source, is wrapped around the bare torso of the infant. The infant and the bili blanket can be covered with clothing and/or a regular blanket. The bili blanket remains on the infant 24 hours a day. Parents can hold and feed the infant with the blanket in place. Blood tests to assess bilirubin levels are used to determine effectiveness of the therapy.

For additional information, watch the video "Bili Blanket Instructions" at https://biliblanketbaby.com/how-to-use/.

- Phototherapy should be administered continuously, except during feeding times or parental visits, when eye patches are removed to allow for bonding.
- Exchange transfusion is used in cases where phototherapy is not effective or severe hemolytic disease is present (Allen, 2015).
  - In this procedure, approximately 85% of the neonate's RBCs are replaced with donor cells.
  - This procedure reduces bilirubin, removes RBCs coated with maternal antibody, corrects anemia, and removes other toxins associated with hemolysis (Hardy et al., 2016).
  - Efforts to prevent Rh hemolytic disease with Rh immunoglobulin (RhoGam) administered to Rh-negative women, along with the use of phototherapy, has diminished the need for exchange transfusion (Hardy et al., 2016).
- Infants discharged before 72 hours of life should be seen for follow-up by a health care provider within 1 to 2 days to

TABLE 17–5   Hyperbilirubinemia Associated With Breastfeeding: A Comparison of Breastfeeding Versus Breast Milk Jaundice

BREASTFEEDING JAUNDICE	BREAST MILK JAUNDICE
Early onset of jaundice (within the first few days of life).	Late onset (after 3–5 days).
Associated with ineffective breastfeeding.	Gradual increase in bilirubin that peaks at 2 weeks of age.
Dehydration can occur.	Associated with breast milk composition in some women that increases the enterohepatic circulation of bilirubin.
Delayed passage of meconium stool promotes reabsorption of bilirubin in the gut.	Treatment: Continued breastfeeding in most infants. In some cases where bilirubin levels are excessively high, breastfeeding may be interrupted and formula feedings are given for several days. This typically results in a decline of the bilirubin level. Breastfeeding is resumed when bilirubin levels decline.
Treatment: Encourage early effective breastfeeding without supplementation of glucose water or other fluids.	

Blackburn, 2013.

TABLE 17–6   Management of Hyperbilirubinemia in the Healthy Term and Near-Term Neonate

AGE (HR)	CONSIDER PHOTOTHERAPY	PHOTOTHERAPY
≤24		
25–48	≥12	≥15
49–72	≥15	≥18
>72	≥17	≥20

AAP, 2004.

assess the neonate's health status and to assess for jaundice.
- Early identification and treatment decrease the risk of bilirubin encephalopathy (Kaplan et al., 2015).

Nursing Actions for Hyperbilirubinemia

- Review maternal and neonatal record for risk factors.
- Assess degree of jaundice every shift with the use of a transcutaneous meter.
  - When meter is not available, in a well-lit area, use your fingers to blanch the neonate's skin on the face, upper trunk, abdomen, thigh, and lower leg and feet. The skin will appear yellow after the pressure is released and before skin returns to normal color.
- Document the assessment findings.
  - How rapidly the degree of jaundice progresses guides the method of treatment.
- Notify the physician if jaundice is present.
  - Prompt treatment is essential to preventing bilirubin toxicity.
- Obtain serum bilirubin levels as per orders.

- The rate of rise of the bilirubin level is critical in determining the treatment needed.
- Ensure adequate hydration by feeding the neonate every 2 to 3 hours to promote excretion of bilirubin in the urine and stool and to compensate for insensible water loss due to phototherapy (Hardy et al., 2016).
- Implement phototherapy as ordered and provide related nursing care.
  - Proper nursing care enhances the effectiveness of phototherapy and minimizes complications.
- Assess for side effects of phototherapy:
  - Eye damage
  - Loose stools
  - Dehydration
  - Hyperthermia
  - Lethargy
  - Skin rashes
  - Abdominal distention
  - Hypocalcemia
  - Lactose intolerance
  - Thrombocytopenia
  - Bronze baby syndrome: Dark gray-brown pigmentation of skin that disappears after phototherapy is discontinued.
- Provide verbal and written discharge instructions about how to identify signs of jaundice in an infant and when to notify the physician.
  - For those infants discharged with mild jaundice, teaching should include measures to assess hydration, excretion of bilirubin, and home management of phototherapy lights if applicable.

CRITICAL COMPONENT

Care of the Neonate Receiving Phototherapy
- Fluorescent lights
  - Fluorescent "bili lights" should be positioned 18 to 20 inches from the infant.

Continued

- Fluorescent lights should be positioned 2 inches from the top of an incubator.
- A photometer should be used to measure irradiance of lamps to facilitate optimal treatment.
- Banks of lights should be covered by Plexiglas.
- The neonate should have only a diaper in place for maximal exposure to light.
- Place eye patches on the neonate to protect eyes from the effects of the light.
- During feedings, remove eye patches and have parent or nurse hold the neonate.
- Change the neonate's position frequently to facilitate increased exposure to the light.
- Vital signs, including temperature monitoring, should be done per agency protocol.
- Monitor I&O. Phototherapy results in increased insensible fluid loss.
- Feedings every 2 to 3 hours are important to provide adequate fluids to compensate for insensible fluid loss and promote excretion of bilirubin.
- Monitor newborn for side effects of phototherapy.

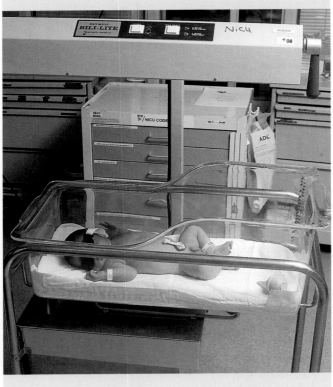

Hardy et al., 2016.

CENTRAL NERVOUS SYSTEM INJURIES

Various types of central nervous system (CNS) injuries can occur among term and premature neonates. Injury can be the result of intracranial hemorrhage (Table 17–7), hypoxia and ischemia

during the prenatal and intrapartal periods and postbirth, systemic chronic fetal compromise such as IUGR, or hypotension that leads to a decreased cerebral perfusion resulting in preventricular leukomalacia (Table 17–8).

Depending on the extent and location of the injury, CNS injuries may result in normal outcomes or serious long-term problems such as seizures, neurological deficits, developmental disability, motor deficits, visual impairments, or death (Verklan, 2015).

Risk Factors

- Prematurity
- Birth trauma
- Breech delivery or other malpresentations
- Precipitous labor
- Difficult labor, traumatic delivery, and use of forceps
- Hypoxia, asphyxia, hypotension, ischemia, respiratory distress. Hypoxic events may be related to:
  - Maternal causes such as cardiac arrest and hypovolemic shock.
  - Uteroplacental causes such as placental abruption, cord prolapse, and uterine hyperstimulation.
  - Fetal causes such as cardiac arrhythmias (deVries, 2015).

Assessment Findings

- Clinical manifestations are specific to the type and extent of the CNS injury (see Tables 17–7 and 17–8).

Medical Management

- Decrease risk for hypoxia, ischemia, and asphyxia during the perinatal and intrapartal periods.
  - Identification and treatment of a compromised fetus may prevent asphyxiation and multiorgan damage (Verklan, 2015).
- Neurological and behavioral evaluation
- Laboratory tests
  - Serum glucose level
  - Electrolyte levels
  - Arterial blood gas analysis
  - Blood, urine, CSF cultures
  - Complete blood count with differential
- Computed tomography (CT) scan, ultrasonography, magnetic resonance image (MRI), and skull radiographs as indicated
- Lumbar puncture for CSF analysis if clinically indicated
- Electroencephalography to confirm occurrence of seizures and to identify presence and severity of brain damage if clinically indicated
- Neurology consultant as indicated
- Medications to treat seizure activity
- Infants with hypoxic-ischemic encephalopathy may require the following medical management and treatment (Verklan, 2015):
  - Resuscitation at the time of delivery
  - Oxygen and ventilator support
  - Monitoring of fluids, electrolytes, and acid-base balance
  - Monitoring of blood volume and blood pressure

TABLE 17–7 Types of Central Nervous System Injuries: Hemorrhages

	SUBDURAL HEMORRHAGE	SUBARACHNOID HEMORRHAGE	INTRACEREBELLAR HEMORRHAGE
Definition	Tear of the dura overlying the cerebellum or cerebral hemispheres.	Intracranial hemorrhage into the cerebrospinal fluid–filled space between the pial and arachnoid membranes on the surface of the brain. Most common neonatal intracranial hemorrhage.	Hemorrhage in the cerebellum from primary bleeding or from extension of intraventricular or subarachnoid hemorrhage into the cerebellum. Occurs more commonly in preterm, LBW neonates.
Pathophysiology	Excessive molding, stretching, or tearing of the falx and tentorium. Stretching or tearing of the vein of Galen or cerebellar bridging veins.	May occur because of trauma in a term neonate or hypoxia in a preterm neonate. Venous bleeding in the subarachnoid space related to ruptured small vessels in the leptomeningeal plexus or bridging veins in the subarachnoid space.	Breech presentation, difficult forceps delivery, external pressure over the occiput History of a hypoxic–ischemic insult Vitamin K deficiency Vascular factors
Manifestations	Symptoms may be delayed for first 24 hours, then: Seizures Decreased level of consciousness Asymmetrical motor function Full fontanel Irritability Lethargy Respiratory abnormalities Facial paralysis	Commonly there are no symptoms. Seizures may occur, starting on day 2 of life. Apnea may occur in preterm neonates.	Manifestations occur within the first 2 days to 3 weeks of life. Apnea Bradycardia Decreasing hematocrit Bloody cerebrospinal fluid
Prognosis	Hydrocephalus Mortality rate 45% Hypoxic–ischemic injury	90% of babies with seizures will have normal follow-up. Abnormal outcome is rare.	Poorer outcome in preterm neonates than in term newborns. Neurological deficits probable.

Verklan, 2015.

- Maintaining perfusion and preventing/treating hypotension
- Evaluating and supporting the renal, hepatic, gastrointestinal, pulmonary, and cardiovascular systems
- Total body cooling or selective head cooling for infants with moderate to severe hypoxic-ischemic encephalopathy to improve survival and neurodevelopment (Harris et al., 2014)

Nursing Actions

- Review maternal prenatal and intrapartal histories for risk factors.
- Perform physical assessment of the neonate, including evaluation of tone, reflexes, and behavior.
- Maintain respiratory support as needed.
- Obtain laboratory tests as per order.
- Ensure that ordered diagnostic tests are completed.
- Assist with diagnostic procedures such as lumbar puncture.
- Administer medications as per order.
- Manage neonates receiving cooling therapy.
- Provide the family with support and information about their infant's status, treatment, and follow-up.

INFANTS OF DIABETIC MOTHERS

Diabetes is the most common chronic medical problem affecting pregnant women (Hay, 2012). Maternal diabetes during pregnancy is associated with poor outcomes for the fetus and neonate

TABLE 17–8   Types of Central Nervous System Injury: Hypoxic–Ischemic Encephalopathy

	HYPOXIC–ISCHEMIC ENCEPHALOPATHY	PERIVENTRICULAR LEUKOMALACIA
Definition	Abnormal neonatal neurological behavior resulting from a hypoxic–ischemic event. Brain edema and massive cellular necrosis. Intraventricular, subdural, or intracerebral hemorrhage.	Necrosis of periventricular white matter resulting from ischemia. Ischemic lesion of arterial origin. Multicystic encephalomalacia with/without hemorrhage into ischemic area.
Risk Factors	Hypoxia, anoxia, decreased blood supply to the brain (ischemia). Acute birth asphyxia (e.g., cord compression). Chronic subacute asphyxia (prenatal or intrapartum). Systemic hypotension. Multiorgan system failure may occur.	Systemic hypotension leading to decreased cerebral blood flow. Apnea and bradycardia, secondary to poor cerebral perfusion. Chorioamnionitis
Clinical Manifestations	Clinical manifestations depend on extent of encephalopathy. Stage I: Mild encephalopathy Hyperalert state Hyperresponsiveness Normal muscle tone and reflexes Increased tendon reflexes Myoclonus present Tachycardia Dilated pupils EEG normal Usually no seizure activity Stage II: Moderate encephalopathy Lethargy and hypotonia Increased tendon reflexes Myoclonus Weak suck Strong grasp Incomplete Moro reflex Seizures Pupils constrict and reactive Abnormal EEG findings Stage III: Severe encephalopathy Level of consciousness deteriorates to comatose Apnea, bradycardia	Acute phase: Lethargy, CNS depression, and hypotension. After 6–10 weeks: Frequent tremors, and startle reflex. Abnormal Moro reflex. Hypertonia, irritability, extension of legs, increased flexion of arms.

TABLE 17–8   Types of Central Nervous System Injury: Hypoxic–Ischemic Encephalopathy—cont'd

	HYPOXIC–ISCHEMIC ENCEPHALOPATHY	PERIVENTRICULAR LEUKOMALACIA
	Mechanical ventilation needed.	
	Seizures occur within 12 hours of life.	
	Severe hypotonia, absent Moro, grasp, and suck reflexes.	
	Pupils unequal; poor light reflex and variable reactivity.	
	Deterioration may occur within 24–72 hours.	
	Death may follow.	
Prognosis	Outcome depends on severity of encephalopathy.	Outcome depends on location and extent of injury.
	20%–50% of asphyxiated babies with hypoxic–ischemic encephalopathy (HIE) will die.	Motor deficits
		Spastic diplegia
	Early seizure activity associated with poorer outcome.	Visual impairments
	Less severe HIE associated with hyperactivity and attention deficit problems.	Lower limb weakness
	Normal outcome may occur.	Intellectual deficits more common when there is upper arm involvement.

Verklan, 2015.

(Armentrout, 2015). Complications of high maternal levels of glucose during pregnancy are:

- Congenital anomalies:
  - Cardiac anomalies, such as transposition of the great vessels, ventricular septal defect, and left to right ventricular wall hypertrophy
  - Skeletal defects, such as sacral agenesis and neural tube defects
  - Small left colon syndrome and renal anomalies (Hay, 2012)
- IUGR, perinatal asphyxia, and SGA due to placental insufficiency (Armentrout, 2015)
- Neurological damage and seizures related to inadequate glucose supply to the brain due to neonatal hyperinsulinism
- Risk of childhood obesity and type 2 diabetes (Hay, 2012)

Assessment Findings

- Macrosomia
  - Increased birth weight due to fetal exposure to elevated maternal glucose levels. In response to high glucose levels, the fetal pancreas produces insulin. Hyperinsulinemia results in increased fat production and growth (Hay, 2012).
- Fractured clavicle and/or brachial nerve damage
  - Macrosomic neonates are at risk for traumatic deliveries, including shoulder dystocia.
- Hypoglycemia
  - Risk of hypoglycemia due to increased levels of fetal and neonatal insulin and decreased circulating glucose after delivery
- Hypocalcemia and hypomagnesemia

- Polycythemia
  - Caused by insulin-induced increases in metabolism that leads to hypoxia (Armentrout, 2015)
- Hyperbilirubinemia
  - Polycythemia increases risk of hyperbilirubinemia.
- Low muscle tone
- Poor feeding abilities
- Respiratory distress
  - Risk for RDS due to delay in surfactant production related to the high maternal glucose levels and fetal hyperstimulation (Armentrout, 2015)

Medical Management

- Assess for complications associated with maternal diabetes.
- Perform laboratory tests such as hematocrit and calcium and magnesium levels
- Perform X-ray exams if clinically indicated for birth trauma related to shoulder dystocia
- Consult the cardiologist if cardiac anomalies are suspected.
- Monitor blood glucose. Abnormal results are confirmed by laboratory analysis of plasma glucose (Armentrout, 2015). If the neonate is hypoglycemic, blood glucose levels should be monitored 30 minutes after feeding to evaluate response to treatment.
- Early (by 1 to 2 hours of age) and frequent oral feedings of breast milk or formula unless the neonate feeds poorly or is too sick to be fed orally. If oral feedings are contraindicated and/or the neonate is hypoglycemic, there are two methods of treatment:
  - 40% dextrose gel is administered by syringe in the neonate's buccal cavity (Bennett, Headtke, & Rowe-Telow, 2015).
  - 10% dextrose and water is administered intravenously.

Nursing Actions

- Assess neonate for signs of respiratory distress, birth trauma, congenital anomalies, hypoglycemia, hypocalcemia, polycythemia, and hyperbilirubinemia.
- Monitor blood glucose per agency protocol.
  - May require intravenous fluids along with feedings to maintain adequate blood glucose levels.
- Provide early and frequent feedings to treat and prevent hypoglycemia.
  - May be passive, lethargic, and difficult to arouse.
  - Oral feeding skills must be assessed and supported.
  - Gavage feedings may be indicated.
- Obtain laboratory tests as per orders.
- Maintain a neutral thermal environment to reduce energy needs.

NEONATAL INFECTION

Infections among neonates are a leading cause of morbidity and mortality. The immune system of a neonate is immature, placing the infant at risk for infection during the first several months of life. Table 17–9 lists maternal, neonatal, and environmental factors that predispose a neonate to infection.

Infections are caused by bacteria, viruses, arboviruses (Zika), fungus, yeast, spirochetes (syphilis), and protozoa (Table 17–10).

Infections may affect specific organ systems such as respiratory, urinary tract, brain, gastrointestinal tract, and skin or local sites such as the umbilical stump and eyes. Depending on the type of infection, neonates may be asymptomatic at birth and develop symptoms within a few days of life, or their initial assessment reveals findings related to an infection such as microcephaly (cytomegalovirus [CMV] and Zika) or prominent rashes (chickenpox and rubella).

Neonatal sepsis can be classified into three categories based on age of onset: early onset, late onset, and very late onset. Early-onset sepsis occurs within the first 7 days of life. It is a serious, overwhelming infection that is typically acquired through vertical transmission from the mother (Leonard & Dobbs, 2015). Late-onset sepsis occurs after 7 days of life and is associated with a lower mortality rate than early-onset sepsis. Very-late-onset sepsis affects premature and very-low-birth-weight babies after 3 months of age. This type of sepsis is related to long-term use of equipment such as indwelling catheters and endotracheal tubes (Leonard & Dobbs, 2015).

Neonates are exposed to infection via vertical or horizontal transmission (Wilson & Tyner, 2015). Vertical transmission, the passing of infection from the mother to the baby, can occur in several ways:

- Transplacental transfer: Infection is transmitted to the fetus through the placenta (e.g., syphilis, CMV, and Zika).
- Ascending infection: Infection ascends into the uterus related to prolonged rupture of membranes.

TABLE 17–9 Risk Factors for Neonatal Infection

MATERNAL FACTORS	NEONATAL FACTORS	ENVIRONMENTAL FACTORS
Poor prenatal nutrition	Prematurity	Length of stay in hospital
Low socioeconomic status	Birth weight <2,500 g	Invasive procedures
Substance abuse	Difficult delivery	Use of humidification in incubator or ventilatory care
History of sexually transmitted infection	Birth asphyxia	Routine use of broad-spectrum antibiotics
Recurrent abortion	Meconium staining	
Lack of prenatal care	Need for resuscitation	
Prolonged rupture of membranes (>12–18 hours)	Congenital anomalies	
Vaginal GBS colonization	Black neonates	
Chorioamnionitis	Male neonates	
Maternal temperature during labor and delivery	Multiple gestation	
Premature labor		
Difficult or prolonged labor		
Maternal urinary tract infection		
Invasive procedures during labor and delivery		
Maternal and/or fetal tachycardia		
Fetal scalp electrode use		

Wilson & Tyner, 2015.

TABLE 17–10   Causes of Neonatal Infection

BACTERIAL	VIRAL	FUNGAL	OTHER
Group B Streptococcus	Rubella	*Candida albicans*	Syphilis
Escherichia coli	CMV	Candidiasis	*Treponema pallidum* (spirochete)
Coagulase-negative	Respiratory syncytial virus		Toxoplasmosis
Staphylococcus	Herpes simplex		Protozoan parasite
Staphylococcus aureus	Hepatitis B		
Viridans streptococci	HIV		
Enterococcus species	Varicella-zoster (chickenpox)		
Group D *Streptococcus*	Zika (arbovirus)		
Pseudomonas species			
Klebsiella			
Listeria monocytogenes			
Hemophilus influenzae			
Neisseria gonorrhoeae			
Chlamydia trachomatis			
Chlamydia			
Mycobacterium tuberculosis			

CRITICAL COMPONENT

Centers for Disease Control and Prevention (CDC) Interim Guidance for Evaluation and Management of Infants With Potential Congenital Zika

- Infants born to mothers who have laboratory evidence of Zika virus infection during pregnancy should receive a comprehensive physical exam, neurological assessment, head ultrasound, standard newborn hearing assessment, and Zika virus testing.
- Testing is recommended for infants born to mothers who have laboratory evidence of Zika virus infection during pregnancy and for infants who have abnormal clinical findings suggestive of congenital Zika syndrome and a maternal epidemiological link suggesting possible exposure during pregnancy, regardless of maternal test results.
- Test infant serum for Zika virus RNA, Zika virus immunoglobulin (Ig) M and neutralizing antibodies, and dengue virus IgM and neutralizing antibodies. The initial sample should be collected either from the umbilical cord or directly from the infant within 2 days of birth, if possible.
- Guideline for testing and clinical management of infants and children with postnatal Zika virus infection is in line with testing and clinical management recommendations for adults.

- Zika testing is recommended during the first 2 weeks after symptom onset to diagnose postnatal Zika virus infection. Serological testing is recommended 2 to 12 weeks after symptom onset.

CDC, 2016.

● Intrapartal exposure: The neonate is exposed to infection during the birth process (e.g., herpes virus).

Horizontal transmission (nosocomial infection) is transmitted from hospital equipment or staff to the neonate (Wilson & Tyner, 2015).

Group B Streptococcus

Group B Streptococcus (GBS) is the primary cause of neonatal meningitis and sepsis in the United States. Approximately 15% to 40% of all pregnant women are asymptomatic carriers of GBS, which is found in the urogenital and lower gastrointestinal tract (Field, 2011). Evidence supports the use of antibiotics during labor among women who have positive cultures for GBS during pregnancy in reducing vertical transmission of GBS and early-onset GBS sepsis (Leonard & Dobbs, 2015). The following are recommendations established by the CDC (2014) to prevent perinatal GBS infection:

● All pregnant women should be routinely screened for vaginal and rectal GBS colonization at 35 to 37 weeks' gestation.

Women who are positive for GBS should be given prophylactic antibiotics at the time of labor or rupture of membranes.

● Women who were GBS positive during pregnancy or who have delivered a previous baby with GBS infection, or women with membrane rupture before 37 weeks' gestation should be given penicillin during the intrapartum period without obtaining a GBS culture.

● If GBS status is unknown at the time of rupture of membranes or labor onset, prophylactic antibiotics should be administered if (1) membranes have been ruptured for 18 hours or more, (2) gestational age is less than 37 weeks, or (3) maternal temperature is 100.4°F (38°C) or higher.

● Women with positive GBS cultures who have a planned cesarean section before rupture of membranes or the onset of labor should not receive routine prophylaxis for perinatal GBS prevention.

● For intrapartum chemoprophylaxis, penicillin G is recommended at an initial dose of 5 million units intravenously (IV), followed by 2.5 million units every 4 hours until delivery. Ampicillin can be used as an alternative and is given at an initial dose of 2 g IV followed by 1 g IV every 4 hours until delivery. Women who are allergic to penicillin but are not at high risk for anaphylaxis are given cefazolin intravenously. Erythromycin or clindamycin may also be used intravenously if the GBS isolate is not resistant to these medications.

● Neonates of women who received intrapartum chemoprophylaxis do not require routine antibiotic administration unless they exhibit signs of sepsis.

● Asymptomatic infants of mothers who received prophylactic antibiotics and who are less than 35 weeks' gestation at the time of delivery should be evaluated with a complete blood count with differential and blood cultures. These neonates should be observed in the hospital for at least 48 hours.

● Infants at any gestational age who exhibit signs of infection should have a complete blood count (CBC) with a differential, blood cultures, and a chest x-ray if respiratory symptoms are present (Leonard & Dobbs, 2015). Antibiotics (ampicillin and gentamicin) should be started immediately after blood cultures are obtained.

● Neonates who are term, who appear to be healthy, and whose mothers received 4 or more hours of antibiotic prophylaxis can be discharged after 24 hours if they meet all other discharge criteria.

Assessment Findings for Neonatal Infections

● Signs of infection in a newborn are often nonspecific and subtle (Table 17–11).
● Laboratory findings suggestive of infection include:
  ● Leukocytosis: An elevated white blood cell (WBC) count (greater than 25,000/mm^3)
  ● Leukopenia: A low WBC count (lower than 1,750/mm^3)
  ● Neutrophilia: Increased neutrophil count
  ● Neutropenia: Decreased neutrophil count (less than 1,500/mm^3) is strongly predictive of infection.
  ● An immature to total neutrophil ratio greater than 0.20 is suggestive of infection.
  ● Thrombocytopenia: Platelet count below 100,000/mm^3 can be related to viral infection or bacterial sepsis (Wilson & Tyner, 2015).

Medical Management

● Laboratory tests to perform if the neonate exhibits signs of infection or is at risk for infection include:
  ● CBC, including a differential to evaluate WBC counts.
  ● Microbial cultures of the blood, urine, and CSF.
● Neonatal sepsis can be diagnosed definitively only with a positive blood culture (Leonard & Dobbs, 2015). Urine and CSF cultures may also be obtained when sepsis is suspected. Other cultures are obtained as clinically indicated (e.g., skin).
  ● C-reactive protein levels may be measured every 12 hours to detect inflammation associated with infection (Wilson & Tyner, 2015).
  ● Polymerase chain reaction testing for bacterial or viral DNA allows for identification of a specific bacterial or viral gene segment (Wilson & Tyner, 2015).

TABLE 17–11 Signs of Neonatal Infection

RESPIRATORY	THERMOREGULATION	CARDIOVASCULAR	NEUROLOGICAL	GASTROINTESTINAL	SKIN	METABOLIC
Apnea	Hypothermia	Bradycardia	Tremors	Poor feeding	Rash	Glucose instability
Grunting	Fever	Tachycardia	Lethargy	Vomiting	Pustules	
Retractions	Temperature instability	Arrhythmias	Irritability	Diarrhea	Vesicles	Metabolic acidosis
Tachypnea		Hypotension	High-pitched cry	Abdominal distention	Pallor	
Cyanosis		Hypertension	Hypertonia	Enlarged liver/spleen	Jaundice	
		Decreased perfusion	Hypotonia		Petechiae	
			Seizures		Vasomotor instability	
			Bulging fontanelles			

- Antibiotic therapy, if indicated for suspected sepsis after cultures are obtained
  - Antibiotics, such as ampicillin and aminoglycosides, that provide broad-spectrum coverage are often started initially (Wilson & Tyner, 2015).
  - If culture results are negative, antibiotics will be stopped after 48 to 72 hours.
  - If sepsis is confirmed, antibiotics continue for 10 to 14 days, and 21 days for meningitis (Wilson & Tyner, 2015).
  - If it is determined the infection is not bacterial in nature, appropriate antiviral or antifungal medications are ordered (Leonard & Dobbs, 2015).
  - The dosage and frequency of medication administration are dependent on the neonate's weight, gestational age, postnatal age, and liver and kidney function (Leonard & Dobbs, 2015).
- Intravenous fluids, parenteral nutrition and/or feedings
- Monitor glucose and electrolytes
- Ventilation as indicated

Nursing Actions

- Assess maternal and neonatal histories for factors that may place a neonate at risk for infection, such as maternal GBS status.
- Monitor vital signs, I&O, and weight.
- Assess neonate for signs of infection (see Table 17–11).
  - Notify the physician if the neonate demonstrates signs of infection. Early recognition and treatment of neonatal infection is important in preventing morbidity and mortality.
- Provide respiratory support as needed.
- Monitor glucose and electrolytes.
- Obtain laboratory tests as per order.
- Assist with diagnostic tests such as lumbar puncture for CSF.
  - CSF is obtained and sent to lab for a Gram stain and culture.
  - Holding the infant still in a flexed position is imperative for a successful lumbar puncture.
- Administer antibiotics as per orders.
- Administer feedings, intravenous fluid, and parenteral nutrition as per orders.
- Utilize standard precautions.
  - Wash hands before handling equipment and caring for the neonate.
  - Implement contact, droplet, or enteric precautions depending on diagnosis.
- Provide parents with information about the neonate's status, infection prevention strategies such as hand washing before contact with the baby, and diagnostic tests and treatments as appropriate.

SUBSTANCE ABUSE EXPOSURE

In the United States, 15.9% of pregnant women smoke cigarettes, 8.5% drink alcohol, and 5.9% use illicit drugs and cannabis (SAMHSA, 2015). The number of heroin users has increased significantly over the past 10 years and approximately three-quarters of those who use heroin report nonmedical use of prescription opioids as well as additional substances such as cocaine, methamphetamines, tobacco, alcohol, and cannabis (SAMSHA, 2015). Effects of perinatal maternal substance use on the neonate are specific to the substance and have both short-term and long-term effects on the developing fetus and neonate (Table 17–12).

Neonatal abstinence syndrome (NAS) is a group of signs and neurological behaviors exhibited by neonates resulting from the abrupt discontinuation of intrauterine exposure to various substances, including heroin, nicotine, alcohol, cannabis, opiates, cocaine, and methamphetamines (American Academy of Pediatrics [AAP], 2013). NAS can occur in 55% to 94% of newborns whose mothers were addicted to or treated with opioids while pregnant (McQueen & Murphy-Oikonen, 2016).

The extent to which a newborn exhibits drug withdrawal is dependent on timing of the last exposure, type of substance, and the half-life of the substance (AAP, 2013). Neonates exposed to alcohol in utero may demonstrate withdrawal symptoms within 3 to 12 hours after birth (AAP, 2012). Neonates exposed to narcotics in utero exhibit withdrawal within 48 to 72 hours after birth. Neonates exposed to barbiturates in utero exhibit withdrawal between days 1 and 14 (AAP, 2012).

CRITICAL COMPONENT

Signs of Neonatal Withdrawal

- Apnea
- Behavior irregularities
- Diarrhea
- Dysmature swallowing
- Excessive crying
- Excessive/frantic sucking
- Excoriated skin
- Fever
- High-pitched cry
- Hyperreflexia
- Hypertonia
- Irritability/restlessness
- Lacrimation
- Nasal congestion
- Poor feeding
- Seizures
- Skin mottling
- Sleep problems
- Sneezing
- Sweating
- Tachypnea
- Tremors
- Vomiting
- Wakefulness
- Weight loss or failure to gain weight
- Yawning

Sherman, 2015b.

TABLE 17–12   Substances Commonly Used During Pregnancy: Signs of Withdrawal and Short- and Long-Term Effects

SUBSTANCE	POSTBIRTH EFFECTS/SIGNS OF WITHDRAWAL	SHORT- AND LONG-TERM EFFECTS
Tobacco	None known	Low birth weight
		IUGR
		Smaller head circumference
		Increased stillbirth
		Cleft palate/lip
		Childhood cancer
		Lower IQ
		Learning difficulties
		Attention deficit disorder
		Increased risk for sudden infant death syndrome (SIDS)
		Increased risk for asthma/respiratory infections
		Inner ear infections
Alcohol	Onset of withdrawal 12 hours after birth	Facial anomalies:
	Hypertonia	Flat upper lip
	Tremors	Flat philtrum
	Weak suck	Short eye openings
	Poor feeding	Low birth weight
	Crying	Failure to thrive
	Increased wakefulness	Microcephaly
	Increased mouthing behavior	Mental retardation
		Poor fine motor skills
		Aggressiveness
		Attention deficit disorder
		Poor short-term memory
		Problem-solving difficulties
		Neurosensory hearing losses
		Gait problems
		Hand-eye coordination problems
		Increased risk of infection
		Lack of understanding of consequences
		Impulsive behavior
		Poor judgment
		Short attention span

TABLE 17–12 Substances Commonly Used During Pregnancy: Signs of Withdrawal and Short- and Long-Term Effects—cont'd

SUBSTANCE	POSTBIRTH EFFECTS/SIGNS OF WITHDRAWAL	SHORT- AND LONG-TERM EFFECTS
Cannabis	Tremors	Social interaction problems
	Altered sleep patterns	Low birth weight
	High-pitched cry	Preterm birth
	Exaggerated startle reflex	IUGR
		Attention deficit disorder
		Impulsiveness
		Poor self-directed responses
		Lower scores on verbal and memory assessments
		Increased risk for SIDS with paternal use
		Congenital anomalies
Cocaine	Tremors	Prematurity
	Hyperreflexia	IUGR
	Hypotonia	Decreased head circumference
	Abnormal state patterns—prolonged periods of being awake/crying	Low birth weight
		Congenital anomalies
	Extreme sensitivity to stimuli/easily distressed	Fetal distress during labor may lead to meconium aspiration
	Depressed interactive behaviors	Cerebrovascular accident, intraventricular hemorrhage
	Poor response to comforting	Increased risk for SIDS
	Short attention to stimuli	Attention deficit and behavioral problems
	Poor suck leading to feeding problems	Cognitive delays
Methamphetamines	Abnormal sleep patterns	IUGR
	Tremors	Reduced brain growth
	Poor feeding	Developmental effects
	State disorganization	Congenital anomalies
	Agitation/lethargy	Increased risk for SIDS
	Weight gain problems	
	Sweating	
	Vomiting	
	With methamphetamine and cocaine use:	
	Frantic first sucking	
	High-pitched cry	
	Loose stools	
	Yawning	
	Fever	
	Hyperreflexia	
	Excoriation	

Continued

TABLE 17–12   Substances Commonly Used During Pregnancy: Signs of Withdrawal and Short- and Long-Term Effects—cont'd

SUBSTANCE	POSTBIRTH EFFECTS/SIGNS OF WITHDRAWAL	SHORT- AND LONG-TERM EFFECTS
Narcotics/Opioids	Hypertonia	Prematurity
Heroin	Tremors	Hypoxia/low Apgar scores
Methadone	Hyperreflexia	IUGR
Morphine	Seizures	Low birth weight
OxyContin	Irritability/restlessness	Microcephaly
	High-pitched cry	Increased risk for meconium stained fluid/meconium aspiration
	Excessive crying	Congenital infections
	Sleep problems	Increased risk for SIDS
	Wakefulness	Increased chromosomal abnormalities (heroin exposure)
	Yawning	
	Nasal congestion	
	Sneezing	
	Lacrimation	
	Sweating	
	Fever	
	Skin mottling	
	Diarrhea	
	Vomiting	
	Poor feeding	
	Dysmature swallowing	
	Excessive/frantic sucking	
	Tachypnea	
	Apnea	
	Excoriated skin	
	Behavior irregularities	
	Weight loss or failure to gain weight	
Inhalants	Fetal dysmorphogenesis syndrome—similar to fetal alcohol syndrome	Developmental delay
	Small for gestational age	Language problems
	Microcephaly	Cerebellar dysfunction
	Deep-set eyes	Hyperactivity
	Small face	
	Low-set ears	
	Micrognathia	
	Spoon-shaped fingertips/small fingernails	

Hudak, 2015; Sherman, 2015b.

Prenatal Alcohol Exposure

Alcohol use during pregnancy can have no effect or it can cause a wide range of problems, including major long-term disabilities (Sherman, 2015b), fetal alcohol syndrome, alcohol-related birth defects, and alcohol-related neurodevelopment disorders.

Fetal alcohol syndrome (FAS) includes a wide spectrum of physical, cognitive, and behavioral abnormalities associated with maternal alcohol use during pregnancy (Hudak, 2015). Signs of FAS include:

- Distinctive facial features: Small eyes, thin upper lip, and short nose.
- Heart defects.
- Joint, limb, and finger deformities.
- Delayed physical growth, both intrauterine and postbirth.
- Vision problems.
- Hearing problems.
- Mental retardation.
- Behavior disturbances, such as short attention span, hyperactivity, and poor impulse control (Hudak, 2015).

Alcohol-related birth defects are congenital anomalies associated with alcohol use during pregnancy that may affect the heart, skeleton, kidneys, eyes, and ears.

Alcohol-related neurodevelopmental disorder involves abnormalities of the central nervous system and include:

- Neurological problems (e.g., poor hand-eye coordination and fine motor skills, and neurosensory hearing loss).
- Decreased cranial size, brain abnormalities.
- Cognitive and behavioral problems (Sherman, 2015b).

Assessment Findings

See Table 17–12.

Medical Management

- Identify neonates at risk.
- Physical assessment of the neonate, including observation for physical and behavioral effects of prenatal substance use.
- Toxicology screening of the neonate's urine and/or meconium.
- Diagnostic tests such as cranial ultrasound and EEG, if indicated by clinical manifestations of withdrawal symptoms
  - Problems such as infection and hypoglycemia may manifest symptoms similar to those of neonatal withdrawal and should be ruled out by the appropriate diagnostic tests (AAP, 2012).
- Use of an assessment tool to quantify the severity of signs and symptoms
  - Use of the tool should be initiated within 2 hours of birth, and neonates should be assessed for signs of withdrawal every 3 to 4 hours (Sherman, 2015b).
  - Use the tool to guide decisions about when a neonate should be evaluated for treatment with medication (McQueen & Murphy-Oikonen, 2016).

- Pharmacological therapy is considered if seizures, excessive weight loss, dehydration, poor feeding, diarrhea, vomiting, fever, and inability to sleep occur (AAP, 2013).
- Medications to treat withdrawal in neonates include:
  - Methadone, morphine, clonidine, and phenobarbital for opioid withdrawal.
  - Benzodiazepines to treat withdrawal from alcohol.
- Frequent, small feedings with a high calorie formula (22 to 24 calories/oz.)
- Monitor feedings, output, and weight daily.
- Patient education regarding substance use and breastfeeding
  - Breastfeeding is contraindicated if a woman is actively using cocaine, methamphetamines, alcohol, heroin, and/or marijuana (AAP, 2012).
  - Breastfeeding is not contraindicated with methadone use (AAP, 2012). Infants of mothers on methadone must be weaned gradually to avoid withdrawal.
  - Women who smoke cigarettes should be advised to quit and be given information about cessation resources. Women who choose to continue to smoke should be taught to avoid smoking around the baby, to smoke immediately after breastfeeding and not before, and to cut down on the number of cigarettes that they smoke (Sherman, 2015b).
- Comprehensive follow-up care for the mother or the foster mother before discharge. Infants exposed to substances prenatally often need long-term interdisciplinary physical and developmental care (Sherman, 2015b).
  - Referrals must be made to the appropriate departments and agencies (Sherman, 2015b). In many health care settings, health care providers obtain a social service consult for women who have a history of substance use. Notification of agencies such as Child Protective Services is dependent on laws of each state. In some states, neonates who are positive for prenatal substance exposure are placed in foster care.

Nursing Actions

- Review maternal history, including risk factors of substance use and history of current or past substance use.
- Assess the neonate, including gestational age.
- Assess for congenital anomalies and physical and behavioral signs of withdrawal/neonatal abstinence syndrome.
- Monitor vital signs.
- Obtain toxicology screening as per order.
  - Clean-catch urine or meconium sample may be ordered.
- Use a scoring tool to assess for signs of withdrawal on neonates who are at high risk for neonatal abstinence syndrome (Fig. 17–8).
  - Notify the physician if the score is outside of what is considered normal.
  - The decision to treat with medication is based on the neonate's score.
- Care for neonates experiencing neonatal abstinence syndrome:

System	Signs and symptoms	Date Time						Comments
		Score						
CENTRAL NERVOUS SYSTEM DISTURBANCES	Crying: Excessive high-pitched	2						
	Crying: Continuous high-pitched	3						
	Sleeps less than 1 hour after feeding	3						
	Sleeps less than 2 hours after feeding	2						
	Sleeps less than 3 hours after feeding	1						
	Hyperactive Moro reflex	2						
	Markedly hyperactive Moro reflex	3						
	Mild tremors: Disturbed	1						
	Moderate-severe tremors: Disturbed	2						
	Mild tremors: Undisturbed	3						
	Moderate-severe tremors: Undisturbed	4						
	Increased muscle tone	2						
	Excoriation (specify area)	1						
	Myoclonic jerks	3						
	Generalized convulsions	5						
METABOLIC, VASOMOTOR, AND RESPIRATORY DISTURBANCES	Sweating	1						
	Fever less than or equal to 101°F (37.2–38.3°C)	1						
	Fever greater than 101°F (38.4°C)	2						
	Frequent yawning (greater than 3)	1						
	Mottling	1						
	Nasal stuffiness	1						
	Sneezing (greater than 3)	1						
	Nasal flaring	2						
	Respiratory rate (greater than 60/min)	1						
	Respiratory rate (greater than 60/min with retractions)	2						
GASTROINTESTINAL DISTURBANCES	Excessive sucking	1						
	Poor feeding	2						
	Regurgitation	2						
	Projectile vomiting	3						
	Loose stools	2						
	Watery stools	3						
	TOTAL SCORE							

FIGURE 17–8 Neonatal Abstinence Scoring Tool.

- Assess feedings and daily weights: Increased activity, decreased sleep, irritability, loose stools, vomiting, and poor feeding behavior may all result in increased caloric needs.
- Provide frequent and small feedings: A higher calorie formula (22 to 24 cal/oz.) can be used to support increased caloric needs.
- Allow the neonate to rest during feedings.
- Position the neonate upright during feedings.
- Utilize nipples that have a slower flow if the neonate has a strong, frantic suck.
- Utilize gavage feedings if the neonate is unable to organize a productive suck.
  - Provide a pacifier to the neonate.
  - Bathe the baby in warm water to treat increased tone and irritability.

- Swaddle neonate with positioning that encourages flexion versus extension (Gomella, Cunningham, & Eyal, 2013).
- Minimize stimuli by providing a quiet environment, with lights dimmed.
- Be sensitive to infant cues that indicate stress; minimize stress-inducing activities.
- Rock the neonate gently (Sherman, 2015b).
- Care for the mother of a neonate with neonatal abstinence syndrome:
  - Provide nonjudgmental, honest, supportive care.
  - Teach what to expect in regard to the neonate's behavior. Educate about strategies that will provide comfort to her infant during withdrawal.
  - Teach her how to feed her infant.

- Observe maternal–newborn interactions and involve the mother in the care of her newborn.
  - Neonates who have been exposed to substances during the prenatal period often exhibit behaviors that interfere with the maternal–newborn relationship, such as irritability, resistance to being comforted, arching while being held, altered sleep states, poor feeding behavior, easily agitated when stimulated, and difficult transitions from one state to another.
  - Characteristics of mothers with a history of substance abuse that may impair the maternal–newborn relationship include lack of sensitivity to infant cues, lack of emotional stability, lack of communication with the infant, and inconsistent/unavailable caregiving.
  - Document all assessments and observations in the medical record per agency protocol (Sherman, 2015b).

CONGENITAL ABNORMALITIES

Congenital anomalies or birth defects affect 1 in every 33 neonates born in the United States (CDC, 2017). They are the leading cause of infant deaths, accounting for 20% of all infant deaths in the United States (Mathews, MacDorman, & Thoma, 2015). Congenital anomalies are the result of chromosomal abnormalities and/or environmental factors. Environmental factors include teratogens such as radiation, illicit substances, alcohol, diseases (e.g., diabetes), medications, and infections such as TORCH (see Chapter 7). Abnormalities range from being undetectable at birth to major and life-threatening.

Assessment Findings

- Table 17–13 lists common congenital anomalies.
- Table 17–14 lists common cardiac anomalies.
- Table 17–15 lists common metabolic disorders.

Nursing Actions

- Nursing care is determined by the type and severity of the anomaly.
- Genetic disease screening is obtained before discharge of the neonate.
- Provide emotional support for parents and family.
- Provide information on support groups.
- Provide information on need for follow-up care.

REGIONAL CENTERS

Women experiencing a high-risk pregnancy may require transfer to a facility that can provide the appropriate level of care after delivery. Many facilities/communities lack the resources to provide care to high-risk mothers and high-risk neonates; thus, regional centers were developed to provide services such as high-risk perinatal care and neonatal intensive care. Transport of a high-risk neonate to a center with a NICU requires coordination between the transferring and receiving hospitals, appropriate preparation, a highly skilled team, and the appropriate equipment (Fig. 17–9). The following are key considerations of neonatal transport:

- During the transport process, the transport team provides care that is an extension of the NICU. The aim is to provide the appropriate amount of support to the neonate to maintain stable condition. The transport process should minimize adverse effects of transfer on the neonate and be carried out in a way that protects the safety of the neonate and the transport team (Bowen, 2015).
- The transport team must be knowledgeable about high-risk neonatal care and assessment. Members of the team may include a neonatal nurse practitioner, neonatologist, resident, fellow, registered nurse, respiratory therapist, and a paramedic or emergency medical technician (Bowen, 2015).
- The transport process is as follows:
  - Once the need for NICU care is identified, arrangements are made to transfer the high-risk neonate.
  - Information pertaining to maternal and neonatal histories is communicated during the referral call.
  - The appropriate team is dispatched with supplies and equipment needed to care for the neonate.
  - The neonate is stabilized before transport.
  - During transport, the infant is kept in an incubator, thermoregulation is maintained, respiratory support and IV therapy are provided, and the following are monitored:
    - Vital signs, oxygen saturation, blood glucose, the neonate's condition, pain status, and response to transport
  - Strategies should be used to provide developmental care during transfer, such as protecting the neonate's eyes from bright lights, using ear protection in noisy vehicles such as helicopters, using a gel mattress to prevent jarring, and using blankets to promote containment.
  - Notify parents when the infant arrives at the receiving facility (Bowen, 2015).

Various vehicles may be used for transport, such as ambulance, helicopter, or fixed-wing aircraft. The type of vehicle that is used will be determined by factors such as the neonate's condition and diagnosis, distance of transport, weather, and cost. Appropriate supplies and equipment based on the neonate's condition must be stocked and checked regularly. Equipment includes:

- Monitoring devices, such as a pulse oximeter, cardiorespiratory monitor, temperature and blood pressure monitors.
- Oxygen tanks and other respiratory supplies, such as endotracheal tubes, bag and mask for resuscitation, nasal cannula, ventilator, and suctioning equipment.
- Medications.
- Intravenous therapy equipment, including pumps.
- Equipment to maintain and assess thermoregulation, such as an incubator, thermometer, heat packs, chemical mattress, and blankets.
- Equipment to perform blood glucose and blood gas monitoring.
- Equipment to perform chest tube insertion or needle aspiration.
- Personal protective equipment, such as gloves and gowns.

TABLE 17–13   Common Congenital Anomalies

TYPE OF ANOMALY	INCIDENCE	DESCRIPTION	TREATMENT
Tracheoesophageal fistula	1 in 4,700 live births	Abnormal opening between the trachea and esophagus	Surgical repair
Diaphragmatic hernia	1 in 4,000 live births	Herniation of abdominal organs through a hole in the diaphragm into the thoracic cavity	Gastric decompression Stabilization Surgical repair
Omphalocele	1 in 5,000–6,000 live births	Herniation of abdominal contents through the umbilicus, which is covered by the peritoneal sac	Surgical repair Staged surgical repair for large defects (abdominal contents returned gradually)
Gastroschisis	1 in 2,000–2,500 live births	Herniation of abdominal contents through a hole in the abdomen often to the right of the umbilicus	Surgical repair Staged surgical repair for large defects
Cleft lip	1 in 1,000 live births	Failure of the mesenchymal masses of the nasal and maxillary prominences to come together	Surgical repair
Cleft palate	1 in 1,500 live births	Failure of the mesenchymal masses in the palate to fuse	Surgical repair
Spina bifida: meningocele Myelomeningocele	1 in 3,000 live births	A sac with meninges and cerebrospinal fluid bulge through defect in undeveloped vertebrae A sac with meninges and nerve tissue bulge through a defect in the spinal column	Surgical repair Surgical repair
Anencephaly	3 in 10,000 live births	Incomplete formation of the cranium and brain	Most babies die within a few days of birth
Developmental dysplasia of the hip	1–2 in 1,000 live births	Dislocation of the femoral head from the acetabulum	Pavlik harness to promote abduction/flexion to stabilize hip Surgery if Pavlik harness is not successful
Polydactyly	2 in 1,000 live births	Extra digits on the hand or foot	Surgery or ligation
Syndactyly	1 in 2,200 live births	Fusion of digits of hand or foot	Surgery depending on extent of anomaly
Talipes equinovarus	1 in 1,000 live births	Sole of the foot is turned in; the back part of the foot is deformed. Also called "clubfoot," usually bilateral.	Casting/splinting Surgery Treatment depends on severity

CDC, 2017; Sterk, 2015.

TABLE 17–14 Common Cardiac Anomalies

TYPE OF ANOMALY	INCIDENCE	DESCRIPTION	TREATMENT
Ventricular septal defect (VSD)	2 in 1,000 live births	Opening in the septum between the right and left ventricles of the heart	Up to 75% of VSDs close without treatment Treat with digoxin and diuretics if congestive heart failure is present. Surgical repair
Atrial septal defect (ASD)	1 in 2,000 live births	Opening in the septum between the right and left atria.	ASDs may close without treatment. Treat congestive heart failure with medication. Surgical repair may be needed.
Coarctation of the aorta	1 in 10,000 live births	Narrowing of the aorta at the transverse aortic arch or in the area of the ductus arteriosus	Medical management of congestive heart failure. Surgical repair
Tetralogy of Fallot	1 in 2,500 live births	Consists of four defects: 1. VSD 2. Aorta overriding VSD 3. Pulmonary stenosis 4. Hypertrophy of the right ventricle	Medical management includes propranolol for cyanotic infants. Prostaglandin E1 may be administered to maintain a patent ductus arteriosus until surgery, for infants with a severe tetralogy of Fallot. Surgical repair
Transposition of great vessels	1 in 3,500 live births	The positions of the great arteries are reversed from the normal position. Aorta emerges from the right ventricle, and the pulmonary artery emerges from the left ventricle.	This defect results in a medical emergency. Stabilization—treat acidosis Administer prostaglandin E1 to maintain a patent ductus arteriosus until surgery is performed.

CDC, 2017; Sadowski, 2015.

DISCHARGE PLANNING

Discharge planning for high-risk neonates involves many considerations since these neonates often require special care and follow-up after release from the hospital. In some cases, infants require long-term evaluation to monitor health issues, growth, and neurodevelopment. Many high-risk conditions, such as prematurity and related complications, perinatal substance use, and congenital anomalies, have long-term or lifelong physical, cognitive, and behavioral consequences. The following are critical components of the discharge process for high-risk neonates (Hummel, 2015):

● When a high-risk neonate is admitted, planning for discharge begins. Parents should be encouraged to be involved with the care of their infant from the time of admission. Care-related teaching with parents should begin as soon after delivery as possible.
● Interdisciplinary teams are often involved in the discharge process. The team may consist of physicians, nurse practitioners, nurses, social workers, occupational therapists, case managers, lactation consultants, respiratory therapists, nutritionists, pharmacists, and home health agency/nursing staff.
● The neonate's condition must be stable (e.g., weight gain, temperature stability, able to tolerate feedings, stable respiratory status) (Fig. 17–10).
● All appropriate examinations and screenings are completed, including an eye exam, genetic disease/metabolic disease screening, critical congenital heart disease screening, and a hearing screening.
● Pass the infant car seat challenge. The AAP recommends that all neonates born before 37 weeks undergo and pass an infant car seat challenge prior to discharge. The preterm neonate can have weaker airways and is thus more susceptible to breathing issues in a semireclined position. For a car seat challenge, the neonate:
  ● Is secured snugly in an appropriate sized car seat at a 45-degree angle for a specified amount of time.
  ● Must maintain adequate oxygenation, heart rate, and respiratory rate during trial.

TABLE 17–15   Common Genetic Disorders of Metabolism

TYPE OF DISORDER	INCIDENCE	DESCRIPTION	TREATMENT
Phenylketonuria	1 in 10,000 live births	Lack of the enzyme needed to convert phenylalanine to tyrosine. If untreated, causes cognitive and physical problems.	Diet that restricts intake of phenylalanine.
Disorders of fatty acid oxidation (e.g., medium chain acyl-CoA-deficiency)	1 in 20,000 live births	18 disorders identified. Impaired fat metabolism leads to hypoglycemia and organ failure.	Hypoglycemia is treated. Fasting is avoided.
Congenital adrenal hyperplasia	1 in 5,000 live births	Cortisol production is inhibited. Adrenal hypertrophy results, with excessive production of adrenal androgens. Electrolyte imbalances common, female infants exhibit ambiguous genitalia.	Steroid administration Corrective surgery for ambiguous genitalia.
Maple syrup urine disease	1 in 200,000	Lack of enzymes needed to metabolize leucine, valine, and isoleucine. These amino acids build up in the blood. Disease is fatal if untreated.	Peritoneal dialysis Low-protein diet
Galactosemia	1 in 40,000 live births	Lack of enzyme that converts galactose to glucose. Inability to metabolize lactose. If untreated, results in liver disease, mental retardation, and cataracts.	Lactose-free or soy formula.

Sterk, 2015.

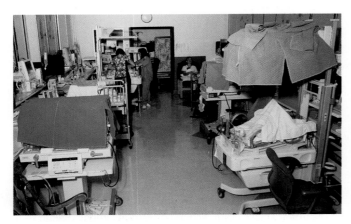

FIGURE 17–9 Neonatal intensive care unit.

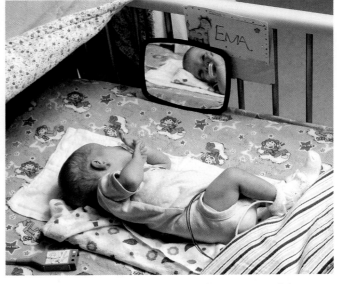

FIGURE 17–10 A 10-week-old neonate, born at 27 weeks' gestation, who will soon be going home.

● Family's readiness to take their infant home. The family's willingness and ability to provide care to their infant with special needs is evaluated, as are their financial resources. In addition, the home setting is assessed for safety and adequacy.

● The educational needs of the family are met. Discharge teaching includes:

　● General infant care, such as bathing, feeding, diapering, and skin care.

　● Safety issues, such as car seat safety, back to sleep positioning for sleep, infant CPR, and babyproofing the house.

　● Instructions on use of required equipment (e.g., apnea monitoring).

- Information on treatments (e.g., oxygen, suctioning) and medications ordered.
- Signs and symptoms of illnesses that need to be reported to the primary care provider.
- Infant growth and developmental milestones.
- Follow-up information, including visits with the pediatrician, immunization schedules, and referrals to the appropriate medical and developmental specialists.

PSYCHOSOCIAL NEEDS OF PARENTS WITH HIGH-RISK NEONATES

The birth of a baby who is premature or has conditions that place him or her at risk for illness or death is a significant stressor for the family. Parents may grieve over the loss of an ideal baby and find the experience of having a baby with complications overwhelming. It is devastating for most parents when the mother is discharged and the baby must remain in the hospital.

Common effects on the parents and family are:

- Delay of attachment process due to the separation of parent and newborn, which can place the newborn at risk for abuse and neglect.
- Guilty feelings by the mother, who may feel she did something wrong to cause her newborn to be ill.
- Emotional distancing of parents from their newborn as a protective mechanism due to fear of their child's death.
- Anger at the loss of control of having an ill or premature newborn.
- Disappointment at not being able to bring their newborn home.
- Disruption of family life; parents needing to return to work, caring for other children, and at the same time wanting to spend time in the hospital with their newborn.

Nursing Actions

- Orient parents to the NICU environment by explaining equipment/monitors used for their newborn.
- Assess parents' comfort level with the NICU environment.
- Provide opportunities for parents to share their concerns and frustrations by developing a trusting rapport with them.
- Provide opportunities for parents to talk about their experiences by asking how they are coping with the experience.
- Provide information regarding their neonate's status to both parents at a level they can understand.
- Inform parents that they should ask any questions they have regarding the condition and care of their neonate.
- Inform parents that they can talk to their neonate's nurse at any time.
- Assess the parents' readiness to care for their neonate and provide opportunities for them to participate in the care of their neonate.
- Encourage parents to touch and hold their neonate as indicated by the neonate's health status.

- Encourage the mother to pump her breasts and bring the milk to the NICU to be used for feeding.
- Review breast milk storage and provide equipment as needed.
- Provide a private area for the mother to breastfeed when the neonate is able to nurse.
- Encourage parents to take photos to share with their family and friends.
- Praise parents for their involvement in the neonate's care.
- Provide information on support groups for parents of preterm neonates or neonates with disabilities.

LOSS AND GRIEF

When an infant dies, parents must work through profound grief associated with the death of their child and the loss of their hopes and dreams for that child and their family. Grief is an individual process, and members of the family will experience it in different ways and in varied time lines. The stages of grief include:

- Avoidance, disbelief, shock, guilt.
- Pain, physical discomfort, depression, difficulty concentrating, anger at self or partner.
- Acceptance and adaptation. Grief persists, but a sense of balance is achieved (Kenner & Boykova, 2015).

Nurses must keep in mind that each person experiences and expresses grief in his or her own way. Culture, religion, and personal experience and beliefs will impact how individuals and families respond to loss. Nurses can help families that are grieving the death of their newborn with the following measures:

- Allow parents to express their feelings by being present and listening.
- Express empathy and condolences. Avoid trite phrases such as "At least you are young; you can have another baby."
- Refer to the baby by name if he or she has been named.
- Provide information about the process of grieving and what to expect physically and emotionally.
- Provide ample opportunity for the parents and family members to spend time with the baby before and after he or she dies.
- Provide parents with memorabilia associated with their baby, such as pictures, blankets, a hat, a lock of hair, ID bracelet, footprints, and crib card.
- Offer to contact the hospital chaplain. Encourage the family to contact their own clergy or spiritual leader. Explore the family's desire for baptism or other religious rites.
- Discuss the family's plan for autopsy, a memorial or funeral, and burial or cremation.
- Encourage the family to accept help and support from others.
- Refer parents to community services and support groups that may assist in facilitating the grief process (Kenner & Boykova, 2015).

Clinical Pathway for the Preterm Infant

	Birth to First Hour	1 to 24 Hours of Age	24 Hours of Age to Discharge
Assessments	Review prenatal record to determine projected gestational age.	Complete gestational assessment as per hospital policy.	Assess every 2–4 hours or per hospital policy.
	Identify risk factors for premature birth.	Assess every 1–2 hours or per hospital policy.	Weigh the neonate every day or per hospital policy.
	Obtain Apgar score at 1 and 5 minutes.		Obtain length and head circumference weekly or per hospital policy.
	Obtain weight, length, and head circumference.		
	Complete neonatal assessment.		
Thermoregulation	Place neonate on preheated radiant warmer and dry gently immediately after birth.	Prevent heat loss by maintaining a neutral thermal environment (NTE).	Prevent heat loss by maintaining an NTE.
	Cover head with warmed hat.	Assess axillary temperature every 1–2 hours or per hospital policy.	Encourage skin-to-skin contact or kangaroo care when neonate is stable.
	Per hospital policy, wrap in dry, warmed blankets, place in a polyethylene wrap, and/or on a chemical mattress for transport to NICU.	Assess for cold stress symptoms.	Dress and wrap neonate when advanced to an open crib.
		Postpone bathing until neonate is stable.	Assess axillary temperature every 2–4 hours or per hospital policy.
	Place in a preheated radiant warmer or a thermoregulated incubator.		Provide heat source when bathing.
	Assess axillary temperature every 15–30 minutes or per hospital policy.		Assess for cold stress symptoms.
			Teach parents to assess temperature and signs of cold stress.
Respiratory	Clear the nose and mouth of mucus with the use of a bulb syringe.	Assess for signs of respiratory distress: grunting, flaring, retractions.	Assess for signs of respiratory distress: grunting, flaring, retractions.
	Immediately after birth, assess neonate for respiratory effort, including apnea, and provide resuscitation as needed.	Assess lung sounds.	Assess lung sounds.
		Administer oxygen as needed.	Administer oxygen as needed.
	Apply pulse oximeter and monitor values.	Provide respiratory support as needed.	Provide respiratory support as needed.
	Assess for signs of respiratory distress: grunting, flaring, retractions.	Monitor pulse oximeter values.	Monitor pulse oximeter values.
	Assess lung sounds.	Obtain chest x-ray and blood gases as ordered.	Obtain chest x-ray and blood gases as ordered.
	Administer oxygen as needed.	Monitor I&O.	Monitor I&O.
	Provide respiratory support as needed.		Obtain daily weights.
	Obtain chest x-ray and blood gases as ordered.		Teach parents signs and symptoms of respiratory distress.
			Teach parents oxygen management if neonate is to be discharged with oxygen.
Cardiovascular	Assess skin color for cyanosis.	Assess skin color for cyanosis.	Assess skin color for cyanosis.
	Assess heart rate at birth, and at 1 and 5 minutes of age.	Assess heart rate and rhythm every 1–2 hours or per hospital policy.	Assess heart rate and rhythm every 2–4 hours or per hospital policy.
	Assess heart rate and rhythm every 15–30 minutes or per hospital policy thereafter.	Continue on cardiorespiratory monitor for continuous observation.	Continue on cardiorespiratory monitor for continuous observation.
	Place on cardiorespiratory monitor for continuous observation.		Teach parents CPR when neonate is close to discharge.

Clinical Pathway for the Preterm Infant—cont'd

	Birth to First Hour	1 to 24 Hours of Age	24 Hours of Age to Discharge
Nutrition	Obtain and monitor blood glucose levels per hospital policy. Obtain intravenous access and administer parenteral nutrition if ordered.	Obtain and monitor blood glucose levels per hospital policy. Administer parenteral and or enteral nutrition as ordered. Encourage mother to begin pumping to supply breast milk for neonate. Encourage kangaroo care to enhance milk supply. Use nonnutritive sucking with tube feedings. Monitor for signs of feeding intolerance. Monitor I&O.	Obtain and monitor blood glucose levels per hospital policy. Administer parenteral and or enteral nutrition as ordered. Encourage kangaroo care to enhance milk supply. Use nonnutritive sucking with tube feedings. Monitor for signs of feeding intolerance. As neonate matures, assess for signs of readiness for oral feedings. Monitor I&O. Monitor daily weights. Teach parents proper techniques for breastfeeding or bottle feeding their neonate.
Sepsis	Obtain maternal history for risk factors. Obtain CBC and blood cultures as ordered. Administer antibiotics as ordered. Assess for signs of sepsis.	Assess for signs of sepsis. Administer antibiotics as ordered.	Assess for signs of sepsis. Administer antibiotics as ordered. Teach parents strategies to prevent infection.

CONCEPT MAP

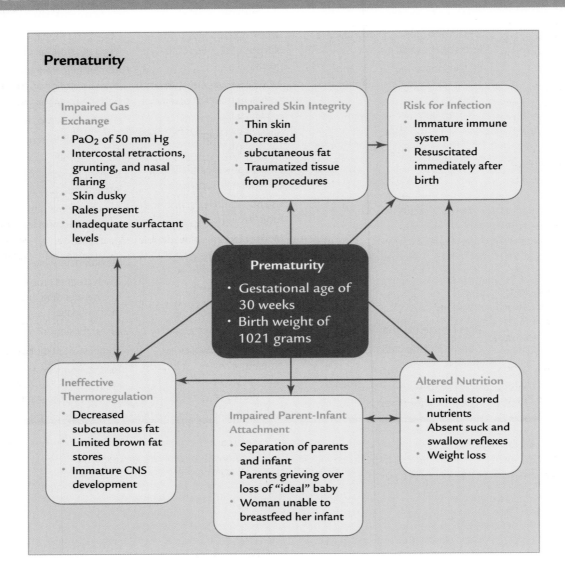

Prematurity

Impaired Gas Exchange
- PaO_2 of 50 mm Hg
- Intercostal retractions, grunting, and nasal flaring
- Skin dusky
- Rales present
- Inadequate surfactant levels

Impaired Skin Integrity
- Thin skin
- Decreased subcutaneous fat
- Traumatized tissue from procedures

Risk for Infection
- Immature immune system
- Resuscitated immediately after birth

Prematurity
- Gestational age of 30 weeks
- Birth weight of 1021 grams

Ineffective Thermoregulation
- Decreased subcutaneous fat
- Limited brown fat stores
- Immature CNS development

Impaired Parent-Infant Attachment
- Separation of parents and infant
- Parents grieving over loss of "ideal" baby
- Woman unable to breastfeed her infant

Altered Nutrition
- Limited stored nutrients
- Absent suck and swallow reflexes
- Weight loss

Problem No. 1: Impaired gas exchange

Goal: Adequate gas exchange

Outcome: PaO_2 is 60 to 70 mm Hg; $PaCO_2$ is 35 to 45 mm Hg; skin color is pink; lung sounds are clear; and no signs of retractions, grunting, or nasal flaring.

Nursing Actions
1. Monitor vital signs, oxygen saturation, and arterial blood gases.
2. Maintain patent airway.
3. Suction airway as indicated.
4. Administer oxygen as per orders.
5. Maintain a neutral thermal environment.
6. Cluster nursing activities.
7. Monitor for adverse effects related to surfactant replacement therapy.

Problem No. 2: Impaired skin integrity

Goal: Intact skin

Outcome: The neonate's skin will be intact and without signs of skin irritation.

Nursing Actions
1. Assess skin for redness, dryness, breakdown, and rashes.
2. Use a neutral pH cleanser and sterile water when bathing. Bathe only soiled body parts.
3. Use adhesives sparingly.
4. Apply emollient to dry areas.
5. Change diapers frequently and apply zinc oxide.
6. Change positions frequently.
7. Use water, air, or gelled mattresses as indicated.

Problem No. 3: Risk of infection

Goal: Be free of infection

Outcome: Neonates will not exhibit signs of infection such as temperature instability, increased apnea, lethargy, feeding intolerance, or purulent drainage.

Nursing Actions

1. Promote hand washing for staff and parents.
2. Assess for signs of infection.
3. Maintain intact skin.
4. Properly prepare sites for invasive procedures.
5. Properly care for invasive lines to maintain sterility.
6. Administer antibiotics as per orders.
7. Encourage use of breast milk for infant feedings.

Problem No. 4: Ineffective thermoregulation

Goal: Stable temperature within normal range

Outcome: Neonate's temperature will be between 97.5°F and 99°F (36.4°C and 37.2°C).

Nursing Actions

1. Keep the neonate dry.
2. Use plastic barriers when indicated.
3. Prewarm radiant warmers, incubators, and linens.
4. Monitor temperature every 2 to 4 hours and adjust environment as needed.
5. Encourage kangaroo care.
6. Keep area free of drafts.
7. Swaddle the neonate when holding outside of warmer or incubator.

Problem No. 5: Altered nutrition

Goal: Growth and weight gain within normal ranges

Outcome: Neonate will gain 20 to 30 grams per day.

Nursing Actions

1. Administer parenteral nutrition, enteral feedings, or oral feedings as per orders.
2. Encourage use of breast milk.
3. Monitor weight daily.
4. Monitor length and head circumference weekly.
5. Monitor the neonate during feedings for signs of feeding intolerance, such as vomiting, regurgitation, and excessive gastric residual.
6. Encourage breastfeeding when indicated.
7. Monitor I&O.
8. Allow for rest periods between feedings.

Problem No. 6: Impaired parent–infant attachment

Goal: Positive parent–infant attachment

Outcome: Parents hold the infant close to the body and the infant appears calm and relaxed; parents spend time each day with the infant and participate in care of the infant; parents respond to infant cues.

Nursing Actions

1. Orient parents to the NICU environment.
2. Provide opportunities for parents to share their concerns and frustrations.
3. Provide opportunities for parents to talk about their experiences of having a high-risk baby.
4. Assess parents' readiness to care for their baby and provide opportunities for participation in their baby's care.
5. Instruct parents on neonatal care.
6. Praise parents for their involvement.
7. Encourage the woman to pump her breast and bring her breast milk for use with infant feeding.
8. Encourage kangaroo holding by both parents.

Case Study

Baby girl Polk is a newly delivered 32 weeks' gestation neonate who is admitted to the NICU. Her mother, Mallory, is a 42-year-old African American single woman. Mallory is a G2 P0 who conceived after three attempts at in vitro fertilization. Mallory was admitted to the birthing unit for preterm labor. She was given magnesium sulfate, ampicillin, and two doses of betamethasone. Her labor continued. When her cervix was 5 cm dilated, a decision was made to discontinue the magnesium sulfate. A few hours after the magnesium sulfate was discontinued, Mallory gave birth spontaneously to a baby girl. The 1- and 5-minute Apgar scores were 7 and 8, respectively. Baby Polk weighed 2,010 g and was assessed at 32 weeks based on the Ballard score.

Detail the aspects of your initial nursing assessment.
List the nursing diagnosis for this neonate.
What are the immediate priorities in the nursing care of Baby Polk?
Discuss the rationale for the selected priorities.
List the anticipated medical care for Baby Polk.

Four hours later:

Baby Polk is on NCPAP. There is an increase in intercostal retractions and expiratory grunting. The results of arterial blood gas tests are P_{CO_2} of 70 and pH of 7.2. CBC indicates an increase in WBC.

Medical orders include initial dose of Survanta after intubation, IV of D10W, glucose monitoring every 4 hours, ampicillin 50 mg/kg, and gentamicin 4 mg/kg.

Based on this additional information, list the nursing diagnosis for this neonate.
List the anticipated medical care.
Discuss the nursing care for this neonate and mother.

One week later:

Baby Polk is extubated and is placed on a high-flow nasal cannula at 1 L. She is tolerating gavage feedings and gaining weight. She is experiencing occasional episodes of apnea and bradycardia.

Discuss the criteria for discharge from the NICU.
Describe the discharge teaching for the care of Baby Polk.

REFERENCES

Allen, M. (2015). *Hyperbilirubinemia: Identification and management in the healthy term and late preterm infant* (3rd ed.). Washington DC: Association of Women's Health, Obstetric and Neonatal Nurses.

American Academy of Pediatrics (AAP). (2004). Management of hyperbilirubinemia in the newborn infant 35 or more weeks of gestation. *Pediatrics, 114,* 297–316.

American Academy of Pediatrics (AAP). (2012). Neonatal drug withdrawal. *Pediatrics, 129,* e540–560. doi:10.1542/peds.2011-3212

American Academy of Pediatrics (AAP). (2013). Prenatal substance abuse: Short and long-term effects on the exposed fetus. *Pediatrics, 131*(3), e10090–1024. doi:10.1542/peds.2012-3931

Armentrout, D. (2015). Glucose management. In M. T. Verklan & M. Walden (Eds.), *Core curriculum for neonatal intensive care nursing* (pp. 162–170). St. Louis, MO: Elsevier Saunders.

Association of Women's Health, Obstetric and Neonatal Nurses (AWHONN). (2013). *Neonatal skin care: Evidence based clinical practice guideline* (3rd ed.). Washington, DC: Association of Women's Health, Obstetric and Neonatal Nurses/National Association of Neonatal Nurses.

Bancalari, E. H., & Walsh, M. C. (2015). Bronchopulmonary dysplasia. In R. J. Martin, A. A. Fanaroff, & M. C. Walsh (Eds.), *Neonatal-perinatal medicine: Diseases of the fetus and infant.* (10th ed., vol. 2, pp. 1157–1169). Philadelphia, PA: Mosby Elsevier.

Benjamin, K., & Furdon, S. (2015). Physical assessment. In M. T. Verklan & M. Walden (Eds.), *Core curriculum for neonatal intensive care nursing* (pp. 110–143). St. Louis, MO: Elsevier Saunders.

Bennett, C., Headtke, E., & Rowe-Telow, M. (2015). Use of dextrose gel reverses neonatal hypoglycemia and decreases admissions to the NICU… Proceedings of the 2015 AWHONN Convention. *Journal of Obstetric, Gynecologic & Neonatal Nursing, 44,* S52–3. doi:10.1111/1552-6909.12614

Blackburn, S. (2013). *Maternal, fetal, & neonatal physiology* (4th ed.). St. Louis, MO: Elsevier.

Bradshaw, W. T. (2015). Gastrointestinal disorders. In M. T. Verklan & M. Walden (Eds.), *Core curriculum for neonatal intensive care nursing* (pp. 583–631). St. Louis, MO: Elsevier Saunders.

Brand, M. C., & Boyd, H. A. (2015). Thermoregulation. In M. T. Verklan & M. Walden (Eds.), *Core curriculum for neonatal intensive care nursing* (pp. 95–109). St. Louis, MO: Elsevier Saunders.

Briere, C., McGrath, J. M., Xiaomei, C., Brownell, E., & Cusson, R. (2016). Direct-breastfeeding in the neonatal intensive care unit and breastfeeding duration for premature infants. *Applied Nursing Research, 32,* 47–51. doi:10.1016/j.apnr.2016.04.004

Bowen, S. L. (2015). Intrafacility and interfacility neonatal transport. In M. T. Verklan & M. Walden (Eds.), *Core curriculum for neonatal intensive care nursing* (pp. 407–425). St. Louis, MO: Elsevier Saunders.

Caplan, M. (2015). Neonatal necrotizing enterocolitis. In R. J. Martin, A. A. Fanaroff, & M. C. Walsh (Eds.), *Neonatal-perinatal medicine: Diseases of the fetus and infant.* (10th ed., vol. 2, pp. 1423–1432). Philadelphia, PA: Mosby Elsevier.

Centers for Disease Control and Prevention (CDC). (2014). Prevention of perinatal group B streptococcal disease. *Morbidity and Mortality Weekly Report, 59,* 1–36.

Centers for Disease Control and Prevention. (2016). *Update: Interim guidance for the evaluation and management of infants with possible congenital zika virus infection—United States, August 2016.* Retrieved from www.cdc.gov/mmwr/volumes/65/wr/mm6533e2.htm?s_cid=mm6533e2_w.

Centers for Disease Control and Prevention. (2017). *Birth defects.* Retrieved from www.cdc.gov/ncbddd/birthdefects.

Cho, E., Kim, S., Kwon, M., Cho, H., Kim, E. H., Jun, E. M., & Lee, S. (2016). The effects of kangaroo care in the neonatal intensive care unit on the physiological functions of preterm infants, maternal–infant attachment, and maternal stress. *Journal of Pediatric Nursing, 31*(4), 430–438. doi:10.1016/j.pedn.2016.02.007

deVries, L. S. (2015). Intracranial hemorrhage and vascular lesions. In R. J. Martin, A. A. Fanaroff, & M. C. Walsh (Eds.), *Neonatal-perinatal medicine: Diseases of the fetus and infant* (10th ed., vol. 2, pp. 886–903). Philadelphia, PA: Mosby Elsevier.

Diehl-Jones, W., & Fraser, D. (2015). Hematological disorders. In M. T. Verklan & M. Walden (Eds.), *Core curriculum for neonatal intensive care nursing* (pp. 662–688). St. Louis, MO: Elsevier Saunders.

Ditzenberger, G. R. (2015). Nutritional management. In M. T. Verklan & M. Walden (Eds.), *Core curriculum for neonatal intensive care nursing* (pp. 172–196). St. Louis, MO: Elsevier Saunders.

Eichenwald, E. (2016). Apnea of prematurity. *Pediatrics, 137*(1). e20153757. doi:10.1542/peds.2015-3757

Field, P. (2011). Group B strep infection in the newborn. *Nursing, 41*(11), 62.

Foster, J. P., Psaila, K., & Patterson, T. (2016). Non-nutritive sucking for increasing physiologic stability and nutrition in preterm infants. *Cochrane Database of Systematic Reviews, 10.* doi:10.1002/14651858.CD001071.pub3

Fraser, D. (2015). Respiratory distress. In M. T. Verklan & M. Walden (Eds.), *Core curriculum for neonatal intensive care nursing* (pp. 447–474). St. Louis, MO: Elsevier Saunders.

Fraser, D., & Diehl-Jones, W. (2015). Ophthalmologic and auditory disorders. In M. T. Verklan & M. Walden (Eds.), *Core curriculum for neonatal intensive care nursing* (pp. 813–831). St. Louis, MO: Elsevier Saunders.

Gomella, T., Cunningham, M., & Eyal, F. (2013). *Neonatology: Management, procedures, on-call problems, diseases, and drugs* (7th ed.). New York, NY: Lange.

Halbardier, B. H. (2015). Fluid and electrolyte management. In M. T. Verklan & M. Walden (Eds.), *Core curriculum for neonatal intensive care nursing* (pp. 146–161). St. Louis, MO: Elsevier Saunders.

Hardy, W., D'Agata, A., & McGrath, J. M. (2016). The infant at risk. In S. Mattson & J. E. Smith (Eds.), *Core curriculum for maternal-newborn nursing* (pp. 363–416). St. Louis, MO: Elsevier Saunders.

Harris, M. N., Carey, W. A., Ellsworth, M. A., Haas, L. R., Hartman, T. K., Lang, T. R., & Colby, C. E. (2014). Perceptions and practices of therapeutic hypothermia in American neonatal intensive care units. *American Journal of Perinatology, 31*(1), 15–20. doi:10.1055/s-0033-1334454

Hay, W. (2012). Care of the infant of the diabetic mother. *Current Diabetes Reports, 12,* 4–15.

Herrmann, K., & Carroll, K. (2014). An exclusively human milk diet reduces necrotizing enterocolitis. *Breastfeeding Medicine, 9*(4), 184–190. doi:10.1089/bfm.2013.0121

Heuchan, A. M., & Clyman, R. I. (2014). Managing the patent ductus arteriosus: Current treatment options. *Archives of Disease in Childhood—Fetal & Neonatal Edition, 99*(5), F431–436. doi:10.1136/archdischild-2014-306176

Hudak, M. L. (2015). Infants with antenatal exposure to drugs. In R. J. Martin, A. A. Fanaroff, & M. C. Walsh (Eds.), *Neonatal-perinatal medicine: Diseases of the fetus and infant* (10th ed., vol. 1, pp. 682–694). Philadelphia, PA: Mosby Elsevier.

Hummel, P. (2015). Discharge planning and transition to home care. *Core curriculum for neonatal intensive care nursing* (pp. 373–406). St. Louis, MO: Elsevier Saunders.

Kaplan, M., Wong, R. J., Sibley, E., & Stevenson, D. K. (2015). Neonatal jaundice and liver disease. In R. J. Martin, A. A. Fanaroff, & M. C. Walsh (Eds.), *Neonatal-perinatal medicine: Diseases of the fetus and infant* (10th ed., vol. 2, pp. 1618–1673). Philadelphia, PA: Mosby Elsevier.

Kaspar, A., & Rubarth, L. B. (2016). Neuroprotection of the preterm infant. *Neonatal Network, 35*(6), 391–395. doi:10.1891/0730-0832.35.6.391

Kenner, C., & Boykova, M. (2015). Families in crisis. In M. T. Verklan & M. Walden (Eds.), *Core curriculum for neonatal intensive care nursing* (pp. 331–347). St. Louis, MO: Elsevier Saunders.

Kochanek, K. D., Murphy, S. L., Xu, J. Q., & Tejada-Vera, B. (2016). Deaths: Final data for 2014. *National Vital Statistics Reports, 65*(4).

Leonard, E. G., & Dobbs, K. (2015). Postnatal bacterial infections. In R. J. Martin, A. A. Fanaroff, & M. C. Walsh (Eds.), *Neonatal-perinatal medicine: Diseases of the fetus and infant* (10th ed., vol. 2, pp. 734–750). Philadelphia, PA: Mosby Elsevier.

Maisels, M. J. (2015). Managing the jaundiced newborn: A persistent challenge. *Canadian Medical Association Journal, 187*(5), 335–343. doi:10.1503/cmaj.122117

March of Dimes. (2016). *Preterm labor and premature birth.* Retrieved from www.marchofdimes.org/complications/preterm-labor-and-premature-birth.aspx.

Martin, J. A., Hamilton, B. E., Osterman, M. J. K., Driscoll, A. K., & Matthews, T. J. (2017). Births: Final data for 2015. *National Vital Statistics Report, 66*(1).

Mathews, T. J., MacDorman, M. F., & Thoma, M. E. (2015). Infant mortality statistics from the 2013 linked birth/infant death data set. *National Vital Statistics Report, 64*(9).

McQueen, K., & Murphy-Oikonen, J. (2016). Neonatal abstinence syndrome. *New England Journal of Medicine, 375,* 2468–2479. doi:10.1056/NEJMra1600879

Natarajan, C. K., Sankar, M. J., Jain, K., Agarwal, R., & Paul, V. K. (2016). Surfactant therapy and antibiotics in neonates with meconium aspiration syndrome: A systematic review and meta-analysis. *Journal of Perinatology, 36,* S49–S54. doi:10.1038/jp.2016.32

Newnam, K. M. (2014). Oxygen saturation limits and evidence supporting the targets. *Advances in Neonatal Care, 14*(6), 403–409. doi:10.1097/ANC.0000000000000150

Ohlsson, A., & Aher, S. (2014). Early erythropoietin for preventing red blood cell transfusion in preterm and/or low birth weight infants. *Cochrane Database of Systemic Reviews, 4*. Art. No:CD004863.

Rankin, M. W., Jimenez, E. Y., Caraco, M., Collinson, M., Lostetter, L., & DuPont, T. L. (2016). Validation of test weighing protocol to estimate enteral feeding volumes in preterm infants. *Journal of Pediatrics, 178,* 108–112. doi:10.1016/j.jpeds.2016.08.011

Sadowski, S. L. (2015). Cardiovascular disorders. In M. T. Verklan & M. Walden (Eds.), *Core curriculum for neonatal intensive care nursing* (pp. 527–582). St. Louis, MO: Elsevier Saunders.

Shah, N. A., & Wusthoff, C. J. (2016). Intracranial hemorrhage in the neonate. *Neonatal Network, 35*(2), 67–72. doi:10.1891/0730-0832.35.2.67

Sharma, D. (2016). Golden 60 minutes of newborn's life. Part 1: Preterm neonate. *Journal of Maternal-Fetal Neonatal Medicine, 29*(22), 1–33. doi:10.1080/14767058.2016.1261398

Sherman, J. (2015a). Care of the extremely low birth weight (ELBW) infant. In M. T. Verklan & M. Walden (Eds.), *Core curriculum for neonatal intensive care nursing* (pp. 427–438). St. Louis, MO: Elsevier Saunders

Sherman, J. (2015b). Perinatal substance abuse. In M. T. Verklan & M. Walden (Eds.), *Core curriculum for neonatal intensive care nursing* (pp. 43–57). St. Louis, MO: Elsevier Saunders.

Spruill, C. T. (2015). Developmental support. In M. T. Verklan & M. Walden (Eds.), *Core curriculum for neonatal intensive care nursing* (pp. 197–215). St. Louis, MO: Elsevier Saunders.

Steinhorn, R. H. (2015). Pulmonary vascular development. In R. J. Martin, A. A. Fanaroff, & M. C. Walsh (Eds.), *Neonatal-perinatal medicine: Diseases of the fetus and infant* (10th ed., vol. 2, pp. 1198–1209). Philadelphia, PA: Mosby Elsevier.

Sterk, L. (2015). Congenital anomalies. In M. T. Verklan & M. Walden (Eds.), *Core curriculum for neonatal intensive care nursing* (pp. 767–794). St. Louis, MO: Elsevier Saunders.

Substance Abuse and Mental Health Services Administration (SAMHSA). (2015). *Behavioral health trends in the United States: Results from the 2014 national survey on drug use and health* (*HHS* Publication No. SMA 15-4927, NSDUH Series H-50). Retrieved from www.samhsa.gov/data/.

Sun, Y., Hellstrom, A., & Smith, L. E. H. (2015). Retinopathy of prematurity. In R. J. Martin, A. A. Fanaroff, & M. C. Walsh (Eds.), *Neonatal-perinatal medicine: Diseases of the fetus and infant* (10th ed., vol. 2, pp. 1767–1774). Philadelphia, PA: Mosby Elsevier.

Verklan, M. T. (2015). Neurologic disorders. In M. T. Verklan & M. Walden (Eds.), *Core curriculum for neonatal intensive care nursing* (pp. 734–766). St. Louis, MO: Elsevier Saunders.

Wilson, D. J., & Tyner, C. I. (2015). Infectious diseases in the neonate. In M. T. Verklan & M. Walden (Eds.), *Core curriculum for neonatal intensive care nursing* (pp. 689–718). St. Louis, MO: Elsevier Saunders.

Wong, D., Abdel-Latif, M. E., & Kent A. L. (2014). Antenatal steroid exposure and outcomes of very premature infants: A regional cohort study. *Archives of Disease in Childhood—Fetal and Neonatal Edition, 99*(1), 12–20. doi:10.1136/archdischild-2013-305713

Women's Health

18

Well Women's Health

Linda L. Chapman, RN, PhD

LEARNING OUTCOMES

Upon completion of this chapter, the student will be able to:

1. Identify factors that place a woman at risk for adverse health conditions.
2. Discuss preventive screenings for women across the life span.
3. Describe how lifestyle factors such as diet, exercise, and cigarette smoking influence women's health.
4. Discuss the effects of obesity on women's health.
5. Discuss the physical and emotional changes related to perimenopause and menopause.
6. Describe the health care needs of lesbians and their barriers to health care.
7. Develop a health promotion teaching plan for an older adult based on the normal physiological changes related to aging.

Nursing Diagnoses

- At risk for adverse health conditions related to lack of knowledge regarding health promotion
- Knowledge deficit related to menopausal changes
- At risk for disturbed sleep pattern related to night sweats
- At risk for falls related to impaired balance

Nursing Outcomes

- The woman will verbalize two lifestyle changes that can reduce her risk for adverse health conditions.
- The woman will verbalize changes related to menopause and methods to decrease menopausal signs and symptoms.
- The woman will verbalize three strategies for improving disturbed sleep pattern.
- The woman will develop a health promotion plan based on her physiological changes related to aging.

HEALTH PROMOTION

Health promotion is a critical component of women's health (Fig. 18–1). Health promotion is defined by the World Health Organization (WHO) as "the process of enabling people to increase control over, and to improve, their health" (WHO, 2017). Based on this definition, nursing care focuses on providing women with information and resources that enable them to increase control over and improve their health.

Risk Reduction

The following are the leading causes of death in females in the United States:

- Heart disease: 22.3%
- Cancer: 21.6%
- Chronic lower respiratory disease: 6%
- Stroke: 6%
- Alzheimer's disease: 5%

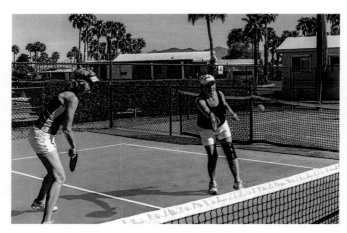

FIGURE 18–1 Health promotion for women of all ages is a critical component for women's health.

- Unintentional injuries/accidents: 3.9%
- Diabetes: 2.7%
- Influenza and pneumonia: 2.2%
- Kidney disease: 1.8%
- Septicemia: 1.6% (CDC, 2017a)

CRITICAL COMPONENT

Heart Attack and Stroke Warning Signs
Heart Attack

Symptoms vary among women and are different from those experienced by men. They can include:

- Uncomfortable pressure, squeezing, fullness, or pain in the center of the chest.
- Pain or discomfort in one or both arms, back, neck, jaw, and/or stomach.
- Shortness of breath with or without chest discomfort.
- Newly developed exercise intolerance.
- Episodic nausea/indigestion.
- Palpitations.
- Abdominal pain.
- Light-headedness.
- Sweating.

Stroke

- Sudden onset of numbness or weakness in the face, arm, and/or leg, especially on one side
- Sudden onset of trouble seeing out of one or both eyes
- Sudden onset of trouble walking, dizziness, loss of balance, or coordination
- Severe headache with no known cause

Department of Health and Human Services (DHHS), 2012.

The leading causes of death in females vary by age groups and race (Table 18–1). Health promotion and risk reduction can prevent or decrease the risk for many of these causes. Actions for reducing risks include:

- Eating a healthy diet that is rich in vegetables, fruits, whole grains, fiber, fat-free or low-fat dairy, and fish, and a diet low in foods that are high in saturated fat and sodium (Fig. 18–2).

The women's diet needs to include 3 cups of low-fat or fat-free milk or low-fat yogurt and/or low-fat cheese for adequate amounts of calcium. This helps to decrease the risk of and/or degree of osteoporosis. Women who cannot get enough calcium in their diets should take a calcium supplement.
- Getting at least 150 minutes of moderate-intensity physical activity per week. This can include brisk walking, swimming, biking, or dancing. Physical activity and weight-bearing exercise improve bone health by slowing bone loss and improving muscle strength and balance. It also helps maintain a healthy weight. Women should consult their health care providers before starting a new exercise program.

CRITICAL COMPONENT

Physical Activity

Physical activity can lower a woman's risk for:

- Heart disease.
- Type 2 diabetes.
- Colon cancer.
- Breast cancer.
- Falls.
- Depression.

CDC, 2015c.

- Receiving the recommended immunization for female adults aged 19 and older (CDC, 2018a):
  - Influenza: annually.
  - Tetanus and diphtheria toxoids/tetanus toxoid, reduced diphtheria toxoid, and acellular pertussis vaccine (Td/Tdap): Substitute Tdap for Td once, then Td every 10 years.
  - Measles, mumps, and rubella vaccine (MMR): 1 dose for adults aged 19 to 59 years; not recommended for adults over age 60 years.
  - Varicella (VAR) vaccine: Adults without evidence of immunity to varicella should receive 2 doses of single-antigen VAR 4 to 8 weeks apart.
  - Herpes zoster vaccine: 1 dose for adults over age 60 years
  - Human papillomavirus (HPV) vaccine: 3 doses for women aged 19 to 26 years

HPV is the most common sexually transmitted virus in the United States. It is the main cause of cervical cancer and genital warts and can cause cancers of the cervix, vulva, vagina, penis, or anus. It can also cause oropharyngeal cancers: cancer in the back of the throat, base of the tongue, and tonsils. There are more than 100 types of HPV:

- Types 6, 11, 40, 42, 53, 54, 61, 72, 73, and 80 cause genital warts.
- Types 6 and 11 are linked to 90% of genital warts cases.
- Types 16, 18, 31, 33, 35, 39, 45, 51, 56, 58, 59, and 60 cause abnormal cells to form on cervix that can develop into cervical cancer.
- Types 16 and 18 are linked to 70% of cervical cancer cases (Qiagen, 2017).

Gardasil, Gardasil 9, and Cervarix are vaccines given to prevent most cases of cervical cancer and genital warts. Gardasil protects

TABLE 18-1   Top 3 Leading Causes of Death in Females by Age Group and Race

AGE	AMERICAN INDIAN/ ALASKA NATIVE	ASIAN OR PACIFIC ISLANDER	BLACK	HISPANIC	WHITE
15–19	• Accidents • Suicide • Homicide	• Suicide • Accidents • Cancers	• Accidents • Homicide • Cancers	• Accidents • Suicide • Cancers	• Accidents • Suicide • Cancers
20–24	• Accidents • Suicide • Homicide	• Accidents • Suicide • Cancers	• Accidents • Homicide • Heart disease	• Accidents • Suicide • Homicide	• Accidents • Suicide • Homicide
25–34	• Accidents • Suicide • Chronic liver disease	• Cancers • Accidents • Suicide	• Heart disease • Accidents • Cancers	• Accidents • Cancers • Suicide	• Accidents • Suicide • Cancers
35–44	• Accidents • Chronic liver disease • Heart disease	• Cancers • Suicide • Accidents	• Cancers • Heart disease • Accidents	• Cancers • Accidents • Heart disease	• Accidents • Cancers • Heart disease
45–54	• Heart disease • Accidents • Cancers	• Cancers • Heart disease • Stroke	• Cancers • Heart disease • Accidents	• Cancers • Heart disease • Accidents	• Cancers • Heart disease • Accidents
55–64	• Cancers • Heart disease • Chronic liver disease	• Cancers • Heart disease • Stroke	• Cancers • Heart disease • Diabetes mellitus	• Cancers • Heart disease • Diabetes mellitus	• Cancers • Heart disease • Accidents
65–74	• Cancers • Heart disease • Diabetes mellitus	• Cancers • Heart disease • Stroke	• Cancers • Heart disease • Stroke	• Cancers • Heart disease • Diabetes mellitus	• Cancers • Heart disease • Chronic lower respiratory diseases
75–84	• Heart disease • Cancers • Chronic lower respiratory disease	• Cancers • Heart disease • Stroke	• Heart disease • Cancers • Stroke	• Heart disease • Cancers • Stroke	• Cancers • Heart disease • Chronic lower respiratory diseases
85+	• Heart disease • Cancers • Alzheimer's disease	• Heart disease • Cancers • Stroke	• Heart disease • Cancer • Stroke	• Heart disease • Cancers • Alzheimer's disease	• Heart disease • Cancers • Alzheimer's disease

Kochanek, Murphy, Xu, & Tejada-Vera, 2016.

against HPV types 6, 11, 16, and 18. Gardasil 9 protects against types 6, 11, 16, 18, 31, 33, 45, 52, and 58. Cervarix protects against types 16 and 18. These vaccines are most effective when given before the person becomes sexually active. Gardasil is recommended for girls and boys aged 11 or 12 years, and Cervarix is recommended for girls and women aged 13 through 26 years.

SAFE AND EFFECTIVE NURSING CARE: Understanding Medication

HPV Vaccine—Gardasil and Gardasil 9
- Indication: Prevention of cancers of the cervix, vulva, vagina, penis, or anus and prevention of genital warts.
- Action: Formation of antibodies to HPV

- Common side effects: Injection site reaction
- Route and dose: Intramuscular; number of doses varies based on age at administration of first dose.
  - Two doses are recommended for person initiating vaccine before age 15 years. Second dose given 6 to 12 months after first dose.
  - Three doses are recommended for persons aged 15 and older. The second dose given 1 to 2 months after first dose; third dose given 6 months after first dose (CDC, 2018a).

Nursing Actions
- Provide information about the vaccine.
- Explain importance of completing the entire series.
- Explain the need for continued routine cervical cancer screening.
- Explain that the vaccine does not prevent STIs.

Vallerand & Sanoski, 2017.

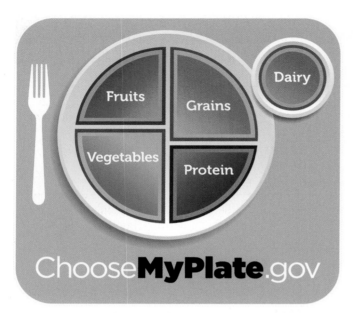

FIGURE 18-2 MyPlate is a tool that can be used when discussing nutrition with a client.

Source: United States Department of Agriculture, http://ChooseMyPlate.gov

- Maintaining a healthy weight.
  - 38.3% of women over age 20 are obese (Ogden, Carroll, Fryer, & Flegel, 2015).
  - 34.4% of women aged 30 to 39 are obese.
  - 42.1% of women aged 40 to 59 are obese.
  - 38.3% of women aged 60 and older are obese (Ogden et al., 2015).
  - Obesity places women at risk for a variety of health problems.

CRITICAL COMPONENT

Obesity

Obesity is defined as a body mass index (BMI) of 30 or higher. Obesity places a woman at higher risk for:
- Hypertension.
- Coronary heart disease.
- Type 2 diabetes.
- Cerebrovascular accident.
- Cholecystitis.
- Sleep apnea.
- Cancer, including endometrial, breast, colon, kidney, gall-bladder, and liver.
- Osteoarthritis of knee, hip, and lower back.
- Abnormal menstrual cycle and infertility.
- High-risk pregnancies related to diabetes and hypertension.

CDC, 2015b.

- Avoiding cigarette smoking and secondhand smoke.
  - Tobacco use is a leading cause of heart disease and cancer.
  - More women die from lung cancer than from cancers of the female genital system (American Cancer Society, 2016c).
  - The estimated number of new cases of cancer in women for 2016 are (American Cancer Society, 2016c):
    - Lung and bronchus: 106,470.
    - Breast: 246,660.
    - Female genital system: 105,890.
- Limiting alcohol consumption.
  - Those who choose to drink alcohol should do so in moderation, which is one drink per day for women.

TABLE 18-2   Recommended Screenings and Immunizations for Women Across the Life Span

SCREENING TESTS	AGES 19–39	AGES 40–49	AGES 50–64	AGES 65 AND OLDER
Blood pressure test	At least every 2 years	At least every 2 years	At least every 2 years	At least every 2 years
Cholesterol test	Start at age 20, get a cholesterol test regularly if at increased risk for heart disease.	Get a cholesterol test regularly if at increased risk for heart disease.	Get a cholesterol test regularly if at increased risk for heart disease.	Get a cholesterol test regularly if at increased risk for heart disease.
Dual-energy x-ray absorptiometry (DXA) scan			Frequency is based on health history and risk for osteoporosis.	Frequency is based on health history and risk for osteoporosis.
Diabetes screening	Screening recommended if blood pressure is higher than 135/80 or if taking medicine for high blood pressure.	Screening recommended if blood pressure is higher than 135/80 or if taking medicine for high blood pressure.	Screening recommended if blood pressure is higher than 135/80 or if taking medicine for high blood pressure.	Screening recommended if blood pressure is higher than 135/80 or if taking medicine for high blood pressure.

TABLE 18-2   Recommended Screenings and Immunizations for Women Across the Life Span—cont'd

SCREENING TESTS	AGES 19–39	AGES 40–49	AGES 50–64	AGES 65 AND OLDER
Mammogram		Discuss with health care provider. (American Cancer Society recommends screening every year for women aged 45–54; women aged 40–45 should have the option to start yearly mammograms.)	Starts at age 50, screening every 2 years. (American Cancer Society recommends screening every year to age 54, then every 2 years age 55 and older.)	Every 2 years through age 74. Age 75 and older, discuss with health care provider. (American Cancer Society recommends screening every 2 years for women age 75 and older if the woman is in good health and expected to live 10 or more years.)
Cervical cancer screening	Get a Pap test every 3 years if woman is 21 or older and has a cervix. If 30 and older, get a Pap test and HPV test together every 5 years.	Get a Pap test and HPV test together every 5 years for women who have a cervix.	Get a Pap test and HPV test together every 5 years for women who have a cervix.	Frequency based on health history.
Pelvic exam	Yearly starting at age 21 or earlier if sexually active.	Yearly	Yearly	Yearly
Chlamydia test	If sexually active, yearly until age 24. Yearly ages 25–39, if new partner or multiple partners.	Yearly if new partner or multiple partners	Yearly if new partner or multiple partners	Yearly if new partner or multiple partners
Sexually transmitted infection (STI) tests	Frequency determined by risk for STI. All pregnant women need to be tested for various STIs.	Frequency determined by risk for STI. All pregnant women need to be tested for various STIs.	Frequency determined by risk for STI.	Frequency determined by risk for STI.
Colonoscopy			Every 10 years starting at age 50; more frequently if at risk for colon cancer	Every 10 years until age 75; more frequently if at risk for colon cancer.
Eye exam	Eye exam if experiencing problems or visual changes.	Baseline exam at age 40, then every 2–4 years.	Every 2–4 years	Every 1–2 years
Hearing test	Every 10 years	Every 10 years	Every 3 years	Every 3 years
Skin exam	Monthly mole self-exam; every 3 years by health care provider starting at age 20	Monthly mole self-exam; yearly by health care provider	Monthly mole self-exam; yearly by health care provider	Monthly mole self-exam; yearly by health care provider
Dental and oral cancer exam	Yearly	Yearly	Yearly	Yearly

American Cancer Society, 2016a; Women's Health, 2013.

- Drinking during pregnancy increases the risk of:
  - Premature birth.
  - Fetal alcohol spectrum disorder.
  - Birth defects such as heart defects and hearing and vision impairments.
  - Low birthweight.
  - Spontaneous abortion.
  - Stillbirth (March of Dimes, 2016).
- Excessive drinking increases a woman's risk for (CDC, 2016a):
  - Infertility.
  - Liver disease.
  - Diabetes.
  - Memory loss and shrinkage of brain.
  - Cancer of the mouth, throat, esophagus, liver, colon, and breast.
  - Heart damage.
- Binge drinking increases the risk for sexual assault, especially for women in college settings (CDC, 2016a).
  - 12% of adult women report binge drinking (5 drinks) 3 times a month.
- Preventing injury from accidents.
  - Motor vehicle crashes are the leading cause of death from injury among younger women.
    - Risk reduction: Wear seat belts, follow speed limits, and do not drink alcohol prior to driving.
  - Injury related to falls are the leading cause of injury, death, and disability for women aged 65 years old or older.
    - Risk reduction: Exercise to improve strength and balance, modify home to reduce fall hazards, wear shoes when walking indoors and outside, and conduct medication assessment to minimize side effects such as dizziness.
- Preventing sexually transmitted illnesses.
  - Use condoms correctly and for all sexual contact.
  - Be in a monogamous relationship—both the woman and her partner have sex only with each other.
  - Both the woman and her partner are screened for sexually transmitted infections (STIs), including HIV, prior to engaging in sexual activities.

Routine Screenings

Screening tests assist the woman's health care provider in identifying potential alterations in health and initiating early interventions. Recommended screenings and immunizations for women are presented in Table 18–2.

Breast Cancer Screening

Early detection of breast cancer when the tumor is small and has not spread provides the best opportunity for successful treatment (American Cancer Society, 2017). Mammograms are recommended for women with average risk for breast cancer; this includes those with no personal or family history of breast cancer and no *BRACA1* or *BRACA2* gene mutation that increases breast cancer risk. MRI screening and mammograms are recommended

for women who are at high risk for breast cancer (American Cancer Society, 2017). Women are considered high risk if they have a known *BRACA1* or *BRACA2* gene mutation and/or a lifetime risk of breast cancer of 20% or greater. Lifetime risk for breast cancer can be calculated using the breast cancer risk assessment tool (www.cancer.gov/bcrisktool). See Table 18–2 for recommended frequency of mammograms and breast MRI. Monthly self-breast exams are no longer recommended, but women should be aware of breast changes that need to be reported to her health care provider (Fig. 18–3).

CRITICAL COMPONENT

Screening Mammograms

A mammogram uses a specially designed low-dose x-ray machine to take an image of the breast to detect abnormal changes. Each breast (one at a time) is placed between the x-ray plate and plastic plate. Pressure is gradually increased to flatten the breast, allowing a clearer picture to be obtained. Women may experience a sense of the breast being squeezed or pinched. The radiologist will compare the present x-ray with previous breast x-rays, looking for changes, lumps/masses, and calcifications. When abnormities are identified on a screening mammogram, further testing is needed; this may include a diagnostic mammogram, ultrasound, MRI, or biopsy. Women with breast implants must inform the mammogram facility, as implants can hide some of the breast tissue. Women should not wear any deodorants, perfume, lotion, or powder under their arms or on their breasts on the day of the appointment. These substances can make shadows on the x-ray.
DHHS, 2013.

Cervical Cancer Screening

Healthy People 2020 objectives for cervical cancer screening are as follows:

- Increase the proportion of women who receive cervical cancer screening based on the most current guideline, from 84.5% to 93% of females aged 21 to 65 years.
- Increase the proportion of women counseled by their provider about Pap tests, from 59.8% to 65.8% of females aged 21 to 65 years (Healthy People 2020, 2017).

Current cervical cancer screening recommendations include the following:

- Women aged 21 to 29 years should have a Pap test every 3 years.
- Women aged 30 to 65 years should be screened with a Pap test combined with an HPV test every 5 years.
- Women older than age 65 years can stop cervical cancer screening if they have not had any precancerous cells found in the previous 20 years.
- Women who had a total hysterectomy should stop screening, unless hysterectomy was due to cervical precancer or cancer (American Cancer Society, 2016b).

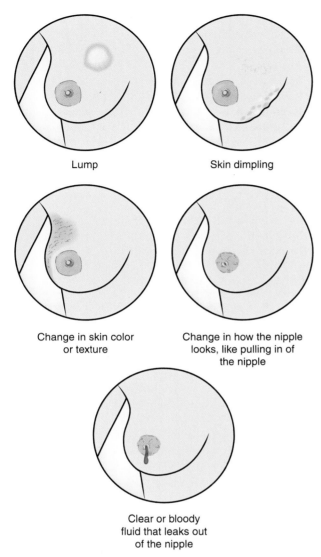

Lump

Skin dimpling

Change in skin color or texture

Change in how the nipple looks, like pulling in of the nipple

Clear or bloody fluid that leaks out of the nipple

FIGURE 18–3 Visual signs of breast cancer.

CRITICAL COMPONENT

Papanicolaou (Pap) Smear

The Pap test is a microscopic examination of cells taken from the cervix. This screening test is primarily used for early detection of cancerous or precancerous cells. During the test, a speculum is inserted into the vagina and both cervical and vaginal specimens are obtained using a synthetic fiber brush and plastic spatula. An abnormal result needs to be followed up with further testing. The best time to get a Pap test is 5 days after the end of the menstrual period. The woman should not douche or use tampons, vaginal creams, spermicide foams, creams, jellies, lubricants, moisturizers, or medications for 48 hours prior to the test. She should not have sexual intercourse for 48 hours prior to the test.

American Cancer Society, 2016b.

REPRODUCTIVE CHANGES ACROSS THE LIFE SPAN

Throughout a woman's lifetime, her body undergoes physical changes related to hormonal changes. Major reproductive changes occur during puberty and before and after menopause.

Puberty

During puberty, a person becomes sexually mature and capable of reproduction. In girls, the onset of puberty usually occurs between ages 8 and 13, accompanied by accelerated growth of the body that usually begins with the feet and ends with the face. Puberty is triggered by the production of gonadotropin-releasing hormone from the hypothalamus, which stimulates the anterior pituitary to release gonadotropins. Gonadotropins stimulate the ovaries to secrete estrogen (Fig. 18–4). Estrogen is responsible for the development of secondary sex characteristics in females, including:

- Enlargement of breasts: growth of the duct system of the mammary glands and erection of nipples.
- Growth of body hair: axillary and pubic hair.
- Widening of the hips.

Menarche, the initial menstrual period, usually occurs 2 to 2.5 years after the beginning of puberty. Puberty is completed when menstruation assumes a regular pattern. For more on the menstrual cycle, see Chapter 3.

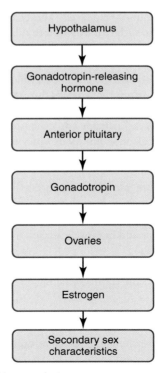

FIGURE 18–4 Hormonal triggers.

Menopause

Menopause is the stage of life that marks the permanent cessation of menstrual activity. This natural biological process usually occurs between ages 35 and 58. Menopause is divided into three stages:

- Perimenopause: Usually in her forties, the woman begins to experience menopausal signs and symptoms that last for 4 to 8 years. During this period of time, the woman experiences irregular menstrual cycles. It is possible for the woman to become pregnant during this stage.
- Menopause: Occurs 12 months after a woman's last menstrual period. Average age in United States is age 51 with a range of 48 to 58 years of age.
- Postmenopause: Refers to the time after menopause.

As a woman enters her late 30s, the quality and quantity of her ova gradually decline, resulting in a gradual decline in the production of estrogen and progesterone. The woman will begin to experience changes in her body related to the decreasing levels of these hormones. These changes are often referred to as signs and symptoms of menopause.

Signs and Symptoms of Menopause

- Irregular periods
  - The time between cycles may become longer or shorter.
  - Menstrual flow may become heavier or lighter.
  - Cycles become anovulatory, and the woman is no longer fertile.
- Hot flashes
  - Hot flashes are the most common symptom of menopause.
  - This symptom is caused by a vasomotor response to changes in the hormonal levels. This change triggers blood vessels near the surface of the skin to dilate, causing an increase of blood supply and subsequent increase of heat to the skin surface.
  - When a woman experiences a hot flash, she feels a sudden sensation of warmth that spreads through her upper body and face. Her neck and face become red, and she begins to sweat and may feel irritable and exhausted.
  - Warm rooms, alcohol, hot foods, spicy foods, caffeine, and stress can trigger a hot flash.
- Night sweats
  - Night sweats are hot flashes that occur while the woman is sleeping.
  - Women who experience night sweats will wake up with their bed linens and nightwear soaked from sweat.
- Sleep disturbances
  - Women may experience altered sleep patterns related to night sweats and difficulty falling asleep and staying asleep.
- Sexual dysfunction
  - Sexual desire and arousal disorders may occur.
  - Some women experience vaginal atrophy as declining estrogen levels cause vaginal tissue to become thinner and drier.
  - Dyspareunia is also related to vaginal dryness.

- Psychological side effects may include:
  - Mood swings.
  - Irritability.
  - Anxiety.
  - Lethargy.
  - Lack of energy.
  - Panic attacks.
  - Forgetfulness.
  - Difficulty coping.
  - Depression.
- Women may also experience:
  - Thinning of hair or hair loss.
  - Food cravings.
  - Dry skin and loss of skin elasticity.
  - Weight gain, especially around the waist and hips.
  - Irregular heartbeat and palpitations.

Treating Menopausal Symptoms

There are three approaches for the treatment of menopausal symptoms: lifestyle changes, alternative medicine, and menopause hormone therapy (MHT).

- Lifestyle changes
  - Get 8 hours of sleep per night.
  - Eat a balanced diet.
  - Women who are overweight or obese should lose weight.
  - Exercise.
  - Avoid caffeine and alcohol.
  - Avoid cigarette smoking and secondhand smoke.
- Alternative medicine
  - Herbal supplements
    - Inform health care provider of herbal supplements used. Black cohosh treatment has no proven benefit and may place the woman at risk for liver toxicity (Allmen, 2016).
  - Acupuncture
  - Biofeedback
  - Hypnosis
- Menopausal hormone therapy (MHT).
  - There are conflicting research findings on the safety of MHT. Women need to talk with their health care providers as to the benefits and risks of MHT.
  - Estrogen alone is prescribed for women who do not have a uterus.
    - Types of preparations are oral, transdermal, and vaginal
  - Estrogen and progesterone therapy are prescribed for women who have a uterus. The use of progesterone with estrogen therapy reduces the risk of endometrial cancer.
    - Types of preparations are oral, transdermal, and progesterone intrauterine device.
  - Dosage of MHT are based on severity of symptoms. Usually started at a middle dose range and increased or decreased as needed. Women in their 60s are usually prescribed lower dose transdermal preparation.
  - Length of use of MHT varies and women may continue using MRT into their 70s (Allmen, 2016).
  - Estrogen is contraindicated for women who have:

- Unexplained vaginal bleeding.
- Liver disease.
- Gallbladder disease.
- Blood-clotting disorders.
- Pulmonary embolism.
- Untreated hypertension.
- Uterine cancer.
- Breast cancer.

CRITICAL COMPONENT

Position Statement: Hormone Therapy

Hormone therapy is the most effective treatment for menopausal symptoms such as hot flashes and vaginal dryness. If women have only vaginal dryness or discomfort with intercourse, the preferred treatments are low doses of vaginal estrogen. Hot flashes generally require a higher dose of hormone therapy that will have an effect on the entire body.

Women who still have a uterus need to take a progestogen (progesterone or a similar product) along with the estrogen to prevent cancer of the uterus. Five years or less is usually the recommended duration of use for this combined treatment, but the length of time can be individualized for each woman.

Women who have had their uterus removed can take estrogen alone. Because of the apparent greater safety of estrogen alone, there may be more flexibility in how long women can safely use estrogen therapy.

North American Menopause Society, American Society of Reproductive Medicine, and the Endocrine Society, 2018.

Treatment for Specific Menopausal Discomforts

- Hot flashes: Avoid alcohol, hot beverages, spicy foods, warm rooms, and smoking; these can trigger hot flashes. Dress in layers, so that the woman can remove clothing as she becomes warm and add clothing as she cools down. Avoid wearing clothing made from wool or synthetics. Use of fans is also helpful.
  - Medications used to treat other conditions that have been shown to decrease hot flashes include low-dose antidepressants such as fluoxetine (Prozac), the antiseizure medication gabapentin (Neurontin), and antihypertensive clonidine (Catapres) (Mayo Clinic Staff, 2015).
- Night sweats: Sleep in cotton nightwear. Use cotton bed linens. Sleep in cool room. Sleep with fan blowing over body. Take a cool shower before bedtime.
- Sleep disturbances: Establish a regular bedtime pattern. Do not watch TV or use the computer in bed. Keep the bedroom dark, quiet, and cool. Wear loose-fitting, breathable garments. Leave cell phone in another room at night. Eat dinner early and avoid alcohol and caffeine close to bedtime.
- Sexual dysfunctions related to vaginal dryness: Use water-based lubricants during sexual intercourse. Use vaginal moisturizers. Use estrogen vaginal cream. Soy flour and flax-seeds in the woman's diet may prevent or decrease the degree of vaginal dryness.

- Physiological: Establish a daily physical exercise program. Limit alcohol consumption. Increase exposure to natural light or use light box to treat seasonal affective disorder.
  - MHT may be prescribed in addition to lifestyle changes.
  - Psychotherapy and medications for depression or anxiety may be used when physiological symptoms have not improved with previously mentioned methods.

Nursing Actions

The focus of nursing actions is patient education. Topics should include:

- Physiological and emotional changes related to menopause, stressing that menopause is a natural phase of a woman's life.
- Discussion of the individual woman's premenopausal symptoms and methods she uses for relief of these symptoms, including medications, lifestyle changes, and alternative medicines.
- Discussion of additional treatments for specific symptoms, including lifestyle changes, medications, and alternative medicine.

OSTEOPOROSIS

Osteoporosis is the loss of bone mass that occurs when more bone mass is absorbed than the body creates. Bone mass in women usually decreases after age 35 at a rate of 0.3% to 0.5%. Osteoporosis affects both men and women, but 80% of Americans diagnosed with osteoporosis are women. Women who experience osteoporosis are at greater risk for vertebral and hip fractures. The Fracture Risk Assessment Tool was developed by WHO to calculate the 10-year probability of fractures. This tool can be viewed at www.shef.ac.uk/FRAX/tool.jsp?locationValue=9.

Osteoporosis is diagnosed with a dual-energy x-ray absorptiometry (DXA) scan, which measures the bone density in the hip, spine, and forearm. These numbers are compared to the average peak density for those of the same sex and race, assigning a number called a T score:

- A T score of −2.5 or below is indicative of osteoporosis.
- A T score of −1 to −2.5 is indicative of osteopenia, which is lower than normal bone density that puts the person at risk for osteoporosis.

Signs and Symptoms

- Back pain related to a fracture or collapsed vertebrae
- Loss of height related to collapsed vertebrae
- Stooped posture related to collapsed vertebrae
- Bone fractures related to bone weakness

Risk Factors for Osteoporosis

Those at higher risk for developing osteoporosis include:

- Caucasian women.
- Thin, small-boned women.
- Those with a family history of hip fractures.

- Current smokers.
- Those with an inactive lifestyle.
- Those deficient in calcium and vitamin D.
  - Vitamin D assists in calcium absorption.
- Those who consume three or more alcohol drinks each day.
- Those who take certain medications, including:
  - Corticosteroids for more than 3 months
  - Aromatase inhibitors
  - Proton pump inhibitors
- Those with a BMI less than or equal to 20 (adult weight under 127 pounds).
- Those with a history of eating disorders such as anorexia.
- Those who have had weight loss surgery.

Risk Reduction

- Maintain a diet high in calcium and vitamin D. This should start around 9 years of age to help form a strong bone matrix and should continue throughout the woman's life based on these guidelines:
  - 1,300 mg of calcium for girls aged 9 to 18 years
  - 1,000 mg of calcium/day for women aged 19 to 50 years (premenopausal)
  - 1,200 mg of calcium for women aged 51 years and older (menopausal)
  - 600 IU of vitamin D/day for girls and women 9 to 70
  - 800 mg/day of calcium for women older than 70 years of age (American College of Obstetricians and Gynecologists [ACOG], 2012b).
- Engage in weight-bearing exercise.
  - Walking, jogging, dancing, and weight lifting three to four times/week
- Avoid smoking.
  - Avoid both firsthand and secondhand smoke.
- Limit alcohol use.
  - Heavy drinking is linked to lower bone density.

CRITICAL COMPONENT

Calcium-Rich Foods
- Canned sardines (3 oz.): 325 mg
- Plain low-fat yogurt (4 oz.): 310 mg
- Cheddar cheese (1.5 oz.): 307 mg
- Orange juice, calcium fortified (8 oz.): 300 mg
- Cheddar cheese (1.5 oz.): 307 mg
- Milk, 2% milk fat (8 oz.): 300 mg
- Almond milk, rice milk, or soy milk: 300 mg
- Salmon (3 oz.): 181 mg
- Kale, frozen (8 oz.): 180 mg

Pharmacotherapy

The American College of Obstetricians and Gynecologists (ACOG) recommends osteoporosis pharmacotherapy for:

- Women who have experienced a fragility or low-impact fracture.
- Women with a DXA T score of less than or equal to –2.5.

- Women with risk factors and with a DXA T score of less than –1.5 (ACOG, 2012b).

Pharmacotherapy includes the drugs in the following sections.

Bisphosphonates

Action: Inhibits resorption of bone, the process where breakdown of bone and release of minerals occurs with the resulting transfer of calcium from the bone fluid to the blood.

Adverse effects: Musculoskeletal aches and pains, gastrointestinal irritation, and esophageal ulcerations.

- Alendronate (Fosamax)
  - Prevention: 5 mg/day or 35 mg/week
  - Treatment: 10 mg/day or 70 mg/week
- Ibandronate (Boniva)
  - Prevention and treatment: 150 mg/month
  - Treatment: 3 mg every 3 months by IV
- Risedronate (Actonel)
  - Prevention and treatment: 5 mg/day
- Zoledronate (Reclast)
  - Prevention: 5 mg every 2 years by IV
  - Treatment: 5 mg every year by IV

CRITICAL COMPONENT

Bisphosphonates
To reduce side effects and to enhance absorption of the oral medication, the woman should:
- Take the medication in the morning on an empty stomach at least 30 minutes before breakfast.
- Take the medication with at least 8 oz. of water (do not take with juice, coffee, or tea, as these can ↓ absorption of medication).
- Take the medication in a sitting or standing position to decrease the risk of the pill becoming lodged in the esophagus where it can cause ulcerations and scarring.
- Remain upright for at least 30 minutes to decrease the risk of reflux of the pill into the esophagus.

Vallerand & Sanoski, 2017.

Estrogen-Receptor Modulators

Action: Binds with estrogen receptors, producing estrogen-like effects on bone and reduces resorption of bone (Vallerand & Sanoski, 2017)

Adverse effects: Venous thromboembolism, leg cramps, and death from stroke

- Raloxifene (Evista)
  - Prevention and treatment: 60 mg/day

Hormone Therapy

- Conjugated estrogen + medroxyprogesterone acetate (Premphase)
  - Prevention: 0.625 mg of conjugated estrogen once daily on days 1 to 14 and 5 mg medroxyprogesterone acetate once daily on days 15 to 28

- Prescribed for women who have a uterus
- Contraindicated for women with known or suspected estrogen-dependent neoplasia
- Conjugated estrogen (Premarin)
  - Prevention: 0.3 to 1.25 mg/day
  - Prescribed for women who do not have a uterus
  - Contraindicated for women with known or suspected estrogen-dependent neoplasia

Other Medications

- Denosumab (Prolia)
- Teriparatide (Forteo)
  - Use with postmenopausal women who are at high risk for fractures; for women with osteoporosis associated with sustained, systemic glucocorticoid
  - Daily subcutaneous injection: 20 mcg

SAFE AND EFFECTIVE NURSING CARE: Understanding Medication

Denosumab (Prolia)
- Indication: Treatment of osteoporosis in individuals who cannot take bisphosphonates, such as people with reduced kidney function.
- Actions: ↓ bone resorption with ↓ occurrence of vertebral and hip fractures
- Route and dose: Subcutaneous; 60 mg every 6 months
- Common side effects: Cystitis, hypocalcemia, hypophosphatemia, hypercholesterolemia, back pain, extremity pain, musculoskeletal pain, dyspnea
- Nursing actions: Encourage woman to have routine dental exam and care since medication places her at risk for osteonecrosis of the jaw.

Vallerand & Sanoski, 2017.

Nursing Actions

The primary nursing action is patient education. A teaching plan should include the following:

- Discussion of risk factors for osteoporosis and fracture related to osteoporosis.
- Information on fall prevention:
  - Remove throw rugs from home.
  - Keep floors clear of objects such as books, paper, shoes.
  - Ensure stairways are well lit.
  - Install grab bars near shower, tub, and toilet.
  - Have annual eye exams and update glasses.
  - Limit alcohol use.
  - Wear shoes inside and outside (CDC, 2015a).
- Reason for bone density assessment and what to expect when having a DXA scan.
- Discussion on foods high in calcium and vitamin D.

- Discussion on physical activity that can decrease risk for osteoporosis.
- Discussion on prescribed medication—explain reason for prescribed medication, dose, route, and side effects.
- Discussion, as needed, on avoiding smoking and use of alcohol.

SPECIFIC POPULATIONS

Nurses who specialize in women's health should be aware of the needs of certain specific populations.

Adolescent Health

Adolescence, ages 12 to 19 years, is a time of physical, cognitive, and psychosocial development.

- Physical: Biological changes that occur include sexual maturity (development of primary and secondary sex changes), increases in height and weight (adolescent female will grow 2 to 8 inches and gain 15 to 55 pounds), and completion of skeletal growth.
- Cognitive: The adolescent moves from being a concrete thinker to thinking abstractly, using logic to solve problems, using deductive reasoning, and planning for the future. Adolescents begin to be concerned with moral and social issues and compare their beliefs with those of their peers.
- Psychosocial: The adolescent is working toward role identity—who they are and who they will be in life. They develop a set of personal moral and ethical values and a greater sense of self-esteem and self-worth as well as a satisfactory sexual identity.

Most adolescents are physically healthy but are at risk for major health problems. Health problems and issues for female adolescents include:

- Unintentional injuries, suicide, and homicides—these are the leading causes of death for females aged 15 to 19.
- Eating disorders—obesity, anorexia, and bulimia.
- Sexually transmitted illnesses—chlamydia and gonorrhea are prevalent in adolescents.
- Teen pregnancies—249,078 babies born to women aged 15 to 19 years (CDC, 2016b).
- Issues related to self-esteem—20% of high school students report being electronically bullied, and 15% report being bullied on school property (CDC, 2018b).
- Menstrual disorders.
- Acne.

The 2015 National Youth Risk Surveillance surveyed high school students throughout the United States from September 2014 to December 2015. The survey's questionnaire focused on six categories of primary health behaviors among youth: behaviors that contribute to unintentional injuries and violence; tobacco use; alcohol and other drug use; sexual behaviors related to unintentional pregnancy and STIs; unhealthy dietary behaviors; and physical inactivity (Kann et al., 2016). Table 18–3 provides a sample of the results for high school females.

TABLE 18-3 Youth Risk Behavior Surveillance (Female)—United States 2015

THE PERCENTAGE OF HIGH SCHOOL FEMALE STUDENTS WHO:	BLACK	HISPANIC	WHITE
Rarely or never wore a bicycle helmet	85.6	90.3	75.3
Rarely or never wore seat belts	7.6	6.3	3.5
Rode with a driver who had been drinking alcohol	21.2	27.3	17.5
Drove when they had been drinking alcohol	5.1	8	5.4
Texted or e-mailed while driving a car	33.1	28.2	45.3
Carried weapons	6.2	7.1	8.1
Carried weapons on school property	2.1	2.9	1.6
Were in physical fights	25.4	18.6	13.5
Were electronically bullied	11.9	16.7	26
Were bullied on school property	15.1	12.4	29.1
Were physically forced to have sexual intercourse	10.3	10.1	9.9
Experienced physical dating violence	12.2	11.4	11.9
Experienced sexual dating violence	11.7	14.2	16.6
Felt sad or hopeless	33.9	46.7	37.9
Seriously considered attempting suicide	18.7	25.6	22.8
Attempted suicide	10.2	15.1	9.8
Currently smoke cigarettes	0.8	2.1	4.4
Currently use smokeless tobacco	2.5	1.1	2.5
Currently use electronic vapor products	25	14.5	24.2
Currently drink alcohol	25.9	35.6	35.3
Drink 5 or more drinks of alcohol in a row	9.9	17.9	18.6
Currently use marijuana	22.1	23.5	18.7
Ever used cocaine	6.6	1.8	3.3
Ever used Ecstasy	2.5	4.1	4
Ever used heroin	1.5	1.9	0.8
Ever had sexual intercourse	37.4	39.8	40.3
Had sexual intercourse with 4 or more persons	9.2	6.7	9.2
Are currently sexually active	35.7	30.1	31.4
Used a condom during last sexual intercourse	46.7	48.3	55.9
Did not eat fruit	5.2	4	4.3
Did not eat vegetables	8.8	7.7	3.7
Drank 2 or more glasses/day of milk	5.8	12.8	17.8
Drank a can or bottle or glass of soda two or more times/day	15	11.4	9
Were physically active at least 60 minutes/day on 5 or more days in last 7 days	33.4	33.1	43.5
Played video or computer games or used computer for 3 or more hours/day	48.4	47.4	38.3
Watched 3 or more hours/day of television	41.5	29.2	18.8

Kann et al., 2016.

Nursing Actions

Nurses working in the middle school and high school settings are ideally positioned to promote healthy behaviors in adolescents. School nurses are often viewed by youth as safe adults to turn to for issues regarding health or body changes or sexual information. School nurses can provide health information and risk reduction information to large groups of adolescents based on the needs of their school's population. They can also advocate for the availability of health resources for youth in their school districts.

Lesbian Health

Lesbian, gay, bisexual, and transgender (LGBT) individuals experience health disparities related to societal stigma, discrimination, and denial of civil rights (Healthy People 2020, 2017). *Healthy People 2010*'s report identified the need for more research to document, understand, and address the factors that contribute to the health disparities in the LGBT communities. A result of this report, *Healthy People 2020* set a goal to improve the health, safety, and well-being of LGBT individuals (Healthy People 2020, 2017).

Lesbians face barriers to quality health care, such as lack of health insurance, fear of negative reaction from health care provider due to sexual orientation, and lack of understanding by health care providers of lesbian health issues. Lesbians see their health care provider less often than do heterosexual women and seek medical care at a later stage than heterosexual women (Dibble & Robertson, 2010). Health issues for lesbians include:

- Cancer: Higher risk for breast, cervical, endometrial, and ovarian cancer because lesbians have higher rates of smoking, alcohol use, and obesity than do heterosexual women (Dibble & Robertson, 2010).
- Obesity: Lesbians tend to have higher body mass than heterosexual women, resulting in higher risk for heart disease and cancer (Eliason & Drabble, 2010).
- Polycystic ovarian syndrome (PCOS): PCOS is a common hormonal reproductive problem of all women. It appears more frequently in lesbians and increases women's risk for menstrual disorders, infertility, abnormal insulin production, and heart disease.
- Osteoporosis: Higher risk for osteoporosis due to smoking, alcohol, and/or antidepressant use.
- Heart disease: Higher risk for heart disease due to higher rates of smoking and obesity.
- Tobacco, alcohol, and substance use: Use of these substances is higher in lesbians compared to heterosexual women.
- Domestic violence: Domestic violence occurs in lesbian relationships. All women need to be screened for domestic violence. There are few agencies that exclusively address domestic violence in lesbian relationships.

Nursing Actions

For some lesbians, family friends replace their family of origin. When attending health-promotion support groups such as weight control, smoking cessation, or Alcoholic Anonymous, lesbians sometimes prefer groups that are primarily lesbian. They are more likely to use alternative health care (Dibble & Robertson, 2010).

Patient education is the primary nursing action to assist lesbians in understanding the importance of health promotion. Primary areas of health promotion education include:

- Routine screening and immunization.
- Exercise to assist in weight control and bone health.
- Healthy diet and weight reduction.
- Smoking cessation and avoiding secondhand smoke.
- Limiting alcohol use.
- Safety planning and resources for women who are experiencing domestic violence.
- Risk deduction for osteoporosis.

SAFE AND EFFECTIVE NURSING CARE: Cultural Competence

ACOG COMMITTEE OPINION: Health Care for Lesbians and Bisexual Women

Lesbians and bisexual women encounter barriers to health care that include concerns about confidentiality and disclosure, discriminatory attitudes and treatment, limited access to health care and health insurance, and often a limited understanding as to what their health care risks may be. Health care providers should offer quality care to all women regardless of sexual orientation. The American College of Obstetricians and Gynecologists endorse equitable treatment for lesbians and bisexual women and their families, not only for direct health care needs, but also for indirect health care issues.

ACOG, 2012a.

Geriatric Health

From conception until death, the human body is aging. Early in life, aging is viewed as a process of developing and maturing. Later in life, it can be viewed as a time of decline of health or loss of function. Health promotion is aimed at minimizing the effects of normal aging and maximizing quality of life for older adults.

Evidence-Based Practice: Effectiveness of Dancing to Improve Older Adults' Health

Hwang, P., & Braun, K. (2015). The effectiveness of dance interventions to improve older adults' health: A systematic literature review. *Alternative Therapies in Health and Medicine, 21,* 64–70.

Eighteen research studies that evaluated the benefits of a dance intervention to the physical health of older adults were systematically reviewed. Styles of dancing included ballroom, contemporary, cultural (Greek, Turkish, Korean, Cantonese, and line dancing), and jazz. Aerobic fitness classes taught to music, such as Zumba, were excluded. Average age of participants in the 18 studies ranged from 52 to 78. Two of the studies targeted older adults with preexisting medical conditions. The review of the 18 articles grouped studies' measurements into six measurement categories: flexibility, muscular strength/endurance/balance, cardiovascular endurance, cognation, and body composition.

The findings of this systematic review of 18 articles "suggest that dance, regardless of its style, can significantly improve muscle strength and endurance, balance and other aspects of functional fitness in older adults" (Hwang & Braun, 2015, p 64).

Age-Related Physiological Changes and Health Promotion

Table 18–4 provides an overview of the common changes that occur in older adults and recommendations for minimizing the effects of these changes.

- Dry skin and itching
  - Causes
    - Decreased fluid intake
    - Decreased humidity
    - Loss of sweat and oil glands
    - Increased time in the sun
    - Smoking
    - Health problems such as diabetes or kidney disease
  - Health promotion
    - Increase fluid intake to 8 or more glasses taken throughout the day.
    - Apply moisturizers/lotions daily.
    - Use a humidifier in dry climates.
    - Use mild soaps and warm water instead of hot water.
    - Limit time in the sun, use sunscreens, and wear protective clothing when in the sun.
- Nutrition
  - Diet is a factor in the development of type 2 diabetes, coronary heart disease, atherosclerosis, stroke, and cancer.
  - Obesity increases the risk for osteoarthritis of the knee, hip, and lower back, which can limit mobility in older adults.
  - Factors that may affect an older adult's ability to eat well include:
    - Living alone
    - Depression—decreased interest in food
    - Mouth pain
    - Limited income
    - Decreased ability to taste food—certain medications can interfere with ability to taste; gum disease and issues with dentures can leave a bad taste in the mouth; alcohol and smoking can alter how food tastes.

TABLE 18–4 Age-Related Physiological Changes and Health Promotion

PHYSIOLOGICAL CHANGES	POTENTIAL EFFECT ON OLDER ADULTS	HEALTH PROMOTION
↓Muscle mass	↓Strength	• Strength training • Healthy diet
↓Total body water & ↓renal tubular secretion and reabsorption	↑Risk for dehydration	• Minimum fluid intake of 8 glasses; intake spread throughout the day
↓Smell and ↓taste	↓Appetite	• Maintain healthy gums and teeth • Use "color" in food presentation to make food more interesting
↓Metabolism	↑Body fat and ↓muscle mass	• ↓Decrease calorie intake • ↑Physical activity • Strength training
↓T-cells	↑Risk for infections	• Healthy diet • Appropriate hand-washing technique to ↓ risk of infections
↓Lung tissue elasticity; ↓Ability to clearing of the tracheobronchial tree	↑Risk for pneumonia	• ↑Physical activity • Healthy diet • Yearly influenza vaccination (PPSV23)
↓T-cells; ↑DNA damage with ↓DNA repair capacity	↑Risk for cancer	• Cancer screening for early detection of cancers
Loss of high-frequency hearing	↓Ability to recognize speech	• Hearing evaluation and treatment for hearing loss
↓Peripheral vision; ↓depth perception; cataracts	↓Eyesight	• Eye evaluation and treatment as indicated • Sunglasses when driving in sunlight
↓Intestinal motility	↑Incidents of constipation	• Daily exercise • Stay hydrated • Include fruit, vegetables in diet, whole grains, and probiotics in diet

TABLE 18–4 Age-Related Physiological Changes and Health Promotion—cont'd

PHYSIOLOGICAL CHANGES	POTENTIAL EFFECT ON OLDER ADULTS	HEALTH PROMOTION
↓Elasticity of bladder wall; Weakening of bladder; Urethra blockage due to prolapsed uterus; cystocele	↑Risk for frequency of urination, urinary incontinence and cystitis	• Kegel exercises • Maintain ideal weight—obesity can contribute to incontinence • Bladder training—gradually delay urination after getting urge • Double voiding • Timed voiding—urinating on a schedule
Muscle weakness in legs; vertigo; balance difficulties; vision changes; dehydration; hypotension; confusion; foot disorders; arthritis of lower extremities	↑Risk for falls	• Fall risk evaluation: develop prevention plan based on evaluation • Home environment: appropriate lighting; remove loose carpets and floor clutter; install grab bars in bathroom • Adjust medications as indicated • Footwear with flat, nonskid soles • Yearly vision evaluations and appropriate eye glasses
Osteoporosis	↑Risk for fractures	• Increase intake of foods high in calcium • Take 600–800 IU of vitamin D • Engage in weight-bearing such as walking • Stop smoking
Deposits of lipofuscin; valves thicken; wall of heart thickens; ↑heart size	↑Risk for cardiovascular disease ↑Risk for hypertension ↑Risk for atrial fibrillation Heart murmurs	• Heart healthy diet • Exercise • Do not smoke • Treatment, as indicated, for diabetes, hypertension, hyperlipidemia
↓Sensitivity of baroreceptors	↑ Risk for orthostatic hypotension	• Slowly rise from sitting or prone positions
Atherosclerosis; cardiovascular diseases; atrial fibrillation	↑Risk for cerebrovascular accident	• Healthy diet low in saturated fats, trans fats, cholesterol and sodium • Treat, as indicated, hypertension, diabetes, peripheral artery disease, atrial fibrillation • ↑Physical activity
↓Hepatic mass and blood flow; ↓glomerular filtration	↑Risk for adverse drug reactions	• Inform health care provider and pharmacist of all medications—prescribed, over-the-counter and herbal—that are being taken • Follow direction for taking medications • Report any physical or mental changes to health care provider
↓Prefrontal cortex and the hippocampus	Alteration in learning, memory, planning, and other complex mental activities	• Prevention or control of hypertension and diabetes • Take 2.4 mcg of vitamin B12; helps the brain, blood, and nervous system • Exercise and physical activity • Healthy diet • Engage in intellectually stimulating activities • Maintaining relationships with family, friends, and community

- Health promotion
  - Take a detailed dietary history that provides information on the woman's eating habits.
  - Assist the woman in identifying ways to modify her diet to enhance her health.
  - Address medical conditions that may interfere with appetite or ability to taste food or chew.
- Mouth care
  - Oral health is important to the overall health of older adults.
  - Healthy teeth and gums facilitate the older adult's ability to eat well and enjoy food.
  - Health promotion
    - Brush teeth twice a day with fluoride toothpaste.
    - Floss once a day.
    - Regular dental checkups every 6 months.
    - Quit smoking.
    - Eat a healthy diet and maintain hydration.
- Medications
  - Older adults are more sensitive to medications, due to slower metabolisms and organ function. The digestive systems, liver, and kidney functions slow as a person ages. These changes affect the degree that drugs are absorbed into the bloodstream, how they react in the organs, and how quickly they are eliminated.
  - Older people take more medications than younger people, which increases possible drug interactions.
  - Health promotion
    - Take medications as directed. Report side effects to health care provider.
    - Make a list of all medications (prescribed, over-the-counter, vitamins, and supplements), including name, dose, and reason for taking them. Bring list to each medical and dental office visit and share information with health care providers.
    - Create a file for all medications with all written information that came with the medication.
    - Check expiration dates and take outdated medication to pharmacy for proper disposal.
- Sexual health
  - Older women are sexually active.
  - Age does not affect the woman's capacity to have an orgasm. The clitoris remains sensitive to stimulation and continues to increase in size when sexually aroused. Intensity of orgasm may decrease as the woman ages.
  - Frequency of sexual intercourse may decrease as a woman ages.
  - Changes related to declining estrogen levels cause vaginal dryness, burning, irritation, itchiness, discharge, and pain on penetration.
  - Decreased libido may be related to decreased levels of estrogen and testosterone. Women in their 60s have two times less testosterone than women in their twenties.
  - Health promotion

- Maintain a physically fit state through exercise and healthy diet. This will promote a more energetic life that can create more energy for sex.
- Local vaginal estrogen applied to the vulva and vagina promotes vaginal health and treats vaginal atrophy and dryness.
- Consider medication for hypoactive sexual desire disorder, prescribed for perimenopausal women who had a normal interest in sex but now feel distress that they have lost this desire.
- Encourage open discussion with her partner, sharing feelings about sex and changes that have occurred in her body and her partner's body.
- Women who do not have a partner or have a partner who is not sexually active should weekly masturbate with or without a vibrator to promote vaginal health. Masturbation increases blood flow to the genital tissues (Allmen, 2016).

SAFE AND EFFECTIVE NURSING CARE: Understanding Medication

Estradiol Cream (Estrace Cream)

- Indication: Management of atrophic vaginitis related to menopause
- Action: Lessens:
  - Dryness and soreness in the vagina
  - Itching, redness, or soreness of the vulva
  - Feeling an urge to urinate more often than is needed or experiencing pain while urinating
  - Pain during sexual intercourse
- Route and dose: Vaginal; 2 to 4 g daily for 1 to 2 weeks, then ↓ to 1 to 2 g for 1 to 2 weeks, then maintenance dose of 1 g 1 to 3 times weekly for 3 weeks, then off for 1 week
- Side effects: Breast pain, enlarged breasts, itching of the vagina or genitals, headache, nausea, stinging or redness of the genital areas, and thick, white vaginal discharge without odor or with a mild odor.
- Nursing actions:
  - Provide instruction on proper administration of medications.
  - Recommend use at bedtime to increase effectiveness of absorption.
  - To limit exposure to male sexual partner, do not use just before vaginal intercourse.
  - Check with health care provider if vaginal estrogen can be used with latex devices like condoms, diaphragms, and cervical caps.

Mayo Clinic Staff, 2015; Vallerand & Sanoski, 2017.

SAFE AND EFFECTIVE NURSING CARE: Understanding Medication

Flibanserin (Addyi)

- Indication: Treatment of premenopausal women with hypoactive sexual desire disorder
- Action: ↑sexual desire with ↓ distress and interpersonal dysfunction
- Route and dose: PO; 100 mg daily (at bedtime)
- Common side effects: Dizziness, drowsiness, hypotension, and nausea
- Nursing actions:
  - Instruct woman not to drink grapefruit juice while taking medication.
  - Instruct woman that alcohol is contraindicated; alcohol can ↑ hypotensive effects.
  - Instruct woman that use of moderate or strong CYP3A4 inhibitors is contraindicated due to risk of severe hypotension and syncope.
  - Do not drive for 6 hours after dose; medication can affect degree of alertness.

Vallerand & Sanoski, 2017.

- Driving
  - A person's eyes change and reflexes slow, which can affect the ability to safely drive a car.
  - Deciding when to give up driving is a difficult decision for older adults since not driving decreases a person's feeling of independence.
  - Health conditions that can interfere with a person's ability to safely drive include (Every Day Health, 2015):
    - Dementia.
    - Visual and hearing changes.
    - Stroke.
    - Parkinson's disease.
    - Arthritis.
    - Diabetes.
    - Certain medications.
  - Health promotion
    - Recommend yearly eye exams and appropriate visual corrections.
    - Do not drink and drive.
    - Avoid driving at night or in bad weather.
    - Limit distractions while driving: turn off radio, avoid conversations with people in the car, and do not text or use cell phone.
    - Do not drive when taking medications that cause drowsiness or delayed reflexes.
    - Wear sunglasses when driving in sunlight.

Nursing Actions

- Discuss age-related physiological and emotional changes.
- Develop an individualized teaching plan based on the woman's age-related changes.
- Provide health-promotion information based on the woman's assessed needs.

CRITICAL COMPONENT

Signs That Driving Is No Longer Safe

It may be time to limit or stop driving if the person:
- Has trouble seeing or following traffic signals, road signs, and pavement markings.
- Stops at green lights or when there is no stop sign.
- Gets confused by traffic signals.
- Runs stop signs and red lights.
- Gets lost in familiar locations.
- Finds dents and scrapes on the car, fence, mailbox, and garage doors.
- Responds more slowly to unexpected situations.
- Has trouble moving foot from gas to brake pedal.

AARP Driver Safety, 2010; Every Day Health, 2015.

CONCEPT MAP

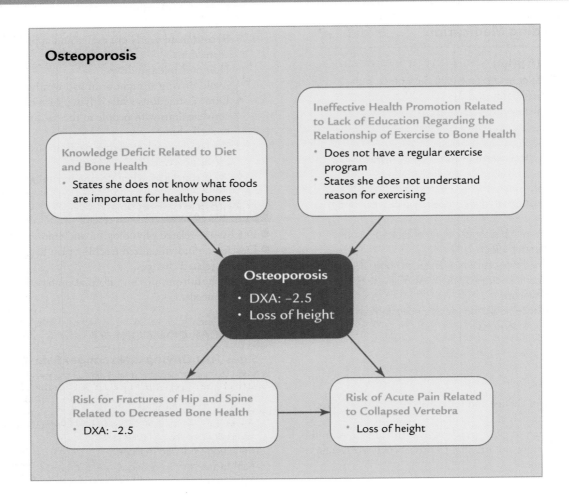

Osteoporosis

Knowledge Deficit Related to Diet and Bone Health
- States she does not know what foods are important for healthy bones

Ineffective Health Promotion Related to Lack of Education Regarding the Relationship of Exercise to Bone Health
- Does not have a regular exercise program
- States she does not understand reason for exercising

Osteoporosis
- DXA: –2.5
- Loss of height

Risk for Fractures of Hip and Spine Related to Decreased Bone Health
- DXA: –2.5

Risk of Acute Pain Related to Collapsed Vertebra
- Loss of height

Problem No. 1: Knowledge deficit related to diet and bone health

Goal: Increased knowledge of the relationship between diet and bone health

Outcome: The woman's diet will include foods high in calcium and foods high in vitamin D.

Nursing Actions
1. Assess diet for calcium and vitamin D using a 24-hour food recall.
2. Explain the relationship of calcium and strong bone matrix.
3. Explain that vitamin D helps with calcium absorption.
4. Assist the woman in identifying foods she prefers that are high in calcium and foods that are high in vitamin D.

Problem No. 2: Ineffective health promotion related to lack of education regarding the relationship of exercise to bone health

Goal: Effective health promotion

Outcome: The woman will develop a regular exercise routine that includes weight-bearing and weight-lifting activities.

Nursing Actions
1. Provide information regarding the causes of osteoporosis.
2. Provide information regarding the relationship of weight-bearing exercise and improved bone mass.
3. Discuss past exercise experiences and identify previous barriers to exercising.
4. Provide information on weight-bearing exercises and weight lifting.
5. Assist the woman in developing an exercise program that reflects her likes and meets the need for improved bone health.

Problem No. 3: Risk for fractures of hip and spine related to decreased bone health

Goal: Remains free of hip or spine fractures

Outcome: The woman will state three ways to improve bone health.

Nursing Actions
1. Explain the relationship between osteoporosis and fractures of hip and spine.
2. Assess the woman's level of knowledge regarding ways to improve bone health.

3. Provide information on nutrition and bone health.

4. Provide information on exercise and bone health.

5. Provide information on prescribed medications for treatment of osteoporosis.

Problem No. 4: Risk of pain related to collapsed vertebrae
Goal: Does not experience collapsed vertebrae
Outcome: The woman will not experience pain related to osteoporosis.

Nursing Actions

1. Provide information on the benefits of calcium and vitamin D in improving bone health.

2. Provide information on the negative effects of smoking and excessive alcohol consumption on bone health.

3. Provide information on the relationship of osteoporosis and fractures of the spine.

4. Assist the woman in developing an action plan for decreasing her risk for fractures of the spine.

Case Study

Kathy is a 65-year-old married woman with three grown children and five young grandchildren. She recently retired from teaching in an elementary school. She is 5 foot 6 inches tall and weighs 170 pounds. Her BP is 124/96. She has a family history of type 2 diabetes, stroke, and colon cancer. She recently had a DXA that indicated osteopenia. She informs you that she spends most of her day watching TV, sewing, and reading. The nutritional assessment reveals that her diet is high in fats and carbohydrates and low in fruits and vegetables.

Based on this knowledge and health needs of older women, list the priority learning needs and state rationale for your selected learning needs.

Describe your teaching plan based on the identified priority learning needs. The plan should include:

- Preparation of the learning environment.
- Methods to assess her learning needs.
- Information that will be shared.
- Methods for evaluating effectiveness of teaching.

REFERENCES

AARP Driver Safety. (2010). 10 signs that it's time to limit or stop driving. Retrieved from www.roadsafeseniors.org/resources/being-safer-road-user/educational-training-resources/10-signs-it's-time-limit-or-stop.

Allmen, T. (2016). *Menopause confidential.* New York, NY: Harper Collins.

American Cancer Society. (2016a). *American Cancer Society guidelines for early detection of cancer.* Retrieved from www.cancer.org/healthy/find-cancer-early/cancer-screening-guidelines/american-cancer-society-guidelines-for-the-early-detection-of-cancer.html.

American Cancer Society. (2016b). *The American Cancer Society guidelines for the prevention and early detection of cervical cancer.* Retrieved from www.cancer.org/cancer/cervical-cancer/prevention-and-early-detection/cervical-cancer-screening-guidelines.html.

American Cancer Society. (2016c). *Cancer facts and figures 2016.* Retrieved from www.cancer.org/acs/groups/content/@research/documents/document/acspc-047079.pdf.

American Cancer Society. (2017). *Breast cancer early detection and diagnosis.* www.cancer.org/cancer/breast-cancer/screening-tests-and-early-detection/breast-mri-scans.html

American College of Obstetricians and Gynecologist (ACOG). (2012a). Committee opinion No. 525: Health care for lesbians and bisexual women. *Obstetrics & Gynecology, 119*(5), 1077–1080.

American College of Obstetricians and Gynecologist (ACOG). (2012b). Osteoporosis. *Obstetrics & Gynecology, 120,* 718–733.

Centers for Disease Control and Prevention (CDC). (2015a). *Check for safety—a home fall prevention checklist for older adults.* Retrieved from www.cdc.gov/steadi/pdf/check_for_safety_brochure-a.pdf

Centers for Disease Control and Prevention (CDC). (2015b). *The health effects of overweight and obesity.* Retrieved from www.cdc.gov/healthyweight/effects/index.html.

Centers for Disease Control and Prevention (CDC). (2015c). *Physical activity and health.* Retrieved from www.cdc.gov/physicalactivity/basics/pa-health/

Centers for Disease Control and Prevention (CDC). (2016a). *Excessive alcohol use and risk to women's health.* Retrieved from www.cdc.gov/alcohol/fact-sheets/womens-health.htm.

Centers for Disease Control and Prevention (CDC). (2016b). *Teen pregnancy.* Retrieved from www.cdc.gov/TeenPregnancy/index.htm

Centers for Disease Control and Prevention (CDC). (2018b). *Preventing bullying.* Retrieved from www.cdc.gov/violenceprevention/pdf/bullying-factsheet.pdf

Centers for Disease Control and Prevention (CDC). (2017a). *Leading causes of death in females, 2014.* Retrieved from www.cdc.gov/women/lcod/2014/race-ethnicity/index.htm.

Centers for Disease Control and Prevention (CDC). (2018a). *Recommended immunization schedule for adults aged 19 years or older by age group, United States, 2018.* Retrieved from www.cdc.gov/vaccines/schedules/downloads/adult/adult-combined-schedule.pdf.

Dibble, S., & Robertson, P. (Eds). (2010). *Lesbian health 101.* San Francisco, CA: UCSF Nursing Press.

Eliason, M., & Drabble, L. (2010). Got a light? Smoking and lesbians. In S. Dibble & P. Robertson (Eds.), *Lesbian health 101.* San Francisco, CA: UCSF Nursing Press.

Every Day Health. (2015). *6 signs it's time to stop driving.* Retrieved from www.everydayhealth.com/senior-health/driving-safety.aspx

Healthy People 2020. (2017). *2020 topics and objectives.* Retrieved from www.healthypeople.gov/2020/topics-objectives.

Hwang, P., & Braun, K. (2015). The effectiveness of dance interventions to improve older adults' health: A systematic literature review. *Alternative Therapies in Health and Medicine, 21,* 64–70.

Kann, L., McManus, T., Harris, W., Shanklin, S., Flint, K., Hawkins, J., . . . Zaza, S. (2016). Youth risk behavior surveillance—United States 2015. *Morbidity and Mortality Weekly Report, 65*(6), 1–174.

Kochanek, M., Murphy, S., Xu, J., & Tejada-Vera, B. (2016). Deaths: Final data 2014. *National Vital Statistic Reports, 65,* 4.

March of Dimes. (2016). *Alcohol during pregnancy.* Retrieved from www.marchofdimes.org/pregnancy/alcohol-during-pregnancy.aspx.

Mayo Clinic Staff. (2015). *Menopause.* Retrieved from www.mayoclinic.org/diseases-conditions/menopause/diagnosis-treatment/drc-20353401

North American Menopause Society, American Society of Reproductive Medicine, and the Endocrine Society. (2018). The experts do agree about hormone therapy. Retrieved from www.menopause.org/for-women/menopauseflashes/menopause-symptoms-and-treatments/the-experts-do-agree-about-hormone-therapy

Ogden, C., Carroll, M., Fryer, B., & Flegel, K. (2015). *Prevalence of obesity in United States, 2011–2014. NCHS data brief. No. 219.* Retrieved from https://www.cdc.gov/nchs/data/databriefs/db219.pdf.

Qiagen. (2107). *High- and low-risk HPV types.* Retrieved from www.thehpvtest .com/about-hpv/high-and-low-risk-hpv-types/?LanguageCheck=1

U.S. Department of Health and Human Services (DHHS), Office of Women's Health. (2013). *Mammograms.* Retrieved from www.womenshealth .gov/a-z-topics/mammograms.

U.S. Department of Health Human Services (DHHS), Office of Women's Health. (2012). *A lifetime of good health.* Retrieved from http://www.hoccprograms. org/guide.pdf.

Vallerand, A., & Sanoski, C. (2017). *Davis's drug guide for nurses* (15th ed.). Philadelphia, PA: F.A. Davis.

Women's Health. (2013). Screening tests for women. Retrieved from www.women-shealth.gov/files/assets/docs/charts-checklists-guides/screening-tests-for-women.pdf

World Health Organization (WHO). (2017). *Health promotion.* Retrieved from www.who.int/topics/health_promotion/en/

Alterations in Women's Health

19

Linda L. Chapman, RN, PhD

LEARNING OUTCOMES

Upon completion of this chapter, the student will be able to:

1. Describe diagnostic procedures commonly used in women's health care.
2. Discuss various causes of menstrual disorders.
3. Describe common alterations in women's health, including medical management and nursing actions.
4. Describe potential complications/disorders related to childbirth trauma.

Nursing Diagnosis

- Deficient knowledge related to lack of information regarding menstrual disorder
- Anxiety related to diagnosis of breast cancer

Nursing Outcomes

- The woman will state causes of menstrual disorder and two possible treatments.
- The woman will appear relaxed and report anxiety related to diagnosis of breast cancer is reduced to a manageable level.

COMMON DIAGNOSTIC PROCEDURES

Table 19–1 provides an overview of the common diagnostic procedures used in women's health care.

HYSTERECTOMY

Hysterectomy is the surgical removal of the uterus and is one of the most common major surgeries for women. The three most prevalent reasons for hysterectomy are leiomyomas (fibroids), endometriosis, and prolapsed uterus. Other reasons include cancer of the reproductive organs, abnormal uterine bleeding, chronic uterine pain, and pelvic inflammatory disease (PID).

Types of Hysterectomy Procedures

The type of hysterectomy is determined by the reason for hysterectomy and the age and health status of the woman. The types are:

- Supracervical hysterectomy or partial hysterectomy: Removal of the uterus (cervix is left in place).
- Total hysterectomy or simple hysterectomy: Removal of the uterus and the cervix.
- Hysterectomy with bilateral salpingo-oophorectomy: Removal of the uterus, cervix, fallopian tubes, and ovaries.
- Radical hysterectomy: Removal of the uterus, cervix, fallopian tubes, ovaries, upper portion of the vagina, and lymph nodes. This is done to treat some cases of reproductive cancer.

TABLE 19–1   Common Diagnostic Procedures

TEST	INDICATION	PROCEDURE
Bone mineral densitometry (BMD)	Diagnose bone loss and osteoporosis. Assess effectiveness of osteoporosis medication therapy. Predict risk of future bone fractures.	Dual-energy x-ray absorptiometry (DXA): Two x-rays of different energy levels are used to measure BMD. The DXA machine (a specially designed x-ray machine) is used. X-ray is usually of the lower spine and hip. Women should not wear metal in area being x-rayed. Women should not take calcium supplements for at least 24 hours before exam.
Breast biopsy and aspiration	Breast abnormality noted by palpation, mammography, or ultrasound. Diagnostic: To distinguish between benign and malignant tumors	Excisional biopsy: The removal of the entire lump or suspicious area. This is done for lumps smaller than 1 inch in diameter. Tissue is examined by a pathologist to determine if cancerous cells are present. Procedure may be done using local or regional anesthesia. Incisional biopsy: The removal of a portion of the tumor. Usually done with tumors larger than 1 inch in diameter. Tissue is examined by a pathologist. Procedure may be done using local or regional anesthesia. Fine-needle biopsy: A fine needle is inserted into the questionable tissue. Fluid is removed from the cyst, or cells are removed from the solid mass. The fluid or cells are examined by the pathologist. Usually done as an office procedure using local anesthesia. Core-needle biopsy: This procedure uses a larger-bore needle to obtain a small cylinder of tissue. Usually done as an office procedure using local anesthesia.
Cervical conization	Abnormal Pap smear Diagnostic: To detect cervical cancer Therapeutic: Treatment of cervical intraepithelial lesions	A cone-shaped portion of cervical tissue is removed. The tissue sample is removed by scalpel, CO_2 laser, or loop electrosurgical excision procedure (LEEP). Tissue is examined by a pathologist.
Colposcopy	Dysplasia, condylomas, and abnormal Pap smear Diagnostic: To rule out cancer of the cervix	The vagina and cervix are exposed with the use of a speculum. Acetic acid is placed on the cervix. A colposcope, an electric microscope with a light, is used to view the cervical area. Abnormal cervical changes are seen as white areas. A biopsy is taken from the whitest area and is evaluated by a pathologist.
Dilation and curettage	Diagnostic: To detect uterine malignancy, to evaluate fertility, and to evaluate dysfunctional uterine bleeding Therapeutic: Treat heavy uterine bleeding, dysmenorrhea, and incomplete abortion	Can be done in the doctor's office, outpatient clinic, or hospital. Metal dilators of increasing sizes are inserted into the cervical os. After the cervix is dilated, curettes are used to scrape and/or remove endometrial tissue. Tissue is evaluated by a pathologist.
Endometrial biopsy	Diagnostic: To determine cause of dysfunctional uterine bleeding and bleeding after menopause	A sample of the endometrium is obtained with the use of a pipelle aspirator, a small hollow plastic tube, which is inserted into the uterus via the cervix. Gentle suction is applied to obtain a sample of the endometrial tissue. The sample is evaluated by a pathologist.

TABLE 19-1   Common Diagnostic Procedures—cont'd

TEST	INDICATION	PROCEDURE
Laparoscopy	Diagnostic: Pelvic adhesions, infertility related to tubal or uterine causes, ectopic pregnancy, ovarian tumors or cysts, PID, and endometriosis Therapeutic: Tubal ligation, retrieval of ova for in vitro fertilization, removal of IUD, removal of adhesions	Gynecologic laparoscopy is used to visualize the internal pelvic contents. A needle is inserted through a small incision into the peritoneal cavity, and the cavity is filled with CO_2 to enhance visualization of the organs. A laparoscope is inserted through a second incision. The laparoscope has a microscope to allow visualization, and it can be used to insert instruments required for procedures.
MRI	Use: To detect tumors of the breast, ovaries, and uterus; evaluate breast implants	MRI is a noninvasive diagnostic scanning technique using magnetic and radio waves to produce an image. The woman lies supine on a table that is slid into the MRI scanner. She must remain motionless during the scan.
Ultrasonography	Breast: Used to distinguish between solid tumors and cysts; detect very small tumors in combination with mammograms; guide interventional procedures such as cyst aspiration Pelvis: Used to detect tumors, cysts, abscesses, bleeding; distinguish between solid tumors and cysts; aid in fertility studies	High-frequency waves of different intensity are delivered by a transducer. Waves are bounced back and converted to electrical energy, which is displayed on a monitor. Breast: The woman should not apply lotion, bath powder, or other substances to the chest or breast the day of the examination. Jewelry and other metal objects must be removed from area of examination. Both breasts are usually examined. Pelvis: Can be either transabdominal or transvaginal. Transabdominal requires a full bladder. Jewelry and other metal objects must be removed from area of examination.

Cancer.Net, 2017; Johns Hopkins, 2017; VanLeeuwen & Smith, 2015.

Surgical and Anesthetic Techniques

- Abdominal hysterectomy: Removal of the uterus and other structures through an abdominal incision. The external incision may be transverse (Pfannenstiel), just above the pubic hairline, or vertical (low midline), below the umbilicus to just above the pubic hairline. Abdominal hysterectomy is usually the preferred technique when the reason for hysterectomy is related to a gynecological cancer. General anesthesia with an endotracheal tube is the preferred anesthetic. When the hysterectomy is for gynecological cancer, in addition to general anesthesia, epidural anesthesia may be used for postoperative pain management.
- Vaginal hysterectomy: The uterus is removed through the vagina. The ovaries and fallopian tubes can also be removed. The woman is placed in a lithotomy position for the operative procedure. A pericervical incision is used. General anesthesia with an endotracheal tube is the preferred anesthetic. Epidural or spinal anesthesia may be used instead of general anesthesia.
- Laparoscope-assisted vaginal hysterectomy (LAVH): The woman is placed in a steep Trendelenburg position. Laparoscope and instruments are inserted through small incisions in the abdomen (Fig. 19–1). The surgeon manually operates the scope and instruments. The uterus is removed through the vagina. The hysterectomy is initiated by laparoscopy

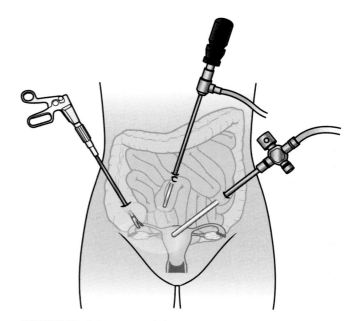

FIGURE 19–1 Laparoscopic hysterectomy.

and subsequent steps are performed vaginally. LAVH carries an increased risk of bladder injury and urinary tract infection. General anesthesia with endotracheal tube is the preferred method due to the CO_2 insufflation required for the laparoscopic procedure and the positioning of the woman during the surgical procedure. CO_2 insufflation causes an increase in intra-abdominal pressure that can cause intraoperative respiratory compromise. The insufflation may also cause cardiovascular compromise from decreased venous return. The steep Trendelenburg position further increases intra-abdominal pressure and may increase risk of aspiration. The woman needs to be monitored for facial and conjunctival edema. If this occurs, extubation following surgery may need to be postponed due to increased risk of laryngeal edema.

- Robotic-assisted laparoscopic hysterectomy: The woman is placed in a steep Trendelenburg position. Three or four small incisions are made near the umbilicus. A laparoscope and robotic instruments connected to a computer are inserted through the incisions into the abdomen. The surgeon controls the movements of the scope and the instruments from a computer station in the operating room. General anesthesia with an endotracheal tube and with muscle relaxation is the preferred method of anesthesia. The surgeon has limited patient access during robotic surgery because of the bulky equipment placed over the patient. Full muscle relaxation is needed to prevent inadvertent patient movement. Due to the deep Trendelenburg position, the woman needs to be monitored for facial and conjunctival edema. If this occurs, extubation following surgery may need to be postponed due to increased risk of laryngeal edema.

Risks Related to Surgical Procedure

- Complication related to anesthesia
- Injury to ureters, bladder, and/or bowel
- Hemorrhage
- Infection
- Deep vein thrombosis/venous thromboembolism

Preoperative Care for Abdominal Hysterectomy

The following medical management and nursing actions are performed prior to an abdominal hysterectomy.

Medical Management

- Physical assessment and health history
- Laboratory tests—complete blood count, type and cross-match, urinalysis
- Electrocardiogram
- NPO 8 hours prior to surgery
- Informed consent obtained
- Antibiotics when indicated

Nursing Actions

- Complete the appropriate admission assessments and required preoperative forms.
- Ensure that all required documents, such as history and physical, current laboratory reports, and consent forms, are in the woman's chart.

- Verify that the woman has been NPO as directed by her physician.
- Complete the surgical checklist, which includes removal of jewelry, eyeglasses/contact lenses, and dentures.
- Explain to the woman and family or support persons what the woman can expect before surgery and after surgery.
- Start an IV line and IV fluid as per orders.
- Administer antibiotics as per orders.
- Have the woman void or insert Foley catheter as per orders.
- Provide emotional support for the woman and her family/support persons.
- Address the woman and/or family's questions and/or concerns.

Postoperative Care for Abdominal Hysterectomy

After abdominal hysterectomy, care includes the following measures.

Medical Management

- IV therapy
- Medications for pain management
- Antibiotic therapy if at risk for infection
- Hormone replacement therapy if ovaries were removed
- Progression of diet within 12 to 24 hours postsurgery
- Foley catheter for 12 to 24 hours postsurgery
- Ambulate once recovered from anesthesia

Nursing Actions

- Monitor vital signs as per protocol.
- Monitor for blood loss—assess for blood on abdominal dressing and perineal pad. The woman will experience small to moderate amounts of vaginal bleeding for several days.
- Monitor level of consciousness and level of sensation and for side effects of anesthesia.
- Assess lung sounds and assist the woman with deep breathing and coughing. Teach the woman to splint her abdomen with a pillow when she coughs.
- Initiate anti-embolism therapy as per orders.
- Assist the woman into a comfortable position and reposition every 2 hours.
- Assess for pain and provide pain relief via prescribed medications, use of relaxation techniques, positioning, and/or soothing environment.
- Assist the woman with ambulation as per orders. Explain to the woman that ambulation decreases her risk for deep vein thrombosis and facilitates return of intestinal peristalsis, which decreases the amount of gas buildup.
- Monitor intake and output.
- DC IV as per orders.
- DC Foley catheter as per orders.
- Assess bowel sounds and advance to a regular diet as per orders.
- Provide opportunities for the woman to ask questions or share her concerns. She may experience emotional symptoms following surgery related to hormonal changes and loss of fertility.

- Provide discharge teaching:
  - Keep the incision area dry, following the surgeon's instructions for bathing and dressing care.
  - Explain that walking is important in helping her to gradually return to her presurgery activity level. The woman needs to follow her surgeon's orders regarding level of activity and heavy lifting.
  - Explain that she may experience light vaginal bleeding for several days.
  - Provide nutritional information—the importance of protein, iron, and vitamin C in the healing process.
  - Provide information on pain management techniques.
  - Instruct the woman not to put anything in the vagina (e.g., do not douche, use tampons, or engage in sexual intercourse) until advised by her surgeon. This will decrease her risk of infections.
  - Instruct the woman to notify health care provider if:
    - Increased pain or pain that is not relieved by medication.
    - Drainage, bleeding, redness, or swelling from the incisional site or increased bleeding from the vagina.
    - Leg/calf pain, swelling, and/or redness.
    - Fever 102.2°F (39°C) or higher, or as instructed by physician

MENSTRUAL DISORDERS

Menstrual disorders are the most common women's reproductive health problem. These include amenorrhea, dysfunctional uterine bleeding, dysmenorrhea, and premenstrual syndrome (Table 19–2). The hypothalamus, pituitary, and ovaries are the main sites of regulation of the menstrual cycle. Normal menstrual cycles occur when the hormone levels and feedback pathway of the hypothalamus-anterior pituitary-ovaries function appropriately. (See Chapter 3 for an overview of the menstrual cycle.)

- Hypothalamus: Secretes gonadotropin-releasing hormone (GnRH), also called luteinizing-hormone-releasing hormone, which simulates the anterior pituitary.
- Anterior pituitary: Secretes follicle-stimulating hormone (FSH) and luteinizing hormone (LH) that stimulates the ovaries.
- Ovaries: The ovarian follicles respond to the increase in FSH by producing increasing amounts of estrogen. LH stimulates the ovaries to release the ova and secrete progesterone. Estrogen and progesterone influence the menstrual cycle.

CHRONIC PELVIC PAIN

Chronic pelvic pain (CPP), a common medical problem for women, is defined as pain in the pelvic region that lasts 6 months or longer, is unresponsive to usual pain treatments, and results in functional or psychological disabilities (International Pelvic Pain Society, 2014). CPP has multiple causes, which can make it difficult to evaluate and treat. Treatment focuses on the underlying cause of pelvic pain. In some cases the cause of pain is unknown,

and treatment focuses on symptom management. Women with CPP experience a variety of symptoms such as:

- Abdominal and/or pelvic pain:
  - Uterine and/or abdominal cramping
  - Sharp pain
  - Steady pain
  - Intermittent pain
  - Pressure or heaviness deep in pelvis
  - Pain during intercourse
  - Pain while having bowel movement
- Difficulty sleeping.
- Constipation.
- Depression.
- Decrease in physical activity.
- Changes in how she relates in her roles as partner, mother, and employee—that is, spending more time in bed, missing work (International Pelvic Pain Society, 2014).

Causes

The causes of CPP can stem from the reproductive, urological, neuromuscular, and/or gastrointestinal systems.

- Reproductive
  - Pelvic inflammatory disease
  - Leiomyoma
  - Adhesions
  - Endometriosis
  - Intrauterine contraceptive device
- Urological
  - Bladder neoplasm
  - Chronic urinary tract infection
  - Kidney stones
- Musculoskeletal
  - Compression fracture of lumbar vertebrae
  - Poor posture
  - Fibromyalgia
- Gastrointestinal
  - Crohn's disease
  - Celiac disease
  - Colitis
  - Irritable bowel syndrome
  - Colon cancer
- Neurological
  - Shingles
  - Degenerative joint disease
  - Herniated disk
- Psychological
  - Personality disorders
  - Depression
  - Sleep disorders
- Other
  - Sexual and/or physical abuse

Medical Management

Medical management of CPP depends on the cause. It can take several weeks to several months of treatment before the woman

TABLE 19–2   Menstrual Disorders

MENSTRUAL DISORDER	DEFINITIONS, SYMPTOMS, SIGNS	PATHOPHYSIOLOGY	MANAGEMENT
Primary amenorrhea	No menses by age 16 and no secondary sex characteristics or no menses by age 13 with secondary sex characteristics	May be related to: • Body build (e.g., minimal levels of body fat) • Heredity (family history of delayed menses) • Pituitary function (lack of secretion of FSH and LH) • Congenital absence of the vagina • 90% of cases have no identifiable cause.	Identify and treat underlying condition (e.g., hormone therapy if related to endocrine dysfunction). Provide emotional support.
Secondary amenorrhea	No menses in 3 months in a woman who has had normal menstrual cycles	May result from: • Lack of ovarian production • Pregnancy • PCOS • Nutritional disturbances • Endocrine disturbances • Uncontrolled diabetes • Heavy athletic activity • Emotional distress	Identify and treat underlying condition (e.g., correct nutritional disorder). Explain cause (e.g., heavy athletic activity).
Menorrhagia	Menstrual bleeding that is excessive in number of days and amount of blood	May result from: • Anovulatory cycle with continued estrogen production • Fibroids are most common anatomic cause. • Inflammatory or infectious cause (e.g., metritis, salpingitis) • Endometrial cause (e.g., hyperplasia, polyps, cancer) • Intrauterine device (IUD)	Endometrial biopsy to assist in diagnosis of underlying cause. Identify and treat underlying condition (e.g., antibiotic therapy if related to infection). If no identifiable cause, short course of contraceptives may be prescribed. Dilation and curettage
Metrorrhagia	Bleeding between periods or after menopause	This is the most significant form of menstrual disorder and warrants immediate investigation. • Occurs with cancerous or benign tumors of the uterus • Associated with IUD and use of oral contraceptives • May be associated with trauma, cervicitis, vaginitis, polyps, ovarian cysts, cervical dysplasia	Endometrial biopsy to rule out endometrial cancer Antibiotics for infection Surgery Chemotherapy

TABLE 19-2   Menstrual Disorders—cont'd

MENSTRUAL DISORDER	DEFINITIONS, SYMPTOMS, SIGNS	PATHOPHYSIOLOGY	MANAGEMENT
Primary dysmenorrhea	Painful menstruation: Cramping usually begins 12–24 hours before onset of flow and lasts 12–24 hours. May experience chills, nausea, vomiting, headaches, irritability, and diarrhea.	Excessive endometrial production of prostaglandin; women with primary dysmenorrhea produce 10 times the amount of prostaglandin. Prostaglandin is a myometrial stimulant and vasoconstrictor.	Explain cause. Prostaglandin inhibitors (ibuprofen) Analgesics Heat to back and lower abdomen Warm bath Exercise Oral contraceptives Diet low in fat and meat products may decrease the duration and intensity of the pain. Biofeedback Acupuncture
Secondary dysmenorrhea	Painful menstruation associated with known anatomic factors or pelvic pathology. Pain can be present at any point of the menstrual cycle.	Related to: • Endometriosis • Pelvic adhesions • Inflammatory disease • Cervical stenosis • Uterine fibroids • Adenomyoma	Identify and treat underlying condition. Same symptomatic measures as in primary dysmenorrhea.
Premenstrual syndrome (PMS)	A combination of emotional and physical symptoms that begin during the luteal phase and diminish after menstruation begins. Symptoms include (but are not limited to) lower abdominal and back pain, bloating, weight gain, breast tenderness, joint and muscle pain, oliguria, diaphoresis, diarrhea, constipation, nausea, vomiting, food cravings, acne, urticaria, headaches, vertigo, fainting, clumsiness, mood swings, depression, irritability, anxiety, lethargy, fatigue, confusion, tension, forgetfulness, sexual arousal or dysfunction.	Etiology is unknown. PMS might be related to: • Hormonal changes related to the menstrual cycle. • Estrogen–progesterone imbalance. • Chemical changes in the brain.	Limit salt intake, caffeine, animal fat, refined sugars, and alcohol. Exercise daily. Sleep 8 hours each night. Ibuprofen for physical symptoms such as cramps, backache, and breast tenderness Herbal remedies such as black cohosh, ginger, and raspberry leaf Commonly prescribed medications are antidepressants, anti-anxiety, diuretics, and oral contraceptives.

University of Maryland Medical Center, 2017.

will begin to feel better. In some cases, the pain does not completely go away (International Pelvic Pain Society, 2014). Treatments may include:

● Pain management, including physical therapy and medications: analgesics (NSAIDs, acetaminophen, opioids), tricyclic antidepressants, neuroleptics (gabapentin, anxiolytics, clonazepam), and muscle relaxants (Flexeril).
● Hormone therapy (for pain management related to menstrual cycle or endometriosis).
● Antibiotics.
● Steroids.
● Laparoscopy surgery to release adhesions.
● Nutrition (avoiding foods that can increase inflammation of colitis or irritable bowel syndrome).
● Psychotherapy to assist the woman in coping with anxiety, depression, and other emotional effects of living with chronic pain.
● Alternative medicine.

Nursing Actions

● Assess and document location, characteristic, frequency, and quality of pain.
● Assess effectiveness of pain interventions.
● Assess level of knowledge regarding cause of pain.
● Provide teaching as indicated by knowledge assessment.
● Provide information regarding diagnostic tests or surgeries.
● Provide information on use of nonpharmacological techniques such as relaxation, guided imagery, heat application, and massage.
● Instruct the woman to use pain-control measures before pain becomes severe.

POLYCYSTIC OVARY SYNDROME

Polycystic ovary syndrome (PCOS), also known as Stein-Leventhal syndrome, is an endocrine disorder that affects 10% of women of childbearing age (Women's Health, 2016). The etiology is not fully understood, but it is believed that there is a genetic component. Women with PCOS often have elevated levels of estrogen, testosterone, and LH and decreased secretions of FSH. These hormonal changes can cause multiple follicular cysts on one or both ovaries (Fig. 19–2). Women with PCOS are at higher risk for:

● Type 2 diabetes: Women with PCOS are at risk for insulin resistance (the body produces insulin but does not use it properly) and hyperinsulinemia (hyperglycemia present despite high levels of insulin). Obesity, which is common with PCOS, further increases the risk for diabetes.
● Cardiovascular disease: Insulin resistance and obesity increase the woman's risk for carotid and coronary atherosclerosis; endocrine changes related to PCOS increases the woman's risk for an increase in low-density lipoprotein cholesterol and a decrease in high-density lipoprotein.

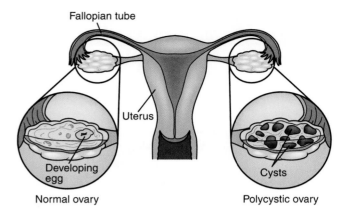

FIGURE 19–2 Polycystic ovary syndrome.

● Hypertension related to insulin resistance.
● Endometrial, ovarian, and/or breast cancer related to high levels of continuous estrogen.
● Dyslipidemia related to endocrine changes.
● Infertility: Anovulation related to increased androgen levels, increased LH, and decreased FSH.
● Pregnancy and birth complications: Spontaneous abortions, gestational diabetes, preeclampsia, and cesarean sections.
● Sleep apnea related to obesity and insulin resistance.
● Metabolic syndrome, which affects about one-third of women with PCOS.

CRITICAL COMPONENT

Metabolic Syndrome

Metabolic syndrome is a group of conditions that increase an individual's risk for heart disease, stroke, and diabetes. To be diagnosed with the syndrome, an individual must have three of the following:

• Abdominal obesity: a waist circumference in women 35 inches or greater
• High triglyceride levels: 150 mg/dL or higher
• Low HDL cholesterol level: 50 mg/dL for women
• Increased blood pressure: Systolic above 130 mm Hg and/or diastolic above 85 mm Hg
• Elevated fasting blood glucose: 110 mg/dL or higher

National Heart Lung and Blood Institute, 2016.

Signs and Symptoms

● Infertility: PCOS is the most common cause of female infertility, usually related to anovulatory menstrual cycles.
● Menstrual disorders: Irregular, infrequent, and/or absent menstrual periods.
● Hirsutism: Increased hair growth on face, chest, stomach, and back.
● Ovarian cysts.
● Obesity.

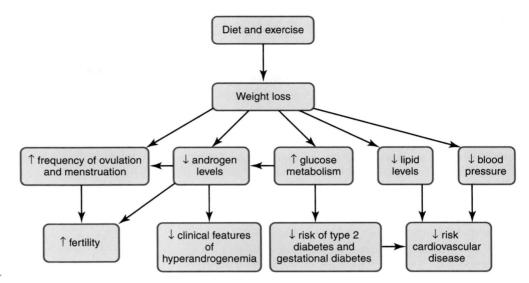

FIGURE 19–3 Effects of weight management in women with PCOS.

- Oily skin and acne.
- Pelvic pain.
- Male-pattern baldness.

Medical Management

- Diet and exercise to assist in weight loss. It also helps:
  - Reduce risk for type 2 diabetes.
  - Decrease levels of androgens.
  - Improve the frequency of ovulation and menstruation.
  - Reduce risk of cardiovascular disease (Fig. 19–3).
- Hormone therapy
  - Low-dose hormonal contraceptives for women who do not wish to conceive. These contraceptives inhibit LH production, decrease testosterone levels, and reduce degree of acne and hirsutism.
- Anti-androgen medications
  - Reduces scalp hair loss, facial and body hair growth, and acne
  - Should not be used by women who are pregnant or attempting pregnancy
- Fertility therapy
  - Medications that induce ovulation, such as Clomid
  - Assisted reproductive technology, such as in vitro fertilization, may be used for women who do not respond to medications.
- Diabetic medications
  - Antidiabetic medications are prescribed to lower blood glucose levels. They also can lower testosterone, which reduces the degree of acne, hirsutism, and abdominal obesity and may help regulate the menstrual cycle and treat infertility.

Nursing Actions

PCOS has both physical and psychological effects. Body image can be negatively impacted by changes stemming from PCOS.

Women need opportunities to share their concerns about PCOS and receive information on methods to decrease or counteract its effects. Areas to discuss with the woman include:

- Risk factors related to PCOS.
- Weight reduction through diet and exercise.
  - Explain the benefits of weight loss on PCOS.
  - Provide information on healthy diet and assist the woman in developing a healthy diet plan.
- Treatment options for hirsutism
  - Laser hair removal
  - Eflornithine HCL cream
- Treatment options for acne and oily skin
  - Evaluation and treatment by dermatologist
- Infertility issues
- Psychological effects of body changes related to PCOS such as depression and increased anxiety.

SAFE AND EFFECTIVE NURSING CARE: Understanding Medication

Eflornithine HCL (Vaniqa)

Indication: Reduction of unwanted facial hair in women.

Action: Inhibits the enzyme ornithine decarboxylase in skin, which decreases synthesis of polyamines.

Common side effects: Burning, rash, stinging, tingling of skin

Route and dosage: Topical. Apply a thin layer to affected areas of the face and adjacent involved areas under the chin and rub in thoroughly. Do not wash for 4 hours following application. Use twice daily at least 8 hours apart.

Vallerand & Sanoski, 2017.

ENDOMETRIOSIS

Endometriosis is a chronic inflammatory disease in which the presence and growth of endometrial tissue is found outside the uterine cavity. The tissue, referred to as endometrial lesions, is usually found in the peritoneal surfaces of reproductive organs and adjacent structures of the pelvis, such as ovaries, fallopian tubes, bladder, bowel, and intestines. The ovaries are the most common site of endometrial lesions, which are estrogen-dependent and thus most commonly occur during the reproductive years. Lesions respond to the changes in estrogen and progesterone levels of the menstrual cycle; each month they build up, break down, and shed as does the endometrial tissue inside the uterus.

The cause of endometriosis is unknown, though the primary theory attributes it to retrograde menstruation that transports endometrial tissue outside the uterine cavity, where it adheres to surrounding organs. Other theories include genetic predisposition, immunologic changes, and hormonal influences (Lobo, Gershenson, Lentz, & Valea, 2017).

Signs and Symptoms

One-third of women with endometriosis are asymptomatic. Symptoms vary depending on the location of the lesions. The degree of symptoms does not correlate with the size of lesions.

Pelvic pain and dysmenorrhea usually begin a few days before menses and stop at the end of menstruation. Other symptoms include:

- Low back pain.
- Pelvic pressure.
- Dyspareunia.
- Infertility.
- Premenstrual spotting and menorrhagia.
- Diarrhea, pain with defecation, and constipation usually present when there are lesions of the bowel.
- Bloody urine and dysuria usually present when there are lesions on the bladder.
- Fixed retroverted uterus.
- Enlarged and tender ovaries.

CRITICAL COMPONENT

Endometriosis

- Abnormal growth of tissue resembling the endometrium that is present outside of the uterine cavity.
- Tissue responds to changes in estrogen and progesterone levels.
  - The tissue grows and thickens during the secretory and proliferative stages of the menstrual cycle.
  - The tissue breaks down and bleeds into the surrounding tissues during the menstrual phase.
- Bleeding into surrounding tissues causes pain and inflammation.
- Scarring, fibrosis, and adhesions result from continued inflammation.

Emotional Impact

The physical symptoms of endometriosis can affect the woman's mental health. The woman may experience anger and grief related to loss of fertility. The pain related to endometriosis can interfere with her social activities, and dyspareunia can affect intimate relationships.

Medical Management

- Analgesic therapy
  - NSAIDs commonly used for pain management.
- Hormonal therapy
  - Goal is to suppress menstruation and further growth of tissue.
  - Common medications include:
    - Oral contraceptive pills
    - GnRH agonists (Lupron, Zoladex, and Nafarelin)
    - Progestins
    - Danazol—this drug has adverse effects on developing fetuses and is not recommended for women who are attempting pregnancy.
- Symptoms usually return within 1 to 5 years after medications are stopped.

SAFE AND EFFECTIVE NURSING CARE: Understanding Medication

Nafarelin (Synarel)

- Indication: Endometriosis
- Action: A synthetic analogue of GnRH. Prolonged use causes a reduction in serum estrone, E_2, testosterone, and androstenedione.
- Side effects: Emotional instability, headaches, vaginal dryness, acne, cessation of menses, impaired fertility, decreased libido, hot flashes
- Route and doses: Intranasal; one spray (200 mcg) in morning in one nostril and one spray (200 mcg) in the other nostril in the evening up to a maximum of 800 mcg/day

Vallerand & Sanoski, 2017.

- Surgical treatment
  - Surgical removal of lesions via laparoscopy procedure and laser treatment is used for women with severe symptoms who are infertile and desire pregnancy. Endometriosis may recur after surgical intervention.
  - Hysterectomy with bilateral salpingo-oophorectomy and removal of adhesions and lesions is used for women with severe symptoms who do not desire pregnancy.
- Assisted reproduction
  - Ovulation induction with intrauterine insemination or in vitro fertilization may be used for infertile women with endometriosis who have not responded to other therapies for infertility (Lobo et al., 2017).

Nursing Actions

- Patient education regarding endometriosis
- Patient education regarding pain management
  - NSAIDs
  - Heat therapy
  - Biofeedback
  - Relaxation techniques
- Emotional support
  - Provide opportunities for the woman to explore her feelings related to living with endometriosis.
- Patient education on prescribed treatment plan
  - Information on medications, including action, side effects, and dosage
  - Information on surgical intervention

INFECTIONS

Infections of the reproductive system and pelvic organs increase a woman's risk for cancer, chronic pain, systemic infections, and infertility. Infections are preventable and treatable. Early interventions decrease the woman's risk for complications related to prolonged or repeated infections of the pelvic region. Infections of the reproductive system and pelvic organs include three types of infections:

- Sexually transmitted infections (STIs)
- Endogenous infections such as bacterial vaginitis
- Iatrogenic infections such as urinary tract infection (UTI) caused by improperly performed medical and/or nursing procedures.

Sexually Transmitted Infections

Sexually transmitted infections, also known as sexually transmitted diseases, are infections that are primarily transmitted through vaginal intercourse, anal intercourse, and oral sex. Table 19–3 summarizes the most common STIs. Chlamydia and gonorrhea are the top two reported STIs and are highest in the female adolescent population (GirlsHealth, 2017).

Women can have an STI and be asymptomatic. Women who are asymptomatic are still at risk for infecting their sexual partner. To decrease the risk of reinfection, treatment needs to be directed at both the woman and her partner.

CRITICAL COMPONENT

Sexually Transmitted Infections

Untreated STIs place a woman at risk for:

- Cervical cancer.
- Pelvic inflammatory disease.
- Infertility due to blocked fallopian tubes.
- Ectopic pregnancy due to blocked fallopian tubes.
- Chronic pelvic pain.

Lesbians and bisexual women are at the same risk for STIs as heterosexual women. The types of sexual behavior that carry a risk for STI between women are:

- Oral-vaginal/vulval contact: Herpes, syphilis, and gonorrhea.
- Digital-vaginal contact: human papillomavirus (HPV), bacterial vaginosis, trichomonas, chlamydia, and gonorrhea.
- Oral-anal contact: Syphilis, herpes, and hepatitis A.
- Genital-genital and genital-body contact: HPV and herpes.
- Insertive sex (sex toys and dildos): Trichomonas, gonorrhea, herpes, and HPV (County of Los Angeles, 2017).

Nursing Actions

- Provide information on transmission and treatment of STI.
- Provide information on methods to decrease risk of STI.
  - Be in a monogamous sexual relationship with a partner who has been screened for STI and is not infected.
  - Use condoms or dental dams correctly every time engaged in sexual activity. Dental dams are polyurethane sheets used between the mouth and vagina or anus during oral sex (Centers for Disease Control and Prevention [CDC], 2016).
  - Talk with partner about STI and the use of condoms before engaging in sexual activities.
  - Talk with your health care provider and your sexual partner about any STI you or your partner presently have or have had in the past.
  - Follow current guidelines for frequency of pelvic exams, Pap tests, and HPV testing.

VAGINITIS

The vaginal flora is a delicate ecosystem primarily composed of various lactobacilli, which inhibit the growth of yeast and bacteria. Vaginitis, an inflammation of the vagina, occurs when the vaginal ecosystem is disrupted. Symptoms of vaginitis include vaginal discharge that can be malodorous, depending on the causative agent; burning; irritation; or itching. The most common types of vaginitis are candida vaginitis, bacterial vaginosis, and trichomoniasis (see Table 19–3).

Candida Vaginitis

Candida vaginitis, also called candidiasis or a yeast infection, is caused by *Candida albicans*. This is a gram-positive fungus that lives on all surfaces of the human body. When the vaginal ecosystem is disturbed, the fungus rapidly grows, causing an infection. Factors that can affect the vaginal ecosystem are:

- Hormonal changes: The presence of candida vaginitis increases before and immediately following the menstrual period due to hormonal changes. High levels of estrogen during pregnancy favor growth of fungus.
- Depressed cell-mediated immunity: Women taking exogenous corticosteroids or who have AIDS are at higher risk for reoccurring candida vaginitis.
- Antibiotic use: Lactobacillus, which inhibits the growth of fungi, is part of the normal vaginal bacteria flora. Certain

TABLE 19–3   Sexually Transmitted Infections (STI)

SDI	CAUSATIVE AGENT	MANIFESTATION/SYMPTOMS	TREATMENT
AIDS	HIV (Viral)	Individual may be asymptomatic for years. Early symptoms: Sore throat, rhinitis, rash Later symptoms: Leukopenia, idiopathic thrombocytopenia, fever, night sweats, weight loss, lymphadenopathy, dry cough Women may also have: candidiasis, BV, PID, and menstrual cycle changes. HIV infection is usually diagnosed via the HIV-1 and HIV-2 antibody tests.	No cure for HIV currently exists. Antiretroviral therapy (ART) is the standard treatment. ART is effective in maintaining the health of HIV-positive women and in reducing the perinatal transmission of the virus.
Chlamydia	*Chlamydia trachomatis* (Bacterial)	Most common bacterial STI in United States and the leading cause of preventable infertility and ectopic pregnancies. Most infected women are asymptomatic; 30% have a mucopurulent cervical discharge. Other symptoms include spotting, urethritis, lower abdominal pain, nausea, fever, dyspareunia. Chlamydia is diagnosed via cultures of cervical epithelial cells. Chlamydia can also live in the throat, rectum, and urethra.	Antibiotic therapy: • Doxycycline 100 mg orally twice a day for 7 days *or* • Azithromycin 1 gm orally given in a single dose • Infected partner needs to be treated to decrease risk of reinfection.
Genital warts/ condylomas	Human papillomavirus (HPV) (Viral)	Painless warty growth in the vagina or on the vulva, perineum, or anal areas	Treatment options include: • Topical application of podofilox, which can be applied by the patient. • Topical application of trichloroacetic acid, which is applied by health care provider. • Cryotherapy. • CO_2 laser surgery. • Electrosurgery. • Surgical removal.
Genital herpes	Herpes simplex virus (HSV), types 1 and 2 (Viral) Is usually spread by having vaginal, oral, or anal sex.	Infected women may have no or minimal symptoms. Symptoms are similar to those of the flu: malaise, muscle aches, and headaches. Other symptoms can include itching and burning feeling in the genital or anal areas, vaginal discharge, feeling of pressure in pelvic area, and lymphadenopathy. Lesions (small red bumps or blisters or open sores) in area where virus entered the body, cervix, vagina. Diagnosis is usually based on patient history and examination.	There is no cure for genital herpes. Treatment plan includes: • Antiviral medications such as acyclovir. • Oral analgesia for symptom management. • Application of cool compresses containing peppermint oil for symptom management. • Use of condoms to prevent spread of virus.

TABLE 19–3   Sexually Transmitted Infections (STI)—cont'd

SDI	CAUSATIVE AGENT	MANIFESTATION/SYMPTOMS	TREATMENT
Gonorrhea	*Neisseria gonorrhoeae* (Bacterial)	Women are commonly asymptomatic. Symptoms include vaginal discharge, menorrhagia, postcoital bleeding, low backache, urinary frequency, dysuria, and pain during sexual intercourse. Gonorrhea is diagnosed via test such as cultures of the cervical discharge.	Recommended therapy is single intramuscular (IM) dose of ceftriaxone given in combination with azithromycin or doxycycline. Infected partner should be treated to decrease risk of reinfection.
Hepatitis B	Hepatitis B virus (HBV) (Viral)	HBV is found in highest concentrations in the blood and lower concentrations in semen, vaginal secretions, and wound exudates. Sexual intercourse is the most common mode of transmission. Women are often asymptomatic. Symptoms include fever, fatigue, loss of appetite, nausea, vomiting, abdominal pain, joint pain, dark-colored urine, clay-colored stools, and jaundice. Symptoms appear 60–150 days after exposure.	There is no specific treatment for acute HBV. Therapy is directed at symptom management. Antiviral medications are used for chronic HBV.
Syphilis	*Treponema pallidum* (Bacterial)	Syphilis progresses in stages: Primary syphilis symptom is a single, painless ulcer (chancre) in the genital area, mouth, or point of contact. Appears 10–90 days after contact. The chancre lasts 4–6 weeks and usually resolves without treatment. Secondary syphilis symptoms include skin rash, fever, sore throat, lymphadenopathy, muscle aches, weight loss, and fatigue. Appears 6 weeks to 6 months after the appearance of the chancre. If not treated, the symptoms resolve on own within 2–10 weeks. Tertiary syphilis: Approximately one-third of infected individuals will develop tertiary syphilis. Without treatment, the bacteria can spread throughout the body, and symptoms are related to damage of internal organs. Screening tests include rapid plasma reagin and Venereal Disease Research Laboratory.	Penicillin G is the treatment of choice. The specific regimen depends on the length of infection. Infected partner should be treated to decrease risk of reinfection.
Trichomoniasis	*Trichomonas vaginalis* (Protozoan)	Most women are asymptomatic. Symptoms appear 5–28 days after exposure. Symptoms include profuse frothy gray or yellow-green vaginal discharge with foul odor; erythema, edema, pruritus of the external genitalia, and pain during sexual intercourse. Small, red ulcerations in the vagina and/or on cervix may be observed during examination. Diagnosis: Microscopic evaluation to confirm trichomoniasis or rapid trichomoniasis test	Metronidazole (Flagyl) is medication of choice. It may be administered as a single dose of 2 g orally or 500 mg orally twice a day for 7 days. Partner needs to be treated at same time and condoms used to prevent future infections. Women should be advised not to drink alcohol for 24 hours after completing metronidazole therapy. The combination of alcohol and medication can cause flushing, nausea, vomiting, headaches, and abdominal cramping.

CDC, 2017a.

broad-spectrum antibiotics, such as penicillin and tetracycline, can destroy lactobacillus, allowing the rapid growth of *C. albicans* (Lobo et al., 2017).

CRITICAL COMPONENT

Prevalence of Candida Vaginitis

Candida vaginitis is common in women of childbearing age. Three out of four women will experience at least one occurrence of candida vaginitis within their lifetime.

Risk Factors

- Suppressed immune system
- Antibiotic therapy
- Steroid therapy
- Diabetes
- Pregnancy
- Menopause

Signs and Symptoms

- Itching and irritation in the vulva and vaginal areas are the primary symptoms.
- White, cheesy vaginal discharge
- Pain with sexual intercourse
- Burning on urination
- Vaginal pH below 4.5

Medical Management

Most vaginal yeast infections can be treated with over-the-counter (OTC) medications. Women often self-diagnose and self-treat. It is important for women to contact their primary health provider if symptoms continue after treatment or are recurrent.

- Diagnosis with a wet smear of vaginal secretions
- Medication: Fluconazole (Diflucan), an antifungal prescription medication, is given when OTCs are not effective or when there is a severe infection. Treatment is a single oral dose of 150 mg. The safety of use during pregnancy has not been established. It is usually compatible with women who are lactating (Vallerand & Sanoski, 2017). Women with reoccurring candida vaginitis may be treated with a 6-month course of fluconazole.

Nursing Actions

- Teach the woman proper use of OTC medications.
- Instruct the woman to notify health care provider if symptoms continue or are recurrent. Women can mistake bacteria vaginitis for candida vaginitis, which has a different treatment plan.
- Instruct the woman to contact health care provider if any of the following occur:
  - Bloody discharge
  - Abdominal pain
  - Fever
- Instruct the woman to wear cotton underwear to decrease risk of recurrent infections.

SAFE AND EFFECTIVE NURSING CARE: Understanding Medication

Use of OTC Medications for Treatment of Candida Vaginitis

- Most vaginal yeast infections can be treated with common OTC remedies:
  - Miconazole (Micon 7, Monistat 3)
  - Tioconazole (Monistat 1, Vagistat-1)
  - Butoconazole (Gynazole-1)
  - Clotrimazole (Mycelex)
- OCTs come in creams and suppositories and are placed in the vagina.
- Length of treatment varies from 1 to 7 days.
- Health care provider needs to be contacted if symptoms continue for more than a week or if symptoms return.
- Before starting an OTC medication, women need to see their health care professional when:
  - It is their first yeast infection.
  - They are 12 years or younger.
  - They are pregnant or breastfeeding.
  - They have reoccurring yeast infections—more than 4/year.
  - They are taking warfarin.
  - They have a suppressed immune system.

Bacterial Vaginosis

Bacterial vaginosis (BV), the most common vaginal infection, occurs when there is a disruption in the normal vaginal flora that includes a decrease in lactobacilli and an increase in organisms such as genital mycoplasma, *Peptostreptococcus*, and *Gardnerella*.

CRITICAL COMPONENT

Bacterial Vaginosis

- Women who experience abnormal vaginal discharge need to be seen by their health care providers since symptoms of BV are similar to those of chlamydia, gonorrhea, candidiasis, and trichomoniasis.
- Women with BV are at greater risk for preterm labor and endometritis.
- BV is more common in lesbians and bisexual women than in heterosexual women.

Risk Factors

- New sexual partner, male or female
- Multiple sexual partners
- Lesbian couples who share sex toys without cleaning them between uses
- Douching can alter the normal vaginal flora.
- Antibiotic therapy can alter the normal vaginal flora.

Signs and Symptoms

- Vaginal odor, often described as fishy.
- Vaginal discharge that is often thin and white or gray; may also be described as milky.

Medical Management

- Microscopic examination of vaginal discharge to rule out other causes such as candidiasis and trichomoniasis
- Gynecological examination to assess the appearance of the vaginal lining and the cervix
- Pharmacological therapy:
  - Metronidazole (Flagyl)—Taken orally in pill form or inserted vaginally in a gel form
  - Clindamycin (Cleocin)—Taken orally in pill form or inserted vaginally in gel form
  - Tinidazole (Tindamax)—Taken orally in pill form
- Male partner does not need to be treated.
- Female partner may need treatment.

Nursing Actions

- Provide education on proper administration, actions, and side effects of medications.
- Instruct women who are taking metronidazole (Flagyl) PO to take with meals and avoid drinking alcohol. The combination of metronidazole (Flagyl) and alcohol can cause severe nausea and vomiting, flushing, tachycardia, and shortness of breath.
- Provide information on signs and symptoms of possible recurrence that the woman should report to health care provider.
- Provide information of risk factors for BV.

Urinary Tract Infections

A urinary tract infection (UTI) is an infection of the urethra, bladder, ureters, and/or kidneys. It is more common in women than men because women have a shorter urethra in close proximity to the vagina and anus. The two most common UTIs are cystitis and urethritis. UTIs are typically ascending infections. Cystitis is usually related to *Escherichia coli*. Urethritis is usually related to STIs such as chlamydia. Untreated cystitis and/or urethritis places women at risk for pyelonephritis. Diagnosis of UTI is usually based on the presenting symptoms and confirmed with a positive urine culture.

Risk Factors

- Young girls and menopausal women related to decreased levels of estrogen
- Suppressed immune system
- Diabetes
- Urinary tract obstructions
- Incomplete or infrequent bladder emptying
- Pregnancy
- Irritation of the urethra during sexual activity can cause bacteria to migrate upward into the urinary tract.
- Allergic reaction to certain ingredients in soaps, vaginal creams, and bubble baths
- Recent urinary procedures such as urinary surgery or urinary cauterization
- Bowel incontinence

Signs and Symptoms

- Dysuria
- Urinary frequency
- Urgency
- Sensation of bladder fullness
- Suprapubic tenderness
- Cloudy, foul-smelling urine
- Backache and pelvic pain
- Low-grade fever

CRITICAL COMPONENT

UTI and Older Women

- Older women are more susceptible to UTI due to:
  - Suppressed immune system.
  - Weakened muscles of the bladder that increases the risk for incomplete emptying of the bladder.
  - Decreased levels of estrogen, which can alter the normal vaginal flora allowing for growth of **E. coli**, which can spread to the urinary tract.
- Older women usually do not present with the common signs of UTI such as fever. When fever does occur, it is related to a serious UTI and needs immediate treatment.
- UTI places stress on the body, and in older women the stress can cause confusion and abrupt changes in behavior.
- Symptoms of UTI in older women can include:
  - Confusion or delirium.
  - Agitation.
  - Hallucinations.
  - Poor motor skills or dizziness.
  - Falling.

Medical Management

Antibiotic therapy is used for uncomplicated UTI. Medications most commonly used are:

- Trimethoprim/sulfamethoxazole (e.g., Bactrim, Septra).
- Ciprofloxacin (e.g., Cipro).
- Nitrofurantoin macrocrystals (e.g., Macrodantin)
- Fosfomycin (e.g., Monurol)

SAFE AND EFFECTIVE NURSING CARE: Understanding Medication

- Trimethoprim/Sulfamethoxazole (Bactrim)
- Indication: Urinary tract infection (also used for treatment of bronchitis, otitis media, pneumonia)
- Action: Inhibits the metabolism of folic acid in bacteria
- Common side effects: Nausea, vomiting, diarrhea, and rashes
- Route and dosage: PO; 160 mg TMP/800 mg SMX every 12 hours for 10 to 14 days

Vallerand & Sanoski, 2017.

Nursing Actions

- Teach women to take full course of antibiotic therapy.
- Provide information on strategies to promote bladder health and ways to decrease risk for developing UTI.
  - Drink 2 to 4 quarts of fluid each day.
  - Void every 2 to 4 hours; avoid postponing urination. When urine remains in the bladder for prolonged periods, bacteria has increased time to multiply.
  - Empty bladder before and after intercourse to flush out bacteria in the urethra.
  - Remain hydrated to keep bacteria flushed out of the urinary tract system.
  - Wipe the urethral meatus and perineum from front to back after voiding.
  - Wear cotton underpants and change daily; avoid tight-fitting underwear and pants.
  - Avoid caffeine and alcohol since these can irritate the bladder.
  - Do not douche or use feminine hygiene products that can alter the normal vagina flora.
  - Avoid harsh soaps, powders, sprays, and bubble baths.
  - Drinking cranberry juice has no proven evidence that it will prevent UTIs. It should not be taken if the woman takes Coumadin, aspirin, or medications that effect the liver (Mayo Clinic, 2016a).
- Teach women about the signs and symptoms of UTI and to report these to their health care providers.

LEIOMYOMA OF THE UTERUS

Leiomyomas of the uterus, also referred to as myomas or uterine fibroids, are benign fibrous tumors of the uterine wall. Leiomyomas are the most common tumors in women. They vary in size, number, and location and are estrogen and progesterone sensitive. Growth of leiomyomas is seen during the reproductive years due to increased levels of estrogen and progesterone. Leiomyomas are usually asymptomatic. The severity of symptoms is related to the number, size, and locations of the myomas.

Risk Factors

- Early menarche
- Heredity: Increased risk when mother or sister has myomas
- Race: Black women more likely to have myomas
- Vitamin D deficiency
- Obesity (Lobo et al., 2017; Mayo Clinic, 2016b)

Signs and Symptoms

- Pelvic pressure from the enlarging mass
- Dysmenorrhea, metrorrhagia, menorrhagia, including risk for anemia related to menorrhagia
- Pelvic pain, backaches, and/or leg pain
- Urinary frequency and urgency when myomas are pressing on the bladder
- Palpation of tumor during bimanual pelvic examination

Medical Management

- Pelvic ultrasound to confirm diagnosis of tumors and rule out pregnancy.
- Routine pelvic examinations every 6 months to assess rate of growth.
- Blood transfusions may be needed for severe anemia related to excessive blood loss.
- Treatment for leiomyomas is based on the size and location of the tumors, the degree to which they interfere with the woman's quality of life, and whether the woman desires pregnancy. Most tumors will shrink after menopause. Treatment options include:
  - GnRH agonists for 3 months to control bleeding and shrink tumor.
  - Uterine artery embolization: Polyvinyl alcohol pellets are injected into selected blood vessels to block the blood supply to the tumor and cause it to shrink.
  - Laser surgery: Laser coagulation vaporizes the fibroids and produces necrosis. It can increase the woman's risk for infertility due to uterine scarring.
  - Myomectomy, removal of the tumor, is common for symptomatic women who desire pregnancy.
  - Hysterectomy is recommended for women who do not desire pregnancy and who are experiencing excess bleeding. Leiomyomas are one of the main indicators for hysterectomy.

Nursing Actions

Nursing actions vary based on the method of medical or surgical treatment. Nurses are most likely to care for women being treated for myomas in the inpatient setting following a hysterectomy.

OVARIAN CYSTS

Ovarian cysts are enclosed sacs that contain fluid, blood, and/or cells that develop inside or on the surface of the ovaries. Ovarian cysts are often discovered during routine pelvic examinations. Most cysts spontaneously disappear either by reabsorption of the fluid within the cyst or by rupturing within 8 weeks (Lobo et al., 2017). Two of the more common types of ovarian cysts are follicular cysts and corpus luteum cysts.

Follicular cysts are the most common type of ovarian cyst. They develop during the follicular phase (first half of the menstrual cycle) when the dominant mature follicle fails to rupture (ovulate) and begins to fill with fluid or when an immature follicle fails to degenerate (Lobo et al., 2017). Follicular cysts are usually asymptomatic. One-quarter of women who have this type of cyst report pain and/or a heavy, achy feeling in the pelvis.

Corpus luteum cysts form from the corpus luteum during the luteal phase (second half of the menstrual cycle). Normally, the corpus luteum forms after ovulation and gradually degenerates if pregnancy does not occur. Occasionally, the corpus luteum seals and fills with fluid or blood and forms a cyst. The woman may experience acute lower abdominal pain and delayed menses followed by menorrhagia (Lobo et al., 2017).

Some cysts rupture and cause intraperitoneal bleeding. Rupture of cysts may be caused by coitus, exercise, lower abdominal trauma, or pelvic exam. The woman with intraperitoneal bleeding will experience sudden and severe abdominal pain and may require surgery and blood transfusions.

Diagnosis is usually based on symptoms and bimanual examination. Ultrasonography may be used to aid in the diagnosis and to rule out pregnancy, but ultrasound cannot provide a definitive diagnosis. It is important to rule out ovarian cancer, and additional tests and procedures may be ordered, such as:

- CA 125 test: This measures the amount of CA 125 (cancer antigen 125) in the blood. Elevated levels occur in women with endometriosis, myomas, PID, and ovarian cancer.
- Laparoscopic surgery to visualize ovaries and/or remove cyst.

Medical Management

- Since most cysts spontaneously disappear either by reabsorption of the fluid within the cyst or by rupturing within 8 weeks, monitoring the condition with repeat pelvic exam in 6 to 8 weeks is the treatment of choice when the symptoms are mild (Lobo et al., 2017).
- NSAIDs used for pain management.

- Oral contraceptives are prescribed to inhibit ovulation to decrease risk of developing additional cysts.
- Surgical removal of cyst is indicated when the cyst:
  - Remains present after several menstrual cycles.
  - Occurs after menopause since postmenopausal women with ovarian cysts have a higher risk for ovarian cancer.
  - Has grown larger.
  - Has an unusual appearance noted on the ultrasound.
  - Causes severe pain.

PELVIC ORGAN PROLAPSE

The pelvic organs are supported by muscles, ligaments, and fascia. When these structures are weakened, pelvic organs can descend into the vagina or against the vaginal wall. This disorder is known as pelvic organ prolapse (POP). POP can affect the bladder, urethra, uterus, and rectum. Common disorders related to POP are uterine prolapse, cystocele, and rectocele (Fig. 19–4). Risk factors for POP are:

- Childbirth trauma related to:
  - Vaginal deliveries.
  - Large babies.
  - Forceps or vacuum deliveries.
  - Poor suturing techniques with repair of episiotomies or lacerations.

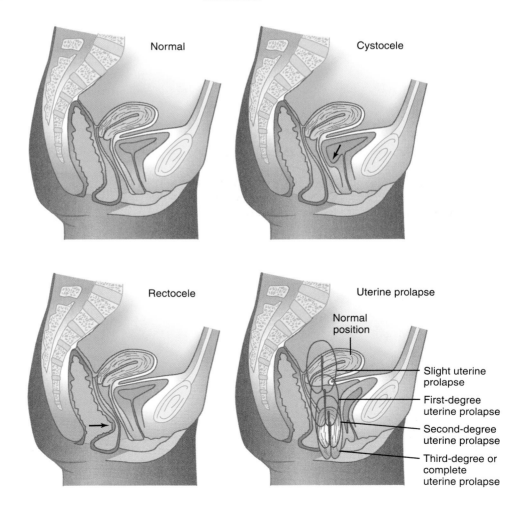

FIGURE 19–4 Cystocele, rectocele, and uterine prolapse.

- Pelvic trauma (i.e., pelvic surgery).
- Stress and strain from heavy lifting, constipation, violent coughing.
- Obesity.
- Menopause: Low levels of estrogen weaken the pelvic floor muscles.

Uterine Prolapse

Uterine prolapse occurs when there is a weakening of the pelvic connective tissue, pubococcygeus muscle, and uterine ligaments, allowing the uterus to descend into the vagina. Degrees of prolapse vary from slight prolapse to third-degree prolapse. Also known as complete uterine prolapse, third-degree prolapse occurs when the uterus has descended out of the vagina (see Fig. 19–4).

Assessment Findings

- Protrusion of uterus into the vagina
- Low backache
- Sensation of heaviness in the pelvis or vagina
- Sensation that the uterus is falling out
- Difficult or painful intercourse

Medical Management

- Vaginal pessary: A rubber or silicone-based ring placed in the vagina to support the uterus; effective for a mild degree of uterine prolapse (Fig. 19–5).
- Surgery, which may include hysterectomy.

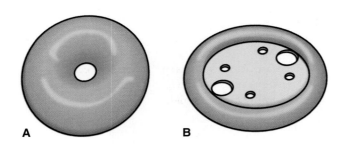

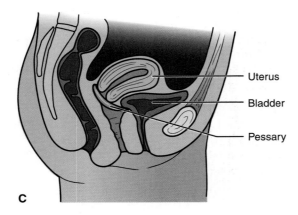

FIGURE 19–5 Vaginal pessary (*A*) Doughnut pessary. (*B*) Ring pessary. (*C*) Inserted pessary.

Nursing Actions

- Explain the importance of Kegel exercises for improving pelvic muscle strength and teach the woman how to do Kegel exercises.
- Instruct the woman on the treatment and prevention of constipation, such as a high-fiber diet and increased fluid intake. This will help in reducing straining during defecation and decrease stress on existing POP.
- Instruct the woman to avoid heavy lifting to decrease stress on pelvic organs.
- Explain the relationship between increased weight and increased risk of prolapsed uterus and discuss weight reduction strategies.
- Provide postoperative care for women having a hysterectomy.

Cystocele and Rectocele

Cystocele, also known as anterior prolapse, is the bulging of the bladder into the vagina. This occurs when the wall between the vagina and bladder weakens and stretches. Rectocele, also known as posterior prolapse, is the bulging of the rectum into the vagina. This occurs when the wall between the vagina and the rectum weakens and stretches.

Assessment Findings for Cystocele

- Bulging mass in the anterior vaginal wall
- Sense of fullness or pressure in the vaginal area
- Degree of bulging increases when straining, coughing, bearing down, lifting, or standing for a prolonged period of time
- Stress incontinence
- Bladder infections
- Urine leakage during intercourse
- Sexual dysfunction such as dyspareunia, vaginal dryness, and irritation (Lobo et al., 2017)

Assessment Findings for Rectocele

- Bulging mass in the posterior vaginal wall
- Straining and prolonged standing can increase the degree of the bulging.
- Irritation of the vaginal mucosa
- Constipation

Medical Management

Medical management is based on degree of bulging, effects on the woman's quality of life, and the woman's overall health. Treatment options include:

- Vaginal pessary to support the bladder.
- Estrogen therapy to improve pelvis muscle strength.
- Surgical repair of the cystocele and/or rectocele.

Nursing Actions

- Explain the importance of Kegel exercises for improving pelvic muscle strength and teach the woman how to do Kegel exercises.
- Instruct the woman on the treatment and prevention of constipation, such as a high-fiber diet and increased fluid intake.

This will help in reducing straining during defecation and decrease stress on existing POP.

- Instruct the woman to avoid heavy lifting to decrease stress on pelvic organs.
- Explain the relationship between increased weight and increased risk of cystoceles/rectoceles and discuss weight-reduction strategies.

URINARY INCONTINENCE

Urinary incontinence is the loss of bladder control and can range from stress incontinence to sudden urge to void followed by uncontrolled voiding. Stress incontinence is leakage of urine when there is an increase in intra-abdominal pressure related to coughing, sneezing, or laughing. Urinary incontinence can have a profound effect on the woman's quality of life by limiting her activities due to the embarrassment of uncontrolled urination.

Risk Factors

- Childbirth
- Aging: Leads to a decrease in estrogen and a weakening of muscles, thus decreasing the ability of the urethra to remain closed.
- Obesity: The risk increases for every 5 units of body mass index (BMI) increase (Lobo et al., 2017).
- Smoking: Causes chronic coughing and places stress on the urinary sphincters.

Assessment Findings

- Leakage of urine when coughing, sneezing, laughing, or lifting
- Sudden and intense urge to void followed by uncontrolled voiding

Medical Management

- Treatment is based on the degree of incontinence and the effect it has on quality of life.
- Behavioral techniques
  - Bladder training: Waiting 5 minutes from feeling the urge to void to urinating and gradually increasing the time between urge to voiding.
  - Scheduled toilet trips: Developing a schedule for voiding and not waiting to feel the urge to void.
  - Limiting alcohol and caffeine use: These act as a bladder stimulant and diuretic.
  - Losing weight.
- Pelvic floor exercises
  - Kegel exercises: Improve pelvic floor muscle strength
- Medications
  - Tolterodine (Detrol) and mirabegron (Myrbetriq): Used to treat overactive bladders
  - Estrogen cream applied to the genital tissues: Improves the tone and tissue in the urethral and vaginal areas
- Medical devices
  - Pessary: Inserted in the vagina; helps hold the bladder in place

- Urethral insert: A small tampon-like disposable plug that the woman inserts into urethra prior to activities that can cause stress incontinence, such as sports or exercise. The plug is removed after the activity and prior to voiding.
- Surgery

SAFE AND EFFECTIVE NURSING CARE: Understanding Medication

Tolterodine (Detrol)

- Action: Inhibits cholinergic mediated bladder contractions → decreased urinary frequency, urgency, and urge incontinence
- Common side effects: Dry mouth, headache, and dizziness
- Route and dosage: PO; 2 mg twice daily

Vallerand & Sanoski, 2017.

Nursing Actions

- Instruct the woman on the importance of Kegel exercises and teach her how to do Kegel exercises.
- Instruct the woman on the treatment and prevention of constipation by increasing fiber in the diet and fluid intake.
- Instruct her to avoid heavy lifting.
- Explain the relationship between increased weight and increased risk of urinary incontinence and discuss weight-reduction strategies.
- Maintain skin integrity by instructing the woman to keep the area clean and dry.
- Encourage the woman to decrease alcohol and caffeine intake, as both cause an increase in urination.
- Provide strategies for retraining the bladder, such as scheduling toileting times and gradually increasing the wait time after she feels the urge to void.

VAGINAL FISTULAS

Vaginal fistulas are abnormal connections between the vagina and bladder, vagina and urethra, and/or vagina and rectum. The fistula provides a pathway for fecal material or urine to enter the vagina. Fistulas can develop as a result of trauma to the tissue related to childbirth, trauma from surgery, pelvic radiation damage, weakened pelvic tissue, and violent coitus or sexual abuse.

Assessment Findings

- Leakage of urine or fecal material from the vagina
- Foul vaginal odor
- Irritation of the vaginal mucosa

Medical Management

- Pelvic, rectal, and perineal skin examinations to determine the location and severity of fistula.

- Small fistulas usually resolve on their own if tissue is allowed to rest.
- Larger fistulas may require surgical repair.

Nursing Actions

- Reinforce teaching and clarify information provided by the primary health care provider.
- Postoperative care:
  - Assess vital signs as per protocol.
  - Assess perineal area for increased bleeding.
  - Assess for pain and use appropriate pain-management techniques.
- Postoperative teaching:
  - Instruct the woman with rectal fistula repair to increase fiber in her diet and increase fluid intake to decrease risk of constipation. Maintaining soft stool decreases trauma to the site and promotes healing.
  - Instruct how to use a sitz bath and explain the importance of sitz baths in promoting healing and comfort.
  - Provide medication information. Antibiotics are usually prescribed.
  - Instruct to notify surgeon when there is an elevated temperature, increased bleeding, or increased pain.

BREAST DISORDERS

Breast disorders include both benign and malignant changes and diseases. Most breast changes and disorders are benign, but the discovery of a breast mass or changes in the breast still evokes feelings of fear and anxiety. Benign and malignant disorders share similar symptoms, so breast changes must be evaluated by the woman's health care provider. The use of mammography, ultrasound, and magnetic resonance imaging (MRI) are important in the early detection and treatment of benign and cancerous disorders of the breast. See Chapter 18 for recommended screening and testing. The three most common breast disorder symptoms are:

- Pain: This is usually related to hormonal changes and is most common in perimenopausal women. Pain can also be associated with cysts of the breast. Fewer than 10% of women with breast cancer will present with pain.
- Discharge from the nipple: This is classified as either spontaneous or elicited. Elicited discharge results from nipple compression or stimulation. Elicited discharge from both nipples that is milky in color and nonbloody is considered normal. Spontaneous discharge or elicited discharge from one nipple or discharge that is bloody needs further evaluation. Nipple discharge is not a common symptom of breast cancer.
- Palpable breast masses are common and are usually benign, but all breast masses must be evaluated to rule out malignancy.

Fibrocystic Breasts

Fibrocystic breast is also referred to as benign breast disease or fibrocystic changes. It is common for breasts to develop fibrous tissue and benign cysts. These changes occur in more than 50% of women between the ages of 20 and 50 years. The cause is not known but it is believed to be related to an imbalance of estrogen and progesterone. The cysts are often tender to touch and fluctuate in size in response to the menstrual cycle. Caffeine intake may exacerbate the condition.

Signs and Symptoms

- Cyclic bilateral breast pain, usually in the upper, outer quadrants of the breasts
- Increased engorgement and density of the breasts
- Increased nodularity of the breasts
- Fluctuation in the size of the cystic areas

Medical Management

- Differentiate between fibrocystic changes and breast cancer using mammography and ultrasound. Health care provider may also aspirate the cyst for evaluation of fluid.
- Management centers on symptom relief:
  - Oral contraceptives
  - Use of OTC pain medications such as NSAIDs and acetaminophen
  - Supportive bra
  - Avoidance of caffeine, smoking, and alcohol
  - Application of heat to the breast

Nursing Actions

- Instruct the woman to follow recommended breast screenings and notify her health care provider if she notes changes in her breasts.
- Provide information on methods of symptom relief, such as heat to breast and use of supportive bra.

Breast Cancer

Breast cancer is the most common cancer in women worldwide. North America has the highest rate of breast cancer, with one in eight women diagnosed at some point in her lifetime. Breast cancer in early stages usually produces no symptoms and cannot be felt on palpation. The woman's prognosis improves with early detection and treatment.

Risk Factors

The major risk factors are:
- Increasing age: The most invasive form of breast cancer is found in women aged 55 and older (American Cancer Society [ACS], 2016a).
- Defects in breast cancer genes *BRCA1* or *BRCA 2*.
- Two out of 10 women diagnosed with breast cancer have a family history of breast cancer (ACS, 2016a).
- Dense breasts (ACS, 2016a).
- Personal history of breast cancer in at least one breast.
- Exposure to head or chest radiation.

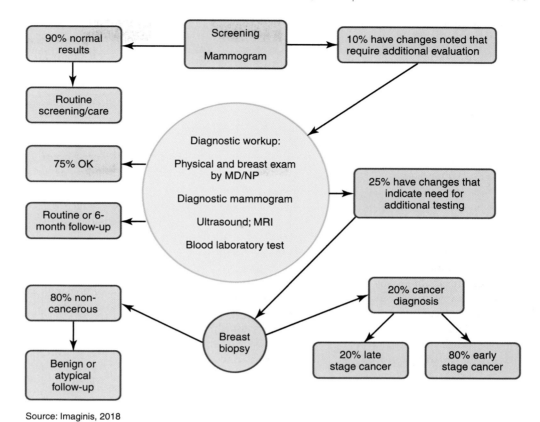

FIGURE 19–6 Breast cancer diagnosis process.

Source: Imaginis, 2018

Additional factors include:

- Excess weight.
- Exposure to estrogen through early onset of menarche, late menopause, or use of hormone therapy.
- Smoking.
- Exposure to carcinogens.
- Excessive use of alcohol.
- Exposure to diethylstilbestrol (DES).

Diagnosis

The screening and diagnostic procedures/tests used in the diagnosis of breast cancer include (Fig. 19–6):

- Diagnostic mammograms create images of the area of concern that provide additional information on size and character of the mass.
- Breast ultrasounds assist in determining if the area of concern is a fluid-filled cyst or solid mass.
- MRI is useful in differentiating benign from malignant tissue, especially in women with dense, fibroglandular breasts; when scar tissue is present from previous breast surgery; and for new tumors in women who have had previous lumpectomy. Yearly screening MRI and mammogram are recommended for women at high risk for breast cancer (ACS, 2016a).
- Breast biopsy can distinguish between benign and malignant tissue.

CRITICAL COMPONENT

Clinical Breast Exam and Breast Self-Exam

Research has not shown a clear benefit of physical breast exams done by either a health professional or by the woman for breast cancer screening. There is very little evidence that these tests help find breast cancer early when women also get screening mammograms. Because of this, a regular clinical breast exam and breast self-exam are not recommended. Still, all women should be familiar with how their breasts normally look and feel and report any changes to a health care provider right away.

ACS, 2016a.

Indicators of Disease Prognosis

- Stages of breast cancer (Table 19–4)
- Presence of hormone receptor levels
- Presence of HER2/neu (human epidermal growth factor receptor 2) in the tumor tissue
- Breast cancer grade, based on how much the cancer cells look like normal cells. A low-grade number means the cancer is slow-growing and less likely to spread, and a high-grade number means it is fast-growing and more likely to spread (ACS, 2016a).

TABLE 19–4   Stages of Breast Cancer

STAGE 0	Ductal carcinoma in situ—cancer cells are limited to a duct and have not invaded into surrounding tissue; this is the earliest form of breast cancer.
STAGE IA	The tumor is 2 cm or less in size, and it has not spread to the lymph nodes or distant sites.
STAGE IB	The tumor is 2 cm or less. There is evidence of micrometastases in one to three axillary lymph nodes. It has not spread to distant sites.
STAGE IIA	The cancer has not spread to distant sites, and one of the following applies: • The tumor is larger than 2 cm and less than 5 cm across; it has not spread to the lymph nodes. • The tumor is 2 cm or less; it has spread to one to three axillary nodes with cancer in the lymph nodes larger than 2 mm across. • The tumor is 2 cm or less, and tiny amounts of cancer are found in the internal mammary lymph nodes. • The tumor is 2 cm or less and has spread to one to three axillary lymph nodes and to internal mammary lymph nodes.
STAGE IIB	The cancer has not spread to a distant site, and one of the following applies: • The tumor is larger than 2 cm and less than 5 cm across; it has spread to one to three axillary lymph nodes, and/or tiny amounts of cancer are found in the internal mammary lymph nodes. • The tumor is larger than 5 cm; it has not grown into the chest wall and has not spread to the lymph nodes.
STAGE IIIA	The tumor has not spread to distant sites, and one of the following applies: • The tumor is 5 cm or less. It has spread to four to nine axillary lymph nodes, or it has enlarged the internal mammary lymph nodes. • The tumor is more than 5 cm but has not invaded the chest wall or skin. It has spread to one to nine axillary nodes or to internal mammary nodes.
STAGE IIIB	The cancer has not spread to distant sites. The tumor has grown into the chest wall or skin, and one of the following applies: • It has not spread to lymph nodes. • It has spread to one to three axillary lymph nodes, and/or tiny amounts of cancer are found in internal mammary lymph nodes. • It has spread to four to nine axillary lymph nodes, or it has enlarged the internal mammary lymph nodes.
STAGE IIIC	The cancer has not spread to distant sites. The tumor is any size, and one of the following applies: • It has spread to 10 or more axillary lymph nodes. • It has spread to lymph nodes under or above the clavicle. • It involves axillary lymph nodes and has enlarged the internal mammary lymph nodes. • It has spread to four or more axillary nodes, and tiny amounts are found in internal mammary lymph nodes.
STAGE IV	The cancer has spread to distant organs or lymph nodes distant from the breast. The most common sites are the bone, liver, brain, or lung.

ACS, 2016g.

CRITICAL COMPONENT

Breast Cancer Screening Tool

• The breast cancer screening tool developed by the National Cancer Institute (NCI) and National Surgical Adjuvant Breast and Bowel Project estimates a woman's risk of developing invasive breast cancer in 5 years and up to age 90. It considers data such as the woman's age, family history of breast cancer, and previous breast biopsies. The tool can be accessed at www.cancer.gov/bcrisktool.

NCI, 2011.

Medical Management

Treatment is determined by stage of cancer. The breast cancer staging system goes from stage 0 (ductal carcinoma in situ, the earliest form of breast cancer) to stage IV (the cancer has metastasized to distant organs or to distant lymph nodes). Medical management includes:

● Surgical interventions:
  ● Lumpectomy: The lump and an area of surrounding normal tissue are removed. This procedure is usually followed by radiation therapy.
  ● Partial or segmental mastectomy: The tumor, the surrounding breast tissue, a portion of the lining of the chest

wall, and some of the axillary lymph nodes are removed. This procedure is usually followed by radiation therapy.

- Simple mastectomy: All the breast tissue along with the area surrounding the nipple and areola are removed. This procedure may be followed by radiation therapy, chemotherapy, or hormone therapy.
- Modified radical mastectomy: The entire breast and several axillary lymph nodes are removed; the chest wall is left intact.
- Some women who have mastectomies choose to undergo breast reconstruction. Breast reconstruction, when desired, is performed by a plastic surgeon at the same time as the mastectomy.
- Radiation therapy, which usually begins 3 to 4 weeks after surgery.
  - External radiation: A radiation therapy machine aims radiation toward the tumor. Treatments are given 5 days a week for 5 to 6 weeks.
  - Internal radiation (mammo site): A radioactive substance sealed in needles, seeds, wires, or a catheter is placed directly into or near the tumor. Treatments are given twice a day for 5 days for a total of 10 sessions.
- Chemotherapy:
  - Oncotype DX test may be performed to determine if the woman is likely to benefit from chemotherapy.
  - Chemotherapy is most commonly used to treat advanced metastatic cancer or to prevent recurrence of cancer.
  - Usually, a combination of two or more drugs is used.
  - Chemotherapy agents may be administered orally or intravenously.
- Hormone therapy:
  - Some breast cancer cells require estrogen to grow and are classified as estrogen-receptor positive. This means that the cancer cells have a protein to which estrogen binds.
  - Antiestrogen medications such as tamoxifen (Nolvadex D) bind to these protein receptors, blocking estrogen binding and reducing the influence of estrogen on the tumor.
  - Fulvestrant (Faslodex) given by injection reduces the number of estrogen receptors on breast tumors.
  - Aromatase inhibitors such as anastrozole (Arimidex) may be used in postmenopausal women whose cancer is classified as estrogen-receptor positive. Aromatase inhibitors interfere with the amount of estrogen produced by the woman's body tissue (not the ovaries) by blocking the conversion of androgens into estrogens.
- Targeted therapy
  - Trastuzumab (Herceptin), a monoclonal antibody that directly targets the HER2 protein of breast tumors, is a treatment option for women with breast cancer that overproduces HER2 (ACS, 2016a).

Nursing Actions

- Provide emotional support to the woman and family, including opportunities for them to share feelings and concerns.

- Provide current, evidence-based information to the woman and family regarding treatment options.
  - Encourage the woman to consider all options and seek other opinions or other professionals if she is not comfortable with recommendations.
- Provide information on methods that address side effects from treatment (Tables 19–5 and 19–6).
- Provide information on nutrition that promotes healing and enhances the immune system.
- Provide information on complementary modalities such as imagery, journal writing, and hypnosis that can be used to diminish side effects from cancer treatment therapies.
- Provide information regarding community resources.
  - Look Good Feel Better is a free program that helps women learn beauty techniques to restore their self-image and cope with appearance-related side effects of cancer treatment. For additional information go to http://lookgoodfeelbetter.org/.
  - Breast cancer support such as American Cancer Society Reach to Recovery Program

CRITICAL COMPONENT

Oncotype DX Test

- The oncotype DX test is a genomic assay that assesses the activity of 21 different genes taken from a tissue sample of the cancer tumor. This test assists the health care provider in determining if the cancer is likely to recur or to benefit from chemotherapy.
- Women with stage I or II, estrogen-receptor-positive (ER+) breast cancer that has not spread to the lymph nodes may benefit from this test in determining type of cancer treatment.

ACS, 2016a.

SAFE AND EFFECTIVE NURSING CARE: Understanding Medication

Tamoxifen (Nolvadex D)

- Indications: Reduces risk of breast cancer in women who are at increased risk for developing breast cancer; treatment of breast cancer
- Action: Competes with estrogen for binding sites in the breast
- Serious side effects: Pulmonary embolism, stroke, uterine malignancies
- Common side effects: Vaginal dryness, hot flashes, joint pain, leg cramps, nausea
- Route and dose: PO; 10 to 20 mg twice daily or 20 mg once daily for 5 years

ACS, 2016a; Vallerand, & Sanoski, 2017.

TABLE 19–5 Management of Radiation Therapy Side Effects

SIDE EFFECT	WAYS TO MANAGE

Diarrhea: Related to damage of healthy cells in large and small intestine	• Drink 8–12 cups of clear liquids.
	  • Gatorade or Pedialyte for electrolyte replacement
	• Eat small frequent meals.
	  • Five to six small meals rather than three large meals
	• Eat foods that provide nourishment without increasing risk for diarrhea.
	  • Foods that are low in fiber, fat, and lactose
	  • Fresh fruit
	  • Cooked vegetables
	• Take antidiarrheal medications such as Imodium A-D.
	• Take care of rectum.
	  • Use baby wipes instead of toilet paper
	  • Take sitz baths

Fatigue: Related to anemia, depression, infection, and medications	• Get 8 hours of sleep per night.
	  • The woman may need more sleep per night than she needed before radiation therapy.
	• Plan time to rest.
	  • Take 10- to 15-minute rest breaks throughout the day.
	  • Take several naps during the day.
	• Decrease daily activities.
	  • The woman may not have enough energy for all the activity she used to do. She should select the activities that are most important to her and limit those that are less important.
	• Exercise
	  • 15–30 minutes of daily exercise improves overall feeling of well-being.
	• Change work schedule.
	  • May need to decrease work hours for a few weeks.
	• Ask family and friends for help at home.

Sexual and fertility changes: Related to damage to healthy tissue of the vagina and ovaries	• Fertility
	  • Women desiring future pregnancies need to talk with health care provider about ways to preserve fertility, such as preserving eggs for future use.
	• Sexual difficulties
	  • Use water or mineral-based lubricant if experiencing vaginal dryness.
	• Vaginal stenosis
	  • Discuss use of vaginal dilators with health care provider.

Skin changes: Related to damage of healthy tissue	• Skin care
	  • Gently wash area; do not rub, scrub, or scratch.
	• Avoid heat and cold.
	  • Wash in lukewarm water.
	  • Do not use heating pads or ice packs.
	• Wear soft and loose-fitting clothes around treatment area.
	• Protect skin from sun.

Urinary and bladder changes: Related to damage of healthy cells of bladder and urinary tract, causing inflammation, ulcers, and infections	• Drink 6–8 cups of fluid per day. • Avoid coffee, black tea, alcohol, and spices. • Report changes to health care provider. • May require antibiotic therapy.

ACS, 2017.

Side effects, except for fatigue, are directly related and limited to the site being treated with radiation therapy (e.g., radiation therapy for breast cancer does not cause diarrhea).

TABLE 19–6 Management of Chemotherapy Side Effects

Anemia	• Eat high-protein foods such as meat, peanut butter, and eggs. • Eat foods high in iron, such as red meats, leafy greens, and cooked dried beans.
Appetite changes	• Eat five or six small meals per day. • Try new food to keep up interest in foods. • Eat with friends and family. • Eat with plastic forks and spoons and use glass pots if food tastes like metal. • Drink milkshakes or eat soup because these are easier to swallow.
Bleeding problems	• Use electric shaver instead of a razor. • Wear shoes all the time (except when sleeping). • Brush teeth with soft toothbrush. • Avoid being constipated.
Constipation	• Eat high-fiber foods such as whole-grain bread, fruits, and vegetables. • Increase fluid intake. • Exercise 15–30 minutes per day.
Mouth and throat changes	• Brush teeth and tongue with soft toothbrush after each meal. • Rinse mouth with solution prescribed. • Use lip balm. • Choose foods that are soft, wet, and easy to swallow.

Cancer Care, 2016.

GYNECOLOGICAL CANCERS

Gynecological cancer includes cancer of the cervix, uterus (endometrium), ovaries, fallopian tubes, vagina, and vulva. Endometrial cancer is the most common reproductive cancer, followed by cervical and ovarian. Cancers of the fallopian tubes, vagina, and vulva are rare. This section will focus on cervical, endometrial, and ovarian cancers.

Cervical Cancer

Prior to the routine use of the Papanicolaou (Pap) smear, which was introduced in the 1950s, cervical cancer was the leading cause of cancer-related deaths in women. It is now ranked as the 16th leading cause of cancer-related deaths (ACS, 2016b). This decrease is attributed to use of Pap smears to detect cervical cancer at an early stage when it can more easily be treated.

Human papillomavirus (HPV), the most common STI, is the primary cause of cervical cancer. Most sexually active people will get the virus at some point. Cervical cancer is typically slow-growing and begins with dysplasia, a precancerous condition that is 100% treatable. However, undetected or untreated precancerous changes can develop into cervical cancer that can spread to the bladder, intestines, lungs, and liver.

Pap tests are used for cervical cytological screening (see Chapter 18 for recommended screenings and immunizations for women across the life span). Women with abnormal cervical cytology screening need further evaluation, since the Pap test is a screening test and not a diagnostic test. A cervical conization is used for definitive diagnosis. Most women who are diagnosed with cervical cancer have not had regular Pap testing or have not followed up on abnormal results.

Risk Factors

● HPV infection (major risk factor)
● Early onset of sexual activity (before age 16)
● Cigarette smoking
● STIs such as genital herpes, chlamydia
● Weakened immune system
● Multiple sex partners
● In utero exposure to DES
● Use of birth control pills for 5 or more years
● Given birth to three or more children

Risk Reduction

See Chapter 18.

Signs and Symptoms

Early stages of cervical cancer usually do not produce symptoms. Symptoms appear when the cancer is advanced and has invaded nearby tissue.

● Vaginal discharge that may be watery, pink, brown, bloody, or foul-smelling
● Leaking of urine or feces from vagina
● Abnormal vaginal bleeding between periods, after intercourse, or after menopause
● Menstrual period that becomes heavier and lasts longer
● Dyspareunia
● Loss of appetite and/or weight
● Fatigue
● Pelvic, back, and/or leg pain

Medical Management

● Cervical cone biopsy to establish diagnosis
● Additional testing to determine if cancer is confined to the cervix or if it has spread to other organs:
  ● Computed tomography (CT) scan
  ● MRI
  ● Positron emission tomography (PET) scan
  ● Intravenous pyelography (IVP)
  ● Chest x-ray
  ● Cystoscopy
  ● Blood studies

TABLE 19–7   Staging and Treatment of Cervical Cancer

STAGES	TREATMENT OPTIONS
Stage 0: Abnormal cells are in the epithelium. These cells may become cancer. Also called carcinoma in situ.	• Conization; LEEP • Laser surgery • Cryosurgery • Total hysterectomy • External radiation
Stage I: Cancer has invaded the cervix and is confined to the cervix. Stage IA$_1$: Cancer is 3 mm deep and 7 mm wide. Stage IA$_2$: Cancer is 3 mm but 5 mm deep and 7 mm wide. Stage IB$_1$: Cancer can only be seen with a microscope and is at least 5 mm deep and 7 mm wide or can be seen without a microscope and is 4 cm. Stage IB$_2$: Cancer is seen without microscope and is 4 cm.	• Total hysterectomy with or without bilateral salpingo-oophorectomy • Conization • Modified radical hysterectomy and removal of lymph nodes • Internal radiation therapy • Combination of internal and external radiation therapy • Radical hysterectomy and removal of lymph nodes • Radical hysterectomy with removal of lymph nodes followed by radiation therapy and chemotherapy • Combination of radiation therapy and chemotherapy
Stage II: Cancer has extended beyond the cervix but not into the pelvic wall. It has invaded the upper but not lower portion of the vagina. Stage IIA: Cancer has spread to the upper two-thirds of the vagina but not to the tissues around the uterus. Stage IIA$_1$: Cancer can be seen without a microscope and is 4 cm. Stage IIA$_2$: Cancer can be seen without a microscope and is greater than 4 cm. Stage IIB: Cancer has spread beyond the cervix to the tissues around the uterus.	• Internal and external radiation therapy and chemotherapy • Radical hysterectomy and removal of lymph nodes • Radical hysterectomy and removal of lymph nodes followed by radiation therapy and chemotherapy
Stage III: Cancer has extended to the lower one-third of the vagina and/or to the pelvic wall and/or has caused kidney problems (may block the flow of urine). Stage IIIA: Cancer has spread to lower one-third of the vagina but not into the pelvic wall. Stage IIIB: Cancer has spread into the pelvic wall and/or has become large enough to block the ureters.	• Radical hysterectomy and removal of lymph nodes followed by internal and external radiation therapy and chemotherapy
Stage IV: Cancer has spread to the bladder, rectum, or other parts of the body. Stage IVA: Cancer has spread to nearby organs such as bladder or rectum. Stage IVB: Cancer has spread to other parts of the body such as liver, lungs, bones, or distant lymph nodes.	• Radical hysterectomy and removal of lymph nodes followed by internal and external radiation therapy and chemotherapy

ACS, 2016c.

● Treatment is based on the stage of cancer and the woman's desire for pregnancy (Table 19–7).

● Chemotherapy is used for cervical cancer that has either metastasized or recurred.

● Angiogenesis inhibitors, such as bevacizumab, are a target drug therapy used with chemotherapy to treat advanced cervical cancer.

Nursing Actions

Patient education and support are critical nursing actions for women with cervical cancer.

● Provide emotional support to the woman and her family.

● Provide information on nutrition that promotes healing and treats/controls side effects from cancer treatments.

- Explain the importance of rest and sleep in the promotion of healing.
- Provide information on community support services.
- Care for women undergoing surgical treatment:
  - Address the woman's and family's questions regarding surgical procedure.
  - Provide preoperative and postoperative care.
- Care for woman undergoing radiation therapy:
  - Provide information on ways to manage side effects related to external radiation (see Table 19–5).
  - Teach the importance of skin care in decreasing risk of tissue breakdown.
  - Instruct the woman to check with health care provider regarding types of lotions and creams to use.
  - Instruct the woman to avoid the use of adhesive tape on the treatment area.
  - Recommend exposing the treatment area to air whenever possible to promote skin integrity.
- Care for woman undergoing chemotherapy:
  - Administer chemotherapy as per orders.
  - Provide information on the management of side effects related to chemotherapy (see Table 19–6).

CRITICAL COMPONENT

Side Effects From External Radiation for Cervical Cancer

Short-term side effects of external radiation to treat cervical cancer include:

- Fatigue.
- Nausea and vomiting.
- Diarrhea.
- Cystitis.
- Bruising.
- Anemia.
- Skin rash.

Long-term side effects include:

- Vaginal stenosis.
- Vaginal dryness.
- Premature menopause.
- Swelling of the legs when pelvic lymph nodes are treated.
- Weakened bones—increased risk for hip fractures.

ACS, 2016e.

Endometrial Cancer

Endometrial cancer is the second most common cancer of the female reproductive system. Diagnosis is established by histological examination of endometrial tissue.

Risk Factors

- Menopausal hormone therapy: Unopposed estrogen therapy in women with a uterus. This can cause endometrial hyperplasia, an increased number of cells in the lining of the uterus.
- Menopause after age 52.
- Obesity affects the synthesis and metabolism of sex hormones and insulin. Obese women tend to have higher levels of estrogen related to the body making additional estrogen in fatty tissue.
- Tamoxifen: Drug used to treat breast cancer
- Nulliparity
- Diabetes
- Polycystic ovarian syndrome

Signs and Symptoms

- Postmenopausal bleeding or abnormal premenopausal bleeding (most common symptom)
- Abnormal vaginal discharge
- Difficult or painful urination
- Dyspareunia
- Pelvic pain or pressure

Stages

- Stage 0: Carcinoma in situ; precancerous lesions confined to the surface layer of the endometrium.
- Stage IA: Cancer cells are in the endometrium and have grown less than halfway through the myometrium.
- Stage IB: Cancer cells are in the endometrium and have grown more than halfway through the myometrium; has not spread beyond the uterus.
- Stage II: Cancer cells have invaded the cervical stroma but have not extended beyond the uterus.
- Stage III: Tumor has spread outside the uterus but is confined to pelvis.
- Stage IV: Tumor has spread outside the pelvis or into the mucosa of the bladder or rectum or distant metastasis (ACS, 2016d).

Medical Management

- Treatment is based on size of tumor, stage of tumor, tumor grade, and whether tumor is affected by estrogen.
- Treatment options
  - Surgery: Hysterectomy, bilateral salpingo-oophorectomy, and pelvic and para-aortic lymph node dissection
  - Radiation therapy
  - Chemotherapy
  - Hormonal therapy (progesterone)

Nursing Actions

- Provide emotional support to the woman and her family.
- Provide information on nutrition that promotes healing and decreases risk for malnutrition.
- Explain the importance of rest and sleep in the promotion of healing.
- Provide preoperative and postoperative care.
- Administer chemotherapy as per orders.
- Provide information on management of side effects from radiation and/or chemotherapy as it applies to the woman (see Tables 19–5 and 19–6).

Ovarian Cancer

There are three main types of ovarian cancers: epithelial, germ cell, and stromal. Ovarian cancer mainly develops in older women, with 50% of new cases affecting women aged 63 years and older. Symptoms of ovarian cancer are often vague, making it difficult to diagnose the disease during early stages. Diagnosis is established by histological examination of the tumor, usually at the time of surgery.

Risk Factors

- Family history of a first-degree relative with ovarian cancer or family history of colorectal or breast cancer
- Personal history of cancer
- Age over 55; risk increases in menopausal women
- Obesity
- First full-term pregnancy after age 35 or never carried pregnancy to full term
- Infertility drugs taken for more than a year
- Tested positive for *BRCA1* or *BRCA2* gene

Signs and Symptoms

Early stages are often asymptomatic or the woman will have vague abdominal, genitourinary, or reproductive symptoms.
- Pressure or pain in the abdomen, pelvis, back, or leg
- Swollen or bloated abdomen
- Urinary urgency and frequency
- Difficulty eating or feeling full quickly (ACS, 2016f)

CRITICAL COMPONENT

Ovarian Cancer Symptom Diary

The four most common occurring early warning signs of ovarian cancer are:

- Bloating.
- Pelvic/abdominal pain.
- Difficulty eating or feeling full quickly.
- Urinary symptoms.

To assist in early detection of ovarian cancer, women may be asked to keep a log of their symptoms for 1 month. They are instructed to record when they experienced any of the four common symptoms, day of the week, and the specific symptom.

　　Women who experience any of these symptoms more than 12 times in 1 month when symptoms first appeared within the past 12 months should be evaluated for possible ovarian cancer. An example of the log is located at www.ovarian.org.uk or download the Ovarian Cancer Action Symptom Diary app.
Ovarian Cancer Action, 2017.

Stages

- Stage I: Cancer cells are found in one or both ovaries.
- Stage II: Cancer cells have spread to other tissue in the pelvis.
- Stage III: Cancer cells have spread outside the pelvis or to the regional lymph nodes.

- Stage IV: Cancer cells have spread to tissue outside the abdomen and pelvis (National Ovarian Cancer Coalition [NOCC], 2017).

Medical Management

- Tests and procedures
  - Transvaginal ultrasound to identify changes in ovaries
  - CT scan and MRI to confirm presence of pelvic mass
  - PET scan to assess for metastasis to other body organs
  - Barium enema x-ray to determine if there is colon and/or rectal involvement
- Stage I: Total abdominal hysterectomy and bilateral salpingo-oophorectomy, omentectomy, biopsy of lymph nodes and other pelvic and abdominal tissues, and chemotherapy when high-grade tumors are present
- Stages II and III: Total abdominal hysterectomy and bilateral salpingo-oophorectomy, omentectomy, and biopsy of lymph nodes and other pelvic and abdominal tissues and chemotherapy with or without radiation therapy
- Stage IV: Surgery to remove as much of the tumor as possible followed by chemotherapy

Nursing Actions

- Provide preoperative and postoperative care.
- Administer chemotherapy as per orders.
- Provide information on management of chemotherapy side effects (see Table 19–6).
- Provide emotional support to the woman and her family.
- Assess for malnutrition and provide nutritional information based on assessment data.

SAFE AND EFFECTIVE NURSING CARE: Patient Education

Nutrition and Cancer Care

Healthy eating habits and good nutrition can help women deal with the effects of cancer and cancer treatments. Protein and calories are essential for healing, fighting infections, and maintaining adequate energy levels. Unfortunately, the side effects of cancer treatments can interfere with women's ability to eat enough food or for their bodies to absorb the nutrients from food, which leads to malnutrition. Suggestions for treating or controlling these side effects are:

- Anorexia: Eat small high-protein and high-calorie meals (i.e., milkshakes, puddings, yogurt, eggs) every 1 to 2 hours versus three large meals.
- Taste changes: Rinse mouth before eating; eat meats with something sweet such as cranberry sauce; use plastic utensils if foods have a metal taste; add spices and sauces to foods.
- Nausea: Eat before cancer treatments; rinse mouth before and after eating; eat foods that are bland, soft, and easy to

digest; do not eat in a room that has cooking odors or that is very warm.
- Diarrhea: Eat broth, soups, bananas, and canned fruit to replace salt and potassium lost by diarrhea; drink at least 8 cups of fluid per day plus at least 1 cup of fluid after each loose bowel movement; avoid greasy foods, high-fiber foods, milk products, and sugar-free candy until cause of diarrhea is identified.

National Cancer Institute, 2017.

INTIMATE PARTNER VIOLENCE

According to the Centers for Disease Control and Prevention, "Intimate partner violence (IPV) includes physical violence, sexual violence, stalking and psychological aggression (including coercive tactics) by a current or former intimate partner, i.e., spouse, boyfriend, girlfriend, dating partner, or ongoing sexual partner" (CDC, 2017b). Approximately 22% of women in the United States will experience IPV during their lifetime (CDC, 2017b). IVP occurs across all socioeconomic, religious, age and ethnic groups, and sexual orientations. Approximately 3% to 9% of women experience IPV during pregnancy (Alhuse, Ray, Sharps, & Bullock, 2015).

Physical violence includes but is not limited to slapping, shaking, choking, burning, and use of weapons. Sexual violence includes but is not limited to forcing a partner to engage in sexual activity against her will or to trade sex for food, money, or drugs. Psychological/emotional violence includes but is not limited to humiliating the woman, controlling what she can and cannot do, isolating her from family and friends, and denying access to money.

Risk Factors

Risk factors for intimate partner violence include individual, relationship, community, and societal factors, such as:

- Low self-esteem.
- Low academic achievement.
- Being an adolescent or young adult.
- Alcohol and/or drug abuse.
- Having few friends.
- Marital conflict.
- Dominance and control of the relationship by one partner over the other (CDC, 2017b).

Characteristics of Abusers

- Extreme jealousy
- Possessiveness
- Extremely controlling behavior
- Blaming partner for anything bad that happens

- Demeaning partner publicly or privately
- Control what the partner wears or how she acts (National Coalition Against Domestic Violence [NCADV], 2017).

CRITICAL COMPONENT

Intimate Partner Violence and Pregnancy
Intimate partner violence during pregnancy is associated with increased incidence of low-birth-weight infants, preterm birth, and neonatal death.

CRITICAL COMPONENT

Signs of Intimate Partner Violence
- Repeated nonspecific complaints
- Overuse of health care system
- Hesitancy, embarrassment, or evasiveness in relating history of injury
- Time lag between injury and presentation for care
- Untreated serious injuries
- Overly solicitous partner who stays close to the woman and attempts to answer questions directed at her
- Injuries of head, neck, face, and areas covered by a one-piece bathing suit; during pregnancy, the breasts and abdomen are particular targets of assault.
- Presence of bruises at various stages of healing

CDC, 2017b.

Nursing Actions

- The American Nurses Association advocates for:
  - Universal screening: All patients are screened for IPV.
  - Routine assessment: A detailed assessment when screening suggests that the woman is at risk for abuse.
  - Documentation of abuse: Documentation is essential for providing a record of abuse and facilitating communication among health professionals.
  - Reporting IPV: Most states have laws requiring mandatory reporting of IPV.
- Common questions asked in an IPV screening tool are:
  - Has your partner ever hit you?
  - Do arguments with your partner result in you feeling bad about yourself?
  - Do you ever feel frightened by what your partner says or does?
  - Do you feel safe in your current relationship?
- When a woman discloses IPV, the nurse should assess to determine urgent safety needs and assist with developing plan of care, provide information regarding IPV and safe shelters, and assist her in developing strategies to protect herself from harm.

CONCEPT MAP

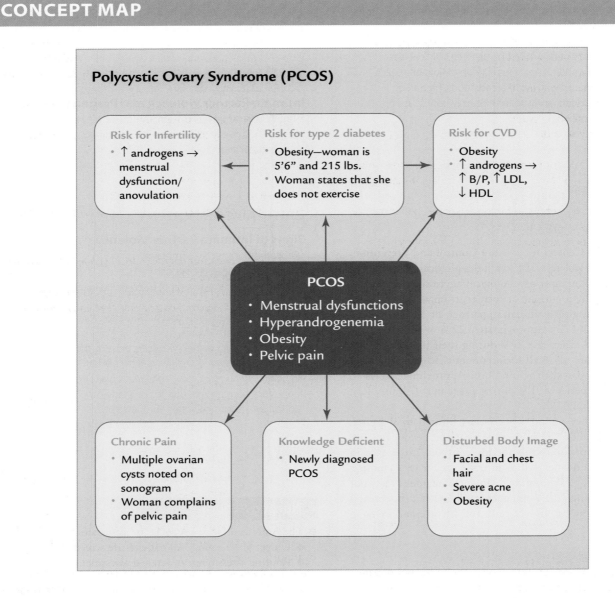

Polycystic Ovary Syndrome (PCOS)

Risk for Infertility
- ↑ androgens → menstrual dysfunction/ anovulation

Risk for type 2 diabetes
- Obesity—woman is 5'6" and 215 lbs.
- Woman states that she does not exercise

Risk for CVD
- Obesity
- ↑ androgens → ↑ B/P, ↑ LDL, ↓ HDL

PCOS
- Menstrual dysfunctions
- Hyperandrogenemia
- Obesity
- Pelvic pain

Chronic Pain
- Multiple ovarian cysts noted on sonogram
- Woman complains of pelvic pain

Knowledge Deficient
- Newly diagnosed PCOS

Disturbed Body Image
- Facial and chest hair
- Severe acne
- Obesity

Problem No. 1: Risk for infertility
Goal: Increased knowledge regarding relationship of PCOS and infertility
Outcome: The woman verbalizes causes of infertility and methods to improve fertility.

Nursing Actions
1. Provide the woman with information on the causes of infertility related to PCOS—anovulation related to increased androgen levels, increased LH, and decreased FSH.
2. Inform the woman that weight loss can improve fertility— weight loss is the first-line treatment for infertility.
   a. Assist woman in developing a weight-management program that includes diet and physical activities.

3. Explain medical options for treating infertility
   a. Treat type 2 diabetes—maintaining normal ranges of serum glucose can regulate menstrual cycle and increase ovulation rates.
   b. Ovulation-inducing medications.

Problem No. 2: Risk for type 2 diabetes
Goal: Serum glucose levels within normal ranges
Outcome: The woman exercises 3 days a week for 30 minutes and eats foods low in carbohydrates and fats.

Nursing Actions
1. Explain that weight loss and exercise improve insulin resistance (the body produces insulin but does not use it properly)

and hyperinsulinemia (hyperglycemia present despite high levels of insulin).
2. Explain the other benefits of a weight-management program that includes diet and exercise:
   a. Improves fertility
   b. Decreases androgen levels
   c. Decreases lipid levels
   d. Decreases blood pressure
3. Assist the woman in developing a weight-management program by:
   a. Asking her to identify the types of physical activities she enjoys and how these can be used in a weight-management program.
   b. Asking her to identify the foods she enjoys and incorporate them into a weight-reduction diet.
   c. Teaching her food groups important in a healthy diet.

Problem No. 3: Risk for cardiovascular disease (CVD)
Goal: ↓B/P; ↓LDL, and ↑HDL
Outcome: The woman exercises 3 days a week for 30 minutes and eats foods low in carbohydrates and fats.

Nursing Actions
1. Explain the importance of weight loss through diet and exercise in decreasing risk for CVD.
   a. Exercise improves cardiopulmonary function, insulin sensitivity, and a decreased BMI.
2. Assist the woman in developing a weight-management program with realistic weight loss and exercise goals.
3. Provide information on prescribed medications for decreasing risk of CVD.

Problem No. 4: Chronic pain
Goal: Decreased pain
Outcome: The woman states her pelvic pain has decreased in frequency and intensity.

Nursing Actions
1. Assess level of pain, location of pain, and frequency of pain.
2. Ask about past pain management techniques and their effectiveness in treating pain related to PCOS.
3. Ask the woman to identify factors that increase or decrease the pain (e.g., lack of sleep, lifting objects).
   a. Discuss ways to decrease factors that increase pain.

4. Assist woman in developing a pain-management program that includes:
   a. Pain diary: List when pain occurs, intensity of pain, how long it lasted, pain-management measures used, and effectiveness of pain management. Instruct her to share this with her health care provider.
   b. Pharmacological: Take medication at start of pain and use adequate amounts as prescribed.
   c. Nonpharmacological: Relaxation techniques, massage, acupressure.

Problem No. 5: Knowledge deficit
Goal: Increased knowledge regarding PCOS
Outcome: The woman develops a plan of action for living with PCOS.

Nursing Actions
1. Ensure that the environment is conducive for learning—quiet room free of distractions.
2. Assess the woman's level of knowledge regarding PCOS.
3. Assist the woman in identifying priority learning needs and address these needs such as:
   a. Causes of PCOS.
   b. Effect of PCOS on her body and mind.
   c. Treatment options.
   d. Ways to cope with changes related to PCOS.
4. Assist the woman in developing a plan of action for living with PCOS.

Problem No. 6: Disturbed body image
Goal: Improved body image
Outcome: The woman verbalizes methods to decrease degree of acne and methods to decrease facial and chest hair.

Nursing Actions
1. Sit with the woman and through active listening, encourage her to express her thoughts and concerns regarding facial and chest hair and acne.
2. Provide information on causes of body changes due to PCOS.
3. Provide information on treatment for acne (i.e., dermatological assessment and prescribed medications).
4. Provide information on hair removal.
5. Refer the woman to PCOS support groups.

Case Study

Katherine is a 70-year-old woman who was recently widowed. She retired from the U.S. Postal Service at age 65. She has three grown children; her daughter lives close to her. She weighs 150 pounds. Her height is 5 foot 6 inches; her height at age 50 was 5 foot 8 inches. Her blood pressure is 124/86. She takes Synthroid and a multivitamin each morning.

Recent lab values are as follows:

Fasting glucose: 110 mg/dL
Hemoglobin: 11.5 g/dL
Hematocrit: 34
RBC: 3.8
WBC: 10.5
EKG: Normal.

She is scheduled for a vaginal hysterectomy and repair of cystocele and rectocele. Her admitting diagnosis is pelvic organ prolapse.

What is pelvic prolapse, and what are cystoceles and rectoceles?
What are the priority preoperative nursing actions for Katherine?
What are the postoperative nursing care actions for Katherine?
Develop a discharge teaching plan for Katherine that includes addressing postoperative care and health promotion.

REFERENCES

Alhuse, J., Ray, E., Sarps, P., & Bullock, L. (2015). Intimate partner violence during pregnancy: Maternal and neonatal outcomes. *Journal of Women's Health, 24*, 100–116.

American Cancer Society (ACS). (2016a). *Breast cancer.* Retrieved from www.cancer.org/cancer/breast-cancer.html.

American Cancer Society (ACS). (2016b). *Cancer facts and figures 2016.* Atlanta, GA: American Cancer Society.

American Cancer Society (ACS). (2016c). *Cervical cancer screening.* Retrieved from www.cancer.org/cancer/cervical-cancer/detection-diagnosis-staging/staged.html.

American Cancer Society (ACS). (2016d). *Endometrial cancer staging.* Retrieved from www.cancer.org/cancer/endometrial-cancer/detection-diagnosis-staging/staging.html

American Cancer Society (ACS). (2016e). *Radiation for cervical cancer.* Retrieved from https://www.cancer.org/cancer/cervical-cancer/treating.html

American Cancer Society (ACS). (2016f). *Signs and symptoms of ovarian cancer.* Retrieved from www.cancer.org/cancer/ovarian-cancer/detection-diagnosis-staging/signs-and-symptoms.html.

American Cancer Society (ACS). (2016g). *Breast cancer stages.* Retrieved from www.cancer.org/cancer/breast-cancer/understanding-a-breast-cancer-diagnosis/stages-of-breast-cancer.html.

American Cancer Society (ACS). (2016h). *Treatment options for cervical cancer, by stage.* Retrieved from www.cancer.org/cancer/cervical-cancer/treating/by-stage.html.

American Cancer Society (ACS). (2017). *Coping with radiation treatment.* Retrieved from www.cancer.org/treatment/treatments-and-side-effects/treatment-types/radiation/coping.html

Cancer Care. (2016). *Understanding and managing chemotherapy side effects.* Retrieved from www.cancercare.org/publications/24-understanding_and_managing_chemotherapy_side_effects.

Cancer.Net. (2017). *Tests and procedures.* Retrieved from www.cancer.net/navigating-cancer-care/diagnosing-cancer/tests-and-procedures.

Centers for Disease Control and Prevention (CDC). (2016). *Dental dam use.* Retrieved from www.cdc.gov/condomeffectiveness/dental-dam-use.html.

Centers for Disease Control and Prevention (CDC). (2017a). *Genital HPV infection—fact sheet.* Retrieved from www.cdc.gov/std/hpv/stdfact-hpv.htm.

Centers for Disease Control and Prevention (CDC). (2017b). *Intimate partner violence.* Retrieved from www.cdc.gov/violenceprevention/intimatepartnerviolence/index.html.

County of Los Angeles Public Health. (2017). *Resources for lesbian and bisexual women.* Retrieved from http://publichealth.lacounty.gov/dhsp/Lesbian-Bisexual.htm

Girls Health. (2017). *Facts about STDs.* Retrieved from www.girlshealth.gov/know-the-facts-first/facts-stds.html

Imaginis. (2017). *Overview of breast cancer diagnosis decision process.* Retrieved from www.imaginis.com/breast-cancer-diagnosis/overview-of-breast-cancer-diagnosis-decision-process.

International Pelvic Pain Society. (2014). *Chronic pelvic pain.* Retrieved from https://www.pelvicpain.org/IPPS/Patients/Patient_Handouts/IPPS/Content/Professional-Patients/Patient_Handouts.aspx?hkey=cffd598e-5453-4b3f-9170-457c59266b50

Johns Hopkins. (2017). *Gynecology tests and procedures.* Retrieved from www.hopkinsmedicine.org/healthlibrary/test_procedures/gynecology/.

Lobo, R., Gershenson, D., Lentz, G., & Valea, F. (2017). *Comprehensive gynecology* (7th ed.). Philadelphia, PA: Elsevier.

Mayo Clinic. (2016a). *Urinary tract infection (UTI).* Retrieved from www.mayoclinic.org/diseases-conditions/urinary-tract-infection/basics/treatment/con-20037892.

Mayo Clinic. (2016b). *Uterine fibroids.* Retrieved from www.mayoclinic.org/diseases-conditions/uterine-fibroids/symptoms-causes/dxc-20212514.

National Cancer Institute. (2011). *Breast cancer risk assessment tool.* Retrieved from https://www.cancer.gov/bcrisktool/.

National Cancer Institute. (2017). *Nutrition in cancer care (PDQ)—patient version.* www.cancer.gov/about-cancer/treatment/side-effects/appetite-loss/nutrition-pdq.

National Coalition Against Domestic Violence (NCADV). (2017). *Signs of an abusive partner.* Retrieved from https://ncadv.org/signs-of-abuse.

National Heart Lung and Blood Institute. (2016). *Metabolic syndrome.* Retrieved from www.nhlbi.nih.gov/health/health-topics/topics/ms.

National Ovarian Cancer Coalition (NOCC). (2017). *Type and stages of ovarian cancer.* Retrieved from http://ovarian.org/about-ovarian-cancer/what-is-ovarian-cancer/types-a-stages.

Ovarian Cancer Action. (2017). *What are the symptoms?* Retrieved from www.ovarian.org.uk/ovarian-cancer/what-are-the-symptoms/.

University of Maryland Medical Center (UMM). (2017). *Menstrual disorders.* Retrieved from www.umm.edu/health/medical/reports/articles/menstrual-disorders.

Vallerand, A., & Sanoski, C. (2017). *Davis's drug guide for nurses* (15th ed.). Philadelphia, PA: F.A. Davis.

VanLeeuwen, A., & Smith, L. (2015). *Davis's comprehensive handbook of laboratory and diagnostic tests with nursing implications* (6th ed.). Philadelphia, PA: F.A. Davis.

Women's Health. (2016). *Polycystic ovary syndrome.* Retrieved from www.womenshealth.gov/publications/our-publications/fact-sheet/polycystic-ovary-syndrome.html

Appendix A AWHONN Quick Guide to Breastfeeding

QUICK CARE GUIDE
BREASTFEEDING SUPPORT: PRENATAL CARE THROUGH THE FIRST YEAR

This Quick Care Guide is based on AWHONN's Breastfeeding Support: Preconception Care Through the First Year Evidence-Based Clinical Practice Guideline, third edition. It is meant to serve as a quick reference for the clinician. Detailed clinical practice guidelines, referenced rationales, and evidence ratings are included in the Guideline. Evidence supporting the benefits of breastfeeding, critical messages, responsibilities, key assessment, and teaching points summarized herein are presented in the Guideline.

BENEFITS OF BREASTFEEDING
Discussions with women who are considering or are undecided about breastfeeding should include description of the following benefits:

For infants:
- Optimal primary source of nutrients necessary for health, growth, immune system, and neuro-development during the first 6 months
- Continued provision of critical nutrients for 6 months and beyond when appropriate complementary foods are added to the diet
- Decreased incidence or severity of infections such as GI and respiratory infections, otitis media, necrotizing enterocolitis, gastroenteritis, and urinary tract infections
- Protective effect against sudden infant death syndrome (SIDS)
- Potential protective effect against childhood and adult-onset diseases such as insulin-dependent diabetes, allergies, asthma, lymphoma, ulcerative colitis, and adult-onset hypertension
- Decreased incidence of gastric reflux and constipation compared with formula feeding
- Potential for enhanced cognitive development, especially in preterm infants
- Potential reduced risk for developing obesity later in life

For women:
- Enhanced uterine involution resulting in less postpartum blood loss and reduced risk of anemia and infection
- Delayed resumption of ovulation that may facilitate family planning
- Association with earlier return to pre-pregnancy weight compared with women who do not breastfeed
- Reduced risk of osteoporosis, ovarian cancer, premenopausal breast cancer, and rheumatoid arthritis
- Enhanced mother–infant attachment, maternal role attainment, and self-esteem
- Potential for reduced risk of metabolic syndrome and cardiovascular disease
- Potential for reduced risk of postpartum depression

For society:
Breastfeeding is less expensive than formula feeding, contributes to significant health care cost savings, and is environmentally sound (friendly).

CRITICAL MESSAGES TO SHARE WITH WOMEN AND THEIR PARTNERS

- Breast and human milk feeding is the norm for feeding all infants, including preterm and other vulnerable newborns. Most women can breastfeed successfully when they are given consistent information and support.
- Breastfeeding can be sustained upon return to work or school.
- Ideally, infants should receive human milk exclusively for the first year of life. During the first 6 months, the infant receives only breast milk; during the second 6 months, as other foods are introduced, the only source of milk given to the infant is breast milk.

RESPONSIBILITIES AND OPPORTUNITIES

- Nurses should support and implement Baby-Friendly Hospital Initiative (BFHI) practices in their workplace.
- Nurses working with breastfeeding women should maintain current, evidence-based knowledge of breastfeeding practice and can be instrumental in initiating or participating in lactation research.
- Nurses and other health care professionals should relay consistent, supportive messages about breastfeeding.
- Nurses working with mothers of preterm and vulnerable newborns should promote and support provision of mother's own milk or banked human milk for this population.
- Breastfeeding support programs should be culturally sensitive, age and developmentally appropriate.
- Practitioners should use the World Health Organization (WHO) growth charts that were developed based on healthy ethnically diverse breastfeeding infants, to assess growth patterns.
- Nursing leaders and educators should advocate for deliberate integration of breastfeeding information into academic and professional education programs to help ensure that health care professionals gain the knowledge needed to promote and support breastfeeding.
- Nurses should advocate for breastfeeding as our cultural norm by supporting breastfeeding promotion legislation and educating society about the benefits of breastfeeding.

QUICK CARE GUIDE

BREASTFEEDING SUPPORT: PRENATAL CARE THROUGH THE FIRST YEAR

Key Assessment Parameters	Key Teaching Points
Preconception and Prenatal Care	
• During the first preconception or prenatal visit, ask the woman whether anyone has explained to her the benefits of breastfeeding for herself and her infant. Assess the woman's knowledge of and experiences with breastfeeding. • Explore the woman's and support person(s) beliefs and attitudes about breastfeeding. • For the woman who is undecided about breastfeeding, continue to explore her concerns and desires during subsequent contacts. • If the woman plans to breastfeed, ask how long she plans to do so and how long she plans to breastfeed exclusively. • Verify presence of support for the woman's decision to breastfeed. • Provide individualized and culturally sensitive education using diverse methodologies. Recommend reliable electronic media and websites. • Review the woman's history. Assess her breasts and nipples for risk factors and physical characteristics that may affect breastfeeding. Refer women with identified breastfeeding risk factors to a lactation specialist as needed. • Encourage women to seek local facilities that follow BFHI principles.	• Educate women about maternal and neonatal benefits of breastfeeding. • Previous breastfeeding experiences, positive or negative, influence choice of feeding method. Some factors, such as perceived insufficient milk supply, can be addressed by education and support that continue throughout pregnancy and the early postpartum period. • Educate significant support persons about the benefits of breastfeeding and ways to support the new mother. • Discuss and correct misconceptions about breastfeeding. Address concerns or ambivalence. • Continue targeted, culturally appropriate education throughout pregnancy. Culture and beliefs can positively or negatively influence the woman's decision to initiate or continue breastfeeding. • Suggest that return to work or school does not mean that the woman must stop breastfeeding. Benefits continue as long as the infant is breastfeeding, even when the infant is being partially breastfed. • Explain that family, friends, health care providers, and peer counselors can help a woman meet her breastfeeding goals. • Discuss community resources that are available to the woman such as support groups, lactation consultants, and La Leche League. • Explain that many physical characteristics do not preclude breastfeeding. Share interventions to address identified problem(s). For example, infants are often able to grasp and pull out inverted nipples during early feedings at the breast. Some women who have had previous breast surgery are able to exclusively breastfeed their infants. • Explain the evidence behind BFHI practices and their relationship with successful breastfeeding.

ASSOCIATION OF WOMEN'S HEALTH, OBSTETRIC AND NEONATAL NURSES

QUICK CARE GUIDE

BREASTFEEDING SUPPORT: PRENATAL CARE THROUGH THE FIRST YEAR	
Key Assessment Parameters	**Key Teaching Points**
Initiating Breastfeeding: Birth Through the First Two Weeks	
<ul><li>Assess intent to breastfeed</li><li>Assess the mother's history of health problems, and assess her and her newborn for events during labor and birth that may interfere with breastfeeding</li><li>Assess parental knowledge and ability to recognize and embrace biologic nurturing, initiate skin-to-skin contact with the newborn, and establish correct infant latch onto the breast.</li><li>Assess parental knowledge of infant states and ability to demonstrate caring for the infant as the infant transitions between states.</li><li>Assess parental knowledge of and ability to respond to infant feeding cues.</li><li>Assess parents' ability to identify signs of adequate milk intake.</li><li>Assess parents' ability to identify and respond to infant cues of satiety.</li><li>Assess parental knowledge about ways to support the mother–infant dyad in a successful breastfeeding experience.</li></ul>	<ul><li>Provide information and support when women express concerns about breastfeeding.</li><li>Educate mothers that many women with certain risk factors, preexisting medical conditions, preconceived perceptions about breastfeeding, or challenging birth experiences can breastfeed successfully with additional support and help.</li><li>Explain the breast crawl and biologic nurturing, and how to facilitate this natural maternal-infant interaction process. Instruct parents how to correctly position infant at breast.</li><li>Facilitate uninterrupted skin-to-skin contact at birth and during hospitalization. Ideally, the first feeding should occur within 1 hour of birth if mother and infant are stable.</li><li>Instruct mother how to identify a correct latch: infant's nose, cheeks and chin should touch the breast. The woman should feel tugging, not pinching or pain, when the infant sucks. The infant is usually held tummy-to-tummy with the mother, and the mother positions her fingers to ensure the lactiferous sinuses are not blocked.</li><li>Teach parents that infant may be sleepy for the first 24 hours. Try to wake the infant every 2–3 hours for feeding. Assure them that waking and feeding the infant should get progressively easier throughout the first 24 hours. Teach parents about infant states and help parents identify how their infant transitions between states.</li><li>Teach early infant feeding cues: rooting, hand-to-mouth movements, sucking movement and sounds, sucking on fingers or hands, mouth opening in response to tactile stimulation and transition between sleep to drowsy and quietly alert state. Crying is a late feeding cue.</li></ul>

QUICK CARE GUIDE

BREASTFEEDING SUPPORT: PRENATAL CARE THROUGH THE FIRST YEAR	
Key Assessment Parameters	**Key Teaching Points**
Initiating Breastfeeding: Birth Through the First Two Weeks (continued)	
	• Teach parents infant cues of satiety: a gradual decrease in the number of sucks, pursed lips, pulling away from breast and releasing the nipple, relaxed body, leg extension, absence of hunger cues, sleep and contented state and small amount of milk seen in mouth. • Parental education should include the following: o Discourage the use of pacifiers until the baby is able to latch on and breastfeed successfully. o Validate that the infant should receive only breast milk unless medically indicated. o Avoid accepting discharge packs containing formula information and samples. • Provide parents with resources to contact after discharge, such as lactation specialists, La Leche League, or breastfeeding support groups. • Recommend follow-up with a health care provider within 48 hours of discharge for all breastfeeding infants.

ASSOCIATION OF WOMEN'S HEALTH, OBSTETRIC AND NEONATAL NURSES

QUICK CARE GUIDE

BREASTFEEDING SUPPORT: PRENATAL CARE THROUGH THE FIRST YEAR	
Key Assessment Parameters	Key Teaching Points
Sustaining Breastfeeding: Two Weeks Through First Year	
<ul><li>Assess how long the woman intends to continue breastfeeding, including her concerns about being successful.</li><li>Assess for the presence of individuals in the woman's life who support her decision to continue breastfeeding.</li><li>Identify factors that may decrease duration of breastfeeding.</li><li>Assess for and identify the mother's perceived challenges to breastfeeding.</li><li>Assess the woman's knowledge of available professional and community resources.</li><li>Discuss options to support continued breastfeeding after returning to work.</li><li>Assess the breastfeeding woman's understanding of techniques to wean her infant.</li></ul>	<ul><li>Define and explain to the mother and her partner the meaning and importance of exclusive breastfeeding, including that the infant receives only breast milk and no other liquid or solid supplements except vitamins, minerals, and medications.</li><li>Explain that exclusive breastfeeding for all infants during the first 6 months of life (except when medically contraindicated) provides adequate nutrition to facilitate optimal growth and development and protection against many newborn and childhood illnesses.</li><li>Discuss the continued benefits of feeding after 6 months, when other foods are introduced into the infant's diet, and that breastfeeding may continue for the first year of life and beyond. Exclusive breastfeeding during this time means that the only source of milk given to the infant continues to be breast milk.</li><li>Describe the influence that support from partners, maternal grandmother, employers, and fellow employees may have on the duration of breastfeeding. Encourage the woman to identify and access her support network or to ask for community support referrals.</li><li>Discuss factors that may negatively influence duration of breastfeeding such as:<ul><li>o Perceived insufficient milk supply</li><li>o Returning to work or school before 2 months postpartum</li><li>o Wanting to leave the infant with another caregiver or have someone else feed</li><li>o Postpartum depression</li><li>o Early introduction of pacifiers</li></ul></li><li>Explain that early introduction of pacifiers may be associated with decreased duration of breastfeeding. As an intervention to decrease the risk of SIDS, pacifiers should be introduced to breastfeeding infants after 1 month of age when breastfeeding is well established.</li></ul>

QUICK CARE GUIDE

BREASTFEEDING SUPPORT: PRENATAL CARE THROUGH THE FIRST YEAR	
Key Assessment Parameters	**Key Teaching Points**
Sustaining Breastfeeding: Two Weeks Through First Year (continued)	

	• Engage adolescent women in discussions about unique concerns, e.g., relatives' advice to quit, embarrassment, modesty, and concern about breastfeeding in public.
	
	 • Explain that pain is a frequently identified barrier to sustaining breastfeeding. Most sources of pain can be treated, and the woman should be encouraged to seek care from her primary care provider or lactation specialist.
	
	 • Help the mother understand that perceived inadequate milk supply is a commonly reported barrier. Describe periods of rapid infant growth (2 weeks, 6 weeks and 3 months) when women may perceive that their milk supply has decreased because their infant is breastfeeding more often.
	
	 • Explore and explain potential and real challenges to breastfeeding such as lack of support for returning to work or school.
	    o Help or encourage women to create a plan for sustaining breastfeeding once they return to employment or school.
	    o Provide the breastfeeding woman with resources for her employer or school administration that highlight how they can provide a supportive breastfeeding environment and benefits to employers when they support breastfeeding such as increased employee productivity and retention.
	
	 • Encourage participation in breastfeeding support groups, regular visits to Women, Infants, and Children (WIC) program office (if the mother participates in WIC) and follow-up phone calls to registered nurses, lactation consultants, or the primary health care provider, as appropriate, to help increase the duration of breastfeeding.

QUICK CARE GUIDE

BREASTFEEDING SUPPORT: PRENATAL CARE THROUGH THE FIRST YEAR	
Key Assessment Parameters	**Key Teaching Points**
Sustaining Breastfeeding: Two Weeks Through First Year (continued)	
	• Encourage use of a double rather than a single pump to decrease the length of time needed to pump. • Encourage women to begin pumping before returning to work. The more experience a woman has with pumping, the more efficient she becomes and the less time pumping will take. • Describe weaning techniques, such as replacing one feeding during the day with solid food, a bottle, or cup depending on the infant's age and stage of development. After the infant has adjusted, replace a second feeding at the opposite time of day. Generally, the first morning and last evening feedings are the last to be stopped.

QUICK CARE GUIDE

BREASTFEEDING SUPPORT: PRENATAL CARE THROUGH THE FIRST YEAR	
Key Assessment Parameters	**Key Teaching Points**
Vulnerable and Preterm Infants	

• Assess the woman's beliefs, attitudes, and knowledge about providing own mother's milk for her vulnerable/preterm infant.
 	
• Assess woman's knowledge about the benefits of skin-to-skin care and non-nutritive sucking.
 	
• Assess the woman's knowledge about and ability to provide human milk via various options including:
  o Milk expression and pumping
  o Newborn oral care
  o Alternative feeding methods
  o Collection, storage, and transport of human milk
 	
• Assess mother and infant's readiness for oral feeding at breast.
 	
• Assess parental knowledge related to the vulnerable/preterm infant's milk intake after discharge.
	• Explain that human milk affords unique advantages for the vulnerable/preterm infant (such as protection from necrotizing enterocolitis, better gastric function, reduced risk for infection, enhanced visual acuity, and enhanced cognitive development), as well as for the woman. Explain that preterm milk is more suitable for the preterm infant than mature or term milk.
	
	• Encourage early and frequent skin-to-skin contact whenever possible in sessions lasting 30 minutes at least once a day. Explain that skin-to-skin contact decreases risk of neonatal infection, hypothermia, and promotes physiologic stability. Skin-to-skin contact may reduce length of stay and is associated with improved growth, increased milk volume and breastfeeding duration, and improved neonatal outcomes.
	
	• Explain that non-nutritive sucking can improve digestion of enteral feedings in preterm infants and aids development of a normal breastfeeding suck pattern.
	
	• Teach the woman to optimize milk yield using the following suggested techniques:
	  o Begin manual expression or pumping within 1-2 hours after birth; when pumping, use an electric, hospital-grade breast pump with double collection kit that mimics infant suckling colostrum whenever possible.
	  o Pump or express milk at the infant's bedside while using relaxation techniques (provide privacy).
	  o Continue to pump for at least 2 minutes after milk droplets stop flowing.
	  o Engage in skin-to-skin contact at least 30 minutes daily, whenever feasible.
	  o Mechanically express 6-8 times per day minimum. If milk volume is inadequate to meet infant needs, milk expression every 2-3 hours (including 1-2 times during the night when prolactin levels are highest) may be warranted.
	  o Individualize the frequency of mechanical expression on the basis of milk output.

-9-

ASSOCIATION OF WOMEN'S HEALTH, OBSTETRIC AND NEONATAL NURSES

QUICK CARE GUIDE

BREASTFEEDING SUPPORT: PRENATAL CARE THROUGH THE FIRST YEAR	
Key Assessment Parameters	**Key Teaching Points**
Vulnerable and Preterm Infants (continued)	
	• Teach procedure for oral care using fresh human milk every 2-3 hours while infant is unable to orally feed.
	• Instruct parents that human milk may be provided to the infant via tube feeding (gavage), cup- or finger-feedings, as well as by bottle.
	• Instruct parents how to properly collect, label, store, and transport human milk to the hospital. Assist parents to identify resources necessary to collect, store, and transport milk.
	• When the infant is medically stable, teach mothers who desire to transition the infant to feeding at breast to put the infant to breast following milk expression to help him or her acclimate to suckling.
	• Demonstrate positions that provide head and shoulder support of the infant, such as the football hold, when infant suction is compromised.
	• Remind the mother to express remaining milk after each breastfeeding session.
	• Explain procedure for and importance of infant test-weighing to provide an accurate estimate of infant milk intake.
	• Discuss that modified demand feedings will likely be needed, coupled with infant test-weighing for a period of time.
	• Emphasize the difference between insufficient milk supply and the infant's ability to consume adequate milk volume.
	• Teach that appropriate follow-up after discharge is critical for the mother of a vulnerable/preterm infant.

Appendix B Recommended Immunization Schedule for Infants and Children Aged 0 to 23 Months

Recommended immunization schedule for infants and children aged 0 to 23 months

Vaccine	Birth	1 mo	2 mo	4 mon	6 mo	9 mo	12 mo	15 mo	18 mo	19–23 mo
Hepatitis B[1] (HepB)	1st dose; see footnote 1	2nd dose			3rd dose					
Rotavirus[2] (RV) RV1 (2-dose series); RV5 (3-dose series)			1st dose	2nd dose	See footnote 2					
Diphtheria, tetanus, & acellular pertussis[3] (DTaP)			1st dose	2nd dose	3rd dose			4th dose		
Haemophilus influenzae type b[4] (Hib)			1st dose	2nd dose	See footnote 4		3rd or 4th dose; see footnote 2			
Pneumococcal conjugate[5] (PCV13)			1st dose	2nd dose	3rd dose		4th dose			
Inactivated poliovirus[6] (IPV:<18 yrs)			1st dose	2nd dose	3rd dose					
Influenza[7] (IIV; LAIV)					Annual vaccination (IIV only) 1 or 2 doses					
Measles, mumps, rubella (MMR)[8]							1st dose			
Varicella[9] (VAR)							1st dose			
Hepatitis A[10] (HepA)							2-dose series; see footnote 10			

(CDC, 2017)

Footnotes

(1) Hepatitis B (HepB) vaccine. (Minimum age: birth)

Routine vaccination:

At birth:

• Administer monovalent HepB vaccine to all newborns within 24 hours of birth.

• For infants born to hepatitis B surface antigen (HBsAg)-positive mothers, administer HepB vaccine and 0.5 mL of hepatitis B immune globulin (HBIG) within 12 hours of birth. These infants should be tested for HBsAg and antibody to HBsAg (anti-HBs) at age 9 through 12 months (preferably at the next well-child visit) or 1 to 2 months after completion of the HepB series if the series was delayed.

• If mother's HBsAg status is unknown, within 12 hours of birth, administer HepB vaccine regardless of birth weight. For infants weighing less than 2,000 grams, administer HBIG in addition to HepB vaccine within 12 hours of birth. Determine mother's HBsAg status as soon as possible and, if mother is HBsAg-positive, also administer HBIG to infants weighing 2,000 grams or more as soon as possible, but no later than age 7 days.

Doses following the birth dose:

• The second dose should be administered at age 1 or 2 months. Monovalent HepB vaccine should be used for doses administered before age 6 weeks.

• Administer the second dose 1 to 2 months after the first dose (minimum interval of 4 weeks); administer the third dose at least 8 weeks after the second dose AND at least 16 weeks after the first dose. The final (third or fourth) dose in the HepB vaccine series should be administered no earlier than age 24 weeks.

• Administration of a total of 4 doses of HepB vaccine is permitted when a combination vaccine containing HepB is administered after the birth dose.

(2) Rotavirus (RV) vaccines. (Minimum age: 6 weeks for both RV1 [Rotarix] and RV5 [RotaTeq])

Routine vaccination:

Administer a series of RV vaccine to all infants as follows:

• If Rotarix is used, administer a 2-dose series at ages 2 and 4 months.

• If RotaTeq is used, administer a 3-dose series at ages 2, 4, and 6 months.

• If any dose in the series was RotaTeq or vaccine product is unknown for any dose in the series, a total of 3 doses of RV vaccine should be administered.

(3) Diphtheria and tetanus toxoids and acellular pertussis(DTaP) vaccine. (Minimum age: 6 weeks. exception: DTaPIPV [Kinrix, Quadracel]: 4 years)

Routine vaccination:

• Administer a 5-dose series of DTaP vaccine at ages 2, 4, 6, 15 through 18 months, and 4 through 6 years. The fourth dose may be administered as early as age 12 months, provided at least 6 months have elapsed since the third dose.

• Inadvertent administration of fourth DTaP dose early: If the fourth dose of DTaP was administered at least 4 months after the third dose of DTaP and the child was 12 months of age or older, it does not need to be repeated.

(4) Haemophilus influenzae type b (Hib) conjugate vaccine. (Minimum age: 6 weeks for PRP-T [ActHIB, DTaP-IPV/Hib (Pentacel), Hiberix, and Hib-MenCY (MenHibrix)], PRPOMP [PedvaxHIB])

Routine vaccination:

• Administer a 2- or 3-dose Hib vaccine primary series and a booster dose (dose 3 or 4, depending on vaccine used in primary series) at age 12 through 15 months to complete a full Hib vaccine series.

• The primary series with ActHIB, MenHibrix, Hiberix, or Pentacel consists of 3 doses and should be administered at ages 2, 4, and 6 months. The primary series with PedvaxHIB consists of 2 doses and should be administered at ages 2 and 4 months; a dose at age 6 months is not indicated.

• One booster dose (dose 3 or 4, depending on vaccine used in primary series) of any Hib vaccine should be administered at age 12 through 15 months.

• For recommendations on the use of MenHibrix in patients at increased risk for meningococcal disease, refer to the meningococcal vaccine footnotes and also to MMWR February 28, 2014/63(RR01):1-13, available at www.cdc.gov/mmwr/PDF/rr/rr6301.pdf.

(5) Pneumococcal vaccines. (Minimum age: 6 weeks for PCV13, 2 years for PPSV23)

Routine vaccination with PCV13:

• Administer a 4-dose series of PCV13 at ages 2, 4, and 6 months and at age 12 through 15 months.

(6) Inactivated poliovirus vaccine (IPV). (Minimum age: 6 weeks)

Routine vaccination:

• Administer a 4-dose series of IPV at ages 2, 4, 6 through 18 months, and 4 through 6 years. The final dose in the series should be administered on or after the fourth birthday and at least 6 months after the previous dose.

(7) Influenza vaccines. (Minimum age: 6 months for inactivated influenza vaccine [IIV], 18 years for recombinant influenza vaccine [RIV])

Routine vaccination:

• Administer influenza vaccine annually to all children beginning at age 6 months. For the 2016–17 season, use of live attenuated influenza vaccine (LAIV) is not recommended.

For children aged 6 months through 8 years:

• For the 2016–17 season, administer 2 doses (separated by at least 4 weeks) to children who are receiving influenza vaccine for the first time or who have not previously received ≥2 doses of trivalent or quadrivalent influenza vaccine before July 1, 2016. For additional guidance, follow dosing guidelines in the 2016–17 ACIP influenza vaccine recommendations (see MMWR August 26, 2016;65(5):1-54, available at www.cdc.gov/mmwr/volumes/65/rr/pdfs/rr6505.pdf).

• For the 2017–18 season, follow dosing guidelines in the 2017–18 ACIP influenza vaccine recommendations.

(8) Measles, mumps, and rubella (MMR) vaccine. (Minimum age: 12 months for routine vaccination)

Routine vaccination:

• Administer a 2-dose series of MMR vaccine at ages 12 through 15 months and 4 through 6 years. The second dose may be administered before age 4 years, provided at least 4 weeks have elapsed since the first dose.

• Administer 1 dose of MMR vaccine to infants aged 6 through 11 months before departure from the United States for international travel. These children should be revaccinated with 2 doses of MMR vaccine, the first at age 12 through 15 months (12 months if the child remains in an area where disease risk is high), and the second dose at least 4 weeks later.

• Administer 2 doses of MMR vaccine to children aged 12 months and older before departure from the United States for international travel. The first dose should be administered on or after age 12 months and the second dose at least 4 weeks later.

(9) Varicella (VAR) vaccine. (Minimum age: 12 months)

Routine vaccination:

• Administer a 2-dose series of VAR vaccine at ages 12 through 15 months and 4 through 6 years. The second dose may be administered before age 4 years, provided at least 3 months have elapsed since the first dose. If the second dose was administered at least 4 weeks after the first dose, it can be accepted as valid.

(10) Hepatitis A (HepA) vaccine. (Minimum age: 12 months)

Routine vaccination:

• Initiate the 2-dose HepA vaccine series at ages 12 through 23 months; separate the 2 doses by 6 to 18 months.

• Children who have received 1 dose of HepA vaccine before age 24 months should receive a second dose 6 to 18 months after the first dose.

(CDC, 2017)

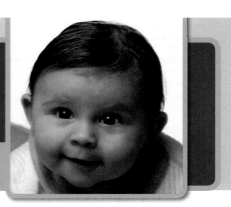

What Does a Safe Sleep Environment Look Like?

Reduce the Risk of Sudden Infant Death Syndrome (SIDS) and Other Sleep-Related Causes of Infant Death

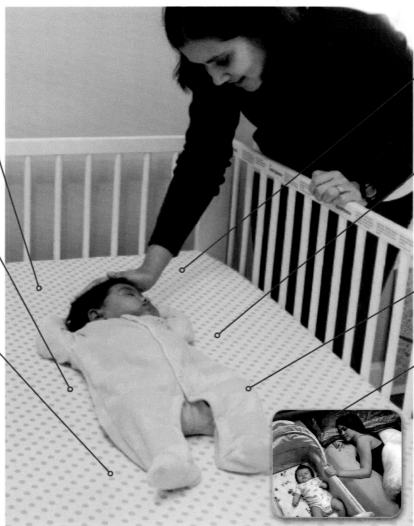

Use a firm sleep surface, such as a mattress in a safety-approved* crib, covered by a fitted sheet.

Do not use pillows, blankets, sheepskins, or crib bumpers anywhere in your baby's sleep area.

Keep soft objects, toys, and loose bedding out of your baby's sleep area.

Do not smoke or let anyone smoke around your baby.

Make sure nothing covers the baby's head.

Always place your baby on his or her back to sleep, for naps and at night.

Dress your baby in sleep clothing, such as a one-piece sleeper, and do not use a blanket.

Baby's sleep area is next to where parents sleep.

Baby should not sleep in an adult bed, on a couch, or on a chair alone, with you, or with anyone else.

*For more information on crib safety guidelines, contact the Consumer Product Safety Commission at 1-800-638-2772 or http://www.cpsc.gov.

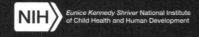
Eunice Kennedy Shriver National Institute of Child Health and Human Development

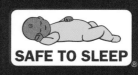
SAFE TO SLEEP

Safe Sleep For Your Baby

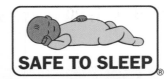

SAFE TO SLEEP®

- Always place your baby on his or her back to sleep, for naps and at night, to reduce the risk of SIDS.

- Use a firm sleep surface, such as a mattress in a safety-approved* crib, covered by a fitted sheet, to reduce the risk of SIDS and other sleep-related causes of infant death.

- Room sharing—keeping baby's sleep area in the same room where you sleep—reduces the risk of SIDS and other sleep-related causes of infant death.

- Keep soft objects, toys, crib bumpers, and loose bedding out of your baby's sleep area to reduce the risk of SIDS and other sleep-related causes of infant death.

- To reduce the risk of SIDS, women should:
  - Get regular health care during pregnancy, and
  - Not smoke, drink alcohol, or use illegal drugs during pregnancy or after the baby is born.

- To reduce the risk of SIDS, do not smoke during pregnancy, and do not smoke or allow smoking around your baby.

- Breastfeed your baby to reduce the risk of SIDS.

- Give your baby a dry pacifier that is not attached to a string for naps and at night to reduce the risk of SIDS.

- Do not let your baby get too hot during sleep.

  * For more information on crib safety guidelines, contact the Consumer Product Safety Commission at 1-800-638-2772 or http://www.cpsc.gov.

- Follow health care provider guidance on your baby's vaccines and regular health checkups.

- Avoid products that claim to reduce the risk of SIDS and other sleep-related causes of infant death.

- Do not use home heart or breathing monitors to reduce the risk of SIDS.

- Give your baby plenty of Tummy Time when he or she is awake and when someone is watching.

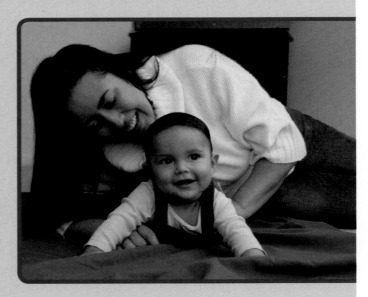

Remember Tummy Time!

Place babies on their stomachs when they are awake and when someone is watching. Tummy Time helps your baby's head, neck, and shoulder muscles get stronger and helps to prevent flat spots on the head.

For more information about SIDS and the Safe to Sleep® campaign:
Mail: 31 Center Drive, 31/2A32, Bethesda, MD 20892-2425
Phone: 1-800-505-CRIB (2742)
Fax: 1-866-760-5947
Website: http://safetosleep.nichd.nih.gov
NIH Pub. No. 12-5759
August 2014

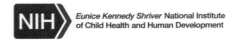

Eunice Kennedy Shriver **National Institute of Child Health and Human Development**

Safe to Sleep® is a registered trademark of the U.S. Department of Health and Human Services.

Appendix D Laboratory Values

LABORATORY VALUE	NONPREGNANT	PREGNANT			NEWBORN
Hemoglobin, g/dL	12–15.8	1st Trimester	2nd Trimester	3rd Trimester	15.2–23.6
		11.6–13.9	9.7–14.8	9.5–15.0	
Hematocrit, %	35.4–44.4	1st Trimester	2nd Trimester	3rd Trimester	46–68
		13.0–41.0	30.0–39.0	28.0–40.0	
Red blood cell count, 10^6 cells/mm^3	3.91–5.11	2.7–4.55			4.51–7.01
White blood cell count, 10^3 cells/mm^3	4.5–11.1	5.6–17			9.1–30.1
Platelets, 10^9/L	150,000–400,000	No significant change			150,000–450,000
Fibrogen, mg/dL	230–500	Increased levels late in pregnancy			200–500
Serum cholesterol, mg/dL	<200	<350			Rises rapidly after birth, reaching adult levels by day 1
Blood glucose, mg/dL		Decreased 10%–20%			<40
Fasting	65–99	<95			
2-hour postprandial	<105	<120			
Total bilirubin, mg/dL	0.3–1.2	No significant change			<24 hours: <6.0 1–2 days: <10 3–5 days: <12

Appendix E Immunization and Pregnancy

Immunization & Pregnancy

Vaccines help keep a pregnant woman and her growing family healthy.

Vaccine	Before pregnancy	During pregnancy	After pregnancy	Type of Vaccine	Route
Hepatitis A	Yes, if at risk	Yes, if at risk	Yes, if at risk	Inactivated	IM
Hepatitis B	Yes, if at risk	Yes, if at risk	Yes, if at risk	Inactivated	IM
Human Papillomavirus (HPV)	Yes, if 9 through 26 years of age	No, under study	Yes, if 9 through 26 years of age	Inactivated	IM
Influenza TIV	Yes	Yes	Yes	Inactivated	IM, ID (18-64 years)
Influenza LAIV	Yes, if less than 50 years of age and healthy; avoid conception for 4 weeks	No	Yes, if less than 50 years of age and healthy; avoid conception for 4 weeks	Live	Nasal spray
MMR	Yes, avoid conception for 4 weeks	No	Yes, give immediately postpartum if susceptible to rubella	Live	SC
Meningococcal: • polysaccharide • conjugate	If indicated	If indicated	If indicated	Inactivated Inactivated	SC IM
Pneumococcal Polysaccharide	If indicated	If indicated	If indicated	Inactivated	IM or SC
Tetanus/Diphtheria Td	Yes, Tdap preferred	Yes, Tdap preferred if 20 weeks gestational age or more	Yes, Tdap preferred	Toxoid	IM
Tdap, one dose only	Yes, preferred	Yes, preferred	Yes, preferred	Toxoid/ inactivated	IM
Varicella	Yes, avoid conception for 4 weeks	No	Yes, give immediately postpartum if susceptible	Live	SC

CS226523B   10/2011

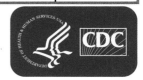

623

Appendix F Cervical Dilation Chart

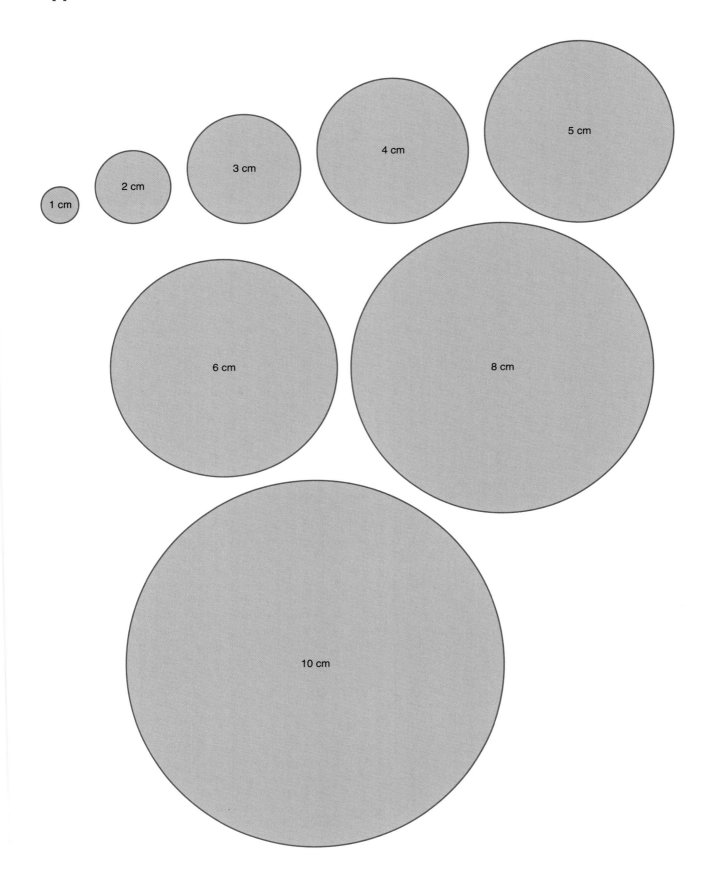

Appendix G Conversions: Approximate Temperature Equivalents

CONVERSIONS: Approximate Temperature Equivalents

°C	°F	°C	°F
35.5	95.9	37.8	100.04
35.6	96.08	37.9	100.22
35.7	96.26	38.0	100.4
35.8	96.44	38.1	100.58
35.9	96.62	38.2	100.76
36.0	96.8	38.3	100.94
36.1	96.98	38.4	102.12
36.2	97.16	38.5	101.3
36.3	97.34	38.6	101.48
36.4	97.52	38.7	101.66
36.5	97.7	38.8	101.84
36.6	97.88	38.9	102.02
36.7	98.06	39.0	102.2
36.8	98.24	39.1	102.38
36.9	98.42	39.2	102.56
37.0	98.6	39.3	102.74
37.1	98.78	39.4	102.92
37.2	98.96	39.5	103.1
37.3	99.14	39.6	103.28
37.4	99.32	39.7	103.46
37.5	99.5	39.8	103.64
37.6	99.68	39.9	103.82
37.7	99.86	40.0	104.0

$$°C = (°F - 32) \times 5/9$$
$$°F = (°C \times 1.8) + 32$$

Appendix H Newborn Weight Conversion Chart

NEWBORN WEIGHT CONVERSION CHART
Pounds and Ounces to Grams

Ounces	Pounds												
	0	1	2	3	4	5	6	7	8	9	10	11	12
0	0	454	907	1361	1814	2268	2722	3175	3629	4082	4536	4990	5443
1	28	482	936	1389	1843	2296	2750	3203	3657	4111	4564	5019	5471
2	57	510	964	1417	1871	2325	2778	3232	3685	4139	4593	5046	5500
3	85	539	992	1446	1899	2353	2807	3260	3714	4167	4621	5075	5528
4	113	567	1021	1474	1928	2381	2835	3289	3742	4196	4649	5103	5557
5	142	595	1049	1503	1956	2410	2863	3317	3770	4224	4678	5131	5585
6	170	624	1077	1531	1984	2438	2892	3345	3799	4252	4706	5160	5613
7	198	652	1106	1559	2013	2466	2920	3374	3827	4281	4734	5188	5642
8	227	680	1134	1588	2041	2495	2949	3402	3856	4309	4763	5216	5670
9	255	709	1162	1616	2070	2523	2977	3430	3884	4337	4791	5245	5698
10	284	737	1191	1644	2098	2551	3005	3459	3912	4366	4819	5273	5727
11	312	765	1219	1673	2126	2580	3034	3487	3941	4394	4848	5301	5755
12	340	794	1247	1701	2155	2608	3062	3515	3969	4423	4876	5330	5783
13	369	822	1476	1729	2183	2637	3091	3544	3997	4451	4904	5358	5812
14	397	850	1304	1758	2211	2665	3119	3572	4026	4479	4933	5386	5840
15	425	879	1332	1786	2240	2693	3147	3600	4054	4508	4961	5415	5868

1 kg = 2.2046 lbs
1 lb = 454 g
1 oz = 28.3 g

Abortion (AB)   The spontaneous or induced termination of a pregnancy prior to 20 weeks' gestation

Abruptio placenta   The separation of the placenta from its site of implantation before delivery

Accelerations   Visually apparent, abrupt increase in FHR 15 beats above baseline for 15 seconds

Acme phase   The peak of intensity of a contraction

Acrocyanosis   Cyanosis of hands and feet in newborn

Active phase   Second phase of labor; cervical dilation above 6 cm

Advocacy   An action taken in response to our ethical responsibility to intervene on behalf of those in our care

Afterpains   Moderate to severe cramp-like pains after birth caused by uterine contractions during the first few postpartum days

Alcohol related birth defects (ARBD)   Congenital anomalies associated with alcohol use during pregnancy

Alcohol related neurodevelopmental disorder (ARND)   Refers to abnormalities of the central nervous system that are associated with prenatal alcohol exposure

Alpha-fetoprotein (AFP)/ α_1-fetoprotein/ Maternal serum alpha fetoprotein (MSAFP)   A glycoprotein produced by the fetus used for assessing for the levels of AFP in the maternal blood as a screening tool for certain developmental defects in the fetus such as fetal neural tube defects (NTDs) and ventral abdominal wall defects

Amenorrhea   Absence of menstruation

Amniocentesis   Diagnostic procedure in which a needle is inserted through the maternal abdominal wall into the uterine cavity to obtain amniotic fluid

Amniotic fluid   Fluid contained within the amniotic sac

Amniotic fluid embolism (AFE)/Anaphylactoid syndrome   A rare, but often fatal complication that occurs during pregnancy, labor and birth, or postpartum in which amniotic fluid which contains fetal cells, lanugo, and vernix enters the maternal vascular system and initiates a cascading process that leads to maternal cardio respiratory collapse and disseminated intravascular coagulation (DIC)

Amniotic fluid index (AFI)   Screening tool that measures the volume of amniotic fluid with ultrasound to assess fetal well-being and placental function

Amniotomy (AROM)   The artificial rupture of membranes

ANA Code of Ethics   Makes explicit the primary goals, values, and obligations of the profession of nursing

Antepartum/antepartal   The time period beginning with conception and ending with the onset of labor

Anticipatory guidance   The provision of information and guidance to women and their families that promotes being informed about and prepared for events to come

Apgar score   A rapid assessment of five physiological signs that indicate the physiological status of the newborn at birth

Assessment   A systematic, dynamic process by which the nurse, through interaction with women, newborns and families, significant others, and health care providers, collects, monitors, and analyzes data; data may include the following dimensions: psychological, biotechnological, physical, sociocultural, spiritual, cognitive, developmental, and economic, as well as functional abilities and lifestyle

Assisted reproductive technologies (ART)   Treatments for infertility that involve the surgical removal of the oocytes and combining them with sperm in a laboratory setting

Asymmetric intrauterine growth restriction   A disproportional reduction in the size of structures and organs; results from maternal or placental conditions that occur later in pregnancy related to impeded placental blood flow

Attachment   Emotional connection that forms between the infant and his or her parents; it is bi-directional from parent to infant and infant to parent

Auscultation   When the Doppler or fetoscope (a listening devise) is used to assess the fetal heart rate by listening

Autonomy   Refers to two concepts that operate as a whole; one is the right of self-determination or the right of the individual to make his or her own choice to accept or reject treatment; the ability to exercise autonomous rights requires and is related to elements in informed consent; the second aspect is concerned with respect of persons, that is, to respect the patient's decision irrespective of the nurses' own values

Ballard maturational score (BMS)   Standardized test to calculate the gestational age of the neonate

Baseline FHR   The average fetal heart rate (FHR) rounded to increments of 5 beats per minute (bpm) during a 10-minute segment between uterine contractions, accelerations, or decelerations

Baseline variability   The fluctuations or variations of the fetal heart rate (FHR) of 2 cycles/min or greater during a steady state in the absence of contractions, accelerations, or decelerations

Beneficence   The obligation to do good; beneficence is concerned not only with doing good but also with removing harm and preventing harm

Bilirubin   The yellow pigmentation derived from the breakdown of red blood cells

Biochemical assessment   Involves biological examination and chemical determination

Biophysical profile (BPP)/ biophysical assessment (BPA)   An ultrasound assessment of fetal status along with a NST

Biophysical risk factors   Factors that originate from the mother or fetus and impact the development or function of the mother or fetus; these risk factors include genetic, nutritional, medical, and obstetric issues

Biparietal diameter (BPD)   The largest transverse measurement and an important indicator of head size; 9.25 cm

Birth rate   Number of live births per 1,000 people

Bishop's score   An assessment of the cervix to assess cervical ripeness

Blastocyst   Stage of embryo development that follows the morula stage; the blastocyst is composed of an inner cell mass referred to as the embryoblast and an outer cell layer referred to as the trophoblast

Bloody show   Brownish or blood-tinged cervical mucus discharge

Body mass index (BMI)   A tool for determining appropriate body weight compared to height

Bonding   Emotional feelings between parent and newborn that begin during pregnancy or shortly after birth; it is unidirectional from parent to newborn

Bradycardia   Baseline FHR of less than 110 bpm lasting for 10 minutes or longer

Braxton-Hicks contractions   Intermittent, painless, and physiological uterine contractions occurring in some pregnancies in the second and third trimesters that do not result in cervical change and are associated with false labor

Breech presentation   The presenting part of the fetus is the buttocks and/or feet

Breast engorgement   Distention of milk glands

Bronchopulmonary dysplasia (BPD)   A chronic lung condition that affects neonates that have been treated with mechanical ventilation and oxygen for problems such as respiratory distress syndrome

Brow presentation   When the fetal head presents in a position midway between full flexion and extreme extension

Brown adipose tissue   Also referred to as brown fat or non-shivering thermogenesis; a highly dense and vascular adipose tissue that is unique to neonates

Caput succedaneum   A localized soft tissue edema of the scalp

Cardinal movements of labor   The positional changes that the fetus goes through to best navigate the birth process

Category I FHR tracings   Normal tracings. Strongly predictive of a well-oxygenated, nonacidotic fetus with a normal fetal acid-base balance

Category II FHR tracings   Indeterminate tracings. Not predictive of abnormal fetal acid-base status, yet there is not adequate evidence to classify them as Category I or III. They require evaluation and continued surveillance

Category III FHR tracings   Abnormal tracings. Predictive of abnormal fetal acid-base status and require prompt evaluation

Cephalic presentation   The presenting part is the head

Cephalhematoma   Hematoma formation between the periosteum and skull with unilateral swelling

Cephalopelvic disproportion (CPD)   A condition in which the size, shape, or position of the fetal head prevents it from passing through the lateral aspect of the maternal pelvis or when the maternal pelvis is of a size or shape that prevents the decent of the fetus through the pelvis; term used when the maternal bony pelvis is not large enough or appropriately shaped to allow for fetal decent

Cervical dilation   This measurement estimates the dilation of the cervical opening by sweeping the examining finger from the margin of the cervical opening on one side to that on the other

Cervical effacement   This measurement estimates the shortening of the cervix from 2 cm to paper thin measured by palpation of cervical length with fingertips

Cervical insufficiency   Describes the inability of the uterine cervix to retain a pregnancy in the absence of the signs and symptoms of clinical contractions, or labor, or both in the second trimester

Cervical ripening   The process of physical softening and opening of the cervix in preparation for labor and birth

Cervix   The neck or lowest part of the uterus; interfaces with the vagina

Cesarean birth   Also referred to as cesarean section or c-section (C/S); an operative procedure in which the fetus is delivered through an incision in the abdominal wall and the uterus

Cesarean delivery on maternal request (CDMR)   A cesarean section that is performed at the request of the woman prior to labor beginning and in the absence of maternal or fetal medical condition that presents a risk for labor

Chadwick's sign   Bluish-purple coloration of the vagina and cervix evident in the first trimester of pregnancy

Childbearing and newborn health care   A model of care addressing the health promotion, maintenance, and restoration needs of women from the preconception through the postpartum period; and low-risk, high-risk, and critically ill newborns from birth through discharge and follow-up, within the social, political, economic, and environmental context of the mother's, her newborn's, and the family's lives

Cholelithiasis   Presence of gallstones in the gallbladder

Chronic pelvic pain (CPP)   Pain in the pelvic region that lasts 6 months or longer and results in functional or psychological disabilities or requires treatment/intervention

Chorionic villi   Projections from the chorion that embed into the decidua basalis and later form the fetal blood vessels of the placenta

Chorionic villus sampling (CVS)   Aspiration of a small amount of placental tissue (chorion) for chromosomal, metabolic, or DNA testing

Circumcision   An elective surgery to remove the foreskin of the penis

Circumoral cyanosis   A benign localized transient cyanosis around the newborn's mouth

Classical cesarean delivery   A vertical midline incision made into the abdominal wall with a vertical incision in the upper segment of the uterus performed for cesarean births

Cleavage   Mitotic cell division of the zygote, fertilized oocyte

Clinical pelvimetry   Measurements of the dimensions of the bony pelvis during an internal pelvic examination for determination of adequacy of the pelvis for a vaginal birth

Cold stress   A term used when there is excessive heat loss that leads to hypothermia and results in the utilization of compensatory mechanisms to maintain the neonate's body temperature

Colic   A term used to describe uncontrollable crying in healthy infants under the age of 5 months

Collaborative working relationships Working together with mutual respect for the accountability of each profession to the shared goal of quality patient outcomes

Colostrum Clear, yellowish breast fluid, which precedes milk production; it contains proteins, nutrients, and immune globulins; produced prenatally as early as the second trimester and prior to lactation in the first days after birth

Combined decelerations A deceleration pattern that has combined features, such as a variable deceleration that is also a late deceleration

Combined spinal epidural analgesia (CSE) Involves the injection of local anesthetic and/or analgesic into the subarachnoid space

Complete abortion Products of conception are totally expelled from uterus

Complete breech A fetal presentation where there is complete flexion of thighs and legs and a buttocks presentation of the fetus

Compound presentation The fetus assumes a unique posture usually with the arm or hand presenting alongside the presenting part

Conception Also known as fertilization; occurs when a sperm nucleus enters the nucleus of the oocyte

Conduction Transfer of heat to cooler surface by direct skin contact such as cold hands of caregivers or cold equipment

Conjugated bilirubin The conjugated form of bilirubin (direct bilirubin) is soluble and excretable

Contraction stress test (CST) Screening tool to assess fetal well-being with EFM in women with nonreactive NST at term gestation; the purpose of the CST is to identify a fetus that is at risk for compromise through observation of the fetal response to intermittent reduction in utero placental blood flow associated with stimulated uterine contractions (UCs)

Convection Loss of heat from the neonate's warm body surface to cooler air currents such as air conditioners or oxygen masks

Coparenting A conceptual term that refers to the ways that parents and/or parental figures relate to each other in the role of parents

Cotyledons Rounded portions, lobes, of the maternal side of the placenta

Couvade syndrome The occurrence in the mate of a pregnant woman of symptoms related to pregnancy, such as nausea, vomiting, and abdominal pain

Cultural stereotyping The practice of making generalizations about a person based on his or her culture

Culturally competent care Providing care to patients and their families that is effective, understandable, and respectful care in a manner that is compatible with their cultural beliefs, practices, and preferred language

Cystitis Infection of the bladder

Cystocele Bulging of the bladder into the vagina

Daily fetal movement count (kick counts) Maternal assessment of fetal movement by counting fetal movements in a period of time to identify potentially hypoxic fetus

Decidua basalis The portion of the decidua that forms the maternal portion of the placenta

Decrement phase The descending or relaxation of the uterine muscle

Descent The movement of the fetus through the birth canal during the first and second stage of labor

Diabetes mellitus (DM) A chronic metabolic disease characterized by hyperglycemia as a result of limited or no insulin production

Diagnosis A clinical judgment about the patient's response to actual or potential health conditions or needs; diagnoses provide the basis for determination of a plan of nursing care to achieve expected outcomes

Diagnostic tests Tests that help to identify a particular disease or provide information which aids in the making of a diagnosis

Diastasis recti/Diastasis recti abdominis A separation of the two rectus abdominis muscle bands at the midline

Dilation The enlargement or opening of the cervical os

Direct bilirubin Conjugated bilirubin

Direct obstetric death Death of a woman resulting from complications during pregnancy, labor/birth, and/or postpartum, and from interventions, omission of interventions, or incorrect treatment

Disseminated intravascular coagulation (DIC) Syndrome in which the coagulation pathways are hyperstimulated; occurs when the body is breaking down blood clots faster than it can form a clot, thus quickly depleting the body of clotting factors and leading to hemorrhage

Diversity A quality that encompasses acceptance and respect related to but not limited to age, class, culture, disability, education level, ethnicity, family structure, gender, ideologies, political beliefs, race, religion, sexual orientation, style, and values

Dizygotic twins Twins resulting from fertilization of two eggs

Doula An individual who provides support to women and their partners during labor, birth, and postpartum. The doula does not provide clinical care.

Dubowitz neurological exam Standardized tool to assess gestational age of neonate

Ductus arteriosus Structure in fetal circulation that connects the pulmonary artery with the descending aorta; the majority of the oxygenated blood is shunted to the aorta via the ductus arteriosus with smaller amounts going to the lungs

Ductus venosus Structure in fetal circulation that connects the umbilical vein to the inferior vena cava. This allows the majority of the high levels of oxygenated blood to enter the right atrium

Duration of contractions Length of a contraction measured by counting from the beginning to the end of one contraction and measured in seconds

Dysfunctional labor Abnormal uterine contractions that prevent the normal progress of cervical dilation or descent of the fetus

Dystocia A long, a difficult, or an abnormal labor

Early decelerations A gradual decrease in FHR, 20–30 bpm below baseline; generally the onset, nadir, and the recovery mirror the contraction

Eclampsia Preeclampsia with the onset of tonic clonic seizure/convulsions which place the mother and fetus at risk for death

Ectoderm The outer layer of cells in the developing embryo

Ectopic pregnancy A pregnancy that develops as a result of the blastocyst implanting somewhere other than the endometrial lining of the uterus; implantation of a fertilized ovum outside the uterus

Effacement The shortening and thinning of the cervix

Effleurage A massage technique using a very light touch of the fingers in two repetitive circular patterns over the gravid abdomen; done by lightly stroking the abdomen in rhythm with breathing during contractions

Elective abortion (EAB) Termination of pregnancy before viability at the request of the woman but not for reasons of the impaired health of the maternal health or fetal disease

Electronic fetal monitoring (EFM) A technique for fetal assessment based on the fact that the FHR reflects fetal oxygenation

Embryo Term used for the developing human from the time of implantation through 8 weeks of gestation

Embryoblast The inner cell mass of the blastocyst which develops into the embryo

Embryonic membranes Two membranes, amnion and chorion, which form the amniotic sac; the chorionic membrane (outer membrane) develops from the trophoblast; the amniotic membrane (inner membrane) develops from the embryoblast; the embryo and amniotic fluid are contained within the amniotic sac

En face Position in which the mother and newborn are face-to-face with eye contact

Endoderm The inner layer of cells in the developing embryo

Endometrial biopsy A biopsy of the endometrial tissue of the uterus to assess for the response of the uterus to hormonal signals that occur during the menstrual cycle

Endometrial cycle Pertains to the changes in the endometrium of the uterus in response to the hormonal changes that occur during the ovarian cycle; this cycle consist of three phases: proliferative phase, secretory phase, and menstrual phase

Endometriosis A chronic inflammatory disease in which the presence and growth of endometrial tissue is found outside the uterine cavity

Endometritis/Metritis An infection of the endometrium that usually starts at the placental site and can spread to encompass the entire endometrium

Endometrium The mucous membrane lining the interior of the uterus

Engagement Occurs when the greatest diameter of the fetal head passes through the pelvic inlet

Engrossment Phenomenon experienced by new fathers who have an intense preoccupation about and interest in their newborn

Entrainment Phenomenon in which the newborn and infant moves his or her arms and legs in rhythm with speech patterns of an adult

Environmental risk factors Risks in the workplace or the general environment that impact pregnancy outcomes; various environmental substances can effect fetal development; examples include exposure to chemicals, radiation, and pollutants

Epidural anesthesia Involves the placement of a very small catheter and injection of local anesthesia and or analgesia between the 4th and 5th vertebrae into the epidural space

Epidural block An anesthetic injected in the epidural space; located outside the dura mater between the dura and spinal canal via an epidural catheter

Episiotomy An incision in the perineum to provide more space for the fetal presenting part at delivery

Epstein's pearls White, pearl-like epithelial cysts on neonate's gum margins and palate

Epispadias An abnormality in which urethral opening is on dorsal side of penis

Erythemia toxicum A rash with red macules and papules (white to yellowish-white papule in center surrounded by reddened skin) that appear in different areas of the body, usually the trunk area. Can appear within 24 hours of birth and up to 2 weeks

Ethical dilemma A choice that has the potential to violate ethical principles

Ethics Based in philosophical discussions of ancient Greek scholars about the nature of good and evil or right and wrong

Ethnocentrism The belief that the customs and values of the dominant culture are preferred or superior in some way

Evaluation The process of determining the patient's progress toward attainment of expected outcomes and the effectiveness of nursing care

Evaporation Loss of heat that occurs when water on neonate's skin is converted to vapors such as during bathing or directly after birth

Evidence-based nursing (EBN) Combining the best research evidence with clinical expertise while taking into account the patients' preferences and their situation in the context of the available resources part of nursing practice

Evidenced-based practice (EBP) The integration of best research evidence, clinical expertise, and patient values in making decisions about the care of patients

Expulsion During this cardinal movement the shoulders and remainder of the body are delivered

Extension This cardinal movement, which is facilitated by resistance of the pelvic floor, causes the presenting part to pivot beneath the pubic symphysis and the head to be delivered; occurs during the second stage of labor

External rotation During this cardinal movement the sagittal suture moves to a transverse diameter and the shoulders align in the anteroposterior diameter; the sagittal suture maintains alignment with the fetal trunk as the trunk navigates through the pelvis

Extremely low birth weight infant (ELBW) An infant who weighs less than 1,000 grams at birth

Face presentation When the fetal head is in extension rather than flexion as it enters the pelvis

False labor Irregular contractions with little or no cervical changes

Family-centered maternity care A model of obstetric care that views pregnancy and childbirth as a normal life event or life transition that is not primarily medical but rather developmental; health care is provided in an inclusive manner, with family and significant others, including children, as an active part of the process; the emphasis is on holistic care, with the focus on the pregnant woman and her well-being, including emotional and psychosocial considerations

Ferguson's reflex   A physiological response of the woman, activated when the presenting part of the fetus is at least at +1 station; it is usually accompanied by spontaneous bearing-down efforts

Ferning   When a sample of fluid in the upper vaginal area is obtained, the fluid is placed on a slide and assessed for "ferning pattern" under a microscope to confirm rupture of membranes

Fertility rate   Total number of live births, regardless of age of mother, per 1,000 women of reproductive age, 15–44 years

Fetal alcohol syndrome (FAS)   Refers to a wide array and spectrum of physical, cognitive, and behavioral abnormalities associated with maternal alcohol use during pregnancy

Fetal attitude or posture   The relationship of the fetal parts to one another; this is noted by the flexion or extension of the fetal joints

Fetal bradycardia   Baseline FHR of less than 110 bpm lasting for 10 minutes or longer

Fetal dystocia   May be caused by excessive fetal size, malpresentation, multifetal pregnancy, or fetal anomalies

Fetal fibronectin (fFN)   A protein detected via immunoassay; a positive test is >50 ng/mL

Fetal heart rate accelerations   The visually abrupt, transient increases (onset to peak <30 sec) in the FHR above the baseline, 15 beats above the baseline and last from 15 seconds to less than two minutes

Fetal heart rate decelerations   Transitory decreases in the FHR baseline; they are classified as early, variable, or late decelerations

Fetal lie   Refers to the long axis (spine) of the fetus in relationship to the long axis (spine) of the woman

Fetal position   Location of the presenting part and specific fetal structures to determine fetal position in relation to maternal pelvis; relation of the denominator or reference point to the maternal pelvis

Fetal presentation   Determined by the part, or pole, of the fetus that first enters the pelvic inlet

Fetoscope   Stethoscope used to auscultate fetal heart rate

Fetus   Term used for the developing human from 9 weeks' gestation to birth

Fidelity   Refers to the faithfulness or obligation to keep promises

First-degree laceration   A laceration that involves the perineal skin and vaginal mucous membrane

First stage of labor   Begins with onset of labor and ends with complete cervical dilation

Flexion   When the chin of the fetus moves toward the fetal chest; flexion occurs when the descending head meets resistance from maternal tissues

Follicular phase   Part of the ovarian cycle; it begins the first day of menstruation and last 12–14 days; during this phase, the graafian follicle is maturing

Footling breech   When either one (single footling) or both (double footling) feet of the fetus present first in the pelvis

Foramen ovale   A structure in fetal circulation; it is an opening between the right and left atria; blood high in oxygen is shunted to the left atrium via the foramen ovale

Forceps   An instrument used to assist with delivery of the fetal head, typically done to improve the health of the woman or the fetus

Foremilk   The milk that is produced and stored between feedings and released at the beginning of the feeding session; it has higher water content

Fourth degree laceration   A laceration that extends into the rectal mucosa and exposes the lumen of the rectum

Fourth stage of labor   Begins with the delivery of the placenta and typically ends within 4 hours or with the stabilization of the mother postpartum

Frank breech   A fetal presentation where there is complete flexion of the thighs and the legs extend over the anterior surfaces of the body

Frequency of contractions   Determined by counting number of contractions in a 10-minute period, counting from the start of one contraction to the start of the next contraction in minutes

Fundus   The upper portion of the uterus

Gate control theory of pain   States that sensation of pain is transmitted from the periphery of the body along ascending nerve pathways to the brain; due to the limited number of sensations that can travel along these pathways at any given time, an alternate activity can replace travel of the pain sensation; thus closing the gate control at the spinal cord and reducing pain impulses traveling to the brain

General anesthesia   The use of IV injection and/or inhalation of anesthetic agents that render the woman unconscious

Genital fistulas   An abnormal connection between the vagina and bladder, rectum, and/or urethra; the fistula provides a pathway for fecal material and/or urine to enter the vagina

Genome   An organism's complete set of DNA

Genotype   Refers to a person's genetic makeup

Gestational carrier   A woman who agrees to bear a genetically unrelated child with the help of assisted reproductive technologies for an individual or couple who intend(s) to be the legal and rearing parent(s), referred to as the intended parent(s)

Gestational diabetes mellitus (GDM)   Any degree of glucose intolerance with the onset or first recognition in pregnancy

Gestational hypertension   A relatively benign disorder without underlying physiological changes in the mother; high blood pressure detected for the first time after mid-pregnancy, without proteinuria; diagnosis is made postpartum

Gestational trophoblastic disease   Refers to a spectrum of placental related tumors in which abnormal trophoblast cells grow inside the uterus after conception

Gestational surrogacy   A woman known as a gestational carrier agrees to bear a genetically unrelated child with the help of assisted reproductive technologies for an individual or couple who intend(s) to be the legal and rearing parent(s), referred to as the intended parent(s)

Glans penis   Tip of the penis

Gonadotoxins   Factors, such as drugs, infections, illness, and heat exposure, that can have an adverse effect on spermatogenesis

Goodell's sign   The softening of the cervix in the first trimester of pregnancy

Gravida   A pregnant woman; also, the number of times a woman has been pregnant (Gravida/Para notation)

Harlequin sign   One side of body is pink and the other side is white

Hegar's sign   The softening of the lower uterine segment (isthmus) in the first trimester of pregnancy

HELLP syndrome   (Hemolysis, **E**levated **L**iver enzymes, and **Low P**latelets) Acronym used to designate the variant changes in laboratory values that is a complication of severe preeclampsia

Hematomas   A collection of blood within the connective tissues; common sites in the postpartum woman are the vagina and perineal areas

Hind milk   The milk produced during the feeding session and released at the end of the session; it has a higher fat content

Hydatiform mole   A benign proliferate growth of the trophoblast in which the chorionic villi develop into edematous, cystic, vascular transparent vesicles that hang in grapelike clusters without a viable fetus

Hydrocele   Enlarged scrotum due to excess fluid

Hyperbilirubinemia   Term used when there is a high level of unconjugated bilirubin in the neonate's blood

Hyperemesis gravidarum   Vomiting during pregnancy that is so severe it leads to dehydration, electrolyte and acid base imbalance, and starvation ketosis

Hyperstimulation   Excessive uterine activity

Hypertonic uterine dysfunction   Uncoordinated uterine activity

Hypospadias   An abnormality in which the urethral opening is on ventral surface of penis

Hypotonic uterine dysfunction   Occurs when the pressure of the UC is insufficient (<25 mmHg) to promote cervical dilation and effacement

Hysterectomy   The surgical removal of the uterus

Hysterosalpingogram   A radiological examination that provides information about the endocervical canal, uterine cavity, and the fallopian tubes

Implantation   The embedding of the blastocyst into the endometrium of the uterus

Implementation   The process of taking action by intervening, delegating, and/or coordinating; women, newborns, families, significant others, or health care providers may direct the implementation of interventions within the plan of care

Inadequate expulsive forces   Occurs in the second stage of labor when the woman is not able to push or bear down

Incompetent cervix   A mechanical defect in the cervix that results in painless cervical dilation and ballooning of the membranes into the vagina followed by expulsion of an immature fetus in the second trimester

Incomplete abortion   Fragments of products of conception are expelled and tissue parts are retained in the uterus.

Increment phase   The ascending or buildup of the contraction which begins in the fundus and spreads throughout the uterus

Indirect bilirubin   Unconjugated bilirubin

Indirect obstetrical death   Death of a woman that is due to a preexisting disease or a disease that develops during pregnancy that is not directly related to obstetrical cause but is aggravated by the changes of pregnancy

Induced abortion   The medical or surgical termination of pregnancy prior to viability

Induction   The deliberate stimulation of uterine contractions before the onset of spontaneous labor

Inevitable abortion   Termination of pregnancy is in progress

Infant mortality   Infant death prior to the first birthday

Infertility   The inability to conceive and maintain a pregnancy after 12 months (6 months for women over 35 years old age) of unprotected sexual intercourse

Intensity   Strength of the contraction and measure by palpation, or internally by an intrauterine pressure catheter (IUPC) in mmHg

Interconceptional interval   The period of time in between pregnancies

Internal rotation   This cardinal movement, the rotation of the fetal head, aligns the long axis of the fetal head with the long axis of the maternal pelvis; occurs mainly during second stage of labor

Internal uterine pressure catheter (IUPC)   This monitoring provides an objective measure of the pressure of contractions expressed as mmHg

Intrahepatic cholestasis of pregnancy (ICP)   A reversible type of hormonally influenced cholestasis characterized by generalized itching, also known as obstetric cholestasis

Intrapartum period   Begins with the onset of regular uterine contractions and lasts until the expulsion of the placenta

Intrauterine growth restriction (IUGR)   A decrease rate of fetal growth usually due to a decrease in cell production related to chronic malnutrition; there are two types of IUGR, symmetric and asymmetric

Involution   The process by which the uterus returns to a prepregnant size, shape, and location; and the placental site heals

Isthmus   The narrower, lower segment of the uterus

Justice   The principle of fairness, that others are entitled to equal treatment or to be treated fairly

Kernicterus   An abnormal accumulation of unconjugated bilirubin in the neonate's brain cells

Labor   The process in which the fetus, placenta, and membranes are expelled through the uterus

Labor augmentation   The stimulation of ineffective uterine contractions after the onset of spontaneous labor to manage labor dystocia

Lacerations   Tears in the perineum that may occur at delivery

Lactation   The production of breast milk

Lanugo   Fine, downy hair that develops after 16 weeks of gestation

Large for gestational age (LGA)   Term used for neonates whose weight is above the 90th percentile for gestational age

Latching-on   Refers to the newborn's ability to grasp the breast and to effectively suckle

Late deceleration A visually apparent gradual decrease of FHR below the baseline. Lowest part of the deceleration occurs after the peak of the contraction

Late maternal death Death of a woman that occurs more than 42 days after termination of pregnancy from a direct or indirect obstetrical cause

Late premature/late preterm Neonate born between 34 and 37 weeks' gestation

Latent phase First phase of labor; the early and slower part of labor with cervical dilation from 0–3 cm

Leiomyomas of the uterus Also referred to as myomas or uterine fibroids; benign fibrous tumor of the uterine wall

Leopold's maneuvers A series of four maneuvers used to palpate a gravid uterus to determine fetal position, presentation, and size

Let-down reflect Also referred to as milk ejection reflex; results in milk being ejected into and through the lactiferous duct system

Leukorrhea A white, odorless, physiological vaginal discharge; increases in pregnancy due to increased mucus secretion by cervical glands

Lightening Term used to describe the descent of the fetus into the true pelvis, which occurs approximately 2 weeks before term in first-time pregnancies

Local An anesthetic injected into perineum at episiotomy site

Lochia Bloody discharge from the uterus that contains sloughed off tissue; it undergoes changes that reflect the healing stages of the uterine placental site

Long-term variability (LTV) The changes in FHR range or fluctuations in the FHR baseline; this term is no longer used

Low birth weight infant (LBW) An infant who weighs less than 2,500 grams but greater than 1,500 grams at birth, regardless of gestational age

Low-lying placenta Placentas near to but not overlying the os are termed low-lying

Luteal phase Part of the ovarian cycle; it begins after ovulation and last approximately 14 days

Macrocephaly Head circumference greater than the 90th percentile

Macrosomia Birth weight above 4,000–4,500 grams

Magnetic resonance imaging (MRI) Diagnostic radiological evaluation of tissue and organs from multiple planes

Mammogram A low-dose x-ray of the breast

Marginal placenta previa The placenta is at the margin of the internal cervical os

Mastitis Inflammation/infection of the breast

Maternal death Death of a woman during pregnancy or within 42 days of termination of pregnancy; the death is related to the pregnancy or aggravated by pregnancy, or management of the pregnancy; it excludes death from accidents or injuries

Maternal phases A process, defined by Reva Rubin, that occurs during the first few weeks of the postpartum period; this process includes three phases: Taking-in, Taking-hold, and Letting-go

Maternal tasks of pregnancy Psychological work done by the pregnant woman toward the development of a positive adaptation to pregnancy and the establishment of a maternal identity

Maternal touch A process, described by Reva Rubin, that new mothers transition through beginning with the first physical contact with their newborns

Meconium stool The first stool eliminated by the neonate; it is sticky, thick, black, and odorless

Medical nutritional therapy (MNT) A cornerstone of diabetes management for all diabetic women; the goal is to provide adequate nutrition, prevent diabetic ketoacidosis, and postprandial euglycemia

Meiosis A process of two successive cell divisions that produces cells that contain half the number of chromosomes (haploid)

Menarche The initial menstrual period

Menopause The permanent cessation of menstrual activity; occurs 12 months after a woman's last menstrual period

Menstrual phase Part of the endometrial cycle; it occurs in response to hormonal changes and results in the sloughing off of the endometrial tissue

Mesoderm The middle layer of cells in the developing embryo

Metritis/Endometritis An infection of the endometrium that usually starts at the placental site and can spread to encompass the entire endometrium

Microcephaly Head circumference below the 10th percentile of normal for newborns gestational age

Milia White papules on the neonate's face; more frequently seen on the bridge of the nose and chin

Missed abortion Embryo or fetus dies during first 20 weeks of gestation but is retained in uterus

Mitotic cell division or mitosis Occurs when a cell (parent cell) divides and forms two daughter cells that contain the same number of chromosomes as the parent cell

Moderately premature Neonate born between 32 and 34 weeks' gestation

Modified BPP Combines a non-stress test with an amniotic fluid index (AFI) as an indicator of short-term fetal well-being and AFI as an indicator of long-term placental function to evaluate fetal well-being

Molding The ability of the fetal head to change shape to accommodate/fit through the maternal pelvis

Mongolian spots Flat bluish discolored areas on the lower back and/or buttock. Seen more often in African American, Asian, Latin, and Native American infants

Monozygotic twins Twins from one zygote that divides in the first week of gestation

Morula 16-cell solid sphere that forms three days following fertilization as a result of mitotic cell division of the zygote

Mottling A benign transient pattern of pink and white blotches on the skin

Multigravida A woman who has been pregnant multiple times

Multipara A woman who has given birth after 20 weeks' gestation multiple times

Multiple gestation A pregnancy with more than one fetus

Myomectomy Surgical removal of fibroids

Myometrium The smooth muscle layer of the uterus

Nadir The lowest point of the deceleration; occurs at the peak of the contraction

Naegele's rule The standard formula for calculating an estimated date of birth based on an LMP (LMP minus 3 months plus 7 days)

Natal teeth Immature caps of enamel and dentin with poorly developed roots

Necrotizing enterocolitis (NEC) A gastrointestinal disease that affects neonates; this disease results in inflammation and necrosis of the bowel, usually the proximal colon or terminal ileum

Neonatal abstinence syndrome Also referred to as neonatal withdrawal; may result from intrauterine exposure to various substances, including opioids such as heroin, methadone, oxycodone, and Demerol; alcohol; Valium; caffeine; and barbiturates

Neonatal period The time period from birth through the first 28 days of life

Neutral thermal environment (NTE) Refers to an environment that maintains body temperature with minimal metabolic changes and/or oxygen consumption

Non-stress test (NST) Screening tool that uses electronic fetal monitoring to assess fetal well-being

Nonmaleficence The obligation to do no harm

Nonreassuring FHR An abnormal FHR pattern that reflects an unfavorable physiological response to the maternal-fetal environment, this term is no longer in common use

Nulligravida A woman who has never been pregnant

Nullipara A woman who has never given birth after 20 weeks' gestation

Obesity Defined by a BMI of ≥30, obesity has long been recognized as a risk factor in pregnancy

Obstetrical emergency An urgent clinical situation that places either the maternal or fetal status at risk for increased morbidity and mortality

Occiput posterior When the occiput of the fetus is in the posterior portion of the pelvis rather than the anterior

Occult prolapse When the cord is palpated through the membranes but does not drop into the vagina

Oligohydramnios Decreased amounts of amniotic fluid (less than 500 mL at term or 50% reduction of normal amounts) during pregnancy

Ominous FHR patterns Fetal heart rates associated with increased risk of fetal acidemia

Oogenesis The formation of a mature ovum (egg)

Open glottis Refers to spontaneous, involuntary bearing down accompanying the forces of the uterine contraction and is usually characterized by expiratory grunting or vocalizations by a woman during pushing

Operative vaginal delivery A vaginal birth that is assisted by a vacuum extraction or forceps

Organogenesis The formation and development of body organs that occurs during the first trimester of pregnancy

Orthostatic hypotension A sudden drop in the blood pressure when the woman stands up from a sitting or lying position

Osteoporosis The loss of bone mass that occurs when more bone mass is absorbed than new body mass is laid down

Outcome A measurable individual, family, or community state, behavior, or perception that is responsive to nursing interventions

Ovarian cycle Pertains to the maturation of ova and consist of three phases: follicular phase, ovulatory phase, and luteal phase

Ovulatory phase Part of the ovarian cycle; it begins when estrogen levels peak and ends with the release of the oocyte (egg) from the mature graafian follicle; the release of the oocyte is referred to ovulation

Oxytocin induction Pharmacological method for induction of labor with oxytocin

Papanicolaou smear A screening test used to identify cervical cancer

Para A woman who has given birth to an infant after 20 weeks' gestation; also, the number of births that occurred after 20 weeks' gestation (Gravida/Para notation) or the number of infants born after 20 weeks' gestation (TPAL notation)

Partial placenta previa The placenta partially covers the internal cervical os

Parturition (or labor) The process in which the fetus, placenta, and membranes are expelled through the uterus

Passage Includes the bony pelvis and the soft tissues of cervix, pelvic floor, vagina, and introitus (external opening to the vagina)

Passenger The fetus

Patent ductus arteriosus (PDA) Occurs when the ductus arteriosus remains open or remains open after birth

Paternal postnatal depression (PPND) Some new fathers experience depression during the first 6 months following childbirth

Peak pressure The maximum uterine pressure during a contraction measured with an IUPC

Pediatric abusive head trauma (PAHT) Also referred to as abusive head trauma or shaken baby syndrome, is a traumatic brain injury that occurs when an infant is violently shaken

Pelvic dystocia Related to the contraction of one or more of the three planes of the pelvis

Pelvic inflammatory disease (PID) A general term that refers to an infection of the uterus, fallopian tubes, and other reproductive organs

Pelvic organ prolapse (POP) The descent of pelvic organs into the vagina or against the vaginal wall

Percutaneous umbilical blood sampling (PUBS) The removal of fetal blood from umbilical cord for fetal blood sampling; also referred to as cordocentesis

Perinatal The time period "around" the birth of a baby; generally refers to the weeks before and after a baby is born, from 28 weeks' gestation to 28 days after birth

Periodic and nonperiodic changes Accelerations or decelerations in the FHR that are related to uterine contractions and persist over time

Persistent pulmonary hypertension (PPHN) Results when the normal vasodilation and relaxation of the pulmonary vascular bed does not occur

Pfannenstiel incision or "bikini cut" A transverse skin incision at the level of the mons pubis with a transverse incision in the lower uterine segment performed for cesarean births

Phenotype Refers to how the genes are outwardly expressed (i.e., eye color, hair color, height)

Phenylketonuria (PKU) An inborn error of metabolism that affects the neonate's ability to metabolize phenylalanine, an amino acid commonly found in many foods such as breast milk and formula

Physiological anemia of pregnancy A relative anemia in mid to late pregnancy due to physiological hypervolemia without a correspondingly proportionate increase in erythrocytes in the maternal system

Pica A craving for and consumption of non-food substances such as starch and clay; can result in toxicity due to ingested substances or malnutrition from replacing nutritious foods with non-food substances

Pilonidal dimple A small pit or sinus in the sacral area at top of crease between the buttocks

Placenta accreta An abnormality of implantation defined by degree of invasion into uterine wall of trophoblast of placenta; invasion of trophoblast beyond the normal boundary

Placenta increta Invasion of trophoblast that extends into myometrium

Placenta percreta Invasion of trophoblast beyond the serosa

Placenta previa Occurs when the placenta attaches to the lower uterine segment of the uterus, near or over the internal cervical os, instead of in the body or fundus of the uterus. All placentas overlying the os (to any degree) are termed previas and those near to but not overlying the os are termed low-lying

Placental reserve Describes the reserve oxygen available to the fetus to withstand the transient changes in blood flow and oxygen during labor

Polycystic ovary syndrome (PCOS) Also known as Stein-Leventhal syndrome, is an endocrine disorder that affects 5%–10% of women of childbearing age that involves multiple follicular cysts on one or both ovaries

Polydactyly Extra digits of hands or feet

Polyhydramnios or hydramnios Increased amounts of amniotic fluid (1,500–2,000 mL)

Position Maternal position during labor and birth

Position of cervix Relationship of the cervical os to the fetal head and is characterized as posterior, mid position, or anterior

Post-term pregnancy One that has a gestational period of 42 completed weeks

Postpartum The 6-week period of time following childbirth

Postpartum blues Also known as baby blues; occurs during the first few weeks postpartum and lasts for a few days; it is a time of heightened maternal emotions with the woman being tearful and irritable with emotional swings

Postpartum chills Episode of shaking and feeling cold that is experienced by most women during the first few hours following birth

Postpartum depression (PPD) A mood disorder characterized by severe depression that occurs within the first 6–12 months postpartum

Postpartum psychosis (PPP) A variant of bipolar disorder and is the most serious form of postpartum mood disorders

Postterm Born after completion of 41 weeks' gestation

Powers Refer to the involuntary uterine contractions of labor and the voluntary pushing or bearing down powers that combine to propel and deliver the fetus and placenta from the uterus

Practice standards Standards that help to guide professional nursing practice; they summarize the nursing profession's best judgment and optimal practice based on current research and clinical practice

Precipitous labor Labor that lasts less than 3 hours from onset of labor to birth

Preconception care Well-woman health care focusing on preparation for and anticipation of a pregnancy, including health promotion, risk screening, and implementation of interventions prior to pregnancy, the goal being to modify risk factors that could negatively impact a pregnancy in order to optimize perinatal outcomes

Preeclampsia Hypertension accompanied by underlying systemic pathology that can have severe maternal and fetal impact; a systemic disease with hypertension accompanied by proteinuria after 20th week of gestation.

Preeclampsia superimposed on chronic HTN Occurs with hypertensive women who develop new onset proteinuria; proteinuria before 20th week gestation or sudden uncontrolled hypertension

Prenatal The entire time period during which a woman is pregnant; includes the antepartum/antepartal and the intrapartal periods

Prenatal care Health care relating to pregnancy that a woman receives during the pregnancy and prior to the onset of labor

Prescriptive behavior Expected behavior of the pregnant woman during the childbearing period

Presenting part The specific fetal structure lying nearest to the cervix

Preterm birth Birth between 20 0/7 weeks of gestation and 36 6/7 weeks of gestation

Preterm infant A late preterm infant is born between 34 and 37 weeks of gestation (34 0/7–36 6/7 weeks). A very preterm infant is born before 32 completed weeks of gestation

Preterm premature rupture of membranes (PPROM) Rupture of membranes with a premature gestation (<37 weeks). Remote from term is from 24–32 weeks' gestation. Near term is 31–36 weeks' gestation

Premature rupture of membranes Rupture of the chorioamniotic membranes before the onset of labor

Previable premature rupture of membranes Rupture of membranes before 23–24 weeks

Prolonged rupture of membranes Rupture of the membranes for greater than 24 hours

Preterm/premature infant An infant born after 20 weeks and before 37 completed weeks of gestation

Primary engorgement An increase in the vascular and lymphatic system of the breasts, which precedes the initiation of milk production; the woman's breasts become larger, firm, warm, and tender and woman may feel a throbbing pain in the breasts

Primigravida   A woman who is pregnant for the first time

Primipara   A woman who has given birth after 20 weeks' gestation one time

Prodromal labor   When contractions are frequent and painful in early labor but ineffective in promoting dilation and effacement

Prolactin   The primary hormone responsible for lactation

Prolapse of the umbilical cord   When the cord lies below the presenting part of the fetus

Proliferative phase   Part of the endometrial cycle; it follows menstruation and ends with ovulation; during this phase the endometrium is preparing for implantation by becoming thicker and more vascular

Prolonged deceleration   A visually apparent abrupt decrease in FHR below baseline that last >2 minutes and <10 minutes

Prolonged rupture of membranes (PROM)   Rupture of membranes longer than 24 hours

Psychosocial risk factors   Maternal behaviors or lifestyles that have a negative response to the mother or fetus; examples include: smoking, caffeine, alcohol/drugs, and psychological status

Pudendal block   An anesthetic injected in the pudendal nerve (close to the ischial spines) via needle guide known as "trumpet"

Pulmonary surfactant   A substance that is composed of 90% phospholipids and 10% proteins that is used in the treatment of respiratory distress syndrome of the neonate

Quad screen   Adds inhibin-A to the triple marker screen to increase detection of Trisomy 21 to 80%

Quickening   A woman's first awareness/perception of fetal movement within her uterus

Radiation   Transfer of heat from neonate to cooler objectives that are not in direct contact with neonate such as cold walls of isolate or cold equipment near neonate

Reassuring FHR   Normal FHR pattern that reflects a favorable physiological response to maternal-fetal environment; this term is no longer in common use

Rectocele   Bulging of the rectum into the vagina

Recurrent abortion   Condition in which two or more successive pregnancies have ended in spontaneous abortion

Respect for others   The principle that all persons are equally valued

Respiratory distress syndrome (RDS)   A life-threatening lung disorder that results from underdeveloped and small alveoli, and insufficient levels of pulmonary surfactant

Resting tone   The pressure in the uterus between contractions

Restrictive behavior   Activities during the childbearing period which are limited for the woman based on cultural practices

Review of systems (ROS)   A component of the health history that includes systematic questioning about health status by body system, typically in a head-to-toe sequence, in order to gather information about current and past medical experiences

Rh factor   A type of antigen on the surface of red blood cells; if a woman's RBCs have the antigen, she is Rh positive, and if they do not have the antigen, she is Rh negative; this is significant and can cause isoimmunization from blood incompatibility if fetal blood enters the maternal system in an Rh positive fetus and an Rh negative mother

Rights approach   The focus is on the individual's right to choose; includes the right to privacy, to know the truth, and to be free from injury or harm

Risk management   A systems approach to the prevention of litigation; it involves the identification of systems problems, and analysis and treatment of risks before a suit is brought

Rupture of the uterus   When there is a partial or complete tear in the uterine muscle

Screening test   A test designed to identify those who are not affected by a disease or abnormality

Second-degree laceration   A laceration that involves skin, mucous membrane, and fascia of perineal body

Second stage of labor   Begins at complete dilation of cervix and ends with delivery of the neonate

Secretory phase   Part of the endometrial cycle; it begins after ovulation and ends with the onset of menstruation; during this phase the endometrium continues to thicken

Septic abortion   A condition in which products of conception become infected during abortion process

Shaken baby syndrome   Also referred to as **pediatric abusive head trauma (PAHT);** a traumatic brain injury that occurs when an infant is violently shaken

Short-term variability (STV)   The changes in the FHR from one beat to the next; is measured with a fetal scalp electrode; this term is no longer used

Shoulder dystocia   Refers to difficulty encountered during delivery of the shoulders after the birth of the head

Shoulder presentation   The presenting part is the shoulder; when the fetal spine is vertical to the maternal pelvis

Small for gestational age (SGA)   A term used for neonate whose weight is below the 10th percentile for gestational age

Social support   Support given by someone with whom the expectant mother has a personal relationship, involving the primary groups of most importance to the individual woman

Sociodemographic risk factors   Variables that pertain to the woman and her family and place an increased risk to the mother and the fetus; examples include income, access to prenatal care, age, parity, marital status, and ethnicity

Sperm antibodies   An immunological reaction against the sperm that causes a decrease in sperm motility

Spermatogenesis   The process in which mature functional sperm are formed

Spinal block   An anesthetic injected in the subarachnoid space

Spontaneous abortion (SAB)   Abortion occurring without medical or mechanical means; also called miscarriage

Spontaneous rupture of the membranes (SROM)   Rupture of the membranes that occurs naturally

Standard   An authoritative statement enunciated and promulgated by the profession and by which the quality of practice, service, or education can be judged

Standards of care Authoritative statements that describe competent clinical nursing practice for women and newborns demonstrated through assessment, diagnosis, outcome identification, planning, implementation, and evaluation

Standards of nursing practice Authoritative statements that describe the scope of care or performance common to the profession of nursing and by which the quality of nursing practice can be judged; standards of nursing practice for women and newborns include both standards of care and standards of professional performance

Standards of professional performance Authoritative statements that describe competent behavior in the professional role, including activities related to quality of care, performance appraisal, resource utilization, education, collegiality, ethics, collaboration, research, and research utilization

Station The level of the presenting part in the birth canal in relationship to the ischial spines; refers to the relationship of the ischial spines to the presenting part of the fetus and assists in assessing for fetal descent during labor

Striae A band of depressed tissue most commonly seen on abdomen, thighs, buttocks, or breasts due to stretching of the skin; synonymous with stretch marks

Stripping the membranes Digital separation of the chorionic membrane from the wall of the cervix and lower uterine segment during a vaginal exam done by a primary care provider to stimulate labor

Subinvolution of the uterus A term used when the uterus does not decrease in size and does not descend into the pelvis

Supine hypotensive syndrome Hypotension resulting from compression of the vena cava when a woman lies supine and the gravid uterus exerts pressure on the inferior vena cava

Symmetric intrauterine growth restriction A generalized proportional reduction in the size of all structures and organs except for heart and brain

Syndactyly Webbed digits of hands or feet

Taboos Cultural restrictions believed to have serious consequences

Tachycardia Baseline FHR of greater than 160 bpm lasting 10 minutes or longer

Tachysystole Abnormally frequent contractions, 5 or more contractions in 10 minutes

Teratogens are any drug, virus, infection, or other exposures that can cause embryo/fetal developmental abnormality

Term birth A birth that occurs after 37 completed weeks of gestation

Therapeutic abortion (TAB) Termination of pregnancy for serious maternal medical indications or serious fetal anomalies

Third-degree laceration A laceration involves skin, mucous membrane, muscle of perineal body, and extends to the rectal sphincter

Third stage of labor Begins immediately after the delivery of the fetus and involves separation and expulsion of the placenta and membranes

Threatened abortion Continuation of pregnancy is in doubt as symptoms indicate termination of pregnancy is in progress

Thrombosis Blood clot within the vascular system

Tocodynamometer An external uterine monitor to measure contractions

TORCH An acronym that stands for **T**oxoplasmosis, **O**ther (hepatitis B), **R**ubella, **C**ytomegalovirus, and **H**erpes Simplex virus

Total placenta previa The placenta completely covers the internal cervical os

Toxoplasma A protozoan parasite found in cat feces and uncooked or rare beef and lamb

Transepidermal water loss (TEWL) Water loss that can occur through the neonate's immature skin

Transition phase Third phase of labor; dilation to 10 cm

Transitional stool Neonatal stools that begin around the 3rd day and can continue for 3 or 4 days; the stool transitions from black to greenish black, to greenish brown, to greenish yellow

Transverse presentation The presenting part is usually the shoulder

Trial of labor after cesarean (TOLAC) When a trial of labor and vaginal birth is attempted in a woman who has had a prior cesarean birth

Triple marker A screening that combines all three chemical markers (AFP, hCG, and estriol levels) with maternal age to detect some trisomies and neural tube defects

Trophic feedings Small volume enteral feedings that are administered to neonates

Trophoblast Outer cell mass of the blastocyst which assists in implantation and becomes part of the placenta

True labor Contractions occur at regular intervals and increase in frequency, duration, and intensity; true labor contractions bring about changes in cervical effacement and dilation

Turtle sign The retraction of the fetal head against the maternal perineum after delivery of the head

Type 1 diabetes mellitus A result of autoimmunity of beta cells of the pancreas resulting in absolute insulin deficiency

Type 2 diabetes mellitus Characterized by insulin resistance and inadequate insulin production

Ultrasonography The use of high-frequency sound waves to produce an image of an organ or tissue

Umbilical artery doppler flow Studies assess the rate and volume of blood flow through placenta and umbilical cord vessels using ultrasound

Umbilical cord The structure that connects the fetus to the placenta; it consists of 2 arteries and 1 vein and is surrounded by Wharton's Jelly

Unconjugated bilirubin A relatively insoluble bilirubin and mostly bound to albumin; also called indirect bilirubin

Undescended testes An abnormality in which testes are not in the scrotum

Urinary incontinence Loss of bladder control

Uterine atony A decreased tone of the uterine muscle postpartum that is the primary cause of immediate postpartum hemorrhage

Uterine fibroids Benign growths of the muscular wall of the uterus

Uterine hypertonus An increasing resting tone $>20-25$ mmHg, peak pressure >80 mmHg or Montevideo units >400

Uterine prolapse   Occurs when there is a weakening of the pelvic connective tissue, pubococcygeus muscle, and uterine ligaments which allows the uterus to descend into the vagina

Uterus   The muscular reproductive organ that contains and supports a pregnancy

Utilitarian approach   This approach suggests that ethical actions are those that provide the greatest balance of good over evil and provides for the greatest good for the greatest number

Utility   The greatest good for the individual or an action that is valued; utility is concerned with the evaluation of risk and benefit or benefit versus burden

Vacuum assisted delivery   A birth involving the use of a vacuum cup on the fetal head to assist with delivery of the fetal head

Vaginal birth after a cesarean (VBAC)   When a trial of labor and vaginal birth is attempted in a woman who has had a prior cesarean birth

Vaginitis   An inflammation of the vagina

Valsalva maneuver   the method of breath holding, closed-glottis pushing

Variable deceleration   A visually apparent abrupt decrease in the FHR below baseline; the decrease is ≥15 bpm lasting ≥15 seconds and <2 minutes in duration

Veracity   The obligation to tell the truth

Vernix caseosa   A protective substance secreted from sebaceous glands that covered the fetus during pregnancy

Very low birth weight infant (VLBW)   An infant who weighs less than 1,500 grams at birth

Very premature/preterm   Neonate born at less than 32 weeks' gestation

Viability   The threshold for viability is at 25, and rarely fewer completed weeks' gestation

Vibroacoustic stimulation (VAS)   Screening tool that uses auditory stimulation (using an artificial larynx) to assess fetal well being with electronic fetal monitoring when NST is non-reactive

Wharton's Jelly   A collagen substance that surrounds the vessels of the umbilical cord and protects the vessels from compression

Zygote   A fertilized oocyte which contains the diploid number of chromosomes (46)

Photo and Illustration Credits

Linda Chapman author photo by Tom Bauer

Chapter 3

Figure 3-1. National Library of Medicine (US). Genetics Home Reference [Internet]. Bethesda (MD): The Library; 2018 Feb 27. Cystic Fibrosis; [cited Feb 28, 2018]. Available from: https://ghr.nlm.nih.gov/condition/cystic-fibrosis#inheritance

Figure 3-2. National Library of Medicine (US). Genetics Home Reference [Internet]. Bethesda (MD): The Library; 2018 Feb 27. Huntington disease; [cited Feb 28, 2018]. Available from: https://ghr.nlm.nih.gov/condition/huntington-disease#inheritance

Figure 3-3. Adapted from National Library of Medicine (US). Genetics Home Reference [Internet]. Bethesda (MD): The Library; 2018 Feb 27. Hemophilia; [cited Feb 28, 2018]. Available from: https://ghr.nlm.nih.gov/condition/hemophilia#inheritance

Figure 3-4. Scanlon, V. and Sanders, T. (2015). *Essentials of Anatomy and Physiology* (7th ed., p. 503). Philadelphia: F.A. Davis.

Figure 3-5. Scanlon, V. and Sanders, T. (2015). *Essentials of Anatomy and Physiology* (7th ed., p. 504). Philadelphia: F.A. Davis.

Figure 3-6. Scanlon, V. and Sanders, T. (2015). *Essentials of Anatomy and Physiology* (7th ed., p. 508). Philadelphia: F.A. Davis.

Figure 3-7. Scanlon, V. and Sanders, T. (2015). *Essentials of Anatomy and Physiology* (7th ed., p. 509). Philadelphia: F.A. Davis.

Figure 3-8. Scanlon, V. and Sanders, T. (2015). *Essentials of Anatomy and Physiology* (7th ed., p. 514). Philadelphia: F.A. Davis.

Figure 3-9. Scanlon, V. and Sanders, T. (2015). *Essentials of Anatomy and Physiology* (7th ed., p. 502). Philadelphia: F.A. Davis.

Figure 3-10. Scanlon, V. and Sanders, T. (2015). *Essentials of Anatomy and Physiology* (7th ed., p. 501). Philadelphia: F.A. Davis.

Figure 3-11. Scanlon, V. and Sanders, T. (2015). *Essentials of Anatomy and Physiology* (7th ed., p. 523). Philadelphia: F.A. Davis.

Figure 3-12. Scanlon, V. and Sanders, T. (2015). *Essentials of Anatomy and Physiology* (7th ed., p. 525). Philadelphia: F.A. Davis.

Figure 3-13. Scanlon, V. and Sanders, T. (2015). *Essentials of Anatomy and Physiology* (7th ed., p. 342). Philadelphia: F.A. Davis.

Figure 3-14. Scanlon, V. and Sanders, T. (2015). *Essentials of Anatomy and Physiology* (7th ed., p. 531). Philadelphia: F.A. Davis.

Figure 3-15. Scanlon, V. and Sanders, T. (2015). *Essentials of Anatomy and Physiology* (7th ed., p. 533). Philadelphia: F.A. Davis.

Chapter 4

Figure 4-1. Scanlon, V. and Sanders, T. (2015). *Essentials of Anatomy and Physiology* (7th ed., p. 533). Philadelphia: F.A. Davis.

Figure 4-2. Ward, S.L. and Hisley, S. (2016). *Maternal-Child Nursing: Optimizing Outcomes for Mothers, Children and Families* (2nd ed., p. 224). Philadelphia: F.A. Davis.

Figure 4-3. Ward, S.L. and Hisley, S. (2016). *Maternal-Child Nursing: Optimizing Outcomes for Mothers, Children and Families* (2nd ed., p. 228). Philadelphia: F.A. Davis.

Figure 4-4. Ward, S.L. and Hisley, S. (2016). *Maternal-Child Nursing: Optimizing Outcomes for Mothers, Children and Families* (2nd ed., p. 230). Philadelphia: F.A. Davis.

Figure 4-6. Ward, S.L. and Hisley, S. (2016). *Maternal-Child Nursing: Optimizing Outcomes for Mothers, Children and Families* (2nd ed., p. 303). Philadelphia: F.A. Davis.

Figure 4-7. U.S. Department of Agriculture. MyPyramid.gov Website. Washington, DC. *Tips for Pregnant Moms - Daily Food Checklist.* https://wicworks.fns.usda.gov/wicworks//Topics/PregnancyFactSheet.pdf

Chapter 5

Figures 5-2 and 5-3. Courtesy of Gwen Ortiz and Randi Willis.

Chapter 6

Figures 6-3 and 6-4. Courtesy of Allbin family.

Chapter 7

Figure 7-7. Adapted from Gilbert, E.S. (2007) *High-Risk Pregnancy and Delivery* (4th ed.). Philadelphia: Mosby Elsevier

Figure 7-9. Dillon, P.M. (2007). *Nursing Health Assessment: A Critical Thinking, Case Studies Approach* (2nd ed., p. 841). Philadelphia: F.A. Davis.

Figure 7-13. Ward, S.L. and Hisley, S. (2016). *Maternal-Child Nursing: Optimizing Outcomes for Mothers, Children and Families* (2nd ed., p. 338). Philadelphia: F.A. Davis.

Chapter 8

Figure 8-4. Ward, S.L. and Hisley, S. (2016). *Maternal-Child Nursing: Optimizing Outcomes for Mothers, Children and Families* (2nd ed., p. 141). Philadelphia: F.A. Davis.

Figure 8-5. Ward, S.L. and Hisley, S. (2016). *Maternal-Child Nursing: Optimizing Outcomes for Mothers, Children and Families* (2nd ed., p. 141). Philadelphia: F.A. Davis.

Figure 8-8B. Ward, S.L. and Hisley, S. (2016). *Maternal-Child Nursing: Optimizing Outcomes for Mothers, Children and Families* (2nd ed., p. 417). Philadelphia: F.A. Davis.

Figure 8-9. Ward, S.L. and Hisley, S. (2016). *Maternal-Child Nursing: Optimizing Outcomes for Mothers, Children and Families* (2nd ed., p. 418). Philadelphia: F.A. Davis.

Figure 8-10. Ward, S.L. and Hisley, S. (2016). *Maternal-Child Nursing: Optimizing Outcomes for Mothers, Children and Families* (2nd ed., p. 418). Philadelphia: F.A. Davis.

Figure 8-11. Ward, S.L. and Hisley, S. (2016). *Maternal-Child Nursing: Optimizing Outcomes for Mothers, Children and Families* (2nd ed., pp. 419–421). Philadelphia: F.A. Davis.

Figure 8-12. Ward, S.L. and Hisley, S. (2016). *Maternal-Child Nursing: Optimizing Outcomes for Mothers, Children and Families* (2nd ed., p. 419). Philadelphia: F.A. Davis.

Figure 8-17A. Ward, S.L. and Hisley, S. (2016). *Maternal-Child Nursing: Optimizing Outcomes for Mothers, Children and Families* (2nd ed., p. 434). Philadelphia: F.A. Davis.

Figure 8-20. Ward, S.L. and Hisley, S. (2016). *Maternal-Child Nursing: Optimizing Outcomes for Mothers, Children and Families* (2nd ed., p. 457). Philadelphia: F.A. Davis.

Figure 8-24. Ward, S.L. and Hisley, S. (2016). *Maternal-Child Nursing: Optimizing Outcomes for Mothers, Children and Families* (2nd ed., p. 416). Philadelphia: F.A. Davis.

Figure 8-25. Dillon, P.M. (2016). *Nursing Health Assessment: The Foundation of Clinical Practice* (3rd ed., p. 393). Philadelphia: F.A. Davis.

Figure 8-26. Ward, S.L. and Hisley, S. (2016). *Maternal-Child Nursing: Optimizing Outcomes for Mothers, Children and Families* (2nd ed., p. 459). Philadelphia: F.A. Davis.

Figure 8-29. Ward, S.L. and Hisley, S. (2016). *Maternal-Child Nursing: Optimizing Outcomes for Mothers, Children and Families* (2nd ed., p. 456). Philadelphia: F.A. Davis.

Figure 8-32. American Academy of Pediatrics and American Heart Association (2016).

Figure 8-33. Wilkinson, J. and Treas, L. (2015). *Fundamentals of Nursing: Theory, Concepts, and Applications* (3rd ed., p. 795). Philadelphia: F.A. Davis.

Figure 8-34A. Ward, S.L. and Hisley, S. (2016). *Maternal-Child Nursing: Optimizing Outcomes for Mothers, Children and Families* (2nd ed., p. 492). Philadelphia: F.A. Davis.

Figure 8-37. Ward, S.L. and Hisley, S. (2016). *Maternal-Child Nursing: Optimizing Outcomes for Mothers, Children and Families* (2nd ed., p. 483). Philadelphia: F.A. Davis.

Concept map created by Sylvia Fisher.

Chapter 10

Figure 10-7. Courtesy of CooperSurgical, Inc. Trumbull, CT.

Figure 10-8. Courtesy of CooperSurgical, Inc. Trumbull, CT.

Figure 10-9. Ward, S.L. and Hisley, S. (2016). *Maternal-Child Nursing: Optimizing Outcomes for Mothers, Children and Families* (2nd ed., p. 517). Philadelphia: F.A. Davis.

Figure 10-10. Ward, S.L. and Hisley, S. (2016). *Maternal-Child Nursing: Optimizing Outcomes for Mothers, Children and Families* (2nd ed., p. 516). Philadelphia: F.A. Davis.

Figure 10-11. Ward, S.L. and Hisley, S. (2016). *Maternal-Child Nursing: Optimizing Outcomes for Mothers, Children and Families* (2nd ed., p. 516). Philadelphia: F.A. Davis.

Figure 10-16. Ward, S.L. and Hisley, S. (2016). *Maternal-Child Nursing: Optimizing Outcomes for Mothers, Children and Families* (2nd ed., p. 531). Philadelphia: F.A. Davis.

Figure 10-17. Ward, S.L. and Hisley, S. (2016). *Maternal-Child Nursing: Optimizing Outcomes for Mothers, Children and Families* (2nd ed., p. 532). Philadelphia: F.A. Davis.

Figure 10-18. Ward, S.L. and Hisley, S. (2016). *Maternal-Child Nursing: Optimizing Outcomes for Mothers, Children and Families* (2nd ed., p. 532). Philadelphia: F.A. Davis.

Occiput posterior. Ward, S.L. and Hisley, S. (2016). *Maternal-Child Nursing: Optimizing Outcomes for Mothers, Children and Families* (2nd ed., p. 421). Philadelphia: F.A. Davis.

Face presentation. Ward, S.L. and Hisley, S. (2016). *Maternal-Child Nursing: Optimizing Outcomes for Mothers, Children and Families* (2nd ed., p. 421). Philadelphia: F.A. Davis.

Shoulder presentation. Ward, S.L. and Hisley, S. (2016). *Maternal-Child Nursing: Optimizing Outcomes for Mothers, Children and Families* (2nd ed., p. 420). Philadelphia: F.A. Davis.

Frank breech. Ward, S.L. and Hisley, S. (2016). *Maternal-Child Nursing: Optimizing Outcomes for Mothers, Children and Families* (2nd ed., p. 420). Philadelphia: F.A. Davis.

Complete breech. Ward, S.L. and Hisley, S. (2016). *Maternal-Child Nursing: Optimizing Outcomes for Mothers, Children and Families* (2nd ed., p. 420). Philadelphia: F.A. Davis.

Footling breech (single). Ward, S.L. and Hisley, S. (2016). *Maternal-Child Nursing: Optimizing Outcomes for Mothers, Children and Families* (2nd ed., p. 420). Philadelphia: F.A. Davis.

Footling breech (double). Ward, S.L. and Hisley, S. (2016). *Maternal-Child Nursing: Optimizing Outcomes for Mothers, Children and Families* (2nd ed., p. 420). Philadelphia: F.A. Davis.

Chapter 11

Figure 11-2. Ward, S.L. and Hisley, S. (2016). *Maternal-Child Nursing: Optimizing Outcomes for Mothers, Children and Families* (2nd ed., p. 492). Philadelphia: F.A. Davis.

Chapter 12

Figure 12-3. Ward, S.L. and Hisley, S. (2009). *Maternal-Child Nursing: Optimizing Outcomes for Mothers, Children and Families* (Enhanced Revised Reprint, p. 478). Philadelphia: F.A. Davis.

Figure 12-5. United States Department of Agriculture. www .ChooseMyPlate.gov.

Chapter 14

Figure 14-3. Ward, S.L. and Hisley, S. (2016). *Maternal-Child Nursing: Optimizing Outcomes for Mothers, Children and Families* (2nd ed., p. 613). Philadelphia: F.A. Davis.

Chapter 15

Figure 15-5. Ward, S.L. and Hisley, S. (2016). *Maternal-Child Nursing: Optimizing Outcomes for Mothers, Children and Families* (2nd ed., p. 647). Philadelphia: F.A. Davis.

Figure 15-8. Reprinted from *Journal of Pediatrics*, 119:418, Ballard, J et al. Copyright 1991, with permission from Elsevier.

Figure 15-10. Ward, S.L. and Hisley, S. (2016). *Maternal-Child Nursing: Optimizing Outcomes for Mothers, Children and Families* (2nd ed., p. 699). Philadelphia: F.A. Davis.

Stork bite. Dillon, P.M. (2007). *Nursing Health Assessment: A Critical Thinking, Case Studies Approach* (2nd ed., p. 859). Philadelphia: F.A. Davis.

Thrush. Dillon, P.M. (2016). *Nursing Health Assessment: The Foundation of Clinical Practice* (3rd ed., p. 413). Philadelphia: F.A. Davis.

Palpating the scrotum. Dillon, P.M. (2016). *Nursing Health Assessment: The Foundation of Clinical Practice* (3rd ed., p. 418). Philadelphia: F.A. Davis.

Checking gluteal folds. Dillon, P.M. (2016). *Nursing Health Assessment: The Foundation of Clinical Practice* (3rd ed., p. 418). Philadelphia: F.A. Davis.

Barlow-Ortolani maneuver #1. Dillon, P.M. (2016). *Nursing Health Assessment: The Foundation of Clinical Practice* (3rd ed., p. 418). Philadelphia: F.A. Davis.

Barlow-Ortolani maneuver #2. Dillon, P.M. (2016). *Nursing Health Assessment: The Foundation of Clinical Practice* (3rd ed., p. 418). Philadelphia: F.A. Davis.

Barlow-Ortolani maneuver #3. Dillon, P.M. (2016). *Nursing Health Assessment: The Foundation of Clinical Practice* (3rd ed., p. 418). Philadelphia: F.A. Davis.

Caput succedaneum. Ward, S.L. and Hisley, S. (2016). *Maternal-Child Nursing: Optimizing Outcomes for Mothers, Children and Families* (2nd ed., p. 679). Philadelphia: F.A. Davis.

Cephalohematoma. Ward, S.L. and Hisley, S. (2016). *Maternal-Child Nursing: Optimizing Outcomes for Mothers, Children and Families* (2nd ed., p. 679). Philadelphia: F.A. Davis.

Epstein's pearls. Dillon, P.M. (2016). *Nursing Health Assessment: The Foundation of Clinical Practice* (3rd ed., p. 414). Philadelphia: F.A. Davis.

Natal teeth. Dillon, P.M. (2016). *Nursing Health Assessment: The Foundation of Clinical Practice* (3rd ed., p. 414). Philadelphia: F.A. Davis.

Heel stick. Ward, S.L. and Hisley, S. (2016). *Maternal-Child Nursing: Optimizing Outcomes for Mothers, Children and Families* (2nd ed., p. 721). Philadelphia: F.A. Davis.

Chapter 16

Figure 16-2. Scanlon, V. and Sanders, T. (2015). *Essentials of Anatomy and Physiology* (7th ed., p. 512). Philadelphia: F.A. Davis.

Figure 16-3. Courtesy of Medela Corporation, McHenry, Illinois.

Chapter 18

Figure 18-2. U.S. Department of Agriculture. www.ChooseMyPlate.gov. Accessed August 13, 2013.

Figure 18-3. U.S. Department of Health and Human Services (2012).

Chapter 19

Figure 19-6. Copyright Imaginis, 2017.

Index

Note: Illustrations are indicated by *f*, tables by *t*, and boxes by *b*.

C

F

Q

R